American Association of Critical-Care Nurses

Core Curriculum for Critical Care Nursing

5th Edition

Edited by

JoAnn Grif Alspach, RN, MSN, EdD, FAAN

Consultant, Staff Development and Competency-Based
Performance Appraisal Systems

Editor, *Critical Care Nurse*
Annapolis, Maryland

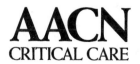

W.B. SAUNDERS COMPANY

A Division of Harcourt Brace & Company

Philadelphia London Toronto Montreal Sydney Tokyo

W.B. SAUNDERS COMPANY
A Division of Harcourt Brace & Company

The Curtis Center
Independence Square West
Philadelphia, Pennsylvania 19106

Library of Congress Cataloging-in-Publication Data

Core curriculum for critical care nursing/American Association of Critical-Care Nurses
[edited by] JoAnn Grif Alspach.—5th ed.

p.   cm.

Includes bibliographical references and index.

ISBN 0-7216-5147-X

1. Intensive care nursing.   I. Alspach, JoAnn.   II. American Association of
   Critical-Care Nurses.   [DNLM: 1. Critical Care—nurses'
   instruction.   2. Critical Care—outlines.   WY 18.2 C796 1998]

RT120.15C63 1998   610.73′61—dc21

DNLM/DLC   97–36175

CORE CURRICULUM FOR
CRITICAL CARE NURSING, 5th edition   ISBN 0–7216–5147–X

Printed in the United States of America.

Last digit is the print number: 9   8   7   6   5   4   3   2   1

This fifth edition of the *Core Curriculum for Critical Care Nursing* is dedicated to the memory of Richard DeAngelis, R.N., M.S., whose contribution of the Cardiovascular chapter of this book in its first four editions will always represent the epitome of devotion, commitment, and competence so characteristic of critical care nurses everywhere.

Contributors

John L. Carty, R.N.C., D.N.Sc., ARNP
Private Practice, Hunter and Associates,
Overland Park, Kansas
Psychosocial Aspects of Critical Care

**Bonnie Mowinski Jennings, R.N.,
D.N.Sc., FAAN; Colonel, U.S. Army
Nurse Corps**
Chief Nurse, Madigan Army Medical Center,
Tacoma, Washinton
Hematologic and Immunologic Systems

**M. Lindsay Lessig, B.S.N., M.S.Ed.,
M.B.A.**
Critical Care Float Nurse, Providence
Medical Center/Seattle, Seattle,
Washington
The Cardiovascular System

Paul M. Lessig, M.D., FACC
Interventional Cardiologist, Swedish Heart
Institute, Swedish Medical Center, Seattle,
Washington
The Cardiovascular System

**Kim Litwack, Ph.D., R.N., CPAN,
CAPA, FAAN**
Associate Professor, College of Nursing,
University of New Mexico, Albuquerque, New
Mexico
The Endocrine System

**Diana L. Nikas, R.N., M.N., CCRN,
CNRN, FCCM**
Neurosurgical Clinical Nurse Specialist,
Harbor-UCLA Medical Center, Torrance,
California
The Neurologic System

Susan L. Smith, R.N., Ph.D.
Director, Clinical Outcomes Assessment,
Emory Hospitals, Atlanta, Georgia
The Gastrointestinal System

**Marilyn Sawyer Sommers, R.N.,
Ph.D., CCRN**
Professor, College of Nursing and Health,
University of Cincinnati, Cincinnati, Ohio
Multisystem

June L. Stark, R.N., B.S.N., M.Ed.
Critical Care Nurse Educator and Project
Manager, Professional Development, St.
Elizabeth's Medical Center, Boston,
Massachusetts
The Renal System

**Robert E. St. John, M.S.N., R.N.,
RRT, CCRN, CS**
Adjunct Assistant Professor of Nursing, Jewish
Hospital College of Nursing and Allied
Health; Adjunct Clinical Instructor of
Nursing, St. Louis University; and
Formerly Pulmonary Clinical Nurse Specialist,
Barnes-Jewish Hospital, St. Louis, Misssouri
The Pulmonary System

Ginger Schafer Wlody, R.N., Ed.D., FCCM
Chair, Department of Performance Improvement, and Ethics Consultant, Carl T. Hayden Veterans Affairs Medical Center, Phoenix, Arizona
Legal and Ethical Aspects of Critical Care Nursing

Stacey Young-McCaughan, R.N., Ph.D., OCN; Lieutenant Colonel, U.S. Army Nurse Corps
Nurse Researcher, Brooke Army Medical Center, San Antonio, Texas
Hematologic and Immunologic Systems

Reviewers

1. THE PULMONARY SYSTEM

   Jill Feldman Malen, R.N., M.S., NS, ANP
   Pulmonary Clinical Nurse Specialist,
   Barnes-Jewish Hospital, St. Louis,
   Missouri

   John P. Lynch, M.D.
   Assistant Professor of Medicine,
   Barnes-Jewish Hospital, St. Louis,
   Missouri

2. THE CARDIOVASCULAR SYSTEM

   Carolyn C. Main, R.N., ARNP, MN
   Cardiology Nurse Practitioner, Minor
   and James Cardiology, Seattle,
   Washington

   James F. Clifton, M.D., FACC
   Director, Noninvasive Cardiology,
   Providence Medical Center, Seattle,
   Washington

   Edward A. Rittenhouse, M.D., FACS
   Thoracic Surgeon, Swedish Cardiac
   Surgery, Seattle, Washington

3. THE NEUROLOGIC SYSTEM

   Maurene Harvey, R.N., M.P.N.
   Critical Care Educator, Consultants in
   Critical Care, Inc., Glendale, California

   Daniel F. Kelly, M.D.
   Division of Neurosurgery, Harbor-
   UCLA Medical Center, and Assistant
   Professor, University of California,
   Los Angeles, School of Medicine,
   Los Angeles, California

4. THE RENAL SYSTEM

   **Charold L. Baer, R.N. Ph.D., FCCM,
   CCRN**
   Professor, Department of Adult Health
   and Illness Nursing, Oregon Health Sci-
   ences University, Portland, Oregon

   Gennaro A. Carpinito, M.D.
   Director of Urology, Boston City Hospi-
   tal, and Associate Professor, Boston
   University School of Medicine, Boston,
   Massachusetts

   James A. Strom, M.D.
   Chief, Division of Nephrology, St.
   Elizabeth's Medical Center, and Associ-
   ate Professor, Tufts University School of
   Medicine, Boston, Massachusetts

5. THE ENDOCRINE SYSTEM

   Leslie Dork, M.S.N., R.N., C.S., CCRN
   Clinical Nurse Specialist, Medical and
   Cardiac Intensive Care, University
   Hospitals, Albuquerque, New Mexico

   Bruce D. Hyman, M.D.
   Assistant Professor of Medicine, Rush
   Medical College, and Assistant At-
   tending Physician in Internal Medicine,
   Rush–Presbyterian–St. Luke's Medical
   Center, Chicago, Illinois

6. HEMATOLOGIC AND IMMUNOLOGIC
   SYSTEMS

   **Linda H. Yoder, R.N., M.B.A., Ph.D.,
   OCN**
   Lt. Col., U.S. Army Nurse Corps, Direc-
   tor of Nursing Research, Department of

Nursing, Brooke Army Medical Center, San Antonio, Texas

Jennifer L. Cadiz, M.D.
Major, U.S. Army Medical Corps; Chief of Hematology Oncology Service, William Beaumont Army Medical Center, El Paso, Texas

7. THE GASTROINTESTINAL SYSTEM

Jackie Looper, R.N.
Manager, GI Services Laboratory, Emory University Hospital, Atlanta, Georgia

John R. Galloway, M.D.
Assistant Professor, Emory University School of Medicine, Emory University, Atlanta, Georgia

8. MULTISYSTEM

Mary Fran Hazinski, R.N., M.S.N., FAAN
Clinical Specialist, Division of Trauma, Departments of Surgery and Pediatrics, Vanderbilt University Medical Center, Nashville, Tennessee

Gary Hecker, R.N., CCRN, CEN, EMT
Doctoral Student, College of Nursing and Health, University of Cincinnati, Cincinnati, Ohio

Robert S. Hoffman, M.D.
Director, New York Poison Control Center, New York, New York

James M. Hurst, M.D.
Associate Professor, Department of Surgery, University of Cincinnati Medical Center, Cincinnati, Ohio

James A. Johnson, M.D., FACS
Alexander Burn Center, Hillcrest Medical Center, Tulsa, Oklahoma

Eric Marsh, M.S.N., R.N.
Trauma Program Manager,

Rainbow Regional Pediatric Trauma Center, Cleveland, Ohio

Andrew Michaels, M.D.
Division of Trauma, Burns, and Emergency Care, University of Michigan Health Center, Ann Arbor, Michigan

Denise A. Sadowski, M.S.N., R.N.
Independent Consultant and Educator, Cincinnati, Ohio

9. PSYCHOSOCIAL ASPECTS OF CRITICAL CARE

Barbara A. Parrett, R.N., M.S.N.
Private Practice, Mental Health, Senior Trainer, Eyemovement Desensitization and Reprocessing, Sacramento, California

James G. Hunter, M.D.
Director, Hunter and Associates Multidisciplinary Mental Health Clinic, Overland Park, Kansas

10. LEGAL AND ETHICAL ASPECTS OF CRITICAL CARE NURSING

John Clochesy, R.N., Ph.D., FAAN, FCCM
Associate Professor and Associate Dean, University of Pittsburgh School of Nursing, Pittsburgh, Pennsylvania

June Levine, R.N., M.S.N., CNA
Vice President for Operations/Nursing, Huntington East Valley Hospital, Glendora, California

Debra Gerardi, R.N., J.D., MPH
Assistant Clinical Instructor, University of California, Los Angeles (UCLA) Department of Surgery, and Unit Director, Wilson Pavilion, UCLA Medical Center, Los Angeles, California

Preface

As a dynamic specialty nursing organization, the American Association of Critical-Care Nurses (AACN) has been continually evolving to better meet the needs of its members and the patients they serve. As the health care industry, health care services, and the traditional boundaries of health care institutions have been altered so rapidly and pervasively, AACN has continued its vital growth and development in order to remain at the forefront of these changes. At this point in its evolution, AACN is engaged in reaffirming and/or redefining its mission, vision, values, and scope of practice in order to distinguish the unique contributions of critical care nursing in a contemporary and enduring manner.

AACN's mission has now been transformed from an emphasis on advancing the art and science of critical care nursing to an emphasis on providing leadership to its members in establishing work and patient care environments that are healing, humane, and respectful and on providing quality resources that maximize nurses' contributions to the care of critically ill patients and their families. AACN's vision of its preferred future remains as it was formulated in 1992: creating a health care system driven by the needs of patients and families, in which critical care nurses make their optimal contribution.

The values that underlie and guide AACN are now articulated more fully and clearly as accountability, advocacy, integrity, collaboration, leadership, stewardship of resources, life-long learning, innovation, and commitment to quality. Its mission, vision, and values are embraced by an ethic of care that acknowledges the interrelatedness and interdependence among individuals, systems, and society and by three ethical principles that provide a basis for decision making: respect for the uniqueness of individuals, beneficence toward others, and justice.

AACN's scope of practice previously included the nurse, the patient, and the critical care environment. Its redefined scope of practice now elegantly presents the Synergy Model to delineate how these elements interrelate in a dynamic, ongoing, and effective manner. The most fundamental premise of the Synergy Model is that patient characteristics drive the competencies that nurses need in order to provide holistic, healing care that achieves optimal patient outcomes.[1] Optimal patient outcomes result when there is synergy between the characteristics of patients and the competencies of nurses. The major components of this model include a set of eight patient characteristics that

---

[1]Villaire, M.: The Synergy Model© of certified practice: Creating safe passage for patients. Crit. Care Nurse 16(4):94–99, 1996.

directly affect their capacity for health: resiliency, vulnerability to stressors, stability, complexity, resource availability, participation in care, participation in decision making, and predictability of illness. The eight nurse competencies represent the capabilities that nurses need in order to meet patients' needs: clinical judgment, advocacy, caring practices, collaboration, systems thinking, response to diversity, clinical inquiry, and facilitation of patient and family learning. A knowledge base of critical care nursing underlies clinical competency and reflects a foundational requirement for the development of these nursing competencies.

The purpose of the *Core Curriculum for Critical Care Nursing* in this, its fifth edition, remains as it was at its inception: to articulate the knowledge base that underlies critical care nursing practice. Each edition of this work attempts to redefine that knowledge base for nurses who practice in this specialty area. Once AACN's design for critical care nursing has been fully developed and its ramifications for practice, education, and certification have been examined, the *Core Curriculum* will be revised once again to reflect those deliberations. In the interim, the fifth edition is presented for your consideration.

A number of similarities exist between the fourth and fifth editions of the *Core Curriculum*. The current edition continues to use the CCRN examination blueprint and task statements to provide direction for determining relevant content and its apportionment throughout the book. Body systems are once again employed to segregate the major content areas into chapters. The subsections related to physiologic anatomy and pathophysiology have also been retained. In addition, we have continued the nursing-oriented emphasis on nursing process and nursing diagnosis that was initiated in the fourth edition. The psychosocial chapter remains organized solely by nursing diagnoses, and the legal and ethical chapter continues to be organized by issues related to these areas of concern.

In addition to the customary changes for revision and updating of general content related to acute and critical care nursing, a number of noteworthy changes and additions exist in this fifth edition of the *Core Curriculum*. The most striking difference in the latest edition is addition of a new chapter on multisystem health problems. This new chapter incorporates content related to the systemic inflammatory response syndrome (SIRS), the multiple organ dysfunction syndrome (MODS), drug and alcohol intoxication, poisoning, burns, hypothermia, and multisystem trauma. The pulmonary chapter includes new coverage on sleep apnea and lung transplantation, as well as extended discussions on new modes of ventilation and oxygen delivery devices, and a brief section on noninvasive respiratory monitoring. The cardiovascular chapter incorporates extensive updating and revision that includes expanded discussion of invasive diagnostic testing, coverage of newer noninvasive diagnostic methods, more detailed coverage of cardiac drugs, treatments and therapies for angina pectoris, newer uses of pacemakers, and coverage of myocarditis, heart transplantation, and cardiac trauma. In addition, the section on dysrhythmias and conduction defects has been extensively reorganized around the clinical effects on heart rate. The neurologic chapter includes additional content related to diagnostic studies, cerebral contusion, cerebral edema, and encephalopathy; the segment on head trauma has been significantly reorganized; the content has been augmented with a number of new illustrations. The renal chapter now covers issues relevant to renal transplantation and updated information on both acute and chronic renal failure. The hematology and immunology chapter has been completely reorganized and now incorporates coverage of thrombocytopenia, hyperviscosity, immunosuppression, and bone marrow transplantation, as well as transplant rejection and graft-versus-host disease. The gastrointestinal chapter has been extensively revised, streamlined, and augmented by the added discussion of liver transplantation, acute fulminant liver failure, and variceal bleeding, and its coverage of radiologic studies, acute pancreatitis, and the nursing diagnoses of altered nutrition and altered oral mucosa has been updated. The psychosocial chapter has new content related to client abuse, as well as coverage of age-related aspects of care. The legal and ethical chapter provides expanded coverage on advanced nursing practice, informed consent, the patient self-determination act, and issues surrounding supervision of unlicensed assistive personnel. To assist readers in locating relevant literature citations, the list of references for each chapter is now subdivided according to specific topic areas.

The contributors, reviewers, and I have made every attempt to provide you with the most current and relevant knowledge base of information related to acute and critical care nursing. We welcome your comments related to this edition and your suggestions for the next edition of the *Core Curriculum.*

Grif Alspach
Annapolis, Maryland

Contents

chapter 3

The Neurologic System   339
Diana L. Nikas, R.N., M.N., CCRN, CNRN, FCCM

PHYSIOLOGIC ANATOMY   339
    Brain   339

chapter 4

The Renal System 464

June L. Stark, R.N., B.S.N., M.Ed.

chapter 5

The Endocrine System 565

Kim Litwack, Ph.D., R.N., CPAN, CAPA, FAAN

chapter 6

Hematologic and Immunologic Systems 601

Stacey Young-McCaughan, R.N., Ph.D.(C), O.C.N.,® Lieutenant
Colonel, U.S. Army Nurse Corps, and Bonnie Mowinski
Jennings, R.N., D.N.Sc., FAAN, Colonel, U.S. Army Nurse
Corps

chapter 7

The Gastrointestinal System 647

Susan L. Smith, R.N., Ph.D.

chapter

... The Pulmonary System

Robert E. St. John, M.S.N., R.N., RRT, CCRN, CS

PHYSIOLOGIC ANATOMY

The Respiratory Circuit

1. The **pulmonary system** exists for the purpose of gas exchange. Oxygen (O_2) and carbon dioxide (CO_2) are exchanged between the atmosphere and alveoli, between the alveoli and pulmonary capillary blood, and between the systemic capillary blood and all the cells of the body
2. **Atmospheric O_2** is consumed by the body through cellular aerobic metabolism, which supplies the energy for life
3. **CO_2**, a by-product of aerobic metabolism, is eliminated primarily through lung ventilation
4. The **respiratory circuit** includes all structures and processes involved in the transfer of oxygen between room air and the individual cell and the transfer of CO_2 between the cell and room air
5. **Cellular respiration** cannot be directly measured but is estimated by the amount of CO_2 produced ($\dot{V}_{CO_2}$) and the O_2 consumed ($\dot{V}_{O_2}$). The ratio of these two values is called the *respiratory quotient* (RQ). The respiratory quotient is normally about 0.8 but changes according to the nutritional substrate being burned (i.e., protein, fats, or carbohydrates). Patients fully maintained on intravenous (IV) glucose alone will have a respiratory quotient approaching 1.0 as a result of the metabolic end product, CO_2
6. **The exchange of O_2 and CO_2** at the alveolar-capillary level (external respiration) is called the *respiratory exchange ratio* (R). This is the ratio of CO_2 produced to O_2 taken up per minute. In homeostasis, the respiratory exchange ratio is the same as the respiratory quotient, 0.8
7. **Proper functioning of the respiratory circuit** requires efficient interaction of the respiratory, circulatory, and neuromuscular systems
8. In addition to its primary function of **O_2 and CO_2 exchange,** the lung also carries out metabolic and endocrine functions as a source of hormones and a site of hormone metabolism. Additionally, the lung is a target of hormonal actions from other endocrine organs

1

. . . .
:
:
: **Steps in the Gas Exchange Process**

1. **Step 1—Ventilation:** volume change, or the process of moving air between atmosphere and the lung alveoli and distributing air within the lungs to maintain appropriate concentrations of O_2 and CO_2 in the alveoli
   a. Structural components involved in ventilation
      i. Lung
         (a) Anatomic divisions: right lung (three lobes: upper, middle, and lower); left lung (two lobes: upper and lower). Lobes are divided into bronchopulmonary segments (ten on right, nine on left). Bronchopulmonary segments are subdivided into secondary lobules
         (b) Lobule: the smallest gross anatomic units of lung tissue, contain primary functional units of the lung (terminal bronchioles, alveolar ducts and sacs, pulmonary circulation). Lymphatics surround the lobule, keep the lung free of excess fluid, and remove inhaled particles from distal areas of the lung
         (c) Bronchial artery circulation: systemic source of circulation for the tracheobronchial tree and lung tissue down to the level of the terminal bronchiole. Alveoli receive their blood supply from the pulmonary circulation
      ii. Conducting airways: The entire area from nose to terminal bronchioles where gas flows, but is not exchanged, is called the *anatomic dead space* (VD_{anat}). The approximate amount is calculated as 2 ml per kilogram (ml/kg) body weight. The airways are a series of rapidly branching tubes of ever-diminishing diameter that eventually terminate in the alveoli
         (a) Nose
            (1) Passageway for movement of air into lung
            (2) Preconditions air by action of cilia, mucosal cells, and turbinate bones
               a) Warms air to within 2% to 3% of body temperature and humidifies it to full saturation before it reaches lower trachea
               b) Filters by trapping particles larger than 6 μm in diameter
            (3) Voice resonance, olfaction, sneeze reflex functions
         (b) Pharynx: posterior to the nasal cavities and mouth
            (1) Separation of food from air is controlled by local nerve reflexes
            (2) Opening of eustachian tube regulates middle ear pressure
            (3) Lymphatic tissues control infection
         (c) Larynx: a complex structure consisting of incomplete rings of cartilage and numerous muscles and ligaments
            (1) Vocal cords: speech function
               a) Narrowest part of the conducting airways in adults
               b) Contraction of muscles of the larynx causes vocal cords to change shape
               c) Vibration of vocal cords produces sound. Speech is a joint function of vocal cords, lips, tongue, soft palate,

and respiration, with control by temporal and parietal lobes of cerebral cortex

    d) Glottis: the opening between vocal cords

  (2) Valve action by the epiglottis helps to prevent aspiration

  (3) Cough reflex: cords close and intrathoracic pressure increases to permit coughing or Valsalva maneuver

  (4) Cricoid cartilage

    a) The only complete rigid ring

    b) Narrowest part of a child's airway

    c) Inner diameter sets the limit for size of endotracheal tubes passed through the larynx

(d) Trachea: a tubular structure consisting of 16 to 20 incomplete, or C-shaped, cartilaginous rings that stabilize the airway and prevent complete collapse with cough

  (1) Begins conducting system, or tracheobronchial tree

  (2) Warms and humidifies air

  (3) Mucosal cells trap foreign material

  (4) Cilia propel mucus upward through airway

  (5) Cough reflex present, especially at point of tracheal bifurcation (carina)

  (6) Smooth muscle innervated by parasympathetic branch of autonomic nervous system

(e) Major bronchi and bronchioles

(f) Terminal bronchioles

  (1) Smooth muscle walls (no cartilage); bronchospasm may narrow lumen and increase airway resistance

  (2) Ciliated mucosal cells become flattened, with progressive loss of cilia toward alveoli

  (3) Sensitive to CO_2 levels: increased levels induce bronchiolar dilation, decreased levels induce bronchiolar constriction

iii. Gas exchange airways: semipermeable membrane permits movement of gases according to pressure gradients. These airways do not contribute to air flow resistance but do contribute to distensibility of the lung. The *acinus* (terminal respiratory unit) is composed of the respiratory bronchiole and its subdivisions (Fig. 1–1)

(a) Respiratory bronchioles and alveolar ducts

  (1) Terminal branching of airways

  (2) Distribution of inspired air

  (3) Smooth muscle layer diminishes

(b) Alveoli and alveolar bud

  (1) The most important structures in gas exchange

  (2) Alveolar surface area is large and depends on body size. The total surface area is about 70 m^2 in a normal adult. The thickness of the respiratory membrane is about 0.6 μm. This fulfills the need to distribute a large quantity of perfused blood into a very thin film to ensure near equalization of O_2 and CO_2

  (3) Alveolar cells

    a) Type I: squamous epithelium, adapted for gas exchange, sensitive to injury by inhaled agents, and structured to prevent fluid transudation into alveoli

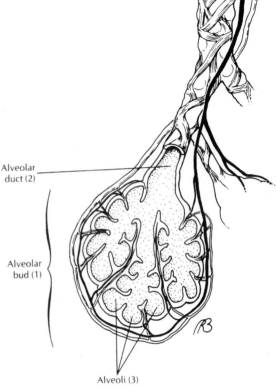

Figure 1–1 • Components of the acinus. (From Eubanks, D. H., and Bone, R. C.: Comprehensive Respiratory Care: A Learning System, 2nd ed. St. Louis, Mosby–Year Book, 1990, p. 168.)

Alveolar duct (2)

Alveolar bud (1)

Alveoli (3)

      b) Type II: large secretory; highly active metabolically; origin of surfactant synthesis and type I cell genesis

      c) Alveolar macrophages phagocytize foreign materials

   (4) Pulmonary surfactant

      a) A phospholipid monolayer at alveolar air-liquid interface that has the property of varying surface tension with alveolar volume

      b) Enables surface tension to decrease as alveolar volume decreases during expiration, thus preventing alveolar collapse

      c) Decreases work of breathing, permits alveoli to remain inflated at low distending pressures, and reduces net forces causing tissue fluid accumulation

      d) Reduction of surfactant makes lung expansion more difficult; the greater the surface tension, the greater the pressure needed to overcome it

      e) Surfactant also detoxifies inhaled gases and traps inhaled and deposited particles

   (5) Alveolar-capillary membrane (alveolar epithelium, interstitial space, capillary endothelium)

      a) Bathed by interstitial fluid; lines respiratory bronchioles, alveolar ducts, and alveolar sacs; forms walls of alveoli

      b) About 1 μm or less in thickness (<1 red blood cell);

permits very rapid diffusion of gases; any increase in thickness diminishes gas diffusion

   c) Total surface area in adult of about 70 m² is in contact with about 60 to 140 ml of pulmonary capillary blood at any one time

   (6) Gas exchange pathway (Fig. 1–2) alveolar epithelium → alveolar basement membrane → interstitial space → capillary basement membrane → capillary endothelium → plasma → erythrocyte membrane → erythrocyte cytoplasm

b. Alveolar ventilation ($\dot{V}_A$): that part of total ventilation taking part in gas exchange and, therefore, the only part useful to the body

   i. Alveolar ventilation is one component of minute ventilation

      (a) Minute ventilation ($\dot{V}_E$): the amount of air exchanged in 1 minute. Equal to exhaled tidal volume ($\dot{V}_T$) multiplied by respiratory rate (RR or f). Normal resting $\dot{V}_E$ in an adult is about 6 L/minute:

$$\dot{V}_T \times RR = \dot{V}_E \ (500 \text{ ml} \times 12 = 6000 \text{ ml})$$

      Tidal volume is easily measured at bedside by hand-held devices or on a mechanical ventilator. Exhaled minute ventilation is a routinely measured parameter

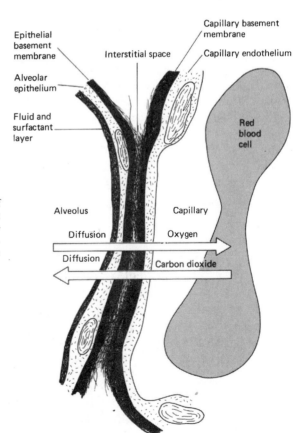

Figure 1–2 • Ultrastructure of the respiratory membrane. (From Guyton, A. C., and Hall, J. E.: Textbook of Medical Physiology, 9th ed. Philadelphia, W. B. Saunders, 1996, p. 508.)

(b) Minute ventilation is composed of both alveolar ventilation ($\dot{V}_A$) and physiologic dead space ventilation ($\dot{V}_D$):

$$\dot{V}_E = \dot{V}_D + \dot{V}_A$$

where $\dot{V}$ = volume of gas per unit of time.

Physiologic dead space ventilation is that volume of gas in the airways that does not participate in gas exchange. It is composed of both anatomic dead space ventilation ($\dot{V}D_{anat}$) and alveolar dead space ventilation ($\dot{V}D_A$)

(c) The ratio of dead space to tidal volume (V_D/V_T) is measured to determine how much of each breath is wasted (i.e., does not contribute to gas exchange). Normal values for spontaneously breathing patients range from 0.2 to 0.4 (20% to 40%)

ii. Alveolar ventilation cannot be directly measured but is inversely related to arterial CO_2 pressure ($PaCO_2$) in a steady state by this formula:

$$\dot{V}_A = \frac{\dot{V}_{CO2} \times 0.863}{PaCO_2}$$

where

$\dot{V}_A$ = alveolar ventilation
$\dot{V}CO_2$ = CO_2 production
$PaCO_2$ = arterial CO_2 pressure
0.863 = correction factor for differences in measurement units and conversion to STPD (standard temperature [0°C] and pressure [760 torr], dry)

iii. Since $\dot{V}CO_2$ remains the same in a steady state, measurement of the patient's $PaCO_2$ reveals the status of the alveolar ventilation

iv. $PaCO_2$ is the only adequate indicator of effective matching of alveolar ventilation to metabolic demand. To assess ventilation, one must measure $PaCO_2$

v. If $PaCO_2$ is low, alveolar ventilation is high and hyperventilation is present

$$\downarrow PaCO_2 = \uparrow \dot{V}_A$$

vi. If $PaCO_2$ is within normal limits, alveolar ventilation is adequate

$$Normal\ PaCO_2 = normal\ \dot{V}_A$$

vii. If $PaCO_2$ is high, alveolar ventilation is low and hypoventilation is present

$$\uparrow PaCO_2 = \downarrow \dot{V}_A$$

c. Defense mechanisms of the lung

i. Although an internal organ, the lung is unique, in that it has continuous contact with particulate and gaseous materials inhaled from the external environment. In the healthy lung, defense mechanisms successfully defend against these natural materials by the following means:

(a) The structural architecture of the upper respiratory tract, which reduces deposited and inhaled materials

(b) The processing system, including respiratory tract fluid alteration and phagocytic activity

(c) The transport system, which removes material from the lung

(d) The humoral and cell-mediated immune responses, which may be the most important bronchopulmonary defense mechanisms

  ii. Loss of normal defense mechanisms may be precipitated by disease, injury, surgery, insertion of endotracheal or tracheostomy tubes, or smoking

 iii. The upper respiratory tract warms and humidifies the inspired air, absorbs selected inhaled gases, and filters out particulate matter. Soluble gases and particles larger than 10 μm are aerodynamically filtered out. Normally, no bacteria are present below the level of the larynx in the respiratory system

  iv. Inhaled and deposited particles reaching the alveoli are coated by surface fluids (surfactant and other lipoproteins) and are rapidly phagocytized by pulmonary alveolar macrophages

   v. Macrophages and particles are transported in mucus by bronchial cilia beating toward the glottis and moving the materials along in a mucus-fluid layer, eventually to be expectorated or swallowed. This process is referred to as the *mucociliary escalator.* Pulmonary lymphatics also drain and transport some cells and particles from the lung

  vi. Antigens activate humoral and cell-mediated immune systems, which add immunoglobins to the surface fluid of alveoli and activate alveolar macrophages

 vii. Disruption or injury to these defense mechanisms predisposes to acute or chronic pulmonary disease

d. Lung mechanics

   i. Muscles of respiration: the act of breathing is accomplished through muscular actions that alter intrapleural and pulmonary pressures, thus changing intrapulmonary volumes

   (a) Muscles of inspiration: during inspiration, the chest cavity enlarges. This enlargement is an active process brought about by contraction of:

   (1) Diaphragm: the major inspiratory muscle

   a) Normal quiet breathing is accomplished almost entirely by this dome-shaped muscle, which divides the chest from the abdomen

   b) Divided into two "leaves": the right and left hemidiaphragms

   c) Downward contraction increases superior-inferior diameter of chest and elevates lower ribs

   d) Innervation is from C3 to C5 level

   e) Normally, accounts for 75% of tidal volume during quiet inspiration

   f) Facilitates vomiting, coughing and sneezing, defecation, and parturition

   (2) External intercostal muscles

   a) Increase the anterior-posterior (A-P) diameter of thorax by elevating ribs

   b) A-P diameter is about 20% greater during inspiration than during expiration *c*) Innervation from T1 to T11

   (3) Accessory muscles in the neck: scalene and sternocleidomastoid

    a) Lift upward on sternum and ribs and increase A-P diameter

    b) Are not used in normal, quiet ventilation

  (b) Muscles of expiration: during expiration, the chest cavity decreases in size. This is a passive act unless forced, and the driving force is derived from lung recoil. Muscles used when increased levels of ventilation are needed are:

   (1) Abdominals: force abdominal contents upward to elevate diaphragm

   (2) Internal intercostals: decrease A-P diameter by depressing ribs

 ii. Pressures within the chest: movement of air into the lungs requires a pressure difference between the airway opening and the alveoli sufficient to overcome the resistance to air flow of the tracheobronchial tree (Table 1–1)

  (a) Air flows into lungs when intrapulmonary air pressure falls below atmospheric pressure

  (b) Air flows out of lungs when intrapulmonary air pressure exceeds atmospheric pressure

  (c) Intrapleural pressure is normally negative with respect to atmospheric pressure as a result of the elastic recoil of the lungs tending to pull away from the chest wall. This "negative" pressure prevents collapse of the lung

  (d) Increased effort (forced inspiration or expiration) may produce much greater changes in intrapulmonary and intrapleural pressures during inspiration and expiration

 iii. Structural components of the thorax

  (a) For protection: sternum, spine, ribs

  (b) Pleura

   (1) Visceral and parietal layers

   (2) Pleural fluid between layers: Allows smooth movement of visceral over parietal layers

   (3) Adherence: normally, the pleural space is a potential space or vacuum and, because of a constant "negative" pressure (less than atmospheric pressure by 4 to 8 mm Hg), any change in the volume of the thoracic cage is reflected by a similar change in the volume of the lungs

TABLE 1–1. Example of Changes in Pressures Throughout the Ventilatory Cycle

Pressures	At Rest (No Air Flow) (mm Hg)	Inspiration (mm Hg)	Expiration (mm Hg)
1. Atmospheric (P_B)	760	760	760
2. Intrapulmonary or intra-alveolar (P_{alv})	760	757	763
3. Intrapleural (P_{pl}) or intrathoracic	756	750	756

(4) Nerve supply: parietal pleura has fibers for pain transmission, but visceral pleura does not

iv. Resistances
(a) *Elastic resistance* (static properties)
(1) The lung, if removed from the chest, collapses to a smaller volume because of lung elastic recoil. This tendency of the lungs to collapse is normally counteracted by the chest wall tendency to expand. The volume of air in the lungs depends on the equal and opposite balance of these forces
(2) Compliance is an expression of the elastic properties of the lung and is the change in volume accomplished by a change in pressure:

$$C_L = \frac{\triangle V}{\triangle P}$$

If compliance is high, the lung is more easily distended; if low, the lung is stiff and more difficult to distend
(b) *Flow resistance* (dynamic properties)
(1) Airway resistance must be overcome to generate flow through the airways
(2) Changes in airway caliber affect airway resistance. Examples would be changes due to bronchospasm or secretions
(3) Flow through the airway depends on pressure differences between the two ends of the tube as well as resistance. The driving pressure for flow in the airways is the difference between atmospheric and alveolar pressures

v. Work of breathing
(a) In order to minimize the work required to maintain a given level of ventilation, the body automatically changes the respiratory pattern
(b) The work performed must be sufficient to overcome the elastic resistance and the flow resistance
(c) In diseased states, the workload increases

e. Control of ventilation: although the process of breathing is a normal rhythmic activity that occurs without conscious effort, it involves an intricate controlling mechanism at the level of the central nervous system (CNS). The basic organization of the respiratory control system is outlined in Figure 1–3
i. Respiratory generator: located in the medulla and composed of two groups of neurons
(a) One group initiates respiration and regulates its rate
(b) One group controls "switching off" inspiration, thus the onset of expiration
ii. Input from other regions of the CNS
(a) Pons: input is necessary for a normal, coordinated breathing pattern
(b) Cerebral cortex exerts a conscious or voluntary control over ventilation
iii. Chemoreceptors: contribute to an important feedback loop that exists to adjust respiratory center output if blood gases are not maintained within normal range

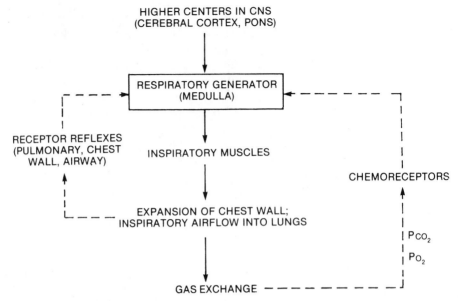

Figure 1-3 • Schematic diagram depicting organization of the respiratory control system. The dotted lines show feedback loops affecting the respiratory generator. (From Weinberger, S. E.: Principles of Pulmonary Medicine, 2nd ed. Philadelphia, W. B. Saunders, 1992, p. 206.)

   (a) Central chemoreceptor: located near the ventrolateral surface of the medulla (but is clearly separate from the medullary respiratory center)

      (1) Responds not directly to blood P_{CO_2} but, rather, the pH of the extracellular fluid (ECF) surrounding the chemoreceptor

      (2) The feedback loop for CO_2 can be summarized as follows:

$$\uparrow \text{arterial } P_{CO_2} \to \uparrow \text{ brain ECF } P_{CO_2} \to \downarrow \text{ brain ECF pH} \to$$
$$\downarrow \text{ pH at chemoreceptor} \to \text{stimulation of central}$$
$$\text{chemoreceptor} \to \text{stimulation of medullary respiratory}$$
$$\text{center} \to \text{increased ventilation} \to \text{decreased arterial } P_{CO_2}$$

   (b) Peripheral chemoreceptors: located in the carotid body and aortic body

      (1) Sensitive to changes in P_{O_2}, with hypoxemia stimulating chemoreceptor discharge

      (2) Minor role in sensing P_{CO_2}

  iv. Other receptors

   (a) Stretch receptors in bronchial wall (Hering-Breuer reflex) respond to changes in lung inflation

      (1) As the lung inflates, receptor discharge increases

      (2) Contribute to the start of expiration

   (b) Irritant receptors located in lining of airways respond to noxious stimuli, such as irritating dust and chemicals

   (c) "J" receptors (juxtacapillary) in alveolar interstitial space

      (1) Cause rapid shallow breathing in response to deformation from increased interstitial volume due to high pulmonary

capillary pressures (such as in congestive heart failure) or inflammation

(2) Stimulation can also cause bradycardia, hypotension, and expiratory constriction of the glottis

(d) Receptors in chest wall (in the intercostal muscles)

(1) Are involved in fine tuning of ventilation

(2) Adjust output of respiratory muscles for the degree of muscular work required

2. **Step 2—Diffusion:** the process by which alveolar air gases are moved across the alveolar-capillary membrane to the pulmonary capillary bed and vice versa. Diffusion occurs down a concentration gradient from a higher to lower concentration. No active metabolic work is required for diffusion of gases to occur. The work of breathing is accomplished by the respiratory muscles and heart, which produce the gradient across the alveolar-capillary membrane

a. The ability of the lung to transfer gases is called the *diffusing capacity* of the lung (D_L). The diffusing capacity measures the amount of gas (O_2, CO_2, carbon monoxide [CO]) diffusing between alveoli and pulmonary capillary blood per minute per mm Hg mean gas pressure difference

b. CO_2 is 20 times more diffusible across the alveolar-capillary membrane than O_2. If the membrane is damaged, its decreased capacity for transporting O_2 into the blood is usually more of a problem than its decreased capacity for transporting CO_2 out of the body. Thus, the diffusing capacity of the lungs for O_2 is of primary importance

c. Diffusion is determined by several variables:

i. Surface area available for gas exchange

ii. Integrity of alveolar-capillary membrane

iii. Amount of hemoglobin in the blood

iv. Diffusion coefficient of gas as well as contact time

v. Driving pressures: the difference between alveolar gas tensions and pulmonary capillary gas tensions (Table 1–2). This is the force that causes gases to diffuse across membranes

(a) During breathing of 100% O_2, the PAO_2 (alveolar oxygen tension) becomes so large that the difference between PAO_2 and $P\bar{V}O_2$ (mixed venous O_2 tension) significantly increases, proportionately increasing the driving pressure

(b) Therefore, hypoxemia due solely to diffusion defects is usually improved by breathing 100% oxygen

d. The A–a gradient ($PAO_2 - PaO_2$) is the alveolar to arterial oxygen pressure difference (i.e., the difference in partial pressure of O_2 in the alveolar gas spaces and the pressure in the systemic arterial blood). This gradient is always a positive number

i. The normal gradient in young adults is less than 10 mm Hg (on

TABLE 1–2. Driving Pressures

Alveolar Gas	Alveolar-Capillary Membranes	Pulmonary Capillaries
PAO_2 104 mm Hg	$\xrightarrow{\text{diffusion}}$	$P\bar{V}O_2$ 40 mm Hg
$PaCO_2$ 40 mm Hg	$\xleftarrow{\text{diffusion}}$	$P\bar{V}CO_2$ 45 mm Hg

room air) but increases with age and may be as high as 20 mm Hg in people over age 60 years

ii. The A–a gradient provides an index of how efficient the lung is in equilibrating pulmonary capillary O_2 with alveolar O_2. It indicates whether gas transfer is normal

iii. A large A–a gradient generally indicates that the lung is the site of dysfunction (except when cardiac right to left shunting is present)

iv. Formula for calculation (on room air)

$$A–a \text{ gradient} = PAO_2 - PaO_2$$

$$PAO_2 = PIO_2 - (PaCO_2 \div 0.8)$$

$$PIO_2 = (PB - 47) \times FIO_2$$

where

47 mm Hg = vapor pressure of water at $37°C$
PIO_2 = pressure of inspired O_2
0.8 = assumed respiratory quotient (ratio of CO_2 produced to O_2 consumed per unit time)
PB = barometric pressure (at sea level, normal PB is 760 mm Hg)
FIO_2 = fraction (percent) of inspired O_2

Therefore,

$$FIO_2 (PB - 47) - (PaCO_2 \div 0.8) - PaO_2 = A–a \text{ gradient}$$

Example of calculation:

$$0.21 (760 - 47) - (40 \div 0.8) - 90 = 10$$

v. Normally, values for A–a gradient increase with age and with increased FIO_2

vi. Pathologic conditions causing increased A–a gradient
   (a) Ventilation-perfusion ($\dot{V}/\dot{Q}$) mismatching
   (b) Shunting
   (c) Diffusion abnormalities

3. Step 3—Transport of gases in the circulation
   a. Approximately 97% of oxygen is transported in chemical combination with hemoglobin (Hb) in the erythrocyte and 3% is carried dissolved in the plasma. PaO_2 is a measurement of the oxygen carried in the plasma and is a reflection of the driving pressure that causes oxygen to dissolve in the plasma and combine with Hb. Thus, O_2 content is related to PaO_2
   b. Oxyhemoglobin (O_2-Hb) dissociation curve (Fig. 1–4)
      i. The relationship between O_2 saturation (and content) and the PaO_2 is expressed in an S-shaped curve that has great physiologic significance. It describes the ability of Hb to bind oxygen at normal arterial O_2 tension levels and release it at lower PO_2 levels
      ii. The relationship between content and pressure of O_2 in the blood is not linear
         (a) The upper flat portion of the curve is the arterial association portion. This protects the body by enabling Hb to load O_2 despite large decreases in PaO_2
         (b) The lower steep portion of the curve is the venous dissociation portion. This protects the body by enabling the tissues to withdraw large amounts of O_2 with small decreases in PaO_2

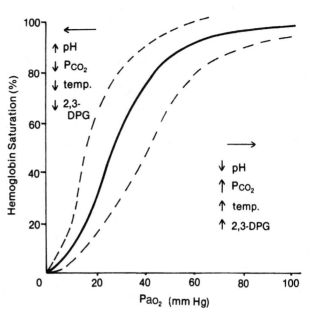

Figure 1–4 • The oxyhemoglobin dissociation curve, relating percent hemoglobin saturation and P_{O_2}. The normal curve is depicted with a solid line; the curves shifted to the right or left (along with the conditions leading to them), with the dotted lines. (From Weinberger, S. E.: Principles of Pulmonary Medicine, 2nd ed. Philadelphia, W. B. Saunders, 1992, p. 10.)

   iii. Hb-O_2 binding is sensitive to O_2 tension. The binding is reversible; affinity of Hb for O_2 changes as the P_{O_2} changes
     (a) When P_{O_2} is increased (as in pulmonary capillaries), O_2 binds readily with Hb
     (b) When P_{O_2} is decreased (as in tissues), O_2 unloads from Hb
   iv. Increase in rate of O_2 utilization by tissues causes an automatic increase in rate of O_2 release from Hb
   v. Shifts of the O_2-Hb curve
     (a) Shifts to the right: more O_2 unloaded for a given P_{O_2}, thus increasing O_2 delivery to tissues. These shifts are caused by:
       (1) pH decrease (acidosis), the *Bohr effect*
       (2) P_{CO_2} increase
       (3) Increase in body temperature
       (4) Increased levels of 2,3-diphosphoglycerate (2,3-DPG)
     (b) Shifts to the left: O_2 not dissociated from Hb until tissue and capillary O_2 are very low, thus decreasing O_2 delivery to tissues. These shifts are caused by:
       (1) pH increase (alkalosis) the Bohr effect
       (2) P_{CO_2} decrease
       (3) Temperature decrease
       (4) Decreased levels of 2,3-DPG
       (5) Carbon monoxide poisoning
     (c) 2,3-DPG is an intermediate metabolite of glucose that facilitates dissociation of O_2 from Hb at tissues. Decreased levels of 2,3-DPG impair O_2 release to tissues. This may occur with massive transfusions of 2,3-DPG–depleted blood
  c. The ability of Hb to release oxygen to the tissues is commonly assessed by the P_{50}
   i. P_{50} = the partial pressure of oxygen at which the hemoglobin is 50% saturated, standardized to a pH of 7.40

ii. Normal P_{50} is about 26.6 mm Hg, with variability based on disease process

d. Each gram of normal Hb can maximally combine with 1.34 ml of O_2 when fully saturated (values of 1.36 or 1.39 are sometimes used)

e. The amount of O_2 transported per minute in the circulation is a factor of both the O_2 content (CaO_2) and the cardiac output. This amount reflects how much O_2 is delivered to the tissues per minute and is dependent on the interaction of the circulatory system (delivery of arterial blood), erythropoietic system (hemoglobin in red blood cells), and respiratory system (gas exchange) according to the following equations:

  i. The O_2 content (CaO_2) is calculated from O_2 saturation, O_2 capacity, and the dissolved O_2

   (a) O_2 capacity is the maximal amount of O_2 the blood can carry. It is expressed in milliliters of O_2 per deciliter (100 ml) of blood (ml/dl) and is calculated by multiplying Hb in grams by 1.34

   (b) O_2 saturation is the percent of Hb actually saturated with O_2 (SaO_2 or $S\bar{v}O_2$) and is usually measured directly. It is equal to the O_2 content divided by the O_2 capacity multiplied by 100

   (c) O_2 content is the actual amount of O_2 the blood is carrying (oxyhemoglobin + dissolved O_2)

$$O_2 \text{ content} = (O_2 \text{ capacity} \times O_2 \text{ saturation}) + (0.0031 \times PaO_2)$$

  ii. Systemic O_2 transport

$$(\text{ml/minute}) = \text{arterial } O_2 \text{ content (ml/dl)} \times \text{cardiac output (L/min)} \times 10 \text{ (conversion factor)}$$

   (a) Normal cardiac output = about 5 to 6 L/minute (range, 4 to 8)

   (b) Normal arterial O_2 content = about 20 ml/dl

   (c) Therefore, systemic O_2 transport averages about 1000 to 1200 ml/minute

f. Focusing only on the O_2 tension of the blood is unwise because an underestimation of the severity of hypoxemia may result. The O_2 content and transport are more reliable parameters because they take into account the Hb concentration and cardiac output

g. Arterial-mixed venous differences in O_2 content ($CaO_2 - C\bar{v}O_2$) is the difference between arterial O_2 content (CaO_2) and mixed venous O_2 content ($C\bar{v}O_2$) and reflects the actual amount of O_2 extracted from the blood during its passage through the tissues

  i. Of the 1000 to 1200 ml of O_2 delivered per minute to the tissues, the cells typically use only about 250 to 300 ml ($\dot{V}O_2$ or O_2 consumption). If $\dot{V}O_2$ remains constant, changes in cardiac output can be related to changes in $CaO_2 - C\bar{v}O_2$ gradient or difference. Mixed venous O_2 values are measured from pulmonary artery catheters

  ii. Normal $CaO_2 - C\bar{v}O_2$ is 4.5 to 6 ml/dl

$$(\text{Hb} \times 1.34) (SaO_2 - S\bar{v}O_2) + (PaO_2 - P\bar{v}O_2) (0.0031)$$

iii. A fall in $C\bar{v}O_2$ resulting in a rise in $CaO_2 - C\bar{v}O_2$ gradient signifies decreased cardiac output and inadequate tissue perfusion

iv. These values are average values because the actual O_2 utilization changes with different tissues. The heart uses almost all the O_2 it receives

h. CO_2 transport: CO_2 is carried in the blood in three forms:

i. Physically dissolved CO_2 ($PaCO_2$), which accounts for 7% to 10% of CO_2 transported in the blood

ii. Chemically combined with Hb as carbaminohemoglobin. This reaction occurs rapidly, and reduced Hb can bind more CO_2 than oxyhemoglobin. Thus, unloading of O_2 facilitates loading of CO_2 *(Haldane effect)* and accounts for about 30% of CO_2 transport

iii. As bicarbonate through a conversion reaction:

$$CO_2 + H_2O \xleftrightarrow{\;CA\;} H_2CO_3 \longleftrightarrow H^+ + (Hb\ buffer) + HCO_3^-$$

(a) This reaction accounts for 60% to 70% of CO_2 in the body

(b) The reaction is slow in the plasma and fast in the red blood cell owing to the enzyme carbonic anhydrase (CA)

(c) When the concentration of these ions increases in the red blood cell, bicarbonate (HCO_3^-) diffuses but H^+ remains

(d) In order to maintain electrical neutrality, chloride diffuses from the plasma (the "chloride shift")

i. Pulmonary circulation (pulmonary artery, arterioles, capillary network, venules, and veins)

i. Pulmonary vessels are peculiarly suited to maintaining a delicate balance of flow and pressure distribution that optimizes gas exchange. They are richly innervated by the sympathetic branch of the autonomic nervous system

ii. In contrast to systemic circulation, pulmonary circulation is a low-resistance system. Pulmonary arteries have far thinner walls than systemic arteries do, and vessels distend to allow for increases in volume from systemic circulation. Intrapulmonary blood volume increases or decreases of approximately 50% occur with changes in the relationship between intrathoracic and extrathoracic pressure

iii. In upright positions, the volume of blood within the pulmonary capillaries is normally equal to the stroke volume of the heart

iv. Pulmonary arteries accompany bronchi within the lung and give rise to a rich capillary network within the alveolar walls. Pulmonary veins are not situated contiguously with the bronchial tree

v. The primary function of the pulmonary circulation is to act as a transport system

(a) Transport of blood through the lung

(1) Flow resistance through vessels is defined by *Ohm's law:*

$$R = \frac{\triangle P}{F}$$

where

$\triangle P$ is the pressure difference between the two ends of the vessel (i.e., upstream and downstream pressures)

F is flow. The driving pressure for flow in the pulmonary

circulation is the difference between the inflow pressure in the pulmonary artery and the outflow pressure in the left atrium

(2) In the lung, the measurement of flow resistance is the pulmonary vascular resistance (PVR)

PVR = mean pulmonary arterial pressure
− mean left atrial (or pulmonary wedge) pressure
÷ cardiac output

(3) About 12% of the total blood volume of the body is in the pulmonary circulation at any one time

(4) Normal pressures in pulmonary vasculature
  a) Mean pulmonary artery pressure: 10 to 15 mm Hg
  b) Mean pulmonary venous pressure: 4 to 12 mm Hg
  c) Mean pressure gradient, therefore, is about 10 mm Hg (considerably less than systemic gradient)
  d) Pressures are higher at the base of the lung than at the apex
  e) Perfusion is better in the dependent areas of the lung

(5) A unique characteristic of the pulmonary arterial bed is that it constricts in response to hypoxia. Diffuse alveolar hypoxia causes generalized vasoconstriction, resulting in pulmonary hypertension. Localized hypoxia causes localized vasoconstriction that does not increase pulmonary hypertension. This localized vasoconstriction directs blood away from poorly ventilated alveoli, thus improving overall gas exchange

(6) Chronic pulmonary hypertension (↑ PVR) can result in right ventricular hypertrophy (cor pulmonale)
  a) Transvascular transport of fluids and solutes
    i) Transvascular fluid filtration in the lung (and in all other organs) is described by the *Starling equation.* Simply stated, this means that fluid and solutes move because of increases or decreases in hydrostatic or osmotic filtration pressures or because of changes in the permeability of the vessel walls to fluids or proteins
    ii) Thus, excess fluid in lung (pulmonary edema) can occur as a result of either a net increase in hydrostatic pressure forces favoring filtration or a decreased resistance to filtration
  b) Metabolic transport
    i) All cardiac output passes through the lung before reaching the systemic circulation. Therefore, the pulmonary circulation can influence the composition of the blood supplying all organs
    ii) Several humoral substances are added, extracted, or metabolized in the lung. Examples are the inactivation of vasoactive prostaglandins, conversion of angiotension I to angiotensin II, and inactivation of bradykinin

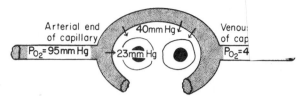

Figure 1–5 • Diffusion of oxygen from a tissue capillary to the cells. (From Guyton, A. C., and Hall, J. C.: Textbook of Medical Physiology, 9th ed. Philadelphia, W. B. Saunders, 1996, p. 514.)

4. **Step 4—Diffusion between systemic capillary bed and body tissue cells**
   a. Pressure gradients allow for diffusion of O_2 and CO_2 among systemic capillaries, interstitial fluid, and cells (Figs. 1–5 and 1–6)
   b. Within the mitochondria of each individual cell, O_2 is consumed through aerobic metabolism. This process produces the energy bonds of adenosine triphosphate (ATP) and the waste products of CO_2 and water

Hypoxemia

Hypoxemia is a state in which the O_2 pressure or saturation of O_2 in arterial blood or both is lower than normal values. Hypoxemia is generally defined as a PaO_2 less than 60 mm Hg or an SaO_2 below 90% at sea level in an adult breathing room air. Disorders that lead to hypoxemia do so through one or more of the following processes:

1. **Low inspired O_2 tension**
   a. Because of reduced ambient pressure (PB) or reduced O_2 concentration of inspired air (FIO_2)
   b. If lungs are normal, the A–a gradient will be normal
   c. Rarely a clinically important cause of arterial hypoxemia. It occurs at high altitudes among healthy humans
2. **Alveolar hypoventilation** ($\uparrow PaCO_2$)
   a. A decrease in alveolar ventilation from disorders of the respiratory center, peripheral nerves that supply muscles of respiration, respiratory muscles of chest wall, or lungs
   b. This causes an increase in $PaCO_2$, resulting in a fall in PAO_2 according to the alveolar air equation
   c. If the lungs are normal, the A–a gradient will be normal. Hypoxemia will improve with ventilation
3. **Mismatching of ventilation ($\dot{V}$) to perfusion ($\dot{Q}$): ($\dot{V}/\dot{Q}$ abnormalities)**
   a. The most common cause of hypoxemia; A–a gradient increased
   b. Ideally, ventilation of each alveolus is accompanied by a comparable amount of perfusion, yielding a $\dot{V}/\dot{Q}$ ratio of 1.00. Usually, however, there is relatively more perfusion than ventilation, yielding a normal $\dot{V}/\dot{Q}$ ratio of 0.8. The normal amount of blood perfusing alveoli ($\dot{Q}$) is 5 L/minute, and the normal amount of air ventilating the alveoli ($\dot{V}$) is

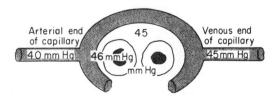

Figure 1–6 • Uptake of carbon dioxide by the blood in the capillaries. (From Guyton, A. C., and Hall, J. C.: Textbook of Medical Physiology, 9th ed. Philadelphia, W. B. Saunders, 1996, p. 515.)

4 L/minute. Figure 1–7 represents a simplification of possible relationships between ventilation and perfusion in the lung

c. When $\dot{V}/\dot{Q}$ is decreased (<0.8), a decrease of ventilation in relation to perfusion has occurred. This is similar to a right-to-left shunt because more deoxygenated blood is returning to the left heart. Low $\dot{V}/\dot{Q}$ ratios and hypoxemia occur together, as good areas of the lung cannot be overventilated to compensate for the underventilated areas. (Hb cannot be saturated more than 100%). Atelectasis, pneumonia, and pulmonary edema are clinical examples of intrapulmonary shunt

d. When $\dot{V}/\dot{Q}$ is increased (>0.8), a decreased perfusion in relation to ventilation has occurred, the equivalent of dead space or wasted

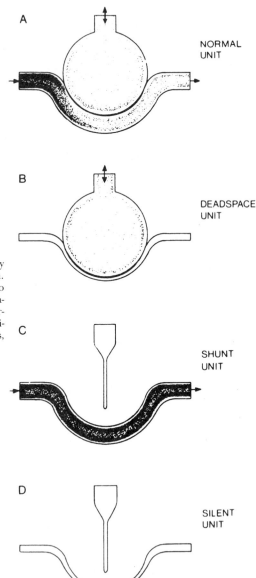

Figure 1–7 • The theoretical respiratory unit. *A,* Normal ventilation, normal perfusion. *B,* Normal ventilation, no perfusion. *C,* No ventilation, normal perfusion. *D,* No ventilation, no perfusion. (From Shapiro, B. A., Peruzzi, W. T., Templin, R., et al.: Clinical Application of Blood Gases, 5th ed. St. Louis, Mosby–Year Book, 1994, p. 22.)

A   NORMAL UNIT

B   DEADSPACE UNIT

C   SHUNT UNIT

D   SILENT UNIT

ventilation. Examples of such disease states are pulmonary emboli and cardiogenic shock

  e. Hypoxemia that is thought to be due to $\dot{V}/\dot{Q}$ mismatch may be corrected by giving the patient a simple incremental FIO_2 test. For example, if the PaO_2 increases significantly in response to an FIO_2 change from 0.30 to 0.60, the primary problem is low $\dot{V}/\dot{Q}$. If the PaO_2 does not increase significantly, a right-to-left shunt exists

4. Shunting

  a. Shunting occurs when a portion of the venous blood does not participate in gas exchange. An anatomic shunt may occur (a portion of right ventricular blood does not pass through pulmonary capillaries) or a portion of pulmonary capillary blood flow may pass adjacent to airless alveoli

  b. Normal physiologic shunting amounts to 2% to 5% of cardiac output (this is bronchial and thebesian vein blood)

  c. Shunting occurs in arteriovenous malformations (AVMs), adult respiratory distress syndrome (ARDS), atelectasis, pneumonia, pulmonary edema, pulmonary embolus, vascular lung tumors, and intracardiac right-to-left shunts

  d. Breathing an increased FIO_2 level does not correct shunting because not all blood comes into contact with open alveoli and the shunted blood passes directly from the pulmonary veins to the arterial blood (venous admixture). The lack of improvement of hypoxemia with O_2 therapy is a hallmark of shunting

  e. Usually, shunting does not result in elevated $PaCO_2$, even though shunted blood is rich in CO_2. Brain chemoreceptors sense elevated $PaCO_2$ and respond by increasing ventilation

  f. Shunting is measured by comparing mixed venous O_2 (from the pulmonary artery catheter) to arterial O_2 ($CaO_2 - C\bar{v}O_2$). The amount of true shunt can be estimated by having the patient breathe 100% O_2 for 15 minutes, thereby eliminating effects of abnormal $\dot{V}/\dot{Q}$ and diffusion defects. Normal shunt is 5 vol% (5 ml/dl)

5. Diffusion defects

  a. Seen in patients with thickened alveolar-capillary membrane, as in pulmonary fibrosis, so that there is a larger distance between alveolar gas and pulmonary capillaries

  b. May be overcome by diffusion because rate of diffusion always depends on the pressure gradient

  c. Is rarely a cause of hypoxemia by itself at rest but may contribute to hypoxemia in patients with $\dot{V}/\dot{Q}$ mismatch and/or shunting caused by disease state or in certain patients during exercise

Acid-Base Physiology and Blood Gases

1. Terminology

  a. *Acid:* a donator of H^+ (hydrogen) ions; any substance with a pH below 7.0

  b. *Acidemia:* the condition of the blood with a pH below 7.35

  c. *Acidosis:* the process, whether metabolic or respiratory, that causes the acidemia

    d. *Base:* an acceptor of H^+ ions; any substance with a pH above 7.0

    e. *Alkalemia:* the condition of blood with a pH above 7.45

    f. *Alkalosis:* the process, whether metabolic or respiratory, that causes the alkalemia

    g. *pH:* the negative logarithm of H^+ ion concentration

       i. Increase in $[H^+]$ = lower pH, more acidic

       ii. Decrease in $[H^+]$ = higher pH, more alkaline

2. Buffering: a normal body mechanism that occurs rapidly in response to acid-base disturbances in order to prevent changes in $[H^+]$ concentration

    a. Bicarbonate (HCO_3^-) buffer system

$$[H^+] + HCO_3^- \leftrightarrow H_2CO_3 \leftrightarrow CO_2 + H_2O$$

    This system is very important because HCO_3^- can be regulated by the kidneys and CO_2 can be regulated by the lungs

    b. Phosphate system

    c. Hb and other proteins

3. Henderson-Hasselbalch equation: defines the relationship between pH, P_{CO_2}, and bicarbonate. Arterial pH is determined by the logarithm of the ratio of bicarbonate concentration to arterial P_{CO_2}. Bicarbonate is regulated primarily by the kidney and P_{CO_2} is regulated by alveolar ventilation:

$$pH = pK + \log \frac{[HCO_3^-]}{Pa_{CO_2}}$$

$$pK = \text{a constant } (6.1)$$

    a. As long as the ratio of HCO_3^- to CO_2 is about 20:1, the pH of the blood will be normal. It is this ratio, rather than the absolute values of each, that determines blood pH

    b. The pH must be maintained within a narrow range of normal because the functioning of most enzymatic systems in the body depends on the hydrogen ion concentration (Fig. 1–8)

4. Normal adult blood gas values (at sea level)

    a. See Table 1–3.

    b. *Note:* Knowledge of blood gas values neither supersedes nor replaces sound clinical judgment

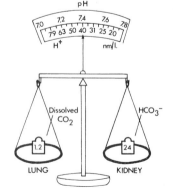

NORMAL ACID-BASE BALANCE

Figure 1–8 • The balance between bicarbonate (24) and dissolved carbon dioxide (CO_2) (1.2 of Pa_{CO_2} = 40) is normally 20:1, and this is usually associated with a pH of about 7.40 and a H^+ concentration of about 40 nmol/L. (From Cherniack, R. M., and Cherniack, L.: Respiration in Health and Disease, 3rd ed. Philadelphia, W. B. Saunders, 1983, p. 85.)

TABLE 1–3. Normal Adult Blood Gas Values (at Sea Level)

	Arterial	Mixed Venous
pH	7.40 (7.35–7.45)	7.36 (7.31–7.41)
Po_2	80–100 mm Hg	35–40 mm Hg
Sao_2	95% or more	70%–75%
Pco_2	35–45 mm Hg	41–51 mm Hg
Hco_3^-	22–26 mEq/L	22–26 mEq/L
Base excess	-2 to $+2$	-2 to $+2$

5. **Effect of altitude on blood gas values**
   a. Po_2 and Sao_2 are lower at high altitudes because of a lower ambient O_2 tension
   b. Normal for 5280 feet (Denver) = Pao_2 of 65 to 75 mm Hg, Sao_2 of 94% to 95%
6. **Respiratory parameter** ($Paco_2$). If the primary disturbance is in the Pco_2, the patient is said to have a respiratory disturbance
   a. $Paco_2$ is a reflection of alveolar ventilation
       i. If increased, hypoventilation is present
      ii. If decreased, hyperventilation is present
     iii. If normal, adequate ventilation is present
      iv. To assess relationships, measurements of both $Paco_2$ and minute ventilation are needed
   b. Respiratory acidosis (elevated $Paco_2$), caused by hypoventilation of any etiology (may be acute or chronic). Treatment generally consists of improving alveolar ventilation
       i. Obstructive lung disease, sleep apnea, and other lung diseases resulting in inadequate excretion of CO_2
      ii. Oversedation, head trauma, anesthesia, and drug overdose
     iii. Neuromuscular disorders, such as Guillain-Barré syndrome, myasthenic crisis
      iv. Pneumothorax, flail chest, or other types of chest wall trauma that interfere with breathing mechanics
       v. Inappropriate mechanical ventilator settings
   c. Respiratory alkalosis (low $Paco_2$) caused by hyperventilation of any etiology. Treatment consists of correcting the underlying cause
       i. Hypoxemia
      ii. Nervousness and anxiety
     iii. Pulmonary embolus, pulmonary edema
      iv. Pregnancy
       v. Excessive ventilation with mechanical ventilator
      vi. Interstitial lung disease
     vii. Response to metabolic acidosis (diabetic ketoacidosis)
    viii. Bacteremia (sepsis), liver disease, or fever
      ix. CNS disturbances, such as brain stem tumors and infections
       x. Respiratory stimulant drugs, such as salicylates, theophylline, catecholamines, and progesterone
7. **Nonrespiratory (renal) parameters** (Hco_3^-). If the primary disturbance is in the bicarbonate level, the patient has a metabolic disturbance
   a. Concentration influenced by metabolic processes

      i. When HCO_3^- is elevated, metabolic alkalosis results:
         (a) Loss of nonvolatile acid
         (b) Gain of HCO_3^-
      ii. When HCO_3^- is decreased, metabolic acidosis results:
         (a) H^+ is added in excess of capacity of kidney to excrete it
         (b) HCO_3^- is lost at rate exceeding capacity of kidney to regenerate it

   b. Causes of metabolic alkalosis (elevated HCO_3^-)
      i. Chloride depletion (vomiting, prolonged nasogastric suctioning, diuretic therapy)
      ii. Cushing's syndrome, hyperaldosteronism, potassium deficiency, renal artery stenosis, licorice
     iii. Exogenous administration of alkali (massive blood transfusions containing citrate, bicarbonate administration, ingestion of antacids)

   c. Causes of metabolic acidosis (decreased HCO_3^-)
      i. Increase in unmeasurable anions (acids that accumulate in certain diseases and poisonings); high anion gap
         (a) Diabetic ketoacidosis, starvation
         (b) Drugs
            (1) Salicylates
            (2) Ethylene glycol
            (3) Methanol alcohol
            (4) Paraldehyde
         (c) Lactic acidosis resulting from tissue hypoperfusion and subsequent anaerobic metabolism (shock, sepsis)
         (d) Renal failure, uremia
      ii. No increase in unmeasurable anions, normal anion gap
         (a) Diarrhea
         (b) Drainage of pancreatic juices
         (c) Ureterosigmoidostomy, long or obstructed ileal conduit
         (d) Rapid intravenous infusion of non-bicarbonate containing solutions causing a dilutional acidosis
         (e) Renal tubular acidosis
         (f) Certain drugs
         (g) Hyperalimentation causing a possible hyperchloremic acidosis

8. Compensation for acid-base abnormalities: a physiologic response of the body to minimize pH changes by maintaining a normal bicarbonate to P_{CO_2} ratio
   a. pH is returned to near normal by changing the component that is not primarily affected
   b. Respiratory disturbances result in kidney compensation, which may take several days to become maximal
      i. Compensation for respiratory acidosis
         (a) Kidneys excrete more acid
         (b) Kidneys increase HCO_3^- reabsorption
         (c) Compensation is slow (days)
      ii. Compensation for respiratory alkalosis
         (a) Kidneys excrete HCO_3^-
         (b) Compensation is slow (days)
   c. Metabolic disturbances result in pulmonary compensation, which begins rapidly but takes a variable amount of time to become maximal

      i. Compensation for metabolic acidosis
- (a) Hyperventilation to decrease $PaCO_2$
- (b) Compensation is rapid (begins in 1 to 2 hours and reaches maximum in 12 to 24 hours)

      ii. Compensation for metabolic alkalosis
- (a) Hypoventilation (limited by the degree of rise in $PaCO_2$)
- (b) Compensation is rapid (minutes to hours)

  d. The body does not overcompensate. Therefore, the acidity or alkalinity of the pH identifies the primary abnormality if there is only one. Abnormalities may be multiple; each is not a discrete entity. Mixed acid-base disturbances often occur

9. **Correction of acid-base abnormalities:** caused by a physiologic or therapeutic response
   a. pH returned to normal by altering component primarily affected; blood gas values are returned to normal
   b. Correction for respiratory acidosis: increase ventilation, treat cause
   c. Correction for respiratory alkalosis: decrease ventilation, treat cause
   d. Correction for metabolic acidosis
      i. Treat underlying cause
      ii. Administer bicarbonate intravenously or orally (given only under specific circumstances)
   e. Correction for metabolic alkalosis
      i. Treat underlying cause
      ii. Direct reduction by isotonic hydrochloric acid (HCl) solution (cautious IV administration required) via central line at a rate no greater than 0.2 mEq/kg/hour)
      iii. Arginine monohydrochloride or ammonium chloride used rarely; acetazolamide (carbonic anhydrase inhibitor–diuretic) used in certain situations

10. **Arterial blood gas (ABG) analysis**
    a. Purpose
       i. Shows end result of what occurs in lung
       ii. Confirms presence of respiratory failure and indicates acid-base status
       iii. Absolutely necessary in monitoring patients in acute respiratory failure and patients on ventilators
    b. Main components: PaO_2, $PaCO_2$, pH, base excess, bicarbonate, SaO_2, O_2 content, Hb. Both FIO_2 and body temperature must be measured for proper interpretation

11. **Guidelines for interpretation of ABGs and acid-base balance**
    a. Examine pH first
       i. If pH is reduced (<7.35), the patient is acidemic
          (a) If $PaCO_2$ is elevated, the patient has respiratory acidosis
          (b) If HCO_3^- is reduced, patient has metabolic acidosis
          (c) If $PaCO_2$ is elevated and HCO_3^- is reduced, the patient has combined respiratory and metabolic acidosis
       ii. If pH is elevated (>7.45), the patient is alkalemic
          (a) If $PaCO_2$ is decreased, the patient has respiratory alkalosis
          (b) If HCO_3^- is elevated, the patient has metabolic alkalosis
          (c) If $PaCO_2$ is decreased and HCO_3^- is elevated, the patient has combined metabolic and respiratory alkalosis

     iii. Expected change in pH for changes in Pa_{CO_2}: a commonly used rule is that the pH rises or falls 0.08 (or 0.1) in the appropriate direction for each change of 10 mm in the Pa_{CO_2}

     iv. If the pH is normal (7.35–7.45), alkalosis or acidosis may still be present as a mixed disorder

  b. Assess hypoxemic state and tissue oxygenation state

     i. Arterial oxygenation is considered compromised when Hb saturation is less than 90% ($Pa_{O_2} < 60$ mm Hg). If the Pa_{O_2} is below 60, hypoxemia is present and should be corrected

     ii. If the patient is receiving supplemental oxygen therapy, Pa_{O_2} values must be interpreted in relation to the FI_{O_2} delivered. One way involves examination of the two as a ratio (Pa_{O_2}/FI_{O_2}). The normal Pa_{O_2}/FI_{O_2} ratio is 286 to 350, although levels as low as 200 may be clinically acceptable. Another way to assess the oxygenation is to use the following formula to calculate A–a arterial P_{O_2} gradient ($PA_{O_2} - Pa_{O_2}$):

$$PA_{O_2} = FI_{O_2} (P_B - 47) - Pa_{CO_2}/R \text{ or } 0.8$$

where

PA_{O_2} = alveolar P_{O_2}
P_B = barometric pressure
47 = vapor pressure mm Hg of water at 37°C
Pa_{CO_2} = partial pressure of arterial CO_2
R = respiratory quotient, ratio of CO_2 production to O_2 consumption ($\dot{V}_{CO_2}/\dot{V}_{O_2}$); assumed to be 0.8

The normal $PA_{O_2} - Pa_{O_2}$ difference is less than 10 to 15 mm Hg. Although it provides an estimate of oxygenation, the gradient does not take into account the normal increasing gradient as a function of increasing FI_{O_2} levels. The higher the FI_{O_2}, the larger the increase in the A–a gradient without changing the level of intrapulmonary shunt or oxygenation

     iii. Excessively high Pa_{O_2} (>100 mm Hg) is generally not necessary and oxygen delivery should be reduced

     iv. Assessment of cardiac output and O_2 transport determines tissue oxygenation. $P\bar{v}_{O_2}$ or $S\bar{v}_{O_2}$ are important guides in evaluating the adequacy of tissue oxygenation

     v. Effectiveness of O_2 transport may be judged clinically by examining the patient carefully for mental status, skin color, urine output, and heart rate. In addition, tests that measure end-organ function are also important tools used by the clinician for assessment

NURSING ASSESSMENT DATA BASE

. . . .

Nursing History

Nursing history consists of the sequence and length of the standard history-taking process and is modified as needed for acutely ill patients

1. **Patient health history:** the patient's interpretation of his or her signs and symptoms and the emotional response to them play a significant role in the development or exacerbation of symptoms
   a. Common symptoms
      i. Dyspnea: the subjective feeling of shortness of breath or breathlessness
         (a) Difficult to quantify objectively
            (1) Count the average number of words the patient is able to speak between breaths
            (2) Ask the patient to rate breathing comfort on a visual analog scale or on a dyspnea scale from 1 to 10
         (b) Emotional problems may cause an increased awareness of respirations and complaints of inability to get enough air, despite normal blood gas values
         (c) Dyspnea caused by increased work of breathing accompanies both obstructive and restrictive lung diseases as well as dysfunction of nerves, respiratory muscles, or thoracic cage
         (d) Question patient regarding exercise tolerance; some dyspnea is normal with exercise but is abnormal if exercise tolerance is decreased
         (e) Assess whether patient's dyspnea is acute or chronic, and determine whether it has recently increased or decreased
         (f) Determine all circumstances under which dyspnea occurs (activities such as walking, stair climbing, eating) as well as how long patient has experienced dyspnea with those activities
         (g) To assess orthopnea or dyspnea when the patient is lying flat, ask how many pillows the patient usually uses for sleep
         (h) Assess for paroxysmal nocturnal dyspnea by asking the patient whether dyspnea has ever awakened him or her from sleep
         (i) Determine whether dyspnea is accompanied by any other symptoms, such as cough, wheezing, or chest pain
         (j) In some patients, it is difficult to differentiate cardiac from pulmonary dyspnea
      ii. Cough: a normal occurrence in some circumstances, as a lung defense mechanism
         (a) Determine whether the cough is acute and self-limiting or chronic and persistent
         (b) Note any change in character and frequency
         (c) Determine timing (both daily and seasonal) and whether cough is accompanied by sputum production, hemoptysis, wheezing chest pain, or dyspnea
         (d) Most common etiologic mechanisms
            (1) Inhaled irritants
            (2) Aspiration
            (3) Airways diseases (i.e., asthma, acute or chronic bronchitis)
            (4) Lung diseases (i.e., pneumonia, lung abscess, tumor)
            (5) Left ventricular failure
            (6) Side effect of medications (i.e., certain angiotensin-converting enzyme [ACE] inhibitors

      iii. Sputum production

          (a) Quantify amount by asking in terms of how many teaspoons or shot glasses of sputum are coughed up daily

          (b) Determine aggravating and alleviating factors

          (c) Assess character of sputum by noting color, odor, and consistency

          (d) Determine whether sputum's current characteristics (quantity and quality) are changed from usual

     iv. Hemoptysis: the expectoration of blood from the lungs or airways

          (a) Determine whether material coughed up is grossly bloody, blood streaked, or blood-tinged (pinkish)

          (b) Try to differentiate from hematemesis. *Hemoptysis* is often frothy, alkaline, and accompanied by sputum; *hematemesis* is nonfrothy, acidic, and dark red or brown in color, with food particles

          (c) Determine approximate amount of hemoptysis using a reasonable measurement guideline, such as number of teaspoons or shot glasses per day. Assess whether all expectorated specimens contain blood or whether this is an isolated event

          (d) Blood may originate from the nasopharynx, airways, or lung parenchyma; blood from these sites remains red because of the contact with atmospheric O_2

          (e) The etiologic mechanisms of hemoptysis fall into three categories by location: airways, pulmonary parenchyma, and vasculature

              (1) Airways disease: most common; bronchitis, bronchiectasis, and bronchogenic carcinoma

              (2) Parenchymal causes: often infectious: tuberculosis (TB), lung abscess, pneumonia

              (3) Cardiovascular disease: mitral stenosis, pulmonary embolism, pulmonary edema, AVM

              (4) Autoimmune disorders: Wegener's granulomatosis, Goodpasture's syndrome

          (f) Suspect neoplasm if hemoptysis occurs in patient without prior respiratory symptoms

      v. Chest pain: as a reflection of the respiratory system, does not originate in the lung, since the lung is free of sensory nerve fibers

          (a) Chest wall pain: arises from the parietal pleura, intercostal muscles, ribs, or overlying skin .

              (1) Well localized

              (2) Often exacerbated by deep inspiration

          (b) Diaphragm pain: often caused by inflammatory process; pain often referred to the ipsilateral shoulder

          (c) Mediastinal pain: caused by mass or air under the mediastinum (pneumomediastinum); pain substernal and dull

  b. Miscellaneous symptoms of respiratory disease: postnasal drip, sinus pain, epistaxis, hoarseness, general fatigue, weight loss, fever, sleep disturbances, night sweats, anxiety and nervousness, appetite depression

  c. Past medical history

      i. Question patient regarding presence of any allergy to either medications or food. Obtain description of type and severity of reaction

     ii. Determine past instances of present illness, with the treatment and outcome. Assess for previous episodes of TB, exposure to TB, or positive TB skin test result. Assess for childhood lung diseases or infections, such as asthma, pneumonia, and whooping cough. Record the treatment given (if any) and length of time patient stayed on medication regimen

   iii. Past surgeries or hospitalizations: dates, hospital, diagnosis, and complications; previous use of O_2 or mechanical ventilation

   iv. Previous chest radiographs: dates, reasons, findings

   v. Previous pulmonary function tests, and results if known

2. Family history (extremely important)

  a. Assess for similar illness or signs and symptoms in patient's parents, siblings, and grandparents

  b. Determine current state of health or cause of death for parents, siblings, and grandparents

  c. There often is a familial history of diseases, such as asthma, cystic fibrosis, bronchiectasis, and alpha₁-antitrypsin deficiency (emphysema)

  d. Determine whether family member ever had TB, with consequent exposure to the patient

3. Social history and habits

  a. Personal status: assess education, socioeconomic class, marital status, general life satisfaction, interests

  b. Health habits:

    i. Smoking

      (a) Determine whether patient is a current or past smoker

        (1) Calculate pack-year history:

$$\text{No. of packs/day} \times \text{No. of years} = \text{pack-years}$$

        (2) Determine whether patient has tried to quit; if so, which methods were used? Assess the patient's desire for information on smoking cessation resources available in the community

      (b) Learn whether patient has smoked marijuana or any other inhaled recreational drug, such as crack cocaine. If so, attempt to quantify the amount of drug use and the frequency

      (c) Determine whether patient chews tobacco. If so, quantify the type chewed and the amount per day

      (d) If patient is a former smoker, determine the time elapsed since the last cigarette

    ii. Drinking habits: determine frequency and amount consumed

      (a) Alcoholic beverages: which type?

      (b) Caffeine-containing beverages

    iii. Eating habits: assess quality of meals (adequacy or excess)

      (a) Determine whether any respiratory symptoms occur with eating (i.e., meal-induced dyspnea or cough)

    iv. Drug history: assess intake of any recreational drugs

    v. Sexual history: question the patient as to sexual activity and orientation

  c. Home conditions: assess economic conditions, housing, any pets and their health. Some respiratory symptoms are exacerbated by allergic response to pet dander and house mite debris found in carpeting and bedding

  d. Occupational history: assess past and present work conditions

    i. Determine whether patient was exposed to heat and cold, industrial
       toxins, or pollutants
    ii. Assess the duration of exposure and whether protective devices were
        used
4. **Medication history** (both prescription and over-the-counter or home remedy)
   a. Current and recent medications, their dose, and the reason for
      prescribing
   b. Assess whether patient is using any inhaled medications
      i. Determine the device used: metered dose inhaler (MDI), Rotohaler,
         Spinhaler, or nebulizer
      ii. Assess frequency of use—on an as-needed (p.r.n.) basis or on a
          regular schedule
      iii. If possible, have the patient demonstrate the technique for inhaling
           medication. Many patients with obstructive lung disease use an
           incorrect technique when inhaling their medication. This results in
           reduced deposition of the drug in the lung, with consequent reduced
           efficacy. Patients should exhale completely then inhale drug slowly
           and deeply, followed by breath holding for 10 seconds if possible

Nursing Examination of Patient

1. **Inspection**
   a. Ensure that the patient is stripped to the waist and, if possible, in the
      seated position
      i. A warm room and good lighting should be available
      ii. The nurse must have a thorough knowledge of anatomic landmarks
          and lines:
          (a) Manubrium, body, and xiphoid process of sternum, right and
              left sternal borders
          (b) Angle of Louis, point of maximal impulse (PMI), suprasternal
              notch
          (c) Interspaces, ribs, costal margins, costal angle, and spinous
              processes
          (d) Pulmonary lobes and areas of contact with chest wall
          (e) Lines: midclavicular, midsternal, anterior-axillary, midaxillary,
              posterior-axillary, vertebral and midscapular
   b. Observe the general condition and musculoskeletal development
      i. State of nutrition, debilitation, and evidence of chronic disease
      ii. Pectus carinatum: the sternum protrudes instead of being lower than
          the adjacent hemithoraces
      iii. Pectus excavatum: the sternum is abnormally depressed between the
           anterior hemithoraces
      iv. Kyphosis: an exaggerated anteroposterior curvature of the spine
      v. Scoliosis: lateral curvature of the spine, causing widened intercostal
         spaces on the convex side and crowding of the ribs on the concave
         side; when accompanied by kyphosis, it is called *kyphoscoliosis.* If
         severe, this condition can result in restrictive lung disease
   c. Observe the A-P diameter of the thorax; the normal A-P diameter is
      approximately one third of the transverse diameter. In patients with
      obstructive lung disease, the A-P diameter may be as great as or greater
      than the transverse diameter (''barrel chest'')

d. Observe the general slope of the ribs
   i. In normal subjects, the ribs are at a 45° angle in relation to the spine
   ii. In patients with emphysema, the ribs are more nearly horizontal
e. Observe for asymmetry
   i. One side may be larger because of tension pneumothorax or pleural effusion
   ii. One side may be smaller because of atelectasis or unilateral fibrosis
   iii. If asymmetry is present, the abnormal side will move less than the other
f. Look for retraction or bulging of interspaces
   i. Retraction of the interspaces, which can be observed during inspiration, indicates more negative intrapleural pressure due to obstruction of inflow of air or increased work of breathing
   ii. Bulging of interspaces may result from a large pleural effusion or pneumothorax, often seen during a forced expiration in patient with asthma or emphysema
g. Observe the ventilatory pattern
   i. Assess level of dyspnea and work of breathing
     (a) Position in which patient can breathe most comfortably. Patients with obstructive lung disease often assume a forward leaning position, resting arms on knees or a bedside table
     (b) Look for use of accessory muscles of breathing
     (c) Note whether patient is using pursed lip breathing
     (d) Observe for flairing of ala nasi during inspiration, as a common sign of air hunger
     (e) Paradoxical movement of diaphragm
   ii. Assess for presence of *inspiratory stridor*—low-pitched or crowing inspiratory sounds that occur when the trachea or major bronchi are obstructed because of:
     (a) Tumor (intrinsic or extrinsic)
     (b) Foreign body
     (c) Severe laryngotracheitis
     (d) Crushing injury
     (e) Goiter
     (f) Scar or granulation tissue
   iii. Observe for *expiratory stridor*—low-pitched crowing sound heard on expiration. Possible causes include:
     (a) Intrathoracic tracheal or mainstem tumor
     (b) Foreign body
   iv. Observe for unusual movements with breathing; on inspiration, the chest and abdomen should expand or rise together. *Paradoxical breathing* occurs with respiratory muscle fatigue. On inspiration, the chest rises and the abdomen is drawn in because the fatigued diaphragm does not descend on inspiration as it should. Instead, the diaphragm is drawn upward by the negative intrathoracic pressure during inspiration
   v. Observe and assess the ventilatory pattern
     (a) *Eupnea:* normal, quiet respirations
     (b) *Bradypnea:* abnormally slow rate of ventilation
     (c) *Tachypnea:* rapid rate of ventilation
     (d) *Hyperpnea:* increase in the depth and, perhaps, in the rate of

ventilation. The overall result is increased tidal volume and minute ventilation

(e) *Apnea:* complete or intermittent cessation of ventilation

(f) *Biot's breathing:* two to three short breaths with long, irregular periods of apnea

(g) *Cheyne-Stokes respiration:* periods of increasing ventilation, followed by progressively more shallow ventilations until apnea occurs. This pattern typically repeats itself. May sometimes occur in normal persons when asleep, it usually indicates

(1) CNS disease

(2) Heart failure

vi. Note splinting of respirations—the act of resisting full inspiration of one or both lungs as a result of pain

h. Other observations

i. General state of restlessness, pain, mental status, fright, or acute distress. Earliest signs of hypoxemia often include change in mental status and restlessness

ii. If O_2 is being administered, record the amount and method of delivery

iii. Inspect extremities

(a) Clubbing of fingers is a sign of a chronic pulmonary or cardiac disease

(b) Cigarette stains on fingers indicate current smoking habit

(c) Lower-extremity edema may indicate right heart failure from possible chronic pulmonary disease and hypoxemia induced pulmonary hypertension

iv. Observe for cyanosis

(a) The fundamental mechanism of cyanosis is an increase in the amount of reduced (deoxygenated) Hb in the vessels of the skin brought about by

(1) A decrease in the O_2 saturation of the capillary blood, or

(2) An increase in the amount of venous blood in the skin as a result of the dilation of venules and capillaries

(b) Visible cyanosis depends on the presence of at least 5 g of reduced Hb per deciliter of blood

(1) This is an absolute, not a relative, value. It is not the percentage of deoxygenated Hb that causes cyanosis but the amount of deoxygenated Hb without regard to the amount of oxyhemoglobin. The presence or absence of cyanosis may be an unreliable clinical sign

(2) In anemia, cyanosis may be difficult to detect because the absolute amount of Hb is too low

(3) Conversely, patients with marked polycythemia tend to become cyanotic at higher levels of arterial O_2 saturation than do patients with normal hemoglobin levels

(c) Discoloration suggestive of cyanosis may occur in situations of abnormal blood or skin pigments (e.g., methemoglobinemia, sulfhemoglobin, argyria)

(d) Factors influencing cyanosis:

(1) Rate of blood flow, perfusion

(2) Skin thickness and color

(3) Amount of Hb

(4) Cardiac output

(5) Perception of examiner

(e) *Central* versus *peripheral* cyanosis

(1) Central cyanosis implies arterial O_2 desaturation or abnormal Hb derivative. Both mucous membrane and skin are affected

(2) Peripheral cyanosis without central cyanosis may result from slowing of perfusion to body area, as in cold exposure, shock, obstruction, or decreased cardiac output. The O_2 saturation may be normal

(f) In carbon monoxide poisoning, the O_2 saturation may be dangerously low without obvious cyanosis because carboxyhemoglobin may cause the skin to turn a cherry-red

v. Assess for neck vein distention, neck masses, and enlarged nodes

vi. Look for signs of superior vena caval syndrome: distention of neck veins and edema of the neck, eyelids, and hands; often seen with lung cancer

2. Palpation

a. Palpate the thoracic muscles and skeleton, feeling for any of the following: pulsations, palpable fremitus, tenderness, bulges, or depressions in the chest wall

b. Expansion of the chest wall

i. Examiner's hands should be placed over lower lateral aspect of the chest, with the thumbs along the costal margin anteriorly or meeting posteriorly in the midline

ii. Movement of the hands is noted on inspiration and expiration. Asymmetry of movement is always abnormal. Reduced chest wall movement is often seen in patients with barrel chest and emphysema

c. Position and mobility of the trachea

i. Deviations of the trachea toward the defect are seen in atelectasis, unilateral pulmonary fibrosis, pneumonectomy, paralysis of the hemidiaphragm, and the inspiratory phase of flail chest

ii. Deviations of the trachea to the side opposite the lesion are seen in neck tumors, thyroid enlargement, tension pneumothorax, mediastinal mass, pleural effusion, and the expiratory phase of flail chest

d. Point of maximal impulse: the location may indicate mediastinal shift

e. Palpation of ribs and chest for tenderness, pain, or air in subcutaneous tissue (crepitus)

f. Vocal fremitus, a palpable vibration of the chest wall, produced by phonation

i. Patients should be instructed to say the word "ninety-nine" loud enough so that the fremitus can be felt with uniform intensity. In clinical practice, some soft-spoken women may need to falsely lower their voice so the fremitus can be felt. The examiner should place his or her hands on the patient's chest wall

ii. Diminished fremitus is a result of any condition that interferes with the transference of vibrations through the chest

(a) Pleural effusion or thickening

(b) Pleural tumors or masses

        (c) Pneumothorax with lung collapse

        (d) Obstruction of bronchus (i.e., owing to sputum plugs or tumors)

        (e) Emphysema

    iii. Increased fremitus is a result of any condition that increases transmission of vibrations through the chest

        (a) Pneumonia, consolidation

        (b) Atelectasis (with open bronchus)

        (c) Pulmonary infarction

        (d) Pulmonary fibrosis

        (e) Secretions with patent airway

g. Pleural friction fremitus

    i. Is produced when inflamed pleural surfaces rub together during respiration

    ii. Produces a "grating" sensation that occurs with the respiratory excursion

    iii. May be palpable during both phases of respiration, but sometimes is felt only during inspiration

h. Rhonchal fremitus

    i. Produced by passage of air through thick exudate, secretions, or an area of stenosis in the trachea or major bronchi

    ii. Unlike friction fremitus, rhonchal fremitus can be relieved by coughing, suctioning, or clearing the secretions from the tracheobronchial tree

i. Subcutaneous emphysema: indicates leak of air under skin from communication with airway, mediastinum, or pneumothorax

    i. May be palpated over the area

    ii. On auscultation, may be mistaken for crackles (rales)

3. Percussion: tapping or thumping of parts of the body to produce sound. The nature of the sound produced depends on the density of the structures immediately under the area percussed

a. Sound vibrations produced by percussion probably do not penetrate more than about 4 to 5 cm below the surface; therefore solid masses deep in the chest cannot be outlined with percussion. In addition, because a lesion must be several centimeters in diameter to be detectable by percussion, only large abnormalities can be located

b. Procedure: accomplished by striking the dorsal distal third finger of one hand that is held against the thorax with the distal tip of the flexed middle finger of the other hand

    i. The striking finger must strike only the stationary finger instantaneously; the striking finger must be withdrawn immediately

    ii. All movement is executed at the wrist

    iii. The examiner must be sensitive to the sounds that are received from the chest wall

    iv. Compare one side of the chest with the other side

    v. For percussion of the posterior chest, the patient should incline the head forward and rest the forearms on the thighs. This posture moves the scapulae laterally

    vi. Percussion begins at the apices and continues downward to the bases, alternating side to side

c. Percussion sounds over the lung

    i. *Resonance:* the sound heard normally over lungs

   ii. *Hyperresonance:* the sound heard over lungs of normal children, in the
apices of the lungs relative to the base in an upright adult, and
throughout lung fields in adults with emphysema or pneumothorax
      (a) Lower in pitch than normal resonance
      (b) Relatively intense and easy to hear
      (c) Indicates increased air (less dense)
  iii. *Tympany:* produced by air in an enclosed chamber; does not occur in
the normal chest, except below the dome of the left hemidiaphragm,
where it is produced by air in the underlying stomach or bowel
      (a) Relatively musical sound
      (b) Usually higher-pitched than that of normal resonance; the
higher the tension within the viscus, the higher the pitch
   iv. *Dullness:* the sound that is heard with lung consolidation, atelectasis,
masses, pleural effusion, or hemothorax
      (a) Short and not sustained
      (b) Soft, not loud
      (c) Similar to a dull ''thud''
      (d) Indicates more dense material (fluid or solid) is present in the
underlying thorax; dullness is normally heard over the liver and
heart
   d. Percussion for diaphragmatic excursion: the range of motion of the
diaphragm may be estimated with percussion
      i. Instruct patient to take a deep breath and hold it
     ii. Determine the lower level of resonance to dullness change (level of
diaphragm) by percussing downward until a definite change in the
percussion note is heard. Mark this spot with a pen
    iii. After instructing patient to exhale and hold the breath, repeat the
procedure
     iv. The distance between the levels at which the tone change occurs is
the diaphragmatic excursion
        (a) Normal diaphragmatic excursion is about 3 to 4 cm; partial
descent or hemidescent of the diaphragm may be related to
paralysis of the diaphragm. Suspect nerve injury in postoperative
patients with these signs following thoracic surgery
        (b) Diaphragm is normally higher on the right than on the left
        (c) The diaphragm is high in
            (1) Conditions that cause an increased intra-abdominal
pressure (pregnancy, ascites)
            (2) Any condition that causes decreased thoracic volume
(atelectasis)
        (d) The diaphragm is fixed and lower than normal in emphysema
        (e) It is difficult to differentiate between an elevated diaphragm and
disease of the thorax that causes dullness to percussion (e.g.,
pleural effusion)
            (1) Paralysis of one or both hemidiaphragms
 4. **Auscultation:** listening to sounds produced within the body
   a. Basic points
      i. The examiner should always compare one lung to the other by
moving stethoscope back and forth across chest starting at the top of
the thorax and moving downward
     ii. The patient should be asked to breathe through the mouth a little

more deeply than usual. Breathing through an open mouth minimizes turbulent flow sounds produced in the nose and throat

iii. The diaphragm of the stethoscope is more sensitive to higher-pitched tones and is thus best for most lung sounds

iv. Stethoscope earpieces should fit snugly to exclude extraneous sounds but should not be so tight that they are uncomfortable

v. The stethoscope tubing should be no longer than 20 inches (the shorter the better). Optimal length is 12 to 14 inches

vi. Place stethoscope firmly on the chest to exclude extraneous sounds and eliminate sounds that may result from light contact with skin or air. Confusing sounds may be produced by:

    (a) Movement of stethoscope on skin or hair

    (b) Breathing on the tubing

    (c) Sliding fingers on tubing or chest piece

    (d) Listening through clothing

b. Normal breath sounds vary according to the site of auscultation

i. *Vesicular* (always normal)

    (a) Soft sounds heard over fields of anterior, lateral, and posterior chest

    (b) Heard primarily during inspiration

ii. *Bronchial* (may be normal or abnormal, depending on location of sounds)

    (a) Heard normally over the trachea

    (b) High-pitched, harsh sound with long and loud expirations

    (c) When heard over lung fields, the sound is abnormal and suggests consolidation

iii. *Bronchovesicular* (may be normal or abnormal, depending on location)

    (a) Heard over large bronchi (near sternum, between scapulae, over right upper lobe apex)

    (b) Abnormal when heard over lung fields; signifies consolidation

c. Abnormalities of breath sounds

i. Absent or diminished sounds caused by decreased air flow (airway obstruction, chronic obstructive pulmonary disease [COPD], muscular weakness, splinting due to pain) or increased insulation blocking the transmission of the sounds to the stethoscope (obesity, pleural disease and fluid, pneumothorax)

ii. Bronchial sounds heard over lung fields suggest consolidation or increased density of lung tissue (e.g., atelectasis, pulmonary infarction, pneumonia, large tumors with no airway obstruction)

d. *Adventitious* sounds: abnormal sounds that are superimposed on underlying breath sounds

i. Evaluate how position and coughing affect adventitious sounds

ii. Terminology

    (a) *Crackles* (rales): signify the opening of collapsed alveoli and small airways

        (1) Described as fine or coarse

        (2) Heard as small pops or crackles; the sound of fine crackles can be mimicked by rubbing a few pieces of hair together near one's ear. The sound of coarse crackles can be mimicked by pulling open Velcro material

          (3) Fine crackles occurring late in inspiration imply conditions that cause restrictive ventilatory defect

          (4) Fine crackles heard early in inspiration are often atelectatic and caused by small airway closure

          (5) Coarse early inspiratory crackles are associated with bronchitis or pneumonia

      (b) *Wheeze:* indicates obstruction to airflow or air passing through narrowed airways

          (1) Continuous high-pitched sound with musical quality; also called "sibilant" wheeze

          (2) Commonly heard during expiration but may be heard during inspiration

          (3) Causative conditions: asthma, bronchitis, foreign bodies or tumors, mucosal edema, pulmonary edema, pulmonary emboli, poor mobilization of secretions

      (c) *Gurgles* (rhonchi) result from air passing through secretions in large airways

          (1) Low-pitched, continuous sounds

          (2) May have snoring quality when very large airways are involved; also called "sonorous" wheezes

          (3) Rhonchi tend to improve or disappear after coughing

      (d) *Pleural friction rub:* indicates inflammation and loss of pleural fluid

          (1) Grating harsh sound in inspiration and expiration; disappears with breath-holding. One can mimic the pleural friction rub sound by cupping a hand over one's ear and rubbing the fingers of the other hand over the cupped hand.

          (2) Heard with pleural infections, infarction, pulmonary emboli, and fractured ribs. Located in area of most intense chest wall pain

      (e) *Mediastinal crunch:* indicates air in pericardium, mediastinum, or both

          (1) Heard synchronously with systole; often associated with pericardial friction rubs

      (f) *Pericardial friction rub*

          (1) Occurs at atrial and ventricular systole; there may be a diastolic component

          (2) Sounds persist with breath-holding; heard most clearly at the left lower sternal border (LLSB)

e. Voice sounds: spoken words are modified by disease in a similar manner as breath sounds, resulting in increased or decreased conduction of sound

  i. Increased conduction occurs when normal lung tissue is replaced with denser more solid tissue; is associated with bronchial breathing

    (a) Bronchophony: the spoken word (e.g., "99") is heard distinctly but the normal sound is muffled

    (b) Egophony: The "E" sound changes to "A"; sound has the quality of sheep bleating

    (c) Whispered pectoriloquy: whispered sounds are heard with clarity, as if the patient is speaking into the diaphragm of one's stethoscope, but the normal sound is muffled

ii. Decreased conduction of sound occurs in the presence of obstructed bronchi, pneumothorax, or large collections of fluid or tissue between the lung and the chest wall

(a) Decreased ability to hear the voice sounds

(b) Is accompanied by decreased fremitus

Diagnostic Studies

1. **Laboratory findings**
   a. Sputum examination
      i. Obtain a specimen through voluntary coughing and expectoration, induction of sputum by inhaling aerosol, nasotracheal or endotracheal suctioning, transtracheal aspiration, or bronchoscopy
      ii. Assess important characteristics
         (a) Color and consistency
         (b) Volume: greater than 25 ml/day is excessive
         (c) Odor: should be odorless
            (1) Foul-smelling may indicate anaerobic putrefactive process
            (2) Musty odor may indicate *Pseudomonas* infection
         (d) Microscopic examination
            (1) Cytologic study for malignant cells
            (2) Smear for bacterial examination (e.g., Gram stain) or fungi
            (3) Sputum cultures to diagnose infection and assess drug resistance
            (4) Special stains on cultures are required for mycobacterial (acid-fast bacilli [AFB]), fungi, *Pneumocystis carinii, Legionella pneumophila*
   b. Pleural fluid examination
      i. Diagnostic thoracentesis or pleural biopsy is performed to obtain specimen
      ii. Determination of transudate versus exudate is based on protein, lactate dehydrogenase (LDH) levels in pleural fluid and blood
      iii. Specimen is examined for cell counts, protein and LDH, glucose, amylase, pH, Gram stain for bacteria, cytology for malignant cells and microorganisms
      iv. Frequently, a biopsy specimen of the parietal pleura is also obtained and the tissue examined by microscopy
   c. Skin tests
      i. For type I hypersensitivity (mediated by immunoglobulin E [IgE]): as in pollens, molds, dusts, grasses
      ii. For type II hypersensitivity (mediated by T lymphocytes): purified protein derivative (PPD) for tuberculosis
      iii. For fungal diseases
   d. Serologic tests are used to determine causative pathogen in bacterial, viral, mycotic, and parasitic diseases

2. **Radiologic findings**
   a. Chest x-ray examination precedes all other studies

      i. Posteroanterior (PA) and lateral views are most commonly used

     ii. Portable anteroposterior (AP) views are used in the intensive care unit (ICU) when the patient cannot be moved. These are generally of lesser quality than an erect PA film because of

        (a) Difficulty in positioning the patient

        (b) Short film distance from the chest; also variable distance in serial films

        (c) Less powerful x-ray generator

        (d) Interference from tubes, lines, and equipment attached to patient

     iii. Lateral decubitus films are used if fluid levels need to be identified (as with pleural effusions and abscesses)

     iv. Oblique views are useful for localizing lesions and infiltrates

      v. Lordotic views enable evaluation of the apical portion of the lung and the middle lobe or lingula and can help determine whether a lesion is anterior or posterior

     vi. Expiratory films are used for visualizing pneumothorax or air trapping

b. Fluoroscopy

      i. Shows movement of pulmonary and cardiac structures, localizes pulmonary lesions, and reveals diaphragmatic motion

     ii. Is used for monitoring during special procedures: catheter insertion, bronchoscopy, thoracentesis, and chest tube placement

     iii. Exposure of patients to radiation is greater during fluoroscopy than during a standard x-ray examination

c. Tomography: provides views at different planes through the lungs

      i. Gives better definition of small or questionable lesions and is particularly useful for determining whether a lesion has calcification within it. Since the advent of computed tomography (CT), however, plain tomography is used less frequently

     ii. CT scan

        (a) Used for scanning axial cross-sections of body

        (b) Particularly useful in detecting subtle differences in tissue density

d. Magnetic resonance imaging (MRI)

      i. Can distinguish tumors from other structures, such as blood vessels, spinal cord involvement, and bronchial walls

     ii. Can differentiate pleural thickening, pleural fluid, and chest wall tumors from each other

e. Pulmonary angiography: visualizes the pulmonary arterial tree through the injection of radiopaque dye

      i. Useful in investigating thromboembolic disease of the lung, congenital abnormalities of the circulation, and delineation of masses

     ii. There are some risks. Pulmonary angiography is dangerous to perform in the presence of pulmonary hypertension; O_2 desaturation has occurred in some patients with injection of contrast medium. Hemodynamic parameters should be measured before the procedure

f. Ventilation-perfusion lung scanning use

      i. Injection or inhalation of radioisotopes is used to obtain information about pulmonary blood flow and ventilation

     ii. Can detect pulmonary emboli and assess regional lung function preoperatively

g. Ultrasonography

      i. Is useful in evaluating pleural disease

      ii. Can detect small amounts of pleural fluid and loculations within the pleural space

      iii. Can distinguish fluid from pleural thickening

      iv. Can localize the diaphragm and detect disease immediately below it, such as a subphrenic abscess

      v. Not useful for defining structures or lesions within the pulmonary parenchyma (the ultrasound beam penetrates air poorly)

3. Other diagnostic studies

  a. Noninvasive tests

    i. Pulmonary function studies

      (a) Purpose

        (1) Classifies pulmonary function as normal or exhibiting a restrictive or obstructive defect

        (2) Detects early disease

        (3) Describes disease in physiologic terms; permits description of patient's condition to others

        (4) Follows up patient in quantitative terms for future comparisons

        (5) Assists in the evaluation of risk of surgery

      (b) Lung volumes and capacities are performed with the patient in the upright position and are compared with predicted ones (Fig. 1–9)

        (1) Volumes: there are four discrete and nonoverlapping lung volumes

          a) Tidal volume (V$_T$): volume of gas inspired and expired during each respiratory cycle

          b) Inspiratory reserve volume (IRV): maximal volume of gas that can be inspired after a tidal breath is taken

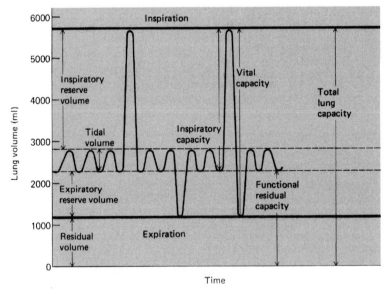

Figure 1–9 • Diagram showing respiratory excursions during normal breathing and during maximal inspiration and maximal expiration. (From Guyton, A. C., and Hall, J. C.: Textbook of Medical Physiology, 9th ed. Philadelphia, W. B. Saunders, 1996, p. 483.)

    c) Expiratory reserve volume (ERV): maximal volume of gas that can be expired from end-expiratory position

    d) Residual volume (RV): volume of gas remaining in lungs at end of a maximal expiration

(2) Capacities: there are four, each of which includes two or more of the primary volumes

    a) Total lung capacity (TLC): volume of gas contained in lung at end of a maximal inspiration

$$TLC = V_T + IRV + ERV + RV$$

    b) Vital capacity (VC): maximal volume of gas that can be expelled from lungs by a forceful effort following a maximal inspiration

$$VC = V_T + IRV + ERV$$

    c) Inspiratory capacity (IC): maximal volume of gas that can be inspired from resting expiratory level

$$IC = V_T + IRV$$

    d) Functional residual capacity (FRC): volume of gas remaining in the lungs at resting end expiration

$$FRC = ERV + RV$$

(c) Ventilatory mechanics: provide information about dynamic lung function. Subjects perform forced breathing maneuvers

(1) Forced expiratory spirograms

    a) FVC: forced vital capacity; reduced in restrictive disease or in obstructive disease if there is air trapping

    b) FEV_t: forced expiratory volume in t (seconds); usually measured at 0.5, 1, and 3 seconds. Reduced in obstructive disease. Most common measure is FEV_1

    c) $FEV_1/VC\%$: forced expiratory volume as a percentage of vital capacity, with t representing time in seconds. Evaluates obstruction to flow

      i) FEV_1/VC: normally $> 75\%$ in adults

      ii) FEV_3/VC: normally $> 95\%$ in adults

    d) FEF: Forced expiratory flows ($FEF_{25\%-75\%}$, $FEF_{75\%-85\%}$, and $FEF_{200-1200}$). These tests assess flows over a range of lung volumes

    e) Values for timed flow studies are decreased out of proportion to vital capacity in obstructive disease

(2) Flow-volume loop studies

    a) Volume and flow during inspiration and expiration are graphically plotted

    b) Obstructive and/or restrictive disease produces abnormal flow-volume loops

(3) Maximum voluntary ventilation (MVV)

    a) Volume of air ventilated with maximal effort over a short period of time

    b) May be used to predict patient's ability to undergo

procedures that require ventilatory reserve (i.e., surgery)

(d) Lung compliance studies assess the distensibility of the lungs; lung compliance is the reciprocal of elastance

    (1) Expressed as increase in volume (V) per increase in transpulmonary pressure (P)

$$C_L = \frac{\Delta V}{\Delta P}$$

    (2) Static compliance (C_{st}) is measured in the absence of air flow

        a) In the patient on a ventilator, it is measured by dividing V_T by plateau pressure (minus PEEP) and is called the *effective static compliance*

        b) Normal values are around 100 ml/cm H_2O

    (3) Dynamic compliance (C_{dyn}) is measured under conditions of flow

        a) In patients on a ventilator, it is measured by dividing V_T by peak inspiratory pressure (minus PEEP) and is called the *effective dynamic compliance*

        b) Normal range is between 40 and 50 ml/cm H_2O

    (4) Compliance is decreased in conditions that make the lungs or thorax stiffer or reduce expansibility. Such conditions include atelectasis, pneumonia, pulmonary edema, fibrotic changes, pleural effusion, pneumothorax, kyphoscoliosis, obesity, abdominal distention, flail chest, and splinting due to pain

    (5) Increases in compliance occur with age or emphysema

    (6) Compliance curves (serial changes in volume plotted against changes in pressure) are useful in monitoring patients on volume ventilators. Determinations of the best pressure-volume combinations for the patient may be made. Comparisons of static and dynamic pressure-volume curves help determine which component (airway, lung, or chest wall) is contributing to changes in compliance

(e) Gas transfer and exchange studies

    (1) Blood gas and acid-base analysis

        a) Fundamental to diagnosis and management of pulmonary problems

        b) See Physiologic Anatomy

    (2) Diffusing capacity (D_L)

        a) Measures the amount of functioning alveolar-capillary surface area available for gas exchange

        b) Values decrease with ventilation-perfusion mismatching and membrane problems and with decreases in pulmonary capillary blood volume

(f) Guidelines for interpretation of pulmonary function testing

    (1) Values are compared with predicted values for age, height, and sex

    (2) Restrictive pulmonary impairment generally results in decreased volumes and capacities

(3) Decreased static lung compliance suggests parenchymal disease

(4) Obstructive defect generally results in decreased tests of dynamic ventilatory function. This may be reversible with use of bronchodilators

(5) COPD with long-term air trapping and destruction of parenchyma results in increased FRC, RV, and TLC

(6) Patient preparation and cooperation are necessary to obtain reliable and valid data for most pulmonary function tests

b. Invasive tests

  i. Lung biopsy

    (a) Needle biopsy is used for diagnosis of malignancy or infection; pneumothorax may be a complication

    (b) Open lung biopsy requires a thoracotomy or thoracoscopic examination but has better diagnostic yields

  ii. Bronchoscopy: insertion of a fiberoptic scope into the airways for direct visualization and possible obtaining of specimens

    (a) Indicated for diagnosis of lung malignancy, evaluation of hemoptysis, removal of foreign body or secretions and sampling an area of lung through either washings, brushings, or biopsy specimens

    (b) After the procedure, patients must be observed for respiratory depression (from drugs used for sedation), decreased ventilation, and hypoxemia

    (c) Supplemental O_2 should be administered during the procedure

    (d) If transbronchial biopsy is performed, hemoptysis or pneumothorax is a possible complication

  iii. Mediastinoscopy is performed for diagnostic exploration of the mediastinum and to obtain biopsy specimens

COMMONLY ENCOUNTERED NURSING DIAGNOSES

Ineffective Airway Clearance related to secretions

1. **Assessment for defining characteristics**
   a. Abnormal breath sounds
   b. Altered rate or depth of respiration
   c. Tachypnea
   d. Cough, effective or ineffective
   e. Cyanosis
   f. Dyspnea
   g. Fever
2. **Expected outcomes**
   a. Breath sounds clear following treatment
   b. Absence of adventitious sounds
   c. Secretions are easily expectorated or suctioned

3. Nursing interventions
   a. Assist the patient to deep breathe
      i. Position the patient to maximize inspiratory muscle length and to maximize ventilation (semi-Fowler's to high Fowler's position, depending on patient comfort)
      ii. Ask the patient to take slow deep breaths, and assess volume for adequacy (i.e., from FRC to TLC) and to sustain breath for several seconds before expiration
      iii. Provide the patient with cues or devices to motivate independent deep-breathing exercises
   b. Position the patient to facilitate coughing
      i. Help the patient to assume a comfortable cough position (i.e., high Fowler's), with knees bent and a light-weight pillow over the abdomen to augment the expiratory pressures and minimize discomfort
      ii. Teach the patient alternate cough techniques, such as controlled cough, forced expiratory technique known as "huff coughing" or quad-assist cough. For a controlled cough, the patient takes a slow maximal inspiration and holds the breath for several seconds, followed by two or three coughs. The huff cough consists of one or two forced exhalations or "huffs" from middle to low lung volumes, with the glottis open
   c. Provide an artificial airway and ventilation if indicated
      i. Oropharyngeal airway
         (a) Purpose: to maintain airway by holding tongue anteriorly
         (b) Technique: correct size measures from the corner of patient's mouth to the angle of the jaw following natural curve of the airway. Apply a jaw lift to help displace the tongue. Rotate the airway 180° before insertion. As the tip of the airway reaches the hard palate, rotate the airway again by 180°, aligning it as before in the pharynx
         (c) Complications: vomiting and aspiration with intact gag reflex; malposition due to improper length; worsen obstruction by pushing tongue back further into pharynx due to incorrect placement. Oral care is more difficult
      ii. Nasopharyngeal airway
         (a) Purpose: useful in facial and jaw fractures when an oral airway cannot be used; more readily tolerated than the oropharyngeal airway
         (b) Complications: nosebleed, nasal mucosa irritation
         (c) Adequate humidification is essential to ensure patency of narrow lumen
         (d) Airway should be taped in place to prevent inadvertent displacement. The tube should be removed periodically to prevent skin breakdown
      iii. Cricothyroidotomy: restricted to extreme emergencies when other methods fail or are unavailable. An incision must be made through the cricothyroid membrane
      iv. Esophageal obturator airway
         (a) For temporary emergency use only
         (b) Usually easier to insert than an endotracheal tube; less training and skill needed

  (c) Risk of aspiration reduced while the tube is in place
  (d) Disadvantages
    (1) Suctioning is difficult
    (2) Stimulates vomiting; do not use if patient is conscious
    (3) If patient vomits during or before passage of tube, the device can be flooded
    (4) Vomiting usually follows removal of the tube. Place patient on his or her side before removing, and be prepared to suction
    (5) The esophagus may be perforated
    (6) Trachea may be intubated inadvertently
  (e) Esophageal gastric obturator airway: allows for gastric suctioning
 v. Endotracheal intubation
  (a) Thorough training and retraining in this procedure are absolute necessities for competency
  (b) Key principles
    (1) Preoxygenate with 100% O_2 for at least 2 minutes if possible
    (2) Check for correct placement of the tube after insertion
      a) Feel air movement through tube opening
      b) Assess for bilateral chest excursion during inspiration and expiration
      c) Auscultate both sides of chest peripherally as well as the abdomen
      d) Use an exhaled CO_2 detector or monitor to determine lung versus esophagus placement
      e) Obtain a chest x-ray study. The tip of the tube should be about 2 to 3 cm above the carina
      f) Provide manual ventilation using a self-inflating resuscitation bag connected to 100% O_2 source set at 10 to 15 L/minute
  (c) Nasotracheal intubation
    (1) Sometimes used when the oral route is not available
    (2) The risk of paranasal sinusitis as well as bleeding is increased
  (d) Nursing care considerations for the intubated patient
    (1) Provide frequent mouth care (absolutely necessary)
    (2) Check placement of the tube immediately after insertion and after tube position adjustments
    (3) Carefully secure the tube to prevent movement and to decrease tracheal damage
    (4) Provide adequate humidity regardless of nasal or oral intubation
    (5) Move oral tubes from one side of the mouth to the other at least daily. Note and document the centimeter (cm) marking on tube at the corner of the lip as a reference point
    (6) Be aware that infection resulting from contaminated equipment or unsterile procedures may develop
    (7) Suction as required according to patient need, not at a routine frequency. Use sterile technique

    a) Use either single use or closed suction catheter system, depending on hospital policy

    b) Provide pre-suctioning and post-suctioning oxygenation with three to five deep inflations using either the manual two-handed technique or the manual demand breath by ventilator of 100% O_2 for 30 seconds

    c) Keep the duration of suctioning brief (10 to 15 seconds) to minimize the amount of O_2 containing air that is evacuated from the lungs. Apply suction only when withdrawing catheter

    d) Monitor the electrocardiogram (ECG) for arrhythmias during and after suctioning; observe for changes in O_2 saturation by pulse oximetry if available

    e) Observe and document amount and description of secretions

  (8) For a prolonged intubation procedure, the person performing the intubation may instill lidocaine into the tube or inject it into the vocal cords to increase patient tolerance

 (e) Tracheal tube cuffs

  (1) Cuff design characteristics

    a) Low sealing pressure; intracuff pressure should not exceed capillary filling pressure of trachea (less than or equal to 25 cm water pressure or 20 mm Hg pressure) to avoid tracheal mucosal injury

    b) Cuff pressure is distributed over large contact area

    c) Large volumes of air accepted with minor increases in balloon tension

    d) Provides sufficient pressure to maintain adequate seal during inspiration and expiration (necessary to allow positive-pressure ventilation and use of PEEP). Also may help prevent pulmonary aspiration of large food particles but does not protect against aspiration of liquids, such as water and enteral formula feedings

    e) Does not distort tracheal wall

  (2) Low-pressure, high-volume cuffs generally meet desired characteristics and have replaced low-residual-volume, high-pressure cuffs

  (3) Principles of cuff inflation and deflation

    a) Inflation of low-pressure cuffs:

     i) Inflate with sufficient air to ensure no leak (minimal occlusive volume [MOV] technique) or only minimal leak during peak inspiration (minimal leak technique [MLT]).

     ii) If increasing amounts of air are needed to obtain a seal, this may be due to tracheal dilation or to a leak in cuff or pilot balloon valve; the condition should be corrected

    b) Routine deflation is not necessary. Periodic deflation may be useful so that patient can breathe around the tube to facilitate speech (often difficult to accomplish when the patient is receiving mechanical ventilation)

 c) Regardless of cuff design or pressure characteristics, all cuff pressures should be routinely measured at least every 8 to 12 hours and whenever the cuff is reinflated or tube position is changed

(f) Key points for extubation

 (1) Criteria for extubation will depend on whether or not the underlying patient condition that led to the need for intubation has improved or reversed to the extent that the artificial airway is no longer necessary. Generally accepted criteria include:

  a) Stable vital signs and hemodynamic parameters

  b) Patient awake and alert

  c) Absence of copius secretions

  d) Ventilatory parameters or measurements (such as maximum inspiratory pressure and negative inspiratory force, spontaneous tidal volume, minute ventilation, and vital capacity) are within acceptable limits

 (2) Postextubation monitoring

  a) Repeat blood gas studies 30 minutes after extubation or sooner as indicated and periodically thereafter

  b) Observe for laryngospasm. Auscultate trachea with stethoscope for stridor, breathing difficulties. Treatment may consist of racemic epinephrine inhalation, steroids to reduce laryngeal edema, and possible reintubation. Postextubation stridor may occur immediately or may take several hours to develop

  c) Monitor the patient's tolerance to extubation by clinical observation, auscultation of breath sounds as well as the neck for stridor, ventilatory measurements, and blood gas studies

vi. Tracheostomy

 (a) Purpose and indications

  (1) To facilitate secretion removal from tracheobronchial tree

  (2) To decrease dead space ventilation

  (3) To bypass upper airway obstruction or as part of surgical intervention requiring alternate airway placement

  (4) To prevent or limit aspiration of oral or gastric secretions (cuffed tubes)

  (5) To aid in patient comfort when assisted or controlled ventilation is needed for an extended period of time

 (b) Principles of care

  (1) Stoma is kept clean and dry

  (2) Frequency of inner cannula tube exchanges with disposable tubes and routine cleaning of inner cannulas with reusable inner cannulas is in accordance with hospital or institutional guidelines

   a) Be prepared for complications during any cleaning procedure

   b) Have the following equipment at the bedside:

i) Self-inflating manual resuscitation bag and mask
ii) Suction equipment (including catheters, oxygen flowmeter and tubing)
iii) Intubation materials
iv) Tracheal tube and stoma cleaning supplies

  c) Be prepared to intubate or otherwise support ventilation

  d) Have an extra tracheostomy tube of same size and type at bedside, and keep a tube obturator at bedside in case the tube must be reinserted emergently

(3) *Uncuffed tubes* are commonly used in children and adult patients with laryngectomies and are sometimes used during the decannulization or weaning process by progressive downsizing of the tube

(4) *Cuffed tubes* are typically used when the patient is receiving artificial ventilation. The tube may be air-filled or a self-inflating foam cuff, depending on the brand

(5) Suctioning is always a sterile procedure except at home, where clean technique may be appropriate

  (c) Weaning from the tracheostomy tube

(1) Criteria (see Extubation Criteria for Endotracheal Tube)

(2) Patient must demonstrate physiologic and psychologic independence from an artificial airway. Techniques include use of:

  a) Cuff deflation periods, with tube opening capped to allow breathing through the upper airway

  b) Tracheostomy button

  c) Fenestrated tube with cuff inflated or deflated, with external tube opening capped or occluded to permit air flow to be directed to upper airway

  d) Progressive downsizing of tube from original size to smaller one

(3) Patient is monitored carefully to see how weaning is tolerated; blood gas studies and clinical observations utilized

(4) Complete sealing of tracheotomy incision may occur within 72 hours of extubation. Patients cannot produce adequate coughing pressure until this is accomplished

  d. Prevent complications of airway intubation

    i. Physiologic alterations caused by airway diversion

      (a) Inspired air is inadequately conditioned and is irritating to delicate pulmonary membranes

      (b) Plastic or metal tubes are foreign bodies. The body responds by increasing production of mucus; ciliary movement is impaired

      (c) Accumulated secretions are a good medium for bacterial growth

      (d) Bypassing the larynx produces aphonia

      (e) Eliminating the glottis from the air route prevents the development of increased intrathoracic pressures, thereby making effective coughing difficult

    ii. Complications during placement of airway

      (a) Endotracheal tube

        (1) Mucous membrane disruption and tooth damage or dislodgment

        (2) With nasotracheal route, one may see:

           a) Nosebleed

           b) Submucosal dissection

           c) Introduction of a polyp or plug from the nose into the lungs, resulting in infection or obstruction

           d) Sinusitis

   (b) Tracheostomy (problems are fewer and less severe if this is an elective procedure done in the operating room)

        (1) Mediastinal emphysema

        (2) Hemorrhage

        (3) Pneumothorax

        (4) Cardiac arrest

        (5) Damage to adjacent structures in the neck

 iii. Complications occurring while tube is in place

   (a) Obstruction due to

        (1) Plugging with secretions that have become dried and inspissated. This is entirely preventable by systemic hydration and proper use of humidification and suctioning

        (2) Herniation of cuff over end of tube

        (3) Kinking of tube

        (4) Cuff overinflation

   (b) Displacement or dislodgment out of the trachea (endotracheal or tracheostomy tube) and inadvertent movement into false passage or pretracheal space (tracheostomy tube)

        (1) Especially hazardous during first 3 to 5 days of tracheostomy. Avoid by using tube of proper length and fixing it securely to patient. Although securing the tube is important, care of the stoma and surrounding skin to prevent skin breakdown or pressure sore from the tube neck plate is also important

        (2) Dislodgment out of trachea into tissue causes mediastinal emphysema, subcutaneous emphysema, and pneumothorax. Diagnosis is determined by reduced or absent air flow movement from tube opening, deterioration in blood gas values and/or vital signs, observations of neck and local tissue swelling with crepitations by palpation, poor chest excursion and respiratory distress, and inability to pass suction catheter properly through the tube

        (3) Low tube placement into one bronchus or at level of carina results in obstruction or atelectasis of the nonventilated lung. Check placement of the endotracheal tube by auscultation, followed by x-ray examination or use of the fiberoptic scope

           a) Displacement into one bronchus. Signs and symptoms are as follows:

              i) Decreased or delayed motion on one side of chest

              ii) Unilateral diminished breath sounds

              iii) Excessive coughing

              iv) Localized expiratory wheeze

　　　　　b) Placement at level of carina. Signs and symptoms are as follows:
　　　　　　　i) Excessive coughing
　　　　　　　ii) Localized expiratory wheeze
　　　　　　　iii) Difficulty in introducing suction catheter
　　　　　　　iv) Bilateral diminished breath sounds
　　　(c) Poor oral hygiene. Mouth care is absolutely essential
　　　(d) Local infection of tracheostomy wound, tracheal tissue, or lungs. Tracheostomy should be treated as a surgical wound and specimens for culture should be obtained if active infection is suspected
　　　(e) Massive hemorrhage resulting from erosion of tracheostomy tube into the innominate vessels; may be fatal. Occurs most often with low placement of tube, excessive "riding" of tube within trachea, or pulling torsion on tube
　　　(f) Disconnection between the tracheal tube and ventilator
　　　　　(1) Most likely to occur when the patient is being turned
　　　　　(2) Adequate alarms on all ventilators are necessary
　　　　　(3) Frequent checking of all connections should be routine
　　　(g) Leaks caused by broken or malfunctioning cuff balloon or pilot valve
　　　　　(1) Diagnosis is confirmed by ability of previously aphonic patient to talk, air movement felt at nose and mouth, pressure changes on ventilator, and decreased exhaled volumes as measured with hand-held portable respirometer or ventilator spirometer
　　　　　(2) It is necessary to remove and replace the tube. Always check cuff for leaks before inserting. Note amount of air required to fill cuff, and compare with later values
　　　(h) Tracheal ischemia, necrosis, dilation
　　　　　(1) As a result of the oval shape of the trachea and round shape of the tube, there is a tendency for erosion in anterior and posterior trachea
　　　　　(2) Diagnosis is indicated by the necessity to use larger and larger amounts of air to inflate the balloon to maintain the seal
　　　　　(3) May progress to tracheoesophageal fistula; this is indicated if food is aspirated through the trachea or air is in the stomach or if a methylene blue dye test is positive
　　　　　(4) Prevention through use of low-pressure cuffs and routine monitoring of cuff pressures
　iv. Early postextubation complications
　　　(a) Acute laryngeal edema
　　　　　(1) Most frequently seen in children
　　　　　(2) In adults, is commonly associated with the use of oversized tube or with preexisting inflammation of upper airway
　　　　　(3) Prevention
　　　　　　　a) Close observation for several hours after extubation
　　　　　　　b) Patient may require supplemental O_2 following prolonged intubation; use of bland aerosol, such as

high humidity via face mask or face tent, is controversial
and of no proven benefit

    (4) Treatment

        a) Oxygen, steroids

        b) Smaller endotracheal tube introduced or tracheotomy
performed

        c) Racemic epinephrine administered via intermittent
positive pressure breathing, since intent is to reduce
subglottic edema by inhalation of potent vasoconstrictor

  (b) Hoarseness

    (1) Common following either short-term or long-term
endotracheal intubation

    (2) Usually disappears during the first week

  (c) Aspiration of food, saliva, or gastric contents if swallowing
mechanism is impaired

    (1) Presence of the tube over extended periods results in loss
of usual protective reflexes of the larynx

    (2) Monitor the patient carefully during feedings: watch for
excessive coughing; start with clear liquids after tube
removal

  (d) Difficult removal of tracheostomy tube

    (1) More frequently seen in infants but occurs in adults as well

    (2) Related to narrow lumen of trachea, which is further
narrowed by swelling

  v. Late postextubation complications

    (a) Fibrotic stenosis of the trachea

      (1) Cause: prolonged use of any tube with rigid inflatable cuff

      (2) Follows earlier ulceration and necrosis of site

      (3) Lesions may become advanced before clinical evidence
appears (dyspnea, stridor). Tracheoesophageal fistula may
form

      (4) Prevention: use of low-pressure cuffs and proper
monitoring of cuff pressures

    (b) Stenosis of larynx

      (1) Cause: discrepancy between anatomy of larynx and size and
shape of the tube

      (2) Treatment

        a) Dilation or surgical intervention

        b) Permanent tracheostomy

4. Evaluation of Nursing Care

  a. On auscultation, adventitious sounds are absent

  b. Patient is able to expectorate secretions

  c. Blood gas values and ventilatory parameters are within acceptable limits

. . . .

Ineffective Breathing Pattern related to respiratory muscle fatigue or impaired respiratory mechanics

1. Assessment for defining characteristics

  a. Dyspnea

  b. Tachypnea

    c. Fremitus

    d. Abnormal ABG values

    e. Cyanosis (late finding)

    f. Cough: effective or ineffective

    g. Nasal flaring

    h. Respiratory depth changes

    i. Assumption of the 3-point position

    j. Pursed lip breathing and prolonged expiratory phase

    k. Increased anteroposterior diameter

    l. Use of accessory muscles

    m. Altered chest excursion

2. Expected outcomes

    a. Respiratory rate and tidal volume are within normal limits for patient, minimal dyspnea

    b. Increased maximal inspiratory pressure and patient reports decreased exertional dyspnea

    c. Patient reports taking antibiotics as needed when sputum color changes (green or yellow)

    d. Patient reports taking bronchodilator medications as prescribed

    e. Patient demonstrates ability to pace activities of daily living (ADL) in line with ventilatory function

3. Nursing interventions

    a. Teach pursed lip breathing, abdominal stabilization, and directed or controlled coughing techniques to minimize energy expenditure of respiratory muscles and to provide optimal care to the mechanically ventilated patient if necessary. Pursed lip breathing forces the patient to breathe slowly and establishes a back pressure in the airway, which helps to stabilize airways and reduce dyspnea sensation, especially after exertion

    b. Evaluate status of inspiratory muscles for training and, if appropriate, initiate inspiratory muscle training

       i. Inspiratory muscle training improves conscious control of respiratory muscles and decreases anxiety associated with increased respiratory effort

       ii. Improved respiratory muscle strength may improve exercise tolerance with less dyspnea

       iii. Monitor oxygen saturation via pulse oximetry as a measure of tolerance during training

    c. Teach patient to monitor color, consistency, and volume of sputum

       i. Respiratory infections increase work of breathing

       ii. Early treatment may speed recovery and thereby reduce work of breathing

    d. Teach patient medication names, dosage, method of administration, schedule, and appropriate behavior should an adverse effect occur. Instruct on consequences of improper use of medications

       i. Beta agonists, anticholinergics, and methylxanthines are commonly prescribed bronchodilators aimed at decreasing air flow resistance and work of breathing

       ii. Patient should be able to perform the proper technique for metered dose inhaler (MDI) self-administration. Often, a spacer attachment is used with the MDI to optimize medication delivery to the lungs. When technique is poor or if the patient is unable to use MDI, assess for need of alternative delivery device, such as a small volume nebulizer

   e. Teach the patient to modify ADL within ventilatory limits

      i. Encourage periodic hyperinflation of lungs with a series of slow deep breaths

      ii. Hyperinflation therapy helps to prevent atelectasis and reduced lung compliance by expanding the alveoli, which are partially closed, and by mobilizing airway secretions

   f. Monitor rate and pattern of respiration, breath sounds, use of accessory muscles of respiration, and sensation of dyspnea. Clinical manifestations of respiratory muscle fatigue include:

      i. Shallow rapid breathing in early stages

      ii. Use of accessory muscles and development of paradoxical breathing pattern

      iii. Active use of expiratory muscles

      iv. Magnified patient sensation of dyspnea

      v. Respiratory alternans

4. Evaluation of nursing care

   a. Rate, depth, and breathing pattern of ventilation remain within normal limits for patient

   b. Patient reports decreased dyspnea at rest and with exertion

   c. When appropriate, patient use of inspiratory muscle training results in improved maximal inspiratory pressures

   d. Patient is able to demonstrate safe administration of inhaled respiratory medications and is aware of side effect monitoring aspects that need to be reported to health care provider

   e. Patient recognizes signs and symptoms to report that may indicate possible respiratory tract infection

. . . .

**Inability to Sustain Spontaneous Ventilation
related to imbalance between ventilatory capacity
and ventilatory demand**

1. Assessment for defining characteristics

   a. Ineffective breathing pattern

   b. Tachypnea or apnea

   c. Accessory muscle use

   d. Arterial Po_2, Pco_2, and pH outside normal limits for patient

   e. Mental status deterioration

   f. Excessive work of breathing; paradoxical breathing pattern

   g. Cyanosis (late finding)

   h. Dyspnea

2. Expected outcomes

   a. Respiratory rate and breathing pattern are normal for the patient

   b. Normalization of arterial pH, Pco_2, and Po_2 to baseline values before acute illness

   c. Decrease in sensation of dyspnea

   d. No air trapping at end of expiration (auto-PEEP)

   e. No ventilator associated nosocomial infections or other complications

3. Nursing interventions

   a. Promote normal rest and sleep patterns. Plan activities to allow rest periods. Rest allows energy reserves to be replenished. Sleep deprivation blunts the patient's respiratory drive

b. Provide an appropriate level of mechanical ventilatory support when necessary

   i. Objectives of mechanical ventilation

     (a) Physiologic objectives

       (1) To support or otherwise manipulate pulmonary gas exchange

         a) Alveolar ventilation (e.g., arterial P_{CO_2} and pH)

         b) Arterial oxygenation (e.g., P_{O_2}, Sa_{O_2}, and C_{O_2})

       (2) To increase lung volume

         a) End-inspiratory lung inflation

         b) Functional residual capacity

       (3) To reduce or otherwise manipulate the work of breathing

     (b) Clinical objectives

       (1) To reverse hypoxemia

       (2) To reverse acute respiratory acidosis

       (3) To relieve respiratory distress

       (4) To prevent or reverse atelectasis

       (5) To reverse ventilatory muscle fatigue

       (6) To permit sedation and/or neuromuscular blockade

       (7) To decrease systemic or myocardial O_2 consumption

       (8) To reduce intracranial pressure

       (9) To stabilize the chest wall

   ii. Major types of mechanical ventilators

     (a) Negative external pressure ventilators: attempt to duplicate spontaneous breathing

       (1) The entire body, up to the neck, is placed within an "iron lung" or tank respirator, while the head and neck protrude to the atmosphere. Beneath the tank, electrically powered bellows create subambient pressure within the tank

       (2) Intermittently applied negative pressure creates a pressure gradient that promotes air entry into the lungs. $\dot{V}_E$ can be altered by changing the negative pressure (and thus the tidal volume) or the respiratory rate, but inspiratory flow rate cannot be adjusted

       (3) Use is restricted to patients with respiratory failure who have normal lung parenchyma (e.g., patients with poliomyelitis)

       (4) Disadvantages

         a) Inability to provide adequate support to patients with lung disease

         b) Available only in controlled mode

         c) Adequate nursing care in tank difficult

       (5) Modified approach to negative-pressure ventilation is the chest cuirass ventilator, consisting of a rigid shell or poncho wrap placed around the rib cage, with a hose attached to a vacuum pump that regulates negative pressure setting as well as ventilating rate

       (6) Regardless of type of negative pressure ventilator, failure to

maintain a proper seal around the chest may result in inadequate alveolar ventilation

(b) Positive-pressure ventilators: the most common type of ventilatory support used in critical care. All apply positive pressure to the airway during the clinician-selected pattern of ventilation

    (1) Response of the breath delivery system to patient efforts

        a) *Triggering:* the initiation of gas delivery. Significant ventilatory loads can be imposed by insensitive or unresponsive ventilator triggering systems. Oversensitive valves can result in spontaneous ventilator cycling independent of patient effort

        b) *Gas delivery:* flow from the ventilator is governed (or limited) by a set flow (flow-limited) or set pressure (pressure-limited) on most machines

        c) *Cycling:* gas delivery can be terminated by set volume, set time, or set flow

    (2) Response of patient efforts to ventilator settings

        a) Altering the activity of mechanoreceptors in the airways, lungs, and chest wall

        b) Altering blood gas tensions

        c) Eliciting respiratory sensations in conscious or semiconscious patients

            i) Result is change in rate (ventilatory demand), depth, and

            ii) Timing of respiratory efforts (synchrony between patient and ventilator) through neural reflexes, chemical (chemoreceptors), and behavioral responses

            iii) Standard modes of mechanical ventilation

                [a] Classified according to initiation of the inspiratory cycle (Fig. 1–10)

                    □ *Spontaneous respiration:* with most ventilators, the patient can be allowed to breathe spontaneously through the ventilator circuit when the ventilator rate is set at zero. Positive airway pressure can be applied when breathing through the circuit

                    □ *Controlled mandatory ventilation* (CMV): the ventilator delivers a preset number of breaths per minute of a predetermined tidal volume. Additional breaths cannot be triggered by the patient. The inability of the patient to trigger a breath beyond the preset rate of the ventilator may lead to patient apprehension and air hunger and is therefore not used clinically. However, it may be desirable to provide complete control of ventilation in certain situations. In these cases, the patient may require chemical sedation, paralysis, or both in order to gain total control of ventilation.

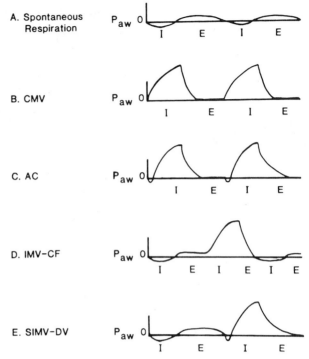

Figure 1-10 • *A–E,* Airway pressure during various modes of ventilation. CMV = controlled mechanical ventilation; AC = assist control; IMV-CF = intermittent mandatory ventilation by a continuous flow circuit; SIMV-DV = synchronized intermittent mandatory ventilation delivered by a demand valve circuit. (From Dantzker, D. R.: Cardiopulmonary Critical Care, 2nd ed. Philadelphia, W. B. Saunders, 1991, p. 269.)

☐ *Assist-Control* (A/C): every breath is supported by the ventilator. A back-up control ventilatory rate is set, but the patient may chose any rate above the set rate. Most ventilators deliver A/C ventilation using volume-cycled or volume-targeted breaths. Pressure-limited or pressure-targeted A/C is available on certain ventilators.
  • Advantages
    — Security of controlled ventilation with support during every breath
    — Ability to increase the level of ventilatory support on demand
  • Risks
    — Excessive patient work of breathing due to improper ventilator settings
    — May be poorly tolerated in awake, nonsedated patients due to dyssynchrony of patient and machine cycle length
    — May be associated with respiratory alkalosis. May potentially worsen air trapping in patients with COPD
    — If pressure-targeted A/C is used, tidal volume may be variable and potentially decreased

□ *Intermittent mandatory ventilation* (IMV): A mode of ventilation and mode of weaning that combines a preset number of ventilator-delivered mandatory breaths of predetermined tidal volume with the capability for intermittent patient-generated spontaneous breaths. A subtype of this mode is called *synchronized intermittent mandatory ventilation* (SIMV), wherein a demand valve is incorporated into the IMV system that senses the start of a patient breath. The demand valve opens, and the mandatory breath is delivered in synchrony with the patient's effort
  • Advantages
    — Patient can perform a variable amount of work with security of preset level of mandatory ventilation
    — SIMV allows for a variation in level of partial ventilatory support from near total support to spontaneous breathing, hence its utility as a weaning tool
  • Risks
    — With IMV, there are risks of ventilator dyssynchrony between patient effort and machine-delivered volume
    — With SIMV, there are risks of hyperventilation and respiratory alkalosis (similar to A/C) excessive work of breathing due to poorly responsive demand valve, worsening dynamic hyperinflation in patients with COPD
□ *Pressure support ventilation* (PSV): A pressure-targeted, flow-cycled, mode of ventilation in which each breath must be triggered by the patient. The application of positive pressure to the airway is set by the clinician. This augmentation to inspiratory effort starts at the initiation of inhalation and typically ends when a minimum inspiratory flow rate is reached. There are two applications for this mode:
  • In conjunction with SIMV, improved patient tolerance and decreased work of spontaneous breaths, especially from demand-flow systems and narrow inner-diameter endotracheal tubes
  • As a stand-alone ventilatory mode for patients under consideration for weaning or during the stabilization period

- Advantages
  - Since patient has significant control over gas delivery, overt dyssynchrony is less likely than with A/C or SIMV
  - Decreased work of breathing roughly in proportion to level of PSV delivered
  - Can be used to compensate for demand valve and endotracheal tube size
- Disadvantages
  - Tidal volume is not controlled
  - Careful monitoring is needed in unstable patients
  - Excessive air leak during inspiration may cause delay in the flow-cycling mechanism of PS
  - Poorly tolerated in some patients with high airway resistance (may improve with adjustment of initial inspiratory flow, which is possible on some ventilators)

☐ *Continuous positive airway pressure* (CPAP): designed to elevate end-expiratory pressure to above atmospheric pressure to increase lung volume and oxygenation. All breaths are spontaneous, and therefore an intact respiratory drive is required. Can be used in intubated as well as nonintubated patients via a face or nasal mask

- Depending on machine type, CPAP is delivered via a continuous flow or demand valve system
- Advantages
  - Offers the benefits of PEEP to spontaneously breathing patients by recruiting and stabilizing previously closed alveoli
  - May help reduce work of breathing in patients with dynamic hyperinflation or auto-PEEP
- Disadvantages
  - May increase inspiratory work of breathing if CPAP levels set too high
  - Increased expiratory work of breathing if PEEP device has high flow resistance

☐ *Bilevel positive airway pressure* (BiPAP, Respironics, Inc.): This noninvasive ventilatory assist device employs a spontaneous breathing mode with the baseline pressure elevated above zero. Unlike CPAP, BiPAP allows separate regulation of inspiratory and expiratory pressures

- Indications
  - Enhanced capabilities of home CPAP used for obstructive sleep apnea
  - A noninvasive method of augmenting alveolar ventilation in hypercapnic respiratory failure
  - A nocturnal support in a variety of restrictive and obstructive disorders
- Application BiPAP is essentially a combination of PSV with CPAP. The differences between inspiratory and expiratory pressures (IPAP and EPAP, respectively) contribute to the total ventilation

iv) Servo-controlled modes of mechanical ventilation
  - [a] Used for both ventilation and for weaning patients by incorporating a feedback system to control a specific variable within a narrow range
    - ☐ *Mandatory minute ventilation* (MMV): ensures delivery of a preset minimum minute volume, with the patient allowed to breathe spontaneously. Should the patient's minute volume fall below the established level, mechanical breaths at a predetermined volume are delivered at a rate sufficient to reach the target level
    - ☐ *Servo-controlled PSV:* a ventilatory support strategy in which the underlying mode is PSV and the targeted parameter is either respiratory rate or tidal volume. If the intended target level is not met, the ventilator modifies either the pressure target level or the way in which the breath is cycled. Depending on the ventilator, examples of these modalities include volume-ensured pressure support (PS), pressure augmentation, volume support, and volume-assisted breaths

v) Alternate modes of mechanical ventilation
  - [a] Ventilatory support strategies aimed at limiting or reducing lung inflation volumes and/or pressures in order to avoid ventilator-associated lung injury
    - ☐ *High-frequency ventilation:* Provides a faster respiratory rate (60 to 3000 breaths/minute) and lower tidal volume (1 to 3 ml/kg) than other ventilator systems, for the purpose of reducing barotrauma and cardiac depression. Three mechanical systems are capable of delivering high-frequency ventilation:

- High-frequency positive-pressure ventilation (HFPPV): time-cycled, volume-limited ventilation that delivers a preset V_T 60 to 100 times per minute
- High-frequency jet ventilation (HFJV): delivers "jets" of high-pressure gas through a small catheter in the trachea or endotracheal tube at frequencies of 60 to 600 breaths/minute
- High-frequency oscillation (HFO) moves a volume of gas to and fro in the airway, without bulk flow at rates of 600 to 3000 cycles/minute (50 Hz) throughout lungs

☐ *Inverse ratio ventilation* (IRV): A ventilatory support strategy that employs a prolonged inspiratory to expiratory (I:E) ratio greater than or equal to 1:1. Breaths are delivered either as pressure-controlled (PC-IRV) or volume-controlled (VC-IRV)

- The major function of prolonged inspiratory time is to allow for recruitment of alveolar units with long time constants
- Increase in mean airway pressure is key to beneficial effects related to oxygenation as well as potential adverse hemodynamic effects (decreased cardiac output)
- Because of abnormal I:E ratio, patient dyssynchrony with ventilator is common and usually requires sedation and/or paralysis
- Auto-PEEP development is common and should be routinely monitored; during PC-IRV, tidal volume varies according to respiratory mechanics

☐ *Differential lung ventilation* (DLV): Each lung is ventilated independently. A double-lumen endobronchial tube is inserted, usually with the distal tip inserted into the left mainstem bronchus, which permits isolation of each lung for the purposes of mechanical ventilation

- Typically, there are two separate ventilators; each has ventilator settings based on the degree of injury for each lung. Machine breaths are delivered synchronously or asynchronously, depending on type of ventilator used
- Meticulous care of endobronchial tube is critical. Malposition may result in tracheal injury, and overinflation of endobronchial tube cuff may result in bronchial rupture.

Sedation or muscle paralysis may be required to avoid agitation and inadvertent tube movement. The tube is left in place for only a limited period of time

- Independent lung ventilation outside the operating room setting is sometimes used for unilateral lung disorders unresponsive to conventional ventilation techniques. This modality is extremely labor-intensive and adequate room space is necessary because two ventilators are used

vi) Guidelines for adjusting ventilator controls and settings during volume-targeted (volume-cycled) ventilation. All are adjusted according to patient's underlying disease process and results of ABG analysis

[a] *Minute ventilation* (usually 6 to 10 L/minute but may be much higher, depending on patient needs)

□ *Tidal volume:* Governed by estimated tidal volume; normally varies from 10 to 15 ml/kg ideal body weight. When there is a clinical concern about lung overinflation and potential stretch injury to the lung tissue, the preset tidal volume may be reduced to 8 to 10 ml/kg. Intentional use of lower tidal volumes may cause an increase in arterial CO_2 levels and is therefore referred to as *permissive hypercapnia.* The use of intermittent sighs during mechanical ventilation is no longer recommended

□ *Respiratory rate:* varies from 8 to 12 per minute for most clinically stable patients; rates above 20 per minute sometimes necessary

□ *Flow rate:* Adjusted so that inspiratory volume delivery can be completed in a time frame that allows adequate time for exhalation. An inspiratory flow rate range of about 40 to 100 L/minute is most commonly employed. Slow flow rates are preferred for optimal air distribution in normal lungs; faster flow rates are beneficial in patients with obstructive lung disease

- Altering the flow rate may improve work of breathing, patient-ventilator synchrony, and comfort of patients who are restless while receiving mechanical ventilation
- Normal I:E ratio is 1:2 to 1:3
- Inspiratory flow of gas from ventilator can be delivered, depending on model, using

one of several flow patterns, such as decelerating, square, or sine wave

[b] *Oxygen concentration*

☐ Initially, the FIO_2 is deliberately set at a high value (often 1.0) to ensure adequate oxygenation. An ABG sample is obtained, and the FIO_2 is adjusted according to the patient's PaO_2 and SaO_2. Inspired partial pressure of O_2 is adjusted so that arterial PaO_2 is acceptable for patient's condition. This is usually greater than 60 mm Hg or an SaO_2 of 90% or greater

☐ Excessively high levels for prolonged periods can cause O_2 toxicity. Use the lowest FIO_2 that achieves an acceptable PaO_2 and SaO_2

☐ Use PEEP as appropriate to reduce the FIO_2 to safe levels

[c] Continuous humidification is mandatory, with inspired air warmed to near body temperature. Standard humidifiers using a water feed system must be monitored closely for water condensation in the tubing and emptied routinely. Heat and moisture exchanges (HME) are sometimes used

[d] Established parameters concerning sensitivity settings (when the patient can trigger machine for "assistance"); adjusted so that minimal patient effort is required, usually -0.50 to -1.5 cm H_2O; certain ventilators allow for flow triggering mechanism and should be set to their maximum sensitivity (1 to 3 L/minute)

[e] Pressure limit alarms should be set at approximately 10 to 15 cm H_2O above the patient's normal peak inflation or airway pressure (PIP)

☐ The goal is to keep PIP below 35 to 40 cm H_2O if possible. The peak inspiratory plateau is equal to or less than 35 cm H_2O

☐ Certain ventilators provide a low airway pressure alarm feature

[f] Check that all other alarms are operational and on at all times

☐ Optimal orders for ventilator settings and parameters

☐ Considerable technical knowledge of machines required along with awareness of pathophysiology of each patient

☐ Consultation of technical manual accompanying each machine needed

vii) Assess the effectiveness of mechanical ventilation on the patient

[a] General measures

  ☐ All patients on life support equipment to be monitored and clinically observed routinely according to institution policy
  - Physical assessment each shift
  - Assessment of ventilator system and current machine settings
  ☐ When medications are to be given, specific orders must be written for clarification. For example, a bronchodilator can be administered continuously by aerosol or via the ventilator circuit by metered dose inhaler
  ☐ Many patients have an arterial line, cardiac monitor, IV line, and urinary catheter if they are on continuous ventilatory support

[b] General monitoring for patients on continuous ventilatory support

  ☐ Hemodynamic monitoring (arterial or pulmonary artery catheter) if indicated
  ☐ Cardiac monitoring, heart sounds, pulses, pulse pressures, ECG as needed or as part of standard ICU routine
  ☐ Pulmonary function studies: vital capacity, negative inspiratory pressure, minute ventilation, maximum voluntary ventilation as required
  ☐ Biochemical, hematologic, and electrolyte studies
  ☐ Cardiac output assessment, blood-volume status
  ☐ Intake/output (I&O), body weight
  ☐ Respiratory pattern assessment, breath sounds, symmetry in chest movement, vital signs
  ☐ Dressings and drainages, tubes, and suction apparatus
  ☐ Neurologic state, level of consciousness, pain, level of anxiety
  ☐ Response to treatments and medications

viii) Ventilatory monitoring of any patient on continuous ventilation

[a] Ventilation checks performed routinely

  ☐ When blood gases are drawn
  ☐ When changes are made in ventilator settings
  ☐ Hourly or more frequently in any unstable patient
  ☐ Routinely throughout each shift

[b] Components of ventilator sheet to be recorded on flow sheet

☐ Blood gas values
  • Record source (e.g., arterial, mixed venous) along with ventilator settings and measurements so that decisions about changes may be made
  • It often is valuable to document patient position at the time of the blood gas drawing, as position changes (side lying, upright, supine) influence ventilation perfusion relationships and, hence, blood gas analysis results
☐ Ventilator settings to be read from machine
  • Ventilator mode (e.g., SIMV or A/C)
  • Tidal volume, machine set rate, pressure support level (if used), preset minute volume, inspiratory flow rate or time and set I:E ratio (depending on mode and ventilator)
  • Temperature of humidification device, temperature of inspired gas
  • O_2 concentration
  • Peak inflation airway pressure limit
  • PEEP level set
  • Alarms on
☐ Ventilator measurements to be taken
  • Peak inflation pressure (PIP), plateau and/or mean airway pressures if requested, and PEEP level (measurement of auto-PEEP may be required in some patients)
  • Fractional percent of inspired oxygen (FIO_2), A–a gradient or PaO_2/FIO_2 ratio, shunt fractions (if ordered)
  • Minute ventilation (exhaled), respiratory rate (both patient and machine), tidal volume (exhaled)
  • Effective compliance, static and dynamic; compliance curves (depending on institutional policy)
  • I:E ratio (displayed), V_D/V_T ratio (if requested)
☐ Respiratory monitoring techniques during mechanical ventilation
  • Pulse oximetry: noninvasive estimate of arterial O_2 saturation (SpO_2) using an infrared light source placed at a finger or another acceptable extremity
    — Useful for trending changes in arterial oxygenation and/or acute desaturation episodes
    — Caution must be exercised not to overrely on normal SpO_2 level to

indicate normal oxygenation in all cases (there are numerous clinical situations that may cause erroneous readings)
- End-tidal CO_2 ($PetCO_2$) monitoring: noninvasive sampling and measurement of exhaled CO_2 tension at the patient-ventilator interface; devices (capnographs) typically employ infrared analysis of respired gas, provide both numerical and graphic display of CO_2 waveform on a breath-by-breath basis or slower speed for trending purposes
  — Normal $PaCO_2$ to $PetCO_2$ gradient is 1 to 5 mm Hg (normal $\dot{V}/\dot{Q}$ matching assumed in lungs)
  — In critically ill patients, gradient may exceed 20 mm Hg
  — Application limited for reliably predicting changes in alveolar ventilation except in patients with normal pulmonary perfusion and $\dot{V}/\dot{Q}$ ratios
  — Multiple clinical uses for patient monitoring using waveform display alone
- Airway pressure monitoring: graphic display of airway pressures generated during the ventilatory cycle
  — This modality requires either a simple transducer or a tubing connection to the ventilator circuit, which is then tied in to standard hemodynamic pressure monitoring module or by ventilator electronic interface directly into physiologic monitor system
  — Displayed airway pressure tracings can be helpful to identify patient-ventilator dyssynchrony, assessment of inspiratory work of breathing, and auto-PEEP detection

c. Prevent development of complications associated with the use of positive pressure ventilation
   i. Cardiac effects
     (a) Decreased cardiac output: caused by decreased venous return to the heart and reduced transmural pressures (intracardiac minus intrapleural pressures). In addition, there are increases in pulmonary vascular resistance and juxtacardiac pressure from the surrounding distended lungs
       (1) Pulse changes, decreased urine output and blood pressure
       (2) Treatment
         a) Trendelenburg position

        b) Fluids to increase preload

        c) Adjustment of volumes delivered by ventilator

        d) Careful PEEP titration

        e) Avoidance of auto-PEEP

    (b) Dysrhythmias possible

        (1) Causes: hypoxemia and pH abnormalities

        (2) Unstable patients on ventilators should have cardiac monitoring

ii. Pulmonary effects

    (a) *Barotrauma* (pneumothorax, pneumomediastinum, subcutaneous emphysema) occurs when a high-pressure gradient between the alveolus and the adjacent vascular sheet causes the overdistended alveolus to rupture. Gas is forced into the interstitial tissue of the underlying perivascular sheet. The gas may dissect centrally along the pulmonary vessels to the mediastinum and into the fascial planes of the neck and upper torso; high inflation volumes, or *volutrauma,* has also been described as an important risk factor

        (1) Positive-pressure ventilation, especially with PEEP, subjects patients to the risk of pneumothorax, particularly if high pressures and volumes are used

        (2) Barotrauma can occur with mainstem intubation, ARDS, COPD, and other patients with acute lung injury

        (3) Diagnosis

            a) Rises in airway peak pressure

            b) Decreased breath sounds and chest movement on the affected side

            c) Restlessness

            d) Vital signs changes

            e) Cyanosis

            f) Chest x-ray changes

    (b) *Atelectasis:* collapse of lung parenchyma from occlusion of air passage, with reabsorption of gas distal to occlusion

        (1) Cause

            a) Obstruction

            b) Possible lack of periodic deep inflations in patients ventilated with small tidal volumes

        (2) Diagnosis

            a) Diminished breath sounds or bronchial breath sounds, rales or crackles

            b) Chest x-ray evidence

            c) A–a gradient increases, PaO_2/FIO_2 ratio decreases

            d) Compliance decreases

        (3) Prevention

            a) Use of adequate tidal volumes

            b) Humidity, vigorous tracheal suctioning based on need

            c) Chest physical therapy, repositioning

    (c) Tracheal damage, tracheoesophageal fistula, vessel rupture

        (1) Cause: excessive tube cuff pressures due to overinflation or reduced tracheal blood flow causing ischemia

        (2) Prevention

        a) Careful monitoring of intracuff pressures or volumes
        b) Avoidance of frequent manipulation and pulling of endotracheal tube
    (d) Oxygen toxicity
        (1) Pathology: impaired surfactant activity, progressive capillary congestion, fibrosis, edema and thickening of interstitial space
        (2) Etiology: prolonged administration of high oxygen concentrations ($FIO_2 > 0.50$)
        (3) Prevention: careful monitoring of blood gases. The goal is to use the lowest FIO_2 possible that achieves adequate oxygenation ($PaO_2 \geq 60$ mm Hg and $SaO_2 \geq 90\%$)
    (e) Inability to wean
        (1) Can occur in any patient, particularly those with COPD, cystic fibrosis, debilitation, malnutrition, and musculoskeletal disorders
        (2) Mechanical ventilation eases the work of breathing for these patients, making the transition off the ventilator (i.e., weaning) difficult
    (f) Hypercapnia–respiratory acidosis
        (1) Caused by inadequate ventilation leading to acute retention of CO_2 and decreased pH
        (2) Patients can tolerate an increased $PaCO_2$ and decreased pH under certain circumstances
        (3) Is corrected by improving alveolar ventilation and treating the underlying cause
    (g) Hypocapnia–respiratory alkalosis
        (1) Caused by hyperventilation, causing increased elimination of CO_2 and increased pH
        (2) If CO_2 is decreased too rapidly, shock or seizures may result, particularly in children. Ventilation should be maintained to produce a normal pH, not necessarily a normal PCO_2
        (3) Treatment
            a) Decrease the respiratory rate
            b) Decrease the tidal volume if inappropriately high
            c) Add mechanical dead space
iii. Fluid imbalance
    (a) Fluid retention: due to overhydration by airway humidification and decreased urinary output because of possible ADH effects. Symptoms include:
        (1) Increased A–a gradient, decreased PaO_2/FIO_2 ratio
        (2) Decreased vital capacity
        (3) Weight gain
        (4) Intake greater than output
        (5) Decreased compliance
        (6) Increased V_D/V_T (dead space/tidal volume) ratios
        (7) Hemodilution (decreased hematocrit and decreased sodium values)
        (8) Increased bronchial secretions
    (b) Dehydration related to decreased enteral or parenteral intake in

relation to urinary and/or gastrointestinal output, and overdiuresis. In addition, insensible losses average 300 to 500 ml/day and increase with fever. Symptoms include:

 (1) Decreased skin turgor
 (2) Intake less than combined outputs
 (3) Decreased body weight
 (4) Hemoconcentration
 (5) Thick, inspissated secretions

(c) Parameters to be monitored

 (1) Daily weight changes (often more accurate than I&O)
 (2) Skin turgor, moistness of oral mucosa
 (3) Hemoglobin and hematocrit values
 (4) Character of pulmonary secretions
 (5) Maintenance of airway humidification

iv. Infection

(a) Patients at risk: debilitated, aged, immobile, early postoperative, immunocompromised

(b) Intubation bypasses normal upper airway defense mechanisms

(c) Ventilatory equipment and therapy may be the carrier, particularly aerosols

(d) Suctioning technique may not be sterile

(e) There may be cross-contamination between patients and staff or autocontamination

(f) Pulmonary patients may have indwelling catheters of various types

(g) Unsterile solutions may be left out in open containers

(h) Patients may be improperly positioned so that aspiration is possible

(i) Preventive measures

 (1) Rigorous hand washing is mandatory and critical
 (2) Isolation techniques as needed
 (3) Routine cultures of patients and machines
 (4) Antibiotics as indicated
 (5) Bronchial hygiene, chest physical therapy as indicated
 (6) Restriction of number of patient contacts (staff and visitors)
 (7) Early recognition and response to clinical and laboratory signs of infection
 (8) Aseptic airway and tracheostomy technique
 (9) Change of ventilator tubing, including humidifier reservoirs, according to institution policy. There is a trend toward extending the time that the ventilator circuit is left in place before a change (e.g., 7 days or longer)
 (10) Emptying and changing of reservoir water according to institution policy. The water in the tubing should be emptied into a waste receptacle every 1 to 2 hours and as needed
 (11) Sterile suction technique using open-suction or closed-suction catheter system
 (12) Avoidance of routine tracheal instillation of normal saline

for lavage purposes (there is no scientific evidence demonstrating benefit)

    v. Gastrointestinal effects

      (a) Complications

        (1) Stress ulcer and bleeding

        (2) Adynamic ileus

        (3) Gastric dilatation from loss of adequate nerve supply; may lead to shock from fluid shifts

      (b) Prevention and treatment

        (1) Routinely auscultate bowel sounds

        (2) Antacids, histamine antagonists

        (3) Hemoccult or Gastroccult and pH stomach aspirate; check stools for blood

    vi. Patient "fighting" the ventilator, displays agitation and distress

      (a) Causes

        (1) Incorrect ventilator setup for patient's needs (e.g., inspiratory flow rate less than patient demand)

        (2) Acute change in patient status

        (3) Obstructed airway, pneumothorax

        (4) Ventilator malfunction

        (5) Acute anxiety

        (6) Acute pain

      (b) Management

        (1) Perform a rapid bedside check of the patient and ventilator

        (2) Disconnect the patient from ventilator, and provide manual ventilation via self-inflating bag with 100% O_2

        (3) Check vital signs, chest expansion, and bedside monitoring equipment

        (4) Suction airway and check patency of endotracheal or tracheostomy tube

        (5) Obtain ABG values

        (6) Sedate the patient if indicated and ordered for acute anxiety, and give analgesics if pain is present. Observe for hypoventilation, and be prepared to adjust the ventilator setting to meet the patient's needs

      (c) Principles for matching ventilator to patient's needs

        (1) Do not assume that patients will adjust to the ventilator; the reverse is desirable

        (2) Vary the cycle frequency, tidal volume, triggering sensitivity, and inspiratory flow rate until the correct combination is achieved

        (3) Provide calm reassurance and moderate sedation as indicated

e. Provide optimal methods for "weaning" patients from continuous mechanical ventilation

    i. Indications for weaning (the term is usually reserved for when ventilatory support is gradually withdrawn, although it includes the overall process of discontinuing ventilator support)

      (a) The underlying disease process is resolved, and signs of the original need for ventilatory support are no longer present

      (b) Patient's strength, vigor, and nutritional status are adequate

(c) Patient does not require more than 5 cm of PEEP or an FIO_2 greater than 0.5 to maintain an acceptable PaO_2 (usually at least 55 to 60 mm Hg)

(d) Stable and acceptable hemodynamic parameters and Hb

(e) Stable and acceptable measurements of arterial blood gases, tidal volume, vital capacity, respiratory rate, minute ventilation, maximum inspiratory and expiratory airway pressures, A–a gradient or PaO_2/FIO_2 ratio, compliance, V_D/V_T ratio is within minimal acceptable range (< 0.6)

(f) Level of consciousness is acceptable

(g) Patient is psychologically prepared, emotionally ready, and cooperative

(h) Predictors of successful weaning and criteria for weaning trial

    (1) Resting minute volume ($\dot{V}E$) of less than 10 L and ability to double this value during a maximum voluntary ventilation (MVV) effort

    (2) Maximum inspiratory pressure (MIP) more negative than minus 20 cm H_2O

    (3) Spontaneous tidal volume (V_T) greater than 5 ml/kg

    (4) Spontaneous respiratory frequency (f) equal to or less than 30 breaths/minute

    (5) Vital capacity above 10 ml/kg body weight

    (6) PaO_2/FIO_2 ratio greater than 200

    (7) f/V_T ratio less than 105 (Rapid Shallow Breathing Index)

    (8) Integrative indices such as the Burns Wean Assessment Program (BWAP) and the CROP index (compliance, rate, oxygenation, and pressure measures)

ii. Principles of weaning

(a) Explain to the patient what will take place. Place the patient in the upright position, if possible, for better lung expansion. Obtain baseline vital signs

(b) To assess patient's ability to ventilate adequately without mechanical assistance, perform ventilatory measurements or weaning parameters while patient is off the ventilator. Measurements include minute ventilation, respiratory rate, tidal volume, maximum inspiratory pressure, vital capacity, and maximum voluntary ventilation

(c) Be prepared to give periodic manual ventilation as needed. Have all equipment at bedside and in working order

(d) Consider placing the patient back on the ventilator with baseline machine settings if signs of poor response to weaning or tiring occur, such as:

    (1) Decreased tidal volume, increased respiratory rate

    (2) Increasing $PaCO_2$ and or decreasing pH

    (3) Patient apprehension

    (4) Diaphoresis, fatigue, decreasing level of consciousness

    (5) Cardiac dysrhythmias, blood pressure or heart rate changes, hemodynamic changes

    (6) O_2 desaturation by blood gas analysis or pulse oximetry

(e) Mechanisms producing a failure to wean may include insufficient ventilatory drive, hypoxemia, high ventilatory requirement, respiratory muscle weakness, low compliance, or excessive work of breathing. The longer it takes to resolve the underlying problem that led to the need for ventilatory support, the more difficult it may be to wean

iii. Techniques of discontinuing ventilator support (T-tube, IMV, PSV, CPAP)

(a) A T-*tube* (also known as the "Briggs," t-piece or t-bar adapter) trial: The patient is disconnected from the ventilator and attached to a high-humidity O_2 or air source by means of a T-shaped airway adapter

    (1) Total unassisted spontaneous breathing occurs, usually for 5 to 60 minutes depending on tolerance, followed by periods of rest

    (2) Optimal duration of the T-tube trial has not been standardized; patients are usually extubated once they can tolerate several hours of unassisted breathing

    (3) ABGs are periodically drawn to assess alveolar ventilation status

    (4) Careful visual observation is required because the ventilator is on standby status and without integral alarms in case of T-tube system disconnection

(b) *Intermittent mandatory ventilation* (IMV): the amount of support being provided by the ventilator is gradually reduced and the amount of respiratory work done by the patient is progressively increased

    (1) The transition period may be several hours to several days, depending on length of time ventilatory support was required as well as institution policy

    (2) The pace of decreasing the IMV rate is determined by clinical assessment and ABG analysis

    (3) Pressure support ventilation (PSV) is often used with IMV in lower amounts (5 to 10 cm H_2O); the IMV rate is reduced while the PSV level is held constant

(c) *PSV* as a stand-alone mode is also used as a means of gradually reducing the level of ventilator support

    (1) The PSV level is initially titrated to a spontaneous tidal volume of 10 to 12 ml/kg and then reduced in 3 to 6 cm H_2O increments based on clinical assessment and ABG analysis

    (2) The PSV is titrated down until a low level of support is reached (5 to 10 cm H_2O)

(d) Continuous positive airway pressure (CPAP) is defined as a method of ventilatory support whereby the patient breathes spontaneously without mechanical assistance against a threshold resistance, with pressure above atmospheric levels maintained at the airway throughout breathing

    (1) The CPAP level is initially set at 3 to 3 cm H_2O

    (2) May be helpful in patients with dynamic hyperinflation and auto-PEEP

    (3) When wean trials are completed, patients are usually extubated from CPAP level at 3 to 5 cm H_2O

(4) In theory, CPAP may prevent or limit the deterioration in oxygenation that often occurs when patients are switched from mechanical ventilation to spontaneous breathing. There are data that refute this concept, however

iv. Treatment of the difficult-to-wean patient

(a) Some patients may pose significant problems when ventilator removal is attempted in terms of costs, health care resources, and ethical dilemmas

(b) Evaluate each patient's inspiratory muscles for training and, if appropriate, initiate inspiratory muscle training (a controversial step as to benefit)

(1) Monitor O_2 saturation with ear or finger or pulse oximeter during training session to verify that patient does not desaturate

(c) Monitor color, consistency, and volume of sputum. A change in sputum characteristics may indicate infection, which may increase the work of breathing

(d) Physical therapy and rehabilitation efforts are very important (both physical and psychologic advantages)

(e) Monitor rate and depth of respiration, breath sounds, use of accessory muscles of respiration, and sensation of dyspnea

(f) Recognize clinical manifestations of respiratory muscle fatigue, including:

(1) Shallow, rapid breathing in early stages (increase f/V_T ratio)

(2) Increased $PaCO_2$ and decreased respiratory rate in late stages

(3) Use of accessory muscles

(4) Magnified sensation of dyspnea

(g) Monitor ratio of inspiratory time/total duration (T_i/T_{tot}) of respiration (an increase in ratio of inspiratory time to total duration of respiration indicates a decrease in respiratory muscle endurance)

(h) Observe for abnormal chest wall motion as an indication of respiratory muscle dysfunction

(1) Paradoxical motion of the chest wall is characterized by expansion of the rib cage and inward motion of the abdomen during inspiration

(2) Asynchronous chest wall motion is characterized by disorganized and uncoordinated respiratory motion

(i) Administer appropriate drug therapy for maintenance of ventilation

(1) Narcotics: morphine sulfate, meperidine, and fentanyl

a) Act as a respiratory depressant; good euphoric agents and excellent analgesics

b) Provide sedation and good control of ventilation without adverse side effects in well-ventilated, well-oxygenated, acid-base–balanced patient, often used in combination with a benzodiazepine for sedative effects

c) The sensation of dyspnea is reduced

d) Large doses may cause increased venous capacitance

e) Drug tolerance may develop with prolonged use

(2) Narcotic antagonists
   a) Used in narcotic overdoses to reverse the effects of narcotics
   b) They are not stimulants but compete with narcotic molecules for cellular receptors in drug-depressed neurons
(3) Benzodiazepines
   a) Diazepam, lorazepam, and midazolam are the most commonly used agents in the critical care setting
   b) Cause CNS depressant effect, which can lead to alveolar hypoventilation and respiratory acidosis, particularly in geriatric patients and in those with liver disease
   c) Severe respiratory depression and apnea can result if used with other CNS depressant drugs
   d) As with any sedation agent, the routine use of a sedation scale (e.g., Ramsay or other) for monitoring and assessing degree of sedation is important
(4) Anesthetic agents
   a) Propofol is a hindered phenolic compound with IV general anesthetic properties. It is used as a sedation agent in the ICU setting. It is unrelated to any of the currently used barbiturate, opioid, or benzodiazepine agents
   b) An IV bolus dose of 0.25 to 1.00 mg/kg is usually required, followed by a continuous infusion rate of 50 to 100 µg/kg/minute. Onset of action is approximately 15 to 60 seconds. The drug has a relatively short half-life
   c) Respiratory and hemodynamic monitoring are essential during continuous infusion
(5) Paralyzing agents: pharmacologic intervention at the myoneural junction, resulting in muscle paralysis. If the patient is conscious, sedation is necessary
   a) Nondepolarizing muscle relaxants administered intravenously
      i) Compete with acetylcholine at receptor site
      ii) Pancuronium, vecuronium, and atracurium are the most common agents used in the critical care setting
      iii) Pancuronium bromide (Pavulon) is regarded by many as the drug of choice for long-term neuromuscular blockade; may cause tachycardia or other adverse hemodynamic effects
      iv) Loading doses given (different for each drug), followed by maintenance doses, with careful monitoring
         [a] Use of peripheral nerve stimulator for determining train-of-four (TOF) at least every 2 hours; the goal is one or two out of four twitches

        [b] Use of end-tidal CO_2 monitoring for visual detection of respiratory efforts; in-line airway pressure graphic monitoring may also be helpful

        [c] Skeletal muscle weakness and disuse atrophy occur when these agents are administered for prolonged periods; full recovery of muscles may take from weeks to months

        [d] Neuromuscular blockade should be stopped at least once daily to assess the patient's underlying level of sedation and also reevaluate the need for continued paralysis

b) Depolarizing muscle relaxant (succinylcholine)

    i) Attaches to muscle cell wall and causes depolarization

    ii) Used primarily for inducing short duration muscle relaxation in anesthesia and endotracheal intubation

    iii) Bolus dose is typically 1.0 to 1.5 mg/kg IV; onset of action approximately 45 to 60 seconds; duration of action after a single dose approximately 2 to 10 minutes

(6) Bronchodilators

    a) Methylxanthines: theophylline, aminophylline (80% theophylline)

        i) Actions: stimulate the CNS, act on the kidney to produce diuresis, stimulate cardiac muscle, and relax bronchial smooth muscle

        ii) Serum levels: therapeutic range, 10 to 20 μg/ml

    b) Beta agonists: stimulate beta receptors in the bronchial smooth muscle, resulting in bronchial smooth muscle relaxation; the most potent bronchodilators currently available

        i) Epinephrine: stimulates $beta_1$ and $beta_2$ receptors; given by inhalation or parenterally, with rapid action either way; duration of action is 0.5 to 2 hours

        ii) Isoproterenol: stimulates both $beta_1$ and $beta_2$; given intravenously, sublingually or inhaled; duration of action is 0.5 to 2 hours

        iii) Metaproterenol: has equal $beta_2$ and $beta_1$ effects; given in inhaled or oral form; duration of action is 3 to 4 hours

        iv) Isoetharine: mainly $beta_2$ effects; given inhaled, with a duration of action of 3 to 4 hours

        v) Terbutaline: mainly $beta_2$ actions; given subcutaneously, orally, or inhaled; duration of action is 2 to 4 hours for subcutaneous route, 3 to 7 hours inhaled; 5 to 8 hours orally; however, side effects are worse with oral doses

        vi) Albuterol: mostly $beta_2$-selective; is given in inhaled

and oral forms; duration of action is 4 to 6 hours
inhaled and 5 to 8 hours in oral form

vii) Bitolterol: mostly beta$_2$-selective; given in inhaled and
oral forms; duration of action is 4 to 8 hours

viii) Pirbuterol: mostly beta$_2$-selective; given by inhalation;
duration of action is 4 to 6 hours

ix) Salmeterol: mostly beta$_2$-selective; given by inhalation;
duration of action of 12 hr; because of the delay in
onset of action, this drug is never to be used in an
acute bronchospasm attack

c) Anticholinergic bronchodilators: block cholinergic
constricting influences on bronchial muscle

i) Work predominantly on large airways

ii) Atropine and ipratropium: given in inhaled forms

d) Antiallergy medications: block IgE-dependent mast cell
release of mediators of bronchoconstriction, such as
histamine and leukotrienes

i) Cromolyn sodium: does not actively bronchodilate
but prevents bronchoconstriction; inhaled liquid by
metered dose inhaler, inhaled powder by Spinhaler
or liquid nasal spray

ii) Nedocromil sodium: given by inhalation aerosol
(similar to cromolyn sodium)

(7) Adrenocorticosteroids: augment the effects of beta agonist
bronchodilators and are anti-inflammatory; often start with
high dose, then taper off. Doses should be kept low to
minimize adrenocortical and pituitary suppression and side
effects

a) Prednisone: oral dose often given once daily, in early
morning to minimize systemic side effects

b) Hydrocortisone: methylprednisolone given IV

c) Inhaled steroids (beclomethasone, flunisolide,
triamcinolone): given after inhaled beta agonists

i) Provide beneficial pulmonary steroid effects with
minimal systemic absorption

ii) When steroids are taken by inhalational route, the
patient must rinse the mouth with water after each
use to prevent a fungal infection (candidiasis) of the
oropharynx or larynx

n. Assist the patient in maintaining adequate nutrition

i. Assess nutritional status

(a) Anthropometric measurements (i.e., weight/height ratio, skinfold
thickness, mid-arm circumference, mid-arm muscle circumference
and creatinine/height index) are reduced in patients with
malnutrition (sometimes these measurements not routinely
obtained in the acute care setting)

(b) Biochemical markers (i.e., albumin, transferrin, prealbumin,
retinol binding protein, total lymphycyte count, and reaction to
skin tests) are reduced in patients with malnutrition

(c) Indirect calorimetry, measurement of energy expenditure by
analysis (measurement of O_2 consumption and CO_2 production)

(1) Limited ability to measure gas exchange on patients receiving supplemental oxygen, especially at FIO_2 levels greater than 0.50, depending on the metabolic measurement system used

(2) Used to more accurately determine a patient's metabolic energy requirements as well as to avoid the consequences of both underfeeding and overfeeding, which may negatively impact the ability to wean off the ventilator

ii. Administer appropriate nutritional therapy to meet the following goals:

(a) Replenish depleted stores of somatic and visceral protein

(b) Promote wound healing

(c) Restore patient to pre-illness weight

(d) Restore patient's immunocompetence and normal nitrogen balance

(e) Successful weaning from the ventilator, when possible

iii. Methods of nutritional support

(a) Oral feedings with appropriate calorie supplements; small, frequent feedings are often more tolerable for dyspneic patients

(b) Enteral feeding solutions via nasogastric, small-bore nasoenteral or gastric feeding tubes for patients who cannot eat but who have functional gastrointestinal tracts

(1) Patients with endotracheal tubes who cannot take oral feedings

(2) Precautions to be taken to avoid pulmonary aspiration

a) Keep the head of the bed raised at least 30 degrees during feedings

b) Check sputum for glucose content with glucose oxidase reagent strips; the presence of blood and other substances may cause false-positive readings

c) Avoid routine use of dyes and food coloring added to enteral formulas; adverse reaction to dyes possible, contamination of food coloring solutions and adverse reactions have been reported, small traces may be difficult to detect in purulent sputum

(c) Total parenteral nutrition (TPN): indicated for patients with a nonfunctional gastrointestinal tract

(1) May be administered peripherally or centrally, depending on vascular access

(2) Substrate concentration (i.e., fats, carbohydrates, and protein) depends on access site, caloric requirements, disease state, and other metabolic parameters

(3) Regardless of route, meticulous care of the IV catheter site and tubing is required in order to prevent infection

iv. General patient care and personal hygienic measures (especially meticulous oral care) usually improve the patient's appetite

4. Evaluation of nursing care

a. The patient is comfortable and well rested on ventilator

b. The patient reports minimal or no significant increase in breathing effort while on the ventilator

c. Acid-base balance and oxygenation parameters are maintained within normal limits

d. No air trapping or auto-PEEP occurs while on mechanical ventilator

e. Ventilator settings are appropriate for the patient's condition
f. No signs of ventilator associated infections or complications are present

. . . .

Impaired Gas Exchange

1. **Assessment for defining characteristics**
   a. Confusion
   b. Somnolence
   c. Restlessness
   d. Irritability
   e. Inability to mobilize secretions
   f. Hypercapnia
   g. Hypoxia
   h. Dyspnea
   i. Cyanosis
   j. Decreased mental acuity
   k. Tachycardia, dysrhythmias
   l. Anxiety
   m. Clinical evidence of hypoxemia
2. **Expected outcomes**
   a. Resolution or improvement of hypoxemia with or without O_2 supplement or mechanical ventilation
   b. Eucapnia or usual compensated $PaCO_2$ and pH levels
   c. Impairment of mental status and restlessness absent or reduced
   d. Patient performs techniques that maximize ventilation-perfusion matching
   e. Patient performs activities of daily living with or without supplemental O_2
   f. Patient can conserve energy by adjusting activities for self-care
   g. Patient expresses feelings of comfort in maintaining air exchange
3. **Nursing interventions**
   a. Assess oxygenation status
      i. Hypoxia-hypoxemia relationships
         (a) Definition of hypoxia: a decrease in oxygenation at the tissue level (a clinical diagnosis); this must be corrected, but in some cases O_2 therapy alone may not correct tissue hypoxia
         (b) Definition of hypoxemia: a decrease in arterial blood O_2 tension (a laboratory diagnosis). A normal PaO_2 alone does not guarantee adequate tissue oxygenation
         (c) Organs most susceptible to lack of oxygen: brain, adrenal glands, heart, kidneys, liver, and retina of eye
         (d) Factors governing effective oxygenation of blood and tissues
            (1) Sufficient O_2 supply in inspired air
            (2) Sufficient ventilation to provide gas exchange between atmosphere and alveoli of lungs
            (3) Ready diffusion of gases across the alveolar-capillary membrane
            (4) Adequate circulation of blood from lungs to tissues; volume of blood and Hb levels must be adequate. A decreasing cardiac output causes a compensatory rise in O_2 extraction at the tissue level

(5) O_2 brought to tissues must be readily released from the Hb molecule and readily diffused into and taken up by various tissues

ii. Assessment of hypoxemia–hypoxia

    (a) Clinical signs and symptoms: restlessness, anxiety, dysrhythmias, apprehension, headache, angina, confusion, disorientation, impaired judgment, hypotension, tachycardia, abnormal respirations, hypoventilation, dyspnea, yawning, cyanosis

    (b) ABG analysis: including oxyhemoglobin saturation, and content; Hb; arteriovenous O_2 content differences (if pulmonary artery catheter is in place)

    (c) Noninvasive O_2 monitoring

        (1) Transcutaneous O_2 tension (TcPO_2: measures O_2 concentration at the skin with an electrode. Heat is applied to improve blood flow. Skin blood flow, thickness, temperature, and skin O_2 consumption are important variables in readings. This technique has been used successfully in neonates, but accuracy decreases as the patient becomes older. Careful calibration as well as monitoring of electrode temperature is critical, as is periodic site rotation to prevent possible blister and further local tissue injury. TcPO_2 normally tends to underestimate PaO_2. With compromised hemodynamic status, PaO_2 may be significantly underestimated

        (2) Pulse oximetry (SpO_2): measures O_2 saturation by using two physical principles. *Spectrophotometry* involves measuring infrared light absorption of Hb (to detect differences between saturated and reduced Hb). *Photoplethysmography* uses light to measure arterial pressure waveforms generated by the pulse in the capillaries (pulse rate and strength) in the tissue of the ear lobe, finger, or other measurement site. Pulse oximeters are generally accurate in SaO_2 range of 70% to 100% but are inaccurate in low blood flow (decreased perfusion due to hypovolemia, hypotension, or vasoconstriction) states. SpO_2 readings are adversely affected by motion of extremity (false pulse rate and waveform artifact), light dilution (interfere with probe ability to detect correct light wavelength), abnormal Hb (the device cannot distinguish between oxyhemoglobin and carboxyhemoglobin and thus overestimates saturation), methemoglobin may cause interference with light absorption, dyes, certain fingernail polish colors, and abnormal skin pigmentation (radiologic vascular dyes, polish, and dark skin pigmentation can interfere with light absorption), and anemia (Hb below 5 g/dl may result in insufficient signal to process readings)

b. Provide O_2 therapy

  i. Areas in nursing care where administration of O_2 may benefit patient

    (a) Before, during, and after tracheal suctioning

    (b) When patient is ambulatory, self-inflating bag and O_2 if the patient is intubated or if tracheostomized and patient's tidal volume is inadequate

    (c) Before any physical activity or nursing care given to cardiac patients with known or suspected oxygenation difficulties

    (d) When transferring an unstable patient with suspected oxygenation deficit

ii. Rationale for use of low-flow O_2 in patient with COPD and chronic CO_2 retention

    (a) Because of decreased sensitivity of central chemoreceptors to blood CO_2 levels, CO_2 no longer serves as a respiratory stimulus, and the only remaining stimulus is hypoxemia. Therefore, high concentrations of O_2 depress the ventilatory drive, leading to depressed minute ventilation and increase in Pa_{CO_2}

    (b) Nursing implications

        (1) Administer only enough O_2 to raise Pa_{O_2} to adequate levels for that patient (~50 to 60 mm Hg)

        (2) Safety lies in controlled low-flow rates, frequent monitoring of blood gases, and careful observation

iii. Principles of O_2 therapy

    (a) Remember the airway; no O_2 treatment is of any use without an adequate or a patent airway

    (b) O_2 is a drug and should be administered in a prescribed dose (the FI_{O_2} is the dose)

    (c) Response to O_2 administration should be interpreted in terms of its effect on tissue oxygenation rather than its effect on the ABG values alone

    (d) The pathology of the disease is the major determinant of the effectiveness of O_2 therapy

    (e) Delivered concentration of gas from any appliance is subject to the condition of the equipment, technique of application, cooperation of the patient, and ventilatory pattern of the patient

    (f) Low-flow O_2 systems do not provide the total inspired gas (the patient is breathing some room air) and therefore are adequate only if tidal volume is adequate, respiratory rates are not excessive, and the ventilator pattern is stable. Variable O_2 concentration of 21% to 90% are provided, but the FI_{O_2} varies greatly with changes in tidal volume and ventilatory pattern

    (g) High-flow O_2 systems provide the entire inspired gas (patient is breathing only the gas supplied by the apparatus) and are adequate only if flow rates exceed inspiratory flow rate and minute ventilation. Both high and low O_2 concentrations may be delivered by high-flow systems (24% to 100% O_2)

iv. Hazards of O_2 therapy

    (a) O_2-induced hypoventilation

        (1) Prevent by use of low-flow rates and concentrations of O_2 (FI_{O_2} of 0.24 to 0.30)

        (2) Patient is at greatest risk when the Pa_{CO_2} is chonically elevated above normal

        (3) O_2 therapy should be used with special caution in patients with COPD with CO_2 retention and other lung diseases resulting in chronic CO_2 retention

    (b) Absorption atelectasis, caused by elimination of nitrogen (nitrogen washout) and effect of O_2 on pulmonary surfactant

(c) Retinopathy of prematurity (retrolental fibroplasia) in neonates
   (1) Fibrotic process behind lens caused by retinal vasoconstriction resulting from high PaO_2
   (2) O_2 concentration should be kept as low as necessary to maintain PaO_2 60 mm Hg or higher
(d) O_2 toxicity
   (1) Caused by lung exposure of too high a concentration (exact level controversial but usually considered to be an $FIO_2 > 0.50$ to 0.70) over an extended time (> 48 to 72 hours)
   (2) May be mild or fatal
   (3) Early signs and symptoms
      a) Retrosternal distress
      b) Paresthesias in extremities
      c) Nausea, vomiting
      d) Fatigue, lethargy, malaise
      e) Dyspnea, coughing
      f) Anorexia
      g) Restlessness
   (4) Late signs and symptoms
      a) Progressive respiratory difficulty
      b) Cyanosis
      c) Dyspnea
      d) Asphyxia
   (5) Pathologic process
      a) Local toxicity to capillary endothelium followed by interstitial edema, which thickens the alveolar-capillary membrane. Type I alveolar cells are destroyed with an exudative response. In the end stages, hyaline membranes form in the alveolar region, followed by fibrosis and pulmonary hypertension
      b) Biochemical changes occur most likely due to overproduction of O_2 free radicals, such as superoxide anion and hydroxyl free radical. These reactive species can produce oxidation reactions that inhibit enzyme functions and/or kill cells. High PO_2 values can also release additional free radicals from neutrophils and platelets, which in turn produce the capillary endothelial damage described
   (6) Both O_2 concentration and duration of O_2 administration are critical (50% O_2 or greater over several days is potentially dangerous)
   (7) Changes seen in O_2 toxicity
      a) Decreased compliance and vital capacity
      b) Increasing A–a gradient, reduced PaO_2/FIO_2 ratio
(e) Prevention of complications caused by O_2 therapy
   (1) O_2 is a potent drug that should be used only when indicated and according to preestablished goals of therapy
   (2) If high concentrations are necessary, the duration of administration should be kept to a minimum and reduced as soon as possible
   (3) The objective is to maintain a PaO_2 of at least 50 to 60 mm Hg

to produce an acceptable SaO_2 of 85% to 90% without causing lung injury or inducing CO_2 retention

(4) Periodic assessment of ABGs is mandatory during initial titration of O_2 therapy as well as whenever pulse oximetry values are in question or inappropriate

(5) Depending on the O_2 delivery device used, the exact concentration of FIO_2 should be measured whenever appropriate with an O_2 analyzer

(6) Patients should never be exposed to dangerous levels of hypoxemia for fear of development of O_2 toxicity. Hypoxia is far more common than O_2 toxicity and must be corrected. Pure O_2 (100%) should never be withheld in an emergency

v. Methods of O_2 delivery (low-flow and high-flow systems)

(a) Masks

(1) General points

a) Useful if O_2 is needed quickly and for short periods

b) Concentrations of 24% to 100% oxygen are delivered, depending on device

(2) Disadvantages

a) Uncomfortable and hot

b) Irritation of skin caused by tight fit

c) Difficult to control FIO_2 precisely, except when the Venturi mask is used

d) Must be removed when patient eats, thereby losing O_2 delivery

(3) Possible complications

a) Patients who are prone to vomit may aspirate

b) Obstruction by flaccid tongue may occur in comatose patients; use oral airway and secure

c) May cause CO_2 retention and hypoventilation if flow is too low and exhalation ports are obstructed

(4) Types of masks

a) Simple

i) 35% to 60% O_2 at 6 to 10 L flows

ii) FIO_2 varies considerably with changes in tidal volume, ventilatory pattern, and inspiratory flow rate and whether mask is loose or tight fitting

b) Partial rebreathing

i) Delivers 35% to 60% O_2 or higher at 6 to 10 L flows

ii) Portion of exhaled breath enters reservoir bag to be rebreathed with incoming 100% O_2 in the next breath

iii) Flows must be adjusted so that reservoir bag does not completely collapse during inspiration; otherwise CO_2 retention may occur

c) Nonrebreathing

i) Delivers 90% or more O_2 concentration, provided there are no leaks in system; one-way valve between reservoir bag and mask prevents rebreathing from 100% O_2 gas source *ii*) An ideal method of delivering a high O_2 gas concentration for short-term purposes

   iii) Reservoir bag must not collapse during inspiration

  d) Air entrainment (Venturi mask)

   i) Adjustments allow for delivery of precise O_2 concentrations of 24% to 50%

   ii) Total air flow must be adequate for ventilatory needs of patient

   iii) Is best suited to patient who must have a consistent FIO_2

(b) Cannula (nasal)

 (1) Low O_2 concentrations are delivered (<40%), but this depends on the patient's tidal volume

  a) FIO_2 can be estimated as a 4% increase in FIO_2 for each liter of O_2 flow; generally not run at flow rates beyond 5 or 6 L/minute

  b) Humidifier is not necessary unless flow rates exceed 4 L/minute

 (2) Advantages

  a) Easy to apply

  b) Light

  c) Economical

  d) Disposable

  e) Patient mobility allowed

 (3) Disadvantages

  a) Easily dislodged

  b) High flow rates uncomfortable (dryness and bleeding)

  c) Skin breakdown possible around ears caused by tubing

(c) Nasal catheter

 (1) Low O_2 concentrations delivered (<40%)

 (2) Catheter should not be forced through the nose; periodic rotation of new catheter to opposite nares at least every 8 hours; rarely used on adults

 (3) Disadvantages

  a) Technique of insertion

  b) Gastric distention

  c) Nasopharyngeal injury

 (4) Eventual delivery of O_2 to blood is not significantly different when either cannula or catheter is used or whether patient's mouth is open or closed. Variability of FIO_2 is caused by O_2 flow-rate setting and patient's rate and depth of respiration

(d) Transtracheal catheter

 (1) This small catheter is percutaneously inserted transtracheally through anterior neck for low-flow O_2 delivery

 (2) Advantages

  a) Economical (less O_2 used to maintain a given SaO_2 than in other methods)

  b) Very cosmetically appealing for some patients (catheter may be concealed by clothing) with improved compliance with therapy

  c) Improved sense of taste, smell, and appetite

  d) Avoidance of nasal and ear irritation

 (3) Disadvantages

      a) Technique of insertion (minor)

      b) Meticulous care needed (major)

      c) Risk of infection

      d) Subcutaneous emphysema if catheter dislodges before transtracheal tract established

      e) Patient must be capable of recognizing and troubleshooting common problems

(e) Reservoir cannula

  (1) Combines concepts of low-flow and reservoir delivery system. Reservoir cannula stores about 20 ml of O_2 during exhalation. Pendant reservoir delivery system is situated over the anterior chest wall

  (2) Advantages

      a) Decreased flow needed for given FIO_2

      b) Reduced O_2 costs

      c) Allows longer periods away from stationary O_2 source

  (3) Disadvantages

      a) Patients may object to appearance of reservoir "mustache" cannula

      b) FIO_2 variability still exists

      c) Amount of O_2 savings varies greatly, depending on individual patient needs

(f) Air entrainment nebulizer

  (1) A pneumatically powered nebulizer device containing sterile water is capable of delivering high-level humidification in the form of an aerosol and heat control as well as O_2 at a preset FIO_2. Dilution of the 100% O_2 source from the flowmeter occurs via a fixed or adjustable air entrainment port located on the nebulizer canister. FIO_2 can be set from 0.21 to 1.0

  (2) Advantages

      a) Ideal for delivering humidification to patient with artificial airway

      b) Delivery of humidified air or O_2 occurs with variety of attachments, including:

         i) Aerosol mask

         ii) Face tent

         iii) Tracheostomy collar

         iv) T-tube or Brigg's adapter

  (3) Disadvantages

      a) Air entrainment nebulizers generate consistent FIO_2 delivery to the patient only when their output flow meets or exceeds the patient's inspiratory flow demands

      b) Because water condensation in large-bore tubing obstructs total flow and decreases air entrainment, FIO_2 increases

      c) Delivered FIO_2 is more variable at O_2 concentrations above 40%

(g) Hyperbaric O_2 therapy

  (1) O_2 is administered at pressures greater than 1 atmosphere

      a) Administered via multiplace (12 or more patients) or monoplace (single patient) chamber

      b) Monitoring systems and ventilators can be adapted to allow treatment of critically ill patient

        (2) Indications: primary treatment for decompression of divers, air or gas embolism, carbon monoxide and/or cyanide poisoning, acute traumatic ischemias (compartment syndrome; crush injury), clostridial gangrene, necrotizing soft tissue infection, ischemic skin grafts or flaps, enhanced healing of problem wounds, refractory osteomyelitis

        (3) Complications: barotrauma, tympanic membrane rupture, pneumothorax, air embolism, O_2 toxicity, fire risk, reversible visual changes, claustrophobia, sudden decompression, radiation necrosis, CNS toxic reaction (rare)

    (h) Other medical gas therapies

        (1) Helium therapy: used as an adjunct in managing large airway obstruction. Because of helium's low density, the driving pressure to move gas in and out of the larger airways is decreased and, therefore, work of breathing is reduced

            a) Administered in prepared gas cylinders of either 80%:20% helium/O_2 mixture or 70%:30%

            b) Because of high diffusibility of helium, gas is generally administered via a nonrebreathing mask; can be used with mechanical ventilator

            c) In nonintubated patient, speech may be distorted during helium administration

        (2) Nitric oxide (NO) therapy: used in the treatment of diseases characterized by pulmonary hypertension and hypoxia. Not approved by the U.S. Food and Drug Administration (FDA) for these applications except as an investigational drug. In very low concentrations (2 to 20 parts per million) mixed with O_2, nitric oxide selectively dilates pulmonary blood vessels, reduces intrapulmonary shunt, and improves arterial oxygenation

            a) Commonly administered via ventilator with special analyzer for precise and stable nitric oxide dose titration, can be given to nonintubated patient through tight-fitting face mask

            b) Toxicity of inhaled nitric oxide possible including: nitrous dioxide production, methemoglobinemia, production of peroxynitrite, platelet inhibition, increased left ventricular filling pressure, rebound hypoxemia and pulmonary hypertension

c. Administer PEEP: a major oxygenation adjunct treatment modality

   i. Pressure above atmospheric is maintained at airway opening at end expiration in order to prevent alveolar collapse at end expiration

   ii. At end of quiet expiration, lung volume is increased; therefore, FRC is increased. Increase in FRC is dependent on both the amount of PEEP used and functional state of the lungs. Alveolar volume is increased, and recruitment of alveoli occurs

   iii. Major goal of PEEP is enhanced O_2 transport by improvement in arterial O_2 tension and saturation. PEEP serves to reduce the shunt effect of collapsed alveoli and may increase PaO_2 dramatically. An important goal of PEEP is to avoid increasing FIO_2, which can lead to O_2 toxicity

   iv. Clinical use of PEEP

    (a) ARDS and diffuse pulmonary infiltrates, characterized by closure of airways or collapse of alveoli at end expiration, resulting in refractory hypoxemia and increased FIO_2 requirements

   (b) Acute respiratory failure that has caused a persistent hypoxemia with an FIO_2 of 0.5 or greater

   (c) Cardiogenic pulmonary edema

   (d) Avoidance of pulmonary O_2 toxicity from high FIO_2 values

   v. Dose: The amount of PEEP is tailored to patient's need; there is no arbitrary upper limit. Determination of optimal level requires accurate assessment of cardiopulmonary function, including measurement and monitoring of peak and mean airway pressures, blood pressure, and cardiac output studies when available. PEEP levels above 10 to 12 cm H_2O are generally considered high

   vi. Side effects of PEEP

   (a) Exacerbation of hemodynamic consequences of positive-pressure breathing. Patients with poor cardiovascular dynamics are at most risk. Adequate intravascular volume is essential

   (1) Venous return may be decreased, resulting in decreased cardiac output. In turn, right ventricular stroke volume may decrease, thus reducing cardiac output and O_2 transport

   (2) Right ventricular afterload is increased because of increased pulmonary vascular resistance when high levels are applied to normal lungs. Important changes may occur in patients with underlying right ventricular dysfunction

   (3) Altered left ventricular function secondary to right ventricular dilation/afterload, causing leftward displacement of the intraventricular septum (decreased left ventricular stroke volume)

   (4) Goal of increased O_2 transport cannot be met if cardiac output decrease is disproportionate to gain in arterial oxygenation (because O_2 transport is a product of O_2 content and blood flow)

   (b) Barotrauma: rupture of lung tissue with high PEEP levels, especially in patients with acute lung injury. Development appears related to high peak inflation pressures and raised mean airway pressures

   vii. Monitoring guidelines

   (a) It is essential to monitor parameters that indicate status of cardiac output and tissue perfusion, including blood pressure, urine output, pulse (central and peripheral), I&O, mental status, skin color and temperature, ABGs (PaO_2 and SaO_2), mixed venous O_2 content ($C\bar{v}O_2$), mixed venous O_2 pressure ($P\bar{v}O_2$), and mixed venous O_2 saturation ($S\bar{v}O_2$). PEEP is adjusted gradually in small increments, with careful evaluation of side effects and patient response

   (b) Patients should have routine arterial pressure monitoring and, if indicated, more complex cardiovascular monitoring (pulmonary artery catheter) available. Urinary output should be closely monitored

   (c) If a significant drop in cardiac output occurs, PEEP may need to be reduced, or vasoactive drug support for blood pressure control may be indicated. Hypovolemia, if present, must be corrected when this is a contributing factor in decreased cardiac output. Short-term inotropic therapy may sometimes be employed to correct decreased cardiac output in the normovolemic patient with known or suspected ventricular dysfunction

(d) PEEP is lost if the patient is disconnected from ventilator for suctioning. For this reason, closed-suction catheter systems are often used in mechanically ventilated patients in order to maintain PEEP levels during suctioning. If a precipitous drop in SpO_2 occurs during suctioning, preoxygenation before the procedure becomes critical

d. Administer continuous positive airway pressure (CPAP)

  i. A nonventilator technique providing a means of maintaining positive pressure during breathing. Similar to PEEP but used in spontaneously breathing patients via a nasal mask. CPAP may also be used in ventilator-dependent patients

  ii. Net result is improved arterial O_2 tensions and saturation levels. Inspired O_2 concentration is reduced

  iii. Used during weaning from mechanical ventilation, in the nonintubated patient for obstructive sleep apnea, and in select pediatric patients

e. Encourage patients to take deep breaths (see Ineffective Airway Clearance)

f. Position patient to facilitate ventilation-perfusion matching ("good side down")

g. Provide rest periods between activities to minimize O_2 demands

h. Alleviate or minimize anxiety that may increase O_2 demands

i. Monitor the patient's response to self-care or any activity. If deterioration exists, provide physical care, including full assistance with turning and transfer, and passive range-of-motion exercises

j. Teach the patient and significant others techniques of self-care, which will minimize O_2 consumption

k. Maintain body temperature at the patient's normal level to avoid extremes, particularly shivering

4. Evaluation of nursing care

a. ABG levels are within normal limits for patient with or without supplemental O_2 or mechanical ventilation

b. Cyanosis and dyspnea are absent

c. Patient performs techniques that maximize ventilation-perfusion matching

d. Patient performs ADL with or without supplemental O_2

e. Fever, chills, and shivering are absent

f. Patient demonstrates energy-conservation techniques for self-care

Ineffective Individual or Family Coping

See Chapter 9.

PATIENT HEALTH PROBLEMS

Acute Respiratory Failure

In a person with acute respiratory failure, the respiratory system cannot carry out its two major functions: (1) delivery of an adequate amount of O_2 into the arterial blood and (2) removal of a corresponding amount of CO_2 from the mixed venous blood. As indicated by the designation "acute," the onset must be relatively sudden; however, the onset can occur over *days,* as is particularly apt to occur in patients with preexisting lung disease, or within *minutes* to *hours,* as in patients without preexisting lung disease.

Acute respiratory failure can be categorized according to the extent to which ABG values are abnormal. Abnormalities can exist in Po_2, Pco_2 or both; the more severe the hypoxemia or hypercapnia, the greater the consensus about categorization. However, interpretation of ABGs must take into consideration two important aspects of the clinical situation: the blood gas values before the onset of acute respiratory failure (which depend on whether previous lung disease was present) and the rapidity with which the abnormalities in the blood gases developed.

As indicated above, the abnormalities in ABGs may be in Po_2 (hypoxemic respiratory failure), or in Pco_2 (hypercapneic respiratory failure), or both. The critical value for the diagnosis based on arterial hypoxemia is a Pao_2 less than 60 mm Hg or Sao_2 less than 90%; lower values can cause a marked decrease in oxyhemoglobin saturation and, therefore, a considerable drop in O_2 content. This is due in part, to the shape or position of the O_2 dissociation curve. The corresponding critical value for diagnosis of acute hypercapnic respiratory failure is a value for arterial Pco_2 above 50 to 55 mm Hg (with an accompanying acidemia: pH < 7.30).

1. **Pathophysiology.** Four major pathophysiologic mechanisms can cause acute respiratory failure (i.e., hypoventilation, ventilation-perfusion mismatching, shunt, and diffusion impairment). Of these, the first three mechanisms are by far the most common, as diffusion limitation is a relatively unimportant cause of clinically significant hypoxemia. These physiologic abnormalities result from structural processes that make up the pathologic background for the abnormalities of gas exchange. The two major processes involved are:
   a. Increase in extravascular lung water
      i. Characterized by severe hypoxemia with normal to low $Paco_2$
      ii. Occurrence in patients with cardiogenic or noncardiogenic pulmonary edema and other parenchymal infiltrates
   b. Impaired ventilation
      i. Characterized by elevated $Paco_2$ and decreased Pao_2
      ii. Occurrence with intrapulmonary (airway disease) or extrapulmonary problems (neuromuscular, chest wall diseases or alterations in respiratory drive). Other causes of respiratory failure include low inspired oxygenation secondary to high altitude or inhalation of toxic gases and low mixed-venous oxygenation secondary to anemia, hypoxemia, inadequate cardiac output, and increased O_2 consumption

2. **Etiologic or precipitating factors (multiple)**
   a. Increase in extravascular lung water (ARDs, pulmonary edema, aspiration, pneumonia, atelectasis)
   b. Impaired ventilation
      i. Intrapulmonary problems: emphysema, chronic bronchitis, asthma, bronchiectasis; especially following sepsis or acute respiratory infection, pulmonary embolism, pneumothorax
      ii. Extrapulmonary problems: pleural effusion, kyphoscoliosis, multiple rib fractures, thoracic surgery, abdominal surgery, peritonitis;

neuromuscular defects such as polio, Guillain-Barré syndrome, multiple sclerosis, myasthenia gravis, brain or spinal injuries, drugs or toxic agents; respiratory center damage or depression: narcotics, barbiturates, tranquilizers, anesthetic agents; cerebral infarction or trauma

3. Nursing assessment data base
    a. Nursing history
        i. Subjective findings
            (a) Patient's chief complaint: most often dyspnea or increased work of breathing
            (b) Other symptoms include:
                (1) Increased pulmonary secretions
                (2) Manifestations of hypoxemia: disorientation, confusion, restlessness, impaired intellectual functioning, tachypnea, tachycardia
                (3) Manifestations of hypercapnia with acidemia: headache, confusion, inability to concentrate, irritability, somnolence, dizziness
        ii. Objective findings
            (a) Etiologic or precipitating factors
                (1) Determine whether the patient has a history of chronic airway obstruction, restrictive defects, neuromuscular defects, or respiratory center damage that might impair ventilation
                (2) Determine whether the patient has any of the conditions that impair gas exchange and diffusion
                (3) Assess for presence of ventilation-perfusion abnormalities
            (b) Family history: determine whether any parents, grandparents, or siblings ever had significant pulmonary disease. One form of emphysema caused by deficiency of the enzyme alpha$_1$-antitrypsin is an inherited disorder
            (c) Social history: check whether the patient is a current or past smoker; calculate pack-year history of smoking (number of cigarettes smoked per day $\times$ years smoked)
            (d) Medication history: obtain list of all prescribed and over-the-counter medications along with their doses and last time patient took the medication. Assess for evidence of noncompliance in taking prescribed medications (i.e., missed doses or overdoses)
    b. Nursing examination of patient
        i. Inspection
            (a) Observe for thoracic abnormalities such as:
                (1) Increased A-P diameter, or barrel chest
                (2) Retraction of thorax
                (3) Pectus carinatum or pectus excavatum
                (4) Spinal deformities
            (b) Inspect ribs and interspaces
                (1) Intercostal retractions indicate increased work of breathing
                (2) Bulging of interspaces on expiration occurs when there is obstruction to air outflow
            (c) Pattern of respiration
                (1) Evidence of increased work of breathing: use of accessory muscles

        (2) Rate, depth, rhythm of breathing

        (3) I:E ratio (normal ratio is 1:2 or 1:3)

        (4) Inspiratory and/or expiratory stridor, indicative of upper airway airflow obstruction

     (d) General observation

        (1) Patient's posture, state of comfort

        (2) Skin color and perfusion: presence of cyanosis, temperature of skin, presence of diaphoresis

        (3) Observe for signs of right heart failure, such as pitting edema of lower extremities, jugular venous distention, and presence of cardiac gallop

        (4) Observe for signs of hypercapnia with acidemia: muscle twitching, asterixis, miosis, papilledema, engorged fundal veins, diaphoresis, hypertension

  ii. Palpation

     (a) Evaluate lung expansion

     (b) Assess vocal fremitus

        (1) Increased fremitus is found with any condition that results in increased density of lung, such as consolidation

        (2) Decreased fremitus is found if there is obstructed major bronchus, fluid in the pleural space or severe COPD with air trapping

  iii. Percussion

     (a) Dullness is heard over more dense lung tissue, such as consolidation or pulmonary edema

     (b) Hyperresonance is heard over chest with air trapping (COPD) or pneumothorax

  iv. Auscultation

     (a) Decreased breath sounds are heard when there is less air movement and less dense lung tissue (COPD)

     (b) Bronchial and bronchovesicular breath sounds are heard over more dense lung tissue (consolidation, atelectasis, pulmonary edema)

     (c) Adventitious sounds

        (1) Crackles or rales

        (2) Rhonchi or gurgles

        (3) Wheezes

     (d) Pleural friction rub: heard when inflamed pleural surfaces rub together

 c. Diagnostic study findings

  i. ABG analysis

     (a) Respiratory failure is defined by ABG measurements as hypoxemic ($\downarrow Pao_2$) and/or hypercapneic ($\downarrow Pao_2$ and $\uparrow Paco_2$)

     (b) Criteria: Pao_2 below 60 mm Hg, $Paco_2$ above 50 mm Hg, or both

        (1) Acute: acidosis, normal or mildly increasing blood buffers (HCO_3^-)

        (2) Chronic: relatively normal pH, elevated blood buffers

  ii. Radiologic findings: depend on primary disease

  iii. Intrapulmonary shunt greater than 15%

4. Nursing diagnoses (see Commonly Encountered Nursing Diagnoses)

 a. Ineffective airway clearance related to secretions

b. Ineffective breathing pattern
c. Impaired gas exchange
d. Inability to sustain spontaneous ventilation
e. Ineffective individual and family coping

. . . .
:
: **Adult Respiratory Distress Syndrome**

ARDS refers to a group of manifestations of an evolving, severe diffuse lung injury, especially to the parenchyma. The acute form of ARDS nearly always occurs suddenly in the presence of certain identifiable risk factors. In some types of acute ARDS, if the patient survives, the injury resolves and recovery is complete. In other patients with acute ARDS, notably the form associated with sepsis (particularly from an abdominal source), there is a high mortality even after the increased permeability pulmonary edema subsides. Instead of healing, the injured lung parenchyma rapidly undergoes organizational changes and a chronic phase evolves

1. **Pathophysiology**
   a. The *acute* phase of ARDS is characterized by damaged integrity of the blood-gas barrier. There is extensive damage to type I alveolar epithelial cells with increased endothelial permeability. Interstitial edema is found along with protein containing fluid leaking into the alveoli. This alveolar fluid also contains erythrocytes and leukocytes in addition to amorphous material comprising strands of fibrin. There also is impaired production and function of surfactant. The resultant physiologic abnormalities are as follows:
      i. Shunting of blood through atelectatic or fluid-filled lung units causes a widening of the alveolar to arterial difference in Po_2; the resultant hypoxemia is resistant to high FIo_2 but is often responsive to PEEP
      ii. The physiologic dead space is increased, frequently exceeding 60% of each breath; consequently, very large minute ventilation may be required to maintain tolerable levels of arterial Pco_2
      iii. The compliance of certain portions of lung parenchyma is reduced. The increased stiffness of the lungs is associated with a decrease in FRC and a requirement for high peak inspiratory pressures during mechanical ventilation. Other portions of the lung have relatively normal specific compliance and, thus, are not as much stiff as they are small
      iv. The resistance to blood flow through the lungs is increased by narrowing or obstruction of the pulmonary vessels. As a result, the pulmonary arterial pressure is often increased even though the pulmonary capillary wedge pressure remains normal or low. Chest radiographs reveal diffuse bilateral infiltrates suggestive of noncardiogenic (low or normal left heart filling pressures) pulmonary edema
   b. The *chronic* phase of ARDS is characterized by thickening of the endothelium, epithelium, and interstitial space. Type I cells are destroyed and replaced by type II cells (neutrophils), which proliferate but do not differentiate into type I cells as normal. The interstitial space is greatly expanded by edema fluid, fibers, and a variety of proliferating cells. Fibrosis commences after the first week. Within the alveoli, the protein-

rich exudate may organize to produce the characteristic "hyaline membrane," which effectively destroys the structure of the alveoli. Resultant physiologic abnormalities are:

   i. Increased vascular resistance

   ii. Hypoxemia from $\dot{V}/\dot{Q}$ mismatch or possible diffusion defect

   iii. Decreased tissue compliance

2. **Etiologic or precipitating factors**

  a. *Direct injury:* pulmonary contusion, gastric aspiration, near-drowning, inhalation of toxic gases and vapors, some infections, fat embolus, amniotic fluid embolus, radiation, bleomycin

  b. *Indirect injury:* septicemia, shock or prolonged hypotension, nonthoracic trauma, cardiopulmonary bypass, drug overdose, head injury, pancreatitis, diabetic coma, multiple blood transfusions

3. **Nursing assessment data base**

  a. Nursing history

    i. Subjective findings

      (a) Client's chief complaint—severe dyspnea

      (b) Other symptoms

        (1) Altered level of consciousness if hypoxemia is severe (i.e., confusion, somnolence, restlessness, irritability, anxiety, decreased mental acuity)

        (2) Production of frothy, pink sputum

    ii. Objective findings

      (a) Patient history: determine whether patient has a history of any of those listed above

      (b) Family history: ARDS is not an inherited disorder

      (c) Social history

        (1) Drug use, particularly heroin or crack cocaine

        (2) Recent alcohol or food intake; assess for signs of aspiration

      (d) Medication history: determine quantities of all medication recently taken, both over the counter and prescription

  b. Nursing examination of patient

    i. Inspection

      (a) Assess work of breathing

        (1) Posture, if patient is seated

        (2) Nasal flaring

        (3) Intercostal retractions

        (4) Use of accessory muscles

      (b) Assess rate and depth of respiration: tachypnea and hyperpnea

    ii. Palpation

      (a) Assess lung expansion: reduced because of low lung compliance

      (b) Assess vocal fremitus: increased because of increased density from diffuse pulmonary edema

    iii. Percussion: dullness to percussion over all lung fields if substantial pulmonary edema is present

    iv. Auscultation

      (a) Bronchovesicular breath sounds over most lung fields resulting from increased density of the lung

      (b) Adventitious sounds: diffuse crackles and gurgles over all lung fields

  c. Diagnostic findings: to exclude other causes of pulmonary edema

      i. ABG analysis

         (a) Hypoxemia is the hallmark of ARDS and is due to intrapulmonary shunting. Hypoxemia is refractory to O_2 therapy (i.e., PaO_2 is below 60 mm Hg or SaO_2 below 90% with FIO_2 above 0.5)

         (b) Respiratory alkalosis occurs in the early phases of ARDS because of hyperventilation

         (c) Hypercapnia is not usually seen initially and is an ominous sign if present

     ii. Chest x-ray: demonstrates diffuse bilateral interstitial and alveolar infiltrates without cardiomegaly or pulmonary vascular redistribution in the acute phase; a fine or coarse reticular pattern evolves in the chronic phase

    iii. Pulmonary function

         (a) Reduced pulmonary compliance

         (b) Reduced FRC secondary to microatelectasis and edema

         (c) Shunt studies demonstrate large right-to-left shunt (usually > 20% of cardiac output) measured during 100% O_2 breathing

         (d) Increased dead space ventilation (V_D/V_T)

         (e) Increased A–a gradient, reduced PaO_2/FIO_2 ratio

     iv. Pulmonary artery occlusive pressure (PAOP) may be normal or low, but pulmonary arterial pressure is often elevated

4. Nursing diagnoses (see Commonly Encountered Nursing Diagnoses)

  a. Impaired gas exchange

      i. Additional nursing interventions

         (a) Change the patient's position every 2 hours to mobilize secretions and allow aeration of all lung fields

         (b) Observe for signs of fluid overload; monitor I&O closely. Pulmonary edema may be minimized by maintaining the lowest intravascular volume compatible with adequate tissue perfusion

         (c) Monitor ABG results; notify physician immediately if PaO_2 drops below 60 mm Hg or if $PaCO_2$ trends upward despite increased patient respiratory efforts. Be prepared for the possibility of endotracheal intubation and mechanical ventilatory support. Consider both conventional and nonconventional modes of mechanical ventilation

         (d) Teach patient such relaxation techniques as imagery and progressive muscle relaxation to decrease demand for oxygen. Be prepared to administer sedation and, if appropriate, paralytic agents

  b. Ineffective individual and family coping

Chronic Obstructive Pulmonary Disease

COPD is an inclusive and nonspecific term referring to a condition in which patients have chronic cough and expectoration and various degrees of dyspnea either at rest or with exertion, with a significant and progressive reduction in expiratory air flow as measured by the forced expiratory volume in 1 second (FEV_1). This air flow abnormality does not show major reversibility in response to pharmacologic agents. Terms such as chronic obstructive airway disease (COAD), chronic obstructive lung disease (COLD), chronic air flow obstruction or chronic airway obstruction (CAO), and chronic airflow limitation (CAL) all mean the same thing.

COPD is usually divided into two subtypes: chronic bronchitis and emphysema. However, other diseases such as cystic fibrosis, bronchiectasis, or bronchiolitis obliterans are associated with chronic air flow limitation. The separate pathophysiology of these subtypes (chronic bronchitis and emphysema) is described here, but many patients exhibit signs and symptoms of both clinical conditions.

1. **Pathophysiology**
   a. *Chronic bronchitis:* a clinical diagnosis defined as the presence of chronic cough with sputum production on a daily basis for a minimum of 3 months per year for not less than two successive years. Many patients exhibit chronic hypoxemia with resultant episodes of cor pulmonale. They may also have reduced responsiveness of the respiratory center to hypoxemic stimuli, a trait that is probably inherited. Some of the pathophysiologic findings of chronic bronchitis are:
      i. Increase in size of the tracheobronchial mucus glands (increased Reid index) and goblet cell hyperplasia, resulting in increased sputum production
      ii. Epithelial mucus cell metaplasia, resulting in a decreased number of cilia. The hypersecretion of mucus and impaired cilia lead to a chronic productive cough
      iii. Increase in bronchial wall thickness with progressive obstruction to air flow (chronic obstructive bronchitis)
      iv. Exacerbations are usually due to infection, with the following clinical picture:
         (a) Increased amount of sputum and retained secretions
         (b) Increased $\dot{V}/\dot{Q}$ abnormalities, which increase hypoxemia, CO_2 retention, and acidemia
         (c) Hypoxemia and acidemia increase pulmonary vessel constriction, raising pulmonary artery pressure and ultimately leading to right heart failure (cor pulmonale)
   b. *Emphysema:* an anatomic alteration of the lung characterized by an abnormal enlargement of the air spaces distal to the terminal, nonrespiratory bronchioles, accompanied by destructive changes in the alveolar walls. Emphysema patients often exhibit increased dyspnea and breathing effort owing to an inherent increased responsiveness to hypoxemia. The resultant clinical picture is typically that of a well-oxygenated and dyspneic patient. The pulmonary abnormalities seen in the emphysema patient are:
      i. Reduction of gas exchange surface of respiratory bronchioles, alveolar ducts, and alveoli
      ii. Increased air trapping, caused by loss of elastic recoil and airway support structures (resulting in increased A-P diameter)
      iii. $\dot{V}/\dot{Q}$ inequality occurs and FRC is increased
      iv. Air sacs are replaced by bullae and capillary area is proportionately diminished
      v. Increased work of breathing results in greater resting O_2 consumption
2. **Etiology or precipitating factors** (chronic bronchitis and emphysema)
   a. Cigarette smoking—the most important factor and major toxic stimulus
   b. Environmental pollution, occupational exposure
   c. Predisposition due to genetic makeup, especially if there is known alpha$_1$-

antitrypsin deficiency. Should be considered in nonsmokers or young patients (< age 50 years) with emphysema

3. Nursing assessment data base
   a. Nursing history
      i. Subjective findings
         (a) Patient's chief complaint: these diseases may present as pure entities, but it is common for patients to have a combination of symptoms of the two
            (1) Chronic bronchitis: chronic cough and sputum production
            (2) Emphysema: dyspnea on exertion (early symptom) and eventual dyspnea at rest
         (b) Other symptoms
            (1) Chronic bronchitis: wheezing, peripheral edema
            (2) Emphysema: weight loss, inability to perform ADL
      ii. Objective findings
         (a) Etiologic or precipitating factors: history of cigarette smoking and environmental or occupational exposure
         (b) Family history of emphysema
         (c) Social history: assess extent of cigarette smoking; calculate pack-year history
         (d) Medication history: determine doses and times of all medications, both over-the-counter and prescription. Assess patient compliance in taking correct dose, adhering to correct schedule, and following proper inhalation technique for inhaled medications
   b. Nursing examination of patient: findings described in terms of the pure entities chronic bronchitis and emphysema, although most patients exhibit some symptoms of both conditions
      i. Inspection
         (a) Chronic bronchitis: observe for signs of right heart failure: peripheral edema, distended neck veins; skin color is dusky or cyanotic. Patients with chronic bronchitis show little sign of respiratory distress or dyspnea at rest
         (b) Emphysema
            (1) Observe thoracic cage for barrel chest appearance. Note posture and work of breathing both at rest and during exercise; use of accessory muscles of respiration is commonly noted.
            (2) Observe for use of pursed lip breathing. Note skin color, usually well-oxygenated and thus pinkish
      ii. Palpation
         (a) Chronic bronchitis
            (1) Note chest expansion; may be normal.
            (2) Assess vocal fremitus; may be normal or increased due to copious secretions in bronchial tree
         (b) Emphysema
            (1) Chest excursion is reduced because patient has hyperinflated lungs and flattened diaphragms from chronic air trapping.
            (2) Vocal fremitus is reduced because of less dense, more hyperinflated lungs
      iii. Percussion
         (a) Chronic bronchitis

(1) May demonstrate resonance if there are no areas of secretion retention or consolidation.

(2) Dullness to percussion is heard in areas of increased lung density (consolidation)

(b) Emphysema: hyperresonance throughout all lung fields

iv. Auscultation

(a) Chronic bronchitis: coarse crackles and gurgles; expiratory wheezes commonly heard

(b) Emphysema: distant, quiet breath sounds due to reduced air movement and air trapping; wheezes heard on occasion

c. Diagnostic study findings

i. Chronic bronchitis

(a) Pulmonary function: reduced FEV_1 and all other measures of expiratory air flow; some reversibility following bronchodilator therapy in selected patients

(b) ABGs: hypoxemia and often hypercapnia with compensated respiratory acidosis

(c) Other laboratory findings: polycythemia on complete blood count (CBC) in some patients

ii. Emphysema

(a) Pulmonary function: increased FRC, residual volume, and TLC. Reduced FEV_1 with $FEV_1/FVC < 75\%$ (greater than 80% is normal) and other expiratory airflow measures with nonreversibility following bronchodilators. Increased lung compliance and decrease in static recoil. Decreased diffusion capacity indicating a reduction in alveolar capillary gas exchange area (not a specific indicator of emphysema, however)

(b) ABGs: may be normal or abnormal, depending on type and severity of $\dot{V}/\dot{Q}$ abnormalities. Hypoxemia, if present, may be mild with normal $Paco_2$; greatest during sleep

(c) Radiologic findings: chest radiographs often show low, flattened diaphragms. In severe emphysema, lung fields may be hyperlucent, with diminished vascular markings and bullae. Disease is most prominent in the upper lung zones except in alpha$_1$-antitripsin deficiency, which may show a basilar predominance. Chest radiographs are of value during acute exacerbation to exclude complications such as pneumonia and pneumothorax

4. **Nursing diagnoses** (see Commonly Encountered Nursing Diagnoses)

a. Ineffective airway clearance

b. Ineffective breathing pattern

c. Impaired gas exchange

i. Additional nursing interventions

(a) Careful administration of O_2 using lowest FIo_2 that produces adequate oxygenation; observe for CO_2 retention with O_2 administration

(b) Observe for signs of fluid overload, monitor I&O closely

(c) Monitor ABGs; notify the physician immediately if Pao_2 drops below patient's known baseline or target level (usually Pao_2 55 to 60 mm Hg or greater) or if $Paco_2$ rises significantly beyond the established baseline value. In the patient with chronic CO_2 retention, monitoring $PaCO_2$ is less important than observing pH changes. Be prepared for the possibility of endotracheal intubation and need for mechanical ventilatory support

   (d) Teach patients to avoid cigarette smoking and other irritants and pollutants
   (e) Teach proper use and administration of inhaled medications
   (f) Following hospital discharge, consider pulmonary rehabilitation program that includes proper exercise training and nutrition
   (g) Consider influenza and pneumococcal vaccine for patient
   (h) For patients with documented alpha$_1$-antitrypsin deficiency receiving alpha$_1$-proteinase inhibitor (Prolastin), provide medication monitoring instruction
   d. Ineffective individual and family coping

Asthma and Status Asthmaticus (Severe Asthmatic Attack)

1. **Pathophysiology**
   a. Asthma: a chronic disease of variable severity characterized by airway hyperreactivity that produces airway narrowing of a reversible nature
      i. Increased responsiveness of airways to various stimuli
      ii. Widespread narrowing of airway with changes in severity; airway closure may occur
      iii. Cellular infiltration and mucosal edema
      iv. Airway hyperreactivity, with smooth muscle contraction and excessive mucus production and diminished secretion clearance
      v. $\dot{V}/\dot{Q}$ abnormalities
      vi. Increased work of breathing and airway resistance
      vii. Hyperinflation of lung, with increase in residual volume (RV)
      viii. Host defect of altered immunologic state
   b. Status asthmaticus: severe asthma attack that is refractory to bronchodilator therapy, including beta-adrenergic agents and IV aminophylline
      i. Severely reduced spirometric values for peak expiratory flow rate (PEFR), FVC, and FEV$_1$
      ii. Hypoxemia is present with a widened alveolar-arterial O_2 tension gradient or reduced PaO_2/FIO_2 ratio
      iii. Airway narrowing from:
         (a) Bronchial smooth muscle spasm minor component
         (b) Inflammation of bronchial walls, which leads to increased mucosal permeability and basement membrane thickening
         (c) Mucus plugging from airways due to increased production and reduced clearance of secretions. The mucus plugging, mucosal edema, and inspissated secretions account for the apparent resistance to bronchodilator therapy in patients with status asthmaticus

2. **Etiologic or precipitating factors for development of an asthma attack**
   a. Respiratory infection
   b. Allergic reaction to inhaled antigen
   c. Inappropriate bronchodilator management
   d. Idiosyncratic reaction to aspirin or other nonsteroidal anti-inflammatory agents (NSAIDs)

    e. Emotional stress
    f. Environmental exposure (air pollution, metabisulfite [food preservative] ingestion)
    g. Exercise
    h. Occupational exposure
    i. Nonselective beta-blocking agents (propranolol, timolol maleate)
    j. Mechanical stimulation (coughing, laughing, and cold air inhalation)
    k. Reflux esophagitis
    l. Sinusitis
3. **Nursing assessment data base**
    a. Nursing history
        i. Subjective findings
            (a) The chief complaint is usually dyspnea, wheezing, cough, and chest tightness
            (b) Severity ranges from intermittent, mild symptoms to severe respiratory symptoms despite intensive therapy
            (c) Other symptoms commonly seen with asthma:
                (1) Physical exhaustion, inability to sleep or rest, anxiety
                (2) Difficulty speaking in sentences
                (3) Thick, tenacious sputum production
        ii. Objective findings
            (a) Etiologic or precipitating factors: determine the presence of one or more causes or precipitating factors
            (b) Family history: determine whether there is a history of asthma in immediate family, grandparents, uncles, and aunts
            (c) Social history
                (1) Assess occupational exposure to dusts, industrial toxins, and heat or cold
                (2) Determine whether the patient smokes tobacco, marijuana, or crack cocaine; the amount; and whether any symptoms relate to cigarette consumption
                (3) Assess patient's recent eating habits for presence of known allergens (i.e., metabisulfites used as a food preservative)
                (4) Evaluate home conditions for presence of potential allergens
                    a) Pet dander
                    b) Carpets or rugs containing house mite debris
                    c) Smoker in the household
                    d) Plants
                    e) Type of humidification or air filtration system
            (d) Medication history: list all prescribed and over-the-counter medications taken in past week. Assess patient compliance in taking correct medications and doses at appropriate times. If patient is using any MDIs, assess the MDI technique if possible. Question the patient regarding any change in symptoms in response to any of the medications
    b. Nursing examination of patient
        i. Inspection
            (a) Observe the A-P diameter of the chest; in severe asthmatics, chronic air trapping may result in barrel chest appearance
            (b) Assess client's work of breathing
                (1) Posture

(2) Respiratory distress at rest

(3) Use of pursed lip breathing

(4) Presence of nasal flairing

(5) Bulging of interspaces on expiration

(6) Diaphoresis

(c) Assess breathing pattern

(1) Prolonged expiration

(2) Expiratory stridor

(3) Rate and depth of respirations—tachypnea and/or hyperpnea

(d) Assess pulse rate, and see if pulsus paradoxus is present; pulse > 110 beats/minute with pulsus greater than 12 mmHg in the presence of tachypnea (respiratory rate > 30/minute) indicates severe episode

(e) Assess for signs of dehydration; dehydration is thought to predispose to mucus impaction secondary to increased bronchial secretion viscosity

ii. Palpation

(a) Assess chest expansion: asthmatic lungs are hyperinflated and often show minimal chest excursion with inspiration

(b) Assess vocal fremitus; may be decreased as a result of decreased density (owing to hyperinflation) of lungs. Rhonchal fremitus may be present if there are copious secretions

iii. Percussion

(a) Hyperresonance is usually heard throughout lung fields

(b) Assessment of diaphragmatic excursion reveals low position of diaphragm and reduced excursion

iv. Auscultation

(a) Prolonged expiration

(b) Expiratory wheezes or rhonchi are heard as air and secretions move through narrowed airways. Sometimes severe wheezing can be heard without a stethoscope

(c) Decreased breath sounds throughout constitute an ominous sign. The asthmatic is then not moving enough air to be audible to the examiner

c. Diagnostic findings

i. Laboratory

(a) Evidence of infection (i.e., positive sputum cultures), elevated white blood cell (WBC) count, fever, increased sputum production

(b) ABG analysis

(1) May initially show low normal or ↓ Pa_{CO_2}, ↑ pH, and ↓ Pa_{O_2} (<60 mm Hg)

(2) In severe asthmatic attacks, there may be progression to a "normal" or increased Pa_{CO_2} level (may be a sign of impending respiratory failure)

(c) Radiologic findings: the chest x-ray study contributes little information; radiograph may be normal or hyperlucent. Its value may be to confirm or rule out a diagnosis of pneumonia, atelectasis, pneumothorax, or other condition that mimics asthma

(d) Pulmonary function: reduced FEV_1 and peak expiratory flow rates. Serial measurements of these parameters with the response to bronchodilators are essential to establish the severity of the obstruction and assess adequacy of response to therapy. In patients requiring hospitalization, PEFR may be less than 60 L/minute initially or does not improve to greater than 50% of predicted value after 1 hour of treatment, and FEV_1 may be less than 30% of predicted value or does not improve to at least 40% of predicted value following 1 hour of aggressive therapy

4. **Nursing diagnoses** (see Commonly Encountered Nursing Diagnoses)
   a. Ineffective airway clearance
      i. Additional nursing interventions
         (a) Administer bronchodilators and monitor therapeutic ranges and clinical response
            (1) Evaluate whether or not patient can properly perform MDI technique
            (2) Salmeterol is contraindicated during an acute asthma attack because of its delayed onset of action; albuterol or some other bronchodilator with a rapid onset of action should be utilized
         (b) Administer fluids and humidification to keep airway secretions thin and easily expectorated
         (c) Provide patient education to avoid allergens and importance of taking medications properly
   b. Ineffective breathing pattern
   c. Impaired gas exchange
      i. Additional nursing interventions
         (a) Close objective monitoring of blood gas levels, acid-base status, and ventilatory parameters (especially FEV_1 or peak flow rates if spirometry is not available)
         (b) Careful monitoring for possible cardiopulmonary arrest in severe cases
   d. Ineffective individual and family coping

Pulmonary Embolism

A pulmonary embolism, an obstruction of the pulmonary arteries by emboli, affects lung tissue, the pulmonary circulation, and the function of the right and left sides of the heart. The degree of compromise correlates with the extent of embolic vascular occlusion and the degree of preexisting cardiopulmonary disease

1. **Pathophysiology**
   a. Most emboli (>90%) arise from deep vein thromboses (DVTs) in the iliofemoral system. Other sites include the right heart and the pelvic area. Nonthrombolic emboli, such as fat, air, and amniotic fluid, also occur but are relatively uncommon
   b. Factors favoring venous thrombosis include (Virchow's triad):
      i. Blood stasis
      ii. Blood coagulation alterations
      iii. Vessel wall abnormalities
   c. Distribution of emboli is related to size of emboli and flow. Very large emboli have an impact in a large artery; however, the thrombus may break up and block several smaller vessels. The lower lobes are frequently involved because they have a high blood flow
   d. Pulmonary infarction (death of the embolized tissue) occurs infrequently.

More often, there is distal hemorrhage and atelectasis but alveolar structures remain viable. Infarction is more likely if the embolus completely blocks a large artery or if there is preexisting lung disease. Infarction results in alveolar filling with extravasated red blood cells and inflammatory cells and causes opacity on the radiograph. Occasionally, the infarct becomes infected, leading to an abscess

   e. Effects of acute pulmonary artery obstruction

      i. Altered gas exchange due to:

        (a) Right-to-left shunting and $\dot{V}/\dot{Q}$ inequalities. Possible etiologic mechanisms for these alterations include:

          (1) Overperfusion of unembolized lung results in low $\dot{V}/\dot{Q}$ ratios

          (2) Eventual reperfusion of atelectatic areas distal to the embolic obstruction

          (3) Development of postembolic pulmonary edema

      ii. The degree of hemodynamic compromise correlates with the degree of vascular occlusion in patients with no underlying heart or lung disease

        (a) Initial hemodynamic consequence is acute reduction in pulmonary vascular cross-sectional area with a subsequent increase in the resistance to blood flow through the lungs

        (b) If cardiac output remains constant or increases, pulmonary arterial pressure must rise

     iii. If cardiac or pulmonary disease exists and has already impaired the pulmonary vascular reserve capacity, a small degree of vascular occlusion will result in greater pulmonary artery hypertension and more serious right ventricular dysfunction

2. Etiologic or precipitating factors for deep venous thrombosis and pulmonary embolism

   a. Congestive heart failure

   b. Acute myocardial infarction

   c. Shock (bacteremia or nonbacteremia)

   d. Obesity

   e. Estrogen administration, pregnancy

   f. Malignancy

   g. Polycythemia vera

   h. Dysproteinemia

   i. Surgery or anesthesia

   j. Prolonged immobilization

   k. Diabetes mellitus

   l. Burns

   m. Trauma (especially fractures of spine, pelvis, or legs) or recent pelvic or lower abdominal surgery

   n. Venous disease of the lower extremity

   o. Previous pulmonary embolus

3. Nursing assessment data base

   a. Nursing history

      i. Subjective findings

        (a) Patient's chief complaint varies considerably, depending on severity and type of embolism. Dyspnea, tachypnea, and chest pain (usually pleuritic) are three subjective complaints common to many clinical situations

        (b) Other symptoms

           (1) Massive pulmonary embolism (>50% vascular occlusion): mental clouding, anxiety, feeling of impending doom and apprehension

           (2) Pulmonary embolism: symptoms may be vague and nonspecific

                a) Tachycardia

                b) Pleuritic chest pain (late finding), diffuse chest discomfort

                c) Hemoptysis suggests pulmonary infarction is present

                d) Anxiety, restlessness, apprehension

                e) Cough

                f) Syncope

                    i) Objective findings

                        [a] Etiologic or precipitating factors: a history of one of the precipitating factors

                        [b] Family history: no familial tendencies for pulmonary emboli but possibly a family history of some of the precipitating factors that increase the risk for pulmonary embolism (i.e., obesity)

                        [c] Social history: assess client's activity level to determine whether immobility is a factor

                        [d] Medication history: determine whether female clients are taking oral contraceptives containing estrogens

b. Nursing examination of patient

  i. Inspection

    (a) Assess chest expansion; may be reduced on affected side because of pleuritic pain

    (b) Observe for signs of increased work of breathing, tachypnea, and dyspnea

    (c) Examine client for petechiae over thorax and upper extremities

    (d) Observe skin for diaphoresis, signs of shock, and cyanosis

    (e) Assess behavior and mental status for mental aberrations, agitation, anxiety, and restlessness

  ii. Palpation

    (a) May elicit asymmetric chest expansion

    (b) Increased fremitus with large hemorrhagic pulmonary infarct

    (c) Pleural friction fremitus may be palpated in clients with pleural inflammation distal to infarct

  iii. Percussion

    (a) Resonance heard throughout lung fields except

    (b) Dullness to percussion over area of infarction

  iv. Auscultation

    (a) Inspiratory crackles (rales) may be heard

    (b) Increased intensity of pulmonic second sound (P_2)

    (c) Fixed splitting of the second heart sound is an ominous finding due to marked right ventricular overload

    (d) Murmur heard over lung field, augmented by inspiration. This murmur is generated by flow through a partially obstructed pulmonary artery. It may be absent initially and then develop as an embolus resolves

    (e) Pleural friction rub

    c. Diagnostic study findings

      i. Laboratory findings

        (a) ABGs may indicate respiratory alkalosis (caused by hyperventilation) and hypoxemia

        (b) The A–a gradient is increased; in a small percentage (6%) of patients, the A–a gradient may be normal

      ii. Radiologic findings

        (a) Chest x-ray is nonspecific, frequently normal. Pleural effusion occurs in 30% to 50% of cases but is small

        (b) Pulmonary angiography: the most definitive test for pulmonary embolism; should be considered when noninvasive tests are equivocal or contradictory or as initial diagnostic test if patient is hemodynamically unstable

      iii. Radionuclide testing

        (a) Lung ventilation-perfusion scan is not definitive but suggestive of pulmonary embolism; less risky than angiography

        (b) Should be performed in all clinically stable patients with suspected pulmonary embolism; about 60% of $\dot{V}/\dot{Q}$ scans will be indeterminant

      iv. The ECG is usually normal but in massive pulmonary embolism may reveal "P pulmonale," right axis deviation, or incomplete or new right bundle branch block. The ECG often demonstrates sinus tachycardia or, less frequently, atrial fibrillation or flutter

      v. Lower-extremity Doppler ultrasonography studies are performed to evaluate for DVT as a possible cause. Negative serial ultrasound scans reduce the likelihood of pulmonary embolism to less than 2%

4. Nursing diagnoses (see Commonly Encountered Nursing Diagnoses)

    a. Ineffective breathing pattern

      i. Additional nursing interventions

        (a) Early ambulation, turning, coughing, deep breathing

        (b) Elastic stockings, pneumatic compression stockings (if not contraindicated during systemic anticoagulation therapy), leg elevation

        (c) Adequate fluid intake

        (d) Administer anticoagulants as ordered; monitor for signs of bleeding

        (e) Administer thrombolytic therapy as ordered

        (f) Administer analgesics to prevent splinting; monitor for respiratory depression

    b. Impaired gas exchange

    c. Ineffective individual and family coping

Chest Trauma

1. Pathophysiology: depends on type and extent of injury. Trauma to chest or lungs may interfere with any of the components involved in inspiration, gas exchange, and expiration

    a. *Blunt injuries.* The chest wall damage must be evaluated in conjunction with the accompanying intrathoracic and intra-abdominal visceral injuries. Injuries seen with blunt trauma include:

     i. Visceral injuries without chest wall damage
- (a) Pneumothorax
- (b) Hemothorax
- (c) Lung contusion
- (d) Diaphragmatic injury
- (e) Aortic rupture
- (f) Rupture of trachea or bronchus
- (g) Cardiac injury

     ii. Soft tissue injuries: possibly a sign of severe underlying damage
- (a) Cutaneous abrasion
- (b) Ecchymosis
- (c) Laceration of superficial layers
- (d) Burns
- (e) Hematoma

     iii. Fracture of sternum: occurs either as a result of direct impact or as the indirect result of overflexion of the trunk

     iv. Rib fractures as a result of overflexion or from straightening. Rib fractures can be unifocal or multifocal. Multiple fractures result in flail chest and are often complicated by injuries to the soft tissues and pleura

     v. Separation or dislocation of ribs and cartilages from an anterior blow to chest

  b. *Penetrating injuries*

     i. Pleural cavity as well as chest wall has been entered. Damage to deeper structures is a serious consequence

     ii. Generally able to predict extent of injury and organs injured by course of wound and nature of penetrating instrument. High-velocity projectiles do more damage than is apparent from the surface

     iii. Injuries seen with penetrating trauma
- (a) Open sucking chest wounds with air entering pleural space during inspiration
- (b) Hemothorax, hemopneumothorax, or chylothorax
- (c) Combined thoracoabdominal injuries (esophageal, diaphragmatic, or abdominal viscus injuries)
- (d) Damage to trachea and large airways
- (e) Wounds of heart or great vessels

2. Etiologic or precipitating factors

  a. Blunt trauma: automobile crashes, falls, assaults, explosives

  b. Penetrating trauma: car crashes, falls, assaults, explosives, bullets, knives, shell fragments, free flying objects, industrial accidents

3. Nursing assessment data base

  a. Nursing history

     i. Subjective findings
- (a) The chief complaint varies with specific injury; tachypnea, dyspnea, pain, and respiratory distress may occur with any injury
- (b) Other symptoms are described according to type of trauma
  - (1) Fractures of ribs, sternochondral junction, or sternum: pain accentuated by chest wall movement, deep inspiration, or touch
  - (2) Flail chest: dyspnea and localized pain

(3) Trauma to lung parenchyma, trachea, or bronchi: hemoptysis and respiratory distress

(4) Contusion to heart: angina

(5) Rupture of aorta and major vessels: dyspnea and backache, intense pain in chest, or back unaffected by respirations

(6) Open sucking chest wound: if the opening in the chest wall is smaller than the diameter of the trachea, the patient may have minimal subjective symptoms. If the opening is larger, more air enters the pleural space, collapsing the lung, resulting in ineffective gas exchange and dyspnea

ii. Objective findings

(a) Etiologic or precipitating factors: a good history describing the traumatic incident is essential. If the patient is not able to answer questions, obtain information from witnesses to the incident regarding blows to the chest, weapon used (if applicable), and position of patient at the moment of impact

(b) Social history: assess recent use of alcohol or drugs, which may have been a causal factor in the trauma

(c) Medication history: assess all medications taken, their doses, and schedule. Determine whether there is a lack of patient compliance with medications; the physiologic result of inadequate or excessive medication can influence level of consciousness, with resultant injury while one is operating machinery or motor vehicles

b. Nursing examination of patient

i. Inspection

(a) Observe skin for ecchymosis, hematomas, abrasions, burns, and lacerations

(b) Observe work of breathing; use of accessory muscles of breathing; intercostal retractions

(c) Observe depth and rate of respirations: patients with rib fractures (or any injury that causes pain) may breathe shallowly to minimize the pain. Tachypnea often accompanies pain and apprehension

(d) Look for asymmetry; may be seen with tension pneumothorax or hemothorax. In flail chest, chest wall movement is paradoxical: sinking in on inspiration and flailing out on expiration

(e) Examine the wound in both respiratory phases

(f) Try to determine intrathoracic or intra-abdominal trajectory of the offending instrument

ii. Palpation

(a) Evaluate chest expansion: often reduced due to pain; is unequal with pneumothorax or hemothorax. With flail chest, there is a fall in the chest cage on inspiration and a rise of the cage on expiration

(b) Palpate for subcutaneous emphysema: may be found in pneumothorax or rupture of trachea or bronchus

(c) Assess for presence of vocal fremitus:

(1) Reduced when air or blood occupies the pleural space: pneumothorax, tension pneumothorax, or hemothorax

(2) Increased in conditions of increased lung density: pulmonary hemorrhage

(d) Palpate position of trachea:

(1) Displaced toward the injured side in pneumothorax

(2) Displaced toward the contralateral side in hemothorax or tension pneumothorax

iii. Percussion

(a) Ipsilateral tympany or hyperresonance is heard in pneumothorax and tension pneumothorax

(b) In rupture of the diaphragm, the left hemidiaphragm is usually involved, resulting in dullness (from fluid-filled bowel) or tympany (from gas-filled bowel) heard over left chest

(c) Dullness to percussion is heard with hemothorax, hemopneumothorax, or parenchymal hemorrhage

iv. Auscultation

(a) Reduced breath sounds are heard in any condition that causes shallow respirations

(b) Diminished or absent breath sounds are heard in pneumothorax, tension pneumothorax, flail chest, hemothorax, or hemopneumothorax

(c) Bronchial breath sounds may be heard with parenchymal hemorrhage

(d) Bowel sounds in chest may be heard with rupture of diaphragm

c. Diagnostic study findings

i. Chest x-ray is performed for all injuries if patient is stable

(a) Rib fractures, parenchymal hemorrhage, hemothorax, or hemopneumothorax is identifiable on chest x-ray

(b) Pneumothorax: expiratory chest films are often used in diagnosis

(c) Tension pneumothorax: shows a shift in the mediastinum to the unaffected side in addition to pneumothorax

(d) Rupture of diaphragm: shows bowel loops in thorax

(e) Rupture of aorta or major vessels: revealed by widening of mediastinum

ii. Bronchoscopy may be used to confirm diagnosis of rupture of trachea or bronchus

iii. Aortography confirms diagnosis of rupture of aorta or other major vessels

iv. ECG is done to evaluate contusion to heart, wherein tachycardia, dysrhythmias, and electrocardiographic changes may be found

4. Nursing diagnoses (see Commonly Encountered Nursing Diagnoses)

a. Ineffective airway clearance

i. Additional nursing interventions

(a) Use suctioning as needed to stimulate cough and clear the airways of blood and secretions

(b) Symptomatic treatment for uncomplicated rib fractures to ensure ability to cough and deep breathe as required

b. Ineffective breathing pattern

i. Additional nursing interventions

(a) Administer analgesia carefully to avoid compromise of ventilation

(b) Monitor water seal chest drainage in treatment of pneumothorax or hemothorax; observe for absence or presence of bubbling observed in the water seal chamber; if suction is ordered, maintain appropriate suction setting

(c) Avoid dependent loops in chest drainage tubing to facilitate drainage; properly secure and tape chest tube insertion site. Observe for signs of leaking pleural fluid or bleeding at insertion site; routinely check system for loose connections

   (d) Assist with emergency decompression of tension pneumothorax with large bore needle into second anterior interspace, or insertion of chest tube

  c. Impaired gas exchange

  d. Impaired individual and family coping

Acute Pneumonia

Pneumonia is an inflammatory process of the alveolar spaces caused by infection

1. **Pathophysiology**
   a. Possible pathogenic mechanisms for development of pneumonia include:
      i. Aspiration
      ii. Inhalation
      iii. Inoculation
      iv. Direct spread from contiguous sites
      v. Hematogenous spread
      vi. Colonization in chronic lung disease (e.g., COPD, cystic fibrosis)
   b. Acquisition of infection depends on the nature of infecting organism, the immediate environment, and the defense status of the host
   c. Important constituents of pulmonary defense system
      i. Upper airway defenses: adversely affected by nasotracheal intubation, endotracheal intubation, tracheostomy suction catheters, and nasogastric tubes
        (a) Nasopharyngeal filtration
        (b) Mucosal adherence
        (c) Bacterial interference
        (d) Saliva
        (e) Secretory IgA
      ii. Lower airway defenses: may be impaired or inactivated by old age, underlying diseases, such as diabetes or chronic bronchitis, hypoxia, pulmonary edema, malnutrition, and drug or O_2 therapy
        (a) Cough reflex
        (b) Mucociliary clearance
        (c) Humoral factors
        (d) Cellular factors
2. **Etiologic or precipitating factors**
   a. Normal host infected with usual organisms
      i. *Streptococcus pneumoniae* (pneumococcus): the most common cause, especially in older patients and those with a variety of chronic diseases
      ii. *Mycoplasma pneumoniae:* spread by droplet nuclei and may occur in epidemics
      iii. *Haemophilus influenzae:* with encapsulated type B organisms, is more likely to cause bacteremia; nontypable *H. influenzae* is seen more in the elderly population
      iv. Viruses: a relatively uncommon cause of pneumonia in adults, accounting for 25% to 50% of nonbacterial pneumonias; influenza A virus is most common cause; others include adenovirus and

coxsackievirus; cytomegalovirus (CMV) and herpes simplex virus (HSV) are often seen in immunocompromised patients

    v. *Chlamydia pneumoniae:* a recently described pathogen that causes a spectrum of illnesses from mild upper respiratory symptoms to pneumonia

    vi. Fungi: *Histoplasma capsulatum* inhalation results in acute severe pulmonary histoplasmosis. Similar reactions in patients infected with blastomycosis, *Cryptococcus,* coccidioidomycosis, *Aspergillus fumigatus,* and *Candida albicans.* Geographic location is important in determining identification of certain organisms

b. Normal host infected with unusual organisms

    i. *Legionella pneumophila* may be sporadic or occur in localized outbreaks in institutions

    ii. *Bacillus anthracis* infects humans who have been in contact with anthrax infected animals

    iii. *Yersinia pestis* causes plague; transmitted from wild animals and their fleas, or via the respiratory route

    iv. *Francisella tularensis* causes pleuropulmonary tularemia, endemic in certain parts of the United States; transmitted by ticks or, possibly, by inhalation from infected animals

    v. Group A *Streptococcus* and *Meningococcus* bacteria reside in the upper respiratory tract; pneumonia occurs in individuals housed in groups, such as in military service. *Streptococcus pyogenes* causes pneumonia typically after outbreaks of viral infections

    vi. *Mycobacterium tuberculosis* or atypical tuberculosis can produce life-threatening pulmonary complications in hosts whose only risk factor is age

c. Abnormal host infected with usual organisms: compromised states can result from presence of chronic underlying disease, poor nutrition, trauma, surgery, or subsequent to immunosuppression

    i. Pneumococcal pneumonia is more severe in this population

    ii. Gram-negative bacilli, such as *Escherichia coli, Pseudomonas aeruginosa, Serratia, Proteus vulgaris, Acinetobacter* and *Klebsiella pneumoniae,* and *Moraxella catarrhalis*

    iii. Anaerobic bacteria, such as *Bacteroides,* cause severe pulmonary infections in the abnormal host

    iv. *Staphylococcus aureus* is seen in diabetic patients, in patients with a recent history of influenza, and institutionalized or hospitalized patients

    v. *K. pneumoniae* causes a virulent, necrotizing pneumonia often seen in alcoholic or otherwise debilitated patients; abscess formation is common

d. Abnormal host infected with unusual organisms

    i. Enterococcal pneumonia is associated with the use of third-generation cephalosporins

    ii. Group B *Streptococcus pneumoniae* is reported in older patients with underlying diseases

    iii. Hospital-acquired *L. pneumophila* occurs in renal transplant patients and those who are debilitated and immunocompromised

    iv. *Legionella micdadei,* the Pittsburgh pneumonia agent, is seen in renal transplant patients during corticosteroid therapy

v. Fungi, including *Aspergillus fumigatus* and *Aspergillus flavum,* are seen mostly in patients who have received high doses of steroids and broad-spectrum antibiotics

vi. *Nocardia asteroides* is seen in renal transplant patients and patients with hematologic malignancies

vii. *Pneumocystis carinii,* typical and atypical mycobacteria, and cytomegalovirus infections are seen in patients with acquired immunodeficiency syndrome (AIDS)

3. Nursing assessment data base

a. Nursing history

i. Subjective findings

(a) Patient's chief complaint varies, depending on organism

(b) Some of more common presentations include:

(1) Pneumococcal pneumonia: abrupt shaking chills or rigor, fever, dyspnea, pleuritic pain, and cough productive of rusty sputum

(2) *Mycoplasma:* fever, myalgias, headache, minimally productive cough, and nonpleuritic chest pain

(3) *H. influenzae:* fever, chills, and cough with purulent sputum

(4) *Klebsiella:* sudden onset, blood-tinged sputum, and tachypnea

ii. Objective findings

(a) Etiology or precipitating factors: determine whether the patient is a normal or abnormal host; assess for presence of above precipitating factors

(b) Family history: not a familial tendency for pneumonia, but there may be a familial tendency for some of the precipitating factors (diabetes or cystic fibrosis)

(c) Social history: assess nutritional habits, smoking habits, and alcohol intake

(d) Medication history: assess all prescribed and over-the-counter medications, doses, and times of administration. Determine patient compliance, especially with antibiotics

b. Nursing examination of patient

i. Inspection

(a) Observe posture and work of breathing; assess use of accessory muscles of breathing

(b) Inspect chest for intercostal retractions

(c) Observe for signs of dyspnea (i.e., nasal flaring)

(d) Assess respiratory patterns; tachypnea and/or hyperpnea often seen

(e) Observe for signs of hypoxemia: duskiness or cyanosis, mental status changes

ii. Palpation

(a) Assess chest expansion: expect to see asymmetric chest movement in unilateral pneumonias caused by pleuritic pain and reduced lung compliance on the affected side

(b) The palpable vibration of the chest wall that results from speech or breathing effort is referred to as *tactile fremitus.* Increased fremitus, often rougher and coarser in feel, occurs in the presence of fluids or a solid mass in the lungs and may be caused by lung consolidation; gentle, more tremulous fremitus can occur with some lung consolidations

  iii. Percussion: dullness or flatness to percussion is heard with consolidation

  iv. Auscultation

    (a) Fine early inspiratory crackles or bronchial breath sounds are heard with areas of consolidation, as in lobar pneumonia; breath sounds may be decreased

    (b) Greater clarity and increased loudness of spoken words are defined as *bronchophony*. Bronchophony is increased in the presence of consolidation

      (1) A whisper heard clearly through the stethoscope is called *whispered pectoriloquy*

      (2) When the intensity of the spoken voice is increased and there is a nasal quality (e's become stuffy broad a's), the auditory quality is called *egophony*

c. Diagnostic study findings

  i. Chest x-ray findings vary with involvement

    (a) Segmental or lobar consolidation

    (b) Multiple infiltrates

    (c) Pleural effusions

    (d) Chest radiograph is particularly helpful in detecting parapneumonic effusions, abcesses, and cavities

  ii. Sputum examination

    (a) Color and consistency typically vary with pathogen

    (b) Initial Gram stain and microscopic examination

      (1) A good sputum specimen contains few (<5) squamous epithelial cells picked up in transit through the upper respiratory tract and can be visualized by low-power field on Gram stain. When the specimen is not expectorated by patient, other means of obtaining sputum include suctioning, transtracheal aspiration, fiberoptic bronchoscopy, needle aspiration of lung, and open lung biopsy

      (2) Expectorated sputum specimens have relatively poor sensitivity and specificity

      (3) Staining demonstrates neutrophils (PMNs) and bacterial agents

      (4) Large numbers of PMNs are seen in most bacterial pneumonias

      (5) Fewer PMNs and more mononuclear inflammatory cells are seen in mycoplasmal and viral pneumonias

    (c) Sputum cultures are done with the initial Gram stain and microscopic examination; however, some bacteria are relatively difficult to grow, and in many cases the initial Gram stain is just as important in making the etiologic diagnosis

  iii. Blood cultures

    (a) Obtaining a blood sample is very important in patient evaluation because of high specificity of a positive culture, especially in hospitalized patients with pneumococcal pneumonia

    (b) Pneumonia patients with documented bacteremia have a poor prognosis

iv. Leukocyte counts
    (a) Often elevated in lobar pneumonia
    (b) May be normal with atypical pneumonia
    (c) May be normal or reduced in the elderly, in immunocompromised patients, in patients with overwhelming infections, and in those with viral infection
v. ABG analysis: may indicate hypoxemia and hypocapnia in lobar pneumonia
vi. Thoracentesis: may be indicated when significant pleural effusion is present

4. **Nursing diagnoses** (see Commonly Encountered Nursing Diagnoses)
  a. Ineffective airway clearance
    i. Additional nursing interventions
      (a) Aseptic technique with hand washing to reduce cross-contamination
      (b) Administer appropriate antibiotic therapy, and monitor response
      (c) Contact isolation or other category as appropriate to prevent spread of infection
      (d) Assess for adequate hydration, administer fluids as ordered
      (e) Assess for presence of pleuritic chest pain reported by patient, pain control may be achieved by anti-inflammatory agents, analgesics, or intercostal nerve blocks
  b. Impaired gas exchange

. . . .

Pulmonary Aspiration

Pulmonary aspiration may result from vomiting or regurgitation. Vomiting is an active mechanism that interrupts breathing, causes the diaphragm to descend, contracts the anterior abdominal wall, elevates the pelvic diaphragm, closes the pylorus, and opens the esophageal sphincter, resulting in material ejected from the stomach. Regurgitation is completely passive and may occur even in the presence of paralyzed muscles. Powerful laryngeal and cough reflexes normally prevent aspiration of gastric contents into the tracheobronchial tree. Any impairment or depression of these normal reflexes increases the risk of pulmonary aspiration

1. **Pathophysiology** (varies with types of aspiration)
  a. Large particles can obstruct major airways and cause immediate asphyxia and death; immediate intervention required
  b. Clear acidic liquid: the pH of aspirated material largely determines the extent of pulmonary injury. As the pH decreases below 2.5 or if the volume of acidic fluid is large, the severity of lung injury increases
    i. A chemical burn destroys type II alveolar cells that produce surfactant and increases alveolar capillary membrane permeability, with subsequent extravasation of fluid and blood into the interstitium and alveoli
    ii. As fluid and blood accumulate in the alveolar space, the lung volume diminishes; thus, both FRC and compliance decrease. Reflex airway closure may also occur
    iii. Alveolar ventilation decreases relative to perfusion, which results in

intrapulmonary shunting. Hypoxia can occur minutes after acid aspiration

   iv. Extensive irritation of the airways by acidic fluid may induce intense bronchospasm

   v. Widespread peribronchial hemorrhage along with pulmonary edema and necrosis may occur

  c. Clear nonacidic liquid: the nature and extent of pulmonary damage depends on the volume of the aspirate and its composition

   i. Aspiration of less acidic or neutral pH liquids can induce hypoxia with acute respiratory decompensation. Reflex airway closure, pulmonary edema, and changes in the characteristics of surfactant may occur. There is little necrosis

   ii. Sequelae are more frequently transient and more easily reversible

  d. Foodstuff or small particles: may produce a severe subacute inflammatory pulmonary reaction with extensive hemorrhage

   i. Within 6 hours of aspiration, there may be extensive hemorrhagic pneumonia

   ii. Extravasation of fluid from the intravascular space into the lungs usually occurs but is generally not as intense or rapid as after acid aspiration

   iii. Severe intrapulmonary shunting may result and arterial Po_2 may be as low as or lower than that seen after the aspiration of acidic liquid

   iv. Arterial Pco_2 is usually much higher after the aspiration of food. This may indicate a higher degree of hypoventilation

   v. Aspiration of acidic foodstuff may produce even more tissue necrosis as a result of the combined effects of acid and foods

  e. Contaminated material: aspiration of material grossly contaminated with bacteria (i.e., bowel obstruction) can be fatal

2. Etiologic or precipitating factors

  a. Aspiration usually occurs in association with specific predisposing conditions

   i. Altered consciousness: drugs, alcohol, anesthesia, seizures, CNS disorders, shock, use of sedatives

   ii. Altered anatomy: tracheostomy, esophageal or tracheal abnormalities, nasogastric or nasointestinal tube, endotracheal tube, intestinal obstruction

   iii. Protracted vomiting or coughing

   iv. Improper positioning of patients, especially if they are receiving enteral hyperalimentation

3. Nursing assessment data base

  a. Nursing history

   i. Subjective findings

    (a) Patient's chief complaint: cough, dyspnea, wheezing are seen with aspiration. With fluids or solid object aspiration, there can be an abrupt onset of acute respiratory distress

    (b) Other symptoms:

     (1) Hypoxemia (mental status changes)

     (2) Increased respiratory secretions, hypotension, tachycardia, tachypnea, fever

   ii. Objective findings

    (a) Etiologic or precipitating factors

(1) Determine the presence of one or more of the above

(2) Obtain detailed description of events leading to onset of symptoms

(b) Social history: assess client's recent oral, alcohol, and drug intake

(c) Medication history

(1) Assess recent intake of all prescription and over-the-counter medications, doses, and schedules

(2) Determine patient compliance with regard to excessive or inadequate dosing, especially with sedatives, analgesics, or anticonvulsants

b. Nursing examination of patient

i. Inspection

(a) Observe posture and work of breathing; assess use of accessory muscles of respiration

(b) Look for retraction of interspaces indicating an obstruction of inflow of air into the airways

(c) Observe for inspiratory stridor caused by foreign body obstruction to large bronchus

(d) Observe respiratory rate; tachypnea usually present

(e) Assess for presence of cyanosis or other signs of hypoxemia

ii. Palpation

(a) Assess tactile fremitus: decreased or absent fremitus with foreign body obstruction of large bronchus a probable finding

(b) Increased fremitus in area of dependent lobe infiltrates and atelectasis a possible finding

iii. Percussion: dullness to percussion in area of infiltrates and atelectasis

iv. Auscultation

(a) Wheezing heard with aspiration of both liquids and solid objects

(b) Crackles and possible wheezing heard in affected lung with aspiration

(c) Absent breath sounds with occluded bronchus

c. Diagnostic study findings

i. Radiographic findings: dependent lobe infiltrates and atelectasis. Gravity-dependent areas of lungs most prone to aspiration include superior segments of lower lobes and posterior segments of upper and lower lobes. If the patient has a nasogastric or nasointestinal tube in place, the examination should verify the proper location and position, particularly if medications and/or enteral formula feedings are being administered

ii. Pulmonary function studies: may show decreased compliance or decreased diffusing capacity

iii. Sputum examination: induced cough or tracheal suction for stain and culture of specimens; cytology sometimes diagnostic. Fiberoptic bronchoscopy is sometimes used for infectious processes

iv. ABG analysis: may demonstrate hypoxemia

v. Open lung biopsy: reserved for patients who are unable to safely undergo transbronchial biopsy

4. Nursing diagnoses (see Commonly Encountered Nursing Diagnoses)

a. Ineffective airway clearance

i. Additional nursing interventions

(a) Avoid the supine position or any position that predisposes to aspiration

(b) Closely monitor characteristics of secretions suctioned or expectorated

(c) If the patient is being nasoenterally fed, carefully monitor the location of the feeding tube and routinely assess for pulmonary aspiration by clinical assessment findings as well as routine testing of tracheal aspirates for the presence or absence of glucose. False-positive readings may be caused by blood or other unknown factors

(d) If endotracheal tube is in place, suction secretions that accumulate above the tube cuff (subglottic secretion removal)

b. Impaired gas exchange

   i. Additional nursing interventions: administer corticosteroids if ordered; they may be of benefit if given immediately after aspiration of acid

Near-Drowning

Near-drowning is defined as immersion in liquid that necessitates the victim's being transported to a hospital emergency department but is not severe enough to result in death within the first 24 hours after submersion

1. Pathophysiology

  a. Electrolyte change: there is a tendency toward hemoconcentration in salt water drownings and hemodilution in fresh water drowning; however, dangerous changes in plasma electrolytes are very unusual

  b. Pulmonary effects: 90% of victims aspirate fluid, and most victims (85%) aspirate less than 25 ml/kg of body weight; however, the water aspirated may contain mud, sand, algae, chemicals, and/or vomitus

    i. In fresh water aspiration, water rapidly enters the circulation; in salt water aspiration, the hypertonic sea water draws fluid from the circulation into the lungs. However, near drowning victims of salt water and fresh water immersion have the same initial pathophysiologic aberrations: major insults include hypoxemia and tissue hypoxia, hypoxic brain injury with cerebral edema, hypercapnia, and acidemia. Hypothermia, pneumonia, and (rarely) disseminated intravascular coagulation (DIC), acute renal failure, and hemolysis may also occur

    ii. Organic and inorganic contents of the aspirated fluid, regardless of the type of water, produce an inflammatory reaction in the alveolar-capillary membrane that leads to an outpouring of plasma-rich exudate into the alveolus, displacement of air, and deposition of proteinaceous material

    iii. There is destruction of surfactant by aspirated water and proteinaceous exudate, resulting in large areas of atelectasis

    iv. Regional hypoxia promotes hypoxic vasoconstriction, which raises pulmonary intravascular pressures, promoting further interstitial fluid flux and frequently giving rise to pulmonary edema

    v. In some patients, hyaline membranes develop on the wall of injured bronchioles, alveolar ducts, and alveoli. This results in reduced compliance and increased dead space:tidal volume ratio, increased respiratory work, and $\dot{V}/\dot{Q}$ mismatch

2. Etiologic or precipitating factors

  a. Fresh water or salt water drowning secondary to young age and inability to swim

  b. Prior alcohol or drug ingestion may be associated with the near-drowning event

  c. Head and neck trauma and loss of consciousness associated with epilepsy, diabetes, syncope, or dysrhythmias

  d. Barotrauma associated with scuba diving

3. Nursing assessment data base

  a. Nursing history

    i. Subjective findings

      (a) Patient's chief complaint: respiratory distress, coughing

      (b) Other symptoms

        (1) Unconsciousness

        (2) Neurologic abnormalities if a period of cerebral anoxia has occurred

    ii. Objective findings

      (a) Etiologic or precipitating factors: determine the presence of one or more of the above factors

      (b) Social history: assess for recent intake of alcohol or drugs; question the patient's expertise in swimming

      (c) Medication history

        (1) Determine all recent prescription and over-the-counter medications taken, their doses, and schedules

        (2) Determine whether any medications were taken in excessive doses, especially sedatives, analgesics, or mood-altering drugs

  b. Nursing examination of patient

    i. Inspection

      (a) Observe posture and work of breathing for signs of labored respirations

      (b) Assess level of consciousness

      (c) Observe for use of accessory muscles of breathing

      (d) Assess respiratory patterns

        (1) Tachypnea in the conscious patient

        (2) Apnea in the unconscious patient

      (e) Observe for intercostal retractions from more negative pleural pressures required to inflate less compliant lungs

      (f) Assess for presence of cyanosis and other signs of hypoxemia

      (g) Assess for presence of hypothermia or fever

    ii. Palpation

      (a) Assess chest expansion: often decreased owing to low lung compliance

      (b) Assessment of vocal fremitus: difficult in dyspneic client; one would expect to see no change or a slight increase bilaterally

    iii. Percussion: dullness to percussion over most lung zones a possible finding because of diffuse pulmonary edema

    iv. Auscultation: diffuse crackles sometimes heard on inspiration bilaterally

  c. Diagnostic study findings

    i. Chest x-ray: aspiration or pulmonary edema

    ii. Laboratory studies

(a) Minimal electrolyte and Hb changes

(b) ABG studies show hypoxemia and metabolic acidosis

(c) Leukocytosis

(d) Coagulation studies: because coagulation disorders, including DIC have been reported in near-drowning victims, screening studies of prothrombin time (PT), activated partial thromboplastin time (aPTT), and platelet count are often done. If these results are abnormal, fibrinogen levels, fibrin split products, and euglobin clot lysis time should be determined

   iii. Electrocardiography: may show dysrhythmias and nonspecific changes. Few victims die of ventricular fibrillation; acidemia, CO_2 retention and hypoxemia result in marked irregular bradycardia, which precedes asystole and cardiac arrest

4. **Nursing diagnoses** (see Commonly Encountered Nursing Diagnoses)

   a. Ineffective airway clearance

      i. Additional nursing interventions: Monitor fluid I&O to avoid fluid overload and worsening pulmonary edema

   b. Impaired gas exchange

      i. Additional nursing interventions

        (a) Monitor arterial blood gases; notify physician immediately if Pa_{O_2} drops and/or Pa_{CO_2} rises

        (b) Be prepared for the possibility of endotracheal intubation, mechanical ventilation, and PEEP

   c. Ineffective individual and family coping

Pulmonary Problems in Surgical Patients

Surgery represents a stress to the respiratory system. Pulmonary problems are the major cause of morbidity after surgery

1. **Pathophysiology**

   a. Changes in pulmonary function occur normally during the immediate postoperative period. These changes are most evident following abdominal or thoracic surgery

      i. Reduction in forced vital capacity (FVC) is consistent with a restrictive defect; is significant but usually temporary

      ii. A reduction in lung volumes, especially FRC, also exists. These changes are due in part to:

        (a) Pain

        (b) Supine position

      iii. Reduced lung compliance is present, resulting in reduced tidal volume and increased respiratory frequency

   b. Microatelectasis is the most common cause of hypoxemia; the increased respiratory frequency leads to respiratory alkalosis

   c. Bacterial invasion of lower airways and reduced clearance postoperatively predispose to respiratory infection

   d. Aspiration of gastric and oropharyngeal contents occurs postoperatively in patients who have a disturbance in consciousness

   e. Arterial hypoxemia due to $\dot{V}/\dot{Q}$ mismatching is common during the postoperative period for normal patients and is exaggerated for COPD patients

2. **Etiologic or precipitating factors**
   a. A history of COPD or cigarette smoking is the most important risk factor. Preoperative hypercapnia is a serious risk factor
   b. Obesity results in decreased vital capacity
   c. The very young and the elderly are at increased risk for postoperative pulmonary complications
   d. People with underlying chronic diseases, with or without malnutrition, are at greater risk
   e. Prolonged anesthesia time increases risk
   f. Thoracic and abdominal surgery are especially hazardous to patients at risk. Maximal inspirations are voluntarily limited because of pain, thereby increasing risk of atelectasis
3. **Nursing assessment data base**
   a. Nursing history
      i. Subjective findings
         (a) Patient's chief complaint: varies with the type of surgery but is often incisional pain
         (b) Other symptoms include cough with or without sputum production and fear or reluctance to cough, deep breathe, and move about after surgery
      ii. Objective findings
         (a) Etiologic or precipitating factors: determine the patient's past medical history for smoking, COPD, cardiovascular disease, and previous pulmonary surgery. Determine type of surgery and anesthesia time
         (b) Family history: not applicable except in relation to contributing to medical history
         (c) Social history
            (1) Assess dietary habits to determine overall nutritional status
            (2) Assess smoking habits and pack-year history
         (d) Medication history
            (1) Determine all recent prescription and over-the-counter medications taken, doses, and schedules
            (2) Determine which medications must be resumed in the immediate postoperative period
   b. Nursing examination of patient
      i. Inspection
         (a) Observe for change in respiratory pattern (i.e., tachypnea or shallow respirations)
         (b) Assess lung expansion, and observe for splinting of respirations caused by incisional pain
         (c) Observe for asymmetry of chest expansion caused by possible unilateral atelectasis
         (d) Observe for signs of respiratory distress and increased work of breathing
      ii. Palpation
         (a) Assess chest expansion for degree and symmetry
         (b) Assess for increased vocal fremitus over area of atelectasis or consolidation
         (c) Assess rhonchial fremitus for presence of secretions in airways
      iii. Percussion

(a) Dullness to percussion sometimes found in areas of consolidation or atelectasis

(b) Assess diaphragm position and excursion to determine whether the patient is able to deep breathe when instructed

iv. Auscultation

(a) Assess for the presence of adventitious sounds

(1) Crackles from small airway collapse due to shallow breathing

(2) Rhonchi or gurgles from secretions in larger airways

(3) Wheezing indicating air flow obstruction

(b) Assess character of breath sounds

(1) Bronchial breath sounds heard with consolidation

(2) Decreased breath sounds with shallow breathing or splinting

c. Diagnostic study findings

i. Preoperative medical evaluation includes chest x-ray, ECG, sputum examination, and pulmonary function tests

(a) FEV_1, FVC, and peak expiratory flow rate (PEFR) are used to predict development of postoperative pulmonary complications

(b) Split pulmonary function studies estimate amount of pulmonary function remaining postoperatively

(c) For patients with abnormal pulmonary function studies, ABG analysis is performed preoperatively. The presence of hypoxemia or CO_2 retention at baseline levels indicates that postoperative ABG levels should be followed closely

(d) Other diagnostic tests may be ordered preoperatively, depending on preexisting pulmonary or cardiac disease. These include:

(1) Cardiac stress test and possible cardiac catheterization if the stress test is positive

(2) CT scan of the chest

(3) $\dot{V}/\dot{Q}$ scan

4. **Nursing diagnoses** (see Commonly Encountered Nursing Diagnoses)

a. Ineffective airway clearance

i. Additional nursing interventions

(a) Preoperatively

(1) Encourage cessation of smoking at least 48 hours before surgery. If surgery can be postponed or is elective, 4 to 6 weeks' cessation prior to surgery may be indicated

(2) Administer bronchodilators as ordered to patients with COPD

(3) Instruct the patient in deep breathing, coughing techniques, ambulation, activity exercises, and active and passive range of motion

(4) Familiarize the patient with respiratory therapy equipment and techniques, such as incentive spirometry, chest physiotherapy, and a monitored postoperative exercise program

(b) Postoperatively

(1) Early ambulation and leg exercises

(2) Chest and abdominal incision support during coughing

(3) Chest physiotherapy and postural drainage

(4) Deep breathing exercises

b. Ineffective breathing pattern related to incisional pain

i. Additional nursing interventions

(a) Administer analgesics as needed, and closely monitor breathing pattern for hypoventilation or splinting

(b) Teach deep-breathing exercises or incentive spirometry

c. Impaired gas exchange

   i. Additional nursing interventions

     (a) Monitor ABGs; notify physician immediately if Pao_2 drops or if $Paco_2$ rises

     (b) Be prepared for the possibility of endotracheal intubation and mechanical ventilation and PEEP

Acute Pulmonary Inhalation Injuries

Inhalation injuries include smoke inhalation, thermal burns, and carbon monoxide poisoning

1. **Pathophysiology**

a. Displacement of oxygen from the environment and inhalation of noxious agents and asphyxiant gases

   i. Effects range from mild irritation of the eyes, throat, and upper respiratory tract to fatal respiratory failure

   ii. Toxic exposure causes irritation and edema of mucous membranes, inflammatory capillary damage, bronchospasm, pulmonary edema (may be delayed up to 24 hours after exposure), and hypoxia

b. Thermal injury to lung tissues produces mucosal sloughing, bronchorrhea, and pulmonary edema

c. Systemic absorption of carbon monoxide or other chemical asphyxiant

   i. Carbon monoxide toxicity is related to dose, duration, alveolar ventilation (activity, cardiac output), and preexisting cardiovascular disease

   ii. Carbon monoxide is normally attached to hemoglobin (COHb) at levels of about 1% but has an affinity for the Hb molecule, which is 200 to 250 times that of O_2. Small amounts of inspired carbon monoxide have major effects on the O_2-carrying capacity of blood and cause severe tissue hypoxia. Elimination of carbon monoxide is via the lungs only

2. **Etiologic or precipitating factors**

a. Exposure to smoke or toxic gases

b. Closed-space injury

c. Prolonged exposure

d. Unconsciousness

e. Preexisting respiratory or cardiovascular disease

f. Solubility of gas

3. **Nursing assessment data base**

a. Nursing history

   i. Subjective findings: patient's chief complaint varies with the type of inhalation. Headache is often seen with carbon monoxide inhalation; cough, wheezing and dyspnea are seen with inhalation of smoke and other noxious agents

   ii. Objective findings

     (a) Etiologic or precipitating factors: determine the presence of one or more of above factors. A careful detailed description of events leading up to and during pulmonary inhalation injury is essential

(b) Social history: assess living conditions, exposure to household product or equipment fumes, if applicable; occupational inhalation exposures; smoking history; recent alcohol or drug use; history of depression or previous suicide attempts

(c) Medication history: determine all prescription and over-the-counter medications, doses and schedules; assess for overdose or missed doses, especially in medications that influence level of consciousness (sedatives)

b. Nursing examination of patient

  i. Inspection

    (a) Observe for facial burns, singed nares, sooty tongue, and pharyngeal and oral blistering (signs of severe exposure)

    (b) Inspect for edema of the lips and face

    (c) Observe for depressed mentation

    (d) Observe for cyanosis

    (e) Observe for cherry-red color to the skin for carbon monoxide poisoning (a rare, late finding)

    (f) Assess work of breathing; use of accessory muscles of respiration

    (g) Assess respiratory patterns—tachypnea

    (h) Observe for dizziness, headache, weakness, nausea and vomiting, diminished visual acuity

  ii. Palpation: assess chest expansion; rapid shallow breathing is due to low compliance of the lungs

  iii. Auscultation: diffuse adventitious sounds are heard bilaterally: wheezes, crackles, and rhonchi

c. Diagnostic findings

  i. Serial carboxyhemoglobin analysis for carbon monoxide poisoning. Healthy nonsmoking individuals have a carboxyhemoglobin level of less than 2%, whereas smokers may have a level of 5% to 10%. Severe carbon monoxide poisoning is present when levels are higher than 20% to 40%. Levels above 60% are associated with coma and death

  ii. Serial ABG analysis

    (a) Carbon monoxide poisoning does not cause a decrease in measured PaO_2 but does impair the O_2-carrying capacity of Hb. Directly measured arterial O_2 saturation (SaO_2) is markedly reduced

    (b) Hypoxemia in thermal injury and toxic exposure with widened A–a gradient or decreased PaO_2/FIO_2 ratio

  iii. Chest radiograph studies

    (a) No change in carbon monoxide inhalation

    (b) Diffuse pulmonary edema in thermal injury and toxic inhalation

  iv. ECG studies: tachycardia, ST segment changes, conduction blocks, atrial or ventricular arrhythmias

  v. Fiberoptic bronchoscopy: performed to rule out and assess life-threatening upper airway injury

4. Nursing diagnoses (see Commonly Encountered Nursing Diagnoses)

a. Ineffective airway clearance

  i. Additional nursing interventions: observe for signs of vocal cord edema and stridor

b. Impaired gas exchange

  i. Additional nursing interventions

(a) Humidified 100% O_2 administration by tight-fitting mask or endotracheal tube for carbon monoxide poisoning to shorten the half-life of carboxyhemoglobin

(b) Hyperbaric oxygenation for carbon monoxide poisoning if the patient presents with neurologic signs or symptoms, ECG changes consistent with ischemia, severe metabolic acidosis, pulmonary edema, or shock. Transfer to a facility should occur only after the patient is stabilized

(c) Observation of carbon monoxide poisoning victim for cognitive, memory, visual, and personality changes

Neoplastic Lung Disease

1. **Pathophysiology:** almost all lung cancers fall within one of four histologic categories: squamous cell carcinoma, small cell carcinoma, adenocarcinoma, and large cell carcinoma. In addition to these, two other forms of neoplastic lung disease are discussed: bronchial carcinoids and malignant mesothelioma

   a. Squamous cell carcinoma: constitutes approximately one third of all bronchogenic carcinomas. These tumors originate in the epithelial layer of the bronchial wall. A series of progressive histologic abnormalities results from chronic or repetitive cigarette smoke-induced injury

   i. Initially, there is metaplasia of the normal bronchial columnar epithelial cells, which are replaced by squamous epithelial cells

   ii. Squamous cells become more atypical until a well-localized carcinoma (carcinoma in situ) develops

   iii. These cells tend to be located in relatively large or proximal airways, most commonly at the subsegmental, segmental, or lobar level. With growth of tumor into the bronchial lumen, the airway may become obstructed and the lung distal to the obstruction frequently becomes atelectatic and may develop a postobstructive pneumonia

   iv. Sometimes a cavity develops within the tumor mass; cavitation is much more common with squamous cell than with other types of bronchogenic carcinoma

   v. Spread beyond the airway usually involves:

      (a) Direct extension to the pulmonary parenchyma or to other neighboring structures

      (b) Invasion of lymphatics, with spread to local lymph nodes in the hilum or mediastinum

   vi. Squamous cell tumors tend to remain within the thorax and to cause problems by intrathoracic complications rather than by distant metastasis. The overall prognosis for 5-year survival is better for patients with squamous cell carcinoma than for patients with any of the other cell types

   b. Small cell carcinoma: comprises about 20% of all lung cancers and consists of several subtypes. These tumors generally originate within the bronchial wall, most commonly at a proximal level

   i. Oat cell carcinoma, the most common subtype, shows a submucosal growth pattern, but the tumor quickly invades lymphatics and submucosal blood vessels. Hilar and mediastinal nodes are involved early in the course of the disease and are frequently the most prominent aspect of the radiographic presentation

      ii. Metastatic spread to distant sites is a common early complication; common sites are brain, liver, bone (and bone marrow), and adrenal glands

     iii. This propensity for early metastatic involvement gives small cell carcinoma the worst prognosis among the four major categories of bronchogenic carcinoma

  c. Adenocarcinoma: accounts for more than one third of all lung tumors, with the majority occurring in the periphery of the lung

      i. The characteristic appearance is the tendency to form glands and to produce mucus

     ii. Usually presents as a peripheral lung nodule or mass. Occasionally, tumors can arise within a relatively large bronchus and therefore may present with complications of localized bronchial obstruction

    iii. May spread locally to adjacent regions of the lung, to pleura, or to the hilar or mediastinal lymph nodes; may metastasize to distant sites: liver, bone, CNS, and adrenal glands. In contrast to small cell carcinoma, it is more likely to be localized at the time of presentation

    iv. Overall prognosis is intermediate between that of squamous cell and small cell carcinoma

  d. Large cell carcinoma: accounts for 15% to 20% of all lung cancers. Is defined by the characteristics that they lack (i.e., the specific features that would otherwise classify them as one of the other three cell types). It is difficult to pinpoint the cells of origin from which these tumors arise

      i. Behavior: similar to that of adenocarcinoma

     ii. Found in the periphery of the lungs, although it tends to be somewhat larger than adenocarcinoma

    iii. Tumor spread and prognosis are the same as with adenocarcinoma

  e. Bronchial carcinoid: viewed as a low-grade malignancy that constitutes approximately 5% of primary lung tumors

      i. Arise in relatively central airways of the tracheobronchial tree from the neurosecretory Kulchitsky cells (K cells).

     ii. In some carcinoid tumors, the histology has more atypical features suggestive of frank malignancy; the overall prognosis for these tumors is poorer than for those without such features

    iii. Patients with bronchial carcinoids are younger than patients with other pulmonary malignancies

    iv. Treatment is surgical resection, if possible, with an excellent prognosis; however, in patients with atypical histology, metastatic disease is commonly found and the prognosis is worse

  f. Malignant mesothelioma

      i. Involves the pleura rather than the airways or pulmonary parenchyma.

     ii. Eventually traps the lung and spreads to mediastinal structures

    iii. No clearly effective form of therapy is available, and fewer than 10% of patients survive 3 years

2. Etiologic or precipitating factors

  a. Smoking is the single most important risk factor for development of carcinoma of the lung. The duration of the smoking history, the number of cigarettes smoked per day, the depth of inhalation, and the amount of each cigarette smoked all correlate with the risk for lung cancer. Each of the four major categories of carcinoma is associated with cigarette smoking; however, the statistical association between smoking and the individual cell types is greatest for squamous cell and small cell carcinomas, which are seen almost exclusively in smokers. Even though smoking increases the risk for adenocarcinoma and large cell carcinoma, these cell types are also observed in nonsmokers. In addition, smoking does not appear to be a risk factor for bronchial carcinoids and malignant mesothelioma

b. Occupational factors

    i. Asbestos, a fibrous silicate used because of its properties of fire resistance and thermal insulation, is the most widely studied of the environmental or occupationally related carcinogens. Carcinoma of the lung is the most likely malignancy to complicate asbestos exposure, although other tumors, especially mesothelioma, are strongly associated with prior asbestos exposure. The risk for development of lung cancer is particularly high in a smoker exposed to asbestos, in which case the two risk factors have a multiplicative effect. There is a long time lapse (> 20 years) after exposure before the tumor becomes apparent

    ii. Other occupational exposures have been implicated in the subsequent development of lung cancer. As with asbestos, there is usually a long latent period of at least two decades from time of exposure until presentation of the tumor. Examples include:

        (a) Arsenic: manufacture of pesticides, glass, pigments, and paints

        (b) Ionizing radiation: uranium miners, gamma radiation, x-rays

        (c) Haloethers: chemical industry workers

        (d) Polycyclic aromatic hydrocarbons: mineral oils, soots, coal tar, and foundry workers

        (e) Synthetic mineral fibers: rock wool or slag wool

        (f) Diesel exhaust

        (g) Crystalline silica

c. Radon decay products

    i. Radon gas is a decay product of naturally occurring uranium in the earth.

    ii. Radon decay products may cause bronchogenic carcinoma or may contribute to cancer risk only when they are inhaled into the respiratory system and interact with pulmonary epithelial or other cells

d. Diet

    i. A number of epidemiologic studies have convincingly shown a relation between greater dietary intake of vegetables and modestly lower risk for lung and other cancers

    ii. Low dietary intake of fruits and vegetables without beta-carotene is associated with increased lung cancer risk

    iii. A low serum level of beta-carotene is associated with risk of later development of lung cancer

e. Nonmodifiable risk factors: gender, race, inherited predisposition

3. **Nursing assessment data base**

a. Nursing history

    i. Subjective findings

        (a) Patient's chief complaint: cough and hemoptysis are the most common symptoms in the patient with lung cancer

        (b) Other symptoms vary, depending on region of tumor involvement

(1) Dyspnea secondary to obstructed bronchus or large pleural effusion

(2) Chest pain from pleural involvement

(3) Dysphagia from tumor involvement of adjacent esophagus

(4) Hoarseness from vocal cord paralysis

(5) Edema of the face and upper extremities from superior vena cava obstruction

(6) Nonspecific symptoms: anorexia and weight loss

  ii. Objective findings

(a) Etiologic or precipitating factors: assess for presence of one or more of the above factors

(b) Family history: although there may be unidentified genetic factors that affect one's susceptibility to environmental carcinogens, there is no clear evidence that a familial tendency exists

(c) Social history: carefully question client regarding all previous occupational exposures, duration of time exposed, and any protective devices used. Assess smoking history, and calculate the number of pack-years.

(d) Medication history: document all prescription and over-the-counter medications taken

b. Nursing examination of the patient

  i. Inspection

(a) Observe for overall nutritional status, weight loss, and wasting

(b) Assess work of breathing and use of accessory muscles of breathing

(c) Assess respiratory patterns: tachypnea

(d) Observe for edema of the face and upper extremities

  ii. Palpation

(a) Evaluate chest expansion: may be decreased on the affected side

(b) Assess vocal fremitus

(1) May be increased if a patent bronchus leads to parenchymal tumor or area of pneumonia

(2) Is absent over the area of pleural involvement

  iii. Percussion

(a) Dullness heard over large tumor near the chest wall or pleural mass

(b) Elevated diaphragm sometimes detected in patients with diaphragmatic paralysis

  iv. Auscultation

(a) Bronchial breath sounds over an area of large tumor or postobstructive pneumonia

(b) Decreased to absent breath sounds with pleural effusion or tumor

c. Diagnostic study findings

  i. Radiologic evaluation

(a) Chest x-ray: may reveal a nodule or mass within the lung, involvement of hilar or mediastinal nodes, or pleural involvement

(b) CT and MRI: help to define the location, extent, and spread of tumor within the chest; can also reveal information about the densities of the lesions

  ii. Bronchoscopy: allows direct examination of the airways

intrabronchially and sampling from the lesion for later cytologic
evaluation
- (a) Forceps biopsy specimens can be used for both histologic and
cytologic analysis
- (b) Bronchial washings are used extensively in the diagnosis of
bronchogenic carcinoma. The usefulness of this technique is
controversial.
- (c) Bronchial brushings for cytologic analysis is an effective diagnostic
procedure, especially when used in combination with forceps
biopsy
- (d) Transbronchial needle aspiration can be useful in the diagnosis of
tumor presenting as submucosal lesion or as a mass that
compresses the bronchial lumen extrinsically. Patients with
necrotic lesions or lesions from which significant bleeding is
anticipated are candidates for this technique

iii. Mediastinoscopy: necessary for staging of lung cancer if the CT scan is
not diagnostic for lymph node involvement

iv. Microscopic examination: cytologic examination can be performed on
sputum, washings, or brushings obtained through the bronchoscope
or on material aspirated from the tumor with a small-gauge needle

v. Staging of lung cancer is based on:
- (a) Size, location, and local complications, such as direct extensions
to adjacent structures or obstruction of the airway lumen
- (b) Mediastinal lymph node involvement
- (c) Distant metastasis

4. **Nursing diagnoses** (see Commonly Encountered Nursing Diagnoses)
   a. Ineffective airway clearance related to postobstructive pneumonia
      i. Additional nursing interventions
         - (a) Suction the patient only if secretions are reachable by catheter
           and the patient is unable to cough; consider chest physical
           therapy
         - (b) Administer antibiotics as ordered, and monitor clinical response
   b. Ineffective breathing pattern related to tumor progression or thoracotomy
      (See nursing diagnoses under Pulmonary Problems in Surgical Patients)
   c. Impaired gas exchange related to altered O_2 supply
   d. Ineffective individual and family coping
      i. Additional nursing interventions
         - (a) Collaborate with social workers in getting another patient with a
           similar diagnosis who has successfully coped with the same
           situation to visit the patient to provide encouragement
         - (b) Provide a referral to hospice care or a similar organization, if
           appropriate

Obstructive Sleep Apnea

1. **Pathophysiology**
   a. Airway obstruction may occur in the upper or lower airways. Acute upper
   airway obstruction is usually due to foreign bodies or trauma. A more
   common and chronic type of upper airway obstruction is obstructive sleep
   apnea. Epidemiologic studies estimate that the condition affects 2% to 4%

of middle-aged adults. *Apnea* is defined as cessation of airflow for more than 10 seconds. *Sleep apnea* is defined as repeated episodes of obstructive apnea and hypopnea during sleep together with daytime sleepiness or altered cardiopulmonary function

b. Upper airway dysfunction and the specific sites of narrowing or closure are influenced by the underlying neuromuscular tone, upper airway muscle synchrony, and the stage of sleep

  i. These events are most prominent during rapid eye movement (REM) sleep secondary to hypotonia of upper airway muscles characteristic of this stage of sleep

  ii. The definitive event in obstructive sleep apnea is posterior movement of the tongue and palate into apposition with the posterior pharyngeal wall, resulting in occlusion of the nasopharynx and oropharynx

  iii. Following the obstruction and resultant apnea, progressive asphyxia develops until there is a brief arousal from sleep, restoration of upper airway patency, and resumption of airflow. The patient quickly returns to sleep, only to experience the sequence of events over and over again

  iv. Patients with sleep apnea are at increased risk for diurnal hypertension, pulmonary hypertension, nocturnal dysrhythmias, right and left ventricular failure, myocardial infarction, and stroke

  v. Hypoxemia, hypercapnia, polycythemia, and cor pulmonale may complicate the late stages of the disease

2. **Etiologic or precipitating factors**

  a. Obesity: increased upper body obesity, reflected by neck circumference, is often characteristic of sleep apnea

  b. Nasal obstruction

  c. Adenoidal or tonsillar hypertrophy (seen in children)

  d. Micrognathia, retrognathia, macroglossia

  e. Vocal cord paralysis

  f. Genetically determined craniofacial features or abnormalities of ventilatory control (CNS) may account for why sleep apnea is common to some families

3. **Nursing assessment data base**

  a. Nursing history

  i. Subjective findings

    (a) Patient's chief complaint: excessive daytime sleepiness

    (b) Other symptoms

      (1) Personality changes or cognitive difficulties related to fatigue

      (2) Automobile or work-related accidents due to fatigue

      (3) Chronic loud snoring

      (4) Morning headaches

      (5) Loss of libido

  ii. Objective findings

    (a) Etiologic or precipitating factors: determine the presence of one or more factors

    (b) Family history: determine whether there is a known history of other family members with documented sleep apnea

    (c) Social history: confirm with family members if patient has snoring, gasping, or choking episodes during sleep or periods when they suspected or witnessed an apnea event (i.e., sleep habits)

(d) Medication history
   (1) Assess all medications taken, doses, and schedules
   (2) Determine whether there is a lack of patient compliance with medicines; the physiologic result of inadequate or excessive medication can influence level of consciousness or may contribute to daytime sleepiness or injury during operation of machinery or a motor vehicle
b. Nursing examination of the patient
   i. Inspection
      (a) Observe for obesity, especially nuchal obesity (neck size ≥ 17 inches in a male, ≥ 16 inches in a female)
      (b) Observe work of breathing, use of accessory muscles; and intercostal retractions
      (c) Observe for signs of hypoxemia (e.g., duskiness or cyanosis, mental status changes)
      (d) Assess for the patient's ability to concentrate and stay awake during routine conversation
      (e) Perform a visual inspection of the nose and throat to assess for infection or blockage; more formal ear-nose-throat (ENT) assessment may be necessary
   ii. Palpation: assess for nasal sinus tenderness as part of evaluation of nasal obstruction caused by sinusitis or other process
   iii. Auscultation
      (a) Assess for upper airway stridor by placing a stethoscope over the trachea
      (b) Wheezing heard with aspiration of solid object creating narrowing of the airway lumen
      (c) Coarse gurgles or rhonchi from secretions in upper airways
      (d) Decreased or absent breath sounds with occluded bronchus
c. Diagnostic study findings
   i. Polysomnography (sleep study)
      (a) A sleep laboratory is the optimum test location for an overnight stay
      (b) Sleep staging, air flow and ventilatory effort, arterial O_2 saturation, ECG, body position, and periodic limb movements are evaluated
   ii. Home evaluation and testing
      (a) Pulse oximetry, portable (home) monitoring of cardiopulmonary channels, such as air flow, ventilatory effort, and heart rate
      (b) Sensitivity and specificity of pulse oximetry alone for diagnosis of sleep apnea is controversial
   iii. ABG analysis alone is not diagnostic of sleep apnea but is performed as part of the diagnostic workup to determine the degree of ventilation and oxygenation impairment at baseline
   iv. Pulmonary function studies may be performed to exclude or confirm concomitant intrinsic lung disease, such as obstructive or restrictive lung disease
4. **Nursing diagnoses**
   a. Ineffective airway clearance related to upper airway obstruction
      i. Additional nursing interventions
         (a) Instruction on modifications of behavioral factors that may contribute to obstructive sleep apnea

        (1) Weight loss (include exercise plan)

        (2) Avoidance of alcohol and sedatives before sleep

        (3) Avoidance of supine sleep position

    (b) Apply nasal CPAP as ordered

        (1) Instruct on proper use and maintenance of equipment

        (2) Teach skin care surrounding the nose area where the mask is applied

        (3) Assess for intolerance to nasal CPAP machine noise and airway pressure

    (c) Instruct on proper care of oral or dental devices if used; side effects include excessive salivation and temporomandibular joint (TMJ) discomfort

    (d) Postoperative monitoring and instruction following surgical treatment or correction for sleep apnea if indicated

    (e) Preoperative and postoperative teaching for patients requiring tracheostomy

        (1) If the neck is thick, decannulation process may be difficult

        (2) Repeat the sleep study or nocturnal oximetry following tracheostomy tube placement, as the patient may still hypoventilate secondary to central sleep apnea or intrinsic lung disease

        (3) Provide tracheostomy tube and stoma care instruction for the patient and family

  b. Ineffective breathing pattern related to upper airway obstruction

  c. Impaired gas exchange related to altered O_2 supply

End-Stage Pulmonary Conditions Eligible for Lung Transplantation

The transplantation of one or both lungs as a treatment for end-stage pulmonary failure has become a commonly accepted practice. Since the initial clinical success of the first single lung transplant in 1983, there have been many clinical advances in a number of areas related to lung transplantation. These include patient and donor selection, operative technique, immunosuppression, and living related lobe transplantation. The number of transplants performed annually and the number of centers performing lung transplants have continued to increase and have broadened the spectrum of diseases treated with lung transplantation.

1. **Pathophysiology:** specific pathophysiologic mechanisms responsible for end-stage pulmonary disease depend on underlying etiologic factors (see next)

2. **Etiologic or precipitating factors:** pulmonary transplantation is appropriate for patients with irreversible, progressively disabling, end-stage pulmonary disease whose life expectancy is projected to be less than 18 months despite the use of appropriate medical or alternative surgical therapies. These include patients with:

  a. Emphysema including alpha 1-antitrypsin deficiency

    i. Patients with COPD and an FEV_1 less than 20% to 25% of predicted, hypercarbia ($PaCO_2$ greater than 50 mm Hg), or a mean pulmonary artery pressure without O_2 greater than 30 mm Hg have a 2-year survival rate of less than 70%

    ii. Usually, patients who receive a transplant have an FEV_1 less than 20% of that predicted

b. Cystic fibrosis
   i. Patients with cystic fibrosis who have an FEV_1 less than 30% of that predicted, a PaO_2 less than 55 mm Hg, or a $PaCO_2$ greater than 50 mm Hg have a 2-year survival rate of approximately 70%
   ii. Women and younger patients with cystic fibrosis have worse survival than men or older patients and should be considered for transplant earlier
c. Pulmonary hypertension (primary and secondary): patients with a mean pulmonary artery pressure greater than 45 mm Hg
d. Idiopathic pulmonary fibrosis or interstitial lung disease
   i. Patients tend to have the highest mortality while awaiting a transplant
   ii. Often these patients have an FEV_1 and FVC less than 50% of that predicted
e. Obliterative bronchiolitis
f. Eosinophilic granuloma
g. Lymphangioleiomyomatosis
h. Sarcoidosis
i. Bronchiectasis
j. Selection criteria for lung transplant recipients
   i. Age equal to or less than 65 years for a single lung transplant
   ii. Age less than 60 years for a bilateral lung transplant
   iii. No other underlying systemic disease such as
      (a) Significant renal or hepatic insufficiency
      (b) Neoplastic disease
   iv. Demonstrated compliance with medical regimens
   v. No evidence of serious psychiatric illness such as
      (a) Functional psychosis or organic brain disease
      (b) Major depression
      (c) Severe characterologic disturbances with a history of self-destructive acts (alcohol, drug abuse)
   vi. No contraindication to immunosuppression
   vii. Abstinence from tobacco longer than 6 months
   viii. No extrapulmonary site of infection
   ix. Ambulatory with rehabilitation potential with O_2 as required
   x. Significant coronary artery disease
3. **Nursing assessment data base**
   a. Nursing history
      i. Subjective findings
         (a) Patient's chief complaint: varies, depending on type of underlying respiratory disorder and degree of disability
         (b) Virtually all patients at the initial screening or clinic visit have some degree of dyspnea and shortness of breath, either at rest or on minimal exertion
      ii. Objective findings
         (a) Etiologic or precipitating factors: identify the presence of one or more factors leading patients to seek information on lung transplantation because of their disease process
         (b) Social history
            (1) Discussion between patient and family with transplant team members about transplant process and opportunity to explore options, ask questions, and voice concerns

        (2) Determination by patient whether or not to proceed with formal evaluation

        (3) Formal evaluation performed on either an inpatient or outpatient basis, depending on degree of pulmonary impairment

b. Nursing examination of the patient

   i. Complete physical examination of the patient utilizes the physical assessment techniques of inspection, palpation, percussion, and auscultation

   ii. Physical findings vary widely, depending on the underlying pulmonary condition and the degree to which pulmonary function is impaired

c. Diagnostic study findings

   i. Pulmonary studies

      (a) Complete pulmonary function studies include:

        (1) Spirometry (includes prebronchodilator and postbronchodilator studies if obstruction is present)

        (2) Lung volumes using nitrogen washout and plethysmography

        (3) Diffusion capacity of carbon monoxide (DLCO)

        (4) Room air ABGs

   ii. Cardiovascular studies

      (a) Echocardiogram with pulse Doppler imaging

      (b) ECG

      (c) Cardiac catheterization except in patients without history of smoking and less than 35 years of age (then only in right side of heart)

   iii. Radiology

      (a) Quantitative $\dot{V}/\dot{Q}$ scan

      (b) Chest radiograph, posteroanterior and lateral

      (c) High-resolution CT of chest (if indicated)

   iv. Infectious disease

      (a) Skin tests: purified protein derivative (PPD), mumps, *Candida*

   v. Other laboratory studies

      (a) Serology: cytomegalovirus (CMV) titer, varicella-zoster (VZ) titer, herpes simplex (HS) titer, Epstein-Barr (EBV) titer

      (b) HIV antigen-antibody, hepatitis screen, blood type and cross-match

      (c) Serum electrolytes, CBC with differential, PT, partial thromboplastin time, platelet count, creatinine clearance, liver function tests, nutritional markers (albumin, total protein), urinalysis

      (d) Thyroid and endocrine function tests, such as thyroid-stimulating hormone (TSH)

   vi. Psychosocial evaluation

   vii. Nutritional assessment

   viii. Assessment of other medical conditions

   ix. Rehabilitation assessment for potential lung transplant candidates (types of tests ordered vary, depending on center)

      (a) Endurance exercise test

      (b) Six-minute walk

      (c) Stair-climbing test

      (d) Treadmill test

        (e) Musculoskeletal assessment

        (f) Chest physiotherapy assessment

        (g) O$_2$ therapy needs

4. Nursing diagnoses

  a. Knowledge deficit about lung transplantation and preoperative and postoperative care

    i. Assessment for defining characteristics

      (a) Patient is unable to describe transplant waiting list procedure

      (b) Patient is unable to describe responsibilities during preoperative preparation

      (c) Patient is unable to anticipate the postoperative recovery responsibilities following transplantation

      (d) Patient and support person or family are unable to describe postdischarge medical care routine as well as anticipated lifestyle changes

    ii. Expected outcomes

      (a) Patient and support person or family understand the particular stresses related to the preoperative waiting phase

      (b) Patient and support person or family are familiar with the proper use and response to a personal beeper they are required to have at all times

      (c) Patient and support person or family understand when to call or notify the transplant team regarding new problems or concerns

      (d) Patient and support person or family understand the operative procedure and the postoperative recovery

    iii. Nursing interventions

      (a) Prepare the patient and support person or family for the preoperative evaluation and waiting period

        (1) Relocation to transplant center for lung transplant

          a) Living arrangements

          b) Support group

          c) Consent forms signed with the surgeon

          d) Medical follow-up and ongoing care while transplantation is awaited

      (b) Conduct preoperative education to patient and support person or family concerning rationale for the preoperative tests, responsibilities of patient while awaiting transplant, operative procedure, and expected postoperative course including activity and medication regimen

        (1) Familiarization with organization or program

          a) Placement on national computerized waiting list

          b) Donor availability, selection, and preparation

          c) Donor-recipient matching for ABO compatibility and size

        (2) Use of beepers for coordination of transplant

          a) Gather information regarding available donor

          b) Notify retrieval team and patient

        (3) Role of transplant nurse coordinator and when to call

        (4) Operative procedures and pre-transplant post-transplant care, including anticipated hospital length of stay

          a) Surgical and anesthetic preparation

          b) Surgical technique

    c) Length of stay in operating room
    d) ICU stay
   (5) Pre-transplant rehabilitation program for conditioning
    a) Goals and expected outcomes
    b) Exercise prescription or O_2 therapy
    c) Intensive supervision and monitoring (i.e., SpO_2)
  (c) Daily self-assessment by patient to report early changes in medical and pulmonary condition
   (1) Progression of endurance training
   (2) Periodic reevaluation of exercise tolerance
 iv. Evaluation of nursing care
  (a) Patient is well informed of transplant program and responsibilities
  (b) Patient is active participant in pulmonary rehabilitation program while awaiting transplantation
b. Potential for postoperative complications following lung transplantation
 i. Assessment for defining charactersitics
  (a) Postoperative bleeding
  (b) Hemodynamic instability (decreased cardiac output, blood pressure)
  (c) Cardiac arrhythmias
  (d) Fluid and electrolyte imbalance
  (e) Hypoxemia
  (f) Infection and lung rejection
  (g) Barotrauma and damage to the airway anastomosis secondary to mechanical ventilation with positive airway pressure and/or ischemia
  (h) Nutritional depletion and gastrointestinal disturbances
  (i) Thoracotomy pain
  (j) Secretion management
 ii. Expected outcomes
  (a) Patient maintains acceptable cardiac output and blood pressures
  (b) Patient maintains homeostatic fluid and electrolyte balance
  (c) Patient is successfully removed from the ventilator postoperatively
  (d) Patient remains free of infection and signs of lung rejection
  (e) Energy and activity level are improved postoperatively
  (f) Pain is well controlled
  (g) There is no significant air leak from chest tubes
  (h) Patient and support person or family demonstrate a good understanding of the plan of care and ICU routine
  (i) ABGs and respiratory mechanics are within normal limits
  (j) Patient demonstrates proper administration of medications and verbalizes side effects
 iii. Nursing interventions
  (a) Monitor systemic and pulmonary arterial (PA) pressures
  (b) Perform hemodynamic profiles as ordered or routinely if the PA catheter is in place
   (1) Identify and correct low cardiac output state if present
   (2) Measure cardiac output, cardiac index (CI), stroke volume (SV), systemic vascular resistance (SVR), and pulmonary vascular resistance (PVR)

   (3) Continuous mixed venous O_2 saturation monitoring to assess relationships between O_2 delivery and uptake
   (4) Titrate vasoactive drugs as necessary
(c) Monitor the ECG for cardiac arrhythmias both at rest and during exercise telemetry postoperatively
(d) Monitor fluid status with particular attention to avoiding volume overload
   (1) Measure urine output (UO) and maintain above 30 cc/hour
   (2) Supply diuretics as indicated
   (3) Monitor blood urea nitrogen (BUN) and serum creatine
(e) Monitor for electrolyte imbalances
(f) Monitor for intrathoracic and/or intra-abdominal bleeding postoperatively
   (1) Assess pleural and mediastinal chest tubes, appropriate suction level as ordered, note color and consistency of drainage, calculate volume and rate of drainage output
   (2) Assess abdomen for distention and tenderness, volume, and consistency of nasogastric drainage
   (3) Transfuse as ordered using Leukopor filters and CMV-negative blood products; autotransfusion set-ups must be routinely available to allow quick response to blood loss
(g) Assess patient's ventilatory and oxygenation status
   (1) Monitor patient's response to mechanical ventilation/O_2 therapy
      a) Observe and record trends in the patient's peak and mean inspiratory airway pressure
      b) Observe and record changes in exhaled tidal volume return compared with preset inspired tidal volume
      c) If a pleural chest tube is present, note absence of air bubbling in the water seal chamber
      d) Monitor the patient's breathing effort and synchrony with the ventilator
      e) Assess and maintain proper location and security of endotracheal tube
   (2) Weaning from mechanical ventilation
      a) Measure vital capacity and negative inspiratory force daily
      b) Ventilator discontinuance; monitor for respiratory muscle fatigue and distress during weaning efforts and after extubation
   (3) Assess pulmonary function: a/A ratio, A–a gradient, ABGs, end-tidal CO_2 monitoring, pulse oximetry; hypoxemia may indicate fluid volume overload, lung infection, or lung rejection
   (4) Assist with bronchoscopy as indicated
   (5) Monitor chest radiographic changes
   (6) Provide pulmonary hygiene, positioning and chest physiotherapy, inhaled bronchodilator treatment as ordered, suctioning based on need
(h) Monitor for infection or rejection in the transplanted lung
   (1) Administer immunosuppression agents as indicated
   (2) Monitor donor and recipient bronchoscopy cultures

      (3) Administer antimicrobial therapy

      (4) Maintain proper isolation procedures

      (5) Observe for clinical and diagnostic signs and symptoms of infection or rejection

          a) Fever, fatigue, decreased exercise tolerance

          b) Chest x-ray changes, increase in respiratory secretions, SpO_2 decreases, $\dot{V}/\dot{Q}$ scan changes, reduced pulmonary function studies

          c) Results of surveillance bronchoscopy (i.e., bronchoalveolar lavage [BAL])

          d) Airway dehiscence

          e) Poor or delayed wound healing, purulent drainage

(i) Perform nutritional assessment to prevent nutritional depletion and complications

      (1) Administer enteral feedings when the gastrointestinal system is intact and the patient is unable to take food by mouth; advance the diet as tolerated

          a) Monitor for aspiration during tube feeding

          b) Match caloric intake with individual nutritional requirements

      (2) Administer TPN when the gastrointestinal tract is not available or nonfunctional

          a) Avoid excessive carbohydrates in order to limit CO_2 production and respiratory workload

          b) Avoid excessive fluids, particularly in patients with renal insufficiency

          c) Consider performing indirect calorimetry to more accurately determine metabolic energy requirements

          d) Maintain sterile technique when caring for venous access devices

(j) Provide adequate thoracotomy pain control according to patient needs

      (1) IV or epidural pain management, patient-controlled analgesics, oral analgesics

      (2) Use care to avoid CO_2 retention

      (3) Consider pain control needs prior to exercise and chest physiotherapy sessions

      (4) Because the early postoperative phase often results in fragmented sleep, confusion, and irritability, the patient may be started on haloperidol and the dose tapered slowly through the recovery phase

(k) Encourage patient participation in inpatient rehabilitation

      (1) Participation in range-of-motion exercises in early postoperative phase (within 12 to 24 hours of surgery)

      (2) Conduct progressive resistance exercises within first 2 to 3 days after transplant surgery if cardiovascular stability is established

      (3) Begin ambulation for short distances; if mechanical ventilation is still required, patients may ambulate short distances with manual resuscitation bag for assisted ventilations

(4) After the patient leaves the ICU, ambulation progresses as rapidly as tolerated

    a) Use of a special walker may be available to hold O_2 tanks and IV pole or pumps, a urinary catheter bag, chest tubes, a portable suction device, and a pulse oximeter

    b) Weaning from O_2 therapy or to level of O_2 flow to maintain SpO_2 equal to or above 92%

    c) Have patient (if able) return to the treadmill for endurance training

        i) Conduct comprehensive education as part of discharge planning process

        ii) Teach patient benefits of participating in outpatient rehabilitation program following discharge

            [a] Progression of endurance program to home exercise program

            [b] Progression of musculoskeletal program

            [c] Improved functional ability to perform ADL

        iii) Instruct on the need for the patient to continue ongoing medical follow-up with private doctor and transplant center

            [a] Periodic pulmonary function studies and O_2 assessment

            [b] Signs and symptoms to report to health care provider

            [c] Recording of laboratory and medication dosages in log book

            [d] Home spirometry and recording in log book

        iv) Teach patient and support person or family about medication regimen

            [a] Teach self-medication administration, such as MDIs

            [b] Teach role of immunosuppression therapy in survival

            [c] Teach medication dose scheduling, monitoring for side effects, and importance of early reporting of adverse reactions to the physician or nurse

        v) Provide psychosocial support throughout the hospital stay, including discharge planning

            [a] Discuss anticipated feelings and issues related to return to independence

            [b] Acknowledge that the support person or family becomes less active

            [c] Encourage self-care activities, such as making one's own appointments and scheduling required laboratory work

            [d] Offer early involvement of hospital or transplant chaplain or pastoral services

iv. Evaluation of nursing care

    (a) Baseline level well documented prior to lung transplant

    (b) Chaplain determines need for referral to the patient's own clergy

(c) Preoperative and postoperative medications are administered appropriately and in a timely manner

(d) Postoperative teaching needs have been met

(e) Patient and support person or family anxiety levels are reduced, and a positive attitude exists toward the future

(f) Cardiac and pulmonary abnormalities are detected and treated early

(g) The transplanted lung is fully expanded bilaterally, and the chest tube is removed

(h) Pain is well controlled

(i) Pulmonary infection or lung rejection is detected and reported early

(j) Wound heals adequately without signs of infection

(k) Lungs are clear to auscultation

(l) Patient and family educational needs are met for general education, medications, exercise, log book, testing, spirometry, and diet

(m) Patient understands outpatient follow-up schedule for tests, rehabilitation, and office visits

References

PHYSIOLOGIC ANATOMY

Ahrens, T.: Changing perspectives in the assessment of oxygenation. Crit. Care Nurs. 13:78–83, 1993.

Dantzker, D. R.: Cardiopulmonary Critical Care, 2nd ed., Philadelphia, W. B. Saunders, 1991.

Epstein, C., and Henning, R.: Oxygen transport variables in the identification and treatment of tissue hypoxia. Heart Lung 22:328–345, 1993.

Guyton, A. C., and Hall, J. E.: Textbook of Medical Physiology, 9th ed. Philadelphia, W. B. Saunders, 1996.

Kacmarek R. M.: Carbon dioxide production, carriage and transport. In Pierson, D. J., and Kacmarek, R. M. (eds): Foundations of Respiratory Care. New York, Churchill Livingstone, 1992.

Misasi, R. S., and Keyes, J. L.: Matching and mismatching ventilation and perfusion in the lung. Crit. Care Nurs. 16:23–38, 1996.

Nelson, L. D.: Assessment of oxygenation: Oxygenation indices. Respir. Care 38:631–640, 1993.

NURSING ASSESSMENT DATA BASE

American Association for Respiratory Care: Clinical practice guideline: Directed cough. Respir. Care 38:495–499, 1993.

Dettenmeir, P. A.: Radiographic Assessment for Nurses. St. Louis, Mosby 1995.

Doering, L. V.: The effect of positioning on hemodynamics and gas exchange in the critically ill: A review. Am. J. Crit. Care 2:208–216, 1993.

COMMONLY ENCOUNTERED NURSING DIAGNOSES

Ackerman, M.: A review of normal saline instillation: Implications for practice. Dimens. Crit. Care Nurs. 15:31–38, 1996.

Adoumie, R., Shennib, H., Brown, R., et al.: Differential lung ventilation: Applications beyond the operating room. J Thorac Cardiovasc Surg 105:229–233, 1993.

Ahrens, T.: Respiratory monitoring in critical care. AACN Clin. Issues Crit. Care Nurs. 4:56–65, 1993.

Aloi, A., and Burns, S. M.: Continuous airway pressure monitoring in the critical care setting. Crit. Care Nurs. 15:66–74, 1995.

American Association for Respiratory Care: Clinical practice guideline: Incentive spirometry. Respir. Care 36:1402–1405, 1991.

American Association for Respiratory Care: Clinical practice guideline: Intermittent positive pressure breathing. Respir. Care 38:1189–1195, 1993.

Barker, A. F., Burgher, L. W., and Plummer, A. L.: Oxygen conserving methods for adults. Chest 105:248–252, 1994.

Branson, R. D., and MacIntyre, N. R.: Dual-control modes of mechanical ventilation. Respir. Care 41:294–305, 1996.

Burns, S. M., and Aloi, A.: Continuous Airway Pressure Monitoring. Aliso Viejo, Calif., American Association of Critical-Care Nurses, 1996.

Burns, S. M., Burns, J. E., and Truwit, J. D.: Comparison of five clinical weaning indices. Am. J. Crit. Care 3:342–352, 1994.

Burns, S. M., Fahey, S., Barton, D., et al.: Weaning from mechanical ventilation: A method for assessment and planning. AACN Clin. Issues Crit. Care Nurs. 2:372–389, 1991.

Chulay, M.: Why do we keep putting saline down endotracheal tubes? It's time for a change in the way we suction. Capsules Comments 2:7–11, 1994.

Clement, J. M., and Buck, E. A.: Weaning from mechanical ventilatory support. Dimens. Crit. Care Nurs. 15:114–129, 1996.

Connolly, M., and Shekleton, M.: Communicating with

ventilator-dependent patients. Dimens. Crit. Care Nurs. 10:115–122, 1991.

Crimlisk, J. T., Horn, M. H., Wilson, D. J., et al.: Artificial airways: A survey of cuff management practices. Heart Lung 25:225–235, 1996.

Crimlisk, J. T., Paris, R., McGonagle, E. G., et al.: The closed tracheal suction system: Implications for critical care nursing. Dimens. Crit. Care Nurs. 13:292–300, 1994.

Eisenberg, P. E.: Pulmonary complications from enteral nutrition. Crit. Care Nurs. Clin. North Am. 3:641–649, 1991.

Esteban, A., Frutos, F., Tobin, M. J., et al.: A comparison of four methods of weaning patients from mechanical ventilation. N. Engl. J. Med. 332:345–350, 1995.

Fiorentini, A.: Potential hazards of tracheobronchial suctioning. Crit. Care Nurs. 8:217–226, 1992.

Gianino, S., and St. John, R. E.: Nutritional assessment of the patient in the intensive care unit. Crit. Care Nurs. Clin. North Am. 5:1–16, 1993.

Godwin, J. E., and Heffner, J. E.: Special critical care considerations in tracheostomy management. Clin. Chest Med. 12:573–583, 1991.

Grap, M. J.: Pulse Oximetry: AACN Research Based Clinical Practice Protocols. Aliso Viejo, Calif., American Association of Critical-Care Nurses, 1996.

Heffner, J. E.: Airway management in the critically ill patient. Crit. Care Clin. 6:533–550, 1990.

Hess, D.: Noninvasive respiratory monitoring during mechanical ventilatory support. Crit. Care Nurs. Clin. North Am. 3:565–574, 1991.

Hess, D., Bigatello, L., Kacmarek, R. M., et al.: Use of inhaled nitric oxide in patients with acute respiratory distress syndrome. Respir. Care 41:424–444, 1996.

Hess, D., and Kacmarek, R. M.: Techniques and devices for monitoring oxgenation. Respir. Care 38:646–671, 1993.

Hill, L.: Peripheral electrical stimulation: Titrating neuromuscular blocking agent levels. Dimens. Crit. Care Nurs. 14:305–314, 1995.

Johnson, M. M., and Sexton, D. L.: Distress during mechanical ventilation: Patient's perceptions. Crit. Care Nurs. 10:48–57, 1990.

Kim, M. J., McFarland, G. K., and McLane, A. M.: Pocket Guide to Nursing Diagnoses, 6th ed. St. Louis, Mosby, 1995.

Knebel, A., Janson-Bjerklie, S., Malley, J., et al.: Comparison of breathing comfort during weaning with two ventilatory modes. Am. J. Respir. Crit. Care Med. 149:14–18, 1994.

Knebel, A., Shekleton, M., Burns, S., et al.: Weaning from mechanical ventilation: Concept development. Am. J. Crit. Care 3:416–420, 1994.

Krafft, P., Fridrich, P., Fitzgerald, R. D., et al.: Effectiveness of nitric oxide inhalation in septic ARDS. Chest 109:486–493, 1996.

Manthous, C. A., Hall, J. B., Caputo, M. A., et al.: Heliox improves pulsus paradoxus and peak expiratory flow in nonintubated patients with severe asthma. Am. J. Respir. Crit. Care Med. 151:310–314, 1995.

Manzano, J. L., Lubillo, S., Henriquez, D., et al.: Verbal communication of ventilator-dependent patients. Crit. Care Med. 21:512–517, 1993.

Marcy, T. W.: Barotrauma: Detection, recognition, and management. Chest 104:578–584, 1993.

Marcy, T. W., and Marini J. J.: Inverse ratio ventilation in ARDS: Rationale and implementation. Chest 100:494–504, 1991.

Marini, J. J.: Pressure-targeted, lung-protective ventilatory support in acute lung injury. Chest 105:109S–114S, 1994.

Passy, V., Prentice, W., and Darnell-Neal, R.: Passy-Muir tracheostomy speaking valve on ventilator-dependent patients. Laryngoscope 103:653–658, 1995.

Peruzzi, W. T.: The current status of PEEP. Respir. Care 41:273–281, 1996.

Pierce, J. D., Wiggens, S. A., Plaskon, C., et al.: Pressure support ventilation: Reducing the work of breathing during weaning. Dimens. Crit. Care Nurs. 12:282–290, 1993.

Pierson, D. J.: Complications associated with mechanical ventilation. Crit. Care Clin. 6:711–724, 1990.

Rappaport, S. H., Shpiner, R., Yoshihara, G., et al.: Randomized, prospective trial of pressure limited versus volume-controlled ventilation in severe respiratory failure. Crit. Care Med. 22:22–32, 1994.

Ruggles, L.: Auto-PEEP: Measurement issues and nursing interventions. Crit. Care Nurs. 15:30–38, 1995.

Shapiro, B. A., Warren, J., Egol, A. B., et al.: Practice parameters for intravenous analgesia and sedation for adult patients in the intensive care unit: An executive summary. Crit. Care Med. 23:1596–1600, 1995.

Shapiro, B. A., Warren, J., Egol, A. B., et al.: Practice parameters for sustained neuromuscular blockade in the adult critically ill patient: An executive summary. Crit. Care Med. 23:1601–1605, 1995.

Shekleton, M. E.: Respiratory muscle conditioning and the work of breathing: a critical balance in the weaning patient. AACN Clin. Issues Crit. Care Nurs. 2:405–414, 1991.

Slutusky, A. S.: ACCP consensus conference: Mechanical ventilation. Chest 104:1833–1859, 1993.

St. John, R. E.: End-Tidal CO_2 Monitoring: AACN Research Based Clinical Practice Protocols. Aliso Viejo, Calif., American Association of Critical-Care Nurses, 1996.

St. John, R. E., and Baker, K. A.: Pressure-controlled inverse ratio ventilation. Crit. Care Nurs. Clin. North Am. 3:621–627, 1991.

Tuxen, D. V.: Permissive hypercapnic ventilation. Am. J. Respir. Crit. Care Med. 150:870–874, 1994.

Weinberger, S. E., and Weiss, J. W.: Weaning from ventilatory support. N. Engl. J. Med. 332:388–389, 1995.

Wood, D. E., and Mathesen, D. J.: Late complications of tracheostomy. Clin. Chest Med. 12:597–609, 1991.

Yang, K. L., and Tobin, M. J.: A prospective study of indexes predicting the outcomes of trials of weaning from mechanical ventilation. N. Engl. J. Med. 324:1445–1450, 1991.

PATIENT HEALTH PROBLEMS

Acute Respiratory Failure

Brochard, L.: Noninvasive ventilation in acute respiratory failure. Respir. Care 41:456–465, 1996

Cole, F. J., and Shouse, B. A.: Alternative modalities of ventilation in acute respiratory failure. Surg Annu 27:55–69, 1995.

MacIntyre, N. R.: Minimizing alveolar stretch injury during mechanical ventilation. Respir. Care 41:318–326, 1996.

Pierson, D. J.: Normal and abnormal oxygenation: Physiology and clinical syndromes. Respir. Care 38:587–599, 1993.

Schuster, D. P.: A physiologic approach to initiating, maintaining, and withdrawing mechanical ventilatory support during acute respiratory failure. Am. J. Med. 88:268–278, 1990.

Adult Respiratory Distress Syndrome

Bernard, G. R., Artigas, A., Brigham, K. L., et al.: Report of the American-European consensus conference on ARDS: Definitions, mechanisms, relevant outcomes and clinical trial coordination. Intensive Care Med. 20:225–232, 1994.

Hudson, L. D., Milberg, J. A., Anardi, D., et al.: Clinical risks for the development of the acute respiratory distress syndrome. Am. J. Respir. Crit. Care Med. 151:293–301, 1995.

Kollef, M. H., and Schuster, D. P.: The acute respiratory distress syndrome. N. Engl. J. Med. 332:27–37, 1995.

Lamm, W. J. E., Graham, M. M., and Albert, R. K.: Mechanism by which the prone position improves oxygenation in acute lung injury. Am. J. Respir. Crit. Care Med. 150:184–193, 1995.

Lewis, J. F., and Jobe, A. H.: Surfactant and the adult respiratory distress syndrome. Am. Rev. Respir. Dis. 147:218–233, 1993.

Russel, J. A., and Phang, P. T.: The oxygen delivery/consumption controversy: Approaches to management of the critically ill. Am. J. Respir. Crit. Care Med. 149:533–537, 1994.

Strieter, R. M., and Kunkel, S. L.: Acute lung injury: The role of cytokines in the elicitation of neutrophils. J Intest Med 42:640–651, 1994.

Walmrath, D., Schneider, T., Schermuly, R., et al.: Direct comparison of inhaled nitric oxide and aerosolized prostacyclin in acute respiratory distress syndrome. Am. J. Respir. Crit. Care Med. 153:991–996, 1996.

Chronic Obstructive Pulmonary Disease

American Thoracic Society: Standards for the diagnosis and care of patients with chronic obstructive pulmonary disease. Am. J. Crit. Care Med. 152:S77–S120, 1995.

Gosselink, R., Troosters, T., and Decramer, M.: Peripheral muscle weakness contributes to exercise limitation in COPD. Am. J. Respir. Crit. Care Med. 153:976–980, 1996.

Asthma and Status Asthmaticus (Severe Asthmatic Attack)

Cherniack, R. M.: Physiologic diagnosis and function in asthma. Clin. Chest Med. 16:567–581, 1995.

Corbridge, T. C., and Hall, J. B.: The assessment and management of adults with status asthmaticus. Am. J. Respir. Crit. Care Med. 151:1296–1316, 1995.

Luna, C. M., Jolly, E. C., and Gene, R. J.: Acute, severe, life-threatening asthma. Clin. Pulmonary Med. 3:119–128, 1996.

Zimmerman, J. L., Dellinger, R. P., Shah, A. N., et al.: Endotracheal intubation and mechanical ventilation in severe asthma. Crit. Care Med. 21:1727–1730, 1993.

Pulmonary Embolism

Fowler, S. B.: Deep vein thrombosis and pulmonary emboli in neuroscience patients. J. Neurosci. Nurs. 27:224–228, 1995.

Roberts, S. L.: Pulmonary tissue perfusion altered: Emboli. Heart Lung 16:128–138, 1987.

Chest Trauma

Gordon, P. A., Norton, J. M., and Merrell, R.: Refining chest tube management: Analysis of the state of practice. Dimens. Crit. Care Nurs. 14:6–12, 1995.

Kovac, A. L.: Upper airway trauma and obstruction: A review of causes, evaluation, and management. Respir. Care 38:351–361, 1993.

Prentice, D., and Ahrens, T.: Pulmonary complications of trauma. Crit. Care Nurs. Q. 17:24–33, 1994.

Acute Pneumonia

American Thoracic Society: Consensus Statement: Hospital-acquired pneumonia in adults: Diagnosis, assessment of severity, initial antimicrobial therapy, and preventative strategies. Am. J. Respir. Crit. Care Med. 153:1711–1725, 1996.

Brooks, K. R., Ong, R., Spector, R. S., et al.: Acute respiratory failure due to *Pneumocystis carinii* pneumonia. Crit. Care Clin. 9:31–48, 1993.

Craven, D. E., and Steger, K. A.: Epidemiology of nosocomial pneumonia: New perspectives on an old disease. Chest 108:1S–16S, 1995.

George, D. L.: Epidemiology of nosocomial pneumonia in intensive care unit patients. Clin. Chest Med. 16:29–44, 1995.

Kollef, M. H., Shapiro, S. D., Fraser, V. J., et al.: Mechanical ventilation with or without 7-day circuit changes: A randomized controlled trial. Ann. Intern. Med. 123:168–174, 1995.

Pulmonary Aspiration

Metheny, N. E.: Minimizing respiratory complications of nasogastric tube feedings: State of the science. Heart Lung 22:213–223, 1993.

Metheny, N. E., McSweeney, M., Wehrle, M. A., et al.: Effectiveness of the auscultatory method in predicting feeding tube location. Nurs. Res. 39:262–267, 1990.

Potts, R. G., Zaroukian, M. H., Guerrero, P. A., et al.: Comparison of blue dye visualization and glucose oxidase test strip methods for detecting pulmonary aspiration of enteral feedings in intubated adults. Chest 103:117–121, 1993.

Torres, A., Serra-Batlles, J., Ros, E., et al.: Pulmonary aspiration of gastric contents in patients receiving mechanical ventilation: the effect of body position. Ann. Intern. Med. 116:540–543, 1992.

Near-Drowning

Fields, A. I.: Near-drowning in the pediatric population. Crit. Care Clin. 8:113–129, 1992.

Modell, J. H.: Drowning. N. Engl. J. Med. 328:253–256, 1993.

Quann, L.: Drowning issues in resuscitation. Ann. Emerg. Med. 22:366–369, 1993.

Wake, D.: Near drowning. Crit. Care Nurs. 11:40–43, 1995.

Pulmonary Problems in Surgical Patients

Brooks-Brunn, J. A.: Postoperative atelectasis and pneumonia. Heart Lung 24:94–115, 1995

Acute Pulmonary Inhalational Injuries

Simmons, K.: Airway care. *In* Scanlan C. L., Spearman, C. B., and Sheldon, R. L. (eds): Egan's Fundamentals of Respiratory Care, 6th ed. St. Louis, Mosby, 1995.

Neoplastic Lung Disease

Arroliga, A. C., and Matthay, R. A.: The role of bronchoscopy in lung cancer. Clin. Chest Med. 14:87–98, 1993.

Beckett, W. S.: Epidemiology and etiology of lung cancer. Clin. Chest Med. 14:1–15, 1993

Dressler, C. M., Bailey, M., Roper, C. R., et al.: Smoking cessation and lung cancer resection. Chest 110:1199–1202, 1996.

Schwartz, R. E., Marrero, A. M., Conlon, K. C., et al.: Inferior vena cava filters in cancer patients: Indications and outcomes. J. Clin. Oncol. 14:652–657, 1996.

Seale, D. D., and Beaver, B. M.: Pathophysiology of lung cancer. Nurs. Clin. North Am. 27:603–613, 1992.

Obstructive Sleep Apnea

Noureddine, S. N.: Sleep apnea: A challenge in critical care. Heart Lung 25:37–42, 1996.

Strollo, P. L., and Rogers, R. M.: Obstructive sleep apnea. N. Engl. J. Med. 334:99–104, 1996.

End-Stage Pulmonary Conditions Eligible for Lung Transplantation

Date, H., Triantafillou, A. N., Trulock, E. P., et al.: Inhaled nitric oxide reduces human lung allograft dysfunction. J. Thorac. Cardiovasc. Surg. 111:913–919, 1996.

Davis, R. D., and Pasque, M. K.: Pulmonary transplantation. Ann. Surg. 221:14–28, 1995.

Howard, D. K., Iademarco, E. J., and Trulock, E. P.: The role of cardiopulmonary exercise testing in lung and heart-lung transplantation. Clin. Chest Med. 15:405–420, 1994.

Lynch, J. P., and Trulock, E. P.: Lung transplantation in chronic airflow limitation. Med. Clin. North Am. 80:657–670, 1996.

Malen, J. F., Ochoa, L. L, Sander, M. C., et al.: Lung transplantation. Crit. Care Nurs. Clin. North Am. 4:111–130, 1992.

Meyer, S. B., Bass, M., Ash, R., et al.: Postoperative care of the lung transplant recipient. Crit. Care Nurs. Clin. North Am. 8:239–252, 1996.

Zorb, S. L.: Lung transplantation overview: The Massachusetts General Hospital experience. Crit. Care Nurs. Clin. North Am. 8:229–237, 1996.

chapter

...The Cardiovascular System

M. Lindsay Lessig, B.S.N., M.S.Ed., M.B.A., and
Paul M. Lessig, M.D., FACC

PHYSIOLOGIC ANATOMY

Gross Anatomy

1. **Heart**
   a. The heart lies in the mediastinum, on and to the left of the midline, resting on the diaphragm
   b. Its long axis is oriented from the right shoulder blade to the left upper quadrant of the abdomen
   c. During inspiration, the heart moves more vertically
   d. During expiration, the heart moves more horizontally
   e. It is oriented more vertically in thin adults and in persons with chronic obstructive pulmonary disease (COPD) and more horizontally in heavier adults
   f. The base, or top wide area, of the heart (atria and great vessels), is located diagonally at the second intercostal space, right/left sternal borders
   g. The apex, or tip, of the heart (junction of the ventricles and ventricular septum) is usually located at the fifth intercostal space, left midclavicular line
   h. The heart weighs approximately 275 g in adult females, 325 g in adult males (± 75 g)
2. **Cardiac silhouette** (seen on chest x-ray) (Figs. 2–1 to 2–4)
   a. *Frontal* view: starting anatomically at top right, moving clockwise (see figs. 2–1 and 2–2):
      i. Superior vena cava: upper right corner
      ii. Aorta "knob"
      iii. Pulmonary artery
      iv. Left atrial appendage (only part of left atrium seen in this view), left ventricle (small portion) seen in left lateral margin
      v. Left ventricular apex: bottom and right lower lateral

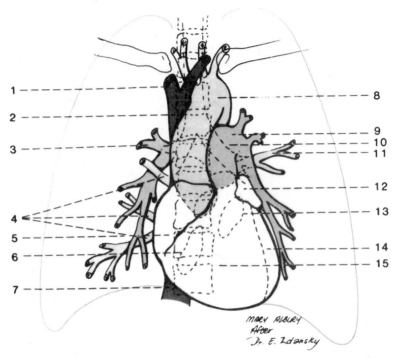

MARY ALBURY
After
Dr. E. Zdansky

1. Right innominate vein
2. Superior vena cava
3. Right main branch of the pulmonary artery
4. Upper and lower lobe veins
5. Right atrium
6. Tricuspid valve
7. Inferior vena cava
8. Arch of the aorta

9. Left main branch of the pulmonary artery
10. Main pulmonary artery
11. Left upper lobe vein
12. Appendage of the left atrium
13. Mitral valve
14. Left ventricle
15. Right ventricle

Figure 2–1 • Cardiac silhouette, posteroanterior view. (From Gedgaudas, E., Moller, J. H., Castaneda-Zuniga, M. D., et al.: Cardiovascular Radiology. Philadelphia, W. B. Saunders, 1985, p. 38.)

Figure 2–2 • Normal thoracicroentgengram, posteroanterior view. (From Gedgaudas, E., Moller, J. H., Castaneda-Zuniga, M. D., et al.: Cardiovascular Radiology. Philadelphia, W. B. Saunders, 1985, p. 38.)

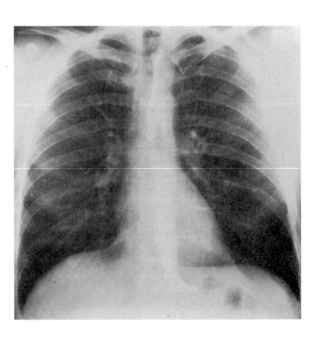

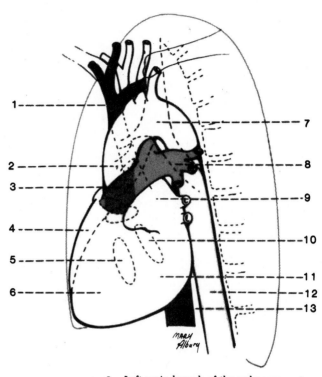

1. Superior vena cava
2. Ascending aorta
3. Main pulmonary artery
4. Right atrium
5. Tricuspid valve
6. Right ventricle
7. Aortic arch

8. Left main branch of the pulmonary artery
9. Left atrium
10. Mitral valve
11. Left ventricle
12. Descending aorta
13. Inferior vena cava

Figure 2-3 • Cardiac silhouette, lateral view. (From Gedgaudas, E., Moller, J. H., Castaneda-Zuniga, M. D., et al.: Cardiovascular Radiology. Philadelphia, W. B. Saunders, 1985, p. 39.)

   vi. Right atrium: right lateral border
   vii. Normal right ventricle is not seen in frontal view
  b. *Lateral* view (see Figs. 2–3 and 2–4)
   i. Heart rests on diaphragm
   ii. Left atrium and right ventricle predominant visually
3. Cardiac skeleton: fibrous skeleton to which heart muscle is attached
  a. Circles all four valves and valve annuli (rings)
  b. Gives support to valves
  c. Offers foundation for ventricular contraction

Structure of Cardiac Wall

1. Pericardium: the fibrous sac that surrounds the heart and roots of the great vessels, enveloping them and containing a small amount (15 to 50 ml) of pericardial fluid. This lubricated space protects the heart from friction, allowing it to easily change volume and size during contractions. The pericardium keeps the heart muscle anchored and girdled within the mediastinum. The two layers of the pericardium are:

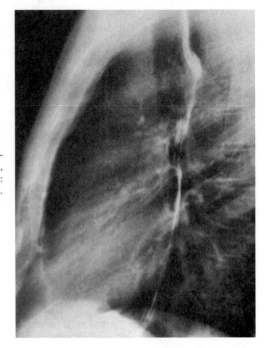

Figure 2–4 • Normal thoracic roentegeno-gram, lateral view. (From Gedgaudas, E., Moller, J. H., Castaneda-Zuniga, M. D., et al.: Cardiovascular Radiology. Philadelphia, W. B. Saunders, 1985, p. 39.)

    a. Fibrous pericardium: the tough, white, outermost layer attached by ligaments to the xiphoid process, vertebral column, and diaphragm

    b. Serous pericardium: the smooth, serous, inner layer that lines the inner surface of the fibrous pericardium

        i. Parietal surface: lines the inner surface of the pericardial sac

        ii. Visceral surface: covers the outer surface of the heart, extending several centimeters onto the great vessels and reflecting back to form the parietal surface

2. Epicardium: equivalent to visceral surface of serous pericardium; the outer surface of the heart muscle and great vessels

3. Myocardium: the muscular, contractile portion of the heart

    a. It is more susceptible to oxygen debt than is skeletal muscle

    b. Muscle fibers extend around the heart in multiple, interlacing layers

4. Endocardium: inner membranous surface, lining chambers of heart; a thin smooth, glistening membrane

5. Papillary muscles: myocardial structures extending into the ventricular chambers and attaching to chordae tendineae

6. Chordae tendineae: strong tendinous attachments from the papillary muscles to tricuspid and mitral valves; serve to prevent eversion of the valves into the atria during systole

· · · · · · · · · · · · · · · · ·

Chambers of the Heart

1. Atria: thin-walled (2 to 3 mm thick), low-pressure chambers

    a. The right atrium and left atrium act as reservoirs of blood for their respective ventricles

b. The right atrium, located above, behind, and to the right of right ventricle, receives systemic venous blood via the superior vena cava, inferior vena cava, and coronary sinus

c. Left atrium—superior, midline, and posterior to other chambers—receives oxygenated blood returning to the heart from the lungs via the pulmonary veins

d. When mitral and tricuspid valves open, there is a rapid filling of blood passively from the atria into the ventricles: approximately 80% to 85% of total filling

e. At the end of diastole, atrial contraction forcefully ("atrial kick") primes the left ventricle with approximately 15% to 20% of blood for ventricular output

2. **Ventricles:** the major "pumps" of the heart

  a. The right ventricle is most anterior of the four cardiac chambers, crescent-shaped

    i. A thin-walled (4 to 5 mm thick), low-pressure system

    ii. Contracts and propels deoxygenated blood into pulmonary circulation via pulmonary artery, the only artery in the body that carries deoxygenated blood

  b. The left ventricle is the main "pump": a conical (ellipsoid) structure posterior and to the left of the right ventricle

    i. A thick-walled (8 to 15 mm thick), high-pressure system

    ii. Squeezes and ejects blood into systemic circulation through the aorta during ventricular systole

  c. The left ventricle could just as easily have been called "the posterior ventricle" and the right ventricle called "the anterior ventricle"

  d. Interventricular septum: functionally more a part of the left ventricle than of the right ventricle, inasmuch as it forms the anterior wall of the left ventricle. Its curved shape protrudes into the right ventricular cavity

Cardiac Valves

1. **Atrioventricular (AV) valves**

  a. Located between the atria and ventricles: tricuspid valve on the right, mitral valve on the left

    i. The tricuspid valve is composed of a large anterior leaflet with two smaller posterior and septal leaflets

    ii. The mitral valve is composed of a long, narrow posterior (mural) leaflet and an oval-shaped anterior (aortic) leaflet

  b. Permit unidirectional blood flow from atria to ventricles during ventricular diastole and prevent retrograde flow during ventricular systole

    i. With ventricular diastole, the ventricles and the papillary muscles relax and the valve leaflets open

    ii. With increased ventricular pressure and systole, the valve leaflets close completely

    iii. The first heart sound (S_1) is produced as the mitral (M_1) and tricuspid (T_1) valves close. M_1 is the initial and major component of S_1

2. **Semilunar valves**

  a. Location

      i. The pulmonary valve is situated between the right ventricle and pulmonary artery. It consists of three semilunar cusps that attach to the wall of the pulmonary trunk. The free borders of the cusps are directed upward into the lumen of the artery. It has no distinct annulus (ring)

     ii. The aortic valve is situated between the left ventricle and aorta. It consists of three slightly thicker valve cusps, the bases of which attach to a valve annulus (fibrous ring)

  b. Permit unidirectional blood flow from the outflow tract during ventricular systole and prevent retrograde blood flow during ventricular diastole

      i. With ventricular systole, valves open when respective ventricle contracts and pressure is greater in the ventricle than in the artery

     ii. After ventricular systole, pressure in artery exceeds pressure in ventricles. This and retrograde blood flow cause valve to close

    iii. The second heart sound (S_2) is produced when aortic (A_2) and pulmonic (P_2) valves close. A_2 is the initial and major component of S_2

Coronary Vasculature (Fig. 2–5)

1. Arteries

  a. Two main arteries branch off at the base of the aorta, supplying blood to the myocardium and the electrical conduction system

  b. Right coronary artery (RCA), 12 to 14 cm long, supplies

      i. Right ventricle

     ii. Right atrium

    iii. Posterior third of the interventricular septum

    iv. Inferior wall of the left ventricle

     v. Branches:

       (a) Acute marginal branch

         (1) Descends from right lateral side of the heart down to the apex

         (2) Supplies the inferior surface of the right ventricle

       (b) Sinoatrial (SA) node in 55% of hearts

       (c) AV node in 90% of hearts

       (d) Posterior wall via the posterior descending artery (PDA) in approximately 85% of hearts (RCA system considered "right-dominant" in these cases)

         (1) Located in the posterior interventricular groove

         (2) Supplies the right ventricle and inferior wall of the left ventricle and the posterior third of the interventricular septum

     vi. Lumen of RCA: 1.5 to 5.5 mm, remaining fairly constant along length until PDA branch

  c. Left coronary artery (LCA)

      i. Left main coronary artery (LMCA)

       (a) Length: usually short, 1 to 25 mm (75% are 6 to 15 mm long)

       (b) Lumen diameter: 3 to 6 mm

       (c) Branches into the left anterior descending and circumflex arteries

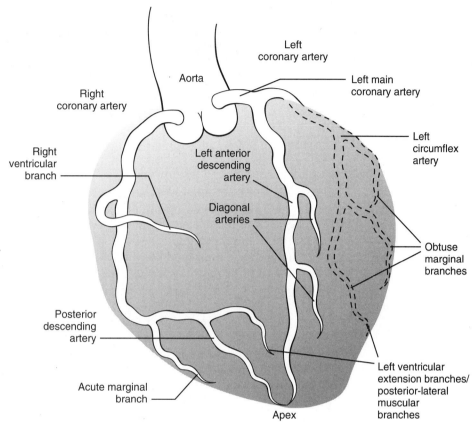

Figure 2–5 • Coronary artery anatomy.

    ii. Left anterior descending (LAD) artery
      (a) Supplies
        (1) Anterior two thirds of the interventricular septum
        (2) Anterior wall of the left ventricle
        (3) Right bundle branch (RBB)
        (4) Anterosuperior division of the left bundle branch (LBB)
      (b) Length: 10 to 13 mm
      (c) Lumen: 2 to 5 mm and tapers at distal ends
      (d) Branches include first diagonal (may have two to six other
          diagonals), first septal perforator (may have three to five other
          perforators)
   iii. Left circumflex (CX) artery also branches from the LMCA
      (a) Left circumflex artery supplies
        (1) AV node in 10% of hearts
        (2) SA node in 45% of hearts
        (3) Lateral posterior surface of left ventricle via the obtuse
           marginal branch (OMB)
        (4) PDA arises from the left circumflex artery in 15% of hearts
           (see description under RCA)
      (b) Major branch is the OMB, which supplies the lateral wall of the
         left ventricle
  d. Coronary collaterals

        i. Networks connecting the right and left coronary arteries exist

          (a) Normally these anastomoses are not visualized, because of their size (20 to 200 μm in diameter)

          (b) They may enlarge significantly over time (1 to 2 mm in diameter), if stenosis of coronary artery occurs

        ii. May provide blood flow beyond obstructed lesions

2. Cardiac veins

    a. Return deoxygenated blood back to the right atrium, mostly through coronary sinus; follow paths similar to those of the arteries and have no valves

    b. Consist of

        i. The great cardiac vein: parallels the LAD and left circumflex arteries; main left ventricular venous drainage system

        ii. The small and middle cardiac veins: both form the coronary sinus that drains into the right atrium

        iii. Thebesian veins: numerous small veins, present mostly in the right atrium and right ventricle, which drain blood directly into these chambers

3. Coronary blood flow

    a. Coronary vascular reserve: Coronary circulation has the ability to increase flow to meet added needs up to approximately six times normal

    b. Coronary blood flow is about 70 to 90 ml/100 g/minute

    c. Myocardial oxygen consumption is 8 to 10 ml/100 g/minute

    d. The heart uses most of the oxygen available in the coronary circulation; little oxygen reserve exists

    e. Indicators of coronary blood flow include

        i. Arterial pressure gradients (left ventricular and aortic diastolic pressures)

        ii. Diastolic filling times

    f. In systole, coronary artery blood flow usually decreases as a result of ventricular compression and contraction

    g. The left ventricle receives coronary blood flow circulation during diastole, whereas the right ventricle receives blood flow during both systole and diastole

    h. Coronary blood flow is reduced by

        i. Decreased tissue perfusion

        ii. Decreased left ventricular diastolic pressures

        iii. Increased myocardial mass

        iv. Mechanical obstruction (stenosis)

· ·

Neurologic Control of the Heart

1. Autonomic nervous system: influences contractility, depolarization/repolarization, rate of conductivity

    a. Sympathetic stimulation: originates in spinal cord; norepinephrine release is main impetus of stimulation to heart; its two effects include

        i. Alpha-adrenergic: causing peripheral arteriolar vasoconstriction

        ii. Beta-adrenergic (both beta$_1$ and beta$_2$)

          (a) Increases SA node discharge, increasing heart rate (positive chronotropy)

          (b) Increases force of myocardial contraction (positive inotropy)

(c) Accelerates AV conduction time (positive dromotropy)
   b. Parasympathetic stimulation: originates in medulla, with action of right vagus nerve (affecting SA node) and left vagus nerve (affecting AV conduction tissue). Acetylcholine release is the main parasympathetic impetus to cardiac effects
      i. Decreases rate of SA node discharge, slowing heart rate (negative chronotropy)
      ii. Slows conduction through AV tissue (negative dromotropy)
   c. Ventricles have mainly sympathetic innervation and only sparse vagal innervation
   d. Under normal conditions, parasympathetic influences predominate in the conducting system (SA node, AV node)
2. **Chemoreceptors**
   a. Afferent impulses located in carotid and aortic bodies
   b. Sensitive to changes in Po_2, Pco_2, and pH, causing changes in heart rate and respiratory rate via stimulation of vasomotor center in medulla
3. **Stretch receptors:** respond to pressure and volume changes
4. **Bainbridge reflex:** stretch receptors located in atria, large veins, venae cavae, and pulmonary artery
   a. Increases in venous return stretch the receptors
   b. Afferent nerve impulses are then transmitted to the vasomotor center in medulla
   c. Medulla increases efferent impulses, increasing sympathetic stimulation (decreasing parasympathetic), thereby increasing heart rate and cardiac output
   d. This enables the heart to pump all the blood returned to it
5. **Respiratory reflex**
   a. On inspiration: intrathoracic pressure decreases, increasing venous return to the heart
   b. Inspiration stimulates stretch receptors in the lungs and thorax
   c. Impulses from these stretch receptors travel (via afferent fibers) to the vasomotor center in the medulla, where they inhibit this center
   d. Inhibition of the medulla's vasomotor center decreases vagal tone; heart rate is increased, allowing the heart to pump out extra blood

Cardiac Muscle Microanatomy and Contractile Properties
(Fig. 2–6):

Cardiac muscle differs from skeletal muscle. It has numerous mitochondria located between individual myofibrils. This provides more adenosine triphosphate (ATP) for the huge metabolic and energy requirements necessary for repetitive muscle action. The two main contractile properties of cardiac muscle are the ability to shorten and to develop force.
1. **Muscle fibers:** a lattice-like arrangement called a functional syncytium
2. **Syncytium:** a network; when one fiber is depolarized, the action potential spreads along the syncytium, stimulating all fibers. The whole syncytium contracts, not just one fiber (all-or-none response)
3. **Sarcomere:** contractile unit
   a. Muscle fiber composed of fibrils; subdivided into overlapping myofilaments made up of contractile and regulatory proteins

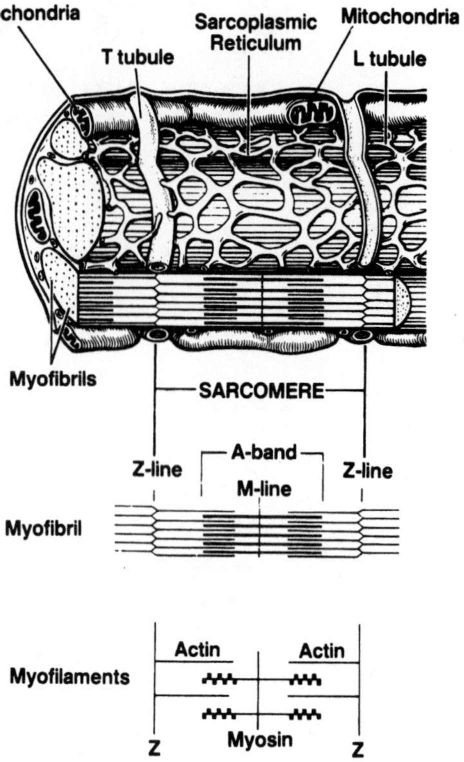

Figure 2-6 • Cardiac microanatomy: the sarcomere. (From Shepard, N., Vaughan, P., and Rice, V.: A guide to arrhythmia interpretation and management. Crit. Care Nurse 2[5]:59, 1982.)

b. The contractile proteins consist of
    i. Myosin: thick filaments, A-band
    ii. Actin: thin filaments
c. Their interactions help produce contraction force and fiber shortening
d. Two regulatory proteins are troponin and tropomyosin
    i. Do not directly aid contraction
    ii. Activate or inhibit actin-myosin interactions
4. **Intercalated discs:** located at end of sarcomeres
    a. Interlock fibers together at ends
    b. Pathway for quick transmission of depolarized impulse
5. **Sarcolemma membrane:** covers individual muscle fibers
6. **Sarcotubular system:** an extensive, tubular, intracellular continuation of sarcolemma
    a. T tubules: transmit action potential rapidly from sarcolemma to all fibrils in muscle
    b. Sarcoplasmic reticulum: houses calcium ions. Action potential in T tubules causes release of calcium from reticulum, resulting in a contraction
7. **Excitation-contraction process**
    a. Myocardial working cells are structured to enable chemical energy to be transformed into mechanical actions
    b. During excitation (depolarization), calcium enters the cell interior across the sarcolemma. A complex enzymatic interaction that includes calcium binding with troponin and the loss of actin-myosin inhibition then occurs. This permits actin and myosin filaments to interact; actin moving inward on myosin

   c. ATP supplies the energy for interactions between actin and myosin

   d. Sarcomeres shorten, resulting in muscle fiber shortening and, subsequently, cardiac muscle contraction

   e. Calcium is then pumped back into the sarcoplasmic reticulum, allowing muscle fiber to relax

Anatomy of the Cardiac Conduction System (Fig. 2–7)

1. SA node

   a. Normal pacemaker of the heart, possessing fastest inherent rate of automaticity (approximately 70 beats/minute)

   b. Located in the right superior wall of the right atrium at junction of the superior vena cava and right atrium

2. Internodal atrial conduction

   a. Impulse is conducted from SA node through the right and left atrial musculature to the AV node

   b. Although the atria do not have specialized high-speed conduction tracts comparable to the ventricular bundles and fascicles, there do appear to be preferred conduction pathways:

      i. Anterior internodal tract (Bachmann's)

      ii. Middle internodal tract (Wenckebach's)

      iii. Posterior internodal tract (Thorel's)

3. Bachmann's bundle: conducts impulses from SA node to LA

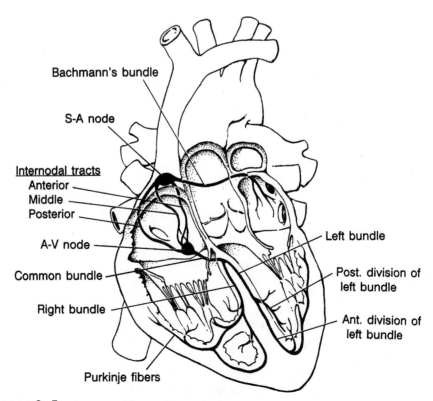

Figure 2–7 • Anatomy of the cardiac conduction system.

4. Atrioventricular node
   a. Delays impulse from atria before it goes to ventricles. This allows time for both ventricles to fill before ventricular systole
   b. Inherent rate of automaticity is approximately 40 beats/minute
   c. Located in right interatrial septum, above tricuspid valve's septal leaflet
5. **Bundle of His** (also known as the common bundle of His): arises from AV node and conducts impulse to bundle branch system. Because of its position, the His bundle is closely related to annuli of tricuspid, mitral, and aortic valves
6. **Bundle branch system:** pathways that arise from bundle of His, and branch at top of interventricular septum
   a. The RBB is the smaller, direct continuation of the bundle of His
      i. Transmits impulse down right side of interventricular septum to the right ventricular myocardium
      ii. The bundle divides into three parts—anterior, lateral, and posterior—which further divide, becoming parts of the Purkinje system (see later description)
   b. The LBB
      i. Larger branch from the bundle of His, transmits impulse to the septum and the left ventricle
      ii. The LBB divides into two main parts:
         (a) The left posterior fascicle transmits impulse over posterior and inferior endocardial surface of the left ventricle
         (b) The left anterior fascicle transmits impulse to anterior and superior endocardial surfaces of the left ventricle
7. **Purkinje system**
   a. Arises from distal portion of bundle branches, forming networks on ventricle's endocardial surface
   b. Transmits impulse into subendocardial and myocardial layers of both ventricles; provides for depolarization (from endocardium to epicardium). Ventricular contraction and ejection of blood out of ventricles follows
   c. Ventricles have their own inherent rate of automaticity of approximately 20 beats/minute

Electrophysiology

1. **Electrophysiologic properties of cardiac muscle cells**
   a. **Excitability:** ability to depolarize and form an action potential when sufficiently stimulated
   b. **Automaticity/rhythmicity:** ability to generate an impulse without an outside stimulus
   c. **Conductivity:** ability to conduct an electrical impulse to neighboring cells, spreading the impulse throughout the heart and achieving total depolarization
   d. **Refractoriness:** temporary inability of depolarized cell to become excited and generate another action potential
2. **Resting membrane potential (RMP):** the electrical potential (charge) of a cardiac muscle cell at rest
   a. RMP for myocardial fibers is -80 to -90 mV (Fig. 2–8)

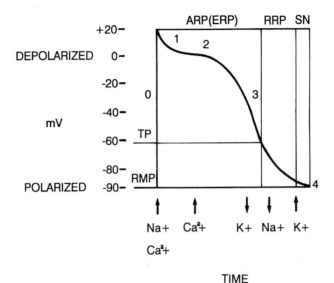

Figure 2–8 • Action potential of a cardiac muscle cell.

   b. The cell ions are composed primarily of sodium, potassium, and calcium
      i. Sodium ion concentration is greater *outside* the cell
     ii. Potassium ion concentration is greater *inside* the cell
    iii. Unbound calcium ion concentration is greater *outside* the cell
3. **Depolarization:** the changing of the electrical charge of a stimulated cell from negative to positive by ions flowing across the cell membrane: sodium moves into a cell, potassium moves out of the cell
4. **Repolarization:** the recovery or recharging of a cell's normal polarity. Sodium moves back out of the cell and potassium moves into the cell. The cell recovers its negative charge
5. **Threshold potential:** the electric voltage level at which cardiac cells become activated and produce an action potential, which leads to muscular contraction
6. **Stimulation of myocardial cells**
   a. Stimulus may be chemical, electrical, or mechanical
   b. When stimulated, electrical charge outside the cell becomes less negative, and depolarization occurs
   c. When threshold potential is reached, changes occur in the membrane
   d. SA and AV nodes achieve threshold potential first
   e. Cell membrane permeability is altered, and specialized channels in the membrane open, allowing for the entry of sodium and calcium ions into the cell
7. **Action potential:** When the cardiac cell changes polarity, the electrical impulse created during that change creates an energy stimulus that travels across the cell membrane: a high-speed, short-lived, self-reproducing current. This activity is represented on the action potential curve (see Fig. 2–8)
   a. *Phase 0:* depolarization: a quick upstroke (several milliseconds) representing initial phase of excitation
   b. *Phase 1:* initial phase of repolarization
   c. *Phase 2:* plateau phase of repolarization: slow inward current of calcium (to a lesser extent, sodium). Potassium diffuses out of the cell

    d. *Phase 3:* last phase of repolarization: outward current of potassium increases and the slow, inward current of sodium and calcium decreases. This causes cell to rapidly repolarize, returning to normal resting membrane potential

    e. *Phase 4:* membrane at resting potential

8. Cardiac pacemaker cells (SA and AV nodes) action potential

    a. Pacer cells, having increased automaticity, spontaneously depolarize in phase 4 without a stimulus. Other cells of the heart, having repolarized and attained phase 4, require another stimulus in order to be depolarized

       i. The rate of automaticity may be altered by increasing or decreasing the slope of phase 4

      ii. Increasing the slope of phase 4 speeds the heart rate; decreasing the slope of phase 4 slows the heart rate

    b. The spontaneous depolarization of pacer cells (SA and AV) is caused by the steady influx of sodium and the efflux of potassium

    c. The SA node has the fastest rate of depolarization

9. Refractoriness of heart muscle

    a. *Absolute refractory period* (effective refractory period): another stimulus to the cell will not produce another action potential (phases 0, 1, and 2 and part of 3 of the action potential curve)

    b. *Relative refractory period:* only a very strong stimulus can initiate an action potential response and cause depolarization (latter part of phase 3)

    c. *Supernormal period:* weak stimulus (one that would not normally elicit an action potential) can evoke an action potential and cause depolarization (occurs at the end of phase 3)

. . . .

Events in the Cardiac Cycle Produced by Depolarization and Repolarization

1. Electroactivity of the heart: ultimately produces muscle contraction and is graphically described in Figure 2–9

2. Diastolic activities: filling phase of ventricles

    a. P wave on the electrocardiogram (ECG): represents atrial depolarization

    b. "a" wave: The pressure rises in the atria

    c. Pressure in the atria is higher than the diastolic pressure in the ventricles, so blood flows from the atria into the ventricles. The ventricles are in diastole

3. Systolic activities: contraction and emptying of ventricles

    a. QRS complex: represents ventricular depolarization

    b. The first phase of ventricular contraction (systole) is called isometric or isovolumetric contraction. Pressure increases, but no blood enters or leaves the ventricles

    c. As pressure rises in the ventricles, the AV valves close, producing the first heart sound (S_1; composed of mitral [M_1] and tricuspid [T_1] components)

    d. "c" wave of the atrial pressure curve: is produced when AV valves are pushed backward toward the atria as ventricular pressure builds

    e. When left ventricular pressure exceeds pressure in the aorta, the aortic valve opens (comparable events in the right ventricle occur with the pulmonic valve)

    f. Blood is rapidly ejected into the aorta (systolic ejection)

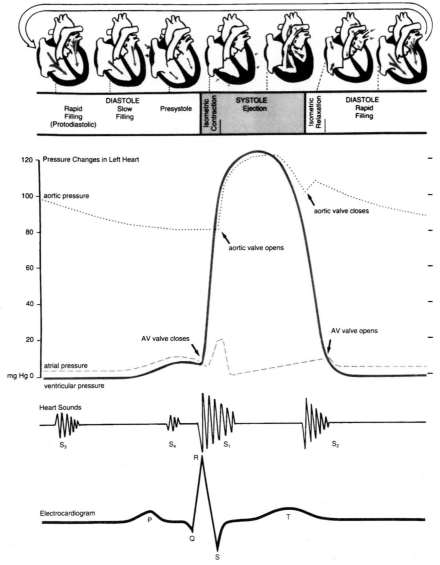

Figure 2–9 • Events in the cardiac cycle. (From Jarvis, C.: Physical Examination and Health Assessment, 2nd ed. Philadelphia, W. B. Saunders, 1996, p. 518.)

   g. Left ventricular pressures decrease, falling below the pressure in the aorta as blood from the left ventricle decreases and ventricular ejection stops

   h. Back flow of blood from the aorta to the left ventricle forces the aortic valve closed and produces the second heart sound (S_2; composed of aortic [A_2] and pulmonic [P_2] components). Comparable events occur in the pulmonary artery, closing the pulmonic valve

   i. Aortic valve closure is represented by the dicrotic notch in the aortic pressure waveform

   j. Repolarization of the ventricles occurs at this time and produces the T wave on the ECG

   k. The aortic valve closes, and pressure in the left ventricle falls rapidly (isometric or isovolumetric relaxation phase): no blood enters the ventricle

l. "v" wave is produced on the atrial pressure curve during isometric relaxation, as a result of the blood's flowing into the atrium from the pulmonary and systemic circuit against closed AV valves

m. When pressure is lower in the ventricles than in the atria, the AV valves reopen to initiate the rapid filling phase during diastole, and the cycle starts over again

Variables Affecting Left Ventricular Function and Cardiac Output

1. **Preload:** force used to stretch the muscle to an initial length
   a. Resting force on myocardium is determined clinically by pressure in ventricles at end of diastole (left ventricular end-diastolic pressure [LVEDP]). End-diastolic wall stress is the true measurement of this force (is difficult to measure)
   b. Preload can be related to a number of variables: fiber length, stretch, volume, wall stress
   c. Increases in preload have the following effects:
      i. Increase the volume of blood returning to the ventricles
      ii. Stretch myocardial fibers, causing more forceful subsequent ventricular contractions
      iii. Increase stroke volume and thus cardiac output
      iv. Increase ventricular work
   d. Muscle fibers can reach a point of stretch beyond which contraction is no longer enhanced; stroke volume then decreases, leading to heart failure
   e. These concepts are described by the *Frank-Starling law* of the heart
   f. Increased preload is seen in
      i. Increased circulating volume
      ii. Mitral insufficiency
      iii. Aortic insufficiency
      iv. Vasoconstrictor use
      v. Atrial kick (normal)
   g. Decreased preload is seen in
      i. Decreased circulating volume
      ii. Mitral stenosis
      iii. Vasodilator use
      iv. Loss of atrial kick

2. **Afterload:** initial resistance that must be overcome by the ventricles in order to develop force and contact, opening the semilunar valves and propelling blood into the systemic and pulmonary circulatory systems (systolic contraction)
   a. Factors affecting afterload include arterial resistance (wall stress and thickness), aortic impedance, end-diastolic pressure, blood viscosity, pulmonary vascular resistance (PVR), blood in aorta
   b. Clinical reflection to measure the afterload: arterial systolic pressure (systemic vascular resistance [SVR]) is utilized because wall stress during systolic contraction cannot be measured
   c. To calculate SVR: mean arterial pressure (MAP) minus central venous

pressure (CVP); this number is divided by cardiac output (CO); the resulting number is then multiplied by 80 and converts into dynes/second/cm^{-5}:

$$\left(\frac{\text{MAP} - \text{CVP}}{\text{CO}}\right) \times 80$$

    d. Dyne: unit of force that would drive a mass of 1 g with a speed of 1 cm/second

    e. Normal SVR = 900 to 1400 dynes/second/cm^{-5}

    f. Excessive afterload: increases left ventricular stroke work, decreases stroke volume, increases myocardial oxygen demands, and may result in left ventricular failure

    g. Increased afterload is seen in

        i. Aortic stenosis

        ii. Peripheral arteriolar vasoconstriction

        iii. Hypertension

        iv. Polycythemia

        v. Arteriolar vasoconstrictor drugs

    h. Decreased afterload seen with use of arteriolar vasodilators

3. Contractility (inotropic state): heart's ability to "squeeze" blood out and change shape from full to empty

    a. There is no accurate way to measure the contractility of the heart directly. Pump performance is the primary way in which it is reflected clinically

    b. Factors that increase the contractile state of the myocardium, shifting the ventricular function curve up and to the left (Fig. 2–10)

        i. Positive inotropic drugs: digitalis, epinephrine, dobutamine

        ii. Increased heart rate (Bowditch's law)

        iii. Sympathetic stimulation (via beta$_1$ receptors)

        iv. Hypercalcemia

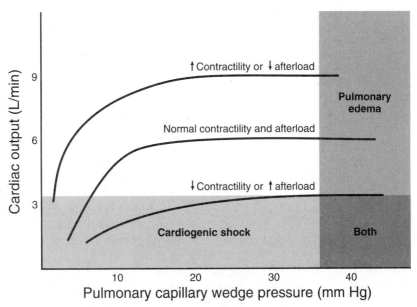

Figure 2–10 • Ventricular function curve. The ventricular function curve is not a Starling curve. It relates all the contributors to cardiac output, except heart rate, to ventricular function. It is an excellent framework for assessment and decision making.

c. Factors that decrease the contractile state of the myocardium, shifting the curve down and to the right (see Fig. 2–10)
   i. Negative inotropic drugs: quinidine, barbiturates, propranolol
   ii. Hypoxia (oxygen saturation <50%)
   iii. Hypercapnia
   iv. Intrinsic depression: cardiac muscle disease or loss of functional myocardial tissue as a result of an infarction
   v. Parasympathetic stimulation (via vagus nerve) has a depressive effect on the SA node, atrial myocardium, and AV junctional tissue. Hence, decreased heart rate results in decreased contractility
   vi. Metabolic acidosis
4. **Heart Rate:** contraction frequency
   a. Influenced by many factors, including
      i. Body position
      ii. Physical activity
      iii. Respiration
      iv. Temperature
      v. Blood volume
      vi. Peripheral vascular tone
      vii. Emotions
      viii. Metabolic status (increased with hyperthyroidism)
   b. Increases cardiac output in normal status
   c. A determinant of myocardial oxygen supply and demand
      i. Increased heart rates increase myocardial oxygen consumption
      ii. Increased heart rates decrease coronary blood flow (less time for filling during diastole)
5. **Cardiac output:** the amount of blood ejected by the left ventricle in 1 minute
   a. Cardiac output is a product of stroke volume (SV) and heart rate (HR):

$$CO = SV \times HR$$

   b. SV is the amount of blood ejected by the left ventricle with each contraction, or the difference between left ventricular end-diastolic volume (LVEDV) and left ventricular end-systolic volume (LVESV):

$$SV = LVEDV - LVESV; 60 \text{ to } 130 \text{ ml}$$

   c. Normal cardiac output = 4 to 8 L/minute
   d. Factors affecting cardiac output:
      i. Changes in heart rate: excessively high heart rates decrease diastolic filling time; ultimately decreasing cardiac output
      ii. Changes in contractility affecting stroke volume
         (a) Increased sympathetic activity causes increased myocardial contractility (positive inotropy) and thus more blood is ejected (increased SV); this increases cardiac output
         (b) Preload: when muscle fibers are stretched as a result of increased preload, force of contraction increases; thus SV and cardiac output increase
         (c) Changes in resistance, such as increased or decreased afterload, decrease SV and cardiac output
      iii. Changes in venous return to heart affect preload
         (a) Reduction in total blood volume decreases venous return and

preload. This causes a fall in cardiac filling, SV, and cardiac output

    (b) Venous constriction decreases venous pooling and increases venous return to the heart. This increases preload, cardiac filling, SV, and cardiac output

  e. Cardiac output decreases as a result of
- i. Arrhythmias
- ii. Hypovolemia
- iii. Mitral stenosis or mitral insufficiency
- iv. Cardiac tamponade
- v. Constrictive pericarditis
- vi. Restrictive cardiomyopathies
- vii. Myocardial infarction with left ventricular failure
- viii. Increased afterload (secondary to aortic stenosis, increased systemic vascular resistance)
- ix. Drugs with negative inotropic effects
- x. Metabolic disorders
- xi. Hypothermia

  f. Cardiac output increases as a result of
- i. Sepsis
- ii. Hyperthyroid states
- iii. Hyperflow states with hepatic or mesenteric shunting

6. Cardiac index (CI)

  a. CI is cardiac output corrected for differences in body size (a cardiac output of 4 L/minute may be adequate for a 100-pound woman but inadequate for a 200-pound man)

  b. Based on body surface area (BSA) estimated from a height and weight nomogram:

$$CI = CO/BSA$$

  c. Normal CI is 2.5 to 4.0 L/minute/m^2

  d. Increased CI is caused by
- i. Exercise
- ii. Mild tachyarrhythmias (in a healthy heart)

  e. Decreased CI is due to
- i. Decreased myocardial contractility (e.g., resulting from myocardial infarction, heart failure, cardiomyopathy, electrolyte imbalances)
- ii. Increased afterload (e.g., resulting from valvular stenosis and pulmonary hypertension)
- iii. Changes in preload (e.g., resulting from hypovolemia or valvular incompetence or stenosis)
- iv. Tachyarrhythmias and irregular rhythms, which decrease diastolic filling time and cause loss of atrial kick

7. Ejection fraction (EF)

  a. Percentage of blood ejected with every beat
- i. Ratio of SV to end-diastolic volume: usually 60% to 75%
- ii. Doesn't become clinically significant until less than 50% of SV
- iii. An increase in afterload can decrease EF without decrease in contractility
- iv. Ischemia can decrease EF

  b. Good reflection of left ventricular performance

8. Ventricular function curve: shows how to relate the contributions of preload, afterload, and contractility (but *not* heart rate) to ventricular function (see Fig. 2–10)

. . . .
: **Systemic Vasculature**

1. **Major functions:** provides tissues with blood, nutrients, and hormones and removes metabolic wastes
2. **Resistance to flow:** depends on diameter of vessels (especially the arterioles), viscosity of the blood, and elastic recoil in vessel walls
3. **Circulating blood volume:** There is approximately 5 L of total circulating blood volume in the adult body. During exercise, increases in cardiac output can circulate at least 25 L/minute (complete cycle occurring every 12 seconds)
4. **Major components of vascular system**
   a. *Arteries*
      i. Strong, compliant, elastic-walled vessels that branch off aorta, carry blood away from heart, and distribute it to capillary beds throughout the body
      ii. A high-pressure circuit
      iii. Able to stretch during systole and recoil during diastole because of elastic fibers located within arterial wall
   b. *Arterioles*
      i. Control systemic vascular resistance and thus arterial pressure
      ii. Have strong, smooth muscular walls innervated by the autonomic nervous system (adrenergic fibers)
         (a) Stimulation causes vascular constriction
         (b) Decreased adrenergic discharge causes vasodilation
      iii. Also controlled by autoregulation (see later description)
      iv. Lead directly into capillaries or first to metarterioles, serving as conduits to supply capillary beds
   c. *Capillary system*
      i. Grass-roots exchange of oxygen and carbon dioxide and solutes between blood and tissues; permits fluid volume transfer between plasma and interstitium
         (a) Gas exchange caused by sum of hydrostatic and colloid osmotic pressures across membrane
         (b) Increased capillary hydrostatic pressure leads to movement of fluid from vessel into interstitium
         (c) Greater capillary osmotic pressure leads to fluid movement from interstitium into vessels
      ii. Plasma protein concentration in capillaries normally is greater than in interstitium. The protein plasma pressure gradient
         (a) Maintains water in vessels
         (b) Prevents edema formation in interstitium
      iii. Albumin accounts for 75% of total plasma osmotic pressure; fibrinogen accounts for a small amount
      iv. Serum albumin is a good indicator of a patient's colloid osmotic pressure
      v. Capillaries lack smooth muscle; lumen diameter is passively controlled by changes in precapillary and postcapillary resistance

      vi. In accordance with Laplace's law, capillaries can handle high internal pressures without rupturing: tension in the wall of the vessel necessary to balance the distending pressure is lessened as the radius of the blood vessel decreases

     vii. Diffusion: gradual molecular mixing of different substances via thermal motion; the process of moving substrates and wastes between blood and tissues in the capillary system

  d. *Venous system*

      i. Stores approximately 65% of total blood volume

     ii. Receives blood from capillaries

    iii. Conducts blood back to heart within a low-pressure system

    iv. Surrounded by skeletal muscles that contract and help compress veins (skeletal muscle pump), sending blood toward the heart

     v. Valves in veins prevent retrograde blood flow

     vi. Venous pressure in lower extremities is normally 25 mm Hg or less

    vii. Swelling and a decrease in blood return are caused by leakage of fluid from circulatory system into the interstitium. They occur in erect, immobile extremities as a gravity effect

Control of Peripheral Blood Flow

1. **Autoregulation:** the ability of the tissues to control their own blood flow

  a. Long-term control: slow changes in blood flow that take days to months to occur

  b. Acute control: rapid changes in blood flow occurring in seconds to minutes

  c. Two hypotheses regarding acute blood flow control include

      i. Vasodilatory theory

       (a) As metabolism increases, oxygen consumption increases and partial pressure of oxygen in tissues decreases

       (b) Oxygen deficit increases production of vasodilator substances (e.g., carbon dioxide, lactic acid, adenosine), dilating arterioles and increasing blood supply

     ii. Oxygen demand theory (nutrient demand theory)

       (a) Oxygen is necessary for vascular contraction

       (b) As oxygen decreases, blood vessels dilate to increase blood flow and the subsequent oxygen level

       (c) Increased tissue metabolic rates create oxygen use increases, decreasing oxygen availability and causing local vasodilation

  d. With acute increases or decreases in arterial pressure, blood flow immediately increases or decreases to adjust for the change and maintain homeostasis

      i. Autoregulation of blood flow is thought to be based on the following two mechanisms:

       (a) Myogenic theory

         (1) As arterial pressure rises, the vessels stretch, stimulating vascular smooth muscle contraction and reducing blood flow to normal

         (2) As pressure decreases, smooth muscles relax

(b) Metabolic theory
   (1) As arterial pressure rises, increased blood flow brings nutrients to the tissues and removes vasodilator substances causing blood vessels to constrict
   (2) Metabolites (adenosine phosphates, prostaglandins, lactic acid, carbon dioxide, potassium) accumulate and cause vasodilation, increasing blood flow to the area that flushes these waste products away
(c) Delicate balance between these two mechanisms: myogenic response → vasoconstriction → decrease in blood supply → local increase in metabolites → vasodilation → wastes removed

2. **Autonomic regulation of vessels**
   a. Vasoconstriction occurs when norepinephrine is released at vasoconstrictor fiber nerve endings when adrenergic sympathetic nervous system is stimulated
      i. Regulates blood flow and arterial pressure in arterioles
      ii. Varies amount of blood stored in veins; venoconstriction causes an increase in venous return to the heart
   b. Vasodilation occurs when acetylcholine is released at vasodilator fiber nerve endings (cholinergic effect by stimulation of parasympathetic nervous system fibers or by inhibition of vasoconstrictor fibers)

3. **Stretch receptors:** baroreceptors (pressoreceptors) to keep mean arterial pressure constant
   a. Receptor sites in arteries (aortic arch, carotid sinus, pulmonary arteries, and atria)
   b. Sensitive to arterial pressures above 60 mm Hg
   c. Activated by elevated blood pressure or blood volume
      i. Respond to stretching of arterial walls
      ii. Impulse transmitted from aortic arch via vagus nerve to medulla
      iii. Sympathetic action inhibited
      iv. Vagal reflex dominates
      v. Result: decreased heart rate and contractility, dilation of peripheral vessels, decreased systemic vascular resistance, blood pressure lowered to normal
   d. Action with decreased blood pressure
      i. Vagal tone decreases
      ii. Sympathetic system becomes dominant
      iii. Result: increases heart rate and contractility, arterial and venous constriction (preserving blood flow to brain and heart) and blood pressure elevated to near normal

4. **Vasomotor center in medulla** (also called cardiac center): consists of two areas: vasoconstrictor and vasodepressor
   a. Vasoconstrictor stimulation causes norepinephrine secretion
      i. Increased heart rate, stroke volume, cardiac output, and, ultimately, arterial blood pressure
      ii. Venoconstriction decreases stores of blood in venous system, increases venous return, and thus increases blood pressure
   b. Vasoconstrictor inhibition stimulates vasodepressor area, causing venodilation
      i. Blood is stored in venous system
      ii. Stroke volume, cardiac output, and arterial pressure decrease

   c. Vasomotor center works with stretch receptors and chemoreceptors in the carotid sinus and aortic arch

      i. Blood pressure increase stimulates carotid sinus, inhibiting vasoconstrictor area

      ii. Vasodilation occurs by stimulation of vasodepressor area

      iii. Chemoreceptors are stimulated by a fall in oxygen saturation or in pH or by rises in carbon dioxide. The vasoconstrictor center is stimulated and causes a rise in arterial pressure

Arterial Pressure

1. **Regulation**
   a. Arterial pressure is controlled by the mechanisms described for systemic blood vessels
   b. The renin-angiotensin-aldosterone system also helps control arterial pressure (see Chapter 4, The Renal System)
      i. Renin: a protease secreted by the kidneys; converts angiotensinogen to angiotensin I
      ii. Renin release from kidney is affected by
         (a) Decreased blood pressure (i.e., hemorrhage, dehydration, diuretics, sodium depletion) → increases in renin secretion
         (b) Rise in sympathetic output → increases in renin secretion
         (c) Fall in sodium concentration → increases in renin secretion
         (d) Increased blood pressure → decreases in renin secretion
      iii. Angiotensin II, the most potent vasoconstrictor known, is subsequently produced when increased renin secretion stimulates its formation. Effects of angiotensin II include
         (a) Arteriolar constriction, increasing systolic and diastolic pressures
         (b) Stimulation of adrenal cortex to secrete aldosterone, causing sodium and water retention
         (c) Increase in extracellular fluid volume, which shuts off the stimulus that initiated the renin secretion, and blood pressure is maintained at a normal level
   c. Renal: fluid volume control factor
      i. As arterial pressure increases, kidneys excrete more fluid
         (a) Causes reduction in extracellular fluid and blood volumes
         (b) Reduces circulating blood volume and cardiac output, leading to normalization of arterial pressure
      ii. As arterial pressure decreases, kidneys retain fluid and sodium, causing increased intravascular volume and cardiac output, leading to normalization of arterial pressure
2. **Factors affecting arterial blood pressure**
   a. Cardiac output
   b. Heart rate
   c. Systemic vascular resistance
   d. Arterial elasticity
   e. Blood volume
   f. Blood viscosity
   g. Age
   h. Body surface area

      i. Exercise

      j. Emotions

      k. Sodium retention

3. **Pulse pressure:** difference between systolic and diastolic pressures, expressed as a numerical value in millimeters of mercury (mm Hg)

      a. A function of stroke volume and arterial capacitance

      b. Normal pulse pressure: 30 to 40 mm Hg

      c. Changes in stroke volume (with exercise, shock heart failure) are reflected in similar changes in pulse pressure

4. **Mean arterial pressure:** average arterial pressure during cardiac cycle, dependent on mean arterial blood volume and elasticity of arterial wall

      a. MAP is calculated by the following formula:

$$\overline{MAP} = Pd + \tfrac{1}{3}(Ps - Pd)$$

where
$\overline{MAP}$ = mean arterial pressure
Pd = diastolic pressure
Ps = systolic pressure
Ps − Pd = pulse pressure
Thus MAP = diastolic pressure + one-third pulse pressure

      b. Example: Blood pressure of 120/60 mm Hg
$\overline{MAP} = Pd + \tfrac{1}{3}(Ps - Pd)$
$\overline{MAP} = 60 + \tfrac{1}{3}(60)$
$\overline{MAP} = 60 + 20$
$\overline{MAP} = 80$

      c. Level of MAP is a function of cardiac output and systemic vascular resistance

NURSING ASSESSMENT DATA BASE

Nursing History

1. **Main complaint:** patient's explanation for seeking medical assistance

2. **History of present illness:** Identify

      a. Description of complaint

      b. Onset: date, time of day, duration, course, precipitating factors

      c. Signs and symptoms: exacerbations, remissions

         i. Discomfort: character, location, radiation, quality, duration, factors that aggravate or produce, factors that alleviate

        ii. Fatigue: with or without activity

       iii. Edema: location, degree, duration

       iv. Syncope and presyncope: time and circumstances of occurrence (postural, nonpostural, activity), provocative events (cough, micturition, head movement)

        v. Dyspnea: orthopnea, paroxysmal nocturnal dyspnea, dyspnea on exertion (determine how much exercise it takes to elicit in number of blocks, flights of stairs)

       vi. Palpitations

      vii. Cough, hemoptysis

     viii. Claudication (how many blocks?)

      ix. Recent weight gains or losses

3. **Past medical history:** Identify all previous illnesses, injuries, surgical procedures

   a. Patient's assessment of general health for last several years

   b. Risk factors: hypertension, hypercholesteremia, smoking, family history, diabetes

   c. Last medical examination, hospitalizations, prior relevant cardiac tests (e.g., echocardiography, catheterization)

   d. Cardiovascular history: coronary artery disease (CAD), myocardial infarctions, angina hypertension, valvular disease, arrhythmias, trauma, peripheral vascular disease, congenital heart defects, heart murmurs, rheumatic fever, cerebrovascular accident (CVA), transient ischemic attacks

4. **Family history:** Identify

   a. State of health or cause of and age at death of immediate family members

   b. Hereditary, familial diseases pertaining to cardiovascular system

      i. Diabetes mellitus

     ii. Hypertension

    iii. Cardiovascular disease

    iv. Family history of sudden death or syncopy

5. **Social history:** Identify

   a. Present and past work experiences

   b. Activity, exercise

   c. Smoking habits (present, past)

   d. Drinking habits

   e. Daily living patterns

   f. Nutrition: types of foods eaten, meals per day, who prepares meals

   g. Support system: relationship with significant others

   h. Cultural issues and language barriers

6. **Medication history:** Identify all prescribed or over-the-counter medications and dosages taken. Determine why and how often the patient is taking each drug, any side effects, compliance issues

7. **Allergies:** Medications, food, environmental, iodine (potential reaction to contrast medium used during cardiac catheterization procedures)

. . . .

Nursing Examination of Patient

These components are often performed in combinations and in different order to help the patient feel comfortable during the examination and be able to participate more readily

1. **Vital signs**

   a. Pulses: Palpate bilaterally

      i. Check rate, rhythm, character and volume, delays

     ii. Describe pulses, using scale of 0 to 3

        (a) 0 = absent pulses

        (b) 1+ = palpable but thready, easily obliterated

        (c) 2+ = normal, not easily obliterated

        (d) 3+ = bounding, easily palpable cannot obliterate

iii. Common sites for palpation of arteries are
   (a) Carotid
   (b) Brachial
   (c) Radial
   (d) Femoral
   (e) Popliteal
   (f) Dorsalis pedis
   (g) Posterior tibialis
iv. Describe pulse characteristics
   (a) Normal pulse character: smooth, rounded
   (b) Pulse deficit: the inability to palpate all the contractions of the heart
      (1) Premature or rapid contractions may not generate a peripheral pulse
      (2) Determine heart rate, compared by feeling radial pulse while auscultating apical pulse, and then record auscultated heart rate
   (c) Pulsus parvus et tardus: small (parvus) pulse with a delayed (tardus) slow upstroke and prolonged downstroke. Noted in
      (1) Aortic stenosis: parvus and tardus
      (2) Mitral stenosis: only parvus
      (3) Constrictive pericarditis: only parvus
      (4) Cardiac tamponade: only parvus
   (d) Pulsus alternans: pulse waves alternate, every other beat is weaker; caused by an impaired myocardium; noted in severe left ventricular failure
   (e) Water-hammer (Corrigan's pulse)
      (1) Abrupt, rapid upstroke followed by rapid downstroke
      (2) Palpated in patients with
         a) Aortic insufficiency
         b) Patent ductus arteriosus
b. Blood pressure
   i. Affected by adrenergic states (anxiety, excitement, fear), position changes, activity
   ii. Sphygmomanometer; key points
      (a) Width of cuff important
         (1) Ideal width is 40% of circumference of arm
         (2) Gives false high reading if too small
         (3) For obese patients, use thigh cuff, 18 cm wide
      (b) Positioning of cuff: no less than 2.5 cm from antecubital fossa
      (c) Falsely low measurement: cuff too large for arm; arm above heart level, inability to accurately hear first Korotkoff sound
      (d) Falsely high measurement: cuff too small for arm, loose cuff not centered over brachial artery, arm below heart level
   iii. Take blood pressure in both arms. More than a 10- to 15-mm Hg difference in systolic pressures indicates diminished arterial flow on side with lower reading (obstruction, dissection)
   iv. Orthostatic blood pressure drop: assess at-risk patients
      (a) Check blood pressure supine, sitting, standing
      (b) Fall of more than 20 mm Hg of systolic pressure signifies orthostatic hypotension

        (c) Caused by vasodilating drugs, volume depletion
- v. Pulsus paradoxus: an exaggeration of normal physiologic response to inspiration (blood pressure lower on inspiration than on expiration)
  - (a) Examine with patient breathing normally
  - (b) Inflate the sphygmomanometer until no Korotkoff sounds are heard. Slowly deflate the cuff until Korotkoff sounds are first heard on expiration; note the pressure reading
  - (c) Continue to deflate the cuff until all sounds are heard during both expiration and inspiration; note this reading
  - (d) Subtract the second reading from the first. This represents the pulsus paradoxus
  - (e) Normally, on inspiration, the difference between inspiration and expiration is less than 11 mm Hg. With pulsus paradoxus, the fall in blood pressure on inspiration is 11 mm Hg or greater
  - (f) Seen in
    - (1) Cardiac tamponade
    - (2) Constrictive pericarditis
    - (3) Emphysema, asthma
    - (4) Hemorrhagic shock

c. Temperature

d. Respirations

2. **General overall appearance:** skin and mucous membranes

   a. Color

   b. Temperature

   c. Moisture

   d. Turgor

   e. Edema: found in dependent areas, pitting versus nonpitting (extremities and sacrum)

   f. Nail bed: color, refill

   g. Angiomas

   h. Petechiae

   i. Cyanosis (circumoral, extremities)

   j. Clubbing of fingers or toes

3. **Neck examination**

   a. Neck veins give important clues regarding fluid status

      i. Jugular veins reflect right atrial and right ventricular filling pressures

     ii. Internal jugular veins are harder to visualize than external jugular veins, but they more accurately reflect pressure and volume changes in the right atrium (central venous pressure)

   iii. Check for distention and pulsation
   - (a) Elevate the head of the bed until you can see jugular waves
   - (b) Shine bright light tangentially to illuminate vessels, if not obvious

   iv. Determine jugular venous pressure
   - (a) The sternal notch is roughly 5 cm above the atrium (when the patient is upright or lying down)
   - (b) Measure distance in centimeters from the sternal notch to the top of the distended neck vein
   - (c) The value obtained plus the 5 cm provides a rough estimate of central venous pressure

    b. Check for hepatojugular reflux

       i. Place patient at 45° angle

      ii. Compress upper right abdomen for 30 to 45 seconds (causes additional venous return from liver to heart)

     iii. If hepatojugular reflex is present, jugular pulses become more pronounced, and the level of filling of the neck veins will rise (signifies inability of the right side of the heart to deal with added volume)

4. Chest examination

    a. Shape and contour of chest

    b. Symmetry

    c. Breathing pattern

5. Cardiac examination

    a. Inspect for visible point of maximal impulse (PMI) of cardiac impulse: easier to see on people with thin chests and in children

    b. Palpate three areas: base, apex, and left sternal border; check for:

       i. Pulsations (e.g., the PMI; the patient *must be supine*)

      ii. Thrills (palpable vibrations, analogous to the sensation felt on the throat of a purring cat) signify turbulence or murmur loud enough to feel (aortic stenosis, mitral stenosis, patent ductus arteriosus, ventricular septal defect)

     iii. A left peristernal lift suggests right ventricular dilatation

     iv. Friction rubs (analogous to sensation felt when rubbing two pieces of leather together): hard to palpate

      v. Apical impulse (the PMI in the *normal* heart): not always easy to palpate

        (a) Normally located at fifth left intercostal space, midclavicular line, and is approximately 2 cm in size

        (b) PMI that can be palpated over two or more intercostal areas signifies diffuse PMI resulting from

           (1) Left ventricular dilatation (left ventricular volume overload)

           (2) Aortic insufficiency, mitral regurgitation, dilated cardiomyopathy

        (c) A forceful, *sustained* apical impulse indicates left ventricular hypertrophy

        (d) Nonsustained but forceful apical impulses are created by high-output states (fever, anemia, anxiety, hyperthyroidism)

    c. Auscultation of heart

       i. Use of stethoscope

         (a) Bell: use to hear low-pitched sounds such as heart sounds S_3 and S_4 and ventricular filling murmurs (i.e., mitral stenosis)

         (b) When using the bell of the stethoscope, do not press or press only hard enough to eliminate air leakage; otherwise, the underlying skin functions as a diaphragm and the low-pitched sounds will not be heard

         (c) Diaphragm: use to hear high-pitched sounds such as heart sounds S_1 and S_2, ejection clicks, opening snaps, and murmurs caused by stenotic valves

         (d) Usual listening positions: supine, left lateral decubitus position, sitting up, and leaning forward

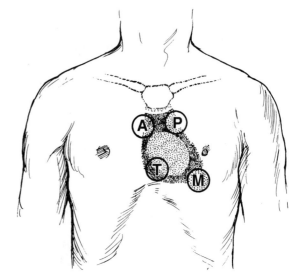

Figure 2–11 • Cardiac examination. Auscultation areas: aortic (A); pulmonic (P); tricuspid (T); mitral (M).

(e) Auscultation areas on the chest (Fig. 2–11)
  (1) Aortic area (second intercostal space, right sternal border)
  (2) Pulmonic area (second intercostal space, left sternal border)
  (3) Tricuspid area (fifth intercostal space, left sternal border)
  (4) Mitral or apical area (fifth intercostal space, left midclavicular line): normal location of heart's apex
ii. Origin of heart sounds: opening and closing of valves (see Fig. 2–9) and rapid acceleration or deceleration of blood produce either low- or high-pitched sounds
iii. Normal heart sounds (Fig. 2–12)
  (a) First heart sound (S_1): produced by mitral and tricuspid valve closure

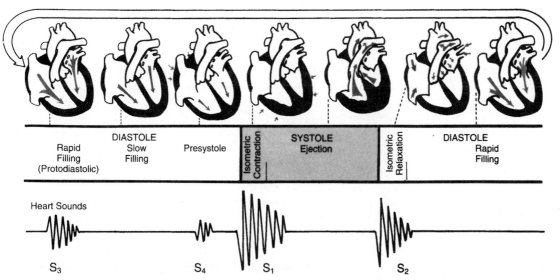

Figure 2–12 • Heart sounds and cardiac cycle. (From Jarvis, C.: Physical Examination and Health Assessment, 2nd ed. Philadelphia, W. B. Saunders, 1996, p. 519.)

(1) Marks the onset of ventricular systole

(2) Left ventricle depolarizes and contracts before right

(3) Listen at apex (heard loudest here)

(4) Component parts of S_1 may be split (mitral component [M_1] before tricuspid component [T_1])

(5) Coincides with carotid artery pulse wave

(b) Second heart sound (S_2): produced by aortic and pulmonic valve closure; usually the loudest heart sound

(1) Marks end of ventricular systole

(2) Listen with diaphragm at base: second intercostal space, left sternal border

(3) Both component parts of S_2 may be heard (aortic component [A_2] before pulmonary component [P_2]), but only at the pulmonic area

(c) Fourth heart sound (S_4)

(1) Normal in many adults

(2) Audible only in sinus rhythms (requires atrial contraction)

(d) Physiologic (normal) split of S_2 (A_2P_2)

(1) P_2 is delayed on inspiration when the right ventricle is slower to contract than the left ventricle; this is because of increased volume loading of the right ventricle in inspiration caused by increased venous return to the heart. This prolongs ejection of blood from the right ventricle and delays pulmonic valve closure, prolonging the time from aortic closure (A_2) to pulmonic closure (P_2). A resulting split occurs between A_2 and P_2 during inspiration

(2) A_2 precedes P_2 and is generally louder

(3) Split of S_2 is heard best over pulmonic area

(4) It may be heard best in normal, quiet respiration when the patient is sitting or standing

iv. Abnormal heart sounds

(a) Fixed splitting of S_2

(1) Persistent splitting of S_2 that does not disappear with expiration (no respiratory variation)

(2) Mainly heard in atrial septal defect

(b) Persistent (wide) splitting of S_2: second heart sound is split on expiration and more widely split on inspiration (as a result of any increase in right ventricular volume or pressure, prolonged right ventricular ejection and delayed pulmonary valve closure, or delay in right ventricular systole (as in right bundle branch block [RBBB]). Seen in

(1) Atrial septal defect

(2) RBBB

(3) Pulmonary hypertension of any cause

(4) Pulmonary stenosis

(5) Ventricular septal defect

(c) Paradoxical splitting (reversed splitting) of S_2 (i.e., P_2 earlier than A_2)

(1) Occurs when left ventricular ejection time is prolonged, resulting in delayed aortic closure; therefore, pulmonic valve closes first

(2) The split widens on expiration and narrows on inspiration (P_2 precedes S_2)

(3) Second component of split (A_2) is louder

(4) The patient's sitting or standing may help in detecting a paradoxic split (or any split)

(5) Seen in

   a) Left bundle branch block (LBBB)

   b) Severe aortic stenosis

   c) Patent ductus arteriosus

(d) Third heart sound (S_3): ventricular gallop

(1) Occurs during the rapid phase of ventricular filling in early diastole; is caused by resistance to ventricular filling, resulting from increased volume load or decreased ventricular compliance

(2) Can normally be heard in children, young adults, and in women during the last trimester of pregnancy (physiologic S_3)

(3) Abnormal when heard in older age groups or in association with disease states (left-sided heart failure, right-sided heart failure, fluid overload)

(4) Sound is low-pitched (heard best with bell)

(5) When originating in the left ventricle, it is heard best at the apex with the patient in the left lateral decubitus position

(6) When originating in the right ventricle, it is heard best along the fourth intercostal space, left sternal border, in inspiration

(7) Heard transiently in patients with mitral insufficiency, ischemia, ventricular failure, tricuspid insufficiency, atrial septal defect

(8) Sounds like "Ken-tuc-KY"

(e) Atrial (presystolic or S_4) gallop

(1) Occurs during atrial contraction, just before S_1 during the late phase of ventricular filling

(2) Occurs when there is volume overload of either ventricle or decreased ventricular compliance

(3) Is often a normal finding in certain adults: trained athletes, older patients

(4) Heard also in patients with

   a) Myocardial ischemia or infarction

   b) Systemic and pulmonic hypertension

   c) Aortic or pulmonary stenosis

   d) Ventricular failure

(5) Heard best

   a) A right-sided S_4 (less common) is usually louder on inspiration, over left lower sternal border

   b) A left-sided S_4 is usually heard best at the apex (does not change with respirations)

(f) Summation gallop

(1) Occurrence of simultaneous atrial (S_4) and ventricular (S_3) gallop

  (2) Heard with tachycardias (which cause shortening of diastole) and heart failure
(g) Extracardiac sounds
  (1) Ejection clicks: sharp, high-pitched sound just after S_1
  (2) Pericardial friction rubs
    a) Are like leather rubbing or new snow crunching
    b) Should be heard with diaphragm (is loudest when the patient is leaning forward) in full expiration
    c) Often have three components (ventricular systole, relaxation, filling)
  (3) Opening snaps: sound produced by a stenotic mitral valve snapping into the open position
  (4) Prosthetic valves: crisp, sometimes metallic clicking, with both opening and closure heard
(h) Murmurs
  (1) Sounds produced by turbulent blood flow. Analyze to determine
    a) Whether murmur is in systole or diastole
      i) Concentrate first on systole. Listen at all areas, starting with the base and moving down the precordium to the apex
      ii) Listen next in diastole, examining all areas
      iii) Listen to all areas with both bell and diaphragm
    b) Characteristics of heart sounds
      i) Ejection murmurs
        [a] Usually rough, extending into or through systole
        [b] Aortic sclerosis, aortic stenosis
      ii) Regurgitant murmurs: are usually a more pure, uniform sound
    c) Site of maximal intensity
    d) Radiation of sound (murmurs radiate in direction of blood flow)
    e) Timing, duration, and location
      i) Systolic ejection murmur: starts after S_1, ends before S_2
      ii) Pansystolic (holosystolic): heard from S_1 through S_2
      iii) Diastolic murmur: starts after S_2, ends before S_1
    f) Effect of respirations on murmur, whether increased or decreased with either inspiration or expiration
    g) Effect of patient position on the murmur's intensity
    h) Characteristic pattern of murmurs
      i) Crescendo: builds up in intensity
      ii) Decrescendo: decreases in intensity
      iii) Crescendo-decrescendo: peaks and then decreases in intensity
    i) Intensity: based on grade of I to VI and recorded with grade over VI to show scale being used
      i) I/VI: barely audible; the clinician can hear only after listening awhile

        ii) II/VI: easily audible

        iii) III/VI: loud; not associated with a thrill

        iv) IV/VI: loud and may be associated with a thrill

        v) V/VI: very loud; can be heard with the stethoscope partly off the chest (tilted); associated with a thrill

        vi) VI/VI: very loud; can be heard with stethoscope off the chest; associated with a thrill

    j) Quality

        i) Blowing

        ii) Musical

        iii) Rough, harsh

        iv) Honking

    k) Pitch

        i) High-pitched

        ii) Low-pitched

(2) Innocent (functional) murmurs

    a) Hemodynamically insignificant, physiologic; usually ejection murmurs

    b) Not associated with cardiovascular disease

    c) Common among children and pregnant women

    d) Found in patients with hyperthyroidism and anemia

    e) Diastolic murmurs are never functional or innocent

(3) Abnormal murmurs (hemodynamically significant)

    a) Systolic

        i) Mitral insufficiency (regurgitation)

            [a] Pansystolic

            [b] Loudest at apex

            [c] Radiates to left axilla

            [d] Intensity varies, grades I to V

            [e] May be associated with thrill at apex and axilla

            [f] Blowing quality, high-pitched

        ii) Tricuspid insufficiency (regurgitation)

            [a] Pansystolic

            [b] Loudest at lower left sternal border

            [c] Variable in intensity (may increase with inspiration)

            [d] Blowing quality, lower pitched

            [e] Radiates to right sternal border, liver

        iii) Aortic stenosis

            [a] Systolic ejection murmur

            [b] There may be crescendo-decrescendo murmur

            [c] Intensity varies; no relation to severity of murmur

            [d] Thrill may be found at second intercostal space, right sternal border

            [e] Radiates to neck and apex

            [f] Harsh in quality, medium or high-pitched

[g] Maximal intensity at base of heart, usually at second intercostal space, right sternal border

iv) Hypertrophic obstructive cardiomyopathy (HOCM) (formerly called idiopathic hypertrophic subaortic stenosis [IHSS]) occurs when septal wall just below aortic valve is hypertrophied

[a] Maximal intensity at second to fourth intercostal spaces, right sternal border

[b] May radiate to apex

[c] Thrill may be found at lower left sternal border

[d] Ejection murmur

[e] Crescendo-decrescendo murmur

[f] Decreases during expiration and squatting, increases with a Valsalva maneuver

v) Pulmonic stenosis

[a] Maximal loudness at second intercostal space, left sternal border

[b] Pulmonary systolic ejection sound (click)

[c] Thrill may be felt at second intercostal space, left sternal border

[d] Harsh

[e] Crescendo-decrescendo

[f] Usually louder on inspiration

[g] Usually grade III to IV intensity

[h] Persistent split of S_2, including expiration: the more severe the stenosis, the more pronounced the split

[i] Louder when patient is supine and during inspiration

vi) Interventricular septal defect

[a] Maximal loudness along lower sternal border

[b] Radiates widely

[c] Thrill usually present at lower left sternal border

[d] Pansystolic or early systolic

[e] Harsh

vii) Patent ductus arteriosus

[a] Continuous systolic and diastolic murmur

[b] Maximal intensity at second intercostal space, left sternal border

[c] Machinery-like murmur

[d] Occasional thrill at second intercostal space, left sternal border

b) Diastolic murmurs

i) Mitral stenosis

[a] Early diastolic and presystolic rumble (if in normal sinus rhythm)

[b] Very low-pitched

[c] May be heard only when patient is lying on left side at PMI with the bell of the stethoscope

[d] Maximal intensity at the apex

[e] When presystolic, usually crescendo

[f] May be associated with an opening snap and accentuated S_1

[g] Intensity is not affected by inspiration

ii) Tricuspid stenosis

[a] Maximal intensity at fourth intercostal space, left sternal border

[b] Intensity should increase on inspiration

[c] Early diastolic

[d] Low-pitched, rumbling

[e] May increase with hepatic compression

[f] May have opening snap

iii) Aortic insufficiency (regurgitation)

[a] Maximal intensity at third to fourth intercostal space, left sternal border, and at apex

[b] Blowing quality, high-pitched

[c] Intensity varies with severity

[d] Radiates to the apex

[e] Thrill uncommon

[f] Pansystolic (unless acute when it is a short, early diastolic murmur)

[g] Decrescendo

[h] Heard best when the patient is sitting up and leaning forward and during exhalation

iv) Pulmonary insufficiency (regurgitation)

[a] Maximal loudness along second intercostal space, left sternal border

[b] Radiates along left sternal border

[c] Decrescendo

[d] High-pitched

[e] Blowing quality

[f] Sometimes increases with inspiration

6. **Extremities examination:** Note the following associated disorders

a. Edema: right-sided heart failure, venous stasis

b. Color, temperature changes: arterial insufficiency (especially if asymmetrically cool)

c. Hair loss: arterial disease

d. Ulcerations: stasis, ischemia

e. Peripheral pulses: check for bruits

f. Motor and sensory function: numbness, foot drop (in advanced peripheral ischemia)

g. Clubbing of nail beds: cyanotic congenital heart defects

h. Varicosities

Diagnostic Studies

1. **Laboratory**

a. Complete blood cell count (CBC), hemoglobin (Hb), hematocrit (HCT)

    b. Clotting profile

       i. Partial thromboplastin time (PTT)

      ii. International normalized ratio (INR): measures effectiveness of anticoagulant therapy

          (a) For atrial fibrillation, therapeutic range for INR is 1.5 to 2.5

          (b) For prosthetic valves, therapeutic range for INR is 2.5 to 3.5

     iii. Activated clotting time (ACT): bedside test done to measure amount of time required for blood coagulation

     iv. Platelet count

    c. Enzymes

       i. Creatine kinase (CK): CK-MB isoenzymes

          (a) Enzyme associated with ATP conversion in contractile muscle tissue; found in heart, brain, skeletal tissues

          (b) MB isoenzymes most sensitive for cardiac tissue

          (c) Rises 4 to 8 hr after onset, peaks 12 to 24 hr after myocardial infarction, returns to normal in ~24 to 48 hr

          (d) A CK-MB concentration greater than 5% of total CK indicates myocardial necrosis

      ii. Cardiac troponin T and I, myoglobin

          (a) Sensitive, earliest cardiac marker enzymes

          (b) Rise less than 6 hr after onset of ischemic symptoms

          (c) Help with quicker decision making in identification, risk stratification, and treatment of patients

     iii. Lactate dehydrogenase isoenzymes (LDH1 and LDH2):

          (a) Enzymes are widespread in body; LDH1 isoenzyme has highest concentration in cardiac, kidney, and red blood cells

          (b) LDH1 rises in 12 to 24 hr, peaks 48 to 72 hr after myocardial infarction, returns to normal in ~7 to 10 days

          (c) An LDH1/LDH2 ratio greater than 1.0 indicates tissue necrosis; may also be seen in hemolyzed sample

    d. Electrolytes, blood urea nitrogen (BUN), creatinine, glucose

    e. Fasting serum lipid profile: normal levels

       i. Total cholesterol level: normal range is 100 to 240 mg/dl; 200 to 240 mg/dl is considered borderline high; less than 200 mg/dl is preferable

      ii. High-density lipoproteins (HDL): normal range is 35 to 45 mg/dl

     iii. Low-density lipoproteins (LDL): normal range is 50 to 160 mg/dl (<130 mg/dl is desirable)

     iv. Triglycerides: normal range is 50 to 160 mg/dl

2. Noninvasive methods of cardiac diagnosis

    a. **Electrocardiography:** records electrical activity of the heart

       i. Basic information

          (a) Identifies

             (1) Basic cardiac rhythm

             (2) Arrhythmias and conduction defects

             (3) Ischemia or infarction

             (4) Electrolyte abnormalities

             (5) Drug effects

             (6) Hypertrophy of ventricles and enlargement of atria

             (7) Anatomic orientation of heart

          (b) ECG paper (Fig. 2–13)

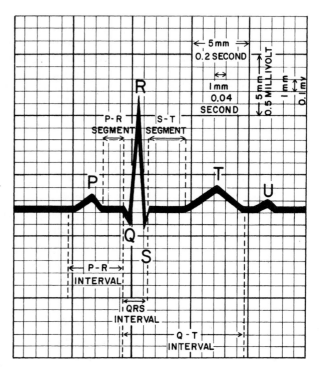

Figure 2-13 • Normal electrocardiogram (ECG) complex.

(1) Time is measured along horizontal axis
  a) Each small (1-mm) box = 0.04 second
  b) Each large (5-mm) box = 0.20 second
  c) Normal speed of paper: 25 mm/second
  d) Measures/records the P wave, QRS complex, and T wave (in time), as well as PR and QT intervals
(2) Voltage is measured in the vertical direction
  a) Each small box (1-mm) = 0.1 mV
  b) Each large box (5-mm) = 0.5 mV
  c) Usual calibration standard is 10 mm = 1 mV
  d) Measures and records amplitude and voltage of P wave, QRS complex, and T wave
  e) Useful in detection of atrial and ventricular hypertrophy
(c) Deflections: the waves of the ECG recording are either above or below the isoelectric line
  (1) Isoelectric line is the straight baseline of the ECG recording, indicating either no electrical forces or none strong enough to generate a wave (segment of ECG from the end of T or U [if U present] wave to the P wave)
  (2) Positive deflections occur when the heart's depolarization wave *moves toward* the positive electrode of the recording lead
  (3) Negative deflections occur when the heart's depolarization wave *moves away from* the positive electrode of the recording lead

(4) Biphasic deflections occur when the heart's depolarization wave is moving both toward and away from the positive electrode. If the wave of depolarization is perpendicular to the positive electrode, waves are small or absent

ii. Cardiac conduction cycle (see Fig. 2–9)

(a) P wave represents atrial depolarization

(1) The right atrium begins depolarization earlier than the left atrium

(2) Normal P wave duration is < 0.10 seconds

(3) Normal amplitude of P wave ≤ 2.5 mm. P waves greater than 2.5 mm in amplitude in any lead are abnormal

(4) "2.5 × 2.5 rule" (handy rule of thumb): a P wave should not be wider than 2.5 mm (left atrial enlargement) or taller than 2.5 mm (right atrial enlargement)

(5) Causes of abnormal P waves

a) Atrial hypertrophy: increased P amplitude or width

b) Right atrial hypertrophy: tall, peaked P waves in leads II, III, or aVF. May show tall or biphasic P waves in V_1 (>2.5 mm in width)

c) Left atrial hypertrophy: wide, notched P waves in limb leads and V_4 to V_6 and/or P waves with broad negative deflection in lead V_1 (larger than 1 mm); P > 2.5 mm in width

(b) PR interval represents time required for atrial depolarization and conduction through AV node

(1) Measure from beginning of P wave to beginning of QRS complex

(2) Normal interval: 0.12 to 0.20 seconds

(3) PR segment represents normal delay of impulse in AV node: electrically silent or isoelectric. A prolonged delay (PR interval > 0.20 seconds) indicates diseased AV node, ischemia, drug effects, or increased vagal tone

(c) A Q wave is present if the first deflection of the QRS is negative

(1) Small physiologic Q waves are usually seen in leads I, aVL, V_5, and V_6, as well as in inferior leads II, III, and aVF

(2) Abnormal when greater than 0.04 second wide (0.03 seconds in inferior leads II, III, and aVF) and more than 25% of R wave amplitude. Large Q waves are usual in leads III, aVR, and V_1

(3) Significant in myocardial infarction, left ventricular hypertrophy

(d) R wave is the first positive deflection occurring in the QRS complex with ventricular depolarization. Prominent R waves may be seen in patients with ventricular hypertrophy, young adults, persons with thin chests, and patients with Wolff-Parkinson-White (WPW) syndrome

(e) S wave is a negative deflection that follows an R wave during ventricular depolarization

(f) QRS complex

(1) Represents entire ventricular depolarization

(2) Measured from onset of Q wave (or R wave if no Q wave is present) to end of QRS

(3) Normal duration: 0.06 to 0.10 second; borderline at 0.11 seconds

(4) Abnormal if 0.12 second or longer; indicative of intraventricular conduction delay; seen in patients with bundle branch blocks (0.12 or greater), WPW syndrome, and hyperkalemia

(5) Atrial repolarization occurs during this time frame but is obscured by QRS

(g) ST segment represents initial ventricular repolarization

(1) Measure immediately after QRS complex to beginning of T wave; normally isoelectric

(2) Prolonged ST segment is caused by hypocalcemia

(3) Elevated ST segment is caused by pericarditis, injury, acute infarctions, left ventricular aneurysms

(4) Depressed ST segment may indicate subendocardial injury or ischemia, electrolyte disturbances, drug effect, or early repolarization, or it may be nonspecific

(h) T wave represents ventricular repolarization

(1) Inverted T waves may be associated with infarctions, ischemia, injury, or hypertrophy

(2) Tall, peaked T waves may be caused by hyperkalemia or acute injury or may be a normal variant

(i) QT interval: represents complete duration of ventricular depolarization and repolarization

(1) Measure from the beginning of the Q wave to the end of the T wave

(2) QT interval varies with heart rate, gender, and age. The corrected QT interval (QTc) takes heart rate into account and provides a normal range corrected for heart rate. In general, a QTc of 0.44 second or more in males and a QTc of 0.45 second in females are considered abnormal

(3) Causes of prolonged QTc include ischemia, electrolyte imbalances (hypocalcemia), hypertrophy, antiarrhythmic drugs (quinidine, procainamide, amiodarone), and congenital prolongation

(4) Prolonged QTc is associated with an increased incidence of polymorphic ventricular tachycardia (torsade de pointes) and, potentially, sudden death

(5) Causes of shortened QTc: acute ischemia, hypercalcemia, and drugs (digitalis)

iii. 12-lead ECG

(a) Standard limb leads (bipolar): two electrodes of opposing polarity ($+/-$) are used to record electrical activity. These bipolar electrodes are placed on patient's arms/legs

(1) Lead I: right arm negative, left arm positive

(2) Lead II: right arm negative, left leg positive

(3) Lead III: left arm negative, left leg positive

(b) Augmented limb leads (unipolar): record electrical activity between one positive electrode (unipolar) and the ECG machine-calculated sum of the other two standard limb electrodes. The wave amplitude is then augmented (enhanced voltage) for ease of visualization

    (1) aVR: right arm positive electrode, normally a negative deflection

    (2) aVL: left arm positive electrode; usually a positive deflection

    (3) aVF: left leg positive electrode; usually a positive deflection

(c) Precordial (chest) leads: record electrical activity between one positive electrode (unipolar) and the ECG machine-calculated sum of the three standard limb electrodes

    (1) V_1: fourth intercostal space, right sternal border

    (2) V_2: fourth intercostal space, left sternal border

    (3) V_3: halfway between V_2 and V_4

    (4) V_4: fifth intercostal space, left midclavicular line

    (5) V_5: level with V_4, left anterior axillary line

    (6) V_6: level with V_4, left midaxillary line

    (7) R waves get progressively larger (normal R-wave progression) moving from V_1 toward V_6. (V_5 is often slightly higher than V_6)

    (8) V_4R: fifth intercostal space, right midclavicular line (for right ventricular infarcts)

(d) Miscellaneous monitoring leads

    (1) Modified chest lead 1 (MCL_1)

        a) Electrode placement (similar to lead V_1)

            i) Positive: fourth intercostal space, right sternal border

            ii) Negative: below left clavicle, midclavicular line

            iii) Ground: below the right clavicle

        b) Typical pattern of PQRST is negative

        c) Helps differentiate ventricular arrhythmias from supraventricular arrhythmias with RBBB aberrancy

            i) When the first beat of a run of ectopic beats has an rsR' or RSR' pattern, an RBBB with aberration is indicated

            ii) Left ventricular ectopy: in the "rabbit ears" configuration, the left peak is taller than the right peak (Rsr' pattern). Other indicators of left ventricular ectopy are R, QR, or qR in this lead

        d) Differentiation between right and left ventricular ectopy is possible

            i) Right ventricular ectopy: negative QRS complex

            ii) Left ventricular ectopy: positive QRS deflection, may also be a biphasic (QR, qR) or monophasic (R) pattern

        e) RBBB and LBBB may be differentiated

            i) RBBB: a classical rSR' pattern

            ii) LBBB: a mostly negative QS or rS pattern

    (2) Lewis lead: used for amplifying P wave

        a) A bipolar chest lead

        b) Negative electrode (right atrium) placed on second intercostal space, right of sternum *c)* Positive electrode (left atrium) placed on fourth intercostal space, right of sternum

      d) Ground electrode placed on fourth intercostal space, right of sternum

      e) Record tracing on lead I

    (3) Esophageal pill leads (a small gelatin capsule enclosing an electrode and attached to a thin wire) or transvenous leads are occasionally helpful in differentiating supraventricular from ventricular rhythms

iv. ECG and rhythm assessment

  (a) Analyze ECG rhythms systematically to include

    (1) Rates (atrial and ventricular)

    (2) Rhythm (regular, irregular, pattern if irregular)

    (3) P wave identification

      a) Relationship to QRS (before, after)

      b) Configuration or morphology

    (4) PR interval measurement

    (5) QRS complex measurement, configuration

    (6) ST segment (isoelectric, depressed, elevated)

    (7) T wave (size, shape, direction)

    (8) Arrhythmia origin: identify if possible

    (9) Possible patient and nursing implications

  (b) Rhythm categories: features and common causes

    (1) Sinus origin

      a) Sinus rhythm (normal sinus rhythm)

        i) Rate: 50 to 100 per minute

        ii) Rhythm: regular

        iii) P waves:

          [a] Normal and upright in leads II, III, aVF

          [b] Precede each QRS complex

          [c] Identical size and shape in any given lead

        iv) PR interval: 0.12 to 0.20 seconds

        v) Hemodynamics: optimum cardiac rhythm

      b) Sinus arrhythmia

        i) Only rhythm varies

        ii) PP or RR intervals vary by more than 0.16 seconds

        iii) Usually related to respiration; RR interval shortens during inspiration (see respiratory reflex, in Neurologic Control of Heart section earlier)

        iv) Causes: normal in children (vagal responses during crying, respirations), healthy young adults; older adults may have SA node disease as cause. Uncommon in middle-aged adults

      c) Sinus bradycardia

        i) Regular rhythm

        ii) Heart rate: less than 50 beats/minute

        iii) PQRST complexes and intervals normal

        iv) Causes: may be normal during sleep and in athletes' hearts; also seen with hypothermia, increased intracranial pressure, decreased sympathetic tone, increased parasympathetic tone, the Valsalva maneuver, carotid massage, vomiting, drugs (beta blockers, calcium channel blockers), hypothyroidism

  v) Hemodynamics: rate dependent; cardiac output is generally not affected until rate is less than 50 beats/minute

d) Sinus tachycardia

  i) Regular rhythm

  ii) Heart rate: 100 to 200 beats/minute (a heart rate over 100 beats/minute is unusual for a resting ECG)

  iii) PQRST complex and intervals normal

  iv) Causes: secondary to anxiety, exercise, pain, hyperthyroidism, shock, anemia, fever, hypoxia, hypercapnia, heat exposure, drugs, heart failure (early sign)

  v) Hemodynamics: depends on atrial rate, contractile state of myocardium, circulating blood volume

e) Sinus block (sinus exit block)

  i) SA node initiates impulse, depolarization of SA node occurs; defect is in conduction to atria

  ii) PQRST not generated because of blocked impulse

  iii) Ventricular rhythm remains regular. Intervals before and after pause are twice (or a multiple of) the normal RR interval

  iv) Sinus Wenckebach is also possible

f) Sinus arrest or sinus pause

  i) SA node fails, no impulse initiated, atrial standstill

  ii) PQRST complex is not seen

  iii) Sinus pause if less than 3.0 seconds long

  iv) Sinus arrest if 3.0 seconds or more long

  v) Pause is usually greater than two regular RR intervals

  vi) Causes of both SA blocks and pauses include increased vagal stimulation (i.e., by suctioning), myocardial infarction, myocarditis, drug effects (e.g., from digitalis)

g) Sick sinus syndrome

  i) Term used for a variety of rhythms, attributed to sinus node dysfunction, that may include

    [a] Inappropriate sinus bradycardia

    [b] Sinus arrest or sinus exit block

    [c] Combinations of SA or AV conduction disturbances

    [d] Paradoxical periods of atrial tachycardias (regular or irregular rhythms) alternating with periods of very slow atrial and ventricular rates (bradycardia-tachycardia syndrome)

  ii) Any or all of these arrhythmias may be documented at various times *iii)* The decreased cardiac output that may result from sick sinus syndrome interferes with cerebral perfusion, causing syncope or presyncope. Other symptoms related to hypoperfusion (fatigue, mentation changes) may also occur

   iv) Other escape pacemakers fail to initiate impulses when the SA node fails

   v) Causes include coronary heart disease, acute myocardial infarction, drugs (e.g., digitalis, beta blockers, antiarrhythmics), aging (this syndrome is seen predominantly in elderly persons)

   vi) Implantation of a permanent pacemaker is the usual therapy

  h) Wandering atrial pacemaker

   i) P waves change shape and direction

   ii) PR interval varies from short to normal

   iii) Thought to be caused by a shifting of focus along an extended sinus node or multiple sinus nodes

   iv) Causes: origin confusing, could be sinus, atrial, nodal. The examiner should check for digitalis toxicity, myocarditis

 (2) Atrial origin

  a) Premature atrial contraction (PACs)

   i) Early atrial impulse, interrupting the inherent regular rhythm

   ii) P waves of ectopic beats are morphologically different from sinus P waves

   iii) PR interval of the PAC may be different. Conduction may be shortened, normal, lengthened, or blocked

   iv) Normal QRS complex if ventricular repolarization was complete; abnormal QRS complex if conducted aberrantly (ventricle partially repolarized); no QRS complex if beat arrived too early during the ventricle's absolute refractory period (i.e., blocked PAC)

   v) Usually no compensatory pause, but may have a partial pause

   vi) Causes: stimulants (caffeine, tobacco, alcohol [ETOH]), hypoxia, drugs, digitalis toxicity, atrial enlargement

  b) Atrial tachycardia

   i) Atrial rate: 100 to 250 beats/minute

   ii) Reentrant type of atrial tachycardia is more common, often occurs as paroxysmal (sudden starts and stops) atrial tachycardia (PAT). The mechanism is a reentry phenomenon occurring in the atrium itself

   iii) P waves best seen in lead V_1

   iv) PP or RR interval is absolutely regular

v) Visible P waves differ from normal; P waves may be buried in preceding T wave

vi) QRS looks normal

vii) Atrial tachycardia resulting from an ectopic focus in the atria is less common. RR interval may vary if associated with AV block

c) Multifocal atrial tachycardia (chaotic atrial tachycardia)

i) Rates vary from 100 to 200 beats/minute

ii) Rhythm varies widely

iii) P-wave morphology changes (three or more in a 10-second strip)

iv) PR intervals vary

v) Origin: several ectopic foci in the atria that initiate impulses

vi) Often associated with chronic pulmonary disease, hypoxia

vii) If rate is less than 100, the rhythm is technically a multifocal (chaotic) atrial rhythm

d) Atrial flutter

i) Atrial rates from 200 to 350 beats/minute

ii) Ventricular rates, along with rhythm, may be constant at 2:1, 3:1, 4:1 (more often) or may vary, if there is a variable AV conduction block

iii) Flutter waves appear as wide, sawtooth waves representing rapid atrial depolarization, persist through QRS complexes, and are best seen in leads II, III, and aVF

iv) Origin: reentry

v) According to the "rule of 150," a supraventricular tachycardia (SVT) at a rate of 150 is atrial flutter with a 2:1 block until proven differently

e) Atrial fibrillation

i) Atrial rates: 350 to 650 beats/minute

ii) Chaotic, disorganized, and rapid atrial activity producing irregular fibrillatory waves of varying amplitude; best seen in V_1 ("whitecaps" in V_1); no P waves on the ECG

iii) Ventricular rhythm is irregular because atrial impulses are randomly conducted through the AV junction

iv) QRS often looks normal, but aberrantly conducted beats are often seen when a long RR interval is followed by a short RR interval, before ventricle is fully repolarized (Ashman's phenomenon)

v) Risk of atrial thrombi with atrial fibrillation

vi) If ventricular rhythm becomes regular ("regularization of atrial fibrillation"), digitalis toxicity should be suspected

(3) AV junctional origin: The AV junction includes cells in the low atrium just above the AV node, the AV node itself, and the bundle of His

a) Premature junctional beats and contractions (PJB, PJC)
  i) Early beat, disrupts rhythm and sinus pacing cadence
  ii) Originates in the AV junction, spreading both antegrade and retrograde
  iii) If origin is high in the AV junction, the atria depolarize in a retrograde manner first (producing an inverted P wave); then the ventricles depolarize. The P wave precedes the QRS and is inverted. The PR interval is shortened (<0.12 second)
  iv) If the origin is low in the AV junction, the ventricles depolarize first, producing a QRS complex, followed by a retrograde P wave
  v) The P wave is inverted in the inferior leads (II, III, aVF)
  vi) When conduction to the atria and ventricles occurs simultaneously, the P wave is buried in the QRS complex
  vii) QRS complex is usually normal
b) Junctional escape rhythm
  i) Rate is 40 to 60 beats/minute
  ii) RR interval is extremely regular
  iii) P-wave morphology as stated in previous section on PJB
  iv) QRS complex is normal
  v) Origin: SA node automaticity is suppressed and the next fastest pacemaker (AV node) takes over
  vi) Common causes: myocardial infarction, ischemia, electrolyte imbalances, atrial myopathy, parasympathetic stimulation, digitalis, other drug effects
  vii) Accelerated junctional rhythm rates are 60 to 100 beats/minute
c) AV junctional tachycardia
  i) An usurping rhythm
  ii) Ventricular rates of 100 to 160 beats/minute
  iii) Rhythm is extremely regular
  iv) P-wave morphology: as stated in earlier section on PJB
  v) QRS complex usually normal, narrow
  vi) Often caused by digitalis toxicity
(4) AV nodal reentrant tachycardia (AVNRT), previously called paroxysmal supraventricular tachycardia (PSVT) or PAT
  a) AV node reentry mechanism
    i) Two or more electrical pathways (one fast with a longer refractory period, one slow with a shorter refractory period) exist and meet proximally and distally
    ii) They include accessory AV pathways or AV nodal pathways

   iii) Impulse goes down one pathway and back up the other pathway (retrograde); caused by refractoriness or structural changes

  b) ECG features:

   i) Impulse often begins abruptly with a PAC

   ii) Atrial and ventricular rates are 170 to 250 beats/minute with regular rhythm

   iii) P waves are retrograde and

    [a] Buried in the QRS complex, not visible (80%)

    [b] Are seen just after the QRS complex (10%)

    [c] Occur just before the QRS complex (10%)

(5) Wolff-Parkinson-White (WPW) syndrome

 a) Abnormal accessory pathways (bypass tracts) exist between the atria and ventricles. Impulse may be conducted rapidly down an anomalous pathway (bypassing the AV node) to stimulate the ventricles (preexcitation)

 b) A fusion complex known as a "delta wave" results when part of the ventricles depolarizes by the normal depolarization pathways through the AV node, whereas some ventricular depolarization is via the bypass tract

 c) A shortened PR interval (<0.12 seconds) occurs, because initial ventricular activation via the anomalous tract bypasses the AV node delay

 d) WPW syndrome is congenital

 e) The delta wave is often intermittently seen

 f) Associated with tachycardias caused by reentry (atrioventricular reciprocating tachycardia [AVRT] or by very rapid atrial fibrillation via the bypass tract. The AVRT associated wtih WPW is almost always narrow (orthodromic, going down the AV node) and rarely wide (antichromic)

 g) Atrial fibrillation associated with the syndrome may be lethal and warrant ablation (radiofrequency or surgical) of the bypass tract

(6) Supraventricular tachycardia

 a) Catch-all term describing any regular tachycardia originating above the bifurcation of the bundle of His for which P waves are not readily discernible and the QRS complex is normal (PSVT, PAT)

 b) Hemodynamic consequences of SVT can be significant because of

  i) Loss of effective atrial contraction (atrial kick); decreasing ventricular filling by approximately 15%, causing cardiac output decrease

  ii) Decreased stroke volume from decreased diastolic ventricular filling time, decreasing cardiac output, blood pressure (BP)

  iii) Coronary artery blood flow diminished, may induce myocardial ischemia *iv)* Myocardial oxygen demands increased, may induce ischemia

  (7) Ventricular origin

   a) Premature ventricular contractions (PVCs)

    i) Usurping, early beat originating from various locations in the ventricles

    ii) Wide, bizarre QRS complexes of varying morphology (>0.12 second) because origin is different and conduction is slow

    iii) Retrograde conduction of the atria may occur

    iv) Compensatory pause usually occurs. SA node rate is not altered, so the next occurring sinus beat that is able to conduct through to the ventricles will produce a normal QRS complex on time

    v) A "full compensatory" pause: RR intervals surrounding the PVC equal two sinus-cycle intervals. To measure,

     [a] Mark off two normal RR intervals (three R waves) with calipers or paper (Fig. 2–14)

     [b] Place the first mark on the QRS complex immediately preceding the PVC; the third mark should fall on the QRS complex of the normal beat immediately following the PVC if fully compensated

    vi) Interpolated PVCs: occur early enough to allow the ventricles to repolarize before the next beat and do not disrupt the rhythm; no compensatory pause is seen

    vii) In the MCL_1 lead, the QRS complex of a PVC originating in the left ventricle is mostly positive; a PVC from the right ventricle is mostly negative

   b) Ventricular escape rhythm

    i) Impulses from higher centers (SA or AV node) either are not generated or are blocked. Ventricles initiate "escape" rhythm that is based on the inherent automaticity of the ventricular tissue

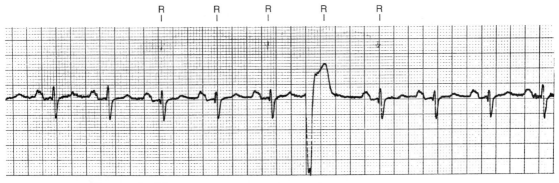

Figure 2–14 • Measuring the compensatory pause of premature ventricular complexes.

       ii) Rate is 20 to 40 beats/minute (usually 20 to 30 beats/minute), rarely less than 20 beats/minute

      iii) Rhythm: usually very regular

      iv) QRS complex: wide, bizarre

      v) No P wave association with QRS complex

c) Accelerated ventricular rhythm (slow ventricular tachycardia)

      i) Rate: 40 to 100 beats/minute

      ii) QRS complex: wide, bizarre

      iii) Usually benign without hemodynamic consequences

      iv) Often seen with acute myocardial infarction

d) Ventricular tachycardia (VT)

      i) Three or more consecutive PVCs

      ii) Sustained or nonsustained (if less than 30 beats)

      iii) RR interval is mostly regular

      iv) QRS complexes wide and bizarre

      v) Rates may be 100 to 250 beats/minute

      vi) Retrograde P waves may be present, but usually there is AV dissociation (diagnostic if seen)

      vii) Fusion beats may be seen and are diagnostic of VT (represent simultaneous ventricular depolarization from the ventricular focus and the normal conduction from above, look like a cross between the normal and ventricular QRS complex)

      viii) SVT with aberration can easily mimic VT

        [a] Check initiating beat of tachycardia; if a PAC, arrhythmia is characteristic of SVT with aberration. If a PVC, is characteristic of VT

        [b] Indicators of VT rather than SVT with aberration

          □ Marked left-axis deviation ($> -30°$)

          □ Left peak of QRS complex is taller than right in lead V_1

          □ An rS configuration in lead V_6

          □ QRS width of more than 0.15 seconds

e) Torsade de pointes (twisting of points)

      i) A form of VT (actually halfway between VT and ventricular fibrillation)

      ii) Irregular and wide QRS complexes undulate and twist on isoelectric axis

      iii) Invariably associated wtih a prolonged QT interval (QTc > 0.46 second)

      iv) Rates from 150 to 250 beats/minute

      v) Usually terminates spontaneously after 5 to 30 seconds but may continue and degenerate into ventricular fibrillation

      vi) Seen with electrolyte imbalances: hypomagnesemia, hypokalemia, or in association with antiarrhythmic drug therapy (quinidine, procainamide, disopyramide, lidocaine) and tricyclic antidepressants

vii) Cardiovert/defibrillate, if hemodynamically unstable

viii) May be terminated by $MgSO_4$ or by speeding the heart rate to shorten the QT interval (through pacing, isoproterenol)

ix) Correct causative factor. Temporary overdrive pacing may be needed until causative factor is removed

x) Does not respond to antiarrhythmic therapy, which may aggravate condition

f) Ventricular fibrillation (V fib)

    i) Uncoordinated chaotic activity of ventricles

    ii) Erratic waveforms with no discernible PQRST complexes

    iii) Coarse V fib: obvious coarse baseline

    iv) Fine V fib: small or barely discernible waveforms, may be mistaken for asystole

g) Ventricular asystole (standstill)

    i) No ventricular activity; no QRS complex

    ii) P waves; seen if sinus rhythm is maintained

(8) Av conduction defects

a) First-degree AV block

    i) Impulse is delayed at the AV junction

    ii) PR interval greater than 0.20 second

    iii) Every sinus beat is conducted to the ventricles, producing a normal QRS complex for every P wave

b) Second-degree AV block: Impulses are not all conducted through the AV node. Some P waves will not be followed by a QRS complex. There are two types:

    i) Type I (Mobitz I or Wenckebach): process located in the AV node; related to infarction, drug effect, or vagal effect

        [a] Progressive delay in conduction through the AV node until a QRS complex is dropped

        [b] PR interval gradually increases until impulse fails to conduct through the AV junctional tissue, producing a dropped QRS complex at varying or constant intervals (grouped beating)

        [c] PR interval is shortest after each dropped beat

        [d] PP interval constant (if sinus rhythm; untrue if sinus arrhythmia)

        [e] RR interval progressively shortens

        [f] P waves and QRS complexes are normal

    ii) Type II (Mobitz II): less common, more serious, involves the bundle branches

              [a] SA node fires regularly, producing a constant PP interval

              [b] An impulse fails to conduct to ventricles (no QRS complex seen)

              [c] PR intervals are constant with conducted beats (unlike those in type I)

              [d] RR interval varies depending on the degree of block (2:1, 3:1)

        iii) Second-degree AV block with 2:1 conduction is a special case and may be either Mobitz I or II

              [a] Narrow, "normal"-looking QRS complex suggests Mobitz I

              [b] Wider QRS complex (i.e., bundle branch block or left ventricular conduction delay) suggests Mobitz II

              [c] Examine other rhythms with same patient; if other examples of clear Wenckebach are seen, the 2:1 is probably Mobitz I, not Mobitz II

    c) Third-degree (complete) AV block: occurs anywhere in the AV node or bundle of His

        i) No conduction of sinus impulses

        ii) Two pacemakers become apparent. Upper: SA node fires normally. Lower: ventricles respond to an escape pacemaker

        iii) Two independent rhythms

        iv) P waves and QRS complexes not associated

        v) PP intervals are regular, rate is typically 60 to 100 beats/minute, if sinus rhythm

        vi) RR interval is usually extremely regular, rate depends on the site and inherent rate of the escape pacemaker

(9) Intraventricular conduction defects

    a) LBBB

        i) RBB is activated first

        ii) Impulse spreads from right ventricle, then back to septum and through the left ventricle distal to the LBBB

        iii) Prolonged activation time of the septum and the left ventricle

        iv) QRS duration prolonged more than .12 seconds (usually more than .13 seconds)

        v) Two or more of the left-sided leads (leads I, aVL, V_5, or V_6) show the RR′ pattern

        vi) Leads V_1 and V_6 afford best views

              [a] V_1 and V_2; a predominately negative complex of QS or rS pattern

              [b] V_6: always positive with broad R wave

              [c] Absence of small Q wave and S wave in leads I, aVL, V_5, and V_6

    b) RBBB

        i) Left ventricle and septum are activated normally; then impulse slowly spreads to the right ventricle

        ii) QRS duration prolonged (>0.12 second)

        iii) V_1 and/or V_2: QRS is triphasic with an rSR′ configuration

        iv) Broad S wave in leads I, aVL, and V_6

        v) Lead V_6: QRS is also triphasic with a qRS configuration

    c) Left anterior fascicular block

        i) Block in the anterior-superior fascicle of the left bundle; the impulse travels through the posterior-inferior fascicle first and then the anterior-superior fascicle

        ii) Produces an exaggerated left axis deviation of more than $-45°$

        iii) Small r and large S waves found in leads II, III, and aVF

        iv) QRS duration: upper limits of normal (0.10 to 0.11 seconds)

        v) Persistent (prominent) S in V_6

        vi) Terminal R in aVR occurs later than terminal R in aVL

    d) Left posterior fascicular block (extremely rare)

        i) Lesion in the posterior-inferior fascicle of the left bundle; the impulse travels through the anterior-superior fascicle first and then to the posterior-inferior fascicle

        ii) Produces an exaggerated right axis deviation of more than 120°

        iii) Small q and tall R waves in leads II, III, and aVF

        iv) Small r waves and large S waves in leads I and aVR

        v) Right ventricular hypertrophy must be excluded clinically before diagnosis of left posterior hemiblock can be made (unless a previous ECG is present to confirm the left posterior fascicular block change)

(c) ECG interpretation of ischemia and infarction (see Myocardial Infarction section later)

(d) ECG changes with potassium imbalances

  (1) Hypokalemia

    a) Prominent U wave (when U-wave height is the same as T-wave height, potassium level is usually ≤3.0 mEq/L)

    b) T-wave amplitude decreased

    c) ST segment depressed

    d) P wave may be prominent

    e) PR interval may be prolonged

    f) Prolonged QTc interval (actually QT-U)

    g) "Stair-stepping" pattern is almost diagnostic ("walk up the stairs" in between the R waves) (Fig. 2–15)

Figure 2–15 • "Stair-stepping" electrocardiographic findings for hypokalemia.

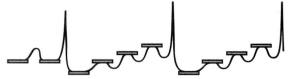

(2) Hyperkalemia
  a) T wave symmetrically peaked (usually ≥10 mm), narrowed, and elevated at serum levels above 5.5 mEq/L
  b) At 6.5 mEq/L and above, the PR interval increases, and the P wave gets smaller or disappears
  c) QRS pattern widens to sine wave at 7.5 mEq/L and above
(e) ECG changes with calcium imbalances
  (1) Hypocalcemia creates a prolonged QTc interval and a prolonged isoelectric ST segment
  (2) Hypercalcemia creates a shortened QTc interval, and the ST segment is shortened or absent
  (3) T waves are generally unchanged
b. *Chest x-ray:* is used to visualize
  i. Cardiac size, position, and chamber size
  ii. Abnormalities of the heart, great vessels, lungs, pleura, and ribs
  iii. Pulmonary vasculature
  iv. Position of catheters, lines, and pacemaker leads
c. *Echocardiography:* one of most important noninvasive tools
  i. High-frequency ultrasound vibrations are emitted via a transducer on the patient's chest or in the esophagus. The returning echo of the sound waves is received. The image is created and recorded for interpretation
  ii. Provides information on
    (a) Chamber size and function, to include
      (1) Left ventricular function: ejection fraction (EF)
      (2) Left ventricular wall motion (shows areas of hypokinesis, akinesis, dyskinesis), wall thickness, cavity size
      (3) Papillary muscle function
      (4) Cardiomyopathy
    (b) Valvular morphology and function
      (1) Cardiac calcifications
      (2) Mitral valve prolapse
      (3) Stenotic valves
      (4) Intracardiac masses to include tumors, thrombi, and valvular vegetations
      (5) Function of prosthetic ball valves
    (c) Congenital defects and shunts (e.g., atrial septal defects, ventricular septal defects)
    (d) Pericardial disease
      (1) Pericardial effusion
      (2) Cardiac tamponade
  iii. M-mode, an early form, is used to measure intracardiac structures with a narrow ultrasound beam, providing a one-dimensional view of the heart. It is used to measure chamber size and wall thickness

    iv. Two-dimensional echocardiography provides real-time imagery of cardiac structures by means of a two-dimensional ultrasound beam, giving a wider view of the heart and its structures

    v. Doppler echocardiography: the change of sound frequencies produced by changes in direction and velocity (the Doppler effect) is used to demonstrate the velocity and direction of blood flow through the heart and great vessels

    vi. Color flow imaging: Doppler signals are processed to depict real-time blood flow superimposed on two-dimensional echocardiogram. Red represents flow towards transducer; blue represents flow away from transducer. Lighter shades mean higher velocity. Used to evaluate shunts, regurgitation, increased velocities

    vii. Stress echocardiography: images obtained before and after exercise or stress induction

       (a) Methods used include treadmill (most common) and pharmacologic stressing (dobutamine)

       (b) Dobutamine: beta$_1$-adrenergic stimulating agent. Increases heart rate and cardiac output, decreases end-systolic volume, increases EF

       (c) Ischemia results in a region of hypokinesis (decreased wall motion)

       (d) Evaluates extent and location of CAD, including ischemic mitral regurgitation

    viii. Transesophageal echocardiography (TEE): transducer placed in esophagus

       (a) Capable of exquisite definition of cardiac structure and function because of its proximity to the heart

       (b) Often used in subjects with poor acoustic penetration of ultrasound from the chest (e.g., patients with COPD, heavy build) and in the operating room to evaluate the results of cardiac surgery

d. *Exercise electrocardiography (exercise stress testing)*

    i. An electrocardiogram performed during exercise

    ii. Indications for exercise testing

       (a) Suspected CAD

       (b) To evaluate response to exercise and functional capacity in patients known to have CAD (such as after myocardial infarction, after angioplasty, undergoing coronary bypass surgery) and to assess risk, severity, and prognosis

       (c) To evaluate effectiveness of revascularization or medical therapy for CAD

       (d) To evaluate arrhythmias, especially exercise-induced ventricular tachycardia

       (e) To monitor patient's progress while enrolled in a cardiac rehabilitation program and to set safe exercise levels

       (f) To evaluate patients with rate-responsive pacemakers

       (g) To screen persons entering physical fitness programs or high-risk professionals (e.g., airline pilots) for CAD

    iii. Contraindications to exercise testing may be

       (a) Acute myocardial infarction

       (b) Unstable (preinfarction) angina (on effort)

    (c) Uncompensated CHF

    (d) Severe aortic stenosis (examiner must listen to patient's heart and carotid arteries before exercise test)

    (e) Uncontrolled arrhythmias: conduction defects greater than those in first-degree AV block

    (f) Severe left main CAD

    (g) Pulmonary embolus, infarct

    (h) Severe illnesses such as fulminant infections, asthma, and renal failure

    (i) Uncontrolled, severe hypertension

    (j) Acute pericarditis or myocarditis

  iv. ECG findings suggestive of ischemia and CAD:

    (a) ST segment depression of 1 mm or greater, 80 milliseconds after the J point (the point where the ST segment "takes off" from the QRS complex) with a flat or down-sloping ST segment from a normal baseline; or 1.5 mm or more at 80 milliseconds with an up-sloping ST depression

    (b) Chest discomfort induced by exercise is very suggestive of CAD, even with a normal ECG response

  v. Findings suggestive of severe coronary heart disease (multivessel or left main coronary artery disease):

    (a) Marked ST segment depression, greater than 2 mm at 80 milliseconds after the J point

    (b) Recovery of ST segment changes or symptoms back to normal takes more than 6 minutes

    (c) Exercise-induced hypotension

    (d) Exercise-induced ventricular tachycardia

  vi. Limitations

    (a) Patient must be able to exercise to at least 85% of the maximum predicted heart rate to have a successful test

    (b) Starting ECG must have normal ST segments at baseline

    (c) Insensitive to single-vessel disease (will miss 40% of such cases: false-negative result)

    (d) False-positive results are frequent in patients at low risk, patients taking digoxin, and patients with left ventricular hypertrophy

e. *Magnetic resonance imaging* (MRI): a safe, diagnostic technique involving no ionizing radiation or contrast agents

  i. Provides a two-dimensional view of cardiovascular structure

  ii. Creates a computer-assisted image derived from measuring tissue proton density

  iii. MRI is used to determine:

    (a) Anatomy of the heart

    (b) Congenital heart defects

    (c) Masses in the myocardium, pericardium

    (d) Ventricular aneurysm

    (e) Aortic dissection

  iv. Safe alternative to x-ray for children and pregnant women

  v. As a magnetic device, it interferes with pacemaker function

  vi. Cannot be used with prosthetic metallic devices (valves, prosthetic joints, etc.)

f. *Ultrafast computed tomography:* a form of computed tomography (CT) in which a rapid electron beam is used to create high-speed imaging
   i. Provides two-dimensional image of cardiovascular structures
   ii. Visualizes coronary calcium, silent atherosclerosis
      (a) Amount of calcium is predictive of multivessel CAD
      (b) The greater the amount of calcium, the greater the likelihood of CAD
   iii. Cost limits use at present
g. *Nuclear medicine:* a radioisotope is injected into a peripheral vein, and its presence or uptake can be imaged. Methods include
   i. Multiple-gated acquisition (MUGA) scan
      (a) Used to measure left ventricular EF
      (b) Very accurate unless patient has an irregular rhythm, in which case multiple images cannot be "gated" (superimposed) with the ECG
   ii. Myocardial scintigraphy (perfusion imaging)
      (a) Involves use of thallium-201 or technetium sestamibi to identify ischemia, infarct, and myocardial viability
      (b) Normal myocardium takes up the isotope from the blood and shows increased uptake on exercise
      (c) Decreased myocardial perfusion results in decreased uptake; ischemic sites show normal uptake at rest and decreased uptake on exercise. Infarcted sites show no uptake at all
      (d) Pharmacologic agents (dipyridamole, adenosine) are used to simulate effects of exercise (potentially induce ischemia) in patients who are unable to exercise
      (e) Normal areas show increased uptake, but areas perfused by diseased arteries do not show increase (hence there is a relative decrease)
      (f) Perfusion imaging is extremely useful when the exercise ECG is nondiagnostic for ischemia
   ii. Infarct-avid imaging (myocardial infarct indicators)
      (a) Technetium-99 pyrophosphate is injected into a peripheral vein
      (b) Infarcted areas of the heart show increased levels of radioactivity as "hot spots." These appear within 4 hours of infarction, may not peak until 12 to 24 hours later, and remain positive for 2 to 7 days
      (c) Limited usefulness in acute myocardial infarction; useful when ECG changes are not definitive or when enzyme levels have already returned to normal
   iv. Clinical uses of nuclear medicine: evaluation of
      (a) Ischemic heart disease: (including risk stratification)
      (b) Left ventricular function
h. *Long-term ambulatory monitoring (Holter)*
   i. ECG continuously recording over at least a 24- to 48-hour period
   ii. Used in documenting
      (a) Arrhythmias not demonstrated by resting or exercise ECG, especially with symptoms of palpitations, syncope, and presyncope
      (b) Efficacy of surgical and medical therapy for arrhythmias
      (c) Pacemaker function

(d) Silent ischemia (if proper recording equipment is used)

iii. Records at least two leads: I and V$_5$ simultaneously

iv. Diary is kept by patient to note symptoms (chest pain, palpitations, syncope) and activities during recording period to correlate with rhythm

3. Invasive methods of cardiac diagnosis

a. *Direct arterial blood pressure monitoring:* catheter inserted into artery and attached to pressure transducer that converts and amplifies arterial pressure to electrical waveform for continuous readings. The radial artery is the most commonly used; the femoral artery, second most often

i. Used when there is a need to be alert to blood pressure trends (e.g., during major cardiac surgery, in critically ill patients, with intra-aortic balloon pump, with potent vasopressors and vasodilators). Also used for ventilated patients, multi–arterial blood gas (ABG) testing, acid-base imbalances

ii. Factors influencing arterial waveforms

(a) Increased blood pressure: more rapid, sharp wave peaks

(b) Decreased blood pressure: more rounded wave, smaller or absent dicrotic notch

(c) Hypovolemia: shape and size of wave varies distinctly as stroke volume varies

(d) Arrhythmias: small, irregular waves; varying stroke volume

iii. Mean arterial blood pressure: more accurate and reliable, not as influenced by extraneous factors, used to calculate resistances (e.g., systemic vascular resistance, pulmonary vascular resistance). See Physiologic Anatomy section earlier

iv. Reference pressure transducer to heart level (phlebostatic axis; see Bedside Hemodynamics section later); radial line should be at same level

v. Allen's test: check adequacy of ulnar circulation before radial catheter insertion

(a) Have patient clench his or her fist tightly

(b) Occlude both radial and ulnar arteries

(c) Have patient open hand

(d) Release pressure over ulnar artery (blanches)

(e) Check for capillary filling

vi. Complications of arterial blood pressure monitoring

(a) Hemorrhage

(b) Emboli: distal arterial (air, clots, fibrin)

(c) Vascular occlusion or spasm

(d) Infection

b. *Central venous pressure monitoring:* single- or multilumen catheter placed in central or peripheral vein, positioned in superior vena cava (inferior vena cava for femoral lines) attached to a pressure transducer to allow for continuous monitoring of central venous pressure

i. CVP: pressure is measured in the great veins, reflects right atrial pressure and, consequently, right ventricular end-diastolic filling (RVEDF) pressures (if no tricuspid obstruction)

ii. Used to monitor blood volume, right ventricular function, and central venous return; access also used for fluid, blood, and medication administration

iii. Vein sites: subclavian, internal or external jugular, femoral, basilic

iv. Normal CVP varies from patient to patient

    (a) Monitor the trends in the CVP readings

    (b) CVP of 2 to 6 mm Hg is considered within normal limits

v. CVP decreases with hypovolemia, venodilation, negative-pressure ventilators, right ventricular assist devices, central venous obstruction (masses), decreased venous return

vi. CVP increases with increased blood volume, right-sided heart failure with venoconstriction, cardiac tamponade, positive-pressure breathing, straining

c. *Bedside hemodynamic monitoring via flow-directed, balloon-tipped catheter capable of thermodilution cardiac output determination* (Figs. 2–16 and 2–17). Various catheters available with other ports for transvenous pacing, mixed venous oxygen saturation measurements, additional fluid and medication administration

    i. Allows for continuous bedside hemodynamic monitoring so that vascular tone, myocardial contractility, intracardiac pressures, cardiac output, and fluid balance can be assessed and effectively managed

    ii. Obtain pressure readings with the patient in a comfortable position (0° to 60°), as long as the transducer is at the same level as the marked phlebostatic axis (intersection of the following two lines)

        (a) Draw a line from the fourth intercostal space at the sternum toward the edge of chest and down to the side

        (b) Draw a second line on the side of chest, halfway between the anterior and posterior portions of the chest (midaxillary), running head to foot

        (c) Mark the intersection of the lines on the side of the chest, and place the transducer at the level horizontal to that mark

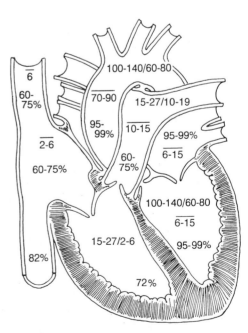

Figure 2–16 • Normal oxygen saturations and pressures in the heart.

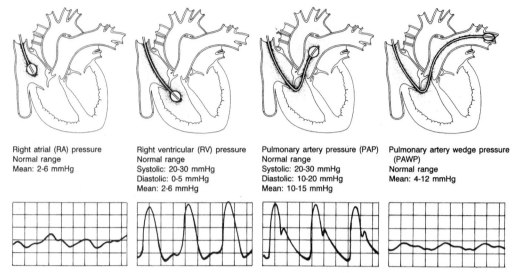

Right atrial (RA) pressure
Normal range
Mean: 2-6 mmHg

Right ventricular (RV) pressure
Normal range
Systolic: 20-30 mmHg
Diastolic: 0-5 mmHg
Mean: 2-6 mmHg

Pulmonary artery pressure (PAP)
Normal range
Systolic: 20-30 mmHg
Diastolic: 10-20 mmHg
Mean: 10-15 mmHg

Pulmonary artery wedge pressure
(PAWP)
Normal range
Mean: 4-12 mmHg

Figure 2–17 • Bedside hemodynamic monitoring via flow-directed, balloon-tipped catheter capable of thermodilution cardiac output determination.

iii. Monitoring right atrial and pulmonary capillary wedge pressures is preferable (instead of only CVP) to assess right and left ventricular dysfunction

iv. Right atrial pressure (RAP) is measured through the proximal port of the catheter

  (a) RAP is the same as right ventricular end-diastolic pressure

  (b) Normal RAP = 2 to 6 mm Hg

  (c) Elevated RAP may indicate

    (1) Intravascular volume overload

    (2) Right ventricular failure

    (3) Tricuspid valve dysfunction (stenosis or regurgitation)

    (4) Pulmonary hypertension, embolism

    (5) Constrictive pericarditis

    (6) Cardiac tamponade

    (7) Left-to-right shunts with right ventricular failure

    (8) Pulmonic stenosis

    (9) Chronic obstructive pulmonary disease

    (10) Right ventricular infarction

  (d) Decreased RAP may indicate

    (1) Hypovolemia (from diuretics, blood loss, burns, vomiting)

    (2) Venodilatation (from nitrates, morphine, hypersensitivity reactions)

v. Right ventricular pressures (RVP): seen when floating catheter into position during insertion

  (a) Catheter must not be left in the right ventricle (VT occurs)

  (b) Normal systolic RVP = 15 to 27 mm Hg and end-diastolic pressure of 2 to 6 mm Hg

  (c) Right ventricular waveform is distinct with sharp upstroke after the QRS and downstroke, no dicrotic notch

  (d) Elevated right ventricular systolic pressures are seen in

    (1) Pulmonary hypertension caused by

      a) Left heart failure (ischemia, left ventricular failure)

    b) Mitral regurgitation, mitral stenosis

    c) Cardiomyopathy

   (2) Pulmonary disease (pulmonary embolism, hypoxemia, COPD)

   (3) Eisenmenger's syndrome: pulmonary hypertension from pulmonary vascular disease; associated with right-to-left shunting, cyanosis

 vi. Pulmonary artery pressures and pulmonary capillary wedge pressure (PCWP) measured through the distal port (see Fig. 2–17)

  (a) Evaluate trends and report significant changes

  (b) Pulmonary artery pressure reflects left- and right-sided heart pressures

  (c) Pulmonary artery systolic pressure represents pressure produced by right ventricle (normal, 15 to 27 mm Hg)

  (d) Increased pulmonary artery pressure is seen with

   (1) Atrial or ventricular septal defects, causing increased pulmonary blood flow as a result of the left-to-right shunt

   (2) Primary pulmonary hypertension, hypoxemia, pulmonary emboli, COPD (increases pulmonary vascular resistance)

   (3) Left ventricular failure and mitral stenosis (increases pulmonary venous pressure), volume overload, decreased left ventricular compliance, ischemia, mitral regurgitation

  (e) Pulmonary artery diastolic pressure generally reflects LVEDP and is used as a measure of left ventricular function and diastolic filling pressures (normal range, 10 to 19 mm Hg)

   (1) Usually 2 to 4 mm Hg higher than mean PCWP or mean LAP

   (2) Correlates fairly well with PCWP in the normal heart, during myocardial infarction, and in left ventricular failure; often used instead of PCWP if obtaining an accurate wedge is impossible

  (f) Pulmonary artery diastolic pressure does not reflect LVEDP with any of the following: in differences between pulmonary artery diastolic pressure and mean PCWP that exceed 4 mm Hg; in heart rates greater than 125 beats/minute; in COPD, adult respiratory distress syndrome, mitral stenosis, or pulmonary embolism (in these instances, the PCWP must be used)

  (g) Pulmonary artery mean: normally less than 10 to 20 mm Hg (used primarily for hemodynamic calculations of pulmonary vascular resistance)

  (h) PCWP (or pulmonary artery wedge pressure [PAWP]) is a reflection of left atrial pressure and is used to assess LVEDP filling pressure = "a" wave

   (1) Balloon of catheter is inflated, wedging in a small branch of the pulmonary artery (see Fig. 2–17)

   (2) PCWP should be 2 to 4 mm Hg less than pulmonary artery diastolic pressure (6 to 15 mm Hg)

   (3) PCWP is elevated in

    a) Left ventricular failure

    b) Constrictive pericarditis

    c) Mitral stenosis or mitral regurgitation

    d) Fluid overload

    e) Ischemia

   (4) PCWP is decreased in

    a) Hypovolemia

    b) Venodilating drugs

 vii. Cardiac output

  (a) Normally 4 to 8 L/minute

  (b) Measured via proximal port by means of thermodilution

   (1) 10-ml of room-temperature 5% dextrose in water (D5W) or 0.9% saline (NS) injectate used (iced solutions, 5 ml, are alternatives)

   (2) Injected at end-expiratory phase of ventilation, in less than 4 seconds

   (3) Attempted three times; readings averaged; falsely high/low readings deleted

   (4) CI, SVR, and PVR are calculated by computer in dynes/second/cm^{-5}:

$$SVR = \frac{MAP - CVP \ (mean)}{CO} \times 80$$

$$PVR = \frac{PA - PCWP}{CO} \times 80$$

  (c) CI: normally 2.5 to 4.0 L/minute/m²

  (d) SVR: normally 900 to 1400 dynes/second/cm^{-5}

  (e) PVR: normally 37 to 250 dynes/second/cm^{-5}

 viii. Complications of hemodynamic monitoring

  (a) Arrhythmias

  (b) Hemorrhage

  (c) Infection

  (d) Thrombi, emboli (air, blood)

  (e) Pneumothorax

  (f) Cardiac perforation

  (g) Electrical microshocks

  (h) Complete heart block

  (i) Pulmonary infarction (balloon left inflated)

 ix. To prevent complications associated with flow-directed balloon-tipped catheters, ensure that

  (a) Balloon is deflated after wedge pressure is obtained, to prevent pulmonary infarction

  (b) Catheter has not wedged when balloon is deflated or has not slipped back into the right ventricle (risk of VT)

  (c) Only 0.8 to 1.5 ml of air is used to inflate the balloon (with 3-ml syringe) (risks of balloon overinflation, possible rupture, and potential emboli or infarctions)

  (d) Catheter is inserted under sterile technique (use catheter guard over the pulmonary artery catheter)

  (e) Introducer sheath is sutured to the skin to prevent catheter migration, which can cause ventricular ectopy; possible perforation of right atrium, right ventricle, or pulmonary artery; or pulmonary infarction because of overwedging

(f) Pressurized, heparinized drip to maintain patency and prevent both clot formation at end of catheter and possible embolization

(g) Distal extremities are evaluated for pulses, swelling, discoloration, and temperature changes indicative of impaired circulation

(h) Electrical equipment in the area is well-grounded and operating correctly (prevent electrically induced ventricular fibrillation)

d. *Cardiac catheterization and angiography:* high-quality coronary images produced by x-ray cineangiography camera or digital imaging. Radiopaque contrast medium is injected into coronary arteries for visualization; recordings are made on video or digital replay. Polaroid-like still photographs are also immediately available for review and documentation.

i. Patients selected include

(a) Asymptomatic patients having

(1) Evidence of significant CAD or severe left ventricular dysfunction on noninvasive tests

(2) Survived a resuscitative effort (VT, V fib)

(b) Symptomatic patients with the following conditions or states

(1) Angina: unstable, variant, or unresponsive to therapy

(2) Atypical chest pain

(3) Post–myocardial infarction

(4) Valvular disease

(5) Congenital heart defects

(6) Aortic disease

(7) Left ventricular failure

ii. Used to identify the following (includes assessing severity and guiding therapy, as needed):

(a) Clinically suspected lesions (e.g., of arteries, valves, muscle tissue, anatomy)

(b) Pathophysiology of cardiac disorders

(c) Left ventricular function

(d) Pressures in cardiac chambers

(e) Cardiac output

iii. Technique

(a) Right heart catheterization performed via the right or left femoral or brachial vein with catheter advanced into the right atrium and then past tricuspid valve into the right ventricle to the pulmonary artery to collect pressure and angiographic data, cardiac outputs, and resistances and to define anatomy

(b) Left heart catheterization performed in a retrograde manner via femoral or brachial artery (or transseptal approach through the right atrium and intra-atrial septum). Catheter is advanced into left ventricle to measure pressure in the chambers and vessels

iv. Left ventriculography: radiopaque contrast medium is injected into left ventricular cavity

(a) Purpose

(1) To evaluate ventricular wall motion and chamber size

a) Akinetic areas: areas of ventricular wall with no motion (e.g., not contracting)

    b) Hypokinetic areas: areas of ventricular wall with less than normal motion in systole
    c) Dyskinetic areas: areas of ventricular wall that bulge during systole
    (2) To determine function, by assessing
        a) End-diastolic volume
        b) End-systolic volume
        c) Stroke volume (modest accuracy)
        d) EF
    (3) To detect ventricular aneurysms
    (4) To evaluate the mitral valve
    (5) To assess prognosis in cardiac surgery
    (6) To demonstrate ventricular shunts
v. Aortography: aorta, aortic valvular insufficiency, saphenous vein grafts, and the aortic arch vessels may be visualized and recorded on film
    (a) Purpose: to determine or diagnose the following
        (1) Aortic valve insufficiency
        (2) Aneurysms or dissections of ascending aorta
        (3) Coarctation of the aorta
        (4) Diseases of the aorta and/or major branches
        (5) Presence of saphenous vein grafts
vi. Coronary arteriography
    (a) Radiopaque contrast material is injected into the ostia of the left and right coronary arteries, allowing for multiple views and recordings of the coronary arterial circulation. Digital computer-assisted technology aids in quantifying results
    (b) Purpose
        (1) To identify extent of significant CAD by noting and grading extent of lesions
            a) 50% of greater lesion: capable of producing ischemia during exercise
            b) 85% or greater lesion: capable of resulting in ischemia at rest
            c) Left main disease (50% or more), three-vessel disease or two-vessel disease (if proximal LAD stenosis is present). Identifies patients whose survival is improved with surgery
            d) Long tubular lesions produce larger degree of flow restriction (at lower percentages) than do discrete lesions
        (2) To guide therapeutic options in ischemic heart disease
        (3) To evaluate atypical angina and coronary arterial spasm (FDA approval withdrawn at present for this use)
        (4) To administer intracoronary thrombolytics
        (5) To perform transcatheter interventional procedures: percutaneous transluminal coronary angioplasty (PTCA), coronary stents, rotational atherectomy
vii. Major complications of cardiac catheterization procedure
    (a) Death: ~0.11% incidence (most frequently seen in left main disease)

(b) Myocardial infarction: ~0.05% incidence

(c) Neurologic events (stroke): ~0.07% incidence

viii. Other complications

(a) Cardiac arrhythmias, bradycardia, conduction disturbances

(b) Hemorrhage or hematoma at insertion site

(c) Arterial perforation, thrombosis, embolus, and dissection

(d) Allergic reactions to contrast medium

(e) Acute renal failure or oliguria caused by contrast medium

(f) Cardiac tamponade (caused by perforation of atrium or ventricle)

(g) Sepsis

(h) Hypovolemia (caused by diuresis from contrast medium)

e. *Intravascular ultrasound* (IVUS): Small ultrasound transducer attached to catheter tip is guided into the coronary artery over a guide wire. Provides high-resolution images. Invaluable in catheterization laboratory for interventional procedures. Assesses

i. Size of lumen, degree of stenosis

ii. Structure of arterial wall

iii. Proper coronary stent placement

iv. Suspected aortic dissections

f. *Electrophysiology studies* (EPS): series of programmed electrical stimuli applied to the heart through pacing electrodes guided under fluoroscopy to record the sequence of activation and to induce arrhythmias

i. Purpose: to reproduce arrhythmias under a controlled environment in order to diagnose and determine the best mode of therapy for control (e.g., medications, pacemaker, ablation procedures)

ii. Patients selected include

(a) Patients who have ventricular or supraventricular tachyarrhythmias that are unresponsive to conventional therapy, in order to guide optimal therapy

(b) Patients at high risk for sudden cardiac death

(c) Patients with unexplained, recurrent syncopal episodes caused by suspected cardiac etiology not demonstrated by noninvasive techniques

(d) Patients who have survived a cardiac arrest without identified etiology

(e) Patients considered for implantable defibrillator

(f) Patients considered for ablation therapy

COMMONLY ENCOUNTERED NURSING DIAGNOSES

Decreased Cardiac Output Due to Cardiac Dysfunction, Either Mechanical or Electrical
(see Patient Health Problems section later)

1. **Assessment for defining characteristics**

a. Fluctuations in patient's hemodynamics: blood pressure, heart rate, cardiac output

b. Arrhythmias observed
c. ECG changes
d. Weakness, fatigue, dizziness
e. Shortness of breath (SOB), dyspnea, rales
f. Cold and clammy skin, cyanosis, pallor
g. Decreased peripheral pulses
h. Decreased or absent urinary output (oliguria or anuria)
i. Jugular vein distention
j. Diminished mentation: loss of consciousness (LOC), orientation
k. Chest pain

2. **Expected outcomes**
a. Decreased work of heart by decreasing myocardial oxygen demands
b. Increased myocardial oxygen supply (minimizing ischemia, size of infarct)
c. Normal hemodynamics: within appropriate range for adequate cardiac output
d. Cardiac rhythms: controlled rate, freedom from arrhythmias
e. Freedom from chest pain
f. Normal urinary output

3. **Nursing interventions**
a. Identify patient's normal blood pressure range
b. Assess blood pressure at regular intervals and with changes in patient condition
c. Assess changes in patient's neurologic status
d. Discuss with physician what drug is to be administered for significant changes in blood pressure
e. Monitor heart rate, rhythm, and patient responses (e.g., blood pressure, mental status, diaphoresis, pain, shortness of breath)
f. Have the patient notify the nurse immediately at onset of chest discomfort and other associated symptoms of distress. Teach patient or the patient's significant other the importance of early recognition and treatment of problems
g. Watch for and identify any ECG changes
   i. Document rhythm strip per unit standards (at least once a shift)
   ii. Obtain 12-lead ECG when new arrhythmia is noted
   iii. Determine patient's response to arrhythmia, verbally and through vital signs
h. Administer appropriate emergency drugs if patient's cardiac rhythm becomes significantly bradycardic or tachycardic, per unit protocols
i. Have emergency equipment readily available, in good working order, fully equipped
j. Be knowledgeable of and prepared to use emergency equipment (defibrillator, transcutaneous pacer, transvenous pacer)
k. Administer cardiopulmonary resuscitation (CPR) and call code if patient is pulseless, in V fib, or in asystole
l. Monitor hemodynamic pressures, cardiac output readings
   i. Notify physician of significant hemodynamic changes
   ii. Collaborate with physician regarding medication needs, management of hemodynamic status
   iii. Be aware of rationale for current therapy, parameters, and goals of care

m. Watch the patient's oxygenation by checking frequent pulse oximetry readings and assessing breath sounds, respirations, and circulation. Administer oxygen as needed

n. Administer fluids as ordered to maintain LVEDP

o. Monitor for heart failure (heart sounds, neck veins)

p. Monitor intake and output (urine output should average at least 30 ml/hour), daily weights

q. Check presence and quality of peripheral pulses

r. Observe for central nervous system disturbances (confusion, restlessness, agitation, dizziness)

s. Check for other signs of perfusion deficits: cool skin, sluggish capillary refilling

t. Place patient in semi-Fowler's position or position of comfort

4. **Evaluation of nursing care**

a. Blood pressure, heart rate, hemodynamics are within normal limits or those set for patient

b. Sinus rhythm is normal on ECG

c. Skin is warm and dry

d. Urinary output is adequate

e. Patient is alert, oriented

f. Patient is comfortable, pain free

. . . .

Acute Pain Related to Coronary Ischemia or to Prolonged Bed Rest

1. **Assessment for defining characteristics**

a. Patient communicates discomfort: describes quality (on a scale of 1 to 10, 10 being worst), intensity, location, radiation, timing, aggravating and alleviating factors (movement, deep inspiration, positioning)

b. Anxiety

c. Diaphoresis

d. Increased blood pressure and heart rate

e. Increase or decrease in respiratory rate

f. Movement: restless or very still

g. Nausea, vomiting

h. Guarding or other protective behavior

i. Dilated pupils

j. ECG changes (ST segment, T waves), tachyarrhythmias

2. **Expected outcomes**

a. Pain or discomfort relieved completely

b. Vital signs stable and within normal limits

3. **Nursing interventions**

a. Have the patient notify the nurse immediately at onset of chest discomfort and other associated symptoms of distress. Teach the patient or the patient's significant other the importance of early recognition and treatment of chest discomfort

b. Collaborate with the physician with regard to medication needs (type, dosages, frequency, route) and titrations or adjustments of medications, depending on the patient's responses (vital signs, pain relief)

c. Document and analyze flow sheet to monitor the patient's pain

i. Assess quality, duration, intensity, frequency

      ii. Assess effectiveness of medications

      iii. Look for trends, drug interactions, and other possible comfort measures

    d. Provide other comfort interventions as appropriate (e.g., back rub, pillow or repositioning, egg crate or other special mattresses)

    e. Alert the physician to continued pain to determine need for further interventions. Cardiac pain means the myocardium is in jeopardy and immediate actions are needed

4. Evaluation of nursing care

    a. Patient is pain free, comfortable (with or without analgesia)

    b. Vital signs are stable

    c. Patient reports pain or discomfort, when it occurs, immediately and clearly to nurse

Activity Intolerance Related to Cardiac Disease or Dysfunction

1. Assessment for defining characteristics

    a. Discomfort: chest, neck, jaw, shoulder, arm

    b. Fatigue, weakness

    c. Dyspnea on exertion

    d. Leg cramps

    e. Increased heart rate

    f. Increased blood pressure

    g. Arrhythmias

    h. ST segment and T-wave changes signifying ischemia

2. Expected outcomes

    a. Progressive ambulation

    b. No complications of bed rest (skin intact, breath sounds clear, no signs of deep vein thromboembolism)

    c. Patient educated as to need for routine exercise and weight control

3. Nursing interventions

    a. Assess and document patient's response to progressive ambulation: to include monitoring heart rate and rhythm, respiration, blood pressure

    b. Long-term benefits of increased activity and risks of inactivity should be discussed with patient and family, and plan of care developed

    c. Assist patient with initial increases in ambulation

    d. Teach patient how to progress safely: correct positioning and use of body, with minimal work for each

      i. Active range of motion

      ii. Dangling

      iii. Transfers from bed to chair or bedside commode

      iv. Ambulation in room

      v. Ambulation in hallway

    e. Ensure that patient is instructed with regard to availability and use of special equipment to assist in ambulation (walkers, canes, wheel chairs), if needed

    f. Plan rest periods between various treatments, nursing activities, visits, and ambulation

    g. Administer pain medication, as needed, before planned ambulation (if patient is pain free, progression in ambulation will be more successful)

    h. If patient becomes unstable (ischemic pain, vital signs beyond set limits, arrhythmias), help him or her back to bed and immediately evaluate need for oxygen, medications (e.g., nitrates, antiarrhythmic), ECG, notification of physician, emergency equipment

    i. Arrange consultations with other health professionals, as appropriate: dietitian for weight control, diet instruction; cardiac rehabilitation nurse for activity plans within the hospital and after discharge; social services to assist with home equipment, home visits, nursing home placements (temporary or permanent)

    j. Encourage patient and family to openly ventilate feelings and ask questions regarding ability to ambulate, life style resumption and changes

4. Evaluation of nursing care

    a. Patient has verbalized and demonstrated understanding of activity capacity and limitations

    b. Patient will achieve ideal body weight

    c. Exercise program is incorporated into patient or significant other's life style

    d. Activity plan includes use of support system and community services, as needed, to achieve desired life style

. . . .

Anxiety Related to Threat of Death, Change in Health Status and Body Image, Threat to Socioeconomic Status

1. Assessment for defining characteristics

    a. Expressed feelings of helplessness, fear, uncertainty, inability to cope, regret, worry

    b. Possible signs of anxiety: restlessness, insomnia, palpitations, increased or erratic respiration, nausea, emesis, anorexia, quivering voice, increased frequency of urination

    c. Complaints or observations of muscle tension, trembling, extraneous movements (e.g., picking at things), wary, rambling speech, inability to focus, very talkative, poor eye contact, self-absorbed

2. Expected outcomes

    a. Verbalizes feelings of anxiety freely

    b. Experiences decrease in perceived anxiety

    c. Demonstrates effective methods of coping with anxiety

    d. Participates in care and discharge planning

    e. Has adequate and appropriate support systems (friends, family, professional help)

3. Nursing interventions

    a. Explain all procedures to patient. Use simple, concise language in a reassuring manner

    b. Assess knowledge level with regard to illness, hospitalization

    c. Evaluate teaching needs (knowledge deficits, misperceptions, misinformation)

    d. Give patient and significant others written information with clear diagrams for reinforcement; verify that the information is understood

    e. Allow patient as much control over environment and activities as feasible

    f. Administer sedatives, sleeping pills as necessary

    g. Maintain calm, reassuring, safe environment

   h. Assist patient in developing realistic goals, stress management ideas
   i. Elicit help from other sources of support: social workers, home health services, family and friends, religious institutions
   j. Encourage family and friends to help with care, if they are supportive and if patient is comforted by this activity

4. Evaluation of nursing care
   a. Decreased symptoms of anxiety
   b. Patient expresses feelings without difficulty
   c. Patient is actively involved in planning care, activities, discharge
   d. Patient verbalizes understanding of illness, medical care, goals

Knowledge Deficit Related to New Diagnosis, Medications, or Treatment Regimens or Related to Lack of Recall, Misunderstanding, or Misinterpretation of Information Regarding Condition and/or Care

This nursing diagnosis should be incorporated into all patient health problems.

1. Assessment for defining characteristics
   a. Patient, family, or significant other asks for information
   b. Verbalizations indicate lack of knowledge or inappropriate or incorrect information
   c. Patient has been noncompliant, resulting in incorrect or inappropriate care at home
   d. Patient is easily agitated, hostile, worried, suspicious (because of misinformation, misunderstanding, or misinterpretation)
   e. Patient is unable to plan realistic goals or home care

2. Expected outcomes
   a. Verbalizes understanding of diagnosis, medications, treatment regimen, follow-up care (to include rationales; risks; when to call physician; dosages, actions, and side effects of medications)
   b. Demonstrates proper techniques for home care and medication administration

3. Nursing interventions
   a. Assess readiness to learn (patient is alert, pain free, not sleep deprived; information is not given immediately after sedatives are administered)
   b. Identify learning needs
   c. Determine best methods for patient to learn (group, one-to-one, videos, computer)
   d. To reinforce learning, use printed materials related to disease, discharge instructions, procedures, medications
   e. Have instruction sheets available in languages other than English, when necessary
   f. Arrange for an interpreter if patient does not understand English (staff, family member, interpretation services)
   g. Document teaching and patient's response
   h. Arrange appropriate consults for cardiac rehabilitation; dietary, occupational, and physical therapy; home health; social work; discharge planning
   i. Schedule practice and return demonstrations of psychomotor skills

4. **Evaluation of nursing care**
    a. Patient or significant other verbalizes understanding of medical condition, therapy received, necessary home care or follow-up, medications, diet, life style changes
    b. Patient or significant other knows where to seek assistance for information and help
    c. Patient or significant other demonstrates proper techniques for various self-care procedures (insulin injections, glucose monitoring) to be accomplished at home

PATIENT HEALTH PROBLEMS

Coronary Artery Disease

A gradual, progressive disease in which the coronary arteries become occluded as a result of atherosclerosis.

1. **Pathophysiology**
    a. Mechanical or chemical injury occurs to the endothelial cells in the intima of the coronary arteries, altering the structure of the cell
    b. Platelets adhere and aggregate at the site of injury, and macrophages migrate to the area as a result of the injury. Lipoproteins enter the intimal layer. These accumulations promote the development over time of a fatty fibrous plaque, or "fatty streak"
    c. This plaque is a pearly white accumulation in the intimal lining, consisting mostly of smooth muscle cells but also collagen-producing fibroblasts and macrophages. These deposits protrude into the lumen, obstructing blood flow
    d. Progressive narrowing of the vessel occurs
    e. This process tends to occur at vessel bifurcations and at the proximal end of the artery
    f. The fatty fibrous plaque can rupture and form either a mural thrombus or an occlusive thrombus
        i. A mural thrombus can partially or totally obstruct the artery. The disrupted plaque and mural thrombus can develop into a more fibrotic, stenotic lesion, changing the plaque's geometry
        ii. An acute, labile, occlusive thrombus can totally obstruct the artery and create clinical complications (myocardial infarction, unstable angina, sudden cardiac death)
        iii. The ruptured plaque, caused by endothelial injury and exposure to blood flow, activates platelet and fibrin formation, enhancing thrombus formation
    g. Coronary blood flow may be further diminished by vasoconstriction (resulting from release of vasoactive materials, impaired vasodilation, and platelet activation)
    h. The atherosclerotic process causes
        i. Decreases in blood flow and oxygen supply to the myocardium
        ii. An imbalance between myocardial oxygen supply and demand, resulting in myocardial ischemia

2. Etiologic or precipitating factors
   a. Heredity: familial component for premature heart disease; myocardial infarction or sudden cardiac death in father less than 55 years of age, mother less than 65 years of age, or other first-degree relatives
   b. Age: CAD is more prevalent among middle-aged and older persons (males, ≥45; females, ≥55 years)
   c. Gender: CAD is more prevalent among men than among women
      i. Before 55 years of age, prevalence is three to four times higher among men than among women (before menopause)
      ii. After 55 years of age, prevalence rates slowly equalize for both sexes; at 75 years of age, they are close to equal
   d. Smoking
      i. Enhances atherogenic progression; decreases HDL cholesterol; influences thrombus formation, plaque instability, arrhythmias
      ii. Dose and duration-dependent: the risk of death from CAD is two to six times higher among smokers than among nonsmokers
   e. Hyperlipidemia: high levels of triglycerides, LDL, and very-low-density lipoproteins are associated with an increased risk of CAD. A 1% increase of total cholesterol correlates with a 2% to 3% increase in risk of coronary heart disease
      i. Triglycerides: higher than 400 mg/dl
      ii. Total cholesterol: 240 mg/dl or higher
      iii. LDL: 160 mg/dl or higher
      iv. HDL: 35 mg/dl or lower
   f. Hypertension
      i. Contributes to direct vascular injury, along with the effects of increased wall stress and oxygen demands
      ii. Approximately 30% of American adults have hypertension (up to three times higher in African-Americans than in the general population)
      iii. Systolic blood pressure higher than 160 and/or diastolic pressure greater than 100 mm Hg (moderate to severe hypertension)
   g. Left ventricular hypertrophy: heart's response to chronic pressure overload; associated with increased risk for cardiovascular events
   h. Thrombogenic risk factors
      i. Enhanced thrombotic state leads to plaque disruption, hemostasis, thrombotic events
      ii. Deficiencies in serum coagulation inhibitors (antithrombin III, protein C, and protein S), elevated plasma fibrinogen, enhanced platelet aggregation
   i. Diabetes mellitus: patients with diabetes mellitus are twice as likely to develop CAD as persons without diabetes mellitus
   j. Obesity: positively associated with an increase in CAD; also contributes to the development of hypertension and diabetes. Fat distribution also plays a role (abdominal or central obesity carries higher risk)
   k. Sedentary life style; studies show a low but positive relationship between inactivity and CAD, mainly resulting from its aggravation of other risk factors
   l. Postmenopausal status: estrogen replacement protects women from vascular injury, increases HDL levels
   m. Other factors that are associated with increased risk that *might* have some benefit if modified and are under further study include

         i. Hyperhomocysteinemia (toxic to vascular endothelium; prothrombotic condition)

         ii. Oxidative stress: oxidized LDL cholesterol dramatically enhances atherogenic process

         iii. Excessive consumption of alcohol: probably because of association with hypertension, cardiomyopathies

3. Nursing assessment data base

  a. Nursing history

      i. Assessment of aforementioned risk factors

      ii. Possible sequelae of CAD include

         (a) Angina pectoris

         (b) Myocardial infarction

         (c) Heart failure

         (d) Sudden cardiac death

         (e) Arrhythmias

         (f) Cardiomyopathy

         (g) Mitral insufficiency

         (h) Ventricular aneurysm or rupture

         (i) Cardiogenic shock

  b. Nursing examination of patient (see Nursing Assessment Data Base section for this chapter): CAD may be asymptomatic and diagnosed because of abnormal findings on testing (stress testing, echocardiography)

  c. Diagnostic study findings

      i. Laboratory

         (a) Fasting lipid profile: total cholesterol, HDL, LDL, triglycerides

         (b) Fasting serum glucose level

      ii. Stress testing: to rule out ischemia, for risk stratification of CAD, for arrhythmia detection, and to assess efficacy of treatment

      iii. Other tests may be appropriate, including echocardiography, dobutamine stress, scintigraphy with exercise or pharmacologic stress, and coronary angiography

4. Nursing diagnoses (see Commonly Encountered Nursing Diagnoses section earlier)

  a. See Nursing Diagnoses sections for each of the possible sequelae of CAD (after identification of CAD, appropriate interventions described in Angina section may be initiated for patients at high risk)

  b. Effective management of therapeutic regimen to decrease modifiable cardiac risk factors

      i. Assessment for defining characteristics: verbalized desire to manage modification of risk factors contributing to CAD progression

      ii. Expected outcomes

         (a) Modifiable risk factors under control and/or improved

         (b) New health practices implemented into life style

         (c) Goals of treatment program met

      i. Nursing interventions

         (a) Provide patient with information regarding risk factors for CAD

         (b) Encourage patient and significant other to quit smoking; provide information and help with regard to risks, methods and programs for stopping, nicotine replacement

        (c) Provide information on lipid-lowering diets that have 30% or less fat, less than 7% saturated fat, less than 200 mg/dl cholesterol
           (1) Goals for lipid management:
               a) LDL < 100 mg/dl
               b) HDL >35 mg/dl
               c) Triglycerides > 200 mg/dl
           (2) Lipid-lowering agents may be necessary; patient should be aware of their uses and side effects
           (3) Diet should include use of monounsaturated and polyunsaturated fats (olive, sunflower, corn oils; soft margarine)
           (4) Vitamins C and E and beta carotene may help slow oxidation of LDL, inhibit platelet aggregation
        (d) If patient is hypertensive, modification will include weight control, routine exercise, moderation of alcohol consumption, moderate sodium restriction
           (1) Goal of blood pressure: 140/90 mm Hg or lower
           (2) Antihypertensive agents may be necessary (diuretics, angiotensin converting enzyme [ACE] inhibitors, beta blockers)
        (e) Weight control should be discussed with patient and a plan for weight loss developed (especially in patients who are <120% their ideal weight for height). Hypertensive patients and/or patients with elevated glucose or triglyceride levels should receive information on achieving ideal body weight
        (f) Exercise and physical activity (after risks are assessed, often after exercise testing in patients over 40 years of age)
           (1) Goal of 30 minutes, three to four times weekly (minimum); preferably 30 to 60 minutes of exercise to include walking, cycling, jogging
           (2) Other opportunities for increased physical activity should be explored with the patient
        (g) Antiplatelet agents (such as acetylsalicylic acid [ASA], 80 to 325 mg/day) may be included in patient's health regimen, if not contraindicated
        (h) Estrogen replacement should be explored for postmenopausal women on an individual basis

Angina Pectoris

Transient myocardial ischemia without cellular death
1. **Pathophysiology:** myocardial oxygen demand outstrips oxygen supply
2. **Etiologic or precipitating factors**
    a. Atherosclerotic coronary artery disease
    b. Hypertension
    c. Aortic valve disease
    d. Anemia
    e. Arrhythmias (especially tachyarrhythmias)
    f. Thyrotoxicosis
    g. Shock

h. Heart failure
i. Coronary artery spasm
j. Precipitating factors
   i. Increased myocardial oxygen demand due to
      (a) Increased heart rate resulting from exertion, tachyarrhythmia, anemia, fever, anxiety, pain, thyrotoxicosis, drugs, digestion, hyperadrenergic states
      (b) Increased contractility resulting from exercise, tachycardia, anxiety, drugs, hyperadrenergic states
      (c) Increased afterload resulting from hypertension, aortic stenosis, drugs (pressors)
      (d) Increased preload resulting from volume overloading, drugs
   ii. Decreased oxygen supply
      (a) CAD (fixed)
      (b) Coronary artery spasm, cold air, drugs (ergots)
      (c) Circulatory diversion (digestion, coronary artery steal)
      (d) Anemia
      (e) Hypoxemia
      (f) Hypovolemia

3. Nursing assessment data base
a. Nursing history
   i. Subjective findings
      (a) Anginal discomfort is any exertional, rest-relieved symptom and may be described as burning, squeezing, aching, heaviness, pressure sensation, smothering, indigestion-like, or "band across the chest." It may occur anywhere between the ears and the umbilicus
      (b) Etiologic or precipitating factors: elicit pertinent information from patient
      (c) Characterize the patient's symptoms
         (1) Duration of discomfort
         (2) Effect of exertion, rest
         (3) Nitrates (if patient has CAD) should decrease and/or alleviate discomfort in minutes
         (4) Location and radiation of the discomfort. Can include chest, neck, jaws, arms, back, epigastrium
         (5) Associated symptoms may include nausea, diaphoresis, palpitations, shortness of breath
         (6) Patient should be asked to quantify the discomfort by using a scale of 1 (the least) to 10 (the worst pain ever experienced by the patient)
         (7) The timing of the discomfort is crucial. Was it with activity, in bed at rest, postprandial? With what kind of activity? How often does it recur?
   ii. Objective findings
      (a) Determine type or form of angina
         (1) Stable angina: angina that has not increased in frequency or severity over time
         (2) Unstable angina: new onset angina or angina that has changed in frequency, severity, or duration or occurs with less exertion or at rest

(3) Prinzmetal's (variant) angina: resting angina caused by coronary artery spasm, associated with transient ST segment elevation

(b) Determine class of angina: Canadian Classification

    (1) Canadian class I: angina produced with strenuous exertion

    (2) Canadian class II: angina produced by walking more than two blocks on a level surface

    (3) Canadian class III: angina produced by walking less than two blocks on a level surface

    (4) Canadian class IV: angina at rest

(c) Other important aspects of history include

    (1) Risk factors for CAD

    (2) Cardiac review of systems

    (3) Medication history

    (4) History of tests, interventions; coronary artery bypass graft (CABG), PTCA

b. Nursing examination of patient (see Nursing Assessment Data Base section earlier)

    i. Inspection

        (a) Frightened

        (b) Minimal movement

        (c) May clutch chest

    ii. Palpation: none

    iii. Auscultation

        (a) Transient mitral regurgitation

        (b) Transient rales

        (c) Transient S_4

c. Diagnostic study findings

    i. Laboratory: CK-MB isoenzymes are not elevated with angina

    ii. ECG: may or may not show evidence of myocardial injury or ischemia (see ECG, Myocardial Infarction section later); transient ST depression and T-wave changes

    iii. Echocardiography: may or may not show transient abnormal wall motion, valve dysfunction, hypertrophy

    iv. Exercise testing: results may or may not be positive for CAD. It is very sensitive for left main artery or three-vessel disease, but it can miss 40% of single-vessel disease

    v. Dobutamine stress echocardiography can demonstrate ischemia, stress-induced wall motion abnormalities, ventricular dysfunction, and ischemic mitral regurgitation

    vi Myocardial scintigraphy (thallium, sestamibi) with exercise or pharmacologic stress (dipyridamole) may demonstrate ischemia, infarction, and left ventricular dysfunction

    vii. Coronary catheterization is used to assess the extent and severity of CAD, as well as to assess valvular and ventricular function. It facilitates risk assessment and guides therapy

4. Nursing Diagnoses (see Commonly Encountered Nursing Diagnoses section earlier)

a. Pain (acute) related to transient, inadequate myocardial oxygen supply due to coronary atherosclerosis or spasm

    i. Additional nursing interventions

(a) Keep goals of treatment in mind: stop ischemia by
    (1) Decreasing myocardial oxygen demand (beta blockers, calcium channel blockers, nitrates)
    (2) Improving myocardial oxygen supply (nitrates, oxygen)
(b) With discomfort: have patient notify nurse, stop activities, return to bed (if up), rest
(c) Administer oxygen per unit protocol
(d) Check vital signs, monitor ECG
(e) Do (or order) 12-lead ECG stat
(f) Ensure that patient has a patent intravenous (IV) line
(g) Administer and titrate medications to reduce or alleviate angina
    (1) Nitroglycerin: rapid-acting nitrate
        a) Action
            i) Relaxes smooth muscle, causing venodilation
            ii) Decreases venous return by systemic pooling of blood, thus decreasing preload
            iii) Reduces myocardial oxygen demand and consumption
            iv) Relieves any associated coronary artery spasm, improving blood flow and oxygenation to myocardium
        b) Indications: angina pectoris, myocardial infarction, left ventricular failure, hypertension
        c) Administration
            i) Administered sublingually every 5 minutes; up to three doses
            ii) Intravenous nitroglycerin to control or prevent ischemia. Can also reduce infarct size. Start IV drip at 5 to 10 μg/minute and titrate every 5 to 10 minutes until pain is relieved or adverse side effects such as hypotension occur. IV solution is readily absorbed into plastic bags and tubing; use special nonabsorbable administration sets, glass bottles. Monitor blood pressure closely. Do not stop nitroglycerin abruptly: wean off by reducing flow 5 to 10 μg/minute every 15 minutes; observe for returning symptoms
            iii) If IV nitroglycerin results in decreased blood pressure, give fluid bolus, place patient in Trendelenburg position
            iv) Nitroglycerin is available also as a spray, an ointment, or a patch. Wear gloves when administering paste: accidental exposure of paste to skin can cause headache symptoms
        d) Side effects include hypotension, headache, sweating, nausea, tachycardia, bradycardia
        e) Patients often develop a tolerance to nitroglycerin's hemodynamic effects after 12 to 24 hr of administration; therefore,
            i) The rate of infusion may need to be adjusted or increased with continued use

    ii) If a nitroglycerin patch is used, the patch can be discontinued for 8 to 12 hr each day (usually during nighttime)

 (2) Beta-adrenergic blockers (e.g., atenolol, metoprolol)

  a) Action: decrease angina

    i) Decrease heart rate and contractility (negatively inotropic, chronotropic)

    ii) Decrease myocardial oxygen demand

    iii) Increase diastolic filling time

    iv) Increase exercise tolerance

  b) Oral administration is usually adequate; IV administration is used with unstable angina

  c) Contraindications: bronchial asthma, heart failure (unless caused by ischemia), AV blocks, hypotension

  d) Side effects

    i) Conduction blocks

    ii) Hypoglycemia, arrhythmias

    iii) Central nervous system effects (decreased energy, decreased libido, nightmares, confusion); rare with cardioselective beta blockers

    iv) Gastrointestinal (diarrhea, nausea, constipation); rare with cardioselective beta blockers

  e) Sudden withdrawal of drug can have rebound effects (including unstable angina, hypertension, myocardial infarction). Gradual withdrawal or adjustment should be made, unless an emergency (e.g., bradycardia) mandates immediate discontinuation

 (3) Calcium channel antagonists

  a) Types

    i) Dihydropyridines (e.g., nifedipine), the most potent vasodilator type, result in reflex tachycardia, necessitating simultaneous use of a beta blocker

    ii) Second-generation dihydropyridines (nicardipine, felodipine, isradipine, amlodipine): more vascular selectivity, longer half-life

    iii) Phenylalkylamines (e.g., verapamil): negative inotropic, dromotropic effects

    iv) Benzothiazepines (e.g., diltiazem): negative inotropic, dromotropic effects (less than those of verapamil)

  b) Actions

    i) Negative inotropic; negative chronotropic and dromotropic effects on SA and AV conductive tissue (except nifedipine)

    ii) Increase angina threshold, reducing ischemia and increasing exercise tolerance

    iii) Powerful vasodilators (e.g., nifedipine) help in management of coronary vasospasm

  c) Uses: angina, hypertension, SVTs

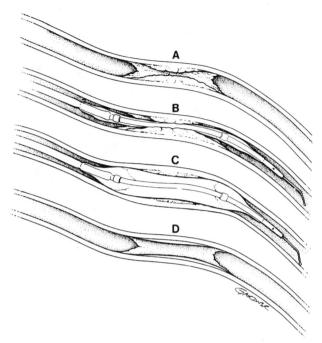

Figure 2–18 • Percutaneous transluminal coronary angioplasty.

       d) Contraindications: aortic valve disease, severe anemia,
           AV blocks, WPW syndrome (verapamil, nifedipine)
    (h) May need to prepare patient and patient's significant other for
         coronary interventions to include emergency cardiac
         arteriography, PTCA, coronary stents, atherectomy, and CABG
    (i) Provide nursing care for patients who require PTCA: used to
         increase the inner diameter of coronary arteries that have been
         stenosed by CAD, to increase coronary blood flow (Figs. 2–18 to
         2–20)

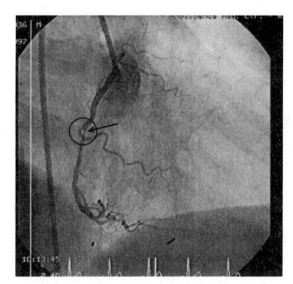

Figure 2–19 • Middle right coronary artery with 80% stenosis before an interventional cardiac catheterization procedure.

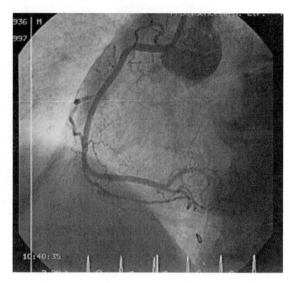

Figure 2-20 • Middle right coronary artery with 0% stenosis after percutaneous transluminal coronary angioplasty and a coronary stent procedure.

(1) Procedure
   a) Performed in cardiac catheterization laboratory
   b) Balloon catheter is placed across the stenosis and inflated
   c) Enlarges the lumen diameter by compressing and splitting the plaque
(2) Indications
   a) Unstable or chronic angina
   b) Acute myocardial infarction
   c) Post CABG with graft stenosis
(3) Selection of patients
   a) Single- or multivessel disease (excluding left main) with at least 50% stenosis
   b) Lesion that is discrete, noncalcific, concentric, and not near bifurcation
   c) Saphenous vein graft stenosis
(4) Potential complications
   a) Acute coronary occlusion resulting from dissection and necessitating emergency CABG in 2% of cases
   b) Contrast medium reaction
   c) Bleeding: hematoma at insertion site, retroperitoneal bleeding, decreased peripheral pulses distal to insertion site
   d) Vasovagal reaction at sheath removal
   e) Restenosis of artery in first 6 months (30% to 40%)
   f) Pseudoaneurysm of femoral artery: should be suspected if there is painful swelling at arterial puncture site
   g) Myocardial infarction (1%)
   h) Arteriovenous fistula (at sheath removal)
(5) Nursing implications
   a) Prepare patient and significant other for the procedure; preparation is similar to that for cardiac catheterization procedure

b) Potential for CABG should be discussed
c) Reassure patient, help decrease anxiety
d) Discuss postprocedure routines
e) Postprocedure nursing care
    i) Observe for complications
    ii) Bed rest for 6 to 8 hours with head of bed elevated no more than 25°
    iii) Affected limb should be kept straight, immobile; soft leg restraint may be used to assist with this. Sandbag can also help remind patient (not really effective in stopping bleeding, may be uncomfortable)
    iv) Patient may be repositioned on side by log-rolling, if procedure site not bleeding
    v) ECG on return from procedure and with chest discomfort
    vi) Monitor vital signs closely
    vii) Monitor pulses, warmth, sensation of affected limb; assess for bleeding and hematoma at femoral site. Document findings on patient flow sheet per unit guidelines
    viii) If there is bleeding or hematoma, hold direct pressure until bleeding has stopped. Mark hematoma and closely watch for signs of increased size. Application of inflatable femoral compression systems may be appropriate for maintaining hemostasis
    ix) Finger foods are easier for patient while head-of-bed elevation is restricted
    x) Assess need for medication for back and groin discomfort
    xi) Maintain IV fluids as ordered and encourage drinking of fluids (to facilitate catheterization dye load excretion by kidneys)
    xii) Ensure adequate output. Foley catheter may be necessary if patient cannot void (within 2 to 4 hours), for patients unable to void in bed at required position, or for patients who are at high risk for bleeding
    xiii) Patient may be on heparin drip after PTCA: monitor PTT or ACT for adequate anticoagulation (ordered parameters). Monitor other sources for bleeding problems (urine, emesis, stools, nosebleeds, neurologic status). Heparin should be stopped 1 to 4 hours before sheath removal
    xiv) Check ACT if sheath is to come out (if <150 seconds, sheath may be removed if patient is stable and without ischemic pain)
f) Postprocedure nursing care during sheath removal
    i) Thoroughly explain removal process to patient

    ii) Medicate patient before removal to diminish discomfort. Medications include morphine or other fast-acting analgesics along with local anesthesia to site

    iii) Have normal saline bolus and atropine (0.5 mg IV) readily available at bedside for vasovagal reactions (hypotension, bradycardia, diaphoresis, nausea)

    iv) Gather all other equipment for removal: suture removal kit; syringes; gloves, goggles, and gown; dressings; sandbag; Doppler device, compression devices, if used (inflatable femoral compression system [Femostop], C-clamp)

    v) Aspirating 5 to 10 ml of blood from each sheath (venous and arterial) ensures that there are no clots on the tip of the sheath to embolize on withdrawal and that any heparin is removed from the patient's system

    vi) Locate arterial pulse. Apply manual, direct pressure just above puncture site (and over arterial pulse) for a minimum of 20 minutes after sheath removal until hemostasis is complete. Pulling the arterial sheath first and then the venous sheath after hemostasis avoids potential risk of arteriovenous fistula

    vii) If using a compression device, follow protocols for safe use during and after sheath removal

g) Postprocedure nursing care after sheath removal

    i) After sheath removal: check vital signs every 15 minutes four times, every 30 minutes four times, and then every hour

    ii) Continue to monitor and document pulses and assess for bleeding or hematoma, promptly treating with direct pressure until hemostasis is complete. Notify physician if bleeding recurs

    iii) Bed rest should be maintained for 6 to 8 hours after sheath removal with head of bed no higher than 30°, with affected leg kept straight

    iv) Auscultate for systolic bruit at site of sheath insertion at least every 8 hours: positive bruit along with localized pain and pulsatile mass suggests possible pseudoaneurysm; notify physician immediately. Surgery or ultrasound-guided compression is necessary for closure

    v) Identify patients at high risk for pseudoaneurysm:
      [a] Obese (difficult to apply direct pressure)
      [b] Sheath size larger than No. 8 French (larger injury to artery)
      [c] Receiving postprocedure anticoagulants (hemostasis problem)
      [d] Elderly (degenerative changes in artery wall)

[e] Females (fat distribution, smaller arteries, potential of multiple punctures during catheterization procedure)

vi) Continue to medicate for discomfort from bed rest

h) Restenosis: major problem related to PTCA (resulting from intimal hyperplasia during healing). Factors associated with increased risk of restenosis: multivessel CAD, proximal LAD stenosis, diabetes, final lumen diameter (less than 100%)

i) Resume heparin, if ordered

j) Administration of glycoprotein IIb/IIIa receptors (abciximab [ReoPro]) may be ordered for high-risk angioplasty patients (including diabetics, females, patients with unstable angina or recent myocardial infarction, those with complex lesion morphology)

  i) Action: inhibits platelet aggregation by preventing fibrinogen and von Willebrand factor from binding to glycoprotein IIb/IIIa receptor sites on platelets

  ii) Administration: started 10 to 60 minutes before the PTCA; a bolus of 0.25 mg/kg is given, with an infusion rate of 10 μg/minute for 12 hours

  iii) Assess patient very closely because of increased risk of bleeding from drug. Additional preventative measures include

    [a] Avoiding intramuscular injections, venipunctures (use heparin lock for drawing blood)

    [b] Limit or avoid use of automatic blood pressure devices

    [c] Place Foley catheter (and nasogastric tube, if needed) before drug administration

    [d] Monitor activated partial thromboplastin time (aPTT) along with platelets (thrombocytopenia, in which platelets <150,000/mm³, is a potential complication)

    [e] Notify physician promptly if blood is observed in urine, stool, emesis

k) Teach the patient discharge activities, symptoms to report (e.g., masses, bleeding, increased localized pain and bruising at site of insertion, tingling or numbness, weakness in the extremities, shortness of breath, chest discomfort), medications, diet, risk factors, and actions to take:

  i) Call 911 and apply pressure for bleeding, swelling, or pain at catheter site

  ii) Limit activities for 2 days

  iii) No driving for 1 day

  iv) Modify medications, diet, risk factors

  v) Discharge follow-up

(j) Provide nursing care for patients who require a coronary stent
  (1) Devices placed intraluminally to achieve maximal lumen size and maintain the patency of the vessel's lumen
    a) Stents are made from various metals
    b) Synthetic materials also being used have the ability to deliver drugs (anticoagulants) and irradiate tissue to reduce restenosis
  (2) Indications
    a) Primary stenting reduces restenosis to 20% in native arteries and grafts
    b) Abrupt closure resulting from dissection after PTCA and lesions at high risk for collapse
    c) Restenosis: post-PTCA
    d) Intimal tears: post-PTCA
  (3) Nursing implications
    a) Same care, precautions as for PTCA
    b) Ensure baseline CBC has been measured and is documented
    c) Administer ASA and other antiplatelet agents as ordered, to include ticlopidine (Ticlid) and abciximab (ReoPro). Ticlopidine features include
      i) Action: as a glycoprotein IIb/IIIa receptor inhibitor, inhibits platelet aggregation
      ii) Dose: 250 mg b.i.d. p.o. with food, for approximately 2 weeks post stent
      iii) Side effects: excess bleeding, rash, diarrhea, gastrointestinal discomfort, neutropenia, bone marrow suppression (with longer use, 1 month or more)
      iv) Interactions: cimetidine decreases efficacy by 50%; ASA is potentiated by drug; serum cholesterol and triglyceride levels are increased
    d) Give patient stent information packet and identification stent card before discharge, and ensure that questions regarding care are answered
(k) Provide nursing care for patients requiring coronary atherectomy: removal of atheromatous material from the artery (debulking)
  (1) Indications: lesions not amenable to PTCA:
    a) Eccentric lesions: directional atherectomy
    b) Calcified lesions: rotational atherectomy
    c) Tubular or long lesions: rotational atherectomy
    d) Ostial lesions: both directional and rotational atherectomy
    e) Long saphenous vein graft (SVG) stenosis: transluminal extraction atherectomy
  (2) Benefits include larger, smoother resultant lumen; decreased incidence of dissection because this procedure does not expand the artery as much as PTCA does, although it is used frequently as an adjunct to PTCA
  (3) Types of atherectomy devices and procedures

a) Directional catheter: a capsule with a cutting chamber on one side and a balloon on the other. The catheter is positioned at the lesion, the balloon is inflated, and the plaque is cut by a rotating cutter and trapped in the chamber for removal. Especially useful in eccentric lesions

b) Rotational atherectomy (Rotablator): flexible catheter with a high-speed, diamond-tipped, rotating burr that ablates plaque and pulverizes atheromatous material into microdebris in the blood stream. Especially useful in calcified or long lesions

c) Transluminal extraction atherectomy; slower rotating cutter that has vacuum suction to withdraw atheromatous debris. Utility limited to SVG stenosis

(l) Provide nursing care for patients who require CABG: surgical revascularization of the myocardium with bypass grafting with the use of saphenous veins or internal mammary arteries

  (1) CABG with SVG

    a) Reversed saphenous vein is used to create a conduit. One end of graft is sewn onto the aorta, and the other end is sewn onto the affected coronary artery distal to the obstruction

    b) Blood flow then bypasses the blockage and is provided to the deprived myocardium

  (2) CABG with either or both internal mammary arteries

    a) The proximal artery remains attached to the subclavian artery, from which it arises, and the distal end is dissected from the anterior chest wall and sewn onto the coronary artery distal to the obstruction

    b) Long-term patency rate is better (>90% at 10 years) than with saphenous veins (40%)

    c) Avoids need for leg incisions if only 1 or 2 vessels require bypass

  (3) Selection of patients (indications)

    a) Prospects of improved longevity better than with long-term medical management

      i) Left main CAD

      ii) CAD × three-vessel with Canadian class III to IV angina

      iii) CAD × two-vessel, if proximal LAD is involved

      iv) CAD with impaired left ventricular function (left ventricular EF < 35%)

    b) Limiting angina, despite maximal tolerable medical management

    c) Occupation requires complete revascularization (i.e., pilot)

    d) Abrupt occlusions after PTCA

    e) Post–myocardial infarction angina or hemodynamic instability

  (4) Complications during surgery

    a) Reoperation to control bleeding: 10% to 15%

   b) Intraoperative stroke: 1% to 2%
   c) Myocardial infarction: 2% to 7%
   d) Death: 1% to 2%
(5) Immediate postoperative complications
   a) Low cardiac output, hypotension: may be due to inadequate volume replacement, fluid shifts (third spacing), hemorrhage. Can decrease systemic perfusion, affecting the kidneys, brain, and heart
   b) Hemorrhage
   c) Hypertension (increased afterload decreases cardiac output)
   d) Cardiac tamponade: suspect if decreased cardiac output/hypotension is present with increased central venous pressures (unless hypovolemic), narrowed pulse pressure, distended jugular veins and pulsus paradoxus, or distant heart sounds
   e) Arrhythmias: caused by electrolyte imbalances, hypoxemia, drug toxicity, hypothermia, anesthesia. Atrial fibrillation is common (approximately 25% of patients)
   f) Respiratory failure: associated with hypoxemia, alveolar hypoventilation
   g) Prerenal azotemia caused by decreased cardiac output, hypovolemia
   h) Electrolyte imbalances: very common, especially hypokalemia, hypocalcemia, hypomagnesemia
   i) Late graft closure: can be prevented by antiplatelet aggregation therapy (ASA, dipyridamole), along with diet, smoking cessation, exercise, and hypertension control
(6) Early extubation (within 6 hours) should be anticipated once patient meets weaning criteria (unless patient has complications necessitating continuation)
(7) Drugs commonly used after CABG
   a) Volume to support blood pressure, preload: albumin, hetastarch, and/or whole and packed red blood cells to increase the preload, elevate CVP, increase systolic blood pressure if it falls below predetermined parameters, and increase HCT
   b) See Heart Failure section later for discussions of medications, interventions used for acute postoperative management of heart failure
   c) Digitalis is often administered prophylactically to prevent complication of atrial fibrillation
   d) ASA, dipyridamole are administered to prevent acute and late graft closure
(8) Intra-aortic balloon pump (IABP) for cardiogenic shock (pump failure); see Heart Failure section later
(9) Patient may require use of ventricular assist device (VAD)
   a) VAD may be used on the left (LVAD), right (RVAD), or both sides of the heart

b) VAD is a pump, bypassing the affected ventricle and allowing the heart to rest and recover

c) LVAD: blood is diverted from the left atrium, bypasses the left ventricle, is sent to the pump, and then returns to the patient via cannulation of the ascending aorta

d) RVAD: blood is diverted from the right atrium, bypasses the right ventricle, is sent to the pump, and then returns to the patient via cannulation of the pulmonary artery

e) The cannula can exit either from the sternal incision, if the chest is not closed, or from a separate parasternal incision

f) Indications for VAD
   i) Cardiogenic shock
   ii) Postcardiotomy ventricular failure
   iii) Patients waiting for transplantation
   iv) Inability to be weaned from cardiopulmonary bypass during cardiac surgery

g) Contraindications to VAD
   i) Prolonged cardiac arrest with severe neurologic damage
   ii) No prospect for patient of being weaned from VAD: irreversible, extensive myocardial damage

h) Complications of VAD
   i) Thromboembolism, hemolysis
   ii) Bleeding
   iii) Renal, respiratory, heart failure
   iv) Air emboli
   v) Infections

i) VAD can be used in combination with IABP

j) Nursing care with VAD
   i) Must be knowledgeable about VAD operation and protocols of use; cardiac perfusionists are most knowledgeable and will be involved
   ii) Frequent assessment of vital signs, hemodynamics, intake and output (I&O) circulation, cardiac output
   iii) Hemodynamics are different: cardiac output measurements are accurate only for LVAD, not RVAD; flow and pressures are not pulsatile
   iv) Monitor for arrhythmias and treat them promptly

k) Weaning criteria
   i) Patient's ventricle shows ability to support cardiac output
   ii) Patient's intrinsic MAP is greater than 60 mm Hg
   iii) CI greater than 1.8 L/minute/m^2
   iv) VAD flow is decreased gradually, allowing patient's heart to take over

ii. Evaluation of nursing care for angina
   (a) Patient has no pain or anginal attacks are less severe

(b) Patient has no complications associated with various angina therapies received

(c) Patient has no arrhythmias

(d) Vital signs and hemodynamics are within normal limits for patient

(e) Patient maintains adequate cardiac output without mechanical support

(f) Laboratory data are within set parameters

(g) Peripheral pulses are present and circulation is good

(h) Urinary output is adequate

(i) Patient is able to provide self-care and follow medical regimen after discharge

b. Decreased cardiac output related to arrhythmias and conduction defects (see Commonly Encountered Nursing Diagnoses section earlier)

    i. Additional nursing interventions

      (a) Observe patient for signs of inadequate myocardial perfusion caused by arrhythmias, heart failure, shock

      (b) Support myocardium through administration of pharmacologic agents, such as antiarrhythmic drugs (see Cardiac Rhythm section later)

    ii. Evaluation of nursing care

      (a) Hemodynamics are normal

      (b) Arrhythmias are controlled or absent

      (c) Patient is free from pain

Myocardial Infarction (MI)

Necrosis of myocardial tissue due to the interruption of coronary perfusion to the myocardium

1. **Pathophysiology:** (see Coronary Artery Disease section earlier)

    a. Blood flow may be obstructed by a thrombus in the coronary artery

    b. Site and amount of necrosis depend on the location of arterial occlusion, on collateral circulation, and on any previous infarctions or disease

    c. The extent of necrosis may be

      i. Transmural: full thickness (endocardium to epicardium)

      ii. Nontransmural: non–Q wave (subendocardial)

2. **Etiologic or precipitating factors**

    a. Atherosclerotic CAD (see Coronary Artery Disease section earlier)

    b. Coronary artery spasm

    c. Coronary artery embolism

    d. Other precipitating factors: acute hypotension, ventricular tachyarrhythmias

3. **Nursing assessment data base**

    a. Nursing history

      i. Subjective findings

        (a) Patient history alone is sufficient to rule out myocardial infarction, even in the absence of ECG changes

        (b) Discomfort in chest that has lasted longer than 30 minutes, is often severe, and is unrelieved by rest or nitrates. May radiate to neck, jaw, arms, and back. These areas may be the only locations of discomfort. Similar to angina in character of discomfort, but usually more severe and longer in duration (see Angina Pectoris section earlier for description of discomfort)

   ii. Objective findings

     (a) Pallor

     (b) Diaphoresis, weakness, lightheadedness

     (c) Vagal effects (bradycardia, vomiting)

     (d) Dyspnea

     (e) Apprehension

     (f) May exhibit complications associated with MI

       (1) Arrhythmias and conduction defects, especially V fib, VT, heart block

       (2) Left heart failure

       (3) Cardiogenic shock

       (4) Systemic or pulmonary thromboembolism

       (5) Mitral insufficiency, papillary muscle rupture

       (6) Ventricular aneurysm or rupture (delayed complication)

       (7) Ventricular septal defect (delayed complication)

       (8) Pericarditis: Dressler's syndrome (occurring 1 to 6 weeks after MI: autoimmune antibody response of body from antigens released with necrotic myocardium. Symptoms include fever, pericardial pain, pleuritis

b. Nursing examination of patient: findings will vary with size and extent of the infarction, patient's status, and history of previous MI

   i. Inspection

     (a) Anxiety

     (b) Pallor, cyanosis, diaphoresis

     (c) Nausea, vomiting

     (d) Arrhythmias evident on ECG

     (e) Shortness of breath

     (f) Ankle edema

   ii. Palpation

     (a) Skin diaphoretic, cool, clammy

     (b) Thrill, heaves, abnormal PMI

     (c) Irregular, slow, fast, and/or thready pulse

   iii. Auscultation: usually normal, but may have

     (a) S_3: diastolic (ventricular) gallop

     (b) S_4: presystolic gallop

     (c) Pericardial friction rub

     (d) Murmurs

     (e) Rales

c. Diagnostic findings

   i. Laboratory findings

     (a) CK-MB isoenzymes elevated within 6 hours (see Nursing Assessment Data Base section earlier)

     (b) Leukocytosis (large MI) due to stress and tissue necrosis; onset several hours after MI pain onset, peaks 2 to 4 days after the infarction. If levels remain high (12,000 to 15,000 cells/mm^3), suspect a possible complication (pericarditis, emboli, infection)

   ii. ECG

     (a) Changes on ECG correlate with location of necrosis (Table 2–1)

TABLE 2–1. Correlation of Coronary Disease Locations with Clinical Manifestations

Location of Occluding Lesion	Clinical Manifestations
Left main coronary artery	Massive left ventricular infarction
Left anterior descending coronary artery	Anterior infarction with Q waves in the precordial (V) leads Septal infarction with Q waves in leads V_1–V_3 Apical infarction Right bundle branch block with left anterior hemiblock Mobitz type II heart block and complete heart block
Left circumflex coronary artery	Lateral or inferolateral infarction True posterior infarction
Right coronary artery	Inferior infarction with Q waves in leads II, III, and aVF AV conduction disturbances (first-degree AV block, Mobitz type I or Wenckebach second-degree AV block) Cardiovascular reflexes (bradycardia, hypotension) Right ventricular infarction evidenced by Elevated systemic venous pressure Decreased cardiac output Minimal to absent pulmonary congestion

Adapted from Conner, R. P.: Coronary artery anatomy: The electrocardiograph—clinical correlation. Crit. Care Nurse 3:72, 1983.

(1) Ischemia: Blood supply to myocardium is inadequate but without cell death. May result in nonspecific depression of ST and/or T segment
(2) ECG signs of MI: necrosis (cell death)
    a) Acute ST elevation
    b) Abnormal Q wave (Fig. 2–21)
        i) More than 0.04 seconds (0.03 seconds for inferior MI)

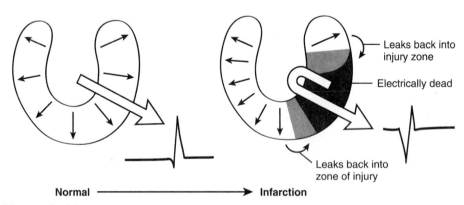

Figure 2–21 • Abnormalities of the initial QRS forces (Q waves): infarction. *Concept:* If a portion of the ventricular myocardium does not contribute its share of electrical forces (i.e., if it is electrically dead), the opposing forces become dominant and a reorientation of initial forces away from the damage zone results, producing a Q wave.

      ii) Appears within hours of transmural MI

(3) Determine location of left ventricular MI. Abnormal Q waves seen in the following specific leads:

    a) Septal MI: leads V_1, V_2

    b) Anterior MI: leads V_3, V_4

    c) Lateral MI: leads V_5, V_6

    d) High lateral MI: leads I, aVL

    e) Inferior MI: leads II, III, aVF

    f) Anteroseptal MI: leads V_1 to V_4

    g) Anterolateral MI: leads V_3 to V_6, I, aVL

    h) Inferolateral MI: leads II, III, aVF, V_5, V_6

(4) Posterior wall infarction

    a) No leads truly reflect posterior surface of heart

    b) Infarction diagnosis is made from reciprocal changes seen in anterior chest leads (V_1 to V_3)

    c) Abnormal, tall R waves seen in V_1 and V_2

    d) ST segment depression in leads V_1 to V_3

    e) Tall T waves in leads V_1 to V_3

(5) Right ventricular infarction

    a) ST elevation seen in lead V_4R

    b) Suspect right ventricular infarction in the setting of inferior wall infarction (often perfused by same coronary artery)

        i) Take 12-lead ECG with left and right precordial leads

        ii) Monitor hemodynamics and note parameters indicative of left and right ventricular infarcts (Table 2–2)

        iii) Observe for signs of heart failure

(6) Non–Q-wave MI (subendocardial infarction): infarction of endocardial surface only, not through entire myocardial wall

    a) No abnormal Q waves

    b) T-wave inversion in leads facing epicardial surface over infarcted area

TABLE 2–2. RV and LV Infarct Hemodynamics

Parameter	Normal	RV Infarct	LV Infarct
RA pressure (CVP)	2–6 mm Hg	↑	Normal
PA systolic (RVP)	15–27 mm Hg	↓	Normal or ↑
PA diastolic	10–19 mm Hg	↓	↑
PCWP	6–15 mm Hg	↓	↑
LVEDP	6–15 mm Hg	↓	↑
CO	4–8 L/min	↓	↓
CI	2.5–4.0 L/min/m²	↓	↓
SVR	900–1400 dynes/sec/cm⁻⁵	↑	↑

RV = right ventricular; LV = left ventricular; RA = right atrial; PA = pulmonary artery; PCWP = pulmonary capillary wedge pressure; LVEDP = left ventricular end-diastolic pressure; CO = cardiac output; CI = cardiac index; SVR = systemic vascular resistance.

       (7) Other causes of Q waves

          a) Normal Q waves; small Q wave in leads I, aVL, V_5, V_6

          b) Normal Q wave in lead III: less than 0.03 seconds, disappears with inspiration

          c) LBBB

          d) Myocarditis, cardiomyopathy

       (8) Determining age of infarction

          a) Acute (hours old): changes in leads over infarct

            i) Hyperacute T wave: first hour

            ii) Elevated ST segment

          b) Recent (hours to days old)

            i) ST segment begins to return to baseline (inferior MI: 95% resolve within 2 weeks; anterior MI: 40% resolve)

            ii) T wave flattens and may then invert

            iii) Q wave persists

          c) Old: abnormal Q wave; ST segments have returned to baseline (T-wave inversion may last days or weeks or may be permanent)

       (9) Serial ECGs are more helpful, along with those done with ischemic pain

    iii. Echocardiography: assesses left ventricular function, wall motion abnormalities, complications such as ventricular septal defect, thrombi, aneurysms

4. Nursing diagnoses (see Commonly Encountered Nursing Diagnoses section earlier)

  a. Pain (acute) related to decreased coronary blood flow that causes myocardial injury and necrosis

    i. Assessment for defining characteristics

      (a) ST elevation associated with prolonged chest pain

      (b) Pain suggests ongoing ischemia and infarction

    ii. Expected outcomes

      (a) Patient will have no pain

      (b) Patient will have adequate hemodynamic parameters

      (c) Arrhythmias will be controlled or absent

    iii. Nursing interventions

      (a) Ensure patient is receiving oxygen at 2 to 4 L/minute or as necessary to maintain adequate oxygen saturation over 90%. Hypoxemia is due to ventilation/perfusion mismatch and left ventricular failure

      (b) Remind patient frequently to notify nurse immediately if discomfort recurs

      (c) Relieve discomfort with analgesics

        (1) Relief of pain decreases elevated sympathetic response and myocardial workload (lowering heart rate, blood pressure) and counters the arrhythmic effect of circulating catecholamines

        (2) Morphine sulfate (MSO_4): 2 to 4 mg IV every 5 minutes to relieve discomfort (up to 30 mg may be required before discomfort is relieved)

                a) Decrease doses in elderly patients and in patients with respiratory disease

                b) Respiratory depression with MSO_4 usually peaks 7 minutes after IV injection and is dose related (not usually a problem in patients with MI)

                c) Orthostatic hypotension usually results from volume depletion: give volume and keep patient in Trendelenburg position

                d) Naloxone, 0.4 mg IV (repeated up to three times in 3-minute intervals), may be given to counteract hypotension, depressed respirations

          (d) Antiemetics may be necessary for the high degree of acute vagal tone with myocardial infarction and the emetic side effects of opiate analgesia

          (e) Anxiolytics (haloperidol) may be used if patient is agitated, delerious, very anxious (sleep deprivation, intensive care unit [ICU] psychosis)

          (f) Flexible visiting hours can assist in relieving anxiety and other stress that can create a situation for pain occurrence (dependent on patient's status, need for rest, procedures, and healthy family dynamics)

          (g) Teaching issues include rationales for all interventions, description of what patient should anticipate experiencing during interventions, how to treat discomfort or pain at home

      iv. Evaluation of nursing care

          (a) No complaints of chest discomfort

          (b) Vital signs within normal limits for patient

          (c) Normal sinus rhythm on ECG

   b. Altered myocardial tissue perfusion secondary to CAD. Patient may be a candidate for *thrombolysis*—intracoronary thrombolytic use via primary PTCA or by intravenous route in emergency department or critical care unit—or may be a candidate for immediate angioplasty

      i. Assessment for defining characteristics

          (a) ST segment elevation associated with prolonged chest pain

          (b) Pain suggests ongoing ischemia and infarction

          (c) The following contraindications to use of thrombolytic therapy are *not* present:

             (1) Recent surgical procedures (within 3 weeks)

             (2) Pregnancy or recent delivery (within 3 weeks)

             (3) History of cerebrovascular disease (within the past 3 months)

             (4) Recent intracranial or intraspinal surgery or head trauma (within the past 2 months)

             (5) Bleeding disorders or recent history of hemorrhage (within the past 2 to 4 weeks)

             (6) Recent organ biopsy (within the past 3 weeks)

             (7) CPR (within the past 3 weeks)

             (8) Current severe, advanced illness

      ii. Expected outcomes

          (a) Patient will have no pain

          (b) Coronary artery flow is restored within 30 to 90 minutes

  (c) Coronary perfusion will be increased, and symptoms will be relieved

  (d) Patient will have adequate hemodynamic parameters

  (e) Arrhythmias will be controlled or absent

  (f) ECG will show ST segment back to baseline

  (g) CK isoenzymes will drop more rapidly than normal, with higher peak as a result of reperfusion

 iii. Nursing interventions

  (a) Facilitate immediate therapy for patient with MI by preparing patient for immediate procedures, and administering medications (Tables 2–3, 2–4)

  (b) Watch for reperfusion arrhythmias. In the initial period after coronary blood flow is restored, ventricular arrhythmias frequently occur. Monitor patient's ECG and watch for hypotension and bradycardia. Give medications as ordered. Be prepared for immediate cardioversion/defibrillation

  (c) Thrombolytic agents may cause bleeding problems in gums, gastrointestinal tract, retroperitoneal cavity, and nervous system and at the insertion site

   (1) Observe insertion site

   (2) Monitor coagulation studies

   (3) Immobilize affected limb

   (4) Watch vital signs, neurologic status closely

  (d) Observe patient for urticaira, fever, bronchospasm, dyspnea, arrhythmias, and flushing (streptokinase and anisoylated plasminogen streptokinase activator complex [APSAC] may cause allergic reactions)

  (e) Be aware of signs of reocclusion: ST segment changes, chest discomfort, arrhythmias, hypotension

 iv. Evaluation of nursing care

  (a) No complaints of chest discomfort

  (b) Vital signs within normal limits for patient

  (c) No signs of bleeding problems

  (d) Coagulation studies are within set or normal parameters

  (e) Normal sinus rhythm on ECG

c. Decreased cardiac output related to ischemic or infarcted myocardium (see Commonly Encountered Nursing Diagnoses section earlier)

 i. Additional nursing interventions

  (a) Rapid recognition and treatment of complications are essential

  (b) Administer appropriate medication therapy for patient with MI as ordered (see Table 2–3)

  (c) Have patient maintain bed rest for the first 12 hours, with use of bedside commode

   (1) Early mobilization is important: use of chair or bedside commode in first 24 hours (improves well-being, lowers risk of pulmonary embolus)

   (2) Increase ambulation in room as tolerated during the first 48 hours

  (d) Instruct patient to avoid Valsalva maneuvers: cause dramatic changes in heart rate and blood pressure (ventricular filling) and can cause arrhythmias (especially important in patient <45 years of age). Stool softeners should be ordered

(e) Earlier "coronary precautions" have been abandoned (i.e., strict bed rest and limitations of physical activity; restrictions of hot and cold fluids; avoidance of vigorous back rubs; assisted eating; and avoidance of caffeine (regular caffeine drinkers have a developed tolerance and can experience withdrawal symptoms of increased heart rate or headaches; several cups of coffee would have no ill effects)

(f) Patient's usual maintenance medications need to be reviewed and potentially adjusted (e.g., diabetic medications)

(g) Keep patient NPO until discomfort or pain is gone, then clear liquids and progress diet

(h) It is important to stress smoking cessation after MI. Patient may need nicotine replacement if he or she is a heavy smoker or showing symptoms of withdrawal

(i) Potential complications with acute MI

    (1) Postinfarction pain (persistent, recurrent)

        a) Common causes: ischemia, pericarditis

        b) When pain is present, an ECG should be obtained and compared with previous ECGs

        c) Pain recurring after infarction suggests ongoing ischemia and should be evaluated promptly

        d) Pericarditis does not occur in first 24 hours

    (2) Heart failure, cardiogenic shock, acute pulmonary edema: Management may include the following:

        a) Bedside hemodynamic monitoring via a pulmonary artery thermodilution catheter

        b) Preload reduction with IV nitroglycerin, diuretics

        c) Afterload reduction with nitroprusside, IABP

        d) Contractility enhanced with dobutamine

        e) Blood pressure maintained with dopamine

        f) Heart rate controlled with beta blockers, cardioversion, atropine, pacemakers

        g) Reperfusion interventions: PTCA, CABG. CABG can be beneficial, especially in patients who have multivessel disease and have undergone unsuccessful interventions (such as PTCA, thrombolytics) and whose symptoms began within 4 to 6 hours earlier

    (3) Right ventricular infarction

        a) Preload is vital for maintaining forward output in right ventricular infarction. Ensure that patient has sufficient volume (normal saline) before giving nitroglycerin because risk of hypotension is high

        b) Inotropic support (dobutamine), when cardiac output fails to improve with volume

        c) AV sequential pacing may be required for increasing cardiac output (blocks are common)

        d) Cardioversion of atrial fibrillation, if patient is hemodynamically unstable

Text continued on page 234

TABLE 2–3. Immediate Management of Acute Myocardial Infarction

Therapy	Rationale	Indications	Contraindications and Caveats	Nursing Considerations
Immediate Management				
Thrombolysis	The **standard therapy** for acute MI: Lowers mortality by 25% Decreases infarct size Increases LV function Benefits greatest if administered within 3 hr of symptom onset	When ST segment is ↑, patient with prolonged ischemic pain Bundle branch block and positive cardiac enzymes for MI No age limit Up to 12 hr if ongoing ischemia For anterior and inferior MI	BP >200 mm Hg systolic or >110 diastolic Prior stroke Recent surgery Intracranial (IC) pathology Lack of ST segment ↑ unless new LBBB ↑ stroke risk with t-PA versus streptokinase (SK) if >70 years old	Detailed history from patient and SO vital to assess for contraindication Close monitoring for bleeding Enzymes after reperfusion: peak elevation is ~12 hr after symptoms Risk of stroke (intracerebral hemorrhage [ICH]) in first day, greater if >65 years old, low body weight (<70 kg), t-PA used, or if hypertension on admission
Primary PTCA	↓ Mortality ↓ Nonfatal MI ↓ Intracranial hemorrhage if PTCA is performed <4 hr after onset of infarction ↓ late costs (lowers readmissions)	High-risk patient (>75 years old, anterior MI, ↑ heart rate, history of prior MI) Cardiogenic shock Hemodynamic instability Contraindication to thrombolytics (bleeding risk)	Must be able to dilate artery within 4 hr of onset of MI Must have immediate availability of CABG surgery	Rapid assessment and preparation of patient and family for PTCA procedure
Ancillary Drug Therapy				
Aspirin	ASA and SK reduces mortality from MI to half that with SK alone ↓ Reinfarction rate, especially if given within 4 hr of onset of symptoms	There is increased platelet activation with thrombolysis; ASA inhibits this	Hypersensitivity to ASA Caution in blood dyscrasia, severe hepatitis	160–325 mg q.d. from presentation for at least 1 yr Watch for evidence of bleeding

Drug	Effects	Indications	Cautions/Adverse Effects	Dosing/Monitoring
Heparin	↑ Patency when used with t-PA Helps decrease formulation of LV thrombi Decreased mortality Decreased incidence of stroke Decreased reinfarction rate Low-dose heparin decreases deep vein thrombi	Patient having PTCA or surgical revascularization procedures Utilized in conjunction with t-PA therapy	↓ Platelets, especially with rethrombosis (incidence of heparin-induced thrombocytopenia is 3%)	70-U/kg bolus IV (at t-PA start), 15 U/kg/hr IV as maintenance Monitor aPTT aPTT goal: 50–75 seconds (1.5–2× control) IV: Treated for no longer than 48 hr, unless risk of emboli 7,500 U subcutaneously b.i.d. (alternative method) May have "rebound effect" with abrupt discontinuation; use of gradual weaning is being studied
Nitrates	↓ Mortality ↓ MI size, LV function, and LV thrombus ↑ LV ejection fraction increases myocardial blood flow by vasodilatation Reduces preload	Acute MI Unstable angina IV over 24–48 hr (in acute MI with pain, heart failure, hypertension)	Severe hypotension No protection against recurrent ischemic events Cautious use with inferior/RV MIs because of need for adequate preload, hypotension risk Beware: IV NTG may interfere with heparin action, requiring higher doses of heparin to achieve aPTT goals while NTG is infusing	12.5–25 μg bolus, then 10–20 μg/min, increasing 5–10 μg every 5–10 min Titrate to ↓ BP (MAP) 10% (30% if patient is hypertensive) Upper limits = severe hypotension Monitor closely Keep systolic BP >90 mm Hg, HR <110 beats/min Half-life is 1–3 min IV (4–5 min subcutaneously) Nitrate tolerance (chronic use) can occur; need planned "drug-free times" Readjust heparin when NTG discontinued

Table continued on following page

TABLE 2–3. Immediate Management of Acute Myocardial Infarction *Continued*

Therapy	Rationale	Indications	Contraindications and Caveats	Nursing Considerations
Beta blockers (metoprolol, antenolol, propranolol)	↓ Mortality ↓ Nonfatal reinfarction May ↓ IC bleeds with thrombolytics Decrease cardiac pain Lower heart rate and contractility, thereby lowering MVO$_2$ requirements Increases perfusion by lengthening diastole	Acute MI, <12 hr since onset of symptoms, if no contraindications Recurring cardiac pain Tachyarrhythmias	Relative contraindications: Severe peripheral vascular disease LV failure (moderate or severe) ↓ HR (<60) Second or third degree AV block PR > 0.24 seconds Hypotension (less than 100 mm Hg systolic) Asthma Severe COPD Insulin-dependent diabetes	IV metoprolol up to 15 mg over 10–15 minutes, then 50–100 mg b.i.d. p.o. IV atenolol, 5 mg, then repeat 5 mg in 10 min, then 100 mg/day p.o.
ACE inhibitors at <24 hr	↓ Mortality ↓ LV failure Decrease ventricular remodeling	Large infarct Anterior Q waves Heart failure, if hemodynamics stable for at least 6 hr Ejection fraction < 40% Given within 24 hr of symptom onset	Hypotension Renal failure Bilateral stenosis of renal arteries Allergy to ACE inhibitors Systolic BP less than 100 mm Hg	Graded dosing schedules: captopril, 6.25 mg p.o., then 12.5 mg 2 hr later, 25 mg 12 hr after, then 50 mg b.i.d. Used for 4–6 weeks after MI, if no complications

Of No Proven Value

Drug	Comments	Indications	Cautions	Dosage
Calcium channel blockers	May ↑ mortality No evidence of benefit acutely No value except in non-Q MI with no revascularization planned	Used for non-Q MI when there are no plans to study or revascularize When beta blockers are contraindicated or unsuccessful for ongoing ischemia or atrial fibrillation (verapamil, diltiazem)	Q-wave infarct Heart failure AV block	
Lidocaine	↓ VF, VT, PVCs No ↓ mortality ↑ Morbidity (asystole, electromechanical dissociation occurrences) CNS toxicity in elderly	VF, VT Wide-complex tachycardias	No longer used prophylactically	1–1.5 mg/kg (75–100 mg) IV bolus, then 0.5–0.75 mg/kg (25–50 mg) IV given every 5–10 minutes if required; total, 3 mg/kg Maintenance: 1–4 mg/min
Magnesium	May decrease mortality, morbidity Preferably given early: <6 hr after symptom onset Has antiplatelet activity, produces systemic/coronary vasodilation	Hypomagnesemia Torsade de pointes (polymorphic VT)		1–2 g IV over 5 min

MI = myocardial infarction; LV = left ventricular; CPR = cardiopulmonary resuscitation; CABG = coronary artery bypass graft; t-PA = tissue plasminogen activator; BP = blood pressure; LBBB = left bundle branch block; SO = significant other; PTCA = percutaneous transluminal coronary angioplasty; ASA = acetylsalicylic acid; IV = intravenous; aPTT = activated partial thromboplastin time; RV = right ventricular; NTG = nitroglycerin; MAP = mean arterial pressure; MVO_2 = myocardial oxygen ventilation rate; AV = atrioventricular; HR = heart rate; COPD = chronic obstructive pulmonary disease; ACE = angiotensin-converting enzyme; VF = ventricular fibrillation; VT = ventricular tachycardia; PVC = premature ventricular contraction; CNS = central nervous system.

TABLE 2–4. Thrombolytic Agents

Thrombolytic Agent	Actions and Indications	Characteristics and Administration	Nursing Considerations
Streptokinase (SK): Protein derived from group C streptococci bacteria	Activates plasminogen into plasmin, which dissolves clot Depletes plasma fibrinogen; fibrinogen breakdown by-products cause an anticoagulant effect	1.5 million U in 30–60 min Half-life: 20 min Effects last 24–36 h Antigenic	Can cause hypotension and reperfusion arrhythmias Rare anaphylactic reactions wtih first use Post-SK use: long-term antibody formation limits second use
Urokinase (UK): Derived from human urine	Direct plasminogen activator	4 ml/minute (6,000 IU/min) for up to 2 hr intra-arterially (average dose required to keep artery open—500,000 IU) Half-life: 20 minutes	Maintain strict bed rest Have separate IV line Higher cost than SK
Tissue plasminogen activator (t-PA), recombinant: human protein manufactured by genetic engineering	Fibrin selective Clot lysis faster than with SK Used in patients with large infarcts, anterior wall infarcts, allergies to SK, previous SK treatment Increased risk of intracranial hemorrhage in elderly	Accelerated, front-loaded dosing: IV 15-mg bolus, then 0.75 mg/kg over 30 minutes (50 mg maximum), then 0.5 mg/kg over 60 minutes (35 mg maximum); total dose is no more than 100 mg Half-life: 6 min Nonantigenic Use with heparin	Higher cost than SK Watch for evidence of bleeding Oozing at IV site should be anticipated

   e) Afterload reduction with sodium nitroprusside, IABP
   f) Patient could be candidate for RVAD
 (4) Left ventricular thrombus: more likely with CK rise of more than 3200 IU/L
 (5) Arrhythmias: atrial fibrillation, VT, V fib, bradyarrhythmias (see Cardiac Rhythm Disorders section later)
 (6) Ventricular septal defects: surgical repair is needed immediately if patient is hemodynamically unstable
 (7) Left ventricular aneurysm
 (8) Acute mitral regurgitation
 (9) Left ventricular free wall rupture
 (10) Papillary muscle rupture
(j) IABP may be necessary for severe hypotension or cardiogenic shock, especially in patients with low cardiac output and

ongoing ischemia (see Heart Failure section later for more detailed coverage of IABP). IABP is used during MI for

(1) Acute mitral regurgitation

(2) Refractory ventricular arrhythmias

(3) Post–MI angina

(4) As a bridge to revascularization

Heart Failure

Heart failure is impaired cardiac function wherein one or both ventricles are unable to maintain an output adequate to meet the metabolic demands of the body. Heart failure can occur either on the right or left side of the heart and is due to either systolic dysfunction (poor contraction), diastolic dysfunction (poor filling), or increased afterload.

"Congestive heart failure" is an imprecise catch-all term. It is a manifestation of cardiac dysfunction but not a diagnosis.

1. **Pathophysiology**
    a. *Left-sided heart failure: systolic dysfunction*
        i. Impaired forward output caused by decreased left ventricular contractility (e.g., CAD, cardiomyopathies) in which the EF is reduced to below normal
        ii. To compensate, the left ventricle dilates and the heart rate increases in an attempt to maintain a normal output. By increasing the stroke volume and heart rate, cardiac output may return toward normal despite a poor EF
        iii. Left ventricular filling pressures rise because of dilatation and/or decreased left ventricular compliance (producing left ventricular disatolic dysfunction)
        iv. Left atrial and pulmonary venous pressures rise, producing pulmonary congestion and edema
            (a) When pulmonary capillary oncotic pressure (30 mm Hg) is exceeded, fluid leaks into pulmonary interstitial space, creating pulmonary edema
            (b) Decreased oxygenation of blood occurs as oxygen exchange is impeded by presence of fluid
        v. Right-sided heart pressure increases as a result of increased pressure in the pulmonary system
        vi. Right-sided heart failure may then occur because of the pulmonary hypertension, resulting in peripheral and organ edema
    b. *Left-sided heart failure: diastolic dysfunction*
        i. A noncompliant, stiff left ventricle has less ability to relax, interfering with adequate filling and resulting in rising diastolic (filling) pressures
        ii. As a consequence, left atrial, pulmonary venous, and pulmonary capillary pressures increase
        iii. Pulmonary artery and right-sided heart pressures elevate, if untreated
        iv. Systolic function is often normal and accounts for the fact that up to 30% of patients with "heart failure" have normal left ventricular systolic function

    c. *Right-sided heart failure: systolic dysfunction*

      i. The right heart is unable to adequately pump blood forward, resulting in a drop in cardiac output

      ii. Right ventricular infarction is the most common cause

      iii. Right ventricular dilatation and elevation of filling pressure develop, resulting in peripheral edema and hypertension

    d. *Right-sided heart failure, diastolic dysfunction:* can occur with right ventricular hypertrophy, cardiomyopathies; analogous to left-sided heart diastolic dysfunction, except that the consequence is peripheral edema, rather than pulmonary, associated with elevated right-sided heart filling pressures (increased jugular venous pressures)

2. **Etiologic or precipitating factors:** see Table 2–5 for factors related to left- and right-sided heart failure

3. **Nursing assessment data base:** patients generally have asymptomatic heart failure for an uncertain time before the recognition of symptoms

    a. Nursing history: see Table 2–6 for clinical findings in left- and right-sided heart failure

    b. Nursing examination of patient (see Table 2–6)

    c. Diagnostic study findings

      i. Laboratory

        (a) HCT, hemoglobin (Hb): for anemia

        (b) Electrolytes

        (c) Renal function: BUN, creatinine

        (d) Liver function: right-sided failure

        (e) Cardiac enzymes (if potential acute MI)

      ii. Radiologic: often normal

        (a) Pulmonary vasculature: edema, fluid

        (b) Cardiac silhouette may show cardiac enlargement: hypertrophy, dilatation

        (c) Enlarged right atrium and right ventricle

        (d) Pleural effusion (left-sided failure)

        (e) Valve calicifications

      iii. ECG

        (a) Nonspecific changes

        (b) For arrhythmias, ischemic disease, conduction abnormalities, drug and electrolyte effects

      iv. Echocardiogram: to assess

        (a) Chamber size: wall thickness

        (b) Systolic and diastolic function (global and regional)

        (c) Thrombus formation

        (d) Valvular function

        (e) Pericardial disease

      v. Radionuclide imaging

        (a) Left and right chamber function and volume assessed

        (b) Ischemia, infarction

      vi. Ultrafast CT and MRI: can be used to assess structural abnormalities, tumors, vascular anomalies, pericardial disease

      vii. Cardiac catheterization: to assess

        (a) Coronary anatomy

        (b) Pressures in right and left chambers

          (1) High filling pressures with or without systolic dysfunction represents diastolic dysfunction

TABLE 2–5. Etiology or Precipitating Factors in Heart Failure

Left-Sided Heart Failure		Right-Sided Heart Failure	Both Sides
Systolic	*Diastolic*		
Ischemic heart disease (50% of all cases)	Coronary artery disease	Left-sided heart failure	Patient noncompliant regarding
Myocardial infarction	Myocardial ischemia	Atherosclerotic heart disease	Medications
Myocardial stunning/ hibernation	Left ventricular hypertrophy	Acute right ventricular myocardial infarction	Dietary restrictions Alcohol (ETOH) use
Coronary artery disease	Cardiomyopathy: hypertrophic, restrictive, dilated	Pulmonary embolism	Medications Negative inotropic agents
Idiopathic dilated cardiomyopathy	Increased circulating volume	Fluid overload, excess sodium intake	Sodium retention
Myocardial contusion	Cardiac tamponade Constrictive	Myocardial contusion Cardiomyopathy	
Aortic insufficiency	pericarditis	Valvular heart disease	
Arrhythmias: ventricular	Left ventricular hypertrophy	Atrial or ventricular septal defect	
tachycardia, atrial fibrillation	Mitral stenosis or insufficiency	Pulmonary outflow stenosis	
Post–pump syndrome	Aortic stenosis or insufficiency	Chronic obstructive pulmonary	
Myocarditis	Age (decreased compliance of	disease: pulmonary hypertension (cor	
Infections: viral, bacterial, fungal	heart muscle) Diabetes mellitus	pulmonale)	
Acute rheumatic fever	Intracardiac shunts	Sleep apnea	
Drug abuse: heroin, alcohol (ETOH), cocaine			
Nutrition deficits: protein, thiamine			
Electrolyte disorders: decreases in calcium, sodium, potassium, phosphate			
Diabetes, thyroid disease			
Drugs suppressing contractility (negative inotropic)			

      (2) Diuretic and IV nitroglycerin use can create a false negative by artificially normalizing the filling pressures

      (3) Ventricular contractility

      (4) Valvular function, cardiac defects

4. **Nursing Diagnoses** (see Commonly Encountered Nursing Diagnoses section earlier)

   a. Decreased cardiac output and altered tissue perfusion related to damaged

TABLE 2–6. Clinical Findings in Heart Failure

Left-Sided Heart Failure		Right-Sided Heart Failure
Systolic	*Diastolic*	
Anxiety	Exercise intolerance	Increased fatigue
Sudden lightheadedness	Orthopnea	Hepatomegaly
Fatigue, weakness, lethargy	Dyspnea, dyspnea on	Splenomegaly
Orthopnea	exertion, paroxysmal	Dependent pitting edema
Dyspnea, dyspnea on	nocturnal dyspnea	Ascites
exertion, paroxysmal	Cough with frothy white/	Cachexia
nocturnal dyspnea	pink sputum (in	Abdominal pain (from
Tachypnea (on exertion)	pulmonary edema)	congested liver)
Cheyne-Stokes (if severe)	Tachypnea (on exertion)	Anorexia, nausea, emesis
Diaphoresis	Basilar crackles, rhonchi,	Weight gain
Palpitations	wheezes	Low blood pressure
Sacral edema, pitting	Pulmonary edema	Oliguria, nocturia
extremities	Symptoms of right-sided	(increased renal
Basilar rales, rhonchi,	heart failure	perfusion/blood volume
crackles, wheezes	Hypoxia, respiratory	when lying in bed)
Skin: cool, moist; cyanosis	acidosis	Venous distention
Hypoxia, respiratory	Elevated pulmonary	Hepatojugular reflux
acidosis	artery diastolic	Fatigue, weakness
Elevated pulmonary artery	pressure, pulmonary	Kussmaul's sign (if
diastolic pressure,	capillary wedge	constriction)
pulmonary capillary	pressure	Murmur of tricuspid
wedge pressure	S_3, S_4 heart sounds	insufficiency
Nocturia	Holosystolic murmur (if	S_3, S_4 heart sounds (right-
Mental confusion	tricuspid, mitral	sided)
Pulse pressure decreased	regurgitation)	Elevated central venous
Pulsus alternans		pressure, and right atrial
Point of maximal impulse		and right ventricular
displaced laterally		pressures
S_3, S_4 heart sounds		
Murmur of mitral		
insufficiency		

myocardium, decreased contractile state, impaired filling, arrhythmias, and conduction defects

    i. Additional nursing interventions

      (a) Provide for rest

        (1) Maintain relaxed, quiet environment

        (2) Organize nursing care to allow for rest period

        (3) Prevent complications of deep vein thrombosis by range-of-motion exercises, TED hose, pneumatic antiembolic stockings

      (b) Monitor ECG and institute appropriate therapy if arrhythmias or conduction defects occur

      (c) Observe for signs and symptoms of decreased cerebral perfusion; if patient is disoriented, protect from injury

      (d) Monitor hemodynamic parameters closely, especially when using vasoactive drugs (often monitoring arterial pressure and hemodynamic pressures with noninvasive BP monitoring, arterial lines, and PA catheter)

(e) Be knowledgeable regarding safe administration of medications commonly used for heart failure

   (1) Dopamine: to support blood pressure and urinary output

      a) Dose-related alpha- and beta-adrenergic and dopaminergic effects

      b) Dopaminergic effects (at low doses of 1 to 2 μg/kg/minute) increase renal and mesenteric blood flow, thereby increasing urinary output

      c) Beta-adrenergic effects (at rates of 2 to 10 μg/kg/minute) increase blood pressure, cerebral and renal perfusion

      d) Alpha-adrenergic effects (at rates of >10 μg/kg/minute) cause peripheral vasoconstriction, increased SVR, increased afterload and blood pressure (possible decrease in cardiac output). Loss of renal and mesenteric dilatation occurs, decreasing renal function

      e) Indications: low cardiac output, hypotension, or renal insufficiency

      f) May cause tachycardia

      g) Check skin for color, temperature, capillary refill; alpha-adrenergic stimulation causes peripheral venoconstriction

      h) Infuse in central line or large vein, using a volumetric infusion pump for safety and accuracy

      i) Extravasation causes tissue necrosis and sloughing. If this occurs, stop infusion, immediately inject phentolamine (Regitine), 5 to 10 mg diluted in 10 to 15 ml of saline solution, around site to lessen deleterious effects of infiltrated dopamine

      j) Close arterial pressure monitoring is important in post-CABG patient

   (2) Dobutamine: to support myocardial contractility

      a) Stimulates beta receptors in the heart muscles

      b) Direct-acting, positive inotropic agent that increases contractility, thereby increasing stroke volume and cardiac output

      c) No beneficial renal effects except from increased cardiac output

      d) Indications: low cardiac output, hypotension caused by cardiogenic shock

      e) Contraindications: hypertrophic cardiomyopathy, severe aortic stenosis

      f) Infused at an IV rate of 2.5 to 10 μg/kg/min

      g) Monitor for tachyarrhythmias, ventricular ectopy

      h) Can decrease blood pressure in low doses usually associated with volume depletion, excessive diuresis, IV nitroglycerin). Check for volume depletion before administering drug

   (3) Amrinone, milrinone (phosphodiesterase inhibitors)

      a) Directly increases myocardial contractility without

increasing the heart rate by increasing cellular levels of cyclic adenosine monophosphate (cAMP)

b) Directly relaxes vascular (both arterial and venous) smooth muscle, producing peripheral vasodilation (decreasing afterload and preload)

c) Amrinone has a half-life of 2 to 5 hr. A typical loading dose is 0.5 to 0.75 mg/kg IV bolus over 2 to 3 minutes followed by a 2- to 20-μg/kg/minute infusion

d) Milrinone (second-generation drug, now used more often than amrinone) has a half-life of 20 to 45 minutes. A loading dose of 50 μg/kg is administered over 10 minutes and followed by a 0.375- to 0.75-μg/kg/minute infusion

e) Untoward effects include tachycardia, arrhythmias, hypotension (to correct hypovolemia)

(4) Sodium nitroprusside: to decrease afterload

a) Primarily decreases afterload via arterial dilatation, also reducing preload and blood pressure and increasing cardiac output

b) Systemic and pulmonary vascular resistance decreases

c) Indication: when cardiac output is diminished as a result of increased systemic vascular resistance (e.g., cardiac surgery, hypertension, heart failure)

d) Contraindications: severe aortic stenosis, coarctation of aorta

e) Action: immediate and very brief; effect ends 1 to 2 minutes after infusion is stopped

f) Monitor blood pressure and hemodynamics closely

g) Rate of infusion is titrated by blood pressure, hemodynamics

h) Initial dose: starting at 0.1 μg/kg/minute

i) Extravasation should be treated with phentolamine (see dopamine earlier); otherwise, necrosis and sloughing of superficial tissue at IV site will occur

(5) IV nitroglycerin: to improve left ventricular function by lowering preload via venodilatation

(6) ACE inhibitor: used for afterload reduction

a) Causes afterload reduction, which decreases left ventricular workload and improves cardiac output

b) Improves heart function and decreases risk of mortality

c) Contraindicated in shock and hyperkalemia when serum potassium level exceeds 5.5 mEq/L

d) Monitor blood pressure, potassium levels (increases K^+ retention), increased creatinine levels

(7) Cardiac glycosides: digitalis

a) Weakly inotropic

b) Primary benefit is for rate control of atrial fibrillation, atrial flutter

(f) Avoid drugs that decrease myocardial contractility

(1) Anti-leukemia drugs (e.g., daunorubicin, doxorubicin)

(2) Disopyramide

(3) Beta blockers are beneficial in patients with ischemic and dilated cardiomyopathy

(g) Placement of IABP may be necessary as a bridge to other interventions. Patient and significant other should be prepared for this procedure

   (1) Purposes of IABP

      a) Decreases afterload

      b) Decreases myocardial oxygen demands

      c) Increases coronary perfusion

      d) Improves cardiac output and tissue perfusion

      e) Can prevent cardiogenic shock, limit size of infarctions

      f) Limits myocardial ischemia if present

   (2) Uses of IABP

      a) Support in acute MI with cardiogenic shock

      b) Circulatory support in post-CABG patients

      c) Support in high-risk cardiac catheterizations

      d) In severe ischemia, as a bridge to revascularization

   (3) IABP is placed percutaneously via the femoral artery into the descending thoracic aorta

   (4) Inflation and deflation of balloon are synchronized with the patient's ECG or arterial pressure waveform

      a) During ventricular diastole, balloon is inflated. Augments diastolic pressures and increases coronary blood flow. Myocardial oxygen supply and contractility are improved

      b) Just before ventricular systole, balloon is deflated. Reduces afterload. Myocardial oxygen demand is decreased.

   (5) Contraindications

      a) Aortic insufficiency

      b) Severe aortic disease

      c) Severe peripheral vascular disease in affected limb

   (6) Complications

      a) Ischemia of limb distal to insertion site: caused by mechanical occlusion of the artery or thromboembolism (10% incidence)

      b) Dissection of aorta

      c) Thrombocytopenia

      d) Septicemia

      e) Infection at insertion site

   (7) Key points in nursing care of patient with IABP

      a) Monitor all vital signs, especially heart rate. IABP timing is based on heart rate: when rate changes dramatically, duration of balloon inflation must be adjusted

      b) Monitor arterial pressures closely and watch volume status: improvement should occur with use

      c) Monitor closely for arrhythmias (especially irregular heart rhythms), which can hamper IABP efficacy

> > > > *d)* Look for signs of improved, effective cardiac output, mental status (if patient is not sedated), urinary output, skin color and warmth, capillary refill
> > > > *e)* Assess peripheral pulses; document presence and changes from baseline. Watch for changes in color, sensation, and temperature
> > > > *f)* Keep a close watch on insertion site for signs of bleeding, hematomas
> > > > *g)* Do not elevate head of bed beyond 15°; patient must keep affected limb straight
> > > > *h)* Assess pulses in upper extremities, especially left arm. Catheter can migrate up and occlude the subclavian artery
> > > > *i)* Heparin anticoagulation is mandatory. Watch for side effects from anticoagulation: abnormal coagulation laboratory results, guaiac-positive stools, or nasogastric secretions and petechiae
> > > > *j)* Be knowledgeable about IABP controls, safeguards, protocols for use
> > > > *k)* Be alert to signs of infection locally or systemically. Prevent infections by following unit protocols for dressing changes and other precautions
> > > > *l)* Prevent complications from immobility (e.g., skin breakdown, respiratory compromise)
> > > (h) LVAD may be necessary in severe left ventricular dysfunction postoperatively
> > > (i) Intubation and mechanical ventilation may be used in patients with hypoventilation and severe hypoxia
> > > (j) Patient will likely need help at home; arrange home services, evaluation of home needs
> > > (k) Provide explanations; begin teaching patient and/or significant other in preparation for discharge (see Commonly Encountered Nursing Diagnoses section, Knowledge Deficits subsection)
> > ii. Evaluation of nursing care
> > > (a) Hemodynamically stable
> > > (b) Arrhythmias controlled or absent
> > > (c) Cardiac output and tissue perfusion adequate
> b. Excess fluid volume caused by ineffective pumping of the heart, increased preload, sodium retention, decreased cardiac output
> > i. Assessment for defining characteristics (see Table 2–6)
> > ii. Expected outcomes
> > > (a) Lungs are clear, according to auscultation and x-ray
> > > (b) Decrease in edema and return to normal weight
> > > (c) Balanced intake and output
> > iii. Nursing interventions
> > > (a) Administer oxygen therapy
> > > (b) Semi–Fowler's position may improve ease of breathing
> > > (c) Monitor intake and output closely
> > > (d) Observe fluid and sodium restrictions closely
> > > (e) Weigh patient daily

(f) Assess patient for signs and symptoms indicating excessive systemic fluid volume (e.g., distended neck veins, crackles, peripheral edema, hepatic or visceral congestion)

(g) Watch laboratory data, particularly arterial blood gases, electrolytes, and especially potassium (patient may be receiving cardiac glycosides, and the potential for toxicity is greater with hypokalemia; patient may become hypokalemic on diuretics)

(h) Observe for changes from initial physical examination to detect worsening of heart failure: increased rales, jugular vein distention

(i) If the patient is on bed rest for prolonged period, institute measures to prevent hazards of immobility

(j) Administer diuretics as ordered. Diuretics decrease intravascular and extravascular fluid volume, and subsequently lower preload
  (1) Loop diuretics (such as furosemide 20 to 80 mg IV) as ordered
  (2) Evaluate for patient response to diuretics: increased urinary output, decreased edema, improved lung sounds and breathing; CVP and PCWP decrease
  (3) Monitor for complications
    a) Electrolyte imbalances, particularly decreased sodium, potassium, and magnesium levels
    b) Renal function (increased creatinine)
    c) Fatigue
    d) Hypovolemia
    e) Nausea, vomiting
    f) Headache
    g) Dry mouth
    h) Muscle cramps
    i) Dizziness

(k) Administer morphine, 3 to 5 mg IV, as ordered to reduce preload
  (1) Induces venodilation; decreases venous return to heart (increased capacitance)
  (2) Reduces pain
  (3) Decreases anxiety
  (4) Decreases myocardial oxygen consumption
  (5) Side effects include decreased respirations (apnea, hypoventilation), bradydysrhythmias, and hypotension

(l) Before discharge, patient and/or significant other should be able to
  (1) Briefly define heart failure and identify life style changes necessary to prevent recurrence
  (2) Identify foods high in sodium and plan to restrict sodium use
  (3) List at least four foods rich in potassium (especially important for patients taking loop diuretics)
  (4) Demonstrate how to take pulse
  (5) List symptoms that indicate worsening of condition, whether from heart failure or from side effects of drugs
  (6) Describe each current medication: name, purpose, dose, frequency, side effects, benefits of compliance

· · · · · · · · · · · · · · ·
:
: **Pericardial Disease**

1. Pathophysiology
   a. *Pericarditis*
      i. Inflammation of the pericardium has a wide variety of etiologies
      ii. It may be acute or chronic (tuberculosis)
      iii. Acute pericarditis is usually viral or idiopathic in etiology
         (a) Produces an acute illness characterized by fever, chest pain (characteristically relieved by sitting up), pericardial friction rub, ST elevation, and little to no pericardial effusion
         (b) Is usually self-limited and responds to nonsteroidal anti-inflammatory drugs (NSAIDs)
         (c) May be recurrent with relapses
   b. *Pericardial effusion*
      i. Results when pericardial fluid is produced too rapidly to be reabsorbed
      ii. If the pericardial fluid accumulates slowly, the pericardium stretches with little increase in intrapericardiac pressure and cardiac filling, and function is not disturbed
      iii. Same etiologies as for pericarditis
      iv. Huge effusions (several liters) may develop slowly without tamponade (especially in uremic pericarditis)
   c. *Cardiac tamponade*
      i. Can be caused by any of the etiologic factors listed in the next section; however, the common causes are few: trauma, iatrogenic trauma (catheter or pacemaker perforation, contusion during CPR), laceration during a pericardiocentesis (postoperative bleeding), aortic dissection, MI with myocardial rupture
      ii. Results when pericardial fluid accumulates too rapidly to allow the pericardium to stretch
      iii. Intrapericardiac pressure rises dramatically
      iv. The increased intrapericardiac pressure exceeds the filling pressures of, first, the right side of the heart (pretamponade) and then both sides of the heart, impairing ventricular filling and output
      v. The CVP and jugular venous pressures rise; may not be seen in marked hypovolemia
      vi. Pulsus paradoxus develops
      vii. Cardiac output falls dramatically
      viii. Compensatory tachycardia develops
      ix. Hypotension and death result in minutes
   d. *Constrictive pericarditis*
      i. Results from chronic scarring of the pericardium after pericarditis of any etiology
      ii. Most common causes are post-traumatic, postpericardiotomy, and postradiation factors; neoplasm; and tuberculosis
      iii. The epicardium becomes thickened with tough and rigid fibrous tissue that may calcify
      iv. This interferes with filling (especially of the right side of the heart) in mid- to late diastole, resulting in decreased cardiac output and increased jugular venous filling pressures

> v. A syndrome of right heart failure with decreased output develops
> vi. The cardiac output usually falls before the PCWP exceeds 25 mm Hg, so that pulmonary edema is not seen
> vii. Death is the usual outcome unless life-saving but high-risk (5% to 15% mortality rate) pericardiectomy is performed

2. Etiologic or precipitating factors

    a. Idiopathic, acute or nonspecific (most common cause)

    b. Infections

        i. Viral: echovirus and coxsackievirus B (the two most common causes of acute pericarditis); adenovirus, enterovirus, influenza, mumps, measles, smallpox

        ii. Bacterial: pneumococci, staphylococci, streptococci, *Pseudomonas* species

        iii. Fungal

        iv. Rickettsial

        v. Tuberculous

    c. Acute myocardial infarction: early (24 to 72 hours after) or delayed (Dressler's syndrome)

    d. Postcardiotomy or post-thoracotomy syndrome (occurs 3 to 7 days after surgery)

    e. Connective tissue diseases such as systemic lupus erythematosus, rheumatoid arthritis, polyarteritis nodosa, and scleroderma

    f. Chest trauma, penetrating (stabbing, rib fractures) or nonpenetrating, including surgical procedures such as pacemaker insertion

    g. Neoplasms (especially metastatic tumors from the lung and breast; melanomas; lymphomas)

    h. Dissecting aortic aneurysms

    i. Radiation therapy to thorax

    j. Systemic disease: uremia, myxedema, sarcoidosis

    k. Immunologic or hypersensitivity reactions: drug reactions (such as those to hydralazine, procainamide, penicillin)

3. Nursing assessment data base

    a. Nursing history

        i. Subjective findings

            (a) Sharp or stabbing precordial pain, increased with inspiration, lying down, swallowing or belching, or turning of thorax; may be relieved by leaning forward

            (b) Associated trapezius ridge pain

            (c) Nonspecific influenza-like complaints such as low-grade fever, joint discomfort, fatigue, weight loss, night sweats

            (d) Weakness, exercise intolerance

        ii. Objective findings

            (a) History of any of the etiologic findings

            (b) Recent history of taking immunosuppressive drugs (e.g., corticosteroids)

            (c) Weight loss

    b. Nursing examination of patient (depending on the severity, may observe any or all of the following symptoms)

        i. Inspection

            (a) Dyspnea with or without pain, orthopnea

            (b) Cough, hemoptysis

        (c) Tachycardia

        (d) Fever

        (e) Anxiety, confusion, restlessness

        (f) Pallor

        (g) Anorexia

        (h) Jugular venous distention

        (i) Kussmaul's sign (rise in CVP on inspiration): seen in patients with constrictive pericarditis

        (j) Flushing, sweating

        (k) Peripheral edema, abdominal swelling or discomfort (constrictive pericarditis) with prominent "Y" descent

    ii. Palpitation

        (a) In cardiac tamponade, pulsus paradoxus develops as the result of the influence of respiration on the beat-to-beat filling of the left ventricle by flow from the pulmonary veins

            (1) During inspiration, there is less pulmonary venous return to the left side of the heart; this decrease is exaggerated by the impaired filling caused by the high intrapericardiac pressure

            (2) May not be seen in states in which left ventricular filling is not solely dependent on pulmonary venous return (aortic insufficiency, ventricular septal defect)

        (b) Decreased or absent peripheral pulses with narrow pulse pressures

        (c) Increased cardiac dullness in large effusions

        (d) Hepatojugular reflux

    iii. Auscultation

        (a) Pericardial friction rub (three components): may be very evanescent

        (b) Heart sounds are often normal except muffled and distant-sounding with effusion

        (c) Pericardial "knock" in constriction

c. Diagnostic study findings

    i. Laboratory

        (a) Moderate leukocytosis, elevated sedimentation rate in acute or chronic pericarditis

        (b) CK isoenzyme levels may be elevated (if associated with MI)

        (c) Blood cultures: to identify causative organisms and their sensitivity to antibiotics

        (d) Antinuclear antibody test: results positive in connective tissue diseases

        (e) Blood urea nitrogen: renal status evaluation

        (f) Purified protein derivative (PPD): tuberculosis

        (g) Pericardiocentesis, especially pericardial biopsy and drainage, may be helpful diagnostically but is not important therapeutically

    ii. ECG

        (a) Acute pericarditis

            (1) Diffuse ST segment concave elevation in all leads except aVR, V_1

            (2) T wave becomes inverted after ST segment is isoelectric again

(3) PR segment depressed

(b) Bradycardia: in uremic patients

(c) Tachycardia: sinus, atrial arrhythmias, atrial fibrillation

iii. Radiologic examination: normal or may show cardiac enlargement that results from pericardial effusion, infiltrates of lungs, left pleural effusion (Dressler's), or masses

iv. Echocardiography: pericardial effusions, wall motion abnormalities, right atrial and right ventricular diastolic collapse (pretamponade)

(a) Respiratory variation in left ventricular inflow of more than 25% (tamponade)

(b) Restriction in ventricular filling (constriction)

v. Cardiac catheterization used to

(a) Evaluate severity of constriction

(b) Assess need for pericardiotomy (constriction)

(c) Differential diagnosis of constriction and restrictive cardiomyopathy (often impossible to differentiate between the two)

(d) Increased right and left ventricular filling pressures with equalization (constriction)

4. **Nursing diagnoses** (see Commonly Encountered Nursing Diagnoses section earlier)

a. Acute pain caused by pericardial inflammation

i. Assessment for defining characteristics (see Nursing History section earlier)

ii. Expected outcomes

(a) Patient can verbalize that pain is alleviated

(b) Laboratory values and clinical findings return to normal

iii. Additional nursing interventions (see Commonly Encountered Nursing Diagnoses section earlier)

(a) Frequently ask patient about pain, discomfort; if pain is present, assess characteristics

(b) Position patient for comfort: sitting up and leaning forward will help to increase comfort

(c) Administer medications to relieve pain, caused by inflammatory process, as ordered (ASA, acetaminophen, anti-inflammatory agents, indomethacin or ibuprofen, analgesics). Pain is often gone or diminished significantly in 24 to 48 hours but may last weeks. Corticosteroids (e.g., prednisone) are used for recurring, severe pain

(d) Administer antimicrobial agents if culture or serologic evidence of susceptible etiologic agent is present

(e) Reassure patients regarding the nonischemic etiology of pain

iv. Evaluation of nursing care

(a) Patient states that pain is less or alleviated

(b) Patient appears more calm, less anxious

(c) Laboratory values show that antimicrobial therapy is effective (e.g., leukocyte count and CBC returning to normal or within normal limits; blood cultures negative)

b. Decreased cardiac output related to potential complications such as tamponade or constriction, arrhythmias, heart failure, and hypotension

i. Assessment for defining characteristics

(a) See Nursing Examination of Patient section earlier
(b) See Diagnostic Findings section earlier
ii. Expected outcomes
(a) Patient shows no signs of tamponade
(b) Patient shows no signs or symptoms of heart failure
(c) Hemodynamics, vital signs, and ECG are within normal limits
iii. Nursing interventions
(a) Monitor patient closely for clinical and hemodynamic changes indicative of tamponade (hypotension, elevated jugular venous pressure, pulsus paradoxus); record and report immediately
(b) Monitor patient for arrhythmias and treat according to unit standards
(c) Monitor for signs and symptoms listed in Nursing Examination of Patient section earlier
(d) Prepare patient for any tests needed to further evaluate status (e.g., x-ray studies, echocardiography, catheterization)
(e) Monitor patient for signs of right-sided heart failure
(f) Keep patient on bed rest
(g) Continually assess patient's level of anxiety; provide quiet, relaxed environment to reduce stress and anxiety and promote rest
(h) Treatment is directed toward the underlying disease
(i) If tamponade occurs
(1) Place patient in Trendelenburg position
(2) Administer oxygen therapy as ordered
(3) Prepare patient for pericardiocentesis
(4) Have emergency equipment readily available, with pericardiocentesis tray always at bedside. Emergency pericardiocentesis (at the bedside) or in the catheterization laboratory is life-saving
(5) Give fluids to increase preload
(6) Collaborate with physician to discontinue any agents that decrease preload (diuretics, nitrates, morphine)
(j) Ensure a patient intravenous line
iv. Evaluation of nursing care
(a) Patient shows no signs or symptoms of tamponade
(b) Hemodynamic pressures and vital signs are within normal limits without pulsus paradoxus
(c) Patient is calm, free from pain
(d) Patient shows no signs or symptoms of heart failure
(e) Cardiac rate and rhythm are normal, without arrhythmias

Myocarditis

Inflammation of the myocardium caused by various microorganisms, chemicals, and drugs. It can be acute or chronic (subacute) and focal or diffuse; it may mimic MI and can lead to severe cardiovascular complications. People of all ages are at risk

1. Pathophysiology
a. Myocardial fibers are inflamed when a virus or some other organism invades and colonizes in the myocardium

b. Interstitial fibrosis develops with infiltrates composed of leukocytes, lymphocytes, macrophages, and plasma. Immune responses to inflammation ensue, and myocardial fibers become injured, hypertrophy, and begin to die

c. Necrosis of the myofibers may be global or spotty

d. There are also vascular responses to the infection that lead to vasculitis and spasm, further contributing to the myocardial fibrosis and necrosis

e. Pericardial involvement often occurs at the same time

f. Contractility and cardiac output decrease, causing progressive intolerance of activity

g. Left ventricular function may be sufficiently impaired to cause heart failure

h. Myocardial injury can continue after active virus infection as a result of persistent immune and autoimmune responses. Small amounts of the virus may remain engulfed in fibrotic and necrotic areas of the heart

2. **Etiologic or precipitating factors**

   a. Causes can include viral, bacterial, rickettsial, parasitic, or mycotic origins

   b. Viral

      i. Most common include coxsackievirus A and B and echovirus

      ii. Others include influenza, cytomegalovirus, human immunodeficiency virus (HIV), viral hepatitis B, mumps, and rubella

   c. Bacterial

      i. *Rickettsia, Salmonella typhi, Coxiella burnetii*

      ii. Diphtheria: most common cause of death

      iii. Tuberculosis

      iv. Streptococci, meningococci, clostridia, staphylococci

   d. Fungal: aspergillosis

   e. Protozoal: Chagas' disease *(Trypanosoma cruzi),* malaria

   f. Pregnancy is a predisposing factor

   g. In Europe and Northern America, viral myocarditis is the most common cause (coxsackievirus B)

3. **Nursing assessment data base**

   a. Nursing history: viral myocarditis is a challenge to diagnose. The responsible virus is hard to identify. The clinical manifestations vary widely but usually present as a dilated cardiomyopathy. Obtaining a careful history is vital

      i. Subjective findings

         (a) Patient may have complaints of "common cold," fever, chills, sore throat, abdominal pain, nausea, vomiting, diarrhea, arthralgia, and myalgia up to 6 weeks before overt symptoms of heart failure

         (b) Chest pain (two thirds of patients) with no evidence of pericarditis. Descriptions by patient identify pain as pleuritic, precordial, or associated with sweating, nausea, or vomiting

         (c) Dyspnea: exertional, paroxysmal nocturnal dyspnea, orthopnea

         (d) Palpitations

         (e) Headache

         (f) Fatigue, weakness

      ii. Objective findings

         (a) History of any infection from the aforementioned or other etiologies

(b) Sudden cardiac death (from ventricular arrhythmias) may be the first manifestation

(c) History of nonsustained ventricular tachycardia

b. Nursing examination of patient

   i. Inspection

      (a) Tachycardia

      (b) Symptoms of heart failure (rapid, fulminant)

      (c) Increased jugular venous pressure

   ii. Palpitation: pulsus alternans (when heart failure is extreme)

  iii. Auscultation

      (a) Narrow pulse pressure

      (b) Hypotension

      (c) S_1 diminished (decreased myocardial contractility)

      (d) S_3 gallop: common

      (e) Murmurs: mitral or tricuspid regurgitation (if ventricular dilatation is present)

      (f) Pericardial friction rub: uncommon

c. Diagnostic study findings

   i. Laboratory

      (a) Pan cultures (blood, throat culture, urine, stool): obtain early to rule out bacterial and fungal etiology

      (b) Slight to moderate leukocytosis with neutrophil response

      (c) Erythrocyte sedimentation rate elevated

      (d) Titers for rickettsia virus

      (e) Obtain tuberculosis skin test

      (f) Blood smears for pericarditis

   ii. Radiologic findings

      (a) Pulmonary congestion

      (b) Cardiomegaly

  iii. ECG

      (a) ST segment is elevated, T waves are inverted

      (b) QTc interval is prolonged

      (c) ST returns to baseline in several days

      (d) T-wave changes may last weeks, months (with severe myocarditis)

      (e) Arrhythmias are seen in one third of patients

         (1) Nonparoxysmal AV nodal tachycardia

         (2) PVCs

         (3) Sinus tachycardia

         (4) Atrial fibrillation

         (5) VT

         (6) SVT

         (7) AV blocks

   iv. Echocardiography

      (a) Diffuse hypocontractility

      (b) Pericardial effusions

      (c) Valvular dysfunction

      (d) Chamber enlargement

   v. Endocardial biopsy: although myocarditis is a nonspecific histologic diagnosis, routine biopsy has no proven utility, because of its high level of insensitivity and numerous false-negative results

vi. EPS: if patient has a history of an episode of sudden death, ventricular fibrillation and/or ventricular tachycardia

4. **Nursing diagnoses** (see Commonly Encountered Nursing Diagnoses section earlier)

  a. Decreased cardiac output related to decreased contractile state from inflammatory process in myocardium

    i. Assessment for defining characteristics (see Nursing Assessment Data Base section earlier)

    ii. Additional nursing interventions

      (a) Ensure adequate oxygenation: check pulse oximetry, maintain oxygen saturations at over 92%. Hypoxia is common with myocarditis

      (b) Observe for signs of cardiac failure; administer afterload reduction agents, diuretics as ordered

      (c) If hemodynamic support is needed, patient may receive IV pressors and inotropic agents. IABP and LVAD may be used to maintain cardiac output as a bridge to transplantation

      (d) Monitor closely for arrhythmias: patient is at high risk for sudden death

      (e) Administer antiarrhythmics as required

      (f) Relieve chest pain promptly

      (g) Immunosuppressive therapy has not proved beneficial for left ventricular function or survival (except for a small number of patients)

    iii. Evaluation of nursing care

      (a) Cardiac output, hemodynamics, and vital signs are within normal limits

      (b) Patient has no arrhythmias

      (c) Patient has no signs or symptoms of heart failure

  b. Activity intolerance caused by diminished cardiac output and pulmonary congestion related to inflammatory process in myocardium

    i. Assessment for defining characteristics

      (a) Exercise intolerance

      (b) Feelings of weakness, fatigue

      (c) Marked sinus tachycardia disproportionate to physical activity

    ii. Expected outcomes

      (a) Progressive (slow) increase in activity tolerance

      (b) Plan of care consistent with patient's responses to activity and set limits

    iii. Nursing interventions

      (a) Maintain bed rest at first (patient needs activities restricted); exception would be bedside commode, if tolerated

      (b) Allow patient to slowly ambulate with assistance

      (c) Monitor heart, respiratory rates, blood pressure, and oxygen saturation with activity

      (d) Patient and significant other need to be instructed about need for progressive increase in ambulation over next 2 months

      (e) Teach patient about symptoms to observe for and report regarding activity tolerance. Patient should be able to monitor pulse

(f) Facilitate and assist with development of an activity and exercise program for patient both in hospital and at home

iv. Evaluation of nursing care

(a) Patient has a developed plan of care for progressive activities and exercise

(b) Support services and significant others are actively involved in patient's rehabilitation

Infective Endocarditis

An acute or chronic (subacute) infection of the heart's endocardial surface, including the valves, chordae tendineae, septum, and mural endothelium. The term *infective* is preferred over *bacterial* because of the variety of microorganisms that can be responsible

1. **Pathophysiology**
   a. Microorganisms invade the body through the blood stream (may be a very transient invasion)
   b. The valves and endothelial surface of the heart can be predisposed to injury. The infecting organisms have an affinity for traumatized areas and preexisting defects, such as valvular disease, prosthetic valves, septal defects, or local trauma (indwelling catheters)
   c. When trauma injury from abnormal hemodynamic or endothelial stress has occurred, deposits of platelets and fibrin form microscopic thrombotic lesions
   d. The affected areas are then amenable to colonization by the microorganisms. Bacteria and organisms from other infections in the body (skin, genitourinary tract, lungs, mouth) attach to the valves and to these thrombotic lesions
   e. As the microorganisms colonize, they cause the deposition of platelet; leukocytes, erythrocytes, and fibrin, forming vegetations. Eventually, valvular tissue is destroyed by the infection, and the valve leaflets may become incompetent, rupture, abscess (ring or annular), or perforate. Mycotic aneurysms may also form as a result of infection
   f. Valves on the left side of the heart are more often affected than valves on the right side, except for infections caused by IV drug use, which involve predominantly the tricuspid and pulmonic valves
   g. The bacteria and microorganisms from the vegetations are circulated systemically, causing bacteremia
   h. Antibody formation increases levels of immune complexes in the blood, causing hypersensitivity reactions (allergic vasculitis) in peripheral parts of the body involving arterioles, vessel walls, and cutaneous tissue
   i. Embolization of the infective material may occur and spread throughout various parts of the body (left-sided vegetation causing systemic emboli; tricuspid valve vegetation causing pulmonary emboli)

2. **Etiologic or precipitating factors**
   a. A wide variety of microorganisms cause endocarditis. Common organisms are
      i. *Streptococcus viridans*: had been most prevalent causative organism in subacute cases (now only ~1/3 of cases)
      ii. *Staphylococcus aureus*: most prevalent causative organism in acute and nosocomial cases

      iii. Gram-negative rods
      iv. *Enterococci faecalis*
      v. *Staphylococcus epidermidis*
      vi. *Streptococcus pneumoniae*
      vii. *Pseudomonas aeruginosa*
      viii. *Candida albicans*
      ix. *Aspergillus fumigatus*
      x. Viral: coxsackievirus, adenovirus

b. Rheumatic valvular disease: was previously most common substrate (now accounts for about 25% to 30% of cases)
c. Open-heart surgical procedures (prosthetic valve replacements)
d. Mitral valve prolapse
e. Congenital heart defects (e.g., patent ductus arteriosus, coarctation of the aorta, ventricular septal defect): about 14% of cases
f. Degenerative valve disease: about 9% of cases
g. Hypertrophic, obstructive cardiomyopathy
h. Genitourinary surgery
i. Gynecologic/obstetric surgery
j. Dental procedures (extractions and, especially, cleaning)
k. Abscesses on skin
l. Invasive tests, monitoring (pulmonary artery catheters)
m. Intravenous drug abuse
n. Prolonged IV therapy (hyperalimentation)
o. Immunosuppressive therapy
p. Inflammatory gastrointestinal disease
q. Previous infective endocarditis

3. **Nursing assessment data base**
  a. Nursing history
    i. Subjective findings: Patient may complain of nonspecific, vague symptoms
      (a) Fever (prolonged, unknown source, sudden onset)
      (b) Chills, night sweats
      (c) Fatigue
      (d) Neurologic dysfunctions: vision losses
      (e) Nausea, vomiting, anorexia, weight loss
      (f) Arthralgias, myalgias
      (g) Back pain (cause unknown)
      (h) Dyspnea
    ii. Objective findings: history of any of the etiologic factors listed
  b. Nursing examination of patient: signs and symptoms are dependent on systemic or local infection, systemic emboli, immune responses
    i. Inspection
      (a) Fever of unknown origin
      (b) Signs and symptoms of heart failure
      (c) Petechiae (caused by emboli or allergic vasculitis) are seen in 20% to 40% of patients on the conjunctivae, neck, chest, abdomen, and mucosa of mouth (usually a sign of a long-standing infection)
      (d) Osler's nodes (resulting from immunologically mediated vasculitis): very tender, reddened, raised nodules on fingers and toe pads

(e) Roth's spots (resulting from emboli or allergic vasculitis): round or oval white spots seen on the retina

(f) Purpuritic pustular skin lesions (caused by emboli)

(g) Janeway's lesions (caused by septic emboli or allergic vasculitis): large, nontender nodules on fingers and toes

(h) Splinter hemorrhages of nails (resulting from emboli or allergic vasculitis)

(i) If patient is monitored with ECG, conduction disturbances may be seen

(j) Decrease or loss of visual fields (resulting from embolization)

(k) Central nervous system disturbances (e.g., hemiplegia, confusion, headache, seizures, transient ischemic attacks, aphasia, ataxia, changes in level of consciousness, psychiatric symptoms) if embolization to the brain has occurred

(l) Hematuria, oliguria, flank pain, hypertension, if kidney is infarcted or abscessed from emboli. Glomerulonephritis is frequently caused by allergic or immunologic reactions; kidney involvement is common

(m) Tachypnea, dyspnea, hemoptysis, sudden pain in chest or shoulder, cyanosis, and restlessness if lung is infarcted

ii. Palpation

(a) Abdominal pain (caused by mesenteric emboli)

(b) Decreased or no pulses in cold limbs (as a result of emboli)

(c) Splenomegaly or pain caused by splenic infarction

(d) Thrills may be palpated if murmurs are present

(e) If heart failure is present, hepatojugular reflux, jugular venous distention, or peripheral edema may be seen

iii. Percussion: If there is associated pericardial effusion, dullness may be percussed in the lower half of the sternum

iv. Auscultation

(a) New murmurs of valvular insufficiency and stenosis (caused by vegetations on the valve leaflets). May also develop later or with therapy and change in character

(b) Decreased or absent breath sounds or adventitious breath sounds if lungs are infarcted

(c) Rales heard if left ventricle fails

c. Diagnostic study findings

i. Laboratory data

(a) Positive blood cultures (several sets initially over a 24-hour period)

(b) Elevated sedimentation rate (immune response)

(c) Anemia (common in subacute endocarditis)

(d) Leukocytosis, thrombocytopenia (associated with splenomegaly)

(e) Proteinuria, microscopic hematuria, pyuria

(f) Rheumatoid factor levels may be elevated, as may circulating immune complex levels

(g) Hyperglobulinemia (common)

(h) Abnormal laboratory values associated with affected organs (e.g., kidneys, lungs, heart)

ii. Chest x-ray may show pleural effusion, pulmonary infiltrates

iii. ECG: signs of infarction if emboli have reached the heart

      iv. Echocardiography: presence of vegetations (higher risk of emboli) on any of the valves; degree of valvular dysfunction and complications (e.g., ruptured chordae tendineae, perforated valve cusps). Transesophageal echocardiography also gives good views of prosthetic valves, mitral valve, aortic valve, ring abscesses

      v. Catheterization: preoperative evaluation, if valve replacement planned. Assess

        (a) Valve dystunction

        (b) Aneurysms, intracardiac shunts

        (c) Underlying CAD

4. Nursing diagnoses (see Commonly Encountered Nursing Diagnoses section earlier)

  a. Decreased cardiac output related to valvular dysfunction, heart failure, and fluid volume excess

    i. Additional nursing interventions

      (a) Assess patient for signs and symptoms of heart failure (caused by damaged valves)

      (b) Monitor for new cardiac murmurs throughout hospitalization. Murmurs may change or appear during course of illness

      (c) Patient may need to be prepared for valve replacement surgery. Valve replacement is indicated if patient has significant damage to valves (to include prosthetic valves), ring or annular abscesses, refractory bacteremia, or heart failure

      (d) Postoperative teaching includes discussion on prophylactic antibiotics (for dental procedures or for bowel or bladder surgery)

  b. Risk of altered body temperature secondary to infection

    i. Assessment for defining characteristics

      (a) Fluctuations in body temperature between above normal and normal

      (b) If patient is hyperthermic, skin may be flushed; patient feels warm to the touch and may be tachypneic and/or tachycardic

    ii. Expected outcomes

      (a) Patient is afebrile

      (b) Patient has negative blood cultures

      (c) Patient is well hydrated, as evidenced by normal skin turgor, balanced intake and output, and moist mucosa

    iii. Nursing interventions

      (a) Monitor vital signs, especially temperature, per unit standards. Persistent or recurring fevers can indicate failure or hypersensitivity to antimicrobial therapy, nosocomial infections, emboli, abscesses, thrombophlebitis, or drug fever

      (b) Assist in reduction of fever (i.e., administer antimicrobials, antipyretics, and cooling measures, as ordered; encourage fluid intake [if no evidence of heart failure])

      (c) Assess patient for signs of dehydration

      (d) Monitor for problems in skin integrity resulting from fever, sweating

      (e) Monitor intake and output, and weigh patient daily

      (f) Draw several blood cultures initially and for temperature spikes (proper technique for blood cultures is vital because of the difficulty in choosing antibiotics to adequately treat microorganisms)

(g) Initiate appropriate antibiotic therapy as soon as possible after initial blood cultures (to halt continued valvular damage and abscess formation). Patient will likely receive prolonged intravenous antibiotic therapy

(h) Check antimicrobial peak and trough serum levels to monitor therapeutic effects and prevent toxicity

(i) Assess for musculoskeletal involvement (arthralgias, back pain, and myalgia are common symptoms). Antibiotic therapy usually helps decrease these symptoms

iv. Evaluation of nursing care

(a) Patient's temperature returns to normal

(b) Blood cultures negative; no signs of active infection

(c) Skin with normal turgor and moist mucous membranes; intake equals output

(d) Cardiac function normal

c. Altered tissue perfusion (potential), secondary to embolization of vegetations on the valves. May be presenting symptom or can happen at any time

i. Assessment for defining characteristics

(a) Patient complains of abdominal pain

(b) Hematuria

(c) Central nervous system dysfunction (e.g., altered level of consciousness, stroke-like symptoms, seizures)

(d) Patient complains of chest pain

(e) Patient exhibits signs of cutaneous embolization (petechiae, splinter hemorrhages, Janeway's lesions)

ii. Expected outcomes

(a) Episodes of systemic embolization have resolved

(b) Affected organs function normally, as evidenced by normal results of diagnostic tests

(c) Adequate circulation to extremities

iii. Nursing interventions: This type of embolization is not treated with anticoagulants unless patient has a previous indication for use (such as prosthetic valve). Anticoagulants have not proved to be beneficial in therapy and may result in the complication of intracranial hemorrhage. Treatment is aimed at the infection and treated with antimicrobials

(a) Assess patient for signs and symptoms of systemic embolization

(b) Monitor LOC: check for signs of cerebral emboli (headache, numbness, weakness, tingling, paralysis, ataxia, sudden blindness, sudden hemiplegia)

(c) Check for petechiae on neck, upper trunk, eyes, and lower extremities

(d) Observe extremities for painful nodes, swelling, erythema, decreased or absent pulses, coolness, and decreased capillary refill

(e) Assess patient for signs and symptoms of myocardial infarction; monitor ECG

(f) Subject all stools to guaiac testing; subject urine and nasogastric aspirations to Hematest

(g) If pulmonary, myocardial, or cerebral embolism occurs, administer oxygen therapy, position patient for comfort and ease of breathing, and administer pain medications as ordered

(h) Surgery for valve replacement will be considered if prosthetic valve is faulty, if native valve is perforated or ruptured, if embolization occurs more than once, if infection is uncontrolled, or if there is persistent heart failure

    iv. Evaluation of nursing care

(a) Patient has no systemic embolization

(b) Patient has no sequelae after embolization: without respiratory distress, abdominal pain, or hematuria; with intact central nervous system; and with normal ECG, laboratory values, negative guaiac test results

Cardiomyopathy

A chronic or subacute disorder of heart muscle. It often involves the endocardial and sometimes the pericardial layers of the heart. The three classifications include dilated (congestive), hypertrophic, and restrictive. It often has unknown, unrecognized causes

1. Pathophysiology

  a. Dilated cardiomyopathy (DCM) (most common type in the United States): usually both left and right ventricles dilate

    i. Myocardial fibers degenerate

    ii. Fibrotic changes occur

    iii. Severe dilatation of the heart occurs; includes atrial and ventricular dilatation, creating global enlargement of the heart

    iv. Systolic and diastolic dysfunction occurs, and contractility decreases, resulting in decreased stroke volume, decreased EF, low cardiac output, and a compensatory increase in heart rate

    v. Mitral annular dilatation is secondary to left ventricular dilatation and results in mitral insufficiency

    vi. Heart failure develops, is often refractory to treatment, and is accompanied by malignant ventricular arrhythmias, which are often the cause of death

    vii. Stasis of blood can cause deep vein thrombosis, pulmonary embolism

    viii. DCM is three times more common in males

  b. Hypertrophic cardiomyopathy (HCM)

    i. Increased mass and thickening of heart muscle, resulting in diastolic dysfunction

    ii. May be caused by concentric hypertrophy or localized hypertrophy often associated with a left ventricular outflow tract dynamic obstruction, referred to as hypertrophic obstructive cardiomyopathy (HOCM; formerly idiopathic hypertrophic subaortic stenosis [IHSS])

    iii. Ventricles become rigid and stiff, restricting filling. Filling volumes are decreased and, therefore, SV decreases

    iv. Left ventricular chamber becomes very small (hypertrophy occurs inwardly at the expense of the left ventricular chamber)

      v. The left atrium becomes dilated

      vi. Contractility may be normal or increased

      vii. The process may continue for years with no obvious problems and delayed onset of symptoms, or it may end with sudden cardiac death as a first sign of the disease process, as a result of malignant ventricular arrhythmias (ventricular fibrillation, ventricular tachycardia)

      viii. The yearly risk of systemic embolization and stroke with HOCM and atrial fibrillation is 20%

  c. Restrictive cardiomyopathy (least common)

      i. Restricted filling of ventricles

      ii. Usually caused by an infiltrative process, most often amyloidosis in adults

      iii. The heart loses its compliance, grows stiff, and cannot distend well in diastole or contract well in systole

      iv. LVEDP increases; contractility decreases, resulting in low cardiac output, heart failure, and death

2. Etiologic or precipitating factors

  a. Dilated cardiomyopathy

      i. Idiopathic

      ii. Viral myocarditis

      iii. Infection: bacterial, parasitic, fungal, protozoal

      iv. Metabolic: chronic hypophosphatemia, thiamine deficiency, protein deficiency

      v. Toxins: alcohol, lead, arsenic, uremia, certain chemotherapeutic drugs, cocaine

      vi. Pregnancy (third trimester) or the postpartum period (common in multiparous women who are older than 30 or have a history of toxemia)

      vii. Neuromuscular disorders: muscular dystrophy, myotonic dystrophy

      viii. Connective tissue disorders: lupus erythematosus, rheumatoid disease, polyarteritis, scleroderma

      ix. Beriberi

      x. Infiltrative disorders: sarcoidosis and amyloidosis

      xi. Familial: 20% of cases

  b. Hypertrophic cardiomyopathy

      i. Idiopathic

      ii. Strong familial component (50% of cases) in HOCM

      iii. Neuromuscular disorders: Friedreich's ataxia

      iv. Metabolic: hypoparathyroidism

      v. Hypertension

  c. Restrictive cardiomyopathy

      i. Idiopathic

      ii. Infiltrative: amyloidosis, sarcoidosis, hemochromatosis, neoplasms

      iii. Endomyocardial fibrosis in children

      iv. Glycogen and mucopolysaccharide deposition

      v. Radiation

3. Nursing assessment data base

  a. Nursing history

      i. Subjective findings

        (a) Ascertain patient's chief complaint and history of present illness

      (b) Patient may complain of angina, syncope, palpitations, dyspnea, orthopnea, fatigue

  ii. Objective findings

      (a) Determine whether there is a familial component (family history of cardiomyopathy or sudden death in young adults)

      (b) Rule out other disease processes, such as hypertension, amyloidosis, and toxemia

      (c) Determine potential etiologic factors such as recent infections, drinking history, current use of medications, pregnancy, and any endocrine disorders

b. Nursing examination of patient (Table 2–7)

c. Diagnostic study findings

  i. Radiologic

      (a) Heart normal or enlarged

      (b) Left atrium enlarged

      (c) Pulmonary congestion

  ii. ECG

      (a) Arrhythmias or conduction defects (e.g., sinus tachycardia, atrial fibrillation, ventricular ectopy, bundle branch blocks)

      (b) High incidence of atrial fibrillation (70% to 80%)

      (c) Evidence of both left atrial and left ventricular enlargement: increased QRS voltage

      (d) Q waves

      (e) LBBB

      (f) Prolonged QTc interval

  iii. Cardiac catheterization: right- and left-sided heart studies

      (a) LVEDP, PCWP, and PAP elevated; cardiac output decreased

      (b) Right ventricular end-diastolic pressure, RAP, and CVP rise in right-sided heart failure or with dilated cardiomyopathy

      (c) Left ventricular outflow tract gradient in HOCM

      (d) Mitral regurgitation

      (e) Rule out CAD

  iv. Echocardiography

      (a) Diastolic dysfunction

      (b) Left ventricular outflow tract pressure gradient (in HOCM)

      (c) Global hypokinesis, left ventricular wall thickening (in dilated cardiomyopathy)

      (d) Systolic anterior motion of the anterior mitral valve leaflet or chordal apparatus (in HOCM)

      (e) Left ventricular hypertrophy (in HOCM)

      (f) Marked, asymmetric septal hypertrophy (in HOCM)

      (g) Left atrial enlargement

      (h) Transesophageal echocardiography (TEE): to evaluate for possible left atrial thrombosis

  v. Radionuclide tests may reveal: increased ventricular volumes, decreased EF in dilated cardiomyopathy, increased uptake in patients with amyloidosis, defects in cardiac wall in patients with neoplasms or sarcoidosis

  vi. EPS and Holter study: to identify ventricular fibrillation and ventricular tachycardia and to guide therapy

TABLE 2–7. Physical Findings Associated with Dilated, Hypertrophic, and Restrictive Cardiomyopathy

Cardiomyopathy	Patient Complaint	Inspection	Palpation	Percussion	Auscultation
Dilated	Dyspnea on exertion, orthopnea, fatigue, palpitations	Clinical manifestations of CHF, dysrhythmias on monitor; conduction defects	Narrow pulse pressure, pulsus alternans, cool skin, +JVD, PMI laterally displaced, left ventricular heave, peripheral edema, hepatomegaly	Cardiac enlargement, dullness in bases of lungs	Irregular heart beat, third and fourth heart sounds, mitral and tricuspid insufficiency, pulmonary rales
Hypertrophic	Dyspnea on exertion, orthopnea, PND, angina, syncope, palpitations	Dyspnea, orthopnea	Forceful and laterally displaced apical impulse, systolic thrill (in HOCM)		Fourth heart sound; a third heart sound may be heard, split-second heart sound, systolic ejection murmur
Restrictive	Fatigue, weakness, dyspnea on exertion, anorexia, poor exercise tolerance	Dysrhythmias, distended neck veins, Kussmaul's sign	Edema, ascites, +HJR, right upper quadrant pain	Cardiac enlargement, pulmonary congestion	Third and fourth heart sounds, mitral and tricuspid insufficiency

PND = paroxysmal nocturnal dyspnea; CHF = congestive heart failure; JVD = jugular venous distention; PMI = point of maximal impulse; HOCM = hypertrophic obstructive cardiomyopathy; HJR = hepatojugular reflex.

4. Nursing Diagnoses (see Commonly Encountered Nursing Diagnoses section earlier)

a. Decreased cardiac output, resulting in altered tissue perfusion, related to depressed ventricular function, arrhythmias, and conduction defects

  i. Assessment for defining characteristics (see Table 2–7)

   (a) Signs of heart failure

   (b) Dysrhythmias, particularly atrial and ventricular on ECG

   (c) Abnormal hemodynamic readings

  ii. Additional expected outcome: patient or significant other will be aware of activities that aggravate symptoms

  iii. Additional nursing interventions

   (a) Potential complications include atrial fibrillation, ventricular arrhythmias, left ventricular failure, infective endocarditis, embolism, ischemia

   (b) Dual-chambered pacing may be used to help improve cardiac output in both dilated and hypertrophic obstructive cardiomyopathy. Prepare patient for the possibility of this procedure, and be knowledgeable about pacemaker procedure, equipment, protocols

   (c) HOCM

    (1) Administer medications to reduce outflow tract obstruction, to improve left ventricular outflow gradient, and to relieve syncope, angina, dyspnea, and arrhythmias (beta blockers such as propranolol; calcium channel blockers such as verapamil and nifedipine; or a type IA antiarrhythmic such as disopyramide)

    (2) Avoid administering isoproterenol, dopamine, or digitalis preparations (in the early stages before heart failure) because they increase contractility and hence worsen the obstruction

    (3) Administer anticoagulants when patient is in atrial fibrillation, and monitor coagulation studies. Observe for signs of bleeding

    (4) Instruct patient to avoid activities that may increase the obstruction, such as strenuous exercise, Valsalva maneuvers, and sitting or standing suddenly

    (5) Because stress aggravates the outflow obstruction, help the patient identify stressors and teach methods of stress reduction

    (6) Avoid agents that decrease preload (nitrates, diuretics, or morphine). Hypovolemia can be very detrimental because the ventricles are very preload dependent for adequate filling

    (7) Because patient is at risk for endocarditis, instruct patient to notify his or her dentist of this risk before any dental or surgical procedures (for prophylactic antibiotics), and instruct in endocarditis prophylaxis

   (d) Dilated cardiomyopathy

    (1) Administer inotropic agents to improve myocardial contractility and decrease degree of heart failure

    (2) Administer diuretics to relieve the pulmonary congestion

        (3) Administer afterload- and preload-reducing agents such as nitroprusside and nitroglycerin to decrease myocardial workload, improve cardiac output, and decrease pulmonary venous pressure

        (4) Judicious use of beta blockers initially in controlled circumstances

          a) Increase cardiac function by slowing or reversing progression of left ventricular dysfunction (due to hyperadrenergic tone)

          b) Increase left ventricular EF

          c) Decrease hospitalization for heart failure

    (e) Restrictive cardiomyopathy: avoid digoxin in patients with cardiac amyloidosis, because it concentrates in the amyloid fibrils and can result in digitalis toxicity

    (f) A patient with end-stage disease may be a candidate for cardiac transplantation (see next section)

  iv. Evaluation of nursing care

    (a) Sequelae of cardiomyopathy are minimized or absent

    (b) Patient or significant other relates measures to prevent endocarditis

    (c) Patient or significant other verbalizes understanding of importance of anticoagulation and monitoring of parameters

b. Impaired gas exchange secondary to pulmonary vascular congestion or pulmonary embolism

  i. Assessment for defining characteristics

    (a) Patients at risk are those in older age groups; immobile patients on bed rest; patients in heart failure, in atrial fibrillation, or who have a dilated myocardium

    (b) Central nervous system symptoms; confusion, somnolence, anxiety, restlessness, irritability

    (c) Hypoxia

    (d) Hypercapnia

    (e) Tachypnea

    (f) Rales

    (g) Hemoptysis

    (h) Inability to remove secretions

    (i) Tachycardia

    (j) Chest discomfort or pain

    (k) Elevated pulmonary artery pressures

    (l) S_3

  ii. Expected outcomes

    (a) Absence or resolution of pulmonary congestion

    (b) Absence or resolution of pulmonary emboli

    (c) Absence of respiratory distress

  iii. Nursing interventions

    (a) Use preventive measures, especially for high-risk patients

      (1) Assist with passive and active exercises while patient is confined to bed

      (2) Apply antiembolism stockings

      (3) Encourage ambulation as tolerated

        (4) Position patient so that angulation at groin and knees is avoided; elevate patient's legs when out of bed. Patient should be instructed not to cross legs or ankles; avoid using knee joint on Gatch bed

        (5) Teach patient to avoid activities that cause straining (Valsalva maneuver)

        (6) Administer anticoagulants as ordered (monitor prothrombin time and PTT; observe for bleeding)

    (b) Monitor vital signs, hemodynamic parameters, and laboratory values, especially ABGs

    (c) Observe for signs and symptoms listed in assessment as defining characteristics

    (d) Administer medications as ordered (e.g., vasodilators, diuretics, anticoagulants, antiarrhythmics, digoxin, potassium replacements)

    (e) Administer supportive measures as situation dictates (e.g., oxygen therapy, pain medications, sedatives, emotional support)

    (f) Teach patient and significant other about benefits of weight reduction, sodium restriction, smoking cessation, exercise

  iv. Evaluation of nursing care

    (a) Patient is hemodynamically stable; vital signs are within set parameters for patient

    (b) Patient has no embolic episodes or pulmonary congestion

    (c) Lungs are clear on auscultation

    (d) Patient is alert and oriented with regard to time, person, and place

    (e) Laboratory values, including ABGs, are within normal limits

    (f) Patient is calm and relaxed

End-Stage Heart Disease

Heart disease has advanced to point where all possible medical or surgical interventions have been exhausted. Life expectancy is less than 24 months. Patient is free of other life-threatening disease; dysfunction of other organ systems is reversible. Heart transplantation is standard of care and is performed on patients of all ages from newborn to 65 years. The mortality rate is as low as 4% from heart transplantation; average survival time is greater than 5 years

1. **Pathophysiology**
   a. Severe left ventricular dysfunction with low cardiac output; EF is less than 25%
   b. See pathophysiology subsection in Heart Failure section

2. **Etiologic or precipitating factors**
   a. Ischemic heart disease and CAD
   b. Dilated cardiomyopathy: idiopathic or secondary to pregnancy or viral infections
   c. Valvular disease
   d. Drug-related myocardial injury
   e. Congenital heart disease
   f. Infection (Chagas' disease)

3. **Nursing assessment data base:** the number of candidates for transplantation far exceeds the number of donor hearts. Careful assessment and selection

are necessary in determining who will potentially return to a functional life after transplantation, as well as to ensure that all conventional remedies have been exhausted

   a. Nursing history

      i. Subjective findings: complaints of dyspnea, angina, low exercise tolerance (bed-to-chair existence, essentially bedridden)

      ii. Objective findings

         (a) Severe heart failure necessitating frequent "tune-ups" and hospitalizations

         (b) Cardiac cachexia: anorexia, weight loss

         (c) Life-threatening arrhythmias

   b. Nursing examination of patient: see Objective Findings just listed

   c. Diagnostic study findings

      i. Cardiac arteriography: before transplantation to ascertain degree of CAD and potential for conventional revascularization

      ii. Cardiac biopsy: to rule out amyloidosis and identify patients with sarcoidosis or myocarditis for possible immunosuppressive therapy

      iii. Hemodynamic assessment

         (a) PVR:

            (1) One cause of perioperative mortality is irreversible pulmonary hypertension

            (2) Donor heart cannot generate pressure high enough to maintain a sufficient pulmonary flow

            (3) Patients with irreversible pulmonary hypertension may be candidates for heart-lung transplantation

            (4) Pharmacologic agents may be used in the catheterization laboratory to evaluate the potential for reversibility of increased PVR

         (b) Assess pulmonary artery pressure, wedge pressure, cardiac output

      iv. EPS: to assess effective antiarrhythmic therapy

4. Nursing diagnoses (see Commonly Encountered Nursing Diagnoses section earlier)

   a. Ineffective family coping: related to ventricular dysfunction, arrhythmias, heart failure, cardiomyopathy, and transplantation process

      i. Assessment for defining characteristics (see applicable sections)

      ii. Expected outcomes

         (a) Patient and family and/or significant other will be prepared for the rigor of waiting for transplantation and the care before and after

         (b) Patient and significant other will participate in plan of care and identify life style changes and support required in coping with transplantation process

         (c) Transplantation will be successful, and patient will tolerate the new heart

      iii. Nursing interventions

         (a) Assess for potential contraindications to transplantation (Table 2–8)

         (b) Collect information on other systemic diseases to evaluate potential for post-transplantation success

            (1) For patients with insulin-dependent diabetes, steroid

TABLE 2–8. Contraindications to Heart Transplantation

Potential Contraindications
    Age > 60 years
    Insulin-dependent diabetes
    Irreversible renal failure
    Malignancy, previous or current
    Familial hypercholesteremia
    Active systemic infection
    Severe obestiy
    History of drug or alcohol abuse
    Recent pulmonary infarction (within 2–3 months)
    Amyloidosis
    Systemic lupus erythematosus
    Severe cerebrovascular/peripheral vascular disease
    Mental illness, emotional instability
    Active peptic ulcer disease
Absolute Contraindications
    Active malignancy
    Cirrhosis of liver
    Severe chronic obstructive pulmonary disease*
    Severe irreversible pulmonary hypertension*

*Potential for heart-lung transplantation.

        therapy after transplantation can increase blood glucose levels

  (2) For patients with renal disease, cyclosporine therapy is nephrotoxic

(c) Assess nutritional status: to optimize potential for post-transplantation success and facilitate the healing process

(d) Assess emotional status: psychiatric history, motivational issues. Transplantation is a major undertaking with a stressful waiting period

(e) Assess ability to comply with a complex lifelong medical regimen: frequent follow-up examinations (to include transvenous endomyocardial biopsies, strict medication protocols, rejection issues)

(f) Assess support system: a strong family, friends, and medical support are needed

(g) Assess financial issues: insurance coverage, costly procedure, drugs, follow-up care

(h) Determine alcohol and drug history

(i) Administer medications, and instruct patient and family with regard to medications as ordered, to include

  (1) IV inotropic drugs (e.g., dobutamine to increase cardiac output, improve renal perfusion)

  (2) Afterload reduction

  (3) Preload reduction: diuretics, nitrates

  (4) Antiarrhythmic therapy

  (5) Anticoagulation: for risk of thromboembolism

(j) Automatic implantable cardiac defibrillator (AICD) with or without pacemaker may need to be placed to prevent sudden death, lethal arrhythmias, bradycardias; teach and prepare patient for this possibility

    (k) Future issues for patient and significant other to be aware of and prepared for
- (1) Need for regular medical examinations
- (2) Home oxygen: may be required for dyspnea, pulmonary congestion
- (3) Home health care: to include intravenous therapy
- (4) Use of indwelling catheters: for infection risks

    (l) Hospitalizations: patient and significant other need to be instructed with regard to
- (1) Possible need for frequent hospital visits for "tune-ups," medication changes, close observation
- (2) Need for hemodynamic monitoring
- (3) High-dose medications
- (4) Mechanical assists: IABP, VAD, ventilators

    (m) Observe for and prevent potential infections (from IV drips, central lines, immunosuppressive therapies)

    (n) Determine potential for patient dependency issues. Discuss with patient and significant other, and formulate plan
- (1) Ensure that patient is allowed to do what he or she can
- (2) Include family in care at home and in hospital
- (3) Arrange for home care
- (4) Emphasize the need to be ready for transplantation immediately. When donor heart becomes available, the donor heart "ischemic time" (time from cross-clamp [donor] to cross-clamp [recipient]) must be less than 5 hr (or the heart will not be usable); therefore the patient must not travel

    (o) Discuss with patient and family the following aspects of pretransplantation, post-transplantation, and follow-up care
- (1) Change in body image with new heart
- (2) Importance of family support
- (3) Unknown waiting period: need for a beeper, availability of donors, donor waiting lists
- (4) Cost: huge financial burden; insurance coverage
- (5) Frequency of check-ups, evaluations, tests
- (6) Possibility of failure to be accepted as a transplantation candidate
- (7) Possibility of rejection reaction after transplantation
- (8) Dependency issues
- (9) Arrange for patient and family to talk with transplantation survivors

    (p) Immediate postoperative cardiac transplant care teaching points:
- (1) Similar to CABG care
- (2) Potential complications include
  - *a)* Bleeding: intrathoracic, pericardial
  - *b)* Right ventricular failure from high pulmonary vascular resistance
  - *c)* Bradycardia: pacemaker may be needed; isoproterenol may be used to treat before temporary pacemaker
  - *d)* Atropine will not help denervated transplanted heart (no vagus innervation)

          e) Vigorous pulmonary toilet is important

    (q) Teaching and communication are of utmost importance, especially with the wide variety of health care professionals with whom the patient and significant other will be involved during this time

  iv. Evaluation of nursing care

    (a) Clear communications among patient, staff, family, transplant teams, physicians

    (b) Patient verbalizes understanding of information given and is able to discuss concerns and questions with health professional team and family

Cardiac Trauma

Trauma to the heart and/or great vessels from penetrating injuries (e.g., knife, gunshot wounds) or nonpenetrating trauma (deceleration, myocardial contusions from falls and motor vehicle crashes). Injury may be to the pericardium, a single chamber, two or more chambers, the great vessels, and/or the coronary arteries

1. Pathophysiology

  a. Penetrating cardiac trauma

    i. Open wound hemorrhages into pericardial space. Hypovolemic shock may be present as a result of hemorrhaging. Most stab wounds (80% to 90%) result in tamponade

    ii. Gunshot wounds → cellular damage to adjacent areas of myocardium

      (a) Myocardial damage is usually extensive, with profuse bleeding

      (b) Often more than one chamber involved

      (c) Embolization is a potential problem when bullets or fragments remain in chambers

    iii. Coronary artery lacerations cause tamponade, MI, death

  b. Nonpenetrating trauma

    i. Deceleration injury is caused by

      (a) Sternal compression

      (b) Impingement of the heart between the sternum and spinal column

      (c) Rupture or dissection of the aorta at the ligamentum arteriosum, where it is anchored

    ii. Blunt aortic trauma creates a shearing force within this vessel

      (a) Causes laceration

      (b) Intimal tear may cause dissections

      (c) Hemorrhage, cardiac tamponade, and subsequent shock are most pressing events

      (d) With cardiac tamponade: decreased ventricular (diastolic) filling volume leads to hypovolemia, hypotension, and death

    iii. Myocardial contusion: direct damage to myocardium causes temporary or permanent myocardial dysfunction

      (a) The right ventricle is the chamber most commonly injured, because of its anatomic position (behind the sternum)

      (b) Right-sided heart afterload increases, if significant pulmonary contusion and adult respiratory distress syndrome have occurred, causing the right chambers to fail and resulting in decreased forward output

(c) Late complications with contusions and lacerations: myocardial fibrosis can cause akinesia or hypokinesia, left ventricular aneurysms, heart failure

2. Etiologic or precipitating factors

a. Blunt trauma
   i. Motor vehicle crashes
   ii. Falls
   iii. Physical assaults, direct blows to chest by fist or objects such as a steering wheel and baseballs
   iv. Kicks from large animals
   v. Blasts, electrical injuries
b. Penetrating trauma
   i. Knives, gunshot wounds, ice picks
   ii. Low-velocity shrapnel, flying objects
   iii. Fractures of ribs and sternum (rare cause)
c. Iatrogenic trauma: invasive catheters

3. Nursing assessment data base

a. Nursing history: history generally provides limited information
   i. Patient is often unconscious
   ii. Have a high index of suspicion when obtaining patient history. Serious cardiac sequelae may have delayed onset (hours to days) after various forms of trauma
   iii. Penetrating wounds are easier to assess than are blunt injuries
   iv. Survival rate is better with stab wounds (they often seal off, if small), depending on clinical condition on arrival to emergency department, on method of injury, and on associated injuries
b. Nursing examination of patient
   i. Inspection
      (a) Symptoms of hemorrhage, shock
      (b) Blunt trauma (aorta): may produce few symptoms
      (c) Most common valve ruptured: aortic. Observe for signs and symptoms of acute aortic insufficiency: cardiogenic shock, chest pain, dyspnea
      (d) Urinary output absent or decreased (aortic rupture)
      (e) Myocardial contusion: may produce subtle signs of chest pain, similar to those of MI
      (f) Inspect trauma patients for associated injuries: head, neck, chest, abdomen
   ii. Palpation
      (a) Jugular venous pressure: increased with tamponade
      (b) Pulses may be decreased in legs
      (c) Discrepancy between pulses in the upper extremities; no femoral pulses (suspect blunt trauma with high-speed automobile crashes, truncal deceleration: sternal, first rib injuries)
   iii. Auscultation
      (a) Isolated upper body hypertension (blunt trauma of aorta)
      (b) New holosystolic murmurs can be heard in ruptured ventricular septum, diastolic murmur in aortic insufficiency
      (c) Pericardial rub: heard in contusions

   c. Diagnostic study findings
      i. Laboratory
         (a) Cardiac isoenzymes: CK isoenzymes often elevated in contusions
         (b) Cardiac tropinin I (cTnI): indicator of myocardial necrosis (normal values: 1.5 to 3.1 ng/ml)
      ii. ECG
         (a) Sinus tachycardia, atrial flutter or fibrillation, premature ventricular contractions, VT, V fib, pulseless electrical activity (PEA)
         (b) Prolonged QTc interval
         (c) Low voltage, electrical alternans (in pericardial effusions)
         (d) RBBB, new R axis deviation: ruptured ventricular septum
         (e) Right precordial ECG lead V_4R: to check signs of right ventricular or RCA damage
         (f) Infarct patterns with coronary artery lacerations
         (g) ST elevations: pericarditis
     iii. Radiologic
         (a) Cardiac silhouette may be enlarged
         (b) Hemothorax
         (c) Rib fractures, pneumothorax, tension pneumothorax
         (d) Pulmonary edema
         (e) Aortic trauma: mediastinal widening; presence of apical cap: extrapleural hematoma, loss of aortic knob, left pleural effusion
     iv. Echocardiography: helps detect lesions in valves and septum, pericardial effusions, tamponade
      v. Transesophageal echocardiography: adds potential for diagnosing aortic dissections
     vi. CT and MRI: for aortic trauma

4. Nursing diagnoses (see Commonly Encountered Nursing Diagnoses section earlier)
   a. Decreased cardiac output related to decreased preload and to myocardial injury caused by cardiac trauma
      i. Assessment for defining characteristics (see Nursing Examination of Patient section earlier)
         (a) Cyanosis, pallor
         (b) Hemodynamic measurements abnormal
            (1) Hypotension
            (2) Increased CVP with tamponade
            (3) Decreased CVP with hypovolemia
            (4) Increased PCWP with infarctions, aortic insufficiency
         (c) Arrhythmias: tachycardias
         (d) Decreased peripheral pulses
      ii. Expected outcomes
         (a) Blood pressure normal
         (b) Hemodynamics stable
         (c) Sinus rhythm, freedom from ectopy and arrhythmias
         (d) Adequate oxygenation
     iii. Nursing interventions
         (a) Rapid assessments of airway, breathing, circulation
         (b) Perform CPR as needed
         (c) Monitor continuously for adequate blood pressure, pulse, hemodynamics

    (d) Ensure adequate oxygenation: use pulse oximetry, check ABG results, evaluate need for intubation or mechanical ventilation (there is a high risk of hypoxemia)

    (e) Listen to breath sounds: check for pneumothorax

    (f) Closely observe for arrhythmias, PEA

    (g) Prepare patient for emergency procedures

      (1) Pericardiocentesis: tamponade

      (2) Chest tube insertion: tension pneumothorax

      (3) Emergency thoracotomy: done at bedside or, if patient is in extremis, in the emergency department

      (4) Emergency surgery in the operating room

    (h) Treat contusion similarly to MI with rest, close monitoring, oxygenation, maintaining fluid balance, treating arrhythmias

   iv. Evaluation of nursing care

    (a) Cardiac output is within set parameters for patient

    (b) No arrhythmias, or arrhythmias controlled by medications and pacemakers

  b. Fluid volume deficit related to hemorrhage, hypovolemic shock

   i. Assessment for defining characteristics

    (a) Decreased urinary output

    (b) Decreased CVP: preload

    (c) Decreased mentation

    (d) Increased pulse rate

    (e) Decreased blood pressure

   ii. Expected outcomes

    (a) Fluid volume (intake and output, preload) and electrolytes are within normal limits

    (b) No signs or symptoms of dehydration

   iii. Nursing interventions

    (a) Monitor vital signs continuously, particularly blood pressure, temperature, heart rate

    (b) Elevate lower extremities to increase preload, if necessary

    (c) Closely watch hemodynamics: CVP, PCWP, MAP

    (d) Maintain strict intake and output measurements to include all losses, plus drainage tubes (nasogastric tube, chest tubes, Jackson-Pratt drains, draining wounds)

    (e) Maintain two large-bore (16-g) IV lines for volume expanders, drugs

    (f) Administer volume expanders as ordered, to include blood, fresh frozen plasma, fluids, crystalloids, colloids (dextran, albumin)

    (g) Monitor fluids and electrolytes: weigh daily

    (h) Observe condition of skin: color, turgor, temperature, refill

    (i) Watch for changes in mental status

    (j) Check urinary specific gravity at least once per shift

   iv. Evaluation of nursing care

    (a) Blood pressure and pulse normal or within set parameters

    (b) Urinary output adequate (>30 ml/hour)

  c. Risk of infection related to foreign body, trauma, surgery

   i. Assessment for defining characteristics

    (a) Elevated temperature

(b) Localized pain, swelling, redness at trauma site

(c) Leukocyte count elevated

ii. Expected outcomes

(a) Wound and incision sites free of signs of infection

(b) Temperature and vital signs within normal limits

(c) Laboratory (CBC, cultures) results normal

iii. Nursing interventions

(a) Check temperature frequently and report if it exceeds set parameters (e.g., 101°F or higher)

(b) Monitor culture and sensitivity reports

(c) Frequently monitor invasive line and wound sites

(d) Keep wounds clean; change dressings per unit standards

(e) Administer antibiotics as ordered and on time, to maintain therapeutic blood levels

(f) Maintain blood and body fluid precautions, good hand-washing technique

(g) Maintain aseptic technique for bedside procedures

(h) Monitor age of invasive lines, IV lines, Foley catheter

iv. Evaluation of nursing care

(a) Temperature less than 100°F

(b) No signs or symptoms of infection

Cardiac Rhythm Disorders

Arrhythmias are divided into cardiac rhythms that are too slow, those that are too fast, and those unable to generate an adequate pulse

Symptomatic Bradycardia: bradycardias, conduction defects, and slow escape rhythms

1. Pathophysiology

a. Dysfunction of SA node: a result of ischemia, infarction, disease, degeneration, defects, or drug effects: SA exit blocks, severe sinus bradycardia, sinus pause/arrest (sick sinus syndrome)

b. Dysfunction of AV node: a result of ischemia, infarction, disease, defects, degeneration, or drug effects leads to AV conduction defects: second-degree, types I (rare) and II: third-degree, complete heart block

i. AV nodal tissue slows or fails to propagate electrical impulses to the ventricles

ii. Slower pacemaker cells in lower sites (junctional, His bundle, ventricular) may escape and take over as the cardiac pacemaker in third-degree blocks

iii. In acute anterior MI, complete heart block develops in 6% to 10% of patients

iv. In inferior MI, ischemia or infarction of the AV node may create a temporary conduction defect, which usually is reversed in less than a week

c. Hypersensitivity of carotid sinus and neurovascular syndromes (dysautonomia)

i. Exaggerated response to vagal stimulation causes slowing of heart rate and conductivity and lowering of blood pressure

ii. Vasodepression can also occur and cause hypotension and decreased sympathetic stimulation, leading to pauses

2. **Etiologic or precipitating factors**
   a. Parasympathetic or vagal stimulation: Valsalva maneuver, nausea, vomiting, suctioning
   b. Aging: structural degeneration of conductive system
   c. MI, ischemic heart disease
   d. Drugs: calcium channel blockers (verapamil, diltiazem); cardiac glycosides (digoxin); beta blockers (propranolol)
   e. Infectious process: endocarditis, myocarditis, typhoid fever, rheumatic fever
   f. Metabolic disorders: myxedema, hypothermia, hypercalcemia
   g. Aortic stenosis
   h. Myocarditis
   i. Tumors
   j. Post–cardiac surgery state
   k. Trauma
   l. Connective tissue disease (sarcoidosis, amyloidosis, systemic lupus erythematous, thyroid disease)
   m. Dive reflex (immersion in cold water)

3. **Nursing assessment data base**
   a. Nursing history
      i. Subjective findings
         (a) Syncope
         (b) Wooziness, lightheadedness
         (c) Fatigue, weakness
         (d) Shortness of breath
         (e) Angina
      ii. Objective findings: history of any etiologies or precipitating factors
         (a) Pauses greater than 3 seconds
         (b) Heart rates less than 40 beats/minute
   b. Nursing examination of patient: Symptoms may be transient, infrequent
      i. Wooziness
      ii. Syncope of presyncope
      iii. Decreased level of consciousness
      iv. Lethargy
      v. Hypotension
      vi. Signs of heart failure, cardiogenic shock
      vii. Dyspnea
      viii. Exercise intolerance
      ix. Decreased cardiac output, cardiac index
   c. Diagnostic study findings
      i. ECG: see salient features of each arrhythmia (see ECG and rhythms section earlier in Nursing Assessment Data Base section)
         (a) Correlation of symptoms with documented ECG is main diagnostic tool
         (b) Pauses documented as 3 seconds or more in duration
         (c) Third-degree heart block with inferior MI: usually narrow QRS complex accompanies bradycardia (higher escape pacemaker)
         (d) Third-degree heart block with anterior MI: wide QRS complex may be observed (lower escape pacemaker)

      ii. Autonomic tests: carotid sinus massage, tilt table testing

     iii. Holter monitoring: to identify arrhythmias not otherwise documented and to correlate with symptoms

     iv. EPS: To test SA and AV node function; may confirm need for permanent pacemaker

4. Nursing diagnoses (see Commonly Encountered Nursing Diagnoses section earlier)

    a. Decreased cardiac output and tissue perfusion related to symptomatic bradycardias

      i. Assessment for defining characteristics

        (a) Heart rate inadequate for maintaining perfusion to vital organs

      ii. Expected outcomes

        (a) Improved hemodynamics via improved heart rate

        (b) Symptoms from bradycardia decreased or absent

     iii. Nursing interventions

        (a) If patient is stable or asymptomatic: monitor closely, notify physician, determine possible causes, have medications and transcutaneous pacemaker equipment readily available (especially if patient is in third-degree block or second-degree AV block type II)

        (b) Ensure good oxygenation: oxygen saturations 92% or greater. Administer oxygen as needed per orders

        (c) Check patency of IV line

        (d) If patient is symptomatic, administer atropine, 0.5 to 1.0 mg IV

           (1) Given every 3 to 5 minutes IV; total IV dosage: up to 0.03 to 0.04 mg/kg

           (2) Effective for marked sinus bradycardia, second-degree and some third-degree blocks

           (3) A dose less than 0.5 mg IV can cause paradoxical bradycardia

        (e) Other potential medications may include dopamine, epinephrine, isoproterenol

        (f) Pacemakers: if patient is unable to maintain adequate cardiac output, a temporary or permanent pacemaker may be indicated

           (1) Purpose: to provide an extrinsic electrical impulse so that depolarization and subsequent contraction occurs

           (2) Main indication: symptomatic bradycardia

TABLE 2–9. Generic Pacemaker Code

I Chamber Paced	II Chamber Sensed	III Response to Sensing	IV Programmability, Rate Modulation	V Antitachyarrhythmia Function
O, none	O, none	O, none	O, none	O, none
A, atrium	A, atrium	T, triggered	P, simple	P, pacing
V, ventricle	V, ventricle	I, inhibited	programmable	S, shock
D, dual	D, dual	D, dual	M, multiprogrammable	D, dual (P and S)
(A and V)	(A and V)	(T and I)		
			R, rate modulation	

From Smith, T. W. (ed.): Cardiovascular Therapeutics: A Companion to Braunwald's Heart Disease. Philadelphia, W. B. Saunders, 1996, p. 346.

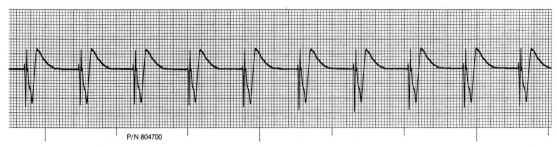

Figure 2–22 • Pacemaker rhythm strip.

(3) Modes of pacing
   a) Asynchronous (fixed rate): impulses are delivered at a predetermined rate, irrespective of any intrinsic electrical activity
   b) Synchronous (demand): impulses are delivered at a predetermined rate only if patient's own heart rate is less than the pacemaker's set rate
   c) Pacemakers that can sense and pace either or both chambers, to provide the normal sequence of atrial and ventricular contraction (AV sequential pacing), are available (Table 2–9; Figs. 2–22 and 2–23)
   d) They can also be rate responsive, increasing the heart rate to meet the demands of increased activity
(4) Components of all pacemakers
   a) Battery
      i) In temporary pacers, battery longevity depends on use and additional capabilities. Batteries should be checked routinely and changed per unit standards
      ii) Permanent pacemaker batteries last approximately 10 years or more, depending on the patient's degree of pacemaker dependency
   b) Lead system: transmit the electrical impulse from the myocardium
      i) Unipolar electrode systems: one pole is the pacing lead tip and the other pole is the pacemaker generator; produce large pacing spikes, which are easily seen on monitors and ECGs

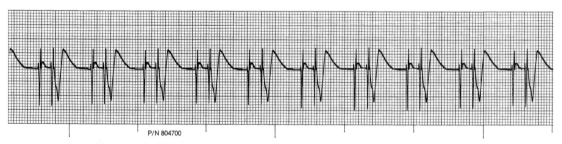

Figure 2–23 • Atrioventricular sequential pacemaker rhythm strip.

        ii) Bipolar electrode systems (most common): both negative and positive electrode poles are at distal end of pacing lead; produce small pacing spikes, which are often not seen on monitors and ECGs

    c) Pulse generator; pacemaker's control box

  (5) Capture threshold level: the minimum pacemaker output setting required to pace heart 100%

    a) Factors that increase threshold: hyperkalemia, hypoxia, drugs (beta blockers, type I antiarrhythmics)

    b) Factors that decrease threshold: increased levels of catecholamines, digitalis toxicity, corticosteroids

(g) Transcutaneous pacemaker: often used as an emergency therapy until a transvenous pacer can be inserted

  (1) One large anterior pacing electrode is ideally placed over the heart, and the other is placed directly posterior on the back

  (2) Pacemaker electrodes are attached to output cable attached to pacing unit. Pacing unit may be either free-standing or part of portable defibrillator unit

  (3) Pacing output and rate are then set

  (4) Patient will need sedation and analgesia because of increased output requirements (50 to 200 mV) for transcutaneous route

  (5) CPR may be performed safely over pacing electrodes, if needed

  (6) Frequent inspection of skin is needed to prevent potential burns, if pacing is prolonged

(h) Transvenous pacemaker: pacing catheter is placed via percutaneous route to the right atrium, right ventricle, or both for pacing. The proximal end of catheter is attached to a pacing generator

  (1) Initial rate is usually set at 60 to 80 beats/minute

  (2) Set output at intermediate output (~5 mA) and decrease until capture is lost (usually at less than 2 mA)

  (3) Set pacing output at two to three times the output required for capture (see Figs. 2–22 and 2–23 for appropriate pacemaker capture)

  (4) Ensure chest x-ray is obtained to rule out pneumothorax, if pacemaker is placed via the subclavian or internal jugular approaches

  (5) Monitor closely for appropriate sensing and pacing

  (6) Sudden loss of capture can signify that pacing electrode has migrated out of position or perforated the right ventricle. Increase the output to attempt recapture and notify physician. Do not attempt to reposition the pacing electrode. Be prepared to use atropine, isoproterenol, or transcutaneous pacing

(i) Epicardial transthoracic pacing: electrode wires are attached to the epicardium (right atrium, right ventricle, or both). Used during cardiac surgery in anticipation of conduction defects or arrhythmias. Proximal ends exit through chest wall in order to be ready for attachment to pulse generator

(1) Electrode wires need to be insulated when not in use

(2) May have one or two right atrial and one or two right ventricle wires and a ground wire

(j) Permanent pacemaker: leads placed in contact with the endocardium. Generator is implanted in a subcutaneous, subclavicular, or abdominal pocket. Capabilities can include sequential placing of the right atrium or the right ventricle or both; programmability and rate responsiveness, to allow for heart rate increases during exercise

(1) During defibrillation, anterior-posterior paddles are preferred, if readily available

(2) Keep defibrillator paddles 1 to 2 inches away from the permanent pacemaker site on chest

(3) Check pacer after defibrillation code is over

(k) Monitor for potential complications of pacemaker insertion

(1) Pneumothorax

(2) Myocardial perforation: can lead to hypotension, tamponade

(3) Hematoma

(4) Arrhythmias (PVCs)

(5) Infections (systemic or local)

(6) Hiccups, muscle twitches (from stimulation of diaphragm, abdomen)

(l) Monitor for potential complications associated with pacemaker functioning

(1) Failure to pace (Fig. 2–24) caused by

a) Battery failure

b) Lead dislodgement

c) Wire fracture

d) Disconnected wire or cable

e) Generator failure

f) Oversensing: no impulse generated because some other activity (often muscular) has been sensed and misinterpreted as a QRS complex

(2) Failure to capture (Fig. 2–25) caused by

a) Lead dislodgement or malposition

b) Battery failure

c) Pacing at voltage below capture threshold

d) Faulty connections

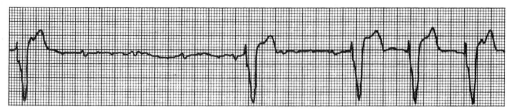

Figure 2–24 • Ventricular demand inhibited (VVI) pacemaker. Failure to discharge (pace) is indicated by lack of a pacemaker spike at appropriate intervals. (From Hudak, C. M., Gallo, B. M., and Benz, J. J.: Critical Care Nursing: A Holistic Approach, 6th ed. Philadelphia, J. B. Lippincott, 1994, p. 228.)

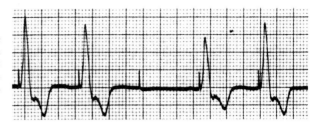

Figure 2-25 • Failure of the pulse generator to capture. (From Phillips, R. E., and Feeney, M. R.: The Cardiac Rhythms, 2nd ed. Philadelphia, W. B. Saunders, 1980, p. 347.)

    e) Lead fracture

    f) Ventricular perforation

(3) Failure to sense (Fig. 2-26): pacemaker may compete with patient's own intrinsic rhythm; caused by

    a) Sensitivity set too high

    b) Battery failure

    c) Malposition of catheter lead

    d) Lead fracture

    e) Pulse generator failure

    f) Lead insulation break

(m) Ensure electrical safety when using temporary pacemakers

    (1) Ensure that all equipment is grounded and in good working order

    (2) Wear gloves when adjusting electrodes

(n) Teaching issues for patients with pacemakers and for significant others include

    (1) Rationales and procedure for pacer placement

    (2) Daily pulse checks at home (permanent pacemaker)

    (3) Symptoms to report: wooziness; fainting; prolonged weakness; fatigue; palpitations; chest pain; difficulty breathing; fever; redness; drainage, or swelling at surgical site; prolonged hiccups; electrical shocks

    (4) Importance of follow-up care: to assess pacemaker function, to adjust pacemaker parameters

    (5) Hazards and interference to avoid: digital pagers and cellular phones, microwaves less than 1 foot away

    (6) Identification bracelet (medical alert)

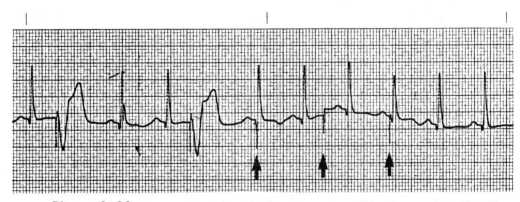

Figure 2-26 • Failure of the pulse generator to sense. Arrows identify pacemaker spikes. (From Boggs, R. L., and Wooldridge-King, M.: AACN Procedure Manual For Critical Care, 3rd ed. Philadelphia, W. B. Saunders, 1993, p. 403.)

(7) Home (telephonic) pacemaker monitoring

    iv. Evaluation of nursing care

       (a) Heart rate is sufficient to maintain stable vital signs and cardiac output; hemodynamics are normal

       (b) Arrhythmias are controlled or absent

       (c) Pacemaker functions properly with no signs of failure to pace, capture, or sense

       (d) Patient or significant other verbalizes understanding of rationale, procedure, and follow-up for pacemaker

Sumptomatic Tachycardia: Rhythms in this section include supraventricular or ventricular tachycardias that cause symptoms necessitating immediate conversion or control

1. Pathophysiology

    a. Increases in normal heart rate with exertion cause cardiac output to increase, with peripheral vascular responses that unload the heart and enhance venous return to the heart

    b. Tachycardia at rest is not accompanied by these beneficial vascular responses

    c. With increased heart rates at rest, the diastolic filling period shortens and cardiac output falls because of decreased ventricular filling

    d. Eventually, blood pressure and pulse pressure drop

    e. Pulmonary venous pressures increase, causing shortness of breath and dyspnea as the results of pulmonary congestion and edema

    f. The heart rate at which cardiac output declines is variable and dependent on the patient's substrate cardiac disease, cardiac reserve, and general health

    g. Myocardial oxygen demands increase and myocardial oxygen supply decreases because of diminished coronary perfusion at rapid heart rates; subendocardial ischemia can result

    h. Loss of atrial systole (kick) also decreases ventricular diastolic filling volumes, stroke volume, and cardiac output in rhythms without the normal atrial-ventricular sequence of contraction

    i. Decreased output can result in end-organ dysfunction (e.g., syncope, presyncope, oliguria)

2. Etiologic or precipitating factors

    a. Supraventricular tachycardias

       i. Acute MI

       ii. Ischemia

       iii. Reentry (most common cause of PSVT)

       iv. Valvular heart disease

       v. Stimulants: alcohol (ETOH), coffee, tobacco

       vi. Congenital heart disease

       vii. Pulmonary disease

       viii. Drug toxicity: digitalis, antidepressants

       ix. WPW (accessory pathway)

       x. Cardiomyopathies

    b. VT: sustained (> 30 seconds)

       i. Acute MI

       ii. Ischemia

       iii. Cardiomyopathies

        iv. Tetralogy of Fallot

        v. Drugs: digitalis, antiarrhythmic agents

        vi. Electrolyte imbalances: low potassium, magnesium

        vii. Hypoxia

        viii. Left ventricular aneurysms

        ix. Congenital long QT syndromes

        x. Valvular heart disease

3. Nursing assessment data base

    a. Nursing history

        i. Dyspnea

        ii. Palpitations

        iii. Shortness of breath

        iv. Angina

        v. Wooziness, syncope

        vi. Weakness, exercise intolerance

    b. Nursing examination of patient

        i. Anxiety

        ii. Mentation changes

        iii. Heart rate exceeds 100 beats/minute

        iv. Jugular venous distention

        v. Polyuria, oliguria

        vi. Hypotension

        vii. Unconsciousness

    c. Diagnostic study findings

        i. ECG

           (a) See ECG features for VT

           (b) See ECG features for SVTs

        ii. Laboratory studies: to ascertain

           (a) Electrolyte imbalances, include magnesium

           (b) ABG: hypoxia, acidosis

           (c) CBC: rule out hemorrhage, infection

        iii. Cardiac catheterization and EPS after patient is stabilized

4. Nursing diagnoses (see Commonly Encountered Nursing Diagnoses section earlier)

    a. Decreased cardiac output and tissue perfusion related to tachyarrhythmias

        i. Assessment for defining characteristics

           (a) Tachyarrhythmias are seen on ECG monitor and/or 12-lead ECG

           (b) Patient is symptomatic (unstable or stable)

        ii. Expected outcomes

           (a) Rhythm termination or control to maintain adequate cardiac output and tissue perfusion

           (b) Patient experiences relief of symptoms related to rapid rhythm

        iii. Nursing interventions

           (a) Identify tachyarrhythmia on monitor or ECG (see Nursing Assessment Data Base, ECG sections earlier for salient features)

           (b) Evaluate stability by rapid assessment of vital signs, level of consciousness, related symptoms

           (c) Ensure adequate airway, breathing, and circulation

           (d) Administer oxygen as needed to provide for oxygen saturations exceeding 92%

(e) If patient is symptomatic and unstable (heart rate is greater than 150 beats/minute), prepare for immediate electrical cardioversion

   (1) Cardioversion is the delivery (to the patient) of a selected amount of electrical energy synchronized with the R wave of the patient's intrinsic rhythm

   (2) The amount of energy required to convert tachyarrhythmias varies from 50 joules (for reentrant tachycardias) to 360 joules (for atrial fibrillation, ventricular fibrillation)

   (3) Explain the entire procedure to the patient and significant other, including risks

   (4) The patient should be asked to sign a consent form, if conditions are not deteriorating too rapidly

   (5) Sedative and anesthetic drugs should be given to the patient before this procedure, if the patient is conscious (an anesthesiologist is often present for elective procedures)

   (6) Hook up the patient to the defibrillator monitor leads; these can be piggybacked into many bedside monitors to gain quick ECG access

   (7) Make sure that the monitor is synchronized to the patient's rhythm: "sync" button should be on, and spikes representing recognition of R wave complexes should be seen on the monitor screen. If spikes are not seen, check gain on machine, try another lead, adjust electrodes

   (8) The code cart and suction equipment should be at bedside. Knowledge of all emergency equipment, including the defibrillator and its safe use, is vital

   (9) Place the defibrillator machine on the left side of the bed if possible, to prevent the operator from leaning over the bed while cardioverting the patient

   (10) If patient goes into ventricular fibrillation, deliver immediate defibrillation; turn off "sync" button, if necessary (most machines default to defibrillation mode after a cardioversion attempt). Remember to turn "sync" back on each time, if repeated cardioversion is necessary

(f) In acute setting, when patient is stable but has very rapid supraventricular rhythm (narrow complex), adenosine may be administered

   (1) Adenosine, 6 mg IV, injected over 3 seconds or less, followed by a dose of 12 mg 1 to 2 minutes later

      a) Adenosine often terminates AV nodal reentry and sinus nodal reentrant tachycardia

      b) It slows conduction to help with arrhythmia identification and potential termination

(g) If stable ventricular tachycardia is recognized or suspected, advanced cardiac life support (ACLS) drugs of choice are

   (1) Lidocaine, 1.0 to 1.5 mg/kg IV push, is given every 5 to 10 minutes to a total of 3 mg/kg if desired; maintenance infusion is 1 to 4 mg/minute IV

(2) Procainamide is a second-line drug for VTs
 a) 20 to 30 mg/minute IV, *slowly* injected
 b) Maximum dose: 17 mg/kg
 c) Other end points for therapy include termination of arrhythmia; severe hypotension; widening of the QRS complex to greater than 50%
 d) If procainamide is successful at terminating VT, a continuous infusion is started at 1 to 4 mg/minute
(3) Bretylium may also be used in uncontrolled VT, if other drugs are ineffective
 a) 5 mg/kg IV in a continuous infusion over 8 to 10 minutes
 b) If effective, finish loading dose with an additional 5 mg/kg IV over 8 to 10 minutes, and then continue infusion at 1 to 2 mg/minute
(h) Treatment of stable SVTs includes
 (1) Atrial fibrillation: the most frequently seen sustained tachyarrhythmia
 a) Main goals are to lower ventricular response rate, decrease symptoms, convert to sinus rhythm if possible
 b) Cardiac glycosides (digitalis) augment parasympathetic tone and lower resting heart rate; not very successful in controlling heart rate during activity
  i) Toxic side effects: any arrhythmia, conduction defects, gastrointestinal upset, visual disturbances, headache, fatigue, restlessness
  ii) To prevent toxicity, reduce dosage in patients with decreased renal and liver function, hypokalemia, hypomagnesemia, hypocalcemia, alkalosis, or hypoxia and in elderly patients
 c) Calcium channel blockers (verapamil, diltiazem) delay AV conduction, prolong refractory period, increase exercise tolerance, reduce symptoms (lower blood pressure, decrease angina)
 d) Beta-adrenergic blockers decrease sympathetic stimulation and lower heart rate at rest as well as during activity and/or stress. May be contraindicated in patients with lung disease or bronchospasm. Preferred with atrial fibrillation occurring after cardiac surgery
 e) Anticoagulation is often used to decrease risk of CVA and thromboembolism in chronic atrial fibrillation and high-risk patients. INR of 2 to 3 is the goal for dose determination. ASA may be used for low risk-patients (young patients without risk factors)
 f) Drugs used to prevent recurrence of atrial fibrillation include
  i) Quinidine, procainamide, disopyramide, propafenone
  ii) Sotalol (beta-adrenergic blocker); watch for prolonged QTc, torsade de pointes, bradyarrhythmias (especially in patients with

electrolyte imbalances or ventricular hypertrophy and in women)

iii) Amiodarone is effective for paroxysmal atrial fibrillation and for prevention of recurrence

g) After CABG: atrial fibrillation is common, usually at days 2 to 10, regardless of previous history of arrhythmia. Beta blockers (for 1 to 2 weeks after surgery) are drugs of choice in treatment. Digitalis may also be used

(2) Atrial flutter: drugs used include quinidine, procainamide, propafenone, sotalol, and amiodarone

(3) Automatic atrial tachycardia (produced by enhanced automaticity in atrial tissue): propafenone

(4) Multifocal atrial tachycardia (MAT): beta blockers (metoprolol), calcium channel blockers, amiodarone have some value

a) Correct the underlying cause

b) MAT is unresponsive to cardioversion

c) Theophyllline levels should be checked (toxicity can cause MAT) because MAT is often seen in respiratory failure

(5) Junctional tachycardia: caused by enhanced automaticity, seen in infants and children after surgery for congenital heart defects and in digitalis toxicity

a) Resistant to drugs, cardioversion

b) Catheter ablation, permanent pacing usually necessary

(6) Paroxysmal SVTs, AVNRT, AVRT, orthodromic (WPW)

a) Vagal maneuvers (gaging, cold water immersion) often terminate arrhythmia. More successful when performed as soon after onset as possible. Patient should be instructed as to safe procedure

b) Adenosine: used for hypotensive patients, for patients in heart failure, in infants, and with beta blocker therapy

c) Calcium channel blockers (verapamil, diltiazem): used especially in patients with bronchospasm, to prevent recurrence

d) Caution with wide complex tachycardias should be exercised (if mechanism for arrhythmia is unknown) because adenosine or calcium channel blockers can cause hypotension, angina, and accelerated conduction through accessory pathways, resulting in very rapid ventricular response rates (>300 beats/minute), ventricular fibrillation, and death

(i) VT

(1) Should be treated if it is

a) Sustained (<30 seconds)

b) Nonsustained but symptomatic (symptoms of diminished output; e.g., angina, shortness of breath, syncope, presyncope) *c)* Nonsustained and asymptomatic but associated with substrate heart disease (ischemia, cardiomyopathy)

     (2) Treatment includes correcting the underlying cause. Choice of antiarrhythmic agent is guided by EPS or some other documentation of efficacy (e.g, serial Holter monitoring)

     (3) Agents commonly used include amiodarone, procainamide, propafenone, mexiletine, sotalol, and occasionally quinidine

(j) Torsade de pointes

     (1) Often seen as a proarrhythmic arrhythmia as a result of antiarrhythmic drug therapy

     (2) Responds to measures that shorten the QT interval (isoproterenol, pacing) and sometimes to magnesium

(k) Patient may need to be prepared for radiofrequency catheter ablation of accessory pathways

     (1) The procedure, done in the EPS laboratory, involves use of a catheter that delivers a low-voltage, high frequency, alternating current that selectively damages abnormal myocardial tissue

     (2) Ablation of the accessory pathway stops retrograde flow of electrical impulses and disrupts reentry circuit

     (3) Uses

          a) Accessory pathways: WPW syndrome

          b) Symptomatic SVT: AVNRT, AVRT with accessory pathway, atrial fibrillation with rapid response, sinus-node reentrant tachycardias, junctional tachycardia, ventricular tachycardias (limited use)

          c) Complications of radiofrequency ablation

               i) Bleeding at catheter site

               ii) Deep vein thrombosis

               iii) Cardiac tamponade

               iv) Myocardial perforation

               v) Infection

               vi) Ischemia

               vii) Stroke

               viii) Complete AV block

               ix) Pulmonary embolism

               x) Pneumothorax

          d) Patient education issues

               i) Procedure description, rationale

               ii) Procedure is lengthy (2 to 4 hours average and up to 10 hours)

               iii) Possible need for a permanent pacemaker

               iv) Postprocedure vital signs and care

               v) Recurrence rate for tachyarrhythmias is 8% to 12%

          e) Monitor patient and procedure site in a manner similar to that for postcoronary intervention (catheterization laboratory) nursing care

(l) Overdrive pacing (antitachycardia) may also be considered for termination of persistent tachycardias (atrial fibrillation, AVNRT, atrial tachycardia, AVRT in selected patients)

(m) Surgical endocardial or epicardial techniques for ablation of the pathways are used in cases in which radiofrequency catheter ablation is not possible and the patient's symptoms are hindering quality of life

(n) AICD

    (1) Device is implanted into patient with sensing leads and defibrillator patches attached to endocardium and to a pulse generator. This is done by either thoracotomy or nonthoracotomy approaches

    (2) Capabilities include

      a) Bradycardia pacing: ventricular demand inhibited (VVI)

      b) Overdrive pacing

      c) Cardioversion: at 25 joules

      d) Defibrillation

      e) ECG storage and event logs (telemetry)

    (3) Indications: recurrent VT/V fib

    (4) Important nursing issues to understand and teach to patient and significant other

      a) If AICD discharges, it is not dangerous to staff, family

      b) Incidence of spontaneous (appropriate or inappropriate) discharges is 75% first year

      c) Concurrent use of antiarrhythmic agents is still necessary to decrease frequency of events

      d) Interrogator units can analyze history of shocks, battery functioning, heart rhythm at time of shock

iv. Evaluation of nursing care

(a) Signs of adequate cardiac output

(b) Tachycardia controlled and terminated

Absent or Ineffective Pulse: All are life-threatening and necessitate immediate intervention, usually CPR

1. Pathophysiology

a. No cardiac output and, subsequently, no tissue perfusion

b. Respirations cease. Patient is clinically dead

c. Rapid state of cell death. Brain cells start to die after 4 to 6 minutes of circulatory collapse. After 10 minutes, some degree of brain death is inevitable

d. V fib: unable to generate organized impulse for muscular contraction

e. Asystole: no electrical activity initiated

f. PEA: electrical activity and conduction occur, with absence of palpable pulse and blood pressure

   i. Caused by lack of ventricular filling volume (hypovolemia, fluid losses, saddle emboli, tamponade)

   ii. Caused by myocardium's inability to effectively contract: lack of oxygen, acidotic states, electrolyte disturbances, physical impairment to contraction (tension pneumothorax), muscular dysfunction resulting from necrosis (MI)

2. Etiologic or precipitating factors
   a. Causes of V fib
      i. MI
      ii. Ischemia
      iii. Myocardial disease: cardiomyopathies, myocarditis
      iv. Anoxia: smoke inhalation, drowning, respiratory failure, airway obstruction
   b. Causes of asystole
      i. Hypokalemia
      ii. Hyperkalemia
      iii. Hypothermia
      iv. Acidosis
   c. Causes of PEA
      i. Hypovolemia: most common cause
      ii. Hypoxia
      iii. Tension pneumothorax
      iv. Acidosis
      v. Acute MI
      vi. Pulmonary embolism
      vii. Hyperkalemia
      viii. Tamponade
      ix. Drug overdose: calcium channel blockers, digitalis, tricyclic antidepressants, beta blockers
      x. Hypothermia
3. Nursing assessment data base
   a. Nursing history
      i. History is often deferred or obtained in conjunction with emergency, life-preserving measures
      ii. Determine whether patient has a history of any of the aforementioned etiologies
   b. Nursing examination of patient
      i. Pulseless
      ii. Unconsciousness or rapidly deteriorating level of consciousness
      iii. No respiration
   c. Diagnostic study findings
      i. ABG: done after immediate actions taken; to check oxygenation, acidosis, ventilation status
      ii. Electrolytes
      iii. ECG: see salient features for each
         (a) In PEA, there is organized electrical activity but no significant cardiac output
         (b) V fib (coarse versus fine)
         (c) Pulseless ventricular tachycardia (very rapid)
4. Nursing diagnoses (see Commonly Encountered Nursing Diagnoses section earlier)
   a. No cardiac output and no tissue perfusion related to ineffective or absent pulse
      i. Assessment for defining characteristics: no pulse, no respiration
      ii. Expected outcomes
         (a) Preservation of life

(b) Patient's response to emergency therapy; rapid restoration of adequate cardiac output and tissue perfusion without brain death

iii. Nursing interventions
   (a) Immediately call cardiac arrest code team
   (b) Assess airway, breathing, and circulation (ABC); perform CPR
   (c) Have crash cart and emergency equipment at bedside
   (d) Defibrillate, as soon as equipment is available, without delay *if patient is in V fib, VT, or asystole* (could be fine ventricular fibrillation)
      (1) Use 200, 300, and 360 joules per ACLS standards
      (2) Be familiar with safe use of defibrillator. Always treat it as if it is a weapon, and visually ensure that everyone at bedside is clear from bed before defibrillating (each time)
   (e) Ensure that CPR is resumed promptly after defibrillation or any assessments
   (f) Emergency medications for V fib (see American Heart Association current ACLS standards for detailed descriptions, algorithms)
      (1) 100% oxygen
      (2) Epinephrine, 1 mg IV push, every 3 to 5 minutes during arrest; start after initial defibrillation
      (3) Lidocaine, 1.0 to 1.5 mg/kg IV push; repeat every 3 to 5 minutes; maximum total dose up to 3 mg/kg IV
      (4) Bretylium, 5 mg/kg IV push; repeat in 5 minutes at 10 mg/kg IV
      (5) Procainamide, sodium bicarbonate, and magnesium may also be used
      (6) Defibrillation is reattempted after each drug intervention
      (7) IV infusions are not hung during immediate arrest; they can be hung only after patient's heart rate and rhythm have been restored and when determination has been made regarding drug effectiveness
   (g) Medications administered for asystole and PEA
      (1) Emergency medications are given in boluses
      (2) Epinephrine, 1 mg IV push, every 3 to 5 minutes during arrest
      (3) Atropine, 1 mg IV, every 3 to 5 minutes (up to 0.03 to 0.04 mg/kg maximum vagolytic dose)
   (h) Automatic external defibrillator (AED) may be the only defibrillator available in some areas of the hospital
      (1) Fully or semi-automatic models
      (2) Cables attached to two adhesive conductive pads
      (3) Machines capable of recording rhythm, analyzing data, yelling "Clear," and delivering electrical shocks
      (4) CPR must be stopped for machine needs to analyze rhythm (takes 15 to 20 seconds), and then it will deliver shocks
      (5) It is important for operator to be familiar with its use. Most problems result from operator difficulties
   (i) AICDs are often used if the patient survives the cardiac arrest

(j) Promptly assess and treat for common causes of PEA
  (1) Administer immediate volume replacement
  (2) Listen for breath sounds; check for pneumothorax
  (3) Ensure proper oxygenation: give 100%
  (4) Hyperventilate patient: respiratory acidosis usually occurs in arrest as a result of inadequate ventilation
  (5) Check ABG results for acidosis
  (6) Assist physician with pericardiocentesis for tamponade, needle decompression of pneumothorax
  (7) Draw blood for drug screens

Mitral Insufficiency

During ventricular systole, blood is partially regurgitated back into the left atrium because of an incompetent mitral valve. This may happen acutely or develop as a chronic condition

1. **Pathophysiology**
    a. With failure of the mitral valve to close completely during ventricular contraction, some fraction of the left ventricular output (often greater than 50%) is ejected backwards into the left atrium
    b. Pressures in the left atrium and pulmonary veins rise (dramatically if the onset is acute), and pulmonary congestion and/or edema results in dyspnea
    c. Forward congestion and/or edema results in chronic fatigue (or hypotension if acute)
    d. The pathophysiology and clinical course vary dramatically, depending on whether the onset is acute or chronic
    e. Acute onset
        i. Left atrial diastolic pressures dramatically increase, along with pulmonary pressures
        ii. The left atrium has no time to compensate and initially remains small and noncompliant (creating high pressures)
        iii. Forward output falls dramatically, and cardiogenic shock develops
        iv. Pulmonary hypertension may develop as a result of high pressures within the pulmonary vascular bed, and pulmonary edema rapidly ensues
    f. Chronic onset
        i. The left atrium has time (often years) to enlarge and develop the compliance to keep its pressure at near normal levels
        ii. Pulmonary artery pressures remain relatively normal
        iii. Eventually the degree of mitral regurgitation may exceed the capacity of the left atrium to compensate, and pulmonary congestion and dyspnea may develop
        iv. The left ventricle compensates for the chronic volume overload by dilating, in an attempt to maintain a normal forward output, while emptying a large volume of its output backwards into the left atrium
        v. Eventually, the left ventricle can dilate to such an extent that it is unable to recover, even after surgical correction of the mitral regurgitation
        vi. Pulmonary venous pressures elevate, with resulting increases in PCWP and secondary pulmonary hypertension

vii. Atrial fibrillation often is seen and occurs secondary to left atrial enlargement

viii. The right ventricle also will progressively hypertrophy, and right-sided heart failure may follow

2. Etiologic or precipitating factors

a. Acute causes

  i. Acute rupture of chordae tendineae as a result of endocarditis or chronic strain on the mitral valve apparatus by mitral valve prolapse, rheumatic heart disease

  ii. Papillary muscle dysfunction or rupture secondary to MI

  iii. Trauma

b. Chronic causes

  i. Rheumatic heart disease

  ii. Congenital malformations of the mitral valve, chordae tendineae, or mitral annulae

  iii. Mitral valve prolapse

  iv. Left ventricular dilatation from other causes

  v. Connective tissue disease, such as Marfan's syndrome

  vi. Infective endocarditis

  vii. Calcified mitral annulus

3. Nursing assessment data base

a. Nursing history

  i. Subjective findings: patient complains of

    (a) Shortness of breath

    (b) Orthopnea

    (c) Paroxysmal nocturnal dyspnea

    (d) Weakness or becoming easily fatigued

    (e) Palpitations

    (f) Symptoms of right ventricular failure

  ii. Objective findings: history of past rheumatic fever, streptococcal infection, endocarditis, ischemia, trauma, mitral valve prolapse

b. Nursing examination of patient

  i. Inspection: if in heart failure, may see

    (a) Tachypnea

    (b) Anxiety

    (c) Diaphoresis

    (d) Cyanosis

    (e) Confusion

    (f) Edema

    (g) Jugular venous distention (in right-sided heart failure)

    (h) Signs of pulmonary edema (frothy, pink sputum)

  ii. Palpation

    (a) Apical impulse (PMI) is laterally displaced, diffuse, and hyperdynamic (in chronic mitral regurgitation)

    (b) An apical systolic thrill may be felt

    (c) Pulse may be irregular if in atrial fibrillation

    (d) Hepatomegaly (late sign)

  iii. Auscultation

    (a) High-pitched blowing holosystolic murmur

      (1) Heard best at the apex with radiation to the axilla

      (2) Begins at S_1 and extends through S_2 (aortic closure)

(b) Rales when pulmonary congestion or edema is present

(c) S$_2$ may be widely split or accentuated (P$_2$) as a result of early closure of aortic valve, because left ventricular ejection time is shortened. The left ventricle empties more quickly because some of its output is moving into the left atrium (rather than the aorta)

(d) Possible S$_3$ at apex

(e) Diastolic flow (rumble) caused by increased flow across the mitral valve during diastole when there is a large amount of mitral regurgitation

  c. Diagnostic study findings

    i. Radiologic

(a) Left atrial and left ventricular enlargement in chronic mitral regurgitation

(b) The left atrium does not enlarge with acute onset

(c) Calcification of mitral valve

(d) Pulmonary edema

    ii. ECG: atrial fibrillation (seen in 75% patients)

    iii. Echocardiography: helps determine the etiology, left ventricular function and dimensions, and the indications for surgery

(a) Degree of insufficiency

(b) Left atrial and left ventricular enlargement in chronic mitral insufficiency

(c) Mitral valve prolapse, mitral annular calcification, flail leaflet, vegetations, rheumatic heart disease

(d) Abnormal regional wall motion if papillary muscle dysfunction is cause

(e) Transesophageal echocardiography: used in guiding mitral valve reconstructive surgery, superior to transthoracic echocardiography in visualizing the mitral valve leaflets

    iv. Cardiac catheterization

(a) Documents severity of mitral regurgitation

(b) Screens for CAD

(c) Documents PCWP and right-sided heart pressures

(d) Can determine regurgitant fraction

4. Nursing diagnoses (see Commonly Encountered Nursing Diagnoses section earlier)

  a. Decrease in cardiac output related to valve dysfunction

    i. Additional nursing interventions

(a) Monitor ECG; watch for arrhythmias. Intervene per unit standards

(b) Administer medications, including nitrates, afterload reduction

(c) Assess patient for signs and symptoms of heart failure

    (1) Acute mitral regurgitation may respond to administration of vasodilators such as nitroprusside

    (2) IABP may be a life-saving procedure in severe cases

(d) Other complications to observe for

    (1) Systemic emboli with atrial fibrillation

    (2) Infective endocarditis

(e) If the valve is to be surgically reconstructed (surgical mitral valvuloplasty) or replaced, patient and significant other must be counseled with regard to the surgery
  (1) Provide explanation of the disease process, preoperative routines, the surgical procedure, including the types of replacement valves to be used and what is to be expected during the immediate postoperative period
  (2) Mitral valve reconstruction shows improved rest and exercise ejection fractions postoperatively (benefits partially the results of preserved chordae tendineae, papillary muscles, valve shape)
  (3) Chronic anticoagulant use is not necessary with reconstruction, if patient is in sinus rhythm
  (4) Postoperative general care for valve repair is similar to postoperative care for most cardiac surgical operations (e.g., CABG) in which a median sternotomy approach is used
  (5) Discharge instructions include the usual postoperative instructions for any heart surgery. If valve was replaced, the importance of endocarditis prophylaxis and chronic anticoagulation must be stressed (if the patient does not comply with these follow-up medications, stroke and possibly death are highly likely)

ii. Evaluation of nursing care
  (a) Hemodynamic stability is evidenced by normal vital signs, lack of arrhythmias, or arrhythmias under control without producing hemodynamic changes
  (b) Patient exhibits an appropriate level of anxiety
  (c) Patient verbalizes an understanding of the preoperative teaching discussed
  (d) Postoperatively, patient is hemodynamically stable; vital signs within normal limits; patient has no other potential complications
  (e) On discharge, patient and significant other relate an understanding of all postoperative care measures, particularly the need for antibiotic prophylaxis when undergoing future surgical or dental procedures and, if necessary, chronic anticoagulant therapy

Mitral Stenosis

A progressive narrowing of the mitral orifice that impedes the flow of blood from the left atrium to the left ventricle during ventricular diastole

1. **Pathophysiology**
   a. Progressive fibrosis, scarring, and thickening of the valve leaflets, usually from rheumatic valvular disease
   b. Extensive fusion of leaflets and chordae tendineae then develops
   c. The area of a normal adult's mitral valve orifice is 3 to 6 cm². In mild mitral stenosis, it is 2 cm² (symptoms may be experienced only with exercise, atrial fibrillation). In severe mitral stenosis, it is 1 cm², with symptoms even at rest

d. Elevation of left atrial pressures results from the obstruction to flow from the left atrium to the left ventricle. As the valve continues to narrow, the left atrium slowly dilates and hypertrophies

e. Intractable atrial fibrillation usually results

f. As atrial pressures elevate, pulmonary capillary hydrostatic pressure rises over the plasma oncotic pressure, and fluid escapes into the pulmonary interstitium and alveoli

g. As the valve orifice narrows to smaller than 1 cm², pulmonary hypertension occurs and right ventricular pressures increase with eventual hypertrophy and dilatation. Right ventricular failure frequently follows

h. The stenotic obstruction impedes forward blood flow and alone is often enough to decrease stroke volume and cardiac output. The loss of atrial kick, which results from the atrial fibrillation, and tachycardia compound the problem, decreasing left ventricular filling time and further decreasing cardiac output

i. Atrial thrombi form, and systemic or cerebral emboli may ensue

2. Etiologic or precipitating factors

a. Rheumatic heart disease (most common cause)

b. Congenital mitral valve disease

c. Tumors of the left atrium (atrial myxoma)

d. Precipitating factors: rheumatic fever, atrial fibrillation, pregnancy (often third trimester

3. Nursing assessment data base

a. Nursing history

    i. Gradual decline in physical activity over the years

    ii. Shortness of breath, dyspnea on exertion

    iii. Paroxysmal nocturnal dyspnea

    iv. Orthopnea

    v. Cough (bronchial irritability), hoarseness

    vi. Hemoptysis (ruptured pulmonary vessels)

    vii. Fatigue

    viii. Palpitations

    ix. Signs and symptoms of right-sided heart failure occur later

    x. Dysphagia (caused by enlarged atrium and displaced esophagus)

    xi. History of

        (a) Systemic emboli

        (b) Rheumatic heart disease

    xii. Objective findings: signs and symptoms of right-sided heart failure occur as late signs

b. Nursing examination of patient; findings depend on the degree of heart failure present

    i. Inspection

        (a) Any of the signs of heart failure

        (b) Jugular vein distention

    ii. Palpation

        (a) May feel right ventricle lift if pulmonary hypertension is present; left ventricular "tap" may be present

        (b) Diastolic thrill present over apical area, depending on the intensity of the murmur

    iii. Auscultation

        (a) S_1 is pronounced

        (b) Low-pitched apical diastolic murmur

        (c) Associated murmur of tricuspid insufficiency may be present if right ventricular failure exists. Listen at left lower parasternal area

        (d) Pulmonary component, S_2, later and louder if pulmonary hypertension exists

        (e) Mitral opening snap present

  c. Diagnostic study findings

     i. Radiologic: chest x-ray film reveals

        (a) Left atrial and right ventricular hypertrophy

        (b) Calcification of mitral valve

        (c) Interstitial edema, pulmonary vascular redistribution to upper lobes of lungs (caused by high PCWP)

     ii. ECG

        (a) Right ventricular hypertrophy pattern (with pulmonary hypertension)

        (b) Atrial fibrillation

        (c) Left atrial enlargement (P mitrale)

    iii. Two-dimensional echocardiography

        (a) Thickened, tethered, and doming (stuck together, "domes") anterior and posterior mitral valve leaflets

        (b) Calculate mitral valve area

        (c) Enlarged left atrium

        (d) Enlarged right ventricle

        (e) Assess degree of pulmonary hypertension, mitral regurgitation, and function of the other valves

    iv. Exercise stress test: used for evaluation of exercise tolerance in mild to moderate disease

     v. Cardiac catheterization

        (a) Severity of disease, calcification of mitral valve area and gradient

        (b) Elevated PCWP

        (c) Elevated RVP and RAP when right ventricular failure is present

        (d) Used to assess function of other valves and rule out CAD

2. Nursing diagnoses (see Commonly Encountered Nursing Diagnoses section earlier)

  a. Decreased cardiac output related to valve dysfunction, mitral insufficiency

  b. Altered tissue perfusion related to systemic or pulmonary emboli from atrial thrombus

     i. Assessment for defining characteristics

        (a) High risk for thrombus formation during atrial fibrillation or heart failure and/or in patients on prolonged bed rest (thrombophlebitis)

        (b) Diminished or absent blood flow with Doppler ultrasound (thrombophlebitis)

        (c) Pulmonary embolism: patient has tachycardia, tachypnea, hypoxia, dyspnea, cough, hemoptysis, elevated pulmonary artery pressure, hypotension, pain in chest, abnormal arterial blood gas values, cyanosis, lung scan positive for emboli

        (d) Central nervous system embolism: patient has symptoms of stroke (e.g., paralysis, weakness, dysphasia, confusion, seizures)

(e) Extremities: patient complains of pain in calf and of cold extremities or unequal temperature of extremities; extremities may exhibit pallor, rubor, or cyanosis; diminished or absent peripheral pulses; capillary refill sluggish and swelling present in affected extremity

(f) Renal: hematuria, oliguria, back pain, rising blood urea nitrogen value

(g) Splenic: pain in left upper quadrant with radiation to left shoulder

(h) Mesenteric: pain in lower abdomen, bloody diarrhea, elevated leukocyte count, and elevated erythrocyte sedimentation rate

ii. Expected outcomes

(a) Absence or resolution of systemic or pulmonary emboli

(b) Patient is hemodynamically stable

iii. Nursing interventions

(a) Assess for signs and symptoms of peripheral systemic emboli (see defining characteristics listed earlier)

(b) Elevate extremities that have thromboemboli

(c) TED hose, pneumatic antiembolism stockings to prevent thrombi formation

c. Other key points

i. Current treatment options include surgical mitral valve replacement, open surgical commissurotomy, and "closed" percutaneous balloon mitral valvuloplasty (BMV)

ii. Medical management is palliative; mechanical correction is eventually required to improve cardiac output and decrease atrial and pulmonary pressures

(a) Diuretics, nitrates: to lower pulmonary congestion, may lower cardiac output

(b) Digitalis, beta-blockade, calcium antagonists: to treat atrial fibrillation, slow ventricular response

(c) Beta-adrenergic blocking agents may increase exercise tolerance by slowing the heart rate and lengthening the diastolic filling period

(d) Anticoagulants: prevent embolization

(e) Prophylaxis for infectious endocarditis during dental procedures

iii. See Mitral Insufficiency section earlier for postoperative nursing issues

Aortic Insufficiency

An incompetent aortic valve causes regurgitation of blood from the aorta to the left ventricle during ventricular diastole

1. **Pathophysiology**

a. The aortic valve can become incompetent as a result of destruction of the cusps (endocarditis), degeneration of the cusps, unhinging of the valvular apparatus (dissection), rheumatic disease, connective tissue disease, congenital heart disease, and trauma

b. When this occurs acutely

i. Increased regurgitation into the left ventricle produces volume overload, *markedly* increasing the LVEDP

ii. Peripheral vasoconstriction develops, because the forward flow of blood is hindered

iii. There is a drop in aortic diastolic pressure that diminishes the coronary blood flow

iv. The compensatory increase in heart rate adds to the already elevated myocardial oxygen demand. Ischemic and sudden cardiac death may occur

c. When this occurs as a chronic process

i. The left ventricle compensates by dilating to increase its stroke volume in order to maintain an adequate forward output (increasing myocardial oxygen demands)

ii. LVEDP increases. Left ventricular myocardial fibers stretch and hypertrophy

iii. As the disease progresses, the left ventricle fails and decompensates; stroke volume and EF decrease. Left ventricular systolic and diastolic pressures increase

iv. A wide pulse pressure develops as a result of low aortic diastolic pressures and high systemic pressures

v. Decreased blood flow to coronary arteries during diastole results in myocardial ischemia

2. **Etiologic or precipitating factors**

a. Infective endocarditis (most common cause of acute aortic insufficiency)

b. Idiopathic calcification of the valve

c. Diseases of the aortic valve and root

d. Congenital malformations (coarctation of aorta, ventricular septal defect, bicuspid aortic valve)

e. Aortic dissection

f. Rheumatic spondylitis

g. Aortic aneurysms (e.g., Marfan's syndrome)

h. Hypertension

i. Trauma: blunt; causing valve rupture

j. Systemic lupus erythematosus

k. Syphilis

l. Rupture of a sinus of Valsalva aneurysm

3. **Nursing assessment data base**

a. Nursing history

i. Subjective findings

(a) Dyspnea (most common symptom): caused by increased LVEDP, pulmonary pressures

(b) Easy fatigability

(c) Paroxysmal nocturnal dyspnea

(d) Orthopnea

(e) Excessive perspiration

(f) Increased force of heartbeat, palpitations

(g) Exertional chest pain (angina): late symptom

(h) Exertional syncope

ii. Objective findings

(a) History of any etiologic factors

(b) History of fever

  b. Nursing examination of patient
    i. Inspection
      (a) Signs and symptoms of left-sided heart failure
      (b) Distinct carotid artery pulsations
      (c) de Musset's sign (nodding of head)
      (d) Flushed appearance
      (e) Müller's sign: uvula bobbing
    ii. Palpation
      (a) Forceful apical impulse, displaced laterally and downward (in chronic forms); apical impulse does not change with acute onset
      (b) Water-hammer pulse: bounding, abrupt rise and fall in carotid arteries and other peripheral pulses
      (c) Systolic thrill: caused by high flow
      (d) Jugular vein distention: when pulmonary hypertension develops
      (e) Positive Quincke's sign: when fingertip is pressed, capillary pulsation of nail beds is visible
    iii. Auscultation
      (a) Very widened pulse pressure, resulting from increased systolic blood pressure, decreased diastolic blood pressure
      (b) Positive Hill's sign: popliteal blood pressure is about 40 mm Hg higher than brachial blood pressure (seen in severe aortic insufficiency)
      (c) High-pitched, blowing, decrescendo, diastolic murmur
        (1) Loudest at lower left sternal border
        (2) Starts right after S_2
        (3) Short (early diastole) with acute aortic insufficiency
        (4) Long (through diastole), if chronic
      (d) S_3 common
      (e) S_4 heard in more severe disease (abnormal left ventricular compliance)
      (f) Rales at bases, if onset is acute
  c. Diagnostic study findings
    i. Radiologic: chest x-ray reveals
      (a) Left ventricular enlargement: normal with mild or acute aortic insufficiency
      (b) Wide mediastinum
      (c) Calcified aortic valve
      (d) Pulmonary vascular redistribution; interstitial pulmonary edema may be present
    ii. ECG
      (a) Left atrial and left ventricular hypertrophy
      (b) Sinus tachycardia (acutely), atrial fibrillation, ventricular arrhythmias, AV blocks (late)
    iii. Echocardiography
      (a) Severity of aortic regurgitation
      (b) Left ventricular cavity dilatation with hyperdynamic wall motion in chronic cases
      (c) Abnormalities of the aortic valve; vegetations
      (d) TEE: to assess ascending and descending thoracic aorta for aneurysms, dissection
    iv. MRI or CT scan: valuable if echocardiography is not feasible or inconclusive regarding aortic dissection

v. Cardiac catheterization
  (a) Hemodynamics
      (1) Increased LVEDP, left atrial pressure
      (2) Increased PCWP
      (3) Increased right-sided heart pressures (late)
  (b) Low systemic diastolic pressures
  (c) Quantifies the degree of insufficiency
  (d) Left ventricular function, EF, other abnormalities
  (e) Coronary anatomy

4. **Nursing diagnoses** (see Commonly Encountered Nursing Diagnoses section earlier)
  a. Decreased cardiac output related to valve dysfunction
      i. Additional nursing interventions
          (a) See Mitral Insufficiency, Nursing Interventions section
          (b) Goals: to lower peripheral systemic resistance; reduce afterload and left ventricular dilatation; to increase EF
          (c) Administer medications prescribed to meet goals: digitalis, diuretics, vasodilators, afterload reduction agents, anticoagulants, oxygen as ordered
          (d) Prepare patient for cardiac surgery if aortic insufficiency is hemodynamically significant and patient is a surgical candidate. Valve replacement is main treatment for the incompetent valve
          (e) Infective endocarditis is the most significant complication to observe for and teach patient about
          (f) Teach patient and significant other about need for adherence to medications and that prophylactic antibiotics will be used to prevent subacute bacterial endocarditis

Aortic Stenosis

The ejection of blood from the left ventricle during systole is impaired because of an obstructive narrowing. Stenosis may be supravalvular, subvalvular, or valvular. Obstructions above the valve are rare and usually congenital. Obstructions below the valve are associated with hypertrophic cardiomyopathy. The most common obstructions in adults are those at the valve itself

1. **Pathophysiology**
  a. The valve becomes thickened and calcified, with fusion of the cusps. Left ventricular afterload gradually increases
  b. A systolic pressure gradient develops between the left ventricle and the aorta
  c. To maintain stroke volume and adequate cardiac output, the left ventricle hypertrophies in a concentric manner
  d. The left ventricle becomes stiff and noncompliant, and the LVEDP increases
  e. Left atrial pressures increase, which increases the pulmonary vascular pressures. Pulmonary congestion develops and eventually increases pressures in the right chambers. Right ventricular failure ensues
  f. Because the left side of the heart has to pump against increased afterload, myocardial oxygen demand is greatly increased. This occurs at the same time that coronary blood flow is being diminished because of the high intracavity pressures

g. Left ventricular hypertrophy and increased LVEDP cause a decrease in subendocardial coronary perfusion, and ischemia results in angina and arrhythmias

h. Forward cardiac output cannot be augmented to meet the requirements of exertion, and exertional syncope may result

i. Complications of aortic stenosis
   i. Sudden cardiac death (high incidence) resulting from ventricular arrhythmias
   ii. Left ventricular failure (diastolic dysfunction)
   iii. Conduction defects
   iv. Infective endocarditis (rare)
   v. Emboli: stroke, vision problems

2. **Etiologic or precipitating factors**
   a. The most common cause: calcific or degenerative aortic stenosis (calcium deposits occur in the cusps of the valve itself; seen in patients 60 years and older)
   b. Rheumatic heart disease (the commissure fuses, leaflets thicken and fibrose; symptoms usually seen in patients in their 50s and 60s), more often associated with mitral valve disease
   c. Congenital heart defects: bicuspid valve (symptoms usually seen in patients in their 40s and 50s), associated with other defects, especially coarctation of the aorta

3. **Nursing assessment data base**
   a. History: often progresses to severe stage with few symptoms noticed. Once symptoms occur, progression may be rapid
      i. Syncope with exertion (transient arrhythmias, decreased cardiac and cerebral perfusion)
      ii. Dyspnea on exertion (pulmonary congestion)
      iii. Angina (caused by left ventricular hypertrophy, increased myocardial demands, lowered coronary blood flow)
      iv. Symptoms of left ventricular failure
      v. Palpitations
      vi. Fatigue or weakness
      vii. History of any etiologic factors
   b. Nursing examination of patient
      i. Inspection
         (a) Anxious
         (b) Labored respiration, tachypnea
         (c) Jugular veins: "a" wave (if right-sided heart failure is present and patient is in sinus rhythm)
      ii. Palpation
         (a) Forceful, sustained apical impulse
         (b) A systolic thrill may be felt in the second or third right intercostal spaces
         (c) Pulsus parvus and tardus (small carotid upstroke and delayed peak)
         (d) Narrow pulse pressure
         (e) Slow radial pulse
      iii. Auscultation
         (a) A harsh, loud systolic ejection murmur loudest at the second right intercostal space, radiating up the neck

          (b) Paradoxical split S_2

          (c) S_3 (in severe left ventricular dysfunction)

          (d) S_4 (with left ventricular hypertrophy)

          (e) Rales (left ventricular failure)

c. Diagnostic study findings

    i. Radiologic

        (a) Cardiac enlargement in late stages

        (b) Pulmonary vascular redistribution, congestion

        (c) Calcified aortic valve

        (d) Dilated ascending aorta

    ii. ECG

        (a) Left ventricular hypertrophy and strain pattern (increased QRS voltage, ST changes)

        (b) Conduction defects: LBBB

        (c) Left axis deviation

        (d) Atrial fibrillation in late stages

    iii. Echocardiography

        (a) Presence and severity of aortic stenosis

        (b) Calcification of aortic area and gradient

        (c) Left ventricular hypertrophy (concentric) and left ventricular function

        (d) Left atrial enlargement

    iv. Cardiac catheterization: used to assess

        (a) Hemodynamics

            (1) Elevated left ventricular systolic pressure and LVEDP

            (2) Elevated PCWP

            (3) Pressure gradient between the left ventricle and the aorta is usually greater than 50 mm Hg

        (b) Calculation of aortic valve area

            (1) Normal: 3.0 to 3.5 cm^2

            (2) In mild aortic stenosis: 1.0 to 1.5 cm^2

            (3) In moderate aortic stenosis: 0.85 to 1.0 cm^2

            (4) In severe aortic stenosis: less than 0.85 cm^2

        (c) CAD

4. Nursing Diagnoses (see Commonly Encountered Nursing Diagnoses section earlier)

a. See Aortic Insufficiency section earlier

b. Decreased cardiac output due to aortic stenosis (other key notes):

    i. Treatment: if patient has symptoms and severe aortic stenosis, surgery is the prime therapy

    ii. Medical management is palliative

        (a) Typical medications ordered include

            (1) Diuretics (can lower cardiac output, inasmuch as the left ventricle is very dependent on preload)

            (2) Vasodilators should be avoided; can cause profound hypotension

            (3) Avoid strenuous activities

            (4) Diet should be low in sodium

            (5) Patient needs to have knowledge of what symptoms to report promptly: patient is at high risk for sudden cardiac death

      iii. Aortic valvuloplasty has proved ineffective

      iv. Surgery: valve replacement with bioprosthetic or metal valves

        (a) CABG often done at the same time

        (b) Lifelong anticoagulants are necessary when prosthetic valves are used

      v. Aortic stenosis (including asymptomatic): increases risks involved with noncardiac surgical procedures

Atrial Septal Defect

A defect in the intra-arterial septum that allows free communication between the right and left sides of the heart at the atrial level. Found in approximately 10% of congenital heart defects. Can result in shortened life span and in morbidity as a result of dyspnea and right-sided heart failure. Paradoxical emboli (right-to-left circulation) can result

1. **Pathophysiology**
   a. Common types of this defect (Fig. 2–27) include
       i. Sinus venosus defect: located high in the septum at the junction of the right atrium and superior vena cava. Frequently associated with partial anomalous pulmonary venous return (PAPVR) of the right upper lobe vein to the superior vena cava. This is the least common type (5% to 10% of atrial septal defects)
       ii) Ostium secundum defect (fossa ovalis): located in the middle of the septum in the area of the foramen ovale. This is the most common type (70%)
       iii. Ostium primum defect (often associated with endocardial cushion defects): located at lower end of the septum, superior to the interventricular septum (20%)
   b. As a result of the defect, flow is from the normally higher pressure left atrium to the right atrium, creating a left-to-right shunt
   c. During diastole, the left-to-right shunt is accentuated, depending on compliance of the atrium and ventricles

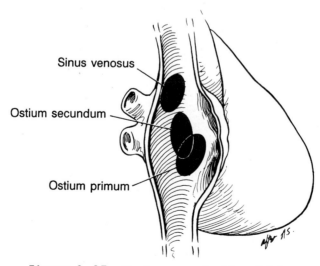

Figure 2–27 • The three types of atrial septal defects.

    d. Right-chamber and pulmonary flow increase because the right chambers handle both the normal systemic venous return from the body and the left-to-right shunt flow through the atrial septal defect

    e. This results in volume overload of the right chambers

    f. The right atrium, right ventricle, and pulmonary artery dilate

    g. The systolic murmur of an atrial septal defect results from increased flow across the normal pulmonic valve (a flow murmur). The diastolic murmur results from increased flow across the tricuspid valve

    h. Pulmonary hypertension and pulmonary vascular disease may develop over time (found in 15% to 20% of adults with this defect). In extreme cases, the shunt may reverse, becoming right to left, which is irreversible (Eisenmenger's syndrome)

    i. Right ventricular dilatation, hypertrophy, and failure can result

    j. Mitral valve anomalies (with cleft leaflets) often occur in endocardial cushion defects (associated with ostium primum defects), resulting in mitral insufficiency

2. Etiologic or precipitating factors

    a. Exact cause unknown

    b. Incidence: twice as common among females

    c. May be due to

        i. Genetic factors

        ii. Maternal and fetal infection during first trimester of pregnancy (e.g., rubella)

        iii. Effects of drugs or medications

        iv. Dietary deficiencies during fetal development

3. Nursing assessment data base: symptoms often develop in the fourth to sixth decade of life

    a. Nursing history

        i. Subjective findings: complaints of

            (a) Mild fatigue

            (b) Exertional dyspnea

            (c) Palpitations

        ii. Objective findings

            (a) More common among women

            (b) History of increased incidence of pulmonary infections during childhood

    b. Nursing examination of patient: presentations vary, depending on the direction of the shunt. When the shunt reverses to right to left, signs and symptoms of severe heart failure will be present with cyanosis

        i. Inspection

            (a) Patient's appearance is generally normal

            (b) Signs of heart failure in older patients

            (c) Cyanosis, clubbing of fingers and toes (with right-to-left shunts)

        ii. Palpation: systolic, hyperdynamic lift along left sternal border, caused by enlarged right ventricle

        iii. Auscultation

            (a) Systolic ejection murmur: heard best in second left intercostal space (at base of heart); caused by increased flow through pulmonic valve

            (b) Fixed split of S_2

(c) An early, low-pitched diastolic murmur may be heard best at lower left sternal border or xiphoid area; is caused by increased blood flow through the tricuspid valve if the shunt flow is large

c. Diagnostic study findings

   i. Radiologic: chest x-ray reveals

     (a) Mild to moderate enlargement of the right atrium, right ventricle, and pulmonary artery

     (b) Increased pulmonary vascular markings

   ii. ECG

     (a) Atrial fibrillation and/or atrial flutter seen in adults, is usually paroxysmal

     (b) PR prolongation

     (c) Incomplete RBBB: rsR', RSR' in V_1

     (d) Left axis deviation in ostium primum defects

   iii. Echocardiography

     (a) Right ventricular enlargement

     (b) The actual defect is occasionally seen with two-dimensional echocardiography, color-flow Doppler studies, and transesophageal echocardiography

     (c) IV injection of contrast medium demonstrates defect by early appearance of contrast medium in the left heart chambers

   iv. Cardiac catheterization: required for quantifying shunt and evaluating hemodynamics, associated heart disease

     (a) Characteristic finding is an increase (step-up) in oxygen concentration in the right atrium

     (b) Increased pulmonary artery pressures may be documented

4. Nursing diagnoses (see Commonly Encountered Nursing Diagnoses section earlier)

a. Activity intolerance related to the atrial septal defect

   i. Additional nursing interventions

     (a) Monitor all vital signs and hemodynamic pressures, and report changes

     (b) Monitor ECG; watch for atrial fibrillation, flutter, AV blocks

     (c) Assess patient for signs and symptoms of heart failure. Administer digitalis, diuretics

     (d) Complications to observe for also include paradoxical embolism, brain abscess, pulmonary infections

     (e) Administer prophylactic antibiotics to prevent endocarditis, which may occur on a cleft mitral valve

     (f) Prepare patient and significant other for possibility of surgical repair, including explanation of the disease process, preoperative routines, surgical procedure, expectations during the immediate postoperative period

     (g) Postoperative care for atrial septal repairs is similar to postoperative care for most cardiac surgical operations in which median sternotomy approach is used; assessment for and prevention of potential complications (atrial fibrillation, embolization) is of utmost importance

b. Potential for infectious process (infective endocarditis) secondary to this congenital heart defect is low (see Infective Endocarditis section earlier)

c. Diminished tissue perfusion related to atrial septal defect; see other key points

      i. Repair of the defect is recommended, to prevent the complications of pulmonary hypertension, heart failure, and early death

     ii. Repair in children may be deferred but should be performed before they enter school (2 to 5 years of age)

   iii. In older children and young adults, the repair should be performed before pulmonary hypertension develops; otherwise, pathophysiologic changes may be irreversible

    iv. A median sternotomy or right thoracotomy approach is used with cardiopulmonary bypass. Defect is patched with pericardial or Dacron patch or is closed with a suture

     v. Transient heart block is the most common complication after closure of septum primum type of defect because of edema or injury to AV bundle. Temporary pacing may be required. Occasionally, heart block may be permanent

    iv. Alternatives to surgery are being explored (e.g., transcatheter closures) and are now being used for selected patients; efficacy remains unproven

   vii. Heart-lung transplantation is the only available option if disease has progressed to include irreversible pulmonary hypertension and pulmonary vascular disease

Ventricular Septal Defect

An abnormal opening between the ventricles occurring in the membranous or muscular portion of the ventricular septum. This is the most common defect seen in children and is frequently associated with other defects

1. Pathophysiology
    a. Common types of this defect (Fig. 2–28)
        i. Perimembranous defects
           (a) Occur in approximately 65% of patients with ventricular septal defect

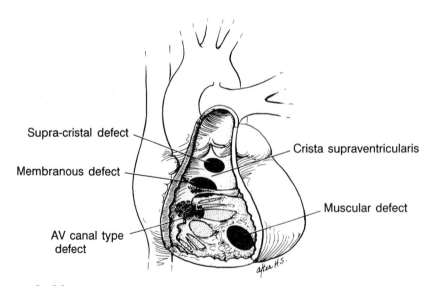

Figure 2–28 • The four common types of ventricular septal defects.

  (b) Located at base of septum under aortic valve
  (c) Aortic insufficiency can result if the valve cusp is poorly supported
ii. Muscular defects
  (a) Occur in 30%
  (b) Occasionally multiple defects
b. Small defects
  i. 75% close spontaneously before affected children are 10 years old (45% by 14 months)
  ii. Generally create no hemodynamic disturbance and no pulmonary hypertension in adults and have low risk of bacterial endocarditis
  iii. Small left-to-right shunt with high pressure gradient between left and right ventricles causes a high-velocity jet and a loud (usually grade IV/VI) murmur
c. Large defects
  i. Left-to-right shunting through the defect as a result of the higher left ventricular pressures
  ii. Increased right ventricular pressures and pulmonary blood flow occurs
  iii. Increased pulmonary blood flow results in increased pulmonary venous return to the left atrium. Left atrial pressures increase along with LVEDP. The left heart chambers are volume overloaded, leading to dilatation, failure, and pulmonary edema
  iv. If defect goes untreated, pulmonary vascular disease and resulting pulmonary hypertension occur as results of increased pulmonary resistance
  v. Over time, the pulmonary hypertension can become irreversible, often exceeding systemic pressures. The shunt then reverses, becoming right to left, with resulting cyanosis (Eisenmenger's syndrome)

2. Etiologic or precipitating factors
a. Precise cause of congenital defect is unknown
b. Factors contributing to congenital defects
  i. Genetic
  ii. Chromosomal (e.g., Down's syndrome)
  iii. Maternal and fetal infections during first trimester of pregnancy (e.g., rubella)
  iv. Effects of drugs and medications (e.g., cocaine use) during fetal development
  v. Dietary deficiencies during fetal development
  vi. Effects of maternal smoking and/or alcohol intake during pregnancy
  vii. High altitudes
c. Acute MI (adult onset): VSD is a serious, but infrequent complication of MI, usually leads to rapid heart failure, shock, and death

3. Nursing assessment data base: effects of large defects often become evident at very early ages (even in infancy). Symptoms are dependent on defect size and patient's age
a. Nursing history
  i. Subjective findings
    (a) Small defects: patients are usually asymptomatic

        (b) Large defects
- (1) Fatigue, exercise intolerance
- (2) Exertional dyspnea
- (3) Angina-like symptoms (caused by pulmonary hypertension)
- (4) Eisenmenger's syndrome

  ii. Objective findings
- (a) Frequently normal growth and development
- (b) In some cases, a history of slow weight gain, small size
- (c) Possible difficulty in feeding
- (d) History of endocarditis
- (e) History of frequent respiratory infections, often with bronchopneumonia
- (f) History of heart murmurs from birth
- (g) Family history of heart defects
- (h) Maternal exposure to infectious process or poor nutrition, drugs, and medications in first trimester

b. Nursing examination of patient: signs vary, depending on shunt direction and size. Right-to-left shunts produce signs and symptoms of severe heart failure and cyanosis

  i. Inspection
- (a) Restless, irritable
- (b) Frail-looking, thin, pale, waxen complexion
- (c) Tachypnea
- (d) Air hunger
- (e) Hemoptysis
- (f) Grunting respirations
- (g) Excessive sweating
- (h) Symptoms of heart failure
- (i) Cyanosis
- (j) Prominent sternum: "pigeon chest" (in older children, a result of large right ventricle while growing)

  ii. Palpation
- (a) Systolic thrill over lower left sternal border
- (b) PMI may be displaced laterally in larger defects
- (c) A lift may be felt over the left sternal border
- (d) Peripheral pulses: rapid, thready

  iii. Auscultation
- (a) Harsh, loud, high-pitched holosystolic murmur
  - (1) Loudest at left sternum, third to fifth intercostal space
  - (2) The louder the murmur, the smaller the defect
  - (3) Nonradiating murmur
- (b) Loud S_2, split but not fixed
- (c) Mitral rumble at apex (from increased flow through mitral valve)
- (d) Possible aortic insufficiency murmurs (membraneous defects) may be heard
- (e) Patient with Eisenmenger's syndrome may not have murmur (with equalization of right- and left-sided heart pressures)
- (f) Rales with failure

c. Diagnostic study findings
  i. Radiologic (large defects)

(a) Left atrium and left ventricle enlarged

(b) Right atrial and right ventricular enlargement in presence of pulmonary artery hypertension

(c) Increased pulmonary vascular markings

(d) Pulmonary artery dilated

ii. ECG

(a) Small defects produce normal ECG

(b) Large defects

(1) Left atrial enlargement and left ventricular hypertrophy

(2) Right ventricular hypertrophy

iii. Echocardiography

(a) Distinguishes shunt flow, increased pulmonary flow, aortic insufficiency, residual shunt flow postoperatively (intra-operative TEE); checks prosthetic patches (postoperatively), aneurysms (postclosure complication)

(b) Chamber enlargement

(c) Shunting can be demonstrated by echocardiographic contrast material and color-flow Doppler studies

iv. Cardiac catheterization: confirms and quantifies shunt; assesses hemodynamics; documents degree of pulmonary hypertension and associated disease (pulmonary stenosis, aortic insufficiency, CAD)

4. **Nursing diagnoses** (see Commonly Encountered Nursing Diagnoses section earlier)

a. Activity intolerance related to ventricular septal defect; see other key points

i. Asymptomatic patients who have no pathologic changes do not require surgery

ii. Patients require surgery when

(a) In severe heart failure: emergency surgery in first 3 months

(b) Ratio of pulmonary to systemic blood flow in the shunt is 1.5:1 or greater

(c) Failure to thrive is evidenced (at 6 months, the prospect of spontaneous closure has diminished considerably)

(d) Repeated, severe respiratory infections, recurrent endocarditis develop

iii. Median sternotomy approach with cardiopulmonary bypass is accepted surgical procedure; prosthetic patch will be placed

iv. Postoperative complications to observe for:

(a) Heart blocks caused by injury of AV node, bundle of His

(b) RBBB

(c) Pulmonary hypertensive crisis: caused by reactive pulmonary vasculature. Increased PVR may lead to right-sided heart failure

(d) Need for antibiotic prophylaxis to prevent infectious endocarditis (if small, residual ventricular septal defect)

v. Teach patients regarding importance of good dental hygiene

Patent Ductus Arteriosus

A persistent patency of the fetal circulation between the aorta and the pulmonary artery that failed to close after birth, seen in 2% of adults

1. **Pathophysiology**
   a. As aorta has higher pressures, blood flows through the patent ductus into the pulmonary artery in a *left-to-right* shunt, and oxygenated blood is recirculated to the lungs (Fig. 2–29)
   b. Resistance in the ductus to the shunting of blood is caused by not only the diameter of the defect but also its length
   c. Left ventricular workload increases, because it handles both the normal cardiac output and the shunt flow. Right-sided heart flow is not increased
      i. Increased blood return to the left atrium and left ventricle overloads the left side of the heart. The left ventricle compensates by enlarging, and symptoms of left-sided heart failure develop
      ii. Pulmonary hypertension may develop over time
   d. Large shunts result in equal pressure in systemic and pulmonary systems (Eisenmenger's syndrome with irreversible pulmonary hypertension)
   e. Increased pulmonary pressures then lead to increased work for the right ventricle (which enlarges and fails)
   f. If obstructive pulmonary vascular lesions develop, the pulmonary artery pressure will rise above the aortic pressure, and the shunt will reverse, becoming right to left. Cyanosis and right-sided heart failure result
   g. Deoxygenated blood is distributed to the left arm and lower parts of the body below the ductus (causing cyanosis and clubbing of toes), whereas the upper parts of the body receive oxygenated blood with no abnormalities
   h. All patients with patent ductus arteriosus are at risk for heart failure and infective endocarditis. Vegetations may embolize to the lungs, leading to infarctions and death
2. **Etiologic or precipitating factors**
   a. During fetal circulation: blood from the pulmonary artery flows through the ductus into the descending aorta in order to bypass the collapsed

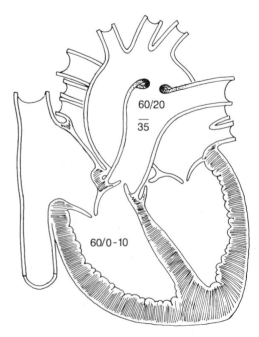

Figure 2-29 • The anatomic defect and associated cardiac catheterization data of a patent ductus arteriosus.

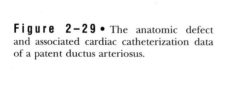

lungs. The ductus functionally closes within 24 to 48 hours after birth but may remain open up to 8 weeks

b. Ductus closure: contraction of smooth muscles in the wall of the ductus results from the increased arterial oxygen tension. If the smooth muscles do not contract, the ductus remains open (i.e., hypoxia at birth). Prostaglandin inhibitors can stimulate closure

c. If the ductus has not closed spontaneously by 3 months, it probably will not

d. Associated anomalies: atrial and ventricular septal defects

e. Very common among premature infants (weighing less than 1000 g) and infants with congenital rubella (acquired during the first trimester)

f. Common among infants with lung disease and infants born at high altitudes (chronic hypoxia)

g. Twice as common among females

3. **Nursing assessment data base:** shunt size and PVR determine hemodynamic effects. Asymptomatic in 50% of cases. Moderate-sized patent ductus arteriosus may not become symptomatic until left ventricular failure and pulmonary hypertension develop (many affected patients are 20 to 30 years of age)

   a. Nursing history: patient may be asymptomatic, and the following may be incidental findings

      i. Subjective findings

         (a) According to parent, child fatigues easily, is irritable, and feeds poorly

         (b) Dyspnea on exertion

         (c) Hoarseness (compression of laryngeal nerve)

         (d) Hemoptysis

         (e) Leg fatigue

         (f) Syncope

         (g) Angina-like pain

      ii. Objective findings

         (a) History of maternal rubella during first trimester

         (b) History of hypoxia at birth

         (c) Failure to thrive; growth and developmental problems

         (d) Inordinately high number of respiratory tract infections

         (e) Deafness, cataracts

         (f) Tachycardia

         (g) Tachypnea

   b. Nursing examination of patient

      i. Inspection

         (a) Signs and symptoms of heart failure

         (b) Cyanosis in lower parts of body and clubbing of toes (if right to left shunting)

         (c) Clubbing, mild cyanosis possible in left fingers (because of entry of unsaturated blood into left subclavian artery)

      ii. Palpation

         (a) Hyperdynamic precordium: left ventricular impulse (overload)

         (b) Bounding, brisk peripheral pulses (especially with large defects)

         (c) Prominent apical impulse

         (d) Systolic thrill in second left intercostal space

       iii. Auscultation
- (a) Loud, rough, continuous machinery-like murmur is indicative of PDA; heard in more than 50% of patients
  - (1) Is loudest high, at left upper sternal border (pulmonic area)
  - (2) Caused by pressure gradient between the aorta and the pulmonary artery
  - (3) Possible mitral flow rumble at apex
- (b) Wide pulse pressure

c. Diagnostic study findings
- i. Radiologic: chest x-ray
  - (a) Left atrial and left ventricular enlargement (in large left-to-right shunts)
  - (b) Increased pulmonary vascular markings, pulmonary edema in failure
  - (c) Enlarged aorta; prominent ascending aorta and aortic knob
  - (d) Central pulmonary artery enlarged
- ii. ECG (in order children, adults)
  - (a) Left atrial enlargement patterns
  - (b) Left ventricular hypertrophy
- iii. Echocardiography: detects the patent ductus arteriosus, reveals enlarged chambers, shows flow from aorta to pulmonary system in diastole. Color-flow Doppler study helps visualize small shunts and associated congenital defects
- iv. Cardiac catheterization: not usually necessary
  - (a) Establishes the aortopulmonary communication and the size and direction of the shunt
  - (b) Assesses pulmonary pressures, resistance, increases in pulmonary artery pressure, PVR (large shunts)
  - (c) Increased pressures will be evident in pulmonary artery with right-to-left shunts

4. **Nursing diagnoses** (see Commonly Encountered Nursing Diagnoses section earlier)
   a. Decreased cardiac output and tissue perfusion related to the pathophysiologic changes of the patent ductus arteriosus
   - i. Additional nursing interventions
     - (a) Postoperative nursing care involves same basic care as for thoracotomy
     - (b) Observe for postoperative complications: uncommon but include recurrent nerve injury, infections, bleeding, and possibility of a hemothorax, pneumothorax, or chylothorax
   b. Potential for infectious process (infective endocarditis) secondary to this congenital heart defect
   c. Other key points regarding management of therapeutic regimen:
   - i. Major risks: infectious endocarditis, left ventricular failure, and Eisenmenger's syndrome
   - ii. Medical management
     - (a) Pharmacologic closure of patent ductus arteriosus (with prostaglandin inhibitors such as indomethacin: effective only in infancy)
     - (b) Control of heart failure with medications

iii. Surgical management

    (a) Surgery is indicated when heart failure is uncontrolled, with failure to thrive or continued patency after 6 months. Surgery should be done before the child goes to school and when diagnosis is made

    (b) Surgery is performed through a small left thoracotomy incision. Once the ductus is reached, it is gently ligated with multiple sutures, or it is divided and closed at the ends with suture ligations

    (c) In adults, calcification and rigidity of ductus make closure much more difficult. A patch may be needed

    (d) Heart-lung transplantation may be indicated in cases of fixed pulmonary hypertension and right-to-left shunting

    (e) Transcatheter closures are being used as alternatives to surgery when feasible. Complications of these procedures are failure to close, emboli, vascular complications, and left pulmonary artery stenosis

Coarctation of the Aorta

A developmental deformity of the aorta, creating a narrowing or infolding of the lumen, which diminishes blood flow. Usually located just beyond the left subclavian artery or just distal to the ligamentum arteriosum. Constitutes 5% to 10% of all congenital heart disease (Fig. 2–30)

1. Pathophysiology

    a. In the fetus, smooth muscle of the ductus arteriosus extends into the aorta. After birth, the tissue contracts to close the duct, the aorta is pulled inward, and abnormal infolding or narrowing occurs

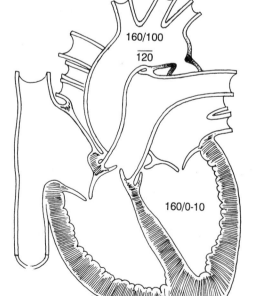

Figure 2–30 • The anatomic defect and associated cardiac catheterization data of a coarctation of the aorta.

  b. Thickening of the aortic medial tissue can form a ridge projecting into the lumen of the aorta, obstructing aortic flow
  c. Fetal development of the aortic arch may also be abnormal, along with formation of other cardiac defects (ventricular septal defect, mitral valve defects, bicuspid aortic valve)
  d. A pressure gradient develops: pressures proximal to the coarctation are increased and pressures distal are decreased
  e. Left ventricular pressures increase, as do pressures in all vessels of the aortic arch
  f. Progressively, the left ventricle dilates, hypertrophies, and can fail because of increased afterload
  g. Cerebral and upper extremity systemic hypertension results from the mechanical obstruction
  h. Collateral circulation develops and supports the lower body and extremities, compensating for decreased blood flow through normal routes. Collaterals involved include internal mammary, internal thoracic, scapular, epigastric, intercostal, lumbar, and thyrocervical arteries
  i. If the coarctation is left untreated, death is caused by consequences of the prolonged hypertension (e.g., strokes, CAD, heart failure, aortic rupture, or dissection). Other complications include bacterial endocarditis, cerebral hemorrhage

2. **Etiologic or precipitating factors:** see Pathophysiology section
3. **Nursing assessment data base:** early in the newborn period, the patient may have heart failure and require intervention. After infancy, many patients are asymptomatic until after 20 to 30 years old. Coarctation is often discovered on routine examinations as the result of hypertension or murmur (a common time is during school physical examinations for sports when affected patients are 6 to 10 years of age)
  a. Nursing history
     i. Subjective findings: patient may complain of headaches, visual disturbances, epistaxis, leg cramps or fatigue (with exercise), dizziness, dysphagia
     ii. Objective findings: unremarkable in the asymptomatic patient
        (a) Cyanosis in preductal coarctation, more noticeable in fingers than in toes
        (b) Critically ill infant may be irritable, may be a poor feeder, may have tachypnea
        (c) Oliguria
        (d) Metabolic acidosis
        (e) Hypotension
  b. Nursing examination of patient
     i. Inspection
        (a) A forceful thrust may be seen at the apex as a result of left ventricular hypertrophy
        (b) Infants may have symptoms of heart failure, lower extremity cyanosis
        (c) In rare cases, the upper body may be more developed (athletic) than the lower body, which may be underdeveloped (thin legs, narrow hips)
     ii. Palpation
        (a) Check simultaneous radial and femoral pulses. Forceful upper

extremity pulses (radial or brachial); typically weak and delayed or absent lower extremity pulses (femoral). Femoral pulses absent in approximately 40% of affected patients (no pulses or weak pulses are a result of narrow pulse pressure, not of low or absent flow)

  (b) Blood pressure in lower extremities is less than that in the upper extremities (opposite of normal). There is often a pressure pulse difference of more than 20 mm Hg. Systolic hypertension is seen in upper extremities

  (c) Blood pressure may vary in both arms, especially if the coarctation is proximal to the left subclavian artery

  (d) Apical thrust

  (e) Suprasternal notch thrill

  iii. Auscultation

    (a) Systolic ejection murmur or click heard best at right upper sternal border if bicuspid aortic valve is present

    (b) Loud S_2 (aortic component)

    (c) S_4 present with left hypertrophy

c. Diagnostic study findings

  i. Radiologic: chest x-ray may be first means of discovery

    (a) Enlarged left ventricle: hypertrophy; cardiomegaly or dilatation

    (b) Notching of ribs (inferior margins of posterior third through eighth ribs), caused by the collateral circulation of the intercostal arteries. Variable finding; usually appears after 6 years of age

    (c) The "3" sign: dilated ascending aorta followed by the constricted area, followed by the poststenotic dilatation

  ii. ECG: may be normal, left ventricular hypertrophy pattern

  iii. Echocardiography: can evaluate aortic and mitral valves, left ventricular hypertrophy: screen for other associated problems. Also useful postoperatively to evaluate surgical outcomes

  iv. MRI: also valuable, confirms diagnosis safely in pregnant patients

  v. Cardiac catheterization (see Fig. 2–30): used to evaluate coronary artery disease, measures the pressure gradients in the aorta. Aortogram shows the location, degree, and character of the aortic lumen narrowing

4. **Nursing diagnoses** (see Commonly Encountered Nursing Diagnoses section earlier)

a. Risk for infection (infective or bacterial endocarditis) secondary to this congenital heart defect

b. Other key points regarding decreased cardiac output and tissue perfusion related to the pathophysiologic changes of the coarctation:

  i. Blood pressure should be recorded in both arms

  ii. Assess simultaneous brachial and femoral pulses

  iii. If patient is asymptomatic, surgery is usually delayed until ages 1 to 5 years but should be performed as soon as possible to avoid hypertension

  iv. Coarctation may be relieved either by PTCA, with or without balloon-expandable stents, or by surgery

  v. The older the patient, the higher the risk of death from surgery

vi Surgical correction often decreases the hypertension and ameliorates the failure

vii. Common causes of death from coarctation in older patients are spontaneous aortic rupture, heart failure, bacterial endocarditis, and cerebral hemorrhage

viii. If surgery is undertaken the operative procedure is performed through a left thoracotomy incision

(a) The coarctation is excised, and either an end-to-end anastomosis, subclavian flap aortoplasty is performed or a tubular prosthetic graft is inserted

(b) Postoperative nursing care involves the basic care for thoracotomy patient

(c) Postoperative complications to watch for are hemothorax, chylothorax, paraplegia (0.5%), paradoxical or persistent hypertension, and, in rare cases, mesenteric vasculitis or bowel infarction; 20% of patients have transient postoperative abdominal pain and/or distention (probably because of the restoration of normal pulsatile blood flow and pressure)

(d) Paradoxical systolic hypertension may occur for the first 24 to 36 hours after surgery; then diastolic pressures may also increase (because of initial elevation in circulating catecholamines) and can cause an increase in renin and angiotensin levels. Paradoxical systolic hypertension is treated with sodium nitroprusside, beta blockers

(e) Other problems include aneurysms and restenosis (especially in neonates and other infants)

(f) Patients need lifelong follow-up monitoring for restenosis, hypertension, valvular disease

Hypertensive Crisis

A life-threatening elevation in blood pressure necessitating emergency reduction (within 1 hour) in order to prevent severe end-organ damage and potentially death if left untreated

1. **Pathophysiology**
   a. Essential hypertension is elevated blood pressure of unknown cause
   b. Secondary hypertension is elevated blood pressure whose cause is known (e.g., renal vascular disease, pheochromocytoma, coarctation of the aorta, pregnancy)
   c. Hypertension produces changes in arterioles (necrosis and inflammation) over time, eventually causing a decrease in blood flow to end organs and potentially permanent damage (Table 2–10)
   d. Accelerated and/or malignant hypertension: diastolic blood pressure higher than 120 mm Hg, associated with rapid vascular injury, retinal exudates and hemorrhages, and papilledema around the optic disc (with diastolic pressures higher than 140 mm Hg)
      i. Arterial dilatation and contraction are caused by large amounts of renin and angiotensin. The turbulent blood flow produced causes microangiopathic hemolytic anemia and intravascular coagulation
      ii. Arterial walls swell with fluid, causing fibrinoid necrosis

TABLE 2–10. The Sequelae of Hypertension: Its Effects on End-Organs That May Lead to Hypertensive Crisis

Hypertension

Enhanced sympathetic stimulation
Effect of renin–angiotension system (increased fluid retention, increased systemic
  vasoconstriction)
Necrosis of arterioles
Decreased blood flow to end-organs

Heart	Brain	Kidney
Tachycardia	Loss of autoregulatory mechanisms	↓ Renal perfusion
↑ Cardiac output	Arterial spasm and ischemia lead to TIAs	↓ Ability to concentrate urine
↓ Perfusion → angina → MI	Weakened vessels → aneurysms → hemorrhage → CVA	↑ BUN, creatinine
CAD		↑ Proteinuria
LV hypertrophy		Kidney failure
LV failure		Uremia
Angina		

TIA = transient ischemic attack; MI = myocardial infarction; BUN = blood urea nitrogen; CVA = cerebrovascular accident; CAD = coronary artery disease; LV = left ventricular; LV failure = left ventricular failure.

e. Hypertensive encephalopathy ensues: sudden, excessive elevation of blood pressure (higher than 250/150 mm Hg) → dysfunction of cerebral autoregulation → vasospasm → ischemia → increased capillary pressure and permeability → cerebral edema and hemorrhage

2. **Etiologic or precipitating factors**
   a. Untreated or uncontrolled essential or secondary hypertension
   b. Patient's poor compliance with antihypertensive medications
   c. Renal dysfunction (acute or chronic renal failure, renal tumors, acute glomerulonephritis, renovascular hypertension caused by acute renal artery occlusion)
   d. Eclampsia of pregnancy
   e. Adrenergic crisis: seen with sharp rise in catecholamine levels (pheochromocytoma, monoamine oxidase [MAO] inhibitor interactions, alpha-adrenergic agonist ingestion, abrupt withdrawal from antihypertensive therapy)
   f. Cardiac or vascular dysfunction: left ventricular heart failure, acute MI, unstable angina, dissecting aortic aneurysm, coarctation of aorta
   g. Cerebral dysfunction: intracerebral or subarachnoid hemorrhage, head injuries, intracranial masses, embolic brain infarction, hypertensive encephalopathy
   h. Postoperative complications: CABG surgery, renal transplantation, peripheral vascular surgery
   i. Pituitary tumors
   j. Adrenocortical hyperfunction
   k. Severe burns

3. **Nursing assessment data base**
   a. Nursing history

      i. Subjective findings

         (a) Patient may be unable to respond to questions; significant other may need to answer history inquiries

         (b) Severe headache

         (c) Epistaxis

     ii. Objective findings

         (a) History of hypertension

         (b) Positive family history for hypertension

         (c) High incidence of essential hypertension among black females

         (d) Medication history positive for MAO inhibitors, oral contraceptives, appetite suppressants, pressor agents, street drugs

         (e) History of any etiologic factor mentioned

         (f) History of coronary artery disease, renal dysfunction

         (g) Uncontrolled intake of sodium in diet

         (h) Risk factors: diabetes, obesity, smoking, hyperlipidemia, stress

  b. Nursing examination of patient

      i. Clinical picture in accelerated and/or malignant hypertension

         (a) Diastolic pressure exceeding 120 mm Hg

         (b) Retinopathy with exudates

         (c) Retinal hemorrhages

         (d) Papilledema of optic disease (in malignant hypertension, diastolic pressure exceeding 140 mm Hg)

         (e) Headache, confusion

         (f) Restlessness, stupor, somnolence

         (g) Epistaxis

         (h) Tachycardia

         (i) Chest discomfort

         (j) Nausea, vomiting

         (k) Rales

         (l) S_3, S_4

         (m) Bruits: carotid, abdominal aorta, femoral area, anteriorly over renal vasculature

         (n) Oliguria, azotemia

     ii. Clinical picture in hypertensive encephalopathy

         (a) Blood pressure exceeding 250/150 mm Hg

         (b) Retinopathy

         (c) Papilledema of optic disc

         (d) Severe headache

         (e) Vomiting

         (f) Decreased LOC

         (g) Transitory focal neurologic signs (e.g., nystagmus)

         (h) Seizures

         (i) Coma

         (j) Diuresis

  c. Diagnostic study findings

      i. Laboratory

         (a) ABG: metabolic acidosis

         (b) CBC: HCT decreased in renal failure; polycythemia seen in renal dysfunction

(c) Electrolytes: hypocalcemia, hyponatremia; aldosteronism causes hypokalemia (in about half of patients)

(d) Blood urea nitrogen and creatinine values elevated in patients with renal disease

(e) Glucose elevated in patients with Cushing's syndrome, pheochromocytoma, or diabetes

(f) Uric acid: hyperuricemia seen in renal failure

(g) Urinalysis: proteinuria indicates possible renal dysfunction; hematuria is seen with malignant nephrosclerosis

(h) Urinary vanillylmandelic acid catecholamines elevated in patients with pheochromocytoma

ii. Radiologic findings

(a) Chest x-ray: cardiomegaly may be seen

(b) Renal arteriography: can demonstrate renal artery stenosis, atherosclerotic lesions, dysplasias

(c) Intravenous pyelography: indicates presence of disease but is unable to differentiate causes

iii. ECG: left ventricular hypertrophy may be seen

iv. CT scan: shows diffuse brain edema with hypertensive crisis

v. Echocardiogram: diastolic function impaired

4. **Nursing diagnoses** (see Commonly Encountered Nursing Diagnoses section earlier): the goal of care is rapid, life-preserving treatment of elevated blood pressure

a. Altered tissue perfusion related to elevated blood pressure caused by accelerated or malignant hypertension

i. Assessment for defining characteristics: see Clinical picture section earlier for types of hypertension

ii. Expected outcomes: blood pressure within limits set for patient; may not be normal values initially. Goal is to lower diastolic to at least 110 mm Hg, MAP by at least 20%

iii. Additional nursing interventions

(a) Ensure that patient has adequate IV access

(b) Administer emergency antihypertensive drugs as ordered

(1) Vasodilators

a) Nitroprusside: 0.5 to 10 μg/kg/minute IV. Titrate every 5 minutes (0.2 μg/kg/minute), drug of choice for hypertensive encephalopathy, cerebral infarction or bleeding, dissecting aortic aneurysm; keep bag and lines protected from light; watch for cyanide toxicity (blurred vision, confusion, tinnitus, seizures)

b) Nitroglycerin: 50 to 100 μg/minute IV; drug of choice for unstable angina and ischemia, left ventricular failure, adrenergic crisis

c) Should provide immediate response

(2) Sympathetic blocking agents

a) Phentolamine (Regitine): 5 to 15 mg/minute IV (test dose: 0.5- to 1-mg bolus); used for pheochromocytoma, overdoses of alpha-adrenergic agents, abrupt withdrawals from hypertensive therapy

b) Labetalol: 20-mg IV bolus, then 20 to 80 mg every 10 minutes; both an alpha- and beta-adrenergic blocking agent, used especially for adrenergic crisis

          (3) ACE inhibitors
               a) Used in presence of left ventricular failure
               b) Captopril: 6.25 to 50 mg orally every 30 to 45 minutes
               c) Enalapril: 1.25 to 5 mg IV every 6 hours
               d) Onset of action for both: 10 to 15 minutes
          (4) Calcium channel blocker
               a) Nifedipine: 10 mg P.O. or sublingual (10 to 20 mg orally every 30 to 45 minutes or sublingually every 15 minutes)
          (5) Beta blockers
               a) Block effects of increased adrenergic tone
               b) Metoprolol: 5 mg IV every 5 minutes up to 15 mg total
               c) Esmolol: 500 µg/kg/minute for 4 minutes, then 50 to 300 µg/kg/minute IV

(c) Administer diuretics (furosemide, ethacrynic acid) as ordered. Watch for volume depletion

(d) Closely monitor patient's response to therapy by frequent assessments of blood pressure, hemodynamics. Titrate IV medications to patient's responses per parameters

(e) Patient should have continuous arterial monitoring while drugs are being titrated and condition is unstable

(f) Watch for side effects of medications

(g) If symptoms of tissue ischemia develop, reduce the speed with which blood pressure is lowered. *Note:* most of the problems that occur in hypertensive crisis occur when treatment is too aggressive for patient to tolerate

(h) Obtain accurate intake and output measurements, along with daily weights

(i) Monitor ECG, observe for arrhythmias: T-wave inversions occur with rapid blood pressure reductions; ischemia is rare

(j) Watch for signs of increased intracranial pressure (from cerebral edema, increased cerebral blood flow caused by medications): changes in mentation or vision; headaches; nausea; vomiting

(k) Intracranial pressure monitoring may be needed

(l) Sudden chest pain may indicate aortic dissection

(m) Reassure patient and family

(n) Create calm, quiet atmosphere, conducive to ample rest for patient

    iv. Evaluation of nursing care
       (a) Blood pressure is within set parameters
       (b) No side effects of medications evidenced
       (c) No signs of cerebral dysfunction or increased intracranial pressures
       (d) ECG in sinus rhythm

b. Potential for fluid volume deficit and hypotension related to diuretic and antihypertensive medications
    i. Assessment for defining characteristics
       (a) Blood pressure is below normal parameters for patient
       (b) Urine output is scant or absent
       (c) Symptoms of hypovolemic shock exist
       (d) Electrolytes are abnormal

  ii. Expected outcomes
   (a) Patient is adequately hydrated
   (b) Urinary output is adequate
   (c) Blood pressure is within set parameters for adequate cardiac output
  iii. Nursing interventions
   (a) Goal is for lowering blood pressure in small doses, to avoid causing hypotension, oliguria, and/or mental changes
   (b) Frequent blood pressure, hemodynamic assessments
   (c) Watch patient's response to drug therapy
   (d) Adjust antihypertensive intravenous medications promptly by titration, dependent on patient's response
   (e) Observe for abnormalities in laboratory test results, especially in electrolytes
  iv. Evaluation of nursing care
   (a) Blood pressure is within set parameters
   (b) Cardiac output is adequate as evidenced by hemodynamic assessments, urinary output, adequate circulation

Aortic and Peripheral Arterial Disease

Diseases of the aorta, cerebral arteries, and peripheral arteries with consequences that include aneurysm formation, dissection, or ischemia in their respective perfusion beds (Figs. 2–31 to 2–33)

1. **Pathophysiology**
 a. *Aortic aneurysm*
  i. The media of the aortic wall develops focal or diffuse weakness at sites of congenital or acquired disease
  ii. Atherosclerosis is the most common cause
  iii. Dilatation, increased pressures, and thinning of the wall all increase wall stress, further weakening and dilating the vessel and producing an aneurysm
  iv. Rupture and death are likely when the diameter exceeds 6 cm (for the thoracic aorta) or 5 cm (for the abdominal aorta)
  v. Complications include dissection, embolization of thrombus, and end-organ disease
  vi. Common sites for aneurysms
   (a) Abdominal aortic aneurysm involving the aorta between the renal and iliac arteries
   (b) Thoracic aortic aneurysm
    (1) Ascending, transverse, or descending aorta
    (2) Most common in men aged 60 to 70 years or older
    (3) Aneurysms of the iliac, femoral, and popliteal arteries
 b. *Aortic dissection*
  i. The intima and media of the thoracic aorta are weakened by atherosclerosis or congenital disease of the media
  ii. Hypertension is a factor in 80% of cases by either causing or contributing to the injury
  iii. A tear develops through the intima into the media and is propagated up and down the aorta by a dissecting column of blood

ANEURYSMS

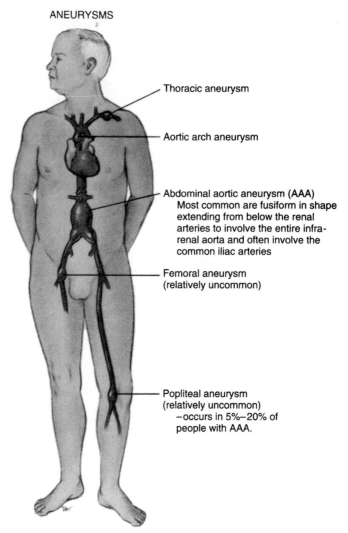

Thoracic aneurysm

Aortic arch aneurysm

Abdominal aortic aneurysm (AAA)
Most common are fusiform in shape
extending from below the renal
arteries to involve the entire infra-
renal aorta and often involve the
common iliac arteries

Femoral aneurysm
(relatively uncommon)

Popliteal aneurysm
(relatively uncommon)
−occurs in 5%−20% of
people with AAA.

Figure 2−31 • Peripheral artery disease: aneurysms. (From Jarvis, C.: Physical Examination and Health Assessment, 2nd ed. Philadelphia, W. B. Saunders, 1996, p. 597.)

    iv. A false channel to the true lumen is created
    v. Some organs may be perfused by the true lumen and some by the false lumen
    vi. Frequently, the dissection extends to the aortic valve, and aortic insufficiency and even bleeding into the pericardium can result
    vii. End-organ ischemia and injury can occur
    viii. Proximal dissections carry a high (80%) mortality rate, but the survival rate with surgical treatment is also high (80% to 85%)
    ix. Distal dissections (distal to the left subclavian artery) can be managed medically with nitroprusside (to lower blood pressure) and beta blockers, unless complications to end-organs or limbs mandate interventions
  c. *Peripheral and cerebral vascular disease*
    i. Atherosclerotic disease develops from the same risk factors and process as those for CAD

OCCLUSIONS

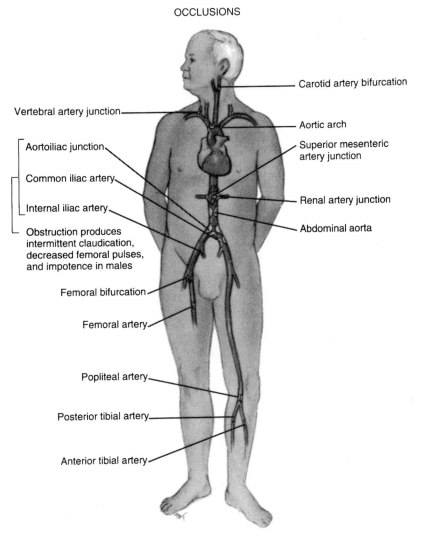

Figure 2–32 • Peripheral artery disease: occlusions. (From Jarvis, C.: Physical Examination and Health Assessment, 2nd ed. Philadelphia, W. B. Saunders, 1996, p. 597.)

     ii. Stenosis and hypoperfusion result, culminating in occlusion and infarction (unless supported by collateral circulation)

    iii. In general, occluded lesions occur at bifurcations

    iv. Common sites for occlusion include the following arteries: carotid, renal, popliteal, aortoiliac, and femoral

2. Etiologic or precipitating factors

    a. Atherosclerosis

    b. Congenital abnormalities (cystic medial necrosis, Marfan's syndrome)

    c. Trauma: blunt trauma can create tears in intima of the thoracic aorta, causing dissecting aneurysms

    d. Severe hypertension

    e. Arteritis

    f. Raynaud's disease

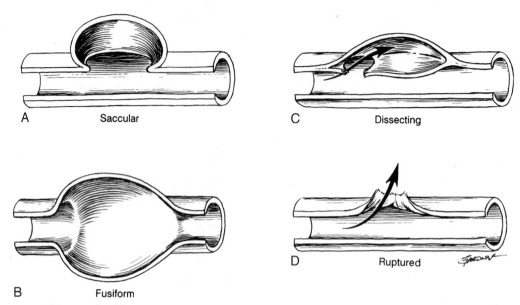

Figure 2–33 • Types of aortic aneurysms: *A,* Sacculated. *B,* Fusiform. *C,* Dissecting. *D,* Ruptured.

3. Nursing assessment data base

    a. Nursing history: manifestations usually do not occur until age 60 or older

        i. Subjective findings: vary with location of aneurysm or occlusion. Patient has complaints of

           (a) Aneurysms (most common)

              (1) Abdominal aortic aneurysm

                a) Pulsation in abdominal area

                b) Dull abdominal or low back pain or ache (impending rupture)

                c) Nausea and vomiting (pressure against the duodenum)

                d) Severe, sharp, sudden abdominal pain: continuous, radiates to back, hips, scrotum, pelvis (rupture)

                e) Syncope

              (2) Thoracic aortic aneurysm

                a) Sudden, tearing chest pain radiating to shoulders, neck, and back

                b) Cough, hoarseness, weak voice resulting from pressure against recurrent laryngeal nerve

                c) Dysphagia caused by pressure on the trachea

                d) Dyspnea resulting from pressure on trachea

              (3) Aortic dissections

                a) Marked by acute severe and instantaneous chest pain (in 90% of cases), radiating to the back, neck, jaw, or abdomen, associated with absence of central pulses and evidence of end-organ injury

                b) "Ripping," "tearing" sensations described

                c) The pain may be differentiated from that of acute MI by its instantaneous, severe onset and the absence of central pulses

                d) Neurologic symptoms are present in 15% of cases

       e) Syncope, presyncope, paralysis, numbness, aphasia

       f) Arm pain

       g) Dyspnea

  (b) Occlusive arterial disease

    (1) Intermittent claudication

       a) Cramping, aching pain; weakness

       b) Pain in the calf (most often) but may also be in foot; severe pain in toes, hips, buttocks, thighs

       c) Reproduced after walking a predictable distance

       d) Relieved with rest, standing still

       e) Hemoptysis

    (2) Nonhealing ulcers

    (3) Impotence

    (4) Severe pain in extremities, pallor, absence of pulses, paresthesias, paralysis (seen in acute thrombosis of abdominal aortic aneurysm)

    (5) Carotid arteries: transient ischemic attacks, monocular visual disturbances, sensory or motor deficits, expressive or receptive aphasia, stroke

    (6) 50% of patients with occlusive arterial disease involving the lower extremities are asymptomatic

  ii. Objective findings

  (a) History of atherosclerosis (CAD, CVA) and hypertension

  (b) Risk factors for atherosclerosis

  (c) Positive family history

  (d) Trauma: blunt, deceleration-type

  (e) History of impotence (seen in severe aortoiliac disease)

b. Nursing examination of patient: the manifestation depends on the organ perfused (e.g., cerebral vascular disease, renal vascular disease, ischemic or infarcted bowel, claudication, ischemic extremities)

  i. Aneurysms: often asymptomatic except for rupture, when patient is in obvious severe pain

  (a) Inspection

    (1) Hypertensive or hypotensive

    (2) Obvious discomfort with rupture or expansion

    (3) Stridor, hoarseness, dysphagia (pressure on esophagus, trachea, pharyngeal nerve)

  (b) Palpation: pulsating abdominal mass

  (c) Auscultation

    (1) Bruits: abdominal aorta; femoral, renal, popliteal arteries

    (2) Murmur of aortic insufficiency, if aneurysm involves aortic ring

  ii. Aortic dissection

  (a) Inspection

    (1) Hypertensive or hypotensive

    (2) Dyspnea

    (3) Stridor, hoarseness, dysphagia (pressure on esophagus, trachea, pharyngeal nerve)

  (b) Palpation

    (1) Wide pulse pressure

    (2) Absence of central pressures (50% of time)

(c) Auscultation: murmur of aortic insufficiency (heard 50% of time)

   iii. Arterial occlusions

     (a) Inspection

       (1) Ulcers, gangrene in extremities

       (2) Pale, mottled extremities on elevation: rubor on dependence of extremities

       (3) Asymmetry of extremities: check calf circumference

       (4) Skin changes due to impaired circulation

       (5) Retinal arterial emboli (carotid disease)

     (b) Palpation

       (1) Weak or absent peripheral pulses

       (2) Cool skin

       (3) Sluggish capillary refill

       (4) Pulsatile mass in popliteal fossa (popliteal aneurysm)

     (c) Auscultation: bruits

  c. Diagnostic study findings

    i. Laboratory

     (a) CBC: decreased HCT and Hb, increased leukocyte count

     (b) BUN and creatinine elevations, proteinuria, hematuria (compromised kidneys)

    ii. Radiologic findings

     (a) Chest x-ray: increased aortic diameter, right deviation of trachea, pleural effusions

     (b) Abdominal films (anteroposterior, lateral views): for abdominal aneurysm

    iii. Doppler ultrasound study

     (a) Amplifies sound generated by vascular blood flow. No sound is transmitted in totally occluded vessels

     (b) Assesses peripheral and cerebrovascular blood flow and velocity

    iv. Aortography: origin and extent of dissection may be seen

    v. CT: lumen diameter, wall thickness, aneurysm size, mural thrombi, and origin and extent of dissection, including blood supply to end organs

    vi. MRI: origin and extent of dissection, aneurysm size

    vii. TEE: assesses presence of dissection in aortic root, proximal ascending aorta, or descending thoracic aorta; aortic insufficiency; pericardial effusion

4. Nursing diagnoses (see Commonly Encountered Nursing Diagnoses section earlier)

  a. Alteration in tissue perfusion related to arterial occlusive disease, aneurysm, dissection, or perioperative complications

    i. Assessment for defining characteristics: see Nursing Assessment Data Base section preceding

    ii. Expected outcomes

     (a) Patient has no pain

     (b) Perfusion to affected extremities is adequate

     (c) No operative complications are experienced

     (d) Patient and significant other verbalize understanding of discharge home care, medications, follow-up, activities, diet, when to call for medical help, symptoms to report

iii. Additional nursing interventions
  (a) Relieve pain by administering ordered analgesics
  (b) Assess peripheral pulses and blood pressure, comparing both sides. Pressure differences exceeding 20 mm Hg in upper extremities indicate possibility of dissection or occluded subclavian, innominate, brachial, or axillary arteries. Pulses may be impossible to assess by palpating and also difficult or impossible with Doppler studies
  (c) Lower blood pressure, if elevated, by promptly administering ordered antihypertensives, beta blockers, nitroprusside
  (d) Monitor hemodynamic pressures, heart rate
  (e) Observe for symptoms of shock
  (f) Provide reassurance, explanations, comfort measures for patient and significant others who are anxious
  (g) A patient with acute arterial occlusion may be eligible for thrombolytic therapy. Intra-arterial thrombolytic therapy with urokinase improves revascularization results, lessens complications, and can decrease need for surgical intervention
  (h) Revascularization interventions are widely used before surgery in peripheral arterial disease
    (1) PTCA is used to open occluded arteries
    (2) Stents are also used to reduce restenosis in both native arteries and grafts
    (3) Atherectomy has been successful
  (i) Prepare patient for surgery: resection, replacement, and/or reconstruction of involved arteries
  (j) Check for a bruit over postoperative graft site
  (k) Monitor hemodynamics postoperatively; watch urinary output
  (l) Watch for signs of bleeding, especially if patient has received thrombolytic therapy
  (m) Teach patient and significant other about peripheral arterial occlusive disease, including
    (1) Smoking cessation: importance, sources of help
    (2) Reduce or control other cardiovascular risk factors: diabetes control, lowered cholesterol levels, controlled hypertension
    (3) Aspirin daily (to lower risk of CVA, MI)
    (4) Activity program: walking
    (5) Good foot care: washing daily, nails trimmed, well-fitting shoes, prompt professional attention to corns, calluses, ulcers
    (6) Weight reduction, if overweight
iv. Evaluation of nursing care
  (a) Palpable pulses felt in affected extremities
  (b) Limbs warm with good color, and brisk capillary refill
  (c) No signs of bleeding
  (d) Patient relaxed and free of pain

Shock

A state in which tissue perfusion to vital body organs is inadequate, frequently because of pathophysiologic alterations of cardiovascular and pulmonary function (see also Chapter 8, Multisystem)

1. **Pathophysiology**
   a. Diminished tissue perfusion deprives the cells of oxygen, nutrients, and, therefore, energy. Cellular dysfunction and potential cell necrosis ensue, because of the lack of oxygenation and resulting acidosis
   b. Cellular dysfunction is reversible at first but leads to organ damage if untreated
   c. Compensatory mechanisms: homeostatic response of the body to hypotension and shock is vasoconstriction to support the blood pressure. This response is appropriate for, and probably evolved from, the need to respond to hemorrhagic shock. It is completely inappropriate and detrimental in the management of cardiogenic shock
      i. Baroreceptor reflex: baroreceptors are activated in the aortic arch and heart. These receptors are volume sensitive, and a drop in mean arterial pressure or blood volume causes decreased stretching of the arterial baroreceptors (they lose their inhibitory effect on the vasomotor center). Sympathetic efferent activity is stimulated and causes secretion of norepinephrine at the vasoconstrictor nerve endings. Parasympathetic activity is decreased at the same time. Vasoconstrictors throughout the body and heart cause
         (a) Arteriolar constriction
         (b) Vasoconstriction
         (c) Increased heart rate
      ii. Transcapillary refill: decreased capillary hydrostatic pressures (from adrenergic vasoconstriction of the precapillary sphincters) cause fluid to be shifted from the interstitial spaces to the intravascular system, increasing blood return to the heart
   d. Decompensation: the body eventually is unable to maintain compensatory mechanisms and
      i. Loss of adrenergic vasoconstriction creates increased cellular permeability. Platelets and white blood cells clump together and obstruct the microvasculature
      ii. Major organs begin to malfunction as they are deprived of oxygen, as a result of hypoxemia and metabolic acidosis (respiratory failure, renal failure, decreased cerebral perfusion, and disseminated intravascular coagulation may also be seen)
2. **Etiologic or precipitating factors**
   a. *Cardiogenic shock:* impaired tissue perfusion as a result of cardiac dysfunction (most common cause of death from MI [10% to 15%])
      i. MI (usually 40% of left ventricle is damaged)
      ii. Myocardial ischemia (left main artery disease, multivessel CAD)
      iii. Cardiomyopathy
      iv. Arrhythmias
      v. Heart failure
      vi. Cardiac tamponade
      vii. Acute valvular dysfunction (acute mitral regurgitation, aortic insufficiency)
      viii. Papillary muscle rupture
      ix. Other severe forms of myocardial injury (trauma)
   b. *Hypovolemic shock:* impaired tissue perfusion resulting from severely diminished circulating blood volume

      i. Hemorrhage: loss of blood, plasma, body fluids as a result of
        (a) Surgery
        (b) Trauma
        (c) Burns
        (d) Severe dehydration (vomiting, diarrhea, diabetic ketoacidosis, diabetes insipidus)
      ii. Internal, extravascular fluid loss: resulting from third-spacing in interstitial space, ascites, ruptured spleen, pancreatitis, hemothorax
      iii. Adrenal insufficiency

  c. *Obstructive shock:* impaired tissue perfusion resulting from some obstruction to blood flow
      i. Pulmonary embolism (see Chapter 1)
      ii. Aortic dissection

  d. *Anaphylactic shock:* impaired tissue perfusion resulting from antigen-antibody reaction that releases histamine into blood stream. Capillary permeability increases, and arteriolar dilatation occurs. Blood return to the heart is decreased dramatically. May be caused by
      i. Contrast media
      ii. Drug reactions
      iii. Blood transfusion reactions
      iv. Food allergies
      v. Insect bites or stings
      vi. Snake bites

  e. *Septic shock* (systemic inflammatory response syndrome): impaired tissue perfusion caused by widespread infection and invasion of microorganisms in the body, causing vasodilatation (see Chapter 8)

  f. *Neurogenic shock:* impaired tissue perfusion caused by damage or dysfunction of the sympathetic nervous system. This type of shock is rare and may be associated with
      i. Trauma
      ii. Anesthesia
      iii. Spinal shock

3. Nursing assessment data base
  a. History and assessments must be done rapidly for immediate life-preserving therapy
  b. Nursing examination of patient: clinical picture of cardiogenic shock
      i. Inspection
        (a) Confused, restless, or obtunded
        (b) Shallow, rapid respiration (may see Cheyne-Stokes respiration)
        (c) Cyanotic
        (d) Neck veins distended (in right ventricular MI and in tamponade)
        (e) Hypotension: systolic blood pressure less than 90 mm Hg by cuff, less than 80 mm Hg by arterial line
        (f) Large differences in cuff pressures and central pressures
        (g) Narrow pulse pressure
        (h) Oliguria
      ii. Palpation
        (a) Cold, clammy extremities
        (b) Low temperature
        (c) Peripheral pulses: thready, rapid, or absent
      iii. Auscultation
        (a) Rales (pulmonary edema)

(b) S_1: soft

(c) S_2: may be paradoxically split

(d) S_3: gallop

(e) Systolic murmur (heard with acute mitral regurgitation, ventricular septal defect, aortic stenosis)

(f) Diastolic murmur of aortic insufficiency may be heard (short in acute aortic insufficiency)

(g) Heart sounds distant in tamponade

iv. Hemodynamics

(a) Elevated CVP with neck vein distention (in right ventricular MI, tamponade)

(b) Decreased cardiac output, CI

(c) Elevated PCWP (>18 mm Hg)

(d) Elevated SVR

c. Clinical picture of hypovolemic shock

i. Inspection

(a) Anxious, irritable

(b) Decreased level of consciousness

(c) Poor capillary refill

(d) Skin: pale, gray

(e) Increased heart rate

(f) Hypotension

(g) Neck veins collapsed

(h) Tachypnea

(i) Urinary output decreased or absent

ii. Hemodynamics

(a) Decreased CVP

(b) Decreased filling pressures

(c) Decreased pulmonary artery pressure, PCWP

(d) Increased PVR, SVR

(e) Decreased cardiac output, CI

d. Clinical picture of anaphylactic shock

i. Inspection

(a) Altered mental status

(b) Stridor, tachypnea, wheezing

(c) Headache

(d) Seizures

(e) Hives, itching

(f) Flushed, warm skin

(g) Nausea, vomiting, diarrhea

(h) Abdominal cramping

(i) Increased heart rate

(j) Hypotension

ii. Auscultation

(a) Upper airway stridor

(b) Wheezing, bronchoconstriction

iii. Hemodynamics

(a) Decreased CVP

(b) Decreased PCWP

(c) Decreased SVR

(d) Variable cardiac output

e. Clinical picture of neurogenic shock
- i. Inspection
  - (a) Mentation changes (restless, confused)
  - (b) Warm and dry skin
  - (c) Bradycardia
  - (d) No sweating (temperature-regulating center altered): risk for overheating, chilling
  - (e) Paralysis
  - (f) Apnea, tachypnea
  - (g) Profound hypotension
  - (h) Nausea, vomiting
  - (i) Decreased urinary output
- ii. Hemodynamics
  - (a) Decreased CVP, PCWP
  - (b) Decreased SVR
  - (c) Decreased cardiac output, CI
  - (d) Decreased pulse oximetry saturations

f. Diagnostic study findings: in hypovolemic and cardiogenic shock
- i. Laboratory
  - (a) ABG
    - (1) Cardiogenic shock: metabolic acidosis on ABG (hypocapnia, hypoxemia)
    - (2) Hypovolemic shock: respiratory alkalosis, metabolic acidosis
  - (b) HCT: decreased with hemorrhage
  - (c) Leukocytosis
  - (d) Abnormal electrolytes: check potassium, sodium, chloride, magnesium
  - (e) CK isoenzymes: elevated in acute MI
- ii. Radiologic findings: chest x-ray assesses for
  - (a) Cardiomegaly
  - (b) Pulmonary congestion
  - (c) Dilated aortic arch (see Aortic Dissection section)
  - (d) Pleural effusion
- iii. ECG
  - (a) Ischemia, infarction
    - (1) Right ventricular infarction: do ECG with right ventricular leads (lead V_4R)
    - (2) Anterior MI commonly associated with cardiogenic shock
    - (3) Prior MI
  - (b) Arrhythmias, conduction defects
  - (c) New right axis deviation: pulmonary embolism
- iv. Echocardiography: check for cause of shock
  - (a) Left and right ventricular dysfunction (wall motion, chamber sizes)
  - (b) Tamponade, pericardial effusions
  - (c) Valve integrity
  - (d) Septal defects
- v. TEE: look for aortic dissection, septal defects, congenital heart defects
- vi. Cardiac catheterization: assesses
  - (a) Hemodynamics

            (b) CAD severity

            (c) Left ventricular function

            (d) Valvular function

            (e) Shunts

            (f) Aortography: dissection, aortic regurgitation

4. Nursing diagnoses (see Commonly Encountered Nursing Diagnoses section earlier)

    a. Decreased cardiac output resulting from impaired contractility in cardiogenic shock

        i. Assessment for defining characteristics

            (a) Hypotension

            (b) See symptoms for associated shock types in the Nursing assessment database section

        ii. Additional nursing interventions (cardiogenic shock)

            (a) Early reperfusion in acute MI is vital: patient will need to be prepared for angiogram and potential interventions such as primary PTCA, thrombolytics, CABG

            (b) Give patient oxygen to maintain oxygen saturation at 92% or greater or per set parameters

            (c) Monitor ABGs, report abnormalities, and correct acidotic states: ensure adequate ventilation and give sodium bicarbonate, as ordered

            (d) Administer drugs as ordered to increase arterial pressure and contractility without increasing myocardial oxygen demands

            (e) IABP may be needed and should be ready to use while patient is being stabilized

            (f) Prepare patient for possible CABG or other cardiac surgery

    b. Fluid deficit related to decreased circulating blood volume (hypovolemic shock): causes include third-spacing (after arrest, sepsis, hemorrhage); excessive diuretics; profuse diaphoresis; extended use of pressor agents

        i. Assessment for defining characteristics

            (a) Decreased urinary output

            (b) Decreased blood pressure

            (c) Decreased venous return

        ii. Expected outcomes

            (a) Maintenance of fluid and electrolyte balances

            (b) Balanced intake and output

            (c) Vital signs: blood pressure and pulse within normal limits for patient

        iii. Additional nursing interventions

            (a) Administer emergency infusions of replacement volume, blood products (whole and packed red blood cells, fresh frozen plasma, platelets), crystalloids, colloids

            (b) Ensure that patient has two patent, large-bore IV lines available: 16-g preferable

            (c) Collaborate with physician in locating source of fluid loss

            (d) Record vital signs at least every hour, more often as warranted

            (e) Monitor heart rate, blood pressure, MAP, CVP, PCWP to evaluate patient response to bleeding and/or fluid losses

            (f) Watch for changes in level of consciousness

            (g) Maintain a strict hourly documentation of all intake and output

            (h) Observe skin condition: color, turgor, temperature

(i) Analyze laboratory results: blood urea nitrogen, HCT, electrolytes; notify physician of abnormal findings

(j) Observe for and identify symptoms associated with volume overload, especially if patient has received large amounts of replacement fluids

(k) Prepare patient for immediate surgery, if necessary

iv. Evaluation of nursing care

(a) Maintenance of fluid volume and electrolyte balance

(b) Vital sign and hemodynamic parameters within normal limits

References

PHYSIOLOGIC ANATOMY

Anderson, R. H., and Becker, A. E.: The Heart: Structure in Health and Disease. New York, Gower Medical Publishing, 1992.

Chatterjee, K., Karliner, J., Rapaport, E., et al. (eds.): Cardiology: An Illustrated Text/Reference. Philadelphia, J. B. Lippincott, 1991.

Cheitlin, M. D., Sokolow, M., and McIlroy, M. B.: Clinical Cardiology, 6th ed. Norwalk, Conn., Appleton & Lange, 1993.

Darovic, G. O.: Hemodynamic Monitoring: Invasive and Noninvasive Clinical Application, 2nd ed. Philadelphia, W. B. Saunders, 1995.

Dracup, K.: Meltzer's Intensive Coronary Care: A Manual for Nurses, 5th ed. Norwalk, Conn., Appleton & Lange, 1995.

Finkelmeier, B. A.: Cardiothoracic Surgical Nursing. Philadelphia, J. B. Lippincott, 1995.

Gedgaudas, E., Moller, J. H., Castaneda-Zunga, W. R., et al.: Cardiovascular Radiology. Philadelphia, W. B. Saunders, 1985.

Giuliani, E. R., Gersh, B. J., and McGoon, M. D. (eds.): Mayo Clinic Practice of Cardiology, 3rd ed. St. Louis, Mosby–Year Book, 1996.

Hudak, C. M., and Gallo, B. M. (eds.): Critical Care Nursing: A Holistic Approach, 6th ed. Philadelphia, J. B. Lippincott, 1994.

Kinney, M. R., and Packa, D. R. (eds.): Andreoli's Comprehensive Cardiac Care, 8th ed. St. Louis, Mosby–Year Book, 1996.

Nettina, S. M. (ed.): The Lippincott Manual of Nursing Practice, 6th ed. Philadelphia, J. B. Lippincott, 1996.

Schlant, R. C., and Alexander, R. W. (eds.): Hurst's The Heart, 8th ed. New York, McGraw-Hill, 1994.

Seidel, H. M., et al.: Mosby's Guide to Physical Examination, 3rd ed. St. Louis, Mosby–Year Book, 1995.

NURSING ASSESSMENT DATA BASE

Bates, B., Bickley, L. S., and Hoeklman, R. A.: A Guide to Physical Examination and History-Taking, 6th ed. Philadelphia, J. B. Lippincott, 1995.

Bishop, M. L., Duben-Engelkirk, J. L., and Fody, E. P.: Clinical Chemistry: Principles, Procedures, Correlations, 3rd ed. Philadelphia, J. B. Lippincott, 1996.

Braunwald, E. (ed.): Heart Disease. A Textbook of Cardiovascular Medicine. Philadelphia, W. B. Saunders, 1997.

Cheitlin, M. D., Sokolow, M., and McIlroy, M. B.: Clinical Cardiology, 6th ed. Norwalk, Conn., Appleton & Lange, 1993.

Dracup, K.: Meltzer's Intensive Coronary Care: A Manual for Nurses, 5th ed. Norwalk, Conn., Appleton & Lange, 1995.

Flavell, C. M.: Women and coronary heart disease. Prog. Cardiovasc. Nurs. 9(4):18–27, 1994.

Harvey, W. P.: Cardiac pearls. Dis. Mon. 40(2):41–113, 1994.

Jarvis, C.: Physical Examination and Health Assessment, 2nd ed. Philadelphia, W. B. Saunders, 1996, pp. 514–598.

Schlant, R. C., and Alexander, R. W. (eds.): Hurst's The Heart, 8th ed. New York, McGraw-Hill, 1994.

Seidel, H. M., Ball, J. W., Dains, J. E., and Benedict, G. W.: Mosby's Guide to Physical Examination, 3rd ed. St. Louis, Mosby–Year Book, 1995.

Swash, M.: Hutchinson's Clinical Methods, 20th ed. Philadelphia, W. B. Saunders, 1995.

Willerson, J. T., and Cohn, J. N.: Cardiovascular Medicine. New York, Churchill Livingstone, 1995.

COMMONLY ENCOUNTERED NURSING DIAGNOSES

Caine, R. M., and Bufalino, P. M. (eds.): Critically Ill Adults: Nursing Care Planning Guides. Baltimore, Williams & Wilkins, 1988.

Carpenito, L. J. (ed.): Nursing Diagnosis: Application to Clinical Practice, 6th ed. Philadelphia, J. B. Lippincott, 1995.

Dressler, D. K., and Gettrust, K. V.: Cardiovascular Critical Care Nursing: Plans of Care for Specialty Practice. Albany, N. Y., Delmare Publishing, 1994.

Kim, M. J., McFarland, G. K., and McLane, A. M.: Pocket Guide to Nursing Diagnoses, 6th ed. St. Louis, Mosby–Year Book, 1995.

Kuhn, R. C: American Association of Critical Care Nurses. In Carroll-Johnson, R. M. (ed.): Classification of Nursing Diagnoses: Proceedings of the Ninth Conference. Philadelphia, J. B. Lippincott, 1995, pp. 209–213.

Hudak, C. M., and Gallo, B. M. (eds.): Critical Care Nursing: A Holistic Approach, 6th ed. Philadelphia, J. B. Lippincott, 1994.

Iyer, P. W., Taptich, B. J., and Bernocchi-Losey, D.: Nursing Process and Nursing Diagnosis, 3rd ed. Philadelphia, W. B. Saunders, 1990.

Sparks, S. M., and Taylor, C. M.: Nursing Diagnosis Reference Manual, 2nd ed. Springhouse, Pa., Springhouse Corp., 1993.

CORONARY ARTERY DISEASE

Cheitlin, M. D., Sokolow, M., and McIlroy, M. B.: Clinical Cardiology, 6th ed. Norwalk, Conn., Appleton & Lange, 1993, pp. 359–405.

Forrester, J. S., Merz, C. N., Superko, R. L., et al.: 27th Bethesda Conference: Matching the intensity of risk factor management with the hazard for coronary disease events. Task Force 4. Efficacy of risk factor management. J. Am. Coll. Cardiol. 27(5):991–1006, 1996.

Furberg, C. D., Hennekens, C. H., Hulley, S. B., et al.: 27th Bethesda Conference: Matching the intensity of risk factor management with the hazard for coronary disease events. Task Force 2. Clinical epidemiology: The conceptual basis for interpreting risk factors. J. Am. Coll. Cardiol. 27(5):976–978, 1996.

Fuster, V., and Chesebro, J. H.: Atherosclerosis, A. Pathogenesis: Initiation, progression, acute coronary syndromes, and regression. In Giuliani, E. R., Gersh, B. J., and McGoon, M.D. (eds.): Mayo Clinic Practice of Cardiology, 3rd ed. St. Louis, Mosby-Year Book, 1996, pp. 1056–1088.

Fuster, V., Fay, W. P., and Chesebro, J. H.: Atherosclerosis, B. Antithrombotic agents in cardiac disease: Platelet inhibitors, anticoagulants, and thrombolytic agents. In Giuliani, E. R., Gersh, B. J., and McGoon, M.D. (eds.): Mayo Clinic Practice of Cardiology, 3rd ed. St. Louis, Mosby-Year Book, 1996, pp. 1089–1132.

Fuster, V., Gotto, A. M., Libby, P., et al.: 27th Bethesda Conference: Matching the intensity of risk factor management with the hazard for coronary disease events. Task Force 1. Pathogenesis of coronary disease: The biologic role of risk factors. J. Am. Coll. Cardiol. 27(5):964–976, 1996.

Kannel, N. M.: Coronary risk factors. In Willerson, J. T., and Cohn, J. N. (eds.): Cardiovascular Medicine. New York, Churchill Livingstone, 1995, pp. 1809–1828.

Pasternak, R. C., Grundy, S. M., Levy, D., and Thompson, P. D.: 27th Bethesda Conference: Matching the intensity of risk factor management with the hazard for coronary disease events. Task Force 3. Spectrum of risk factors for coronary heart disease. J. Am. Coll. Cardiol. 27(5):978–990, 1996.

Ridker, P. M., Manson, J. E., Gaziano, J. M., and Hennekens, C. H.: Primary prevention of ischemic heart disease. In Smith, T. W. (ed.): Cardiovascular Therapeutics: A Companion to Braunwald's Heart Disease. Philadelphia, W. B. Saunders, 1996, pp. 1–21.

Smith, S. C., Blair, S. N., Criqui, M. H., et al.: Preventing heart attack and death in patients with coronary disease. Circulation 92:2–4, 1995.

Taylor, A. L., and Mueller, S. D.: Coronary artery disease in women. In Willerson, J. T., and Cohn, J. N. (eds.): Cardiovascular Medicine. New York, Churchill Livingstone, 1995, pp. 1715–1726.

Willerson, J. T., Cohen, L. S., and Maseri, A.: Pathophysiology and clinical recognition. In Willerson, J. T., and Cohn, J. N. (eds.): Cardiovascular Medicine. New York, Churchill Livingstone, 1995, pp. 333–365.

ANGINA PECTORIS

Ashmed, O.: Angina. In Rakel, R. E. (ed.): Saunders Manual of Medical Practice. Philadelphia, W. B. Saunders, 1996, pp. 227–228.

Barbiere, C. C.: A new device for control of bleeding after transfemoral catheterization. Crit. Care Nurse 15(1):51–54, 1995.

Boggs, R. L., and Wooldridge-King, M. (eds.): AACN Procedure Manual for Critical Care, 3rd ed. Philadelphia, W. B. Saunders, 1993.

Brezina, K., Murphy, M., and Stonner, T.: Care of the patient receiving ReoPro following angioplasty. J. Invas. Cardiol. 6(Suppl. A):38A–42A, 1995.

Caine, R. M., and Bufalino, P. M. (eds.): Critically Ill Adults: Nursing Care Planning Guides. Baltimore, Williams & Wilkins, 1988, pp. 51–54.

Califf, R. M., and the EPIC Investigators: Use of a monoclonal antibody directed against the platelet glycoprotein IIb/IIIa receptor in high-risk coronary angioplasty. N. Engl. J. Med. 330:956–961, 1994.

Coombs, V. J., and Brinker, J. A.: Primary angioplasty in the acute myocardial infarction setting. AACN Clin. Issues 6(3):387–397, 1995.

Darovic, G. O.: Hemodynamic Monitoring: Invasive and Noninvasive Clinical Application. 2nd ed. Philadelphia, W. B. Saunders, 1995.

Deelstra, M. H.: Coronary rotational ablation: An overview with related nursing interventions. Am. J. Crit. Care 2(1):16–23, 1993.

Fischman, D. L., Leon, M. B., Baim, D. S., et al.: A randomized comparison of coronary stent placement and balloon angioplasty in the treatment of coronary artery disease. N. Engl. J. Med. 331:496–501, 1994.

Frishman, W. H. (ed.): Current Cardiovascular Drugs, 2nd ed. Philadelphia, Current Medicine, New York, Churchill Livingstone, 1995.

Gardner, E., Joyce, S., Iyer, M., et al.: Intracoronary stent update: Focus on patient education. Crit. Care Nurse 16(2):65–75, 1996.

Goldstein, S.: Beta-blockers in hypertensive and coronary heart disease. Arch. Intern. Med. 156:1267–1276, 1996.

Gregory, S., and Fowler, S.: Removing femoral sheaths. A new nursing skill. Am. J. Nurs. Suppl. 96(5):12–14, 1996.

Hudgins, C., and Sorenson, G.: Directional coronary atherectomy: A new treatment for coronary artery disease. Crit. Care Nurse 14(1):61–65, 1994.

Jurran, N. B., Smith, D. D., Rouse, C. L., et al.: Survey of current practice patterns for percutaneous transluminal coronary angioplasty. Am. J. Crit. Care 5(6):442–448, 1996.

Karfonta, T., and Mielcarek, F.: Pseudoaneurysm of the femoral artery following cardiac intervention: Identification and management. Prog. Cardiovasc. Nurs. 9(4):13–17, 1994.

Kellen, J. C., Ettinger, A., Todd, L., et al.: The cardiac arrhythmia suppression trial: Implications for nursing practice. Am. J. Crit. Care 5(1):19–25, 1996.

Khan, M. G.: Cardiac Drug Therapy, 4th ed. Philadelphia, W. B. Saunders, 1995.

LeWinter, M. M., and Sobel, B. E.: Chronic angina: Stable. In Smith, T. W. (ed.): Cardiovascular Therapeutics: A Companion to Braunwald's Heart Disease. Philadelphia, W. B. Saunders, 1996, pp. 85–111.

Logan, P.: What you need to know about interventional cardiology. Nursing 25(9):32II–32JJ, 32LL, 32NN, 1995.

Madsen, K.: Converting cardiac surgery patient from dopamine to dobutamine. Crit. Care Nurse 14(1):103–108, 1994.

Noureddine, S. N.: Research review: Use of activated clotting time to monitor heparin therapy in coronary patients. Am. J. Crit. Care 4(4):272–277, 1995.

Opie, L. H.: Pharmacologic options for treatment of ischemic disease. In Smith, T. W. (ed.): Cardiovascular Therapeutics: A comparison to Braunwald's Heart Disease. Philadelphia, W. B. Saunders, 1996, pp. 22–56.

Penney, C. L.: Learning how to remove femoral sheaths. Nursing 25(5):32QQ–32SS, 1995.

Perra, B. M.: Managing coronary atherectomy patients in a special procedure unit. Crit. Care Nurse 15(3):57–59, 63–68, 1995.

Pesola, D. A., Pesola, H. R., and Pesola, G. R.: Advantages for the use of the activated clotting time (ACT). Am. J. Crit. Care 4(5):414–415, 1995.

Smith, S. M.: Current management of acute myocardial infarction. Dis. Mon. 41(6):363–433, 1995.

Théroux, P.: Management of unstable angina. In Smith, T. W. (ed.): Cardiovascular Therapeutics: A Companion to Braunwald's Heart Disease. Philadelphia, W. B. Saunders, 1996, pp. 112–122.

Turner, D. M., and Turner, L. A.: Right ventricular infarction: Detection, treatment, and nursing implications. Crit. Care Nurse 15(1):22–28, 1995.

Waksman, R., King, S. B., Douglas, J. S., et al.: Predictors of groin complications after balloon and new-device coronary intervention. Am. J. Cardiol. 75:886–889, 1995.

Warth, D. C., Leon, M. B., O'Neill, W., et al.: Rotational atherectomy multicenter registry: Acute results, complications and 6-month angiographic follow-up in 709 patients. J. Am. Coll. Cardiol. 24:641–648, 1994.

Wong, S. C., and Leon, M. B.: Intracoronary stents. Curr. Opin. Cardiol. 10(4):404–411, 1995.

MYOCARDIAL INFARCTION

Birnbaum, Y., and Kloner, R. A.: Clinical aspects of myocardial stunning. Coron. Artery Dis. 6(8):606–612, 1995.

Blaufarb, I. S., and Sonnenblick, E. H.: The renin-angiotensin system in left ventricular remodeling. Am. J. Cardiol. 77(13):8C–16C, 1996.

Bowlby, H., Hisle, K., and Clifton, G. D.: Heparin as adjunctive therapy to coronary thrombolysis in acute myocardial infarction. Heart Lung 24(4):292–304, 1995.

Califf, R. M.: Acute myocardial infarction. In Smith, T. W. (ed.): Cardiovascular Therapeutics: A Companion to Braunwald's Heart Disease. Philadelphia, W. B. Saunders, 1996, pp. 127–170.

Chesebro, J. H., Knatterud, G., Roberts, R., et al.: Thrombolysis in Myocardial Infarction (TIMI) trial, phase I: A comparison between intravenous tissue plasminogen activator and intravenous streptokinase. Circulation 76:142–154, 1987.

Clem, J. R.: Pharmacology of ischemic heart disease. AACN Clin. Issues 6(3):404–417, 1995.

Effat, M. A.: Pathophysiology of ischemic heart disease: An overview. AACN Clin. Issues 6(3):369–374, 1995.

Ferrari, R., and Visioli, O.: Particular outcomes of myocardial ischaemia: Stunning and hibernation. Pharmacol. Res. 31(3–4):235–241, 1995.

Frishman, W. H. (ed.): Current Cardiovascular Drugs, 2nd ed. Philadelphia, Current Medicine, New York, Churchill Livingstone, 1995.

Gahart, B. L., and Nazareno, A. R.: Intravenous Medications: A Handbook for Nurses and Allied Health Professionals, 13th ed. St. Louis, Mosby-Year Book, 1996.

Gaw-Ens, B.: Informational support for families immediately after CABG surgery. Crit. Care Nurse 14(1):41–50, 1994.

Glogar, D., Yang, P., and Sturer, G.: Management of acute myocardial infarction: Evaluating the past, practicing in the present, elaborating the future. Am. Heart J. 132:465–470, 1996.

Grines, C. L., Brodie, B. R., Ivanhoe, R., et al.: Six-month clinical and angiographic follow-up after direct angioplasty for acute myocardial infarction. Final results from the Primary Angioplasty Registry. Circulation 90(1):156–162, 1994.

Gross, S. B.: Early extubation: Preliminary experience in the cardiothoracic patient population. Am. J. Crit. Care 4(4):262–266, 1995.

GUSTO Angiographic Investigators: The effects of tissue plasminogen activator, streptokinase, or both on coronary-artery patency, ventricular function, and survival after acute myocardial infarction. N. Engl. J. Med. 329:1615–1622, 1993.

Hochman, J. S., Boland, J., Sleeper, L. A., et al.: Current spectrum of cardiogenic shock and effect of early revascularization on mortality: Results of an International Study. Circulation 91:873–881, 1995.

Holmes, D. R., Bates, E. R., Kleinman, N. S., et al.: Contemporary reperfusion therapy for cardiogentic shock: The GUSTO-I trial experience. J. Am. Coll. Cardiol. 26(3):668–674, 1995.

ISIS-2 (Second International Study Group of Infarct Survival) Collaborative Group: Randomized trial of intravenous streptokinase, oral aspirin, both, or neither among 17,187 cases of suspected myocardial infarction. Lancet 2(8607):349–360, 1988.

Julian, D. G., and Braunwald, E. (eds.): Management of Acute Myocardial Infarction. Philadelphia, W. B. Saunders, 1994.

Kayser, S. R., and Trujillo, T.: The role of magnesium in cardiovascular disease. Prog. Cardiovasc. Nurs. 9(4):37–40, 1994.

Kellen, J. C., Ettinger, A., Todd, L., et al.: The cardiac arrhythmia suppression trial: Implications for nursing practice. Am. J. Crit. Care, 5(1):19–25, 1996.

Mendelson, M. A., and Hendel, R. C.: Myocardial infarction in women. Cardiology 86(4):272–285, 1995.

O'Neill, W. W., Brodie, B. R., Ivanhoe, R., et al.: Primary coronary angioplasty for acute myocardial infarction (the Primary Angioplasty Registry). Am. J. Cardiol. 73:627–634, 1994.

Oz, M. C., Rose, E. A., and Levin, H. R.: Selection criteria for placement of left ventricular assist devices. Am. Heart J. 129(1):173–177, 1995.

Pfeffer, M. A.: LV remodeling after acute myocardial infarction. Annu. Rev. Med. 46:455–466, 1995.

Reeder, G. S.: Acute myocardial infarction: Enhancing the results of reperfusion therapy. Mayo Clin. Proc. 70(12):1185–1190, 1995.

Riegel, G., Thomason, T., Carlson, B., and Gocka, I.: Are nurses still practicing coronary precautions? A national survey of nursing care of acute myocardial infarction patients. Am. J. Crit. Care 5(2):91–98, 1996.

Ryan, T. J., Anderson, J. L., Antman, E. M., et al.: ACC/AHA guidelines for the management of patients with acute myocardial infarction. J. Am. Coll. Cardiol. 28(5):1328–1428, 1996.

Seelig, M. S., and Elin, R. J.: Is there a place for magnesium in the treatment of a myocardial infarction? Am. Heart J. 132:471–477, 1996.

Sirois, J. G.: Acute myocardial infarction. Emerg. Med. Clin. North Am. 13(4):759–765, 1995.

Tootill, D. M.: Thrombolytic therapy: Nursing strategies for successful patient outcomes. Prog. Cardiovasc. Nurs. 10(1):3–12, 1995.

Topol, E. J., George, B. S., Kereiakes, D. J., et al.: Insights derived from the Thrombolysis and Angioplasty in Myocardial Infarction (TAMI) trials. J. Am. Coll. Cardiol. 12(6, Suppl. A):24A–31A, 1988.

Topol, E. J., and Nissen, S. E.: Our preoccupation with coronary luminology: The dissociation between clinical and angiographic findings in ischemic heart disease. Circulation 92(8):2333–2341, 1995.

Turner, D. M., and Turner, L. A.: Right ventricular myocardial infarction: Detection, treatment, and nursing implications. Crit. Care Nurs 15(1):22–27, 1995.

Young, G. P., and Hoffman, J. R.: Thrombolytic therapy. Emerg. Med. Clin. North Am. 13(4):735–758, 1995.

HEART FAILURE

Beattie, S., and Pike, C.: Left ventricular diastolic dysfunction. Crit. Care Nurs 16(2):37–50, 1996.

Cash, L. A.: Heart failure from diastolic dysfunction. Dimen. Crit. Care Nurs. 15(4):170–177, 1996.

Cheitlin, M. D., Sokolow, M., and McIlroy, M. B.: Clinical Cardiology, 6th ed. Norwalk, Conn., Appleton & Lange, 1993, pp. 320–357.

Cohn, J. N.: Heart failure. In Willerson, J. T., and Cohn, J. N. (eds.): Cardiovascular Medicine. New York, Churchill Livingstone, 1995, pp. 947–978.

Dahlen, R., and Roberts, S. L.: Acute congestive heart failure: Preventing complications. Dimen. Crit. Care Nurs. 15(5):226–241, 1996.

Dracup, K.: Heart failure secondary to left ventricular systolic dysfunction. Nurse Pract. 21(9):56–68, 1996.

Dunbar, S. B., and Dracup, K.: Agency for health care policy and research: Clinical practice guidelines for heart failure. J. Cardiovasc. Nurs. 10(2):85–88, 1996.

Guidelines for the evaluation and management of heart failure. Report of the American College of Cardiology/ American Heart Association Task Force on Practice Guidelines (Committee on Evaluation and Management of Heart Failure). J. Am. Coll. Cardiol. 26(5):1376–1398, 1995.

Hudak, C. M., and Gallo, B. M. (eds.): Critical Care Nursing: A Holistic Approach, 6th ed. Philadelphia, J. B. Lippincott, 1994.

Kelly, R. A., and Smith, T. W.: The pharmacology of heart failure drugs. In Smith, T. W. (ed.): Cardiovascular Therapeutics: A Companion to Braunwald's Heart Disease. Philadelphia, W. B. Saunders, 1996, pp. 176–199.

Poole-Wilson, P. A., Colucci, W. S., Massie, B. M., et al. (eds.): Heart Failure: Scientific Principles and Clinical Practice. New York, Churchill Livingstone, 1997.

Redfield, M. M.: Evaluation of congestive heart failure. In Giuliani, E. R., Gersh, B. J., and McGoon, M. D. (eds.): Mayo Clinic Practice of Cardiology, 3rd ed. St. Louis, Mosby, 1996, pp. 569–587.

Stevenson, L. W., and Colucci, W. S.: Management of patients hospitalized with heart failure. In Smith, T. W. (ed.): Cardiovascular Therapeutics: A Companion to Braunwald's Heart Disease. Philadelphia, W. B. Saunders, 1996, pp. 199–209.

PERICARDIAL DISEASE

Cheitlin, M. D., Sokolow, M., and McIlroy, M. B.: Clinical Cardiology, 6th ed. Norwalk, Conn., Appleton & Lange, 1993.

Finkelmeier, B. A.: Cardiothoracic Surgical Nursing. Philadelphia, J. B. Lippincott, 1995.

Schlant, R. C., and Alexander, R. W. (eds.): Hurst's The Heart, 8th ed. New York, McGraw-Hill, 1994, pp. 1649–1662.

Shabetai, R.: Etiology, pathophysiology, clinical recognition and treatment. In Willerson, J. T., and Cohn, J. N. (eds.): Cardiovascular Medicine. New York, Churchill Livingstone, 1995, pp. 1011–1040.

Shabetai, R.: Treatment of pericardial disease. In Smith, T. W. (ed.): Cardiovascular Therapeutics: A Companion to Braunwald's Heart Disease. Philadelphia, W. B. Saunders, 1996, pp. 742–750.

Spodick, D. H.: Diseases of the precordium. In Chatterjee, K., Karliner, J., Rapaport, E., et al. (eds.): Cardiology: An Illustrated Text/Reference. Philadelphia, J. B. Lippincott, 1991, pp. 10.52–10.63.

MYOCARDITIS

Baughman, K. L., and Hruban, R. H.: Treatment of myocarditis. In Smith, T. W. (ed.): Cardiovascular Therapeutics: A Companion to Braunwald's Heart Disease. Philadelphia, W. B. Saunders, 1996, pp. 243–253.

Cheitlin, M. D., Sokolow, M., and McIlroy, M. B.: Clinical Cardiology, 6th ed. Norwalk, Conn., Appleton & Lange, 1993, pp. 585–637.

Cherian, G., and Abraham, M. T.: Myocarditis. In Chatterjee, K., Karliner, J., Rapaport, E., et al. (eds.): Cardiology: An Illustrated Text/Reference. Philadelphia, J. B. Lippincott, 1991, pp. 10.84–10.97.

Davies, M. J., and Ward, D. E.: How can myocarditis be diagnosed and should it be treated? Br. Heart J. 68:346–347, 1992.

Edwards, W. D., and Holmes, D. R.: Cardiomyopathy and biopsy. In Giuliani, E. R., Gersh, B. J., and McGoon, M. D. (eds.): Mayo Clinic Practice of Cardiology, 3rd ed. St. Louis, Mosby-Year Book, 1996, pp. 678–688.

Einsley, R. D., Renlund, D. G., and Mason, J. W.: Myocarditis. In Willerson, J. T., and Cohn, J. N. (eds.): Cardiovascular Medicine. New York, Churchill Livingstone, 1995, pp. 894–916.

Finkelmeier, B. A.: Cardiothoracic Surgical Nursing. Philadelphia, J. B. Lippincott, 1995.

Mason, J. W., O'Connell, J. B., Herskowitz, A., et al.: A clinical trial of immunosuppressive therapy for myocarditis. The Myocarditis Treatment Trial Investigators. N. Engl. J. Med. 333(5):269–275, 1995.

O'Connell, J. B., and Renlund, D. G.: Myocardial diseases. In Willerson, J. T., and Cohn, J. N. (eds.): Cardiovascular Medicine. New York, Churchill Livingstone, 1995, pp. 1591–1605.

Olinde, K. D., and O'Connell, J. B.: Inflammatory heart disease: Pathogenesis, clinical manifestations, and treatment of myocarditis. Annu. Rev. Med. 45:481–490, 1994.

Schlant, R. C., and Alexander, R. W. (eds.): Hurst's The Heart, 8th ed. New York, McGraw-Hill, 1994.

INFECTIVE ENDOCARDITIS

Bansal, R. C.: Infective endocarditis. Med. Clin. North Am. 79(5):1205–1240, 1995.

Bruce, M. S.: Endocarditis. In Rakel, R. E. (ed.): Saunders Manual of Medical Practice. Philadelphia, W. B. Saunders, 1996, pp. 265–267.

Cheitlin, M. D., Sokolow, M., and McIlroy, M. B.: Clinical Cardiology, 6th ed. Norwalk, Conn., Appleton & Lange, 1993, pp. 564–583.

Dajani, A. S., Taubert, K. A., Wilson, W., et al.: Prevention of bacterial endocarditis. J.A.M.A. 277:1794–1801, 1997.

Durack, D. T.: Prevention of infective endocarditis. New Engl. J. Med. 332:38–44, 1995.

Gregoratos, G.: Infective endocarditis. *In* Chatterjee, K., Karliner, J., Rapaport, E., et al. (eds.): Cardiology: An Illustrated Text/Reference. Philadelphia, J. B. Lippincott, 1991, pp. 9.73–9.89.

Karchmer, A. W.: Treatment of infectious endocarditis. *In* Smith, T. W. (ed.): Cardiovascular Therapeutics: A Companion to Braunwald's Heart Disease. Philadelphia, W. B. Saunders, 1996, pp. 718–730.

Matthews, D.: The prevention and diagnosis of infective endocarditis: The primary care provider's role. Nurse Pract. 19(8):53–60, 1994.

Nunley, D. L., and Perlman, P. E.: Endocarditis. Changing trends in epidemiology, clinical and microbiologic spectrum. Postgrad. Med. 93(5):235–238, 241–244, 247, 1993.

Seidel, H. M., Ball, J. W., Dains, J. E., and Benedict, G. W.: Mosby's Guide to Physical Examination, 3rd ed. St. Louis, Mosby–Year Book, 1995.

Snelson, C., Cline, B. A., and Luby, C.: Infective endocarditis: A challenging diagnosis. Dimen. Crit. Care Nurs. 12(1):4–16, 1993.

CARDIOMYOPATHY

Chadi, B. H.: Cardiomyopathy. *In* Rakel, R. E. (ed.): Saunders Manual of Medical Practice. Philadelphia, W. B. Saunders, 1996, pp. 252–255.

Cheitlin, M. D., Sokolow, M., and McIlroy, M. B. (eds.): Clinical Cardiology, 6th ed. Norwalk, Conn., Appleton & Lange, 1993.

Gilbert, E. M., and Bristow, M. R.: Idiopathic dilated cardiomyopathy. *In* Schlant, R. C., and Alexander, R. W. (eds.): Hurst's The Heart, 8th ed. New York, McGraw-Hill, 1994, pp. 1609–1619.

Kasper, E. K., Agema, W. R. P., Hutchins, G. M., et al.: The causes of dilated cardiomyopathy: A clinicopathologic review of 673 consecutive patients. j. Am. Coll. Cardiol. 23:586–590, 1994.

Maron, B. J., and Roberts, W. C.: Hypertrophic cardiomyopathy. *In* Schlant, R. C., and Alexander, R. W. (eds.): Hurst's The Heart, 8th ed. New York, McGraw-Hill, 1994, pp. 1621–1635.

Nishimura, R. A., Guilliani, E. R., and Brandenburg, R. O.: Hypertrophic cardiomyopathy. *In* Giuliani, E. R., Gersh, B. J., and McGoon, M. D. (eds.): Mayo Clinic Practice of Cardiology, 3rd ed. St. Louis, Mosby-Year Book, 1996, pp. 689–711.

Olney, B. A.: Restrictive cardiomyopathy. *In* Giuliani, E. R., Gersh, B. J., and McGoon, M. D. (eds.): Mayo Clinic Practice of Cardiology, 3rd ed. St. Louis, Mosby, 1996, pp. 712–726.

Rodeheffer, R. J., and Gersh, B. J.: Cardiomyopathy and biopsy. *In* Giuliani, E. R., Gersh, B. J., and McGoon, M. D. (eds.): Mayo Clinic Practice of Cardiology, 3rd ed. St. Louis, Mosby–Year Book, 1996, pp. 636–667.

Shabetai, R.: Dilated cardiomyopathy. *In* Chatterjee, K., Karliner, J., Rapaport, E., et al. (eds.): Cardiology: An Illustrated Text/Reference. Philadelphia, J. B. Lippincott, 1991, pp. 10.2–10.17.

Siegel, R. J., and Darovic, G. O.: Cardiomyopathies and pericardial diseases. *In* Darovic, G. O. (ed.): Hemodynamic Monitoring: Invasive and Noninvasive Clinical Application, 2nd ed. Philadelphia, W. B. Saunders, 1995, pp. 759–788.

Wigle, E. D.: Hypertrophic cardiomyopathy. *In* Chatterjee, K., Karliner, J., Rapaport, E., et al. (eds.): Cardiology: An Illustrated Text/Reference. Philadelphia, J. B. Lippincott, 1991, pp. 10.18–10.37.

END-STAGE HEART DISEASE

Aaronson, K. D., Schwartz, J. S., Goin, J. E., and Mancini, D. M.: Sex differences in patient acceptance of cardiac transplant candidacy. Circulation 91(11):2753–2761, 1995.

Bove, L. A., Mancini, M. G., Duris, L., et al.: Nursing care of patients undergoing dynamic cardiomyoplasty. Crit. Care Nurse 15(3):96–100, 102–104, 1995.

Davenport, Y.: Advanced technology within the cardiac transplant process. Intens. Crit. Care Nurs. 11(3):170–174, 1995.

Dressler, D. K.: Transplantation in end-stage heart failure. Crit. Care Nurs. Clin. North Am. 5(4):635–648, 1993.

Farrar, D. J., and Hill, J. D.: Univentricular and biventricular Thoratec VAD support as a bridge to transplantation. Ann. Thorac. Surg. 55:276–282, 1993.

Frazier, O. H., and Macris, M. P.: Progress in cardiac transplantation. Surg. Clin. North Am. 74(5):1169–1182, 1994.

Futterman, L. G., and Lemberg, L.: Cardiomyoplasty: A potential alternative to cardiac transplantation. Am. J. Crit. Care 5(1):80–86, 1996.

O'Connell, J. B., Gunnar, R. M., Evans, R. W., et al.: 24th Bethesda Conference: Cardiac transplantation. Task Force 1: Organization of heart transplantation in the U.S. J. Am. Coll. Cardiol. 22(11):8–14, 1993.

Schroeder, J. S.: Indications for cardiac transplantation. Heart Dis. Stroke 3(6):345–349, 1994.

Stevenson, L. W., Warner, S. L., Steimle, A. E., et al.: The impending crisis awaiting cardiac transplantation. Modeling a solution based on selection. Circulation 89(1):450–457, 1994.

Thompson, C. J.: Denervation of the transplanted heart: Nursing implications for patient care. Crit. Care Nurs. Q. 17(4):1–14, 1995.

Vargo, R., and Dimengo, J. M.: Surgical alternatives for patients with heart failure. AACN Clin. Issues Crit. Care Nurs. 3(2):244–259, 1993.

Vollman, M. W.: Dynamic cardiomyoplasty: Perspectives on nursing care and collaborative management. Prog. Cardiovasc. Nurs. 10(2):15–22, 1995.

CARDIAC TRAUMA

Bearden, C. R.: Myocardial contusion: A case study of a myocardial infarction. Crit. Care Nurs. Q. 17(3):14–20, 1994.

Cheitlein, M. D.: Cardiovascular injury as the internist sees it. *In* Chatterjee, K., Karliner, J., Rapaport, E., et al. (eds.): Cardiology: An Illustrated Text/Reference. Philadelphia, J. B. Lippincott, 1991, pp. 12.13–12.25.

Cheitlin, M. D., Sokolow, M., and McIlroy, M. B.: Clinical Cardiology, 6th ed. Norwalk, Conn., Appleton & Lange, 1993, pp. 690–692.

Christensen, M. A., and Sutton, K. R.: Myocardial contusion: New concepts in diagnosis and management. Am. J. Crit. Care 2(1):28–34, 1993.

Craven, A.: Trauma. *In* Hudak, C. M., and Gallo, B. M.

(eds.): Critical Care Nursing: A Holistic Approach, 6th ed. Philadelphia, J. B. Lippincott, 1994, pp. 964–975.

Daleiden, A.: Clinical manifestations of blunt cardiac injury: A challenge to the critical care practitioner. Crit. Care Nurs. Q. 17(2):13–23, 1994.

Finkelmeier, B. A.: Cardiothoracic Surgical Nursing. Philadelphia, J. B. Lippincott, 1995, pp. 339–349.

Kshettry, V. R., and Bolman, R. M. 3rd: Chest trauma. Assessment, diagnosis and management. Clin. Chest Med. 15(1):137–146, 1994.

Lichtenberg, R., Dries, D., Ward, K., et al.: Cardiovascular effects of lightning strikes. J. Am. Coll. Cardiol. 21(2):531–536, 1993.

Malangoni, M. A., McHenry, C. R., and Jacobs, D. G.: Outcome of serious blunt cardiac injury. Surgery 116(4):628–633, 1994.

Rosenthal, M. A., and Ellis, J. I.: Cardiac and mediastinal trauma. Emerg. Med. Clin. North Am. 13(4):887–902, 1995.

Smith, A., and Fitzpatrick, E.: Penetrating cardiac trauma: Surgical and nursing management. J Cardiovasc. Nurs. 7(2):52–70, 1993.

CARDIAC RHYTHMS

Symptomatic Bradycardia

ACC/AHA Task Force Report: Guidelines for implantation of cardiac pacemakers and antiarrhythmia devices: A report of the American College of Cardiology/American Heart Association Task Force on assessment of diagnostic and therapeutic cardiovascular procedures (Committee on Pacemaker Implantation). J. Am. Coll. Cardiol. 18(1):1–13, 1991.

Caine, R. M., and Bufalino, P. M. (eds.): Critically Ill Adults: Nursing Care Planning Guides. Baltimore, Williams & Wilkins, 1988, pp. 168–179.

Cummins, R. O.: American Heart Association Textbook of Advanced Cardiac Life Support. Dallas, American Heart Association, 1994.

Dracup, K.: Meltzer's Intensive Coronary Care: A Manual for Nurses, 5th ed. Norwalk, Conn., Appleton & Lange, 1995, pp. 275–299.

Dreifus, L. S., Fisch, C., Griffin, J. C., et al.: ACC/AHA Task Force Report. Guidelines for implantation of cardiac pacemakers and antiarrhythmia devices. J. Am. Coll. Cardiol. 18(1):1–13, 1991.

Hayes, D. L.: Pacemaker electrocardiography. In Furman, S., Hayes, D. L., and Holmes, D. R.: A Practice of Cardiac Pacing. Mount Kisco, N.Y., Futura, 1993, pp. 318–321.

Manion, P. A.: Temporary epicardial pacing in the postoperative cardiac surgical patient. Crit. Care Nurse 13(2):30–38, 1993.

Prystowsky, E. N., and Klein, G. J.: Cardiac Arrhythmias: An Integrated Approach for the Clinician. New York, McGraw-Hill, 1994.

Rardon, D. P., Mitrani, R., Klein, L. S., et al.: Management of bradyarrhythmias. In Smith, T. W. (ed.): Cardiovascular Therapeutics: A Companion to Braunwald's Heart Disease. Philadelphia, W. B. Saunders, 1996, pp. 346–351.

Toledo, L. W.: Electronic dysrhythmia treatments. Parts 1 and 2. NurseWeek 1996, Pt. 1, vol 11, issue 5, pp. 1–5; Pt. 2, vol 11, issue 6, pp. 1–7. Available at http:www.nurseweek.com.

Symptomatic Tachycardia

Baker, B. M., Smith, J. M., and Cain, M. E.: Nonpharmacologic approaches to the treatment of atrial fibrillation and atrial flutter. J. Cardiovasc. Electrophysiol. 6(10):972–978, 1995.

Belz, M. K., Wood, M. A., and Ellenbogen, K. A.: Pacemakers and implantable cardioverter defibrillators in the intensive care setting. In Shoemaker, W. C., Ayres, S. M., Grenvik, A., and Holbrook, P. R. (eds.): Textbook of Critical Care, 3rd ed. Philadelphia, W. B. Saunders, 1995, pp. 513–519.

Bubien, R. S., Knotts, S. M., and Kay, G. N.: Radiofrequency catheter ablation: Concepts and nursing implications. Cardiovasc. Nurs. 31(3):17–23, 1995.

Chapman, E. L., Strawn, R. M., and Stewart, B. P.: Differentiating between ventricular tachycardia and supraventricular tachycardia in the clinical setting. Focus Crit. Care 19(2):140–145, 1992.

Cummins, R. O.: American Heart Association Textbook of Advanced Cardiac Life Support. Dallas, American Heart Association, 1994.

DiMarco, J. P.: Drug treatment of supraventricular tachycardias. In Smith, T. W. (ed.): Cardiovascular Therapeutics: A Companion to Braunwald's Heart Disease. Philadelphia, W. B. Saunders, 1996, pp. 277–294.

Finkelmeier, B. A.: Ablative therapy in the treatment of tachyarrhythmias. Crit. Care Nurs. Clin. North Am. 6(1):103–110, 1994.

Ganz, L. I., and Friedman, P. L.: Supraventricular tachycardia. N. Engl. J. Med. 332:162–173, 1995.

Golner, B., Jadonath, R., Merkatz, K., et al.: Radiofrequency catheter ablation as a primary therapy for supraventricular tachycardia. J. Invas. Cardiol. 7(4):107–112, 1995.

Guaglianone, D. M., and Tyndall, A.: Comfort issues in patients undergoing radiofrequency ablation. Crit. Care Nurse 15(1):47–50, 1995.

Hamdam, M., and Scheinman, M.: Current approaches in patients with ventricular tachyarrhythmias. Med. Clin. North Am. 79(5):1097–1120, 1995.

Miles, W. M., Klein, L. S., Mitrani, R., et al.: Nonpharmacologic treatment of supraventricular tachycardias. In Smith, T. W. (ed.): Cardiovascular Therapeutics: A Companion to Braunwald's Heart Disease. Philadelphia, W. B. Saunders, 1996, pp. 294–309.

Rausmussen, M. J., and Mangan, D. B.: Third generation antitachycardia pacing implantable cardioverter-defibrillators. Dimens. Crit. Care Nurs. 13(6):284–291, 1994.

Stevenson, W. G., and Friedman, P. L.: Drug treatment of ventricular tachycardia. In Smith, T. W. (ed.): Cardiovascular Therapeutics: A Companion to Braunwald's Heart Disease. Philadelphia, W. B. Saunders, 1996, pp. 309–333.

Teplitz, L.: Transcatheter ablation of tachyarrhythmias: An overview and case studies. Prog. Cardiovasc. Nurs. 9(3):16–31, 1994.

Pulseless Electrical Activity

ACC/AHA Task Force Report: Guidelines for implantation of cardiac pacemakers and antiarrhythmia devices: A report of the American College of Cardiology/American Heart Association Task Force on assessment of diagnostic and therapeutic cardiovascular procedures (Committee on Pacemaker Implantation). J. Am. Coll. Cardiol. 18(1):1–13, 1991.

Arteaga, W. J., and Windle, J. R.: The quality of life of

patients with life-threatening arrhythmias. Arch. Intern. Med. 155:2086–2091, 1995.

The AVID Investigators: Antiarrhythmics versus Implantable Defibrillators (AVID)—Rationale, design and methods. Am. J. Cardiol. 75:470–475, 1995.

Belz, M. K., Wood, M. A., and Ellenbogen, K. A.: Pacemakers and implantable cardioverter defibrillators in the intensive care setting. In Shoemaker, W. C., Ayres, S. M., Grenvik, A., and Holbrook, P. R. (eds.): Textbook of Critical Care, 3rd ed. Philadelphia, W. B. Saunders, 1995, pp. 513–519.

Cummins, R. O.: American Heart Association Textbook of Advanced Cardiac Life Support. Dallas, American Heart Association, 1994.

Davidson, T., VanRiper, S., Harper, P., et al.: Implantable cardioverter-defibrillators: A guide for clinicians. Heart Lung 23(3):205–215, 1994.

Gilman, J. K., Jalal, S., and Niccarelli, G. V.: Predicting and preventing sudden death from cardiac causes. Circulation 90(2):1083–1092, 1994.

Kendall, M. J., Lynch, K. P., Hjalmarson, A., et al.: Beta-blockers and sudden cardiac death. Ann. Intern. Med. 123(5):358–367, 1995.

Molchany, C. A., and Peterson, K. A.: The psychosocial effects of support group intervention on AICD recipients and their significant others. Prog. Cardiovasc. Nurs. 9(2):23–29, 1994.

Stewart, J. A.: Delayed in-hospital defibrillation. Ann. Emerg. Med. 27(1):5–6, 1996.

MITRAL INSUFFICIENCY

Carabello, B. A.: Management of valvular regurgitation. Curr. Opin. Cardiol. 10(2):124–127, 1995.

Cheitlin, M. D., Sokolow, M., and McIlroy, M. B.: Clinical Cardiology, 6th ed. Norwalk, Conn., Appleton & Lange, 1993, pp. 427–435.

Fenster, M. S., and Feldman, M. D.: Mitral regurgitation: An overview. Curr. Prob. Cardiol. 20(4):193–280, 1995.

Hess, O. M., Scherrer, U., Nicod, P., et al.: Mitral valve disease. In Willerson, J. T., and Cohn, J. N. (eds.): Cardiovascular Medicine. New York, Churchill Livingstone, 1995, pp. 202–224.

Rakel, R. E. (ed.): Saunders Manual of Medical Practice. Philadelphia, W. B. Saunders, 1996.

McGoon, M. D., Hartzell, V., and Scaff, M. D.: Mitral regurgitation. In Giuliani, E. R., Gersh, B. J., and McGoon, M. D. (eds.): Mayo Clinic Practice of Cardiology, 3rd ed. St. Louis, Mosby–Year Book, 1996, pp. 1450–1469.

O'Sullivan, C. K.: Mitral regurgitation as a complication of MI: Pathophysiology and nursing implications. J. Cardiovasc. Nurs. 6(4):26–37, 1992.

Treasure, C. B.: Recognition and management of mitral regurgitation. Heart Dis. Stroke 2(4):346–354, 1993.

MITRAL STENOSIS

Carabello, B. A., and Crawford, F. A.: Therapy for mitral stenosis comes full circle. N. Engl. J. Med. 331:1014–1015, 1994.

Cheitlin, M. D., Douglas, P. S., and Parmley, W. W.: 26th Bethesda Conference: Recommendations for determining eligibility for competition in athletes with cardiovascular abnormalities. Task Force 2: Acquired valvular

heart disease. Med. Sci. Sports Exerc. 26(10, Suppl):S254–S259, 1994.

Finkelmeier, B. A.: Cardiothoracic Surgical Nursing. Philadelphia, J. B. Lippincott, 1995, pp. 24–25.

Hess, O. M., Scherrer, U., Nicod, P., and Chesler, E.: Mitral valve disease. In Wilkerson, J. T., and Cohn, J. N. (eds.): Cardiovascular Medicine. New York, Churchill Livingstone, 1995, pp. 202–205.

Nishimura, R. A., Brandenburg, R. O., Giuliani, E. R., and McGoon, D. C.: Mitral stenosis. In Giuliani, E. R., Gersh, B. J., and McGoon, M. D.: Mayo Clinic Practice of Cardiology, 3rd ed. St. Louis, Mosby–Year Book, 1996, pp. 1435–1447.

Rakel, R. E.: Saunders Manual of Medical Practice. Philadelphia, W. B. Saunders, 1996, pp. 256–258.

Rapaport, E.: Recognition and management of mitral stenosis. Heart Dis. Stroke 2(1):64–68, 1993.

Thibault, G. E.: Clinical problem-solving. Studying the classics. N. Engl. J. Med. 333(10):648–652, 1995.

AORTIC INSUFFICIENCY

Cheitlin, M. D., Sokolow, M., and McIlroy, M. B.: Clinical Cardiology, 6th ed. Norwalk, Conn., Appleton & Lange, 1993, pp. 439–475.

Mangion, J. R., and Tighe, D. A.: Aortic valvular disease in adults: A potentially lethal clinical problem. Postgrad. Med. 98(1):127–135, 140, 1995.

McGoon, M. D., Fuster, V., and Shub, C.: Aortic regurgitation. In Giuliani, E. R., Gersh, B. J., and McGoon, M. D. (eds.): Mayo Clinic Practice of Cardiology, 3rd ed. St. Louis, Mosby–Year Book, 1996, pp. 1418–1434.

AORTIC STENOSIS

Cheitlin, M. D., Sokolow, M., and McIlroy, M. B.: Clinical Cardiology, 6th ed. Norwalk, Conn., Appleton & Lange, 1993, pp. 438–453.

Mangion, J. R., and Tighe, D. A.: Aortic valvular disease in adults: A potentially lethal clinical problem. Postgrad. Med. 98(1):127–135, 140, 1995.

Olson, L. J., and Shub, C.: Aortic valvular stenosis. In Giuliani, E. R., Gersh, B. J., and McGoon, M. D. (eds.): Mayo Clinic Practice of Cardiology, 3rd ed. St. Louis, Mosby–Year Book, 1996, pp. 1398–1417.

Shah, A.: Aortic valve disease. In Rakel, R. E. (ed.): Saunders Manual of Medical Practice. Philadelphia, W. B. Saunders, 1996, pp. 259–261.

ATRIAL SEPTAL DEFECT

Galloway, A. C., Colvin, S. B., and Spencer, F. C.: Atrial septal defects, atrioventricular canal defects, and total anomalous pulmonary venous return. In Sabiston, D. C., and Spencer, F. C. (eds.): Surgery of the Chest, 6th ed. Philadelphia, W. B. Saunders, 1995, pp. 1387–1398.

Nugent, E. W., Plauth, W. H., Edwards, J. E., and Williams, W. H.: The pathology, pathophysiology, recognition, and treatment of congenital heart disease. In Schlant, R. C., and Alexander, R. W. (eds.): Hurst's The Heart, 8th ed. New York, McGraw-Hill, 1994, pp. 1768–1772.

Wang, Y.: Pathophysiology, clinical recognition and treatment. In Willerson, J. T., and Cohn, J. N. (eds.): Cardiovascular Medicine. New York, Churchill Livingstone, 1995, pp. 87–90.

VENTRICULAR SEPTAL DEFECT

Bach, D. S., and Armstrong, W. F.: Echocardiography. *In* Willerson, J. T., and Cohn, J. N. (eds.): Cardiovascular Medicine. New York, Churchill Livingstone, 1995, pp. 138–140.

Gersony, W. M.: Ventricular septal defect and left-sided obstructive lesions in infants. Curr. Opin. Pediatr. 6(5):566–569, 1994.

Guntheroth, W. G.: Ductus arteriosus and ventricular septal defect in adults. *In* Chatterjee, K., Karliner, K., Rapaport, E., et al. (eds.): Cardiology: An Illustrated Text/Reference. Philadelphia, J. B. Lippincott, 1991, pp. 11.51–11.76.

Nugent, E. W., Plauth, W. H., Edwards, J. E., and Williams, W. H.: The pathology, pathophysiology, recognition, and treatment of congenital heart disease. *In* Schlant, R. C., and Alexander, R. W. (eds.): Hurst's The Heart, 8th ed. New York, McGraw-Hill, 1994, pp. 1768–1772.

Oliver, S.: Ventricular septal defects. A case study and discussion. Intens. Crit. Care Nurs. 10(3):195–198, 1994.

Pacifico, A. D., and Kirlin, J. K.: Surgical treatment of ventricular septal defect. *In* Sabiston, D. C., and Spencer, F. C. (eds.): Surgery of the Chest, 6th ed. Philadelphia, W. B. Saunders, 1995, pp. 1446–1461.

Ramaciotti, C., Vetter, J. M., Bornemeier, R. A., and Chin, A. J.: Prevalence, relation to spontaneous closure, and association of muscular ventricular septal defects with other cardiac defects. Am. J. Cardiol. 75(1):61–65, 1995.

Wang, Y.: Congenital heart disease in the adult: Pathophysiology, clinical recognition and treatment. *In* Willerson, J. T., and Cohn, J. N. (eds.): Cardiovascular Medicine. New York, Churchill Livingstone, 1995, pp. 93–98.

PATENT DUCTUS ARTERIOSUS

Cheitlin, M. D., Sokolow, M., and McIlroy, M. B.: Clinical Cardiology, 6th ed. Norwalk, Conn., Appleton & Lange, 1993, pp. 383–391.

Gaynor, J. W., and Sabiston, D. C.: Patent ductus arteriosus, coarctation of the aorta, aortopulmonary window and anomalies of the aortic arch. *In* Sabiston, D. C., and Spencer, F. C. (eds.): Surgery of the Chest, 6th ed. Philadelphia, W. B. Saunders, 1995, pp. 1275–1281.

Nugent, E. W., Plauth, W. H., Edwards, J. E., and Williams, W. H.: The pathology, pathophysiology, recognition and treatment of congenital heart disease. *In* Schlant, R. C., and Alexander, R. W. (eds.): Hurst's The Heart, 8th ed. New York, McGraw-Hill, 1994, pp. 1768–1772.

Rao, P. S., and Sideris, E. B.: Transcatheter occlusion of patent ductus arteriosus: State of the art. J. Invas. Cardiol. 8(7):278–288, 1996.

Wang, Y.: Congenital heart disease in the adult: Pathophysiology, clinical recognition and treatment. *In* Willerson, J. T., and Cohn, J. N. (eds.): Cardiovascular Medicine. New York, Churchill Livingstone, 1995, pp. 93–98.

COARCTATION OF THE AORTA

Bashore, T. M., and Lieberman, E. B.: Aortic/mitral obstruction and coarctation of the aorta [Review]. Cardiol. Clin. 11(4):617–641, 1993.

Finkelmeier, B. A.: Cardiothoracic Surgical Nursing. Philadelphia, J. B. Lippincott, 1995, pp. 62–63.

Gaynor, J. W., and Sabiston, D. C.: Patent ductus arteriosus, coarctation of the aorta, aortopulmonary window and anomalies of the aortic arch. *In* Sabiston, D. C., and Spencer, F. C. (eds.): Surgery of the Chest, 6th ed. Philadelphia, W. B. Saunders, 1995, pp. 1281–1295.

Greenberg, S. B.: Coarctation of the aorta: Diagnostic imaging after corrective surgery [Review]. J. Thorac. Imag. 10(1):36–42, 1995.

Perloff, J. K.: Congenital heart disease in the adult: Clinical approach [Review]. J. Thorac. Imag. 9(4):260–268, 1994.

Rao, P. S.: Coarctation of the aorta [Review]. Semin. Nephrol. 15(2):87–105, 1995.

Waines, C. A., Fuster, V., and McGoon, D. C.: Coarctation of the aorta. *In* Giuliani, E. R., Gersh, B. J., and McGoon, M. D. (eds.): Mayo Clinic Practice of Cardiology, 3rd ed. St. Louis, Mosby–Year Book, 1996, pp. 1572–1579.

HYPERTENSIVE CRISIS

Bines, A. S., and Landron, S. L.: Cardiovascular emergencies in the post anesthesia care unit. Nurs. Clin. North Am. 28(3):493–505, 1993.

Gifford, R. W.: Treatment of patient with systemic arterial hypertension. *In* Schlant, R. C., and Alexander, R. W. (eds.): Hurst's The Heart, 8th ed. New York, McGraw-Hill, 1994, pp. 1443–1445.

Herrera, C. R.: Hypertension. *In* Rakel, R. E. (ed.): Saunders Manual of Medical Practice. Philadelphia, W. B. Saunders, 1996, pp. 220–221.

Kaplan, N. M.: Clinical Hypertension, 6th ed. Baltimore, Williams & Wilkins, 1994, pp. 281–297.

Lasater, M.: Combining vasoactive infusion for maximal cardiac performance in the postoperative period. Crit. Care Nurs. Q. 16(2):11–16, 1993.

Nash, C. A., and Jensen, P. L.: When your surgical patient has hypertension. Am. J. Nurs. 94(12):38–45, 1994.

Porsche, R.: Hypertension: Diagnosis, acute antihypertension therapy, and long-term management. AACN Clin. Issues 6(4):515–525, 1995.

Teplitz, L.: Hypertensive crisis: Review and update. Crit. Care Nurs 13(6):20–27, 30–33, 35–37, 1993.

SHOCK

Alpert, J. S., and Becker, R. C.: Pathophysiology, diagnosis and management of cardiogenic shock. *In* Schlant, R. C., and Alexander, R. W. (eds.): Hurst's The Heart, 8th ed. New York, McGraw-Hill, 1994, pp. 907–925.

Chadi, B.: Shock. *In* Rakel, R. E. (ed.): Saunders Manual of Medical Practice. Philadelphia, W. B. Saunders, 1996, pp. 211–214.

Franklin, C. M., Darovic, G. O., and Dan, B. B.: Monitoring the patient in shock. *In* Darovic, G. O.: Hemodynamic Monitoring: Invasive and Noninvasive Clinical Application, 2nd ed. Philadelphia, W. B. Saunders, 1995, pp. 441–499.

Gerish, B. J., Chesebro, M. D., and Clements, I. P.: Acute myocardial infarction management and complications. *In* Giuliani, E. R., Gersh, B. J., and McGoon, M. D. (eds.): Mayo Clinic Practice of Cardiology, 3rd ed. St. Louis, Mosby–Year Book, 1996, pp. 1300–1306.

Kinney, M. R., and Packa, D. R. (eds.): Andreoli's Comprehensive Cardiac Care, 8th ed. St. Louis, Mosby–Year Book, 1996.

Mathias, C. J., and Gunnar, R. M.: Autonomic dysfunction, hypotension and shock. *In* Willerson, J. T., and Cohn, J. N. (eds.): Cardiovascular Medicine. New York, Churchill Livingstone, 1995, pp. 1263–1212.

O'Neal, P. V.: How to spot early signs of cardiogenic shock. Am. J. Nurs. 94(5):36–40, 1994.

AORTIC AND PERIPHERAL ARTERIAL DISEASE

Gerhard, M., Baum, P., and Raby, K. E.: Peripheral arterial-vascular disease in women: Prevalence, prognosis, and treatment. Cardiology 86(4):349–355, 1995.

Goerdt, C.: Peripheral artery disease. *In* Rakel, R. E. (ed.): Saunders Manual of Medical Practice. Philadelphia, W. B. Saunders, 1996, pp. 286–287.

Harris, L. M., and Ricotta, J. J.: Peripheral arterial embolus. *In* Cameron, J. L. (ed.): Current Surgical Therapy, 5th ed. St. Louis, Mosby-Year Book, 1996, pp. 707–711.

Hill, E. H.: Perioperative management of patients with vascular disease. AACN Clin. Issues Crit. Care 6(4):547–561, 1995.

Karch, A. M.: Pain, pills, and possibilities: Drug therapy in peripheral vascular disease. AACN Clin. Issues Crit. Care 6(4):614–630, 1995.

Krenzer, M. E.: Peripheral vascular assessment: Finding your way through arteries and veins. AACN Clin. Issues Crit. Care 6(4):631–644, 1995.

Marin, M. L., and Veith, F. J.: Endovascular stents and stented grafts for the treatment of aneurysms and other arterial lesions. Adv Surg 29:93–109, 1996.

Poskus, D. B.: Revascularization in peripheral vascular disease: Stents, atherectomies, lasers, and thrombolytics. AACN Clin. Issues Crit. Care 6(4):536–546, 1995.

Rooke, T. W., and Hirsch, A. T.: Peripheral vascular diseases. *In* Willerson, J. T., and Cohn, J. N. (eds.): Cardiovascular Medicine. New York, Churchill Livingstone, 1995, pp. 1162–1181.

Spittell, J. A., Jr.: Peripheral arterial disease. Dis. Mon. 40(12):641–700, 1994.

Wheeler, E. C., and Brenner, Z. R.: Peripheral vascular anatomy, physiology, and pathophysiology. AACN Clin. Issues Crit. Care 6(4):505–514, 1995.

White, C. J., and Ramee, S. R.: Options for percutaneous coronary and peripheral revascularization. Med. Clin. North Am. 76(5):1109–1124, 1992.

Willerson, J. T., Raval, B., Sweeney, M. S., et al.: Diseases of the aorta. *In* Willerson, J. T., and Cohn, J. N.: Cardiovascular Medicine. New York, Churchill Livingstone, 1995, pp. 1113–1162.

Williams, G. M.: Abdominal aortic aneurysm. *In* Cameron, J. L. (ed.): Current Surgical Therapy, 5th ed. St. Louis, Mosby-Year Book, 1996, pp. 616–635.

.... The Neurologic System

Diana L. Nikas, R.N., M.N., CCRN, CNRN, FCCM

PHYSIOLOGIC ANATOMY

Brain

1. **Coverings**
   a. Scalp
      i. Galea aponeurotica: freely movable, dense, fibrous tissue that covers the skull and absorbs the force of external trauma
      ii. Fatty and vascular layer: subcutaneous layer between the skin and galea. Contains blood vessels that contract poorly when injured
      iii. Subaponeurotic space: the space beneath the galea that contains diploic and emissary veins
   b. Skull
      i. Anatomy: a rigid cavity that houses and protects the brain; has a volume of 1400 to 1500 ml (Fig. 3–1)
      ii. Bones: frontal, parietal, temporal, and occipital
      iii. Composition: an inner table and an outer table of solid bone, separated by a diploic space made of cancellous bone. This arrangement provides maximal strength with an economy of weight
      iv. Fossae: three depressions in base of skull—anterior, middle, and posterior (Fig. 3–2)
   c. Meninges (Fig. 3–3)
      i. Dura mater
         (a) Outermost covering of the brain that consists of two layers of tough fibrous tissue
         (b) Outer layer forms periosteum of bone
         (c) Inner layer forms the falx cerebri and tentorium cerebelli
         (d) Meningeal arteries and venous sinuses lie within clefts formed by separation of the inner and outer layers of the dura mater
      ii. Arachnoid mater
         (a) A fine, fibrous, elastic layer that lies between the dura mater and pia mater
         (b) Subarachnoid space

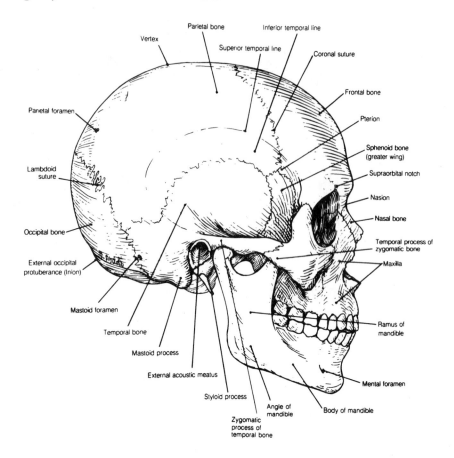

Figure 3-1 • The skull as seen from the side. (From Hall-Craggs, E. C. B.: Anatomy as a Basis for Clinical Medicine. Baltimore, Williams & Wilkins, 1995.)

      (1) Lies between the arachnoid mater and the pia mater; forms the subarachnoid cisterna at base of the brain

      (2) Contains conducting arteries of the brain (circle of Willis)

      (3) Contains cerebrospinal fluid (CSF), which completely surrounds the brain and spinal cord and acts as a shock absorber

      (4) Contains arachnoid villi: projections of the arachnoid mater that serve as channels for absorption of CSF into venous system. Pacchionian bodies are large arachnoid villi distributed along the superior sagittal sinus

   iii. Pia mater

     (a) A delicate layer that adheres to surface of the brain and spinal cord

     (b) Follows sulci and gyri of the brain and carries branches of the cerebral arteries with it

     (c) Choroid plexus formed by blood vessels of the pia mater

2. Divisions of the brain

  a. Cerebrum

     i. Telencephalon: two cerebral hemispheres separated by a longitudinal fissure; joined by the corpus callosum

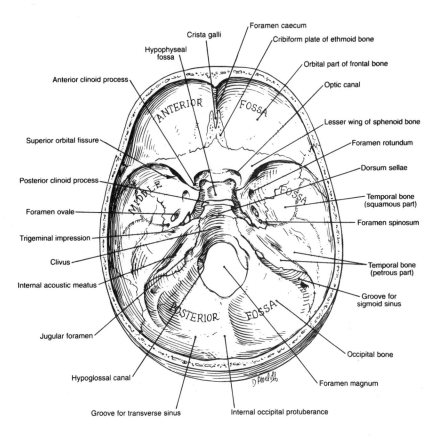

Figure 3–2 • Base of the skull showing the cranial fossae. (From Hall-Craggs, E. C. B.: Anatomy as a Basis for Clinical Medicine. Baltimore, Williams & Wilkins, 1995.)

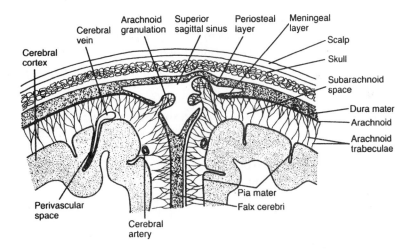

Figure 3–3 • A transverse section through the calvaria, the superior sagittal sinus, and the falx cerebri. Note the relationships among the cerebral cortex and the meninges, the dura mater, the arachnoid, and the pia mater. Arachnoid granulations pierce the dura mater, providing the points of exit for cerebrospinal fluid (CSF) from the subarachnoid space. Arachnoid trabeculae span the CSF-filled subarachnoid space. The pia mater closely adheres to the surface of the brain, held tightly by a glial membrane. (From Burt, A. M.: Textbook of Neuroanatomy. Philadelphia, W. B. Saunders, 1993.)

    (a) Functional localization in cortex

       (1) Frontal lobe: responsible for voluntary motor function (origin of pyramidal motor system) and higher mental functions, such as judgment and foresight, affect, and personality

       (2) Temporal lobes: responsible for hearing, sensory speech in the dominant hemisphere, vestibular sense, behavior, and emotion

       (3) Parietal lobe: responsible for sensory function, sensory association areas, and higher-level processing of general sensory modalities (e.g., stereognosis)

       (4) Occipital lobe: responsible for vision and interpretation of visual stimuli

       (5) Corpus callosum: commissural fibers that transfer learned discriminations, sensory experience, and memory from one cerebral hemisphere to the other

       (6) Cerebral dominance: in right-handed and about 85% of left-handed people, the left cerebral hemisphere is dominant for verbal, linguistic, mathematical, and analytic functions. The nondominant hemisphere is thought to be concerned with geometric, spatial, visual, and musical functions

   (b) Basal ganglia (basal nuclei) (Fig. 3–4)

       (1) Anatomy: includes the caudate, putamen, globus pallidus, claustrum, subthalamic, and substantia nigra nuclei

       (2) Functions: exert regulating and controlling influences on motor integration; suppress muscle tone; and influence postural reflexes. A major center of the extrapyramidal motor system

  ii. Diencephalon (Fig. 3–5)

    (a) Thalamus: anatomically forms lateral walls of the third ventricle; is subdivided into several nuclei

       (1) Certain nuclei receive specific sensory input for general senses, taste, vision, and hearing and relay it to cerebral cortex

       (2) Other nuclei participate in affective aspects of brain function; are functionally related to association areas of cortex; or have a role in motor function and ascending reticular activating system

    (b) Hypothalamus: forms ventral part of the diencephalon, facing the third ventricle medially. Hypothalamic nuclei interconnect with each other and with the limbic system, midbrain, thalamus, and pituitary gland. It regulates:

       (1) Temperature (anterior and posterior hypothalamus)

       (2) Food and water intake (ventromedial and lateral regions)

       (3) Behavior: as part of limbic system, it is concerned with aggressive and sexual behavior; may be involved with sleep along with other central nervous system (CNS) structures

       (4) Autonomic responses: *parasympathetic* responses are elicited by stimulation of anterior hypothalamus; *sympathetic*

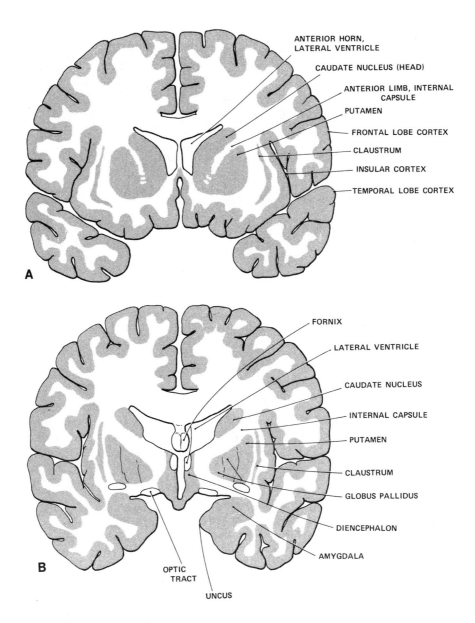

ANTERIOR HORN,
LATERAL VENTRICLE

CAUDATE NUCLEUS (HEAD)

ANTERIOR LIMB, INTERNAL
CAPSULE

PUTAMEN

FRONTAL LOBE CORTEX

CLAUSTRUM

INSULAR CORTEX

TEMPORAL LOBE CORTEX

A

FORNIX

LATERAL VENTRICLE

CAUDATE NUCLEUS

INTERNAL CAPSULE

PUTAMEN

CLAUSTRUM

GLOBUS PALLIDUS

DIENCEPHALON

AMYGDALA

B

OPTIC
TRACT

UNCUS

Figure 3–4 • Two coronal sections through the cerebral hemispheres. *A*, Section through the rostral part of the frontal lobe to show the relationship of the basal ganglia to the surrounding telencephalic structures. *B*, Section through the caudal part of the frontal lobe showing the location of the basal ganglia lateral to the diencephalon. (From Gilman, S., and Newman, S. W.: Manter and Gatz's Essentials of Neuroanatomy and Neurophysiology, 8th ed. Philadelphia, F. A. Davis, 1992.)

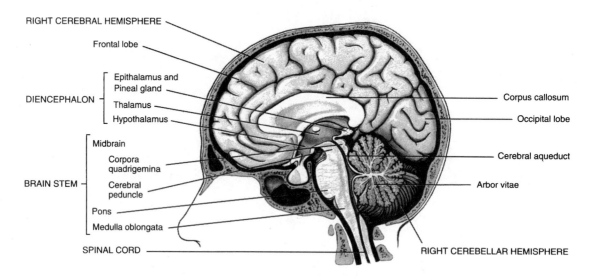

Figure 3–5 • Midsagittal section of the brain showing the major portions of the diencephalon, brain stem, and cerebellum. (From Applegate, E. J.: The Anatomy and Physiology Learning Systems Textbook. Philadelphia, W. B. Saunders, 1995.)

responses may be elicited by stimulation of posterior and lateral hypothalamic nuclei

(5) Hormonal secretion of the pituitary gland (see Chapter 5, The Endocrine System)

  a) Posterior pituitary gland (neurohypophysis): stores and releases antidiuretic hormone (ADH) and oxytocin, which are produced by the supraoptic and paraventricular nuclei, respectively, of the hypothalamus

  b) Increased serum osmolarity or decreased extracellular fluid volume stimulates ADH synthesis and release. ADH causes increased reabsorption of water from the distal tubule and the collecting duct of the nephron of kidney

  c) Oxytocin stimulates contraction of the uterus under appropriate circumstances and ejection of milk from the lactating breast

  d) Anterior pituitary gland (adenohypophysis): hormonal secretion from the anterior pituitary is under control of pituitary releasing and inhibiting factors produced in the hypothalamus and transported to the anterior pituitary via a pituitary portal system (see Chapter 5)

iii. Limbic system (Fig. 3–6)

  (a) Composed of cingulate and parahippocampal gyri, hippocampal formation, dentate gyrus, part of the amygdaloid nucleus, hypothalamus, epithalamus, various nuclei of the thalamus, olfactory cortex, fornix, and anterior commissure

  (b) Responsible for affective aspects of emotional behavior as well as visceral responses accompanying them; also involved in some aspects of memory

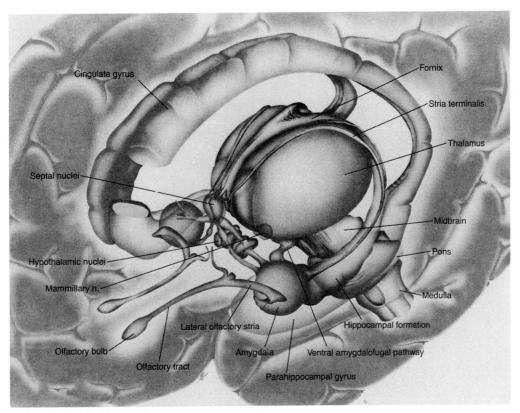

Figure 3–6 • Structures of the limbic system. (From Hendelman, W. J.: Student's Atlas of Neuroanatomy. Philadelphia, W. B. Saunders, 1987.)

b. Brain stem (Fig. 3–7)
  i. Midbrain (mesencephalon): located between the diencephalon and pons
    (a) Contains nuclei of the third (oculomotor) and fourth (trochlear) cranial nerves
    (b) Contains motor and sensory pathways
    (c) Tectal region (inferior and superior colliculi): concerned with auditory and visual systems
    (d) Connected to the cerebellum via superior cerebellar peduncles
  ii. Pons: located between midbrain and medulla; on the ventral surface it appears to form a bridge connecting the right and left cerebellar hemispheres
    (a) Contains nuclei of the fifth (trigeminal), sixth (abducens), seventh (facial) cranial nerves, and some eighth cranial nerve (acoustic) nuclei
    (b) Middle cerebellar peduncles on the basal surface of the pons provide extensive connections between the cerebral cortex and cerebellum, thus ensuring maximal motor efficiency
    (c) Contains motor and sensory pathways (e.g. corticospinal tracts)
  iii. Medulla: located between the pons and spinal cord
    (a) Contains nuclei of the eighth (acoustic), ninth (glossopharyngeal), tenth (vagus), eleventh (spinal accessory), and twelfth (hypoglossal) cranial nerves

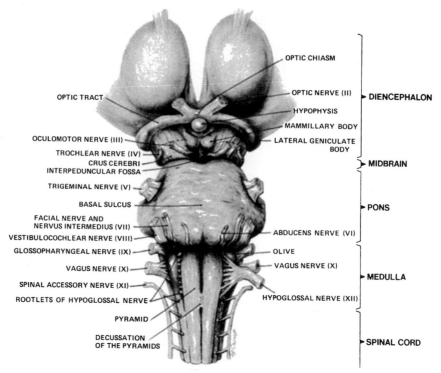

Figure 3–7 • The ventral surface of the human brain stem and diencephalon. (From Gilman, S., and Newman, S. W.: Manter and Gatz's Essentials of Neuroanatomy and Neurophysiology, 8th ed. Philadelphia, F. A. Davis, 1992.)

      (b) Motor and sensory tracts of spinal cord continue into medulla

      (c) Attached to the cerebellum via inferior cerebellar peduncles

    iv. Reticular formation (Fig. 3–8): diffuse cellular network in brain stem, with axons projecting to thalamus, cortex, spinal cord, and cerebellum

      (a) *Ascending* reticular activating system is essential for arousal from sleep, alert wakefulness, focusing of attention, and perceptual association. Destructive lesions of the upper pons and midbrain produce coma

      (b) *Descending* reticular system may inhibit or facilitate activity of motor neurons controlling skeletal musculature

    v. Respiratory and cardiovascular centers have been identified within the brain stem

  c. Cerebellum: lies in the posterior fossa posterior to the brain stem; separated from the cerebrum by tentorium cerebelli

    i. Influences muscle tone in relation to equilibrium, locomotion, posture, and nonstereotyped movements

    ii. Especially important in synchronization of muscle action

    iii. Input is from spinal, brain stem, and cerebral centers; output is via descending pathways (e.g., corticospinal, vestibulospinal, and reticulospinal tracts)

3. Cerebral blood supply (Fig. 3–9)

  a. Arterial system: supplied by the internal carotid and vertebral arteries

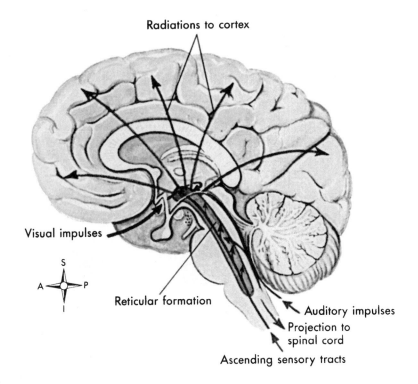

Radiations to cortex

Visual impulses

S
A ←◆→ P
I

Reticular formation

Auditory impulses
Projection to
spinal cord

Ascending sensory tracts

Figure 3−8 • Reticular activating system. Consists of centers in the brain stem reticular formation plus fibers that conduct to the centers from below and fibers that conduct from the centers to widespread areas of the cerebral cortex. Functioning of the reticular activating system is essential for consciousness. (From Thibodeau, G. A., and Patton, K. T.: Anatomy and Physiology. St. Louis, Mosby-Year Book, 1993.)

 i. Circle of Willis: anastomosis of arteries at the base of the brain formed by the short segment of the internal carotid and anterior and posterior cerebral arteries that are connected by an anterior communicating artery and two posterior communicating arteries. This anastomosis may permit collateral circulation if one of the carotid or vertebral arteries becomes occluded

 ii. Internal carotid system: internal carotid arteries arise from common carotid arteries. Branches of this system include:

  (a) Anterior cerebral arteries: supply medial aspect of the frontal and parietal lobes and corpus callosum

  (b) Anterior communicating artery: connects the right and left anterior cerebral arteries

  (c) Middle cerebral arteries: supply most of the lateral surfaces of frontal, temporal, and parietal lobes; the largest branch of the internal carotid arteries

  (d) Posterior communicating arteries: connect the posterior cerebral arteries with the internal carotid arteries

 iii. Vertebral system: vertebral arteries arise from the subclavian arteries and join at the lower border of the pons to form the basilar artery. Branches of this system include:

  (a) Posterior cerebral arteries (PCAs): termination of branches of

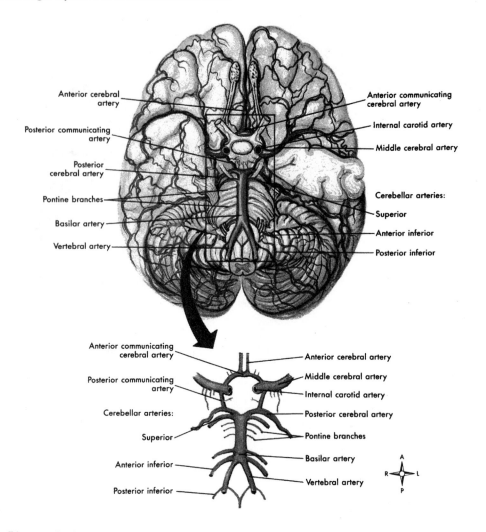

Figure 3-9 • Arteries at the base of the brain. The arteries that compose the circle of Willis are the two anterior cerebral arteries, joined to each other by the anterior communicating cerebral artery, and the posterior cerebral arteries, joined by the posterior communicating arteries. (From Thibodeau, G. A., and Patton, K. T.: Anatomy and Physiology. St. Louis, Mosby-Year Book, 1993.)

the basilar artery that supply the posterior parietal lobe and inferior portion of the temporal and occipital lobes
- (b) Superior cerebellar artery (SCA) and anterior inferior cerebellar (AICA) artery: branches of the basilar artery that supply brain stem
- (c) Posterior inferior cerebellar arteries (PICAs): branches of vertebral arteries that supply the posterior and inferior portions of the cerebellum
- (d) Anterior spinal artery: supplies anterior one half to three quarters of the spinal cord and medial aspect of the brain stem
- iv. Meningeal arteries: branches of the external carotid arteries that supply the dura mater
  - (a) Anterior meningeal artery: a branch of the ophthalmic artery that supplies the anterior portion of the dura, over the tips of the frontal lobes

       (b) Middle meningeal artery: a branch of the maxillary artery that supplies most of the dura (i.e., posterior portion of the frontal lobe, all of the temporal and parietal lobes, and part of the occipital lobe)

       (c) Posterior meningeal artery: supplies the dura mater of the occipital lobe. Arises from the occipital and vertebral arteries

       (d) Pia mater and arachnoid mater: derive their blood supply from the internal carotid and vertebral arteries

     v. Cerebral blood flow (CBF)

       (a) CBF varies with changes in cerebral perfusion pressure (CPP) and diameter of the cerebrovascular bed. CPP is the difference between mean arterial pressure (MAP) and intracranial pressure (ICP):

$$CPP = MAP - ICP$$

         (1) Normal MAP is 80 to 100 mm Hg
         (2) Normal ICP is 5 to 10 mm Hg
         (3) Normal CPP is 70 to 95 mm Hg

       (b) Diameter of the cerebrovascular bed is influenced by:
         (1) Autoregulation: an alteration in diameter of resistance vessels (arterioles) that maintains constant blood flow over a range of perfusion pressures by means of vasodilatation or vasoconstriction. Under normal circumstances, the limits of autoregulation are MAPs between 50 and 150 mm Hg
         (2) Increases in $Paco_2$ cause vasodilatation while decreases in $Paco_2$ cause vasoconstriction leading to increases or decreases in CBF, respectively
         (3) Hypoxemia also leads to vasodilation and increased CBF, although this effect is less powerful than $Paco_2$ changes

       (c) CBF is also influenced by stimulation of various areas of the brain. Seizure activity can increase CBF as much as four times to the involved areas of the brain

  b. Venous system: the cerebrum has external veins that lie in subarachnoid space on surfaces of hemispheres, and it has internal veins that drain the central core of cerebrum and lie beneath the corpus callosum (Fig. 3–10)

     i. Both external and internal venous systems empty into venous sinuses that lie between dural layers

       (a) Superior sagittal sinus: lies in attached border of the falx cerebri. Superior cerebral veins empty into it

       (b) Straight sinus: lies in midline attachment of the falx cerebri to the tentorium. Drains system of internal cerebral veins

       (c) Transverse sinuses: lie in the bony groove along the fixed edge of the tentorium cerebelli. Usually continuous with the straight sinus

       (d) Sigmoid sinuses: receive blood from the transverse sinuses and flow into the jugular foramina to form the internal jugular veins

       (e) Inferior sagittal sinus: lies along the free border of the falx cerebri. Receives blood from medial aspects of the hemispheres

       (f) Emissary veins: connect dural sinuses with veins outside the cranial cavity

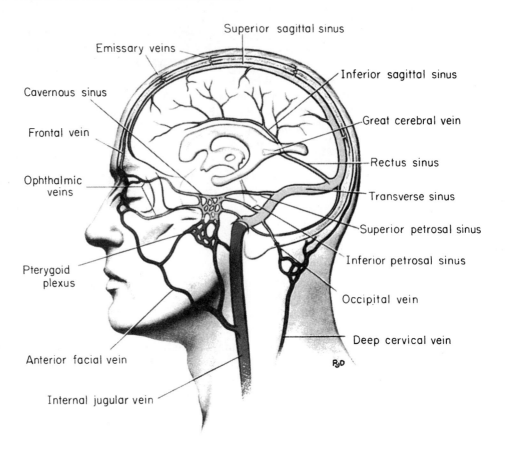

Figure 3–10 • The cranial dural venous sinuses and their principal connections with extracranial venous sinuses. The sigmoid portion of the transverse sinus continues as the internal jugular vein. (From Parent, A.: Carpenter's Human Neuroanatomy. Baltimore, Williams & Wilkins, 1996.)

      ii. Internal jugular veins: collect blood from the large dural venous sinuses

4. Ventricular system and CSF (Fig. 3–11)
  a. A communicating system within the brain, composed of four cavities containing CSF
    i. Lateral ventricles: the largest of the ventricles; one lies in each cerebral hemisphere. The anterior (frontal) horn of the lateral ventricles lies in the frontal lobe; the body extends back through the parietal lobe to the posterior (occipital) horn, which extends into the occipital lobe. The inferior (temporal) horn lies in the temporal lobe
    ii. Third ventricle: lies in midline between two lateral ventricles. Lateral walls are formed by the two thalami
    iii. Fourth ventricle: lies in posterior fossa and is continuous with the aqueduct of Sylvius superiorly and the central canal inferiorly
  b. Functions
    i. CSF cushions the brain and spinal cord and decreases their effective weight
    ii. Displacement of CSF out of the cranial cavity (and, to an extent, increased reabsorption of CSF) compensates for changes in intracranial volume/pressure

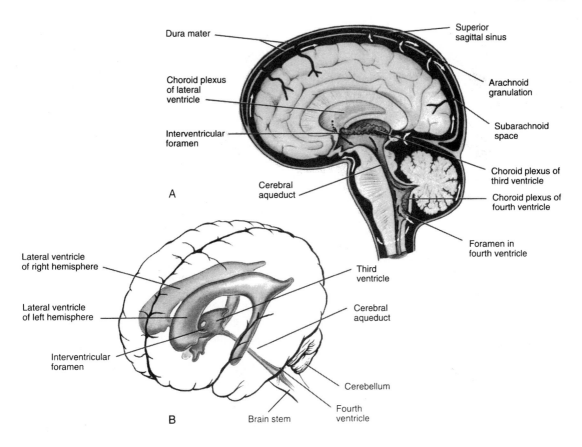

Figure 3–11 • Ventricular system. *A*, Circulation of cerebrospinal fluid. *B*, Ventricles of the brain. (Modified from Applegate, E. J.: The Anatomy and Physiology Learning Systems Textbook. Philadelphia, W. B. Saunders, 1995.)

c. Properties
  i. Clear, colorless, odorless
  ii. Specific gravity: 1.007
  iii. pH: 7.35
  iv. Chloride: 120 to 130 mEq/L
  v. Sodium: 140 to 142 mEq/L
  vi. Glucose: 60% of serum glucose level
  vii. Protein
    (a) Lumbar: 15 to 45 mg/dl
    (b) Cisternal: 10 to 25 mg/dl
    (c) Ventricular: 5 to 15 mg/dl
  viii. Cells
    (a) White blood cells (WBCs): 0 to 5/mm³
    (b) Red blood cells (RBCs): 0/mm³
  ix. Ventricular system and subarachnoid space contain approximately 125 to 150 ml of CSF; rate of synthesis is estimated to be 500 ml/day. CSF is distributed as follows:
    (a) 90 ml in lumbar subarachnoid space
    (b) 25 ml in ventricles
    (c) 35 ml in rest of subarachnoid space

x. Pressure: 80 to 180 mm water, measured at the lumbar level, with the patient in the lateral decubitus position

d. Formation

i. Choroid plexus: tuft of capillaries covered by epithelial cells. Principal source of CSF; found within all ventricles

ii. Most of the CSF (95%) is produced in the lateral ventricles; remainder is formed in third and fourth ventricles

iii. Small amounts may be produced by blood vessels of brain and meningeal linings

iv. Process of osmosis across walls of choroid plexus believed to be responsible for most of the CSF produced, although composition differs from a simple ultrafiltrate of plasma. Active transport of Na^+, K^+, and Cl^- creates an osmotic gradient favoring movement of water across epithelial cells of choroid plexus into the ventricles

e. Circulation of CSF (Fig. 3–12)

i. CSF circulates from lateral ventricles through the interventricular foramen (foramina of Monro) to the third ventricle and, via the aqueduct of Sylvius, to the fourth ventricle

ii. From the fourth ventricle, CSF circulates to the cisterna and subarachnoid space via the foramina of Luschka and Magendie

f. Absorption

i. Arachnoid granulations consist of numerous arachnoid villi located along the superior sagittal sinus and other large sinuses

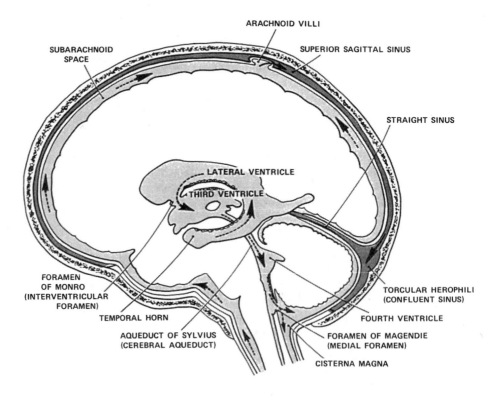

Figure 3–12 • Diagram of the circulation of the cerebrospinal fluid. (From Gilman, S., and Newman, S. W.: Manter and Gatz's Essentials of Neuroanatomy and Neurophysiology, 8th ed. Philadelphia, F. A. Davis, 1992.)

    ii. Most CSF is absorbed via arachnoid villi that project from the subarachnoid space into the dural sinuses

    iii. Hydrostatic pressure gradient between the CSF and venous sinus is one factor that determines CSF absorption

5. Cells of the nervous system (Fig. 3–13)

    a. Neurons: transmitters of nerve impulses (information)

        i. 10 billion in the central nervous system (CNS)

        ii. Functions include:

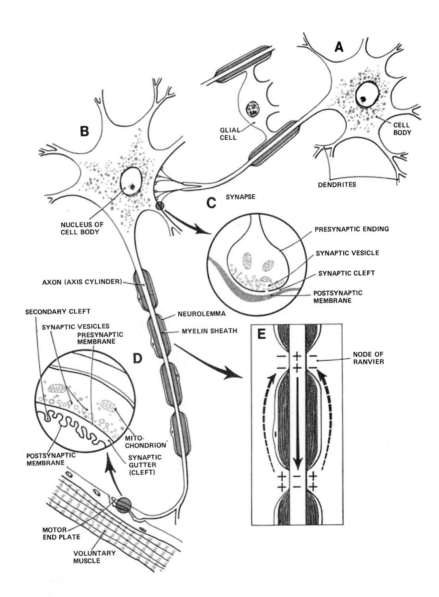

Figure 3–13 • Neurons of the central nervous system (CNS). Neuron *A* is confined to the CNS and terminates on neuron *B* at a typical chemical synapse *(C)*. Neuron *B* is a ventral horn cell; its axon extends into a peripheral nerve and innervates a striated (voluntary) muscle at the myoneural junction (motor end-plate) *(D)*. *E,* The action potential is moving in the direction of the *solid arrow* inside the axon; the *dashed arrows* indicate the direction of flow of the action current. (From Gilman, S., and Newman, S. W.: Manter and Gatz's Essentials of Neuroanatomy and Neurophysiology, 8th ed. Philadelphia, F. A. Davis, 1992.)

(a) Receiving input from other neurons, primarily via dendrites and cell body

(b) Summation of inhibitory or excitatory postsynaptic potentials, eventually leading to an *action potential* (AP)

(c) Conducting action potentials along the axon-to-axon terminal

(d) Transferring information by synaptic transmission to other neurons, muscle cells, or gland cells

iii. Components of each cell

(a) Cell body (soma or perikaryon): carries out metabolic functions of cell; contains nucleus and cytoplasmic organelles (i.e., neurofibrils, neurofilaments, microtubules, Nissl material, endoplasmic reticulum, mitochondria, Golgi apparatus)

(b) Dendrites (see Fig. 3–13*A*): extensions of cell body that conduct impulses toward cell body. The dendritic zone is the receptive area of the neuron. Each neuron may have numerous dendrites

(c) Axon hillock (see Fig. 3–13*B*): thickened area of cell body from which the axon originates

(d) Axon: conducts impulses away from the cell body; usually myelinated. Outside the brain, axons are also covered with neurilemma. Each neuron possesses one axon

(e) Myelin sheath: a white protein-lipid complex that surrounds some axons; laid down by Schwann cells in the peripheral nervous system and by oligodendrocytes in the CNS

(f) Nodes of Ranvier (see Fig. 3–13*E*): periodic constrictions along the axon, where it is not covered by myelin. Impulse is conducted from node to node (saltatory conduction) and thus is more rapid and efficient

(g) Synaptic knobs (terminal buttons or axon telodendria) (Fig. 3–13*C, D*): contain vesicles in which neurotransmitter substances are stored

iv. Neuroglial cells: form supporting structure for the CNS

(a) About 10 times as numerous as neurons

(b) Four types:

(1) Microglia: no special function known under normal conditions, but they phagocytize tissue debris when nervous tissue is damaged

(2) Oligodendroglia: responsible for myelin formation. Seem to have a symbiotic relationship with nerve cells within the CNS

(3) Astrocytes: function uncertain. Send many end-feet to blood vessels, provide nutrients for neurons, and contribute to basic structure of the blood-brain barrier. Constitute structural and supporting framework for nerve cells and capillaries

(4) Ependyma: specialized glial tissue lining ventricles of the brain and central canal of the spinal cord

6. Brain metabolism

a. Carbohydrate

i. The brain has high metabolic energy requirements and utilizes glucose as its principal source of energy in production of adenosine triphosphate (ATP), necessary in cellular processes

      ii. Although glycogen is present in small amounts, glycolysis is not sufficient to maintain adequate production of ATP

     iii. Glucose serves as major contributor in building amino acids and fatty acids, and is source of carbon dioxide (CO_2), which helps to regulate pH

     iv. Hypoglycemia depresses cerebral metabolism and may lead to convulsions, coma, and death

      v. Hyperglycemia contributes to cell death of injured brain cells. May cause intracellular dehydration with resultant cerebral dysfunction

b. Oxygen

      i. Cerebral oxygen (O_2) consumption averages about 49 ml/minute, or about 20% of total-body resting O_2 consumption

     ii. Constant supply of O_2 is essential to normal brain function; cytotoxic cerebral edema results within seconds of anoxia

     iii. Basal cerebral energy requirements are usually met by oxidative metabolism of glucose (the Krebs cycle), but the rate of glycolysis increases markedly during hypoxia in an attempt to maintain functional neuronal activity

c. Blood-brain barrier: special permeability characteristics of brain capillaries and choroid plexus that act to limit transfer of certain substances into extracellular fluid (ECF) or CSF of the brain. Is thought to be due to unique membranous ultrastructure of endothelial cells of vessels in the brain with "tight" junctions and the end-feet projections of astrocytes

      i. Water, CO_2, O_2, and glucose cross cerebral capillaries with ease. Uptake of other substances, such as ions, is much slower

     ii. Maintains homeostatic environment of neurons in the CNS by determining level of metabolism and ionic composition of tissue fluids

     iii. Of clinical significance in treatment and diagnosis of CNS disease. The blood-brain barrier is often disrupted in injured tissue, leading to increased permeability

     iv. The blood-CSF barrier permits selective transport from blood to ventricular system. Substances placed into CSF diffuse readily into interstitial fluid of brain

d. Vitamins: several vitamins are essential for normal CNS functioning. Because these vitamins function as coenzymes, deficiencies cause neurologic symptoms, probably by reducing activity of one or more enzyme systems

      i. Thiamine (vitamin B_1): important in formation of compounds of the Krebs cycle. Deficiencies cause necrosis of cell bodies of cranial nerve nuclei in the brain stem and in areas of the diencephalon

     ii. Vitamin B_{12}: deficiencies lead to combined subacute degeneration of the spinal cord and peripheral nerves, although the exact mechanism is not clearly established

     iii. Pyridoxine (B_6): seizures appear to be the principal reaction to deficiency

     iv. Nicotinic acid: deficiencies cause pellagra, characterized by dermatitis and disturbances in mentation

e. Cerebral neurotransmitters: chemical mediators of nerve impulse transmission

      i. Acetylcholine (Ach): found in cholinergic fibers of the autonomic nervous system (ANS) and nerves to skeletal muscles. May also be involved in drinking behavior

    ii. Norepinephrine (NE): found in the adrenergic fibers of the ANS and produced in the locus coeruleus nucleus of the brain stem. Implicated in feeding behavior, temperature control, and sleep, particularly paradoxical, or rapid eye movement (REM) sleep

    iii. Dopamine (DA): found in the substantia nigra and corpus striatum. Acts as an inhibitory transmitter (e.g., inhibits release of prolactin). Found in decreased amounts in Parkinson's disease. Associated with eating and drinking behavior and, possibly, with sexual behavior

    iv. Gamma-aminobutyric acid (GABA): found at some synaptic junctions and in substantia nigra. Acts as an inhibitory transmitter. Found in decreased amounts in patients with Huntington's chorea

    v. Serotonin (5-HT): produced in raphe nuclei of the brain stem. Also found in high concentrations in hypothalamus, midbrain, and caudate nucleus. Implicated in sleep behavior, particularly slow-wave, and possibly REM sleep

    vi. Glutamate: a neuroexcitatory transmitter substance. Released in large amounts when brain cells are injured by mechanical trauma or hypoxia–ischemia. Hypoxic-ischemic changes are attributed in part to glutamate, which affects the hippocampus in particular

        (a) Glutamate is a potent and rapidly acting neurotoxin by activating N-methyl-D-aspartate (NMDA) receptor complex

        (b) Neurotoxicity may be mediated by the influx of calcium through NMDA receptors

        (c) Produces cellular swelling due to entry of sodium chloride and water

        (d) Neurotoxicity may be blocked by NMDA receptor antagonists

7. Synaptic transmission of impulses

    a. Nerve impulse: nerve cells that are excited by electrical, chemical, or mechanical stimuli produce an impulse that is transmitted (or conducted) along the nerve fibers in an active, self-propagating process requiring expenditure of energy. This mechanism allows one part of the body to "communicate" with other parts

    b. Synapse: a junction between one neuron and the next that permits unidirectional conduction of an impulse from presynaptic to postsynaptic neurons (Fig. 3–13C)

    c. Excitatory neurotransmitter: a substance secreted by presynaptic knobs or vesicles (usually located at axon terminal) that excite a postsynaptic neuron. Released when a cell membrane is polarized by a nerve impulse

    d. Depolarization: causes increase in permeability of a cell membrane, resulting in intracellular flow of sodium ions

        i. Increased levels of intracellular Na^+ cause a decrease in resting membrane potential (RMP)

        ii. RMP is the voltage difference across a cell membrane, with inside negative to outside

        iii. A change in RMP is called the *excitatory postsynaptic potential* (EPSP)

    e. Action potential: if transient voltage change that occurs with depolarization is of sufficient magnitude (i.e., threshold level), an action potential occurs. Once initiated, it is self-propagated and spreads like a wave over the membrane

f. Summation: simultaneous excitation of successively greater numbers of excitatory presynaptic terminals (or rapidly successive discharges from same presynaptic terminal) that cause progressive increase in postsynaptic potential
   i. Facilitation: if summated postsynaptic potential is less than its threshold for excitation, a neuron is said to be facilitated but not excited. No action potential occurs
   ii. Rate of discharge of neuron depends on summated postsynaptic potential in relation to threshold for excitation
      (a) *Complete* refraction: a neuron is incapable of producing an action potential. Limits frequency of impulses that a cell can generate
      (b) *Relative* refraction: a neuron can be excited again but only with summation above the threshold
g. Repolarization
   i. At peak of action potential, a cell membrane again becomes impermeable to Na^+, and the RMP is reestablished
   ii. Cell also becomes more permeable to K^+, and RMP returns with aid of the Na^+-K^+ pump, which pumps Na^+ out of the cell and K^+ into the cell
h. Inhibition
   i. Inhibitory postsynaptic potential (IPSP)
      (a) Hyperpolarization of the cell membrane is caused by secretion of an inhibitory transmitter (perhaps gamma-aminobutyric acid [GABA]) by presynaptic terminals of inhibitory neurons
      (b) Results in increase in negativity of RMP caused by increased permeability of cells to K^+ and Cl^-
      (c) Causes decreased excitability and inhibition of impulse transmission
   ii. Presynaptic inhibition: causes inhibition by reducing amount of neurotransmitter substance released from excitatory presynaptic endings, thus reducing to subthreshold levels the magnitude of EPSP they produce

Spine and Spinal Cord (Fig. 3–14)

1. Vertebral column
   a. Composed of 33 vertebrae
      i. Cervical
         (a) Seven vertebrae that support muscles of head and neck
         (b) Smallest of all of the vertebrae
         (c) Atlas (first cervical vertebra): articulates with the occipital bone superiorly and with axis inferiorly
         (d) Axis (second cervical vertebra)
            (1) Articulates with the atlas and allows for rotation of the head
            (2) Odontoid process (dens): a projection of the axis that articulates with the atlas
      ii. Thoracic
         (a) Twelve vertebrae
         (b) Articulate with ribs and support muscles of chest

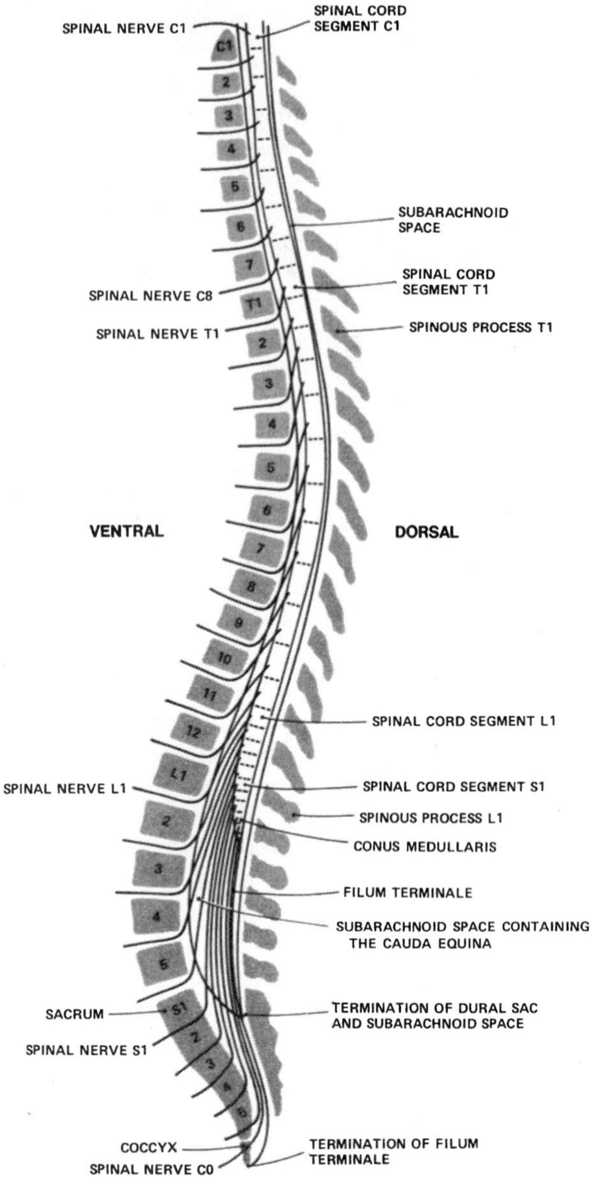

Figure 3-14 • Relationship of the spinal cord segments and spinal nerve roots to the dural sac and vertebrae of the spinal column. The bodies of the individual vertebrae on the ventral side of the spinal cord are numbered. The spinous processes of the vertebrae are dorsal to the spinal cord. (From Gilman, S., and Newman, S. W.: Manter and Gatz's Essentials of Neuroanatomy and Neurophysiology, 8th ed. Philadelphia, F. A. Davis, 1992.)

iii. Lumbar
   (a) Five vertebrae that support the back muscles
   (b) Largest and strongest of the vertebrae
   (c) Site of most herniated intervertebral discs
iv. Sacral: five vertebrae fused to form a large triangular bone (the sacrum)
v. Coccygeal: four rudimentary vertebrae with rudimentary bodies, articulating facets, and transverse processes
b. Typical vertebra
   i. Body: solid portion of the vertebra, lying anteriorly
   ii. Arch: made up of:
      (a) Spinous process

(b) Transverse processes, one on either side of the spinous process

(c) Lamina, which connects the spinous process to the transverse process

iii. Articular processes: portions of the vertebra that come into contact with vertebrae above and below

iv. Intervertebral foramina: openings through which spinal nerves pass

v. Spinal foramina: openings through which the spinal cord passes

vi. Intervertebral disc

(a) Layer of fibrocartilage between bodies of adjoining vertebrae

(b) Acts as a shock absorber

(c) Composed of the anulus fibrosus (tough outer layer) and the nucleus pulposus (gelatinous inner layer)

2. Spinal cord

a. Location: extends from the superior border of the atlas (first cervical vertebra) to the upper border of the second lumbar vertebra

i. Continuous with the medulla oblongata

ii. Conus medullaris: caudal end of the spinal cord

iii. Central canal: opening in the center of the spinal cord that contains CSF and is continuous with the fourth ventricle

iv. Filum terminale: a non-neural filament that extends from the conus medullaris to its attachment to the first coccygeal segment; no known functional significance

b. Meninges: continuous with layers covering the brain

i. Pia mater: vascular, attached to spinal cord, spinal roots, and filum terminale

ii. Arachnoid mater: extends to second sacral level, where it merges with the filum terminale

(a) Subarachnoid space: contains CSF and surrounds the spinal cord

(b) Lumbar cistern: the subarachnoid space between the conus medullaris and the second sacral level

iii. Dura mater: surrounds arachnoid and merges with filum terminale. Ends as a blind sac at the second sacral vertebra

c. Gray matter (Fig. 3–15)

i. An H-shaped, internal mass of gray substance surrounded by white matter

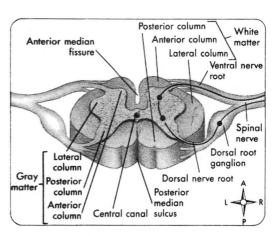

F i g u r e 3 – 1 5 • Spinal cord. Transverse section of the spinal cord shown in the broader view. (From Thibodeau, G. A., and Patton, K. T.: Anatomy and Physiology. St. Louis, Mosby-Year Book, 1993.)

     ii. Anterior gray column (anterior horn): contains cell bodies of efferent or motor fibers

    iii. Lateral column: contains preganglionic fibers of the autonomic nervous system. Is prominent in the upper cervical, thoracic, and midsacral regions

    iv. Posterior gray column (posterior horn): contains cell bodies of afferent or sensory fibers

d. White matter (see Fig. 3–15)

     i. Composed of three longitudinal columns (funiculi): anterior, lateral, and posterior

    ii. Contains mostly myelinated axons

    iii. Funiculi contain tracts (fasciculi) that are functionally distinct (i.e., they have the same or a similar origin, course, and termination) and are classified as:

     (a) Ascending or sensory tracts: pathways to the brain for impulses entering the cord via the dorsal root of the spinal nerves

     (b) Descending or motor tracts: transmit impulses from the brain to motor neurons of the spinal cord and exit via the ventral root of the spinal nerves

     (c) Short ascending and descending fibers that begin in one area of the spinal cord and terminate in another

    iv. Each tract is named to indicate:

     (a) The column in which it travels

     (b) Location of its cells of origin

     (c) Location of axon termination

     v. Ascending (sensory) tracts of clinical significance (Fig. 3–16)

     (a) Fasciculus gracilis and fasciculus cuneatus: posterior white columns

      (1) Fibers enter the dorsal root of the spinal nerve and ascend in the posterior funiculus

      (2) Tracts convey position and vibratory sense, joint and two-point discrimination, tactile localization

     (b) Lateral spinothalamic tract

      (1) Originates in the posterior horn; crosses over via the anterior white commissure to the contralateral funiculus before ascending to the thalamus

      (2) Conveys pain and temperature sensation

     (c) Anterior spinothalamic tract

      (1) Originates in the posterior horn; crosses over to the opposite side of the cord via the anterior white commissure and ascends to the thalamus in anterolateral funiculus

      (2) Conveys light touch, pressure, and sensation to pain and temperature

     (d) Dorsal and ventral spinocerebellar tracts

      (1) Originate in the posterior horn; ascend to the cerebellum via lateral funiculus. The dorsal tract is uncrossed; the ventral tract is crossed

      (2) Convey proprioceptive data that influence muscle tone and synergy

     (e) Spinotectal tract

      (1) Originates in cells of the posterior horn

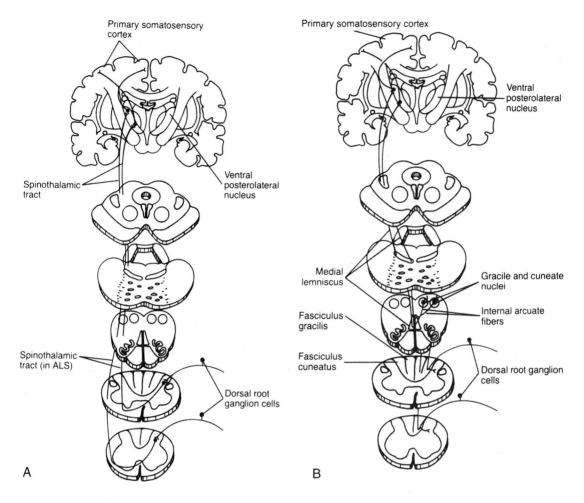

Figure 3-16 • *A,* Simplified schematic diagram of the course of the spinothalamic tract, from the spinal cord to the primary somatosensory cortex. The spinothalamic, spinotectal, and spinoreticular tracts make up the anterolateral system (ALS). *B,* Course of the ascending doral column/medial lemniscal pathway, from the spinal cord to the primary somatosensory cortex. (From Burt, A. M.: Textbook of Neuroanatomy. Philadelphia, W. B. Saunders, 1993.)

   (2) Transmits general sensory information to the tectum (roof) of the midbrain

  vi. Descending (motor) tracts of clinical significance

   (a) Rubrospinal tract

    (1) Originates in the red nucleus of the midbrain; receives fibers from the cerebellum and descends in the lateral funiculus

    (2) Conveys impulses to control muscle tone and synergy

   (b) Ventral and lateral corticospinal tracts (Fig. 3–17)

    (1) Originate in the cerebral cortical motor areas and descend in the lateral and anterior funiculi

    (2) Carry impulses for voluntary movement

   (c) Tectospinal tract

    (1) Originates in the superior colliculus; descends in the anterior funiculus

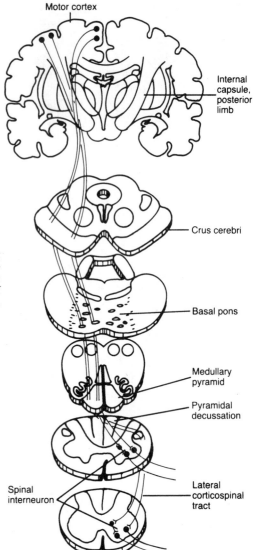

Figure 3–17 • Course of the descending lateral corticospinal tract from the motor cortex to the cervical and lumbar levels of the spinal cord. (From Burt, A. M.: Textbook of Neuroanatomy. Philadelphia, W. B. Saunders, 1993.)

(2) Mediates optic and auditory reflexes (e.g., reflexive head turning in response to visual or auditory stimuli)

    e. Upper and lower motor neurons (Fig. 3–18)

        i. Lower motor neurons (LMNs) are spinal and cranial motor neurons that directly innervate muscles. Lesions of spinal or cranial nerve motor neurons cause flaccid paralysis, muscular atrophy, and absence of reflex responses

        ii. Upper motor neurons (UMNs) in the brain and spinal cord activate lower motor neurons. UMN lesions are associated with spastic paralysis, increased tone, hyperactive reflexes, clonus, Babinski's sign, and Hoffman's reflex

3. Reflexes (Fig. 3–19)

    a. Monosynaptic reflex arc

        i. Stimulation of large afferent nerve fibers sends impulses to the spinal cord through the dorsal roots of the spinal nerve

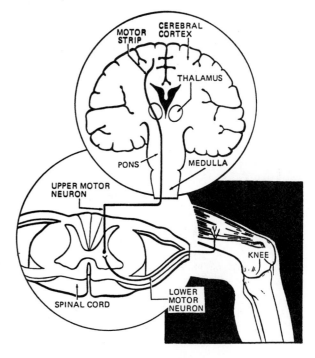

Figure 3-18 • Upper and lower motor neurons. (From Snyder, M., and Jackle, A.: Critical Care Nursing Focus. Bowie, Md., Robert J. Brady Co., 1981.)

      ii. Impulse synapses with anterior motor neurons, sending out an efferent discharge that is confined to axons supplying muscle from which the afferent impulse originated

  b. Polysynaptic reflex arc

      i. Stimulation of small afferent axons of muscle nerves causes synapses with interneurons, leading to asynchronous discharge of motor neurons

      ii. Polysynaptic discharge is distributed in motor axons supplying ipsilateral flexor muscles and contralateral extensor muscles

  c. Law of reciprocal innervation: impulses that excite motor neurons supplying a particular muscle also inhibit motor neurons of antagonistic muscles

Peripheral Nervous System

1. Spinal nerves

  a. Thirty-one symmetrically arranged pairs of nerves, each possessing a sensory (dorsal) root and a motor (ventral) root: eight cervical pairs, 12 thoracic pairs, five lumbar pairs, five sacral pairs, one coccygeal pair

  b. Fibers of the spinal nerve

      i. Meningeal branches: carry sensory and vasomotor innervation to spinal meninges

      ii. Motor fibers: originate in the anterior gray column of the spinal cord, form ventral root of spinal nerve and pass to skeletal muscles

      iii. Sensory fibers: originate in the spinal ganglia of the dorsal roots; peripheral branches distribute to visceral and somatic structures as mediators of sensory impulses to the CNS

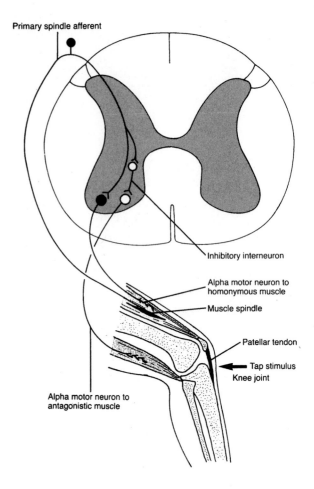

Figure 3–19 • The tendon reflex. The inhibitory interneurons are open: the excitatory neurons and excited lower motor neurons are solid. (From Burt, A. M.: Textbook of Neuroanatomy. Philadelphia, W. B. Saunders, 1993.)

iv. Autonomic fibers
  (a) Sympathetic
     (1) Originate from cells that lie between the posterior and anterior gray columns from the first thoracic to the second lumbar cord segment
     (2) Innervate viscera, blood vessels, glands, and smooth muscle
  (b) Parasympathetic
     (1) Arise from neurons of the third, seventh, ninth, and tenth cranial nerves and sacral cord segments S2–4
     (2) Pass to pelvic and lower abdominal viscera and smooth muscles and glands of head
 v. Cauda equina: spinal nerves arising from the lumbosacral portion of the spinal cord contained within the lumbar cistern
c. Dermatomes (Fig. 3–20): area of the skin supplied by dorsal roots (sensory innervation) of a single spinal nerve
d. Plexuses: network of spinal nerve roots
  i. Cervical
    (a) Composed of anterior rami of C1–4
    (b) Has cutaneous, motor, and phrenic branches
  ii. Brachial
    (a) Composed of anterior rami of C5–8 and T1

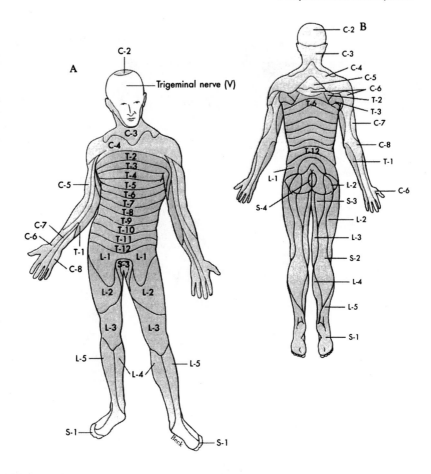

Figure 3–20 • Dermatome distribution of spinal nerves. *A*, Front of the body. *B*, Back of the body. C = cervical spinal nerves; T = thoracic spinal nerves; L = lumbar spinal nerves; S = sacral spinal nerves. (From Thibodeau, G. A., and Patton, K. T.: Anatomy and Physiology. St. Louis, Mosby-Year Book, 1993.)

        (b) Includes circumflex, musculocutaneous, ulnar, median, and radial nerves

    iii. Lumbar

        (a) Composed of anterior rami of L1–4

        (b) Includes lateral femoral cutaneous, femoral, and genitofemoral branches

    iv. Sacral

        (a) Composed of anterior rami of L4–5 and S1–4

        (b) Includes sciatic and pudendal branches

2. Neuromuscular transmission (Fig. 3–21)

  a. Physiologic anatomy

      i. Motor end-plate (neuromuscular junction): specialized region where motor axon loses its myelin sheath and splays out in a flattened plate close to the muscle fiber membrane

     ii. Synaptic cleft: space between the nerve terminal and the muscle fiber membrane

    iii. Synaptic gutter: area of the muscle fiber membrane characterized by

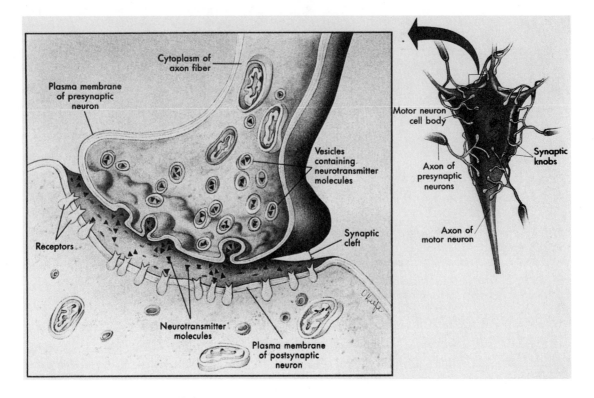

Figure 3–21 • Structure of a synapse. The synaptic knob, or axon terminal, of a presynaptic neuron, the plasma membrane of a postsynaptic neuron, and a synaptic cleft are shown. On arrival of an action potential at a synaptic knob, neurotransmitter molecules are released from vesicles in the knob into the synaptic cleft. The combining of neurotransmitter and receptor molecules in the plasma membrane of the postsynaptic neuron initiates impulse conduction in the postsynaptic neuron. (From Thibodeau, G. A., and Patton, K. T.: Anatomy and Physiology. St. Louis, Mosby-Year Book, 1993.)

  numerous folds, which increase the surface area available for a neurotransmitter substance to act

  iv. Vesicles: structures of nerve terminal that store and release the neurotransmitter substance acetylcholine (ACh)

 b. Release of ACh: when action potential reaches the neuromuscular junction, vesicles release ACh into the synaptic cleft. Amount released depends on the magnitude of action potential and presence of calcium. ACh attaches to receptor sites on the postjunctional muscle membrane and increases its permeability to Na^+ and K^+

 c. End-plate potential: motor-nerve action potential caused by depolarization owing to Na^+ influx and K^+ efflux. Differs from action potential, in that it is local (i.e., nonpropagated) and graded, rather than all-or-nothing

 d. Muscle contraction: action potentials are subsequently formed on either side of the end-plate and conducted in both directions along muscle fiber, initiating a series of events that result in muscle contraction

 e. Acetylcholinesterase (AChE): catalyzes hydrolysis of ACh to choline and acetic acid and thus limits duration of ACh action on the end-plate and ensures production of only one action potential. ACh is then resynthesized in presence of choline acetylase and coenzyme A acetate

3. Cranial nerves (Fig. 3–22)
    a. Olfactory nerve (I)
        i. Receptors are located in nasal mucosa. The axons from these cells form the olfactory nerve, which passes to the olfactory bulb, which then forms the olfactory tract
        ii. A sensory nerve responsible for smell
    b. Optic nerve (II)
        i. Fibers originate from ganglion cells of the retina. At the optic chiasm, optic nerve fibers from the nasal half of the retina cross; those from the temporal half do not. Fibers continue as optic tracts to lateral geniculate bodies of the thalamus and then as geniculocalcarine tracts to the occipital cortex
        ii. A sensory nerve responsible for vision
    c. Oculomotor nerve (III)
        i. Nuclei are located in the midbrain. Preganglionic parasympathetic fibers originate in the Edinger-Westphal nucleus and accompany other oculomotor fibers into the orbit, where they terminate in ciliary ganglion. Postganglionic fibers pass to the constrictor pupillae

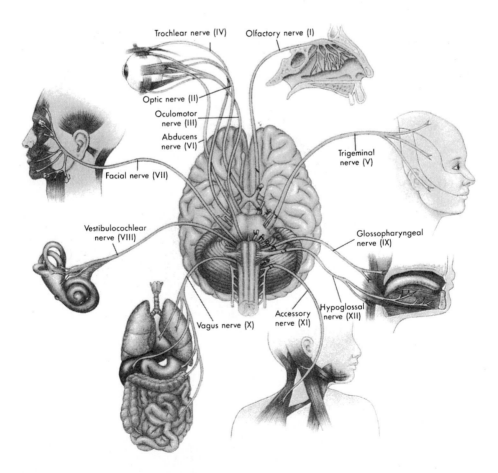

Figure 3–22 • Cranial nerves. Ventral surface of the brain showing attachment of the cranial nerves. (From Thibodeau, G. A., and Patton, K. T.: Anatomy and Physiology. St. Louis, Mosby-Year Book, 1993.)

and ciliary muscles of the eye to cause pupillary constriction in response to light

    ii. Motor fibers supply extraocular muscles

       (a) Inferior rectus (depresses and adducts the eye)

       (b) Medial rectus (adducts the eye)

       (c) Superior rectus (elevates and adducts the eye)

       (d) Inferior oblique (elevates and abducts the eye)

       (e) Levator palpebrae (raises the upper eyelid)

d. Trochlear nerve (IV)

    i. Originates caudal to oculomotor nucleus in the midbrain. It is the only cranial nerve to originate from the dorsal aspect of the brain stem

    ii. Supplies the superior oblique muscle, which intorts the eye when abducted and depresses the eye when adducted

e. Trigeminal nerve (V)

    i. Sensory fibers arise from cells in the semilunar ganglion. The nerve is attached to the lateral aspect of the pons. Motor fibers leave the pons ventromedial to sensory roots

    ii. Three sensory divisions

       (a) Ophthalmic branch provides sensation to the forehead, upper eyelid, cornea, conjunctiva, nose, temples, paranasal sinuses, and part of the nasal mucosa

       (b) Maxillary branch provides sensation to the upper jaw, teeth, upper lip, upper cheek, hard palate, maxillary sinuses, and nasal mucosa

       (c) Mandibular branch provides sensation to the lower jaw, teeth, lip, buccal mucosa, tongue, part of the external ear, and auditory meatus

       (d) All three divisions contribute sensory fibers to the meninges

    iii. Motor fibers innervate muscles of mastication

       (a) Temporalis

       (b) Masseter

       (c) Medial and lateral pterygoid muscles

f. Abducens nerve (VI)

    i. Emerges at the caudal border of the pons near the midline. Enters the orbit with cranial nerves III and IV

    ii. Supplies the lateral rectus muscle, which abducts the eye

g. Facial nerve (VII)

    i. Fibers originate in the caudal portion of the pons at the junction of the pons and medulla, lateral to cranial nerve VI

    ii. Motor portions of nerve innervate all muscles of facial expression as well as salivary and lacrimal glands. The sensory portion of the nerve conveys taste from the anterior two thirds of the tongue

h. Acoustic nerve (VIII) (vestibulocochlear nerve)

    i. Nerve emerges from the brain stem at the pontomedullary junction. Two divisions included:

       (a) Cochlear nerve: fibers from cells in the spiral ganglion end either in the organ of Corti (peripheral fibers) or in the ventral and dorsal cochlear nuclei in the medulla (central fibers). Fibers from these nuclei synapse in the medial geniculate nuclei of the thalamus and then on the auditory cortex of the temporal lobe

(b) Vestibular nerve: fibers from cells in the vestibular ganglion pass to semicircular canals and saccules (peripheral fibers) and vestibular nuclei in brain stem (central fibers)

    ii. Cochlear nerve is responsible for hearing; vestibular nerve aids in maintaining equilibrium and coordinating head and eye movements

i. Glossopharyngeal nerve (IX)

    i. Sensory fibers arise from cells at the back of the tongue, the pharynx, and the palate and enter the medulla behind the facial nerve. Motor fibers originate from the nucleus in the medulla to innervate the stylopharyngeus muscle

    ii. Sensory fibers provide sensation to the pharynx, soft palate, and posterior third of tongue. They also supply special receptors in the carotid body and carotid sinus, which are concerned with reflex control of respiration, blood pressure, and heart rate

    iii. Motor fibers participate with the vagus nerve in swallowing mechanism

j. Vagus nerve (X)

    i. Sensory fibers originate in cells in ganglia just below the jugular foramen and enter the medulla just behind the glossopharyngeal nerve. Motor fibers leave the medulla and join the sensory part of the nerve. Parasympathetic fibers are distributed to the abdominal and thoracic viscera

    ii. Sensory fibers provide sensation to the palate and pharynx (along with IX) and to larynx (X alone)

    iii. Motor fibers innervate palatal muscles, pharyngeal muscles (along with IX), and laryngeal muscles

    iv. Postganglionic parasympathetic fibers inhibit the heart rate and adrenal secretion; they stimulate gastrointestinal peristalsis and gastric, hepatic, and pancreatic glandular secretion

k. Spinal accessory nerve (XI)

    i. Motor fibers arise from the lateral surface of the medulla and upper cervical spinal cord

    ii. Supplies the trapezius (elevates shoulders) and sternocleidomastoid muscles; tilts, turns, and thrusts head forward

l. Hypoglossal nerve (XII)

    i. Motor fibers originate in the ventromedial sulcus of the medulla

    ii. Innervates muscles of the tongue

4. Autonomic nervous system (Fig. 3–23)

a. Structure

    i. Composed of two neuron chains

    ii. Preganglionic cell bodies are located within the lateral gray column of the spinal cord or the homologous motor nuclei of the cranial nerves

    iii. Most preganglionic axons are myelinated and synapse on cell bodies of postganglionic neurons located outside the CNS

    iv. Axons of postganglionic neurons terminate on visceral effectors

b. Divisions

    i. Sympathetic (thoracolumbar)

        (a) Preganglionic axons leave the spinal cord in the ventral roots of T1 and L2 and pass to:

            (1) Paravertebral sympathetic ganglion chain via white rami

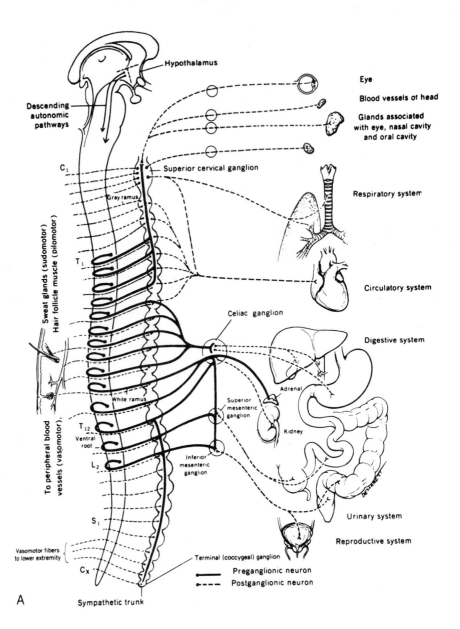

Figure 3–23 • Autonomic nervous system. *A*, Sympathetic division. The preganglionic neurons are cholinergic; most of the postganglionic neurons are adrenergic. The white communicating rami (preganglionic fibers) are limited to spinal levels T1 through L2 or L3. The gray communicating rami (postganglionic fibers) are presented at all spinal levels.

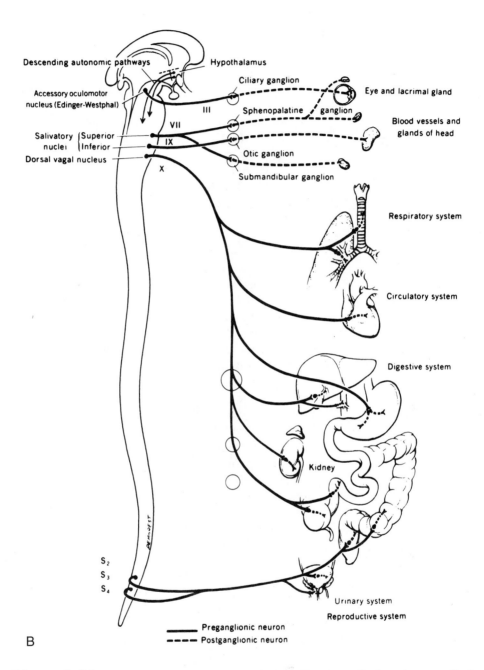

Figure 3-23 • *(Continued) B,* Parasympathetic division. The preganglionic and postganglionic neurons are cholinergic. Preganglionic fibers exit from the brain stem with cranial nerves III, VII, IX, and X and from the sacral levels of the spinal cord. (From Noback, C. R., and Demarest, R. J.: The Human Nervous System, 3rd ed. New York, McGraw-Hill, 1984.)

communicantes, ending on cell bodies of the postganglionic neurons

    (2) Collateral ganglia, ending on postganglionic neurons close to the viscera

(b) Postganglionic axons pass to:

    (1) Viscera via sympathetic nerves

    (2) Gray rami communicantes, and are distributed to autonomic effectors in areas supplied by these spinal nerves

(c) Segmental distribution of sympathetic fibers

    (1) T1: up the sympathetic chain to the head

    (2) T2: into neck

    (3) T3–6: thorax

    (4) T7–11: abdomen

    (5) T12, L1–2: legs

(d) Functions

    (1) Generally antagonistic to parasympathetic activity

    (2) Can synapse with many postganglionic fibers

    (3) Sympathetic stimulation dilates pupils and bronchioles, relaxes smooth muscles of the gastrointestinal (GI) tract, increases blood pressure by constricting blood vessels, increases heart rate, increases secretion of the adrenal medulla

    (4) Brought into widespread activity under emergency conditions ("fight or flight" response); gives rise to mass responses of body systems

ii. Parasympathetic (craniosacral)

(a) Preganglionic cell bodies are in the gray matter of the brain stem and middle three segments of the sacral cord

(b) Preganglionic fibers end on short postganglionic neurons located on or near visceral structures

(c) Supplies visceral structures in the head via oculomotor (III), facial (VII), and glossopharyngeal (IX) cranial nerves and those in the thorax and upper abdomen via the vagus nerves

(d) Sacral outflow supplies the pelvic viscera via the pelvic branches of S2–4

(e) Gives rise to localized reactions rather than mass action of sympathetic stimulation

(f) Parasympathetic stimulation

    (1) Constricts pupils

    (2) Contracts smooth muscle of stomach, intestine, and bladder

    (3) Slows heart rate

    (4) Stimulates secretion of most glands

c. Chemical mediation: the ANS is divided into *cholinergic* and *adrenergic* divisions based on chemical mediator (i.e., the neurotransmitter substance that is released)

i. Cholinergic neurons release acetylcholine and include:

(a) All preganglionic neurons except sympathetic preganglionic neurons to adrenal medulla

(b) Parasympathetic postganglionic neurons

(c) Sympathetic postganglionic neurons to the sweat glands and skeletal muscle blood vessels (vasodilator)

   ii. Adrenergic neurons release norepinephrine and include:

     (a) Sympathetic postganglionic endings, except as noted earlier

     (b) Sympathetic preganglionic neurons to the adrenal medulla

     (c) Constrictor fibers of skeletal muscle blood vessels

NURSING ASSESSMENT DATA BASE

Nursing History

1. **Patient health history**
   a. Current and significant past medical history of all major systems, including traumatic injury
   b. Chronologic sequence of onset and development of each neurologic symptom
   c. Factors that relieve or exacerbate symptoms
   d. Difficulties with activities of daily living (ADL)
   e. Childhood diseases
2. **Family history**
   a. Diabetes mellitus
   b. Cardiac disease
   c. Hypertension
   d. Cancer
   e. Neurologic disorders (e.g., stroke, aneurysms, arteriovenous malformations, seizures)
3. **Social history and habits**
   a. Smoking: past, present, amount, and duration of use
   b. Illicit drug use or abuse: particularly cocaine and amphetamines
   c. Alcohol intake: past, present, amount, and duration of use
   d. Type of work
   e. Hobbies, recreation
4. **Medication history**
   a. Anticonvulsants
   b. Tranquilizers, sedatives
   c. Anticoagulants
   d. Aspirin
   e. Cardiac, including antihypertensive

Nursing Examination of Patient

1. **Inspection**
   a. General cerebral functions: mental status examination
      i. General behavior and appearance
      ii. Consciousness or awareness, attention span, memory, insight, orientation, and calculation

      iii. Intellectual capacity appropriate for educational level

      iv. Emotional state

      v. Thought content, judgment: illusions, hallucinations, delusions

      vi. Conversation: stream of talk, sentence structure

b. Speech

      i. *Dysphonia*: difficulty producing the voice sound

      ii. *Dysarthria*: difficulty with articulation

      iii. *Dysprosody*: difficulty with stress of syllables, inflections, pitch of voice, rhythm

      iv. *Dysphasia*: difficulty in expression or understanding of words (dominant hemisphere function, usually the left)

c. Head and face

      i. Face: for gestalt, mobility, emotional expression

      ii. Eyes: for ptosis, symmetry, and width of palpebral fissures

      iii. Contours: nose, mouth, chin, and ears for signs of congenital or acquired abnormalities

      iv. Hair: scalp, eyebrows, or beard for signs of congenital or acquired abnormalities, such as endocrine disorders

      v. Head: for abnormalities in shape or symmetry

d. Cranial nerves

      i. Olfactory nerve (I): test each nostril separately. Ask patient to identify familiar nonirritating odors, such as cloves, coffee, and perfume. Loss of sense of smell is called *anosmia*

      ii. Optic nerve (II)

        (a) Visual acuity may be tested with a Snellen chart or grossly with newsprint

        (b) Inspect optic fundi with an ophthalmoscope

        (c) Determine visual fields by confrontation. The patient covers one eye and fixates on an object in the distance with the other eye. Bring your finger from periphery into the patient's field of vision. By positioning yourself about 18 to 24 inches directly in front of the patient and positioning your finger halfway between you and the patient, you can compare the patient's visual fields with yours. Test each eye individually

        (d) Unilateral blindness (Fig. 3–24*A*) is caused by lesions of the eye, retina, or optic nerve

        (e) Bitemporal hemianopsia (Fig. 3–24*B*) is caused by lesions affecting the optic chiasm (e.g., pituitary tumors)

        (f) Left (or right) homonymous hemianopsia (Fig. 3–24*C*) is caused by lesions of the right (or left) optic tract

        (g) Left (or right) homonymous hemianopsia with macular sparing (Fig. 3–24*D*) is caused by lesions of the geniculocalcarine tract

      iii. Oculomotor nerve (III)

        (a) Examine shape of pupils: Irregularly shaped pupils can be caused by direct trauma, cataracts, or other ocular dysfunction

        (b) Describe size of the pupils in millimeters. Pupil size represents a balance between parasympathetic and sympathetic innervation. Unequal pupils *(anisocoria)* results from:

          (1) Disruption of parasympathetic fibers of the oculomotor nerve and/or compression of the nucleus by mass lesions

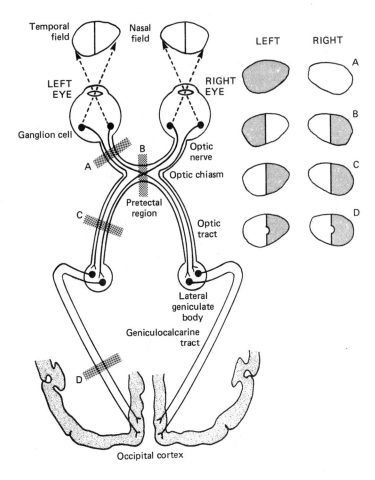

Figure 3–24 • Visual pathways. Lesions at the points marked by the letters cause the visual field defects shown in the diagrams on the right. Occipital lesions may spare the fibers from the macula (as in D) because of the separation in the brain of these fibers from the others subserving vision. (From Ganong, W. F.: Review of Medical Physiology, 14th ed. Norwalk, Conn., Appleton & Lange, 1989.)

or tentorial herniation, causing the ipsilateral pupil to dilate

(2) Disruption of sympathetic pathways (e.g., cervical spinal cord injury) resulting in a constricted pupil on the ipsilateral side (Horner's syndrome)

(c) Direct light reflex: constriction of the pupil when stimulated by light. This tests the afferent limb of CN II and efferent limb of CN III. Lost with oculomotor (parasympathetic) or optic nerve injury but retained with sympathetic disruption

(d) Consensual light reflex: constriction of the opposite pupil when light stimulates eye. This differentiates lesions of CN II from lesions of CN III. A blind eye (CN II lesion) does not have a direct light reflex; it has a consensual light reflex if CN III and midbrain connections are intact

(e) Cortical blindness does not affect either direct or consensual reflexes

(f) Accommodation reflex: convergence of eyes, constriction of pupils, and thickening of lens. Occurs when a person looks at a close object

iv. Oculomotor nerve (CN III), trochlear nerve (CN IV), and abducens nerve (CN VI)

(a) Check range of extraocular movements (EOMs) by having the patient's eyes following your finger through all fields of gaze. Observe for nystagmus at rest and during ocular movements

(b) Ask the patient whether double vision is experienced in any visual field. Determine whether diplopia is caused by CN III, by CN VI, or (when the patient looks down) by CN IV dysfunction

v. Trigeminal nerve (V)

(a) Sensory examination

(1) Test forehead, cheeks, and jaw on each side of face. Use a wisp of cotton for a light touch, a pin for a pinprick, test tubes of hot and cold water for temperature

(2) Corneal reflex: touch the cornea of each eye with a wisp of cotton. Observe for reflex blinking. This tests the afferent limb of CN V and the efferent limb of CN VII of the reflex arc

(b) Motor examination

(1) Ask the patient to clench his or her teeth

(2) Palpate the masseter and temporal muscles; assess strength of masseter muscles by pushing down on mandible (chin) against patient's resistance

(3) Assess the patient's ability to chew

vi. Facial nerve (VII)

(a) Ask the patient to raise his or her eyebrows, frown, smile, open eyes against resistance. Note strength and symmetry of facial muscles

(b) Test taste on the anterior two thirds of the tongue by applying salt and sugar to both sides of the tongue. Ask the patient to identify the taste prior to closing of the mouth

vii. Acoustic nerve (VIII) (vestibulocochlear nerve)

(a) Cochlear (hearing)

(1) Hearing acuity: cover one ear, and test the other with a watch or a whisper. If a deficit is suggested, proceed to steps (2) and (3)

(2) Weber's test: place the stem of a tuning fork on the midline vertex of the skull. Normally, there is no lateralization of sound. When sound is referred to the better-hearing ear, decreased hearing is due to impaired function of cochlear nerve

(3) Rinne's test: place a tuning fork on the mastoid bone. When sound is no longer heard, place it in front of the ear. Because air conduction is normally greater than bone conduction, middle ear disease is suspected in a patient who can hear the tuning fork better when it is placed on the mastoid bone

(b) Vestibular (balance)

(1) Patient complaints of vertigo, nausea, and anxiety; nystagmus; postural deviation; pallor; sweating;

hypotension; and vomiting. All may indicate vestibular nerve dysfunction

    (2) Caloric irrigation test: position the patient 30° up from the supine position to bring the semicircular canals to a vertical plane. After checking to ensure an unoccluded ear canal and an intact tympanic membrane, irrigate the canal with cold water. When the pathway from the vestibular portion of CN VIII to CN III and CN VI is intact, the response in an awake patient will consist of vertigo, nausea, and horizontal nystagmus (fast component) toward the unirrigated side, postural deviation, and past-pointing to the irrigated side. In a patient with impaired vestibular function, some or all of these responses may be abnormal

viii. Glossopharyngeal nerve (IX) and vagus nerve (X)

    (a) Ask the patient to open his or her mouth and say "Ah." Observe for symmetric elevation of the palatal arch

    (b) Gag reflex: stroke the palatal arch with a tongue blade. The palate should elevate, and the patient should have a gag response. This tests the afferent limb of CN IX and the efferent limb of CN X

    (c) Speech: appraise articulation. If a defect is suspected, having patient say "Kuh, Kuh, Kuh"; "La, La, La"; "Mi, Mi, Mi" tests the competency of the soft palate (CN IX), tongue (CN XII), and lips (CN VII), respectively

    (d) Swallowing: if the patient is dysarthric or dysphagic, assess the ability to swallow water. If the patient is unable to follow commands, observe the ability to handle secretions

    (e) Carotid sinus reflex: pressure over the carotid sinus normally produces slowing of the heart rate and fall in blood pressure

    (f) Hoarseness: may indicate damage to the vagus nerve. Laryngoscopic examination may be indicated

ix. Spinal accessory nerve (XI)

    (a) Inspect sternocleidomastoid muscle (SCM) and trapezius muscle for size and symmetry

    (b) Ask the patient to turn his or her head to one side. Place your hand on patient's cheek and the other on patient's shoulder for stability. Instruct the patient to resist your attempt to forceably turn the head back to midline. Palpate opposite the SCM muscle. Repeat on other side

    (c) Ask the patient to push the head forward against your hand. Assess the strength of both SCM muscles

    (d) Ask the patient to shrug his or her shoulders upward against resistance of your downward pressure on the shoulders. Note strength and contraction of the trapezius muscles

x. Hypoglossal nerve (CN XII)

    (a) Inspect the tongue for atrophy while the patient is at rest

    (b) Check alignment of the tongue when it is protruded by comparing the median raphe with the notch between the medial incisors

    (c) Have the patient protrude the tongue and push it to right and left. Have the patient press the tongue against the inside of the cheek while you assess its strength

e. Motor system

   i. Observe size and contour of muscles: note atrophy, hypertrophy, asymmetry, joint malalignments, or involuntary movements, such as fasciculations, tics, tremors, and abnormal positions

   ii. Palpate muscles if tenderness or spasm is suspected or if the muscles seem atrophic or hypertrophic

   iii. Strength testing

     (a) Shoulder girdle: press down on patient's arms after the patient abducts them to shoulder height. Check for scapular winging

     (b) Upper extremities: test biceps, triceps, wrist dorsiflexion, hand grasps, strength of finger abduction and extension

     (c) Lower extremities: test hip flexors, abductors and adductors, knee flexors and extensors (deep knee bend), foot dorsiflexors, foot plantar flexors, invertors, evertors

     (d) Abdominal muscles: observe for umbilical migration as patient does a sit-up

     (e) Note whether weakness follows a distributional pattern, such as proximal-distal, right-left, or upper-lower extremity

     (f) Grade strength on a scale of 0 to 5

       (1) 0 = flaccid, no muscular contraction

       (2) 1 = contraction of muscle felt or seen

       (3) 2 = movement through full range of motion with gravity removed

       (4) 3 = movement through full range of motion against gravity

       (5) 4 = movement against resistance but can be overcome

       (6) 5 = full strength against resistance

   iv. Muscle tone: note whether *rigidity* (increased muscular resistance throughout range of motion of joint), *spasticity* (increased muscular resistance to brisk movement of joint), or *hypotonia* (flaccidity) is elicited by passive motion

   v. Muscle stretch reflexes: elicited by percussing a tendon with a reflex hammer, which causes stretch of muscle spindles and subsequent contraction of muscle fibers. Compare response on one side with the other

     (a) Hyperreflexia may indicate interruption of UMN pathways between cerebrum and LMNs

     (b) Areflexia is most commonly caused by lesions of LMNs

     (c) Reflexes commonly tested include:

       (1) Biceps (C5–6)

       (2) Brachioradialis (C5–6)

       (3) Triceps (C7–8)

       (4) Finger flexion (C7–T1)

       (5) Quadriceps (patellar) (L2–4)

       (6) Achilles (ankle jerk) (L5–S1–3)

   vi. Superficial reflexes: tested by stroking the skin with a moderately sharp object. These reflexes will be lost or abnormal with UMN lesions

     (a) Plantar (S1–2): Babinski sign

(1) Stroking the lateral aspect of the sole of the foot normally causes flexion of the great toe

(2) An abnormal response is extension of the great toe (Babinski sign)

(3) Other methods may elicit an extensor-plantar response, but all indicate UMN pathology

(b) Clonus: oscillation of the foot between flexion and extension when brisk pressure is applied to the sole

f. Cerebellar function

   i. Testing depends on the patient's ability to perform volitional movements (i.e., the motor system related to area being tested must be intact). For example, a hemiplegic or comatose patient cannot perform cerebellar function tests because of the inability to perform voluntary movements

   ii. Four major clinical signs of dysfunction and tests used to detect these dysfunctions are

(a) Dystaxia or ataxia (intention tremor or incoordination of volitional movements)

(1) Observe for swaying when the patient stands with feet together, first with eyes open, then closed (Romberg test)

(2) Gait or truncal dystaxia: swaying while sitting, wide-based gait while walking, and inability to perform tandem (heel-to-toe) walking

(3) Arm dystaxia: detected by

   a) Finger-to-nose test. Asking the patient to touch his or her nose, then your finger

   b) Rapid-alternating movement test. Asking the patient to slap his or her thigh first with palm and then with back of the hand in quick alternating movements.

(4) Leg dystaxia: detected by the heel-to-shin test. Ask the patient to run his or her heel from the opposite knee down the shin

(b) Hypotonia (lack of muscle tone)

(1) Inspect the patient for "rag doll" postures and gait

(2) Lack of muscular resistance when the examiner passively moves the patient's extremity

(3) Patient's leg continues to swing like a pendulum after muscle stretch reflex is elicited

(4) Postural dysequilibrium may be elicited by rebound tests: wrist-slapping and arm-pulling. Movement is not checked and overshooting occurs

(c) Nystagmus (jerky, oscillatory eye movements)

(1) Have the patient follow your finger through fields of gaze

(2) Nystagmus results from lesions of the cerebellum, vestibular system, or brain stem pathways and each pathway has different clinical characteristics

(d) Dysarthria (inability to articulate speech sounds): See the test for CN IX and CN X. May result from dysfunction of CN VIII, CN IX, CN X, or CN XII or cerebellar dysfunction that interferes with coordination of the muscles innervated by these nerves

g. Sensory system
  i. Tested with patient's eyes closed. One side of the body is compared with the other
  ii. Determine whether the distribution of sensory loss is dermatomal, related to peripheral nerves or central pathway, or nonorganic
  iii. Broad dermatomal areas are
    (a) C3–4: "cape" area of shoulders
    (b) C5–T1: surface of arms
    (c) T2 abuts on C4 over "cape" area of shoulders
    (d) T4: nipple line
    (e) T10: umbilicus
    (f) L5: great toe
    (g) S1: small toe
    (h) S4–5: perianal area
  iv. Superficial sensory modalities: functions of the spinothalamic tracts (anterior and lateral). Responses are recorded as normal, abnormal (either increased or decreased), or absent. A dematomal chart may be used to precisely describe the sensory level
    (a) Light touch: touch the patient's hands, trunk, and feet with a wisp of cotton
    (b) Pain: using a pin, gently touch the patient's hands, trunk, and feet. The patient is asked to distinguish sharp from dull and to compare it with the sensation on a normal part of the body such as the face. Both sides are tested. Use a clean safety pin for each patient, and take care not to pierce or scratch the skin
    (c) Temperature: Test perception with test tubes of hot and cold water
    (d) Testing of either pain or temperature is sufficient because both functions are carried in the same tracts
  v. Deep sensory modalities
    (a) Posterior columns (fasciculus gracilis and fasciculus cuneatus) of the spinal cord. May test either function as both columns are carried in the same tract
      (1) Vibration: apply a vibrating tuning fork to the bony prominences and soft tissue, and ask the patient to report when vibration is felt. Apply a fork to a toe or finger, and place your finger under the digit. The patient should report feeling vibration of the tuning fork for a longer time than you do
      (2) Proprioception (position sense): ask the patient to close his or her eyes, and report whether the finger or toe is being moved up or down
    (b) Cortical discriminatory sensation: receptors, sensory pathways, and primary receptive cortical area must be intact for accurate interpretation of the following tests. Performing the tests accurately thus enables one to assess association portions (parietal lobe) of the cortex. Deficits are called *agnosias* (not knowing):
      (1) *Stereognosia*: ask the patient, without aid of vision, to identify familiar objects placed in his or her hand. The inability to identify objects is *astereoognosia*

    (2) *Topognosia*: ask the patient to identify which finger you are touching and whether it is on right or left side. Deficits may be called *finger agnosia, atopognosia,* or "right-left disorientation"

    (3) *Graphognosia*: ask the patient to identify numbers or letters traced on the skin of the palm or fingers. Inability to discern what is written is *agraphognosia*

    (4) Tactile inattention: inability of a patient to identify that he or she has been touched on both sides of the body simultaneously

    (5) *Anosognosia*: inability of a person with a left hemiparesis and sensory loss to recognize the deficit; also referred to as "neglect"

h. Assessment of patient with altered state of consciousness

  i. Consciousness is an awareness of self and environment. Disturbances in consciousness can result from extensive bilateral cerebral lesions or from injury to the diencephalon or pontomesencephalic (pons/midbrain) reticular formation or metabolic abnormalities. Unilateral lesions of the cerebrum and lesions of the medulla or spinal cord do not cause coma

  ii. Level of consciousness

    (a) Determine stimuli necessary to arouse the patient

      (1) Does patient respond when name is called?

      (2) Does patient have to be touched or shaken?

      (3) Are painful stimuli necessary to arouse the patient?

      (4) Does patient have no response to any stimulus?

    (b) Describe the patient's behavior once the patient is aroused

      (1) Is patient oriented or confused?

      (2) Is patient restless, irritable, combative?

      (3) Does patient follow verbal commands?

    (c) Describe the patient's verbal response

      (1) Is patient's speech clear, garbled, or confused?

      (2) Does patient use inappropriate words?

      (3) Does patient make incomprehensible sounds?

      (4) Does patient have any verbal response?

    (d) Determine patient's best motor response

      (1) Does patient obey verbal commands?

      (2) Does patient localize or withdraw from noxious stimuli?

      (3) Does patient exhibit abnormal flexor or extensor posturing?

      (4) Is there no response at all to stimuli—that is, is patient flaccid?

    (e) Chart the responses to the above assessment parameters in detail to provide a clear picture of the patient's level of consciousness. Avoid such terms as "stuporous," "obtunded," "semi-comatose," and "comatose" because patients do not fit neatly into one defined area

  iii. Glasgow Coma Scale (GCS): this standardized tool assesses many of the same areas of level of consciousness as just described. It has become widely accepted as the way of describing the level of consciousness because of the high degree of inter-rater reliability.

Limitations of the GCS include the inability to assess eye opening in patients with periorbital swelling, the loss of verbal response in patients who are intubated, and the lack of brain stem reflex assessment. In addition, the level of consciousness may be depressed by factors such as hypoxia, hypotension, hypothermia, alcohol intoxication, postictal state, and administration of sedatives and narcotics, thereby exaggerating the severity of injury if the GCS is determined prior to resuscitation efforts. The patient's responses are graded and the scores for the best eye opening, verbal and motor categories are summed. The GCS scores range from 3 to 15, with a score of 15 being normal

(a) Eye opening: assesses arousal state
  (1) "Spontaneously" (GCS = 4): patient opens eyes without stimulation
  (2) "To voice" (GCS = 3): patient opens eyes when spoken to
  (3) "To pain" (GCS = 2): patient opens eyes when noxious stimuli are applied
  (4) "None" (GCS = 1): patient does not open eyes to any stimulus

(b) Best verbal response: assesses content of consciousness in terms of ability to produce speech as a function of consciousness and in terms of quality of speech
  (1) "Oriented" (GCS = 5): patient can state his or her name, where he or she is, and the date
  (2) "Confused" (GCS = 4): patients cannot state either who they are, where they are, or the date
  (3) "Inappropriate words" (GCS = 3): patients speak words with no specific intent at communicating
  (4) "Incomprehensible sounds" (GCS = 2): patients grunt, groan, or make other sounds
  (5) "None" (GCS = 1): patients make no attempt at vocalizing. Causes may include intubation, speaking only a foreign language, inability of very young children to respond, or global aphasia. These examples do not indicate total loss of brain function

(c) Best motor response: record best motor response of the patient's arms. Assesses both arousal and content of consciousness
  (1) "Obeys" (GCS = 6): patient follows simple commands, such as "Hold up two fingers"
  (2) "Localizes" (GCS = 5): patient attempts to remove noxious stimuli. Is assessed by applying pressure to the supraorbital ridge or trapezius muscle
  (3) "Withdraws" (GCS = 4): patient's arm or leg is pulled away from painful stimuli of examiner, who applies pressure to nail beds
  (4) "Abnormal flexion" (GCS = 3): adduction, internal rotation, and rigid flexion of the hand and arm, with the hand clenched and the thumb grasped in the hand (decorticate posturing) upon painful stimuli from examiner
  (5) "Abnormal extension" (GCS = 2): adduction, internal

rotation, and rigid extension; the patient's thumb is grasped in a clenched fist (decerebrate posturing)

    (6) "Flaccid" (GCS = 1): patient exhibits no motor movements of any kind to any stimulation

iv. Motor ability

    (a) If the patient can follow verbal commands, assess strength and tone of extremities, as described previously

    (b) If the patient is unable to follow verbal commands, assess motor ability by observing which extremities he or she moves spontaneously or in response to noxious stimuli

    (c) *Hemiparesis* or *hemiplegia* may also be detected by lifting both of the patient's arms off the bed and releasing them simultaneously. The hemiparetic side will fall more quickly and more limply than the normal side

    (d) *Paratonia* is increased muscular resistance of any part of body to passive movement. It usually accompanies diffuse forebrain dysfunction; when it is seen unilaterally, however, it is associated with lesions of frontal lobe and increased ICP

    (e) Flexor posturing (decorticate rigidity) consists of flexion and adduction of the upper extremity, with extension, internal rotation, and plantar flexion in the lower extremity. Is associated with lesions of the cerebral hemispheres, internal capsule, or the upper part of the brain stem

    (f) Extensor posturing (decerebrate rigidity) is characterized by extension, adduction, and hyperpronation of the upper extremities and plantar flexion of the lower extremities. A result of lesions at the pontomesencephalic level

    (g) Muscle stretch reflexes: may be diminished initially after acute intracranial injury caused by cerebral shock. Hyperreflexia and appearance of Babinski reflexes reflect an upper motor neuron lesion. Clonus may also be present

v. Cranial nerves: testing is limited in patients who are unable to cooperate

    (a) The optic nerve (II) is tested indirectly by pupillary light reflexes

    (b) Oculomotor nerve (III)

        (1) Describe shape of the pupil. An oval-shaped pupil may accompany tentorial herniation and increased ICP

        (2) Describe direct light reflex as brisk, sluggish, or nonreactive

        (3) Describe consensual light reflex as "present" or "absent." It remains intact when the oculomotor nerve and midbrain connections are intact

    (c) Oculomotor (III) and abducens (VI) nerves

        (1) In patients who open their eyes spontaneously or in response to stimuli, determine whether they can move their eyes side to side or up and down (more difficult to elicit) in response to verbal or noxious stimuli

        (2) If the patient looks toward a noxious stimulus (e.g., when pressure is applied to the base of the nail bed), you can determine whether the eyes are able to move medially (CN III) and laterally (CN VI) and confirm that CN III and CN VI are intact. If, however, the right eye moves medially but

the left eye stays midline or does not move completely laterally, the patient has a left sixth nerve palsy

(d) Trigeminal (V) and facial (VII) nerves
   (1) The corneal reflex cannot be tested in the uncooperative patient
   (2) For an alternate method for testing the V–VII arc, apply pressure to supraorbital ridge and observe for facial grimacing, which will be decreased or absent on same side as UMN lesion of CN VII

(e) Vestibular portion of CN VIII and its connections via the medial longitudinal fasciculus with CN III and CN VI provide information regarding integrity of the brain stem. Can be tested by oculocephalic or oculovestibular reflexes
   (1) Oculocephalic reflex (doll's eye test): in a comatose patient who has intact connections between CN VIII and CN III and CN VI, brisk turning of patient's head will cause the eyes to move in the opposite direction. This is described as "doll's eyes present." Absent doll's eyes result in the eyes remaining in a fixed position. *Caution:* Before performing this maneuver, be sure that a cervical spine injury has been ruled out
   (2) Oculovestibular reflex (caloric irrigation test): When the pathway from the vestibular portion of CN VIII to CN III and CN VI is intact, a normal coma response (showing the connections between VIII and III and VI to be intact) consists of nystagmus and deviation of the eyes toward the irrigated ear. An abnormal response (showing the brain stem pathways to be impaired) the eyes stay in midposition

(f) Cranial nerves IX and X are tested by the gag reflex, usually accomplished by observing the patient's response to suctioning or movement of the endotracheal tube

vi. Vital signs
   (a) Temperature
      (1) Hyperthemia increases metabolic needs of an already compromised CNS and should be vigorously combated. It usually indicates infection, extreme restlessness, or seizure activity
      (2) Hypothermia, if extreme, can lead to cardiac dysrhythmias. Moderate hypothermia (32° to 34°C) may be helpful in controlling increased ICP and improving outcome in head-injured patients. See Head Trauma section
   (b) Respirations
      (1) Hypercapnia or hypoxia leads to vasodilatation, increased cerebral blood volume (CBV), increased cerebral blood flow, and, in patients with compromised intracranial dynamics, increased ICP
      (2) Respiratory dysrhythmias often correlate with lesions at various levels, although effects are variable and influenced by other factors. *Note:* Intubated patients will not likely demonstrate the following respiratory patterns
         a) Posthyperventilation apnea: a patient with metabolic or

structural forebrain disease will have a period of apnea after taking deep breaths sufficient to lower $PaCO_2$ below normal. This response is abolished in sleep or obtundation

    b) Cheyne-Stokes respiration: a pattern that alternately crescendos to hyperpnea and decrescendos to apnea. Associated with bilateral lesions of cerebral hemispheres, basal ganglia, or metabolic lesions

    c) Central neurogenic hyperventilation: sustained, regular, rapid, and deep hyperpnea. Is seen in patients with lesions of midbrain, often secondary to transtentorial herniation and midpontine lesions

    d) Apneustic breathing: an end-inspiratory pause, often followed with expiratory pauses. Indicates injury to respiratory mechanisms at the mid-pontine or caudal-pontine level

    e) Ataxic breathing (Biot's): completely irregular pattern with both deep and shallow breaths occurring randomly. Represents disruption of medullary inspiratory and expiratory neurons and thus occurs with lesions of the posterior fossa

    f) Cluster breathing: disorganized sequence of breaths with irregular periods of apnea. Is seen with lesions of the caudal pons or rostral medulla

(3) Pulse and blood pressure

    (a) Although of vital importance in overall assessment and care of critically ill patients, pulse and blood pressure are notoriously unreliable parameters in CNS disease. When changes do occur, they are usually seen late in the course of increasing ICP and thus are of limited clinical use

    (b) Cushing's reflex is an increase in systolic pressure greater than the increase in diastolic pressure. This reflex leads to widening pulse pressure and occasionally to reflex slowing of the pulse. It is sometimes seen in patients experiencing periods of increased ICP

2. Palpation
  a. Skull for lumps, depressions, tenderness
  b. Carotid and temporal arteries
  c. Motor system: palpate muscles if tenderness or spasm is suggested by the history or if muscles seem atrophic or hypertrophic
  d. Muscles may also be palpated during strength testing
  e. Testing for muscle tone also involves palpation to the extent that the resistance or lack of resistance to movement is noted when an extremity is moved through the range of motion

3. Percussion: muscle strength reflex testing involves percussion of tendons to elicit the response. Practically speaking, percussion of the CNS is confined to the sinuses or mastoid processes to assess for tenderness

4. Auscultation: auscultate the great vessels, eyes, temples, and mastoid processes for bruits

. . . .
:
: **Diagnostic Studies**

1. **Laboratory Studies**
   a. Blood
      i. Complete blood count (CBC), differential, erythrocyte sedimentation rate (ESR)
      ii. Chemistries including osmolality
      iii. Electrolytes
      iv. Clotting profile including prothrombin time (PT), partial thromboplastin time (PTT), D-dimer, fibrinogen
      v. Arterial blood gases (ABGs)
      vi. Toxicology: alcohol, drugs
   b. Urinalysis
   c. CSF
      i. Compare with normal values
      ii. Wassermann test
      iii. Culture and sensitivity
2. **Radiologic Studies**
   a. Skull series: bone windows of the computed tomography (CT) scan have essentially replaced skull radiographs as the study of choice in diagnosis of abnormalities of the skull and sinuses. However, in the absence of CT scanning, skull radiographs may still be useful in diagnosis of fractures, identification of skull abnormalities, preparation for surgical repair of cranial defects, and illustration of the status of cranial sutures
   b. Spine series: used to assess vertebral alignment, diagnose fractures, dislocations, or degenerative processes of vertebrae. CT is often used as an adjunct to further delineate abnormalities
   c. CT scan
      i. Principle: an x-ray beam is projected through a narrow section of the brain or spine, and detectors at opposite side record transmission readings from tissues. Readings are fed into a computer that derives absorption (or attenuation) of x-ray by tissues in the path of the beam. The computer prints out a digital picture that is converted to a black and white image and displayed on oscilloscope or x-ray film. Denser tissue (e.g., bone) absorbs more x-rays and appears whiter on final image. The scan may be repeated after the patient has received an intravenous contrast agent that enhances tissues with disruption of the blood-brain barrier
      ii. Clinical uses
         (a) Brain: Valuable in diagnosis of almost all intracranial pathology and of particular value in head trauma. Used alone or in conjunction with magnetic resonance imaging (MRI) in detecting intracranial mass lesions. Bone windows provide exquisite detail of the bony architecture of the skull
         (b) Spine: Useful in diagnosis of mass lesions and trauma to the spine. Fractures, dislocations, degenerative changes, and congenital abnormalities may be seen
      iii. Preprocedure and postprocedure care: No specific preprocedure care necessary. If contrast enhancement is used, quantity and specific

gravity of urine will be increased for approximately 8 hours after the scan

   d. CT myelography

      i. Principle: CT examination of spinal canal after injection of a radiopaque substance into subarachnoid space, usually in lumbar area. If a block is seen, the contrast material will also be injected into the subarachnoid space above the lesion at C1–C2 to assess the extent of the abnormality

      ii. Clinical use: diagnosis of intervertebral disc disease, spinal cord tumors, and other diseases of or injuries to spinal cord

      iii. Preprocedure and postprocedure care: patient may complain of headache after the scan and is usually required to lie flat for 4 to 24 hours

   e. Cerebral angiography

      i. Principle: a contrast material is injected into one or more arteries in order to obtain radiographic visualization of intracranial and extracranial circulation

      ii. Clinical uses: diagnosis of vascular abnormalities, such as aneurysms, arteriovenous malformations, vasospasm, and vascular tumors as well as cerebral vasculitis, moyamoya disease, and venous thrombosis. Aids in diagnosis of other intracranial abnormalities that cause stretching and displacement of vessels or change in their diameter

      iii. Preprocedure and postprocedure care: the patient may be premedicated and should be well hydrated. Blood pressure should be under control. After the scan, the injection site is checked for bleeding or hematoma formation. Pressure dressings or ice may be applied. A major complication is stroke caused by dislodging of an atherosclerotic plaque from the wall of an artery or a thrombus that has formed at the end of the catheter

   f. Radioisotope brain scan

      i. Principle: a radioactive substance is introduced into blood, and brain is scanned to determine areas that have accumulated the substance. In some disorders, radioisotope accumulates in abnormal areas of brain probably owing to a breakdown in blood-brain barrier or increased vascularity of the lesion

      ii. Clinical uses

        (a) Screening for presence of brain tumors

        (b) Evaluation of cerebrovascular disease and some infectious processes

        (c) Often used in conjunction with other diagnostic procedures

      iii. Preprocedure and postprocedure care: radioisotope is injected at varying time intervals prior to scanning. No specific postprocedure care or complications

3. Other diagnostic studies

   a. MRI

      i. Technique: magnetic fields and radiofrequencies are used to create signals that generate an MR image. The magnetic field may be altered to emphasize different characteristics of normal and abnormal tissue. A paramagnetic enhancing agent, gadolinium, is used to enhance some lesions

      ii. Clinical uses

(a) Brain: because MRI focuses on the hydrogen ion (i.e., water), brain edema and infarcted tissue are readily detected. Rapidly moving protons in blood emit little signal, and altered flow patterns can be detected by measurement of intensity variations. MRI is generally superior to CT in detecting brain tumors, infectious lesions, and vascular lesions, although cerebral angiography is usually needed to further delineate vascular lesions. The addition of gadolinium further defines areas of increased vascularity or blood-brain barrier disruption

(b) Spine: MRI is far superior to CT in defining lesions such as cysts, vascular abnormalities, and tumors in and around the spinal cord and canal. Degenerative processes, such as disc disease and stenosis, are also readily diagnosed

iii. Preprocedure and postprocedure care: all metal objects must be removed from the patient prior to scanning. Patients should be told of the need to lie very still and that they will be in a small, confined space. If the patient is claustrophobic, sedation may be needed to obtain adequate images. The machine makes a loud, clunking noise that some patients find disturbing. No specific postprocedure care or complications

b. Magnetic resonance angiography (MRA)

i. Principle: the appearance of flowing blood is influenced by factors such as flow velocity, flow configuration, type of scanning sequence used, and direction of flow. MRA depicts flow relationships rather than the lumina of the blood vessels

ii. Clinical uses

(a) Visualizing larger vessels

(b) Screening of neck vessels for abnormalities (although it typically overemphasizes degree of stenosis)

(c) Demonstrating patency of major veins and venous sinuses

(d) Identifying aneurysms and vascular malformations

iii. Preprocedure and postprocedure care: same as with MRI

c. Lumbar puncture, cisternal puncture

i. Principle: a needle is placed into the subarachnoid space below the conus medullaris, usually at the L4–5 interspace (or cisterna magna with a cisternal puncture)

ii. Clinical uses

(a) To obtain CSF for laboratory examination

(b) To measure or reduce CSF pressure

(c) To provide a route for administration of medications

(d) To prepare patients for other diagnostic studies (e.g., myelography)

iii. Preprocedure and postprocedure care

(a) Lumbar puncture: Contraindicated in patients with increased ICP, as it may lead to herniation of brain stem. Infection, headache, or backache may be complications of the procedure. Patients are usually required to lie flat for a few hours after the procedure

(b) Cisternal puncture: Injury to the brain stem may occur and may lead to changes in vital signs or to shock. Hemorrhage or infection may also occur. Patients are usually kept lying flat for 4 to 6 hours

d. Electroencephalography (EEG)
   i. Principle: recording of electrical activity of brain by electrodes attached to scalp. Voltage fluctuations have rhythmicity, depending on the area of the cerebrum being recorded and age and level of alertness of the patient
   ii. Clinical uses
      (a) Most helpful in diagnosis of seizures, space-occupying lesions, and (on occasion) coma
      (b) Although not legally necessary, used to aid in diagnosis of cerebral death
      (c) Monitors burst-suppression activity in patients in barbiturate-induced therapeutic coma for intractable intracranial hypertension in order to titrate the minimum amount of barbiturate necessary to attain burst-suppression without causing loss of electrical activity
   iii. Preprocedure and postprocedure care: preprocedure care varies, depending on the institution and type of EEG (e.g., sleep EEG). Postprocedure care includes washing conductive paste from hair. No risks involved

e. Electromyography (EMG)
   i. Principle: needle electrodes record electrical potentials from contracting muscle fibers. These are displayed on an oscilloscope
   ii. Clinical use: aids in diagnosis of lower motor neuron disease or muscle disorders caused by denervation or myopathy
   iii. Preprocedure and postprocedure care: there is no risk to patient, although needle electrodes are uncomfortable. Because of muscle damage from the needle electrodes, the creatine phosphokinase (CPK) is elevated to approximately two times normal for 6 to 48 hours after the procedure

f. Nerve conduction velocity
   i. Principle: a large motor nerve trunk is stimulated with electrode, and a response is recorded in one of its muscles. Alternately, a pure sensory fiber may be stimulated and the response recorded from the same nerve along its course. The distal latency, the amplitude in millivolts of the negative phase of the response, and the velocity of impulse conduction can be calculated from distance and time elapsed between stimulus and response
   ii. Clinical use: diagnosis of peripheral neuropathies and nerve compression
   iii. Preprocedure and postprocedure care: there is no risk to patient, although needle electrodes are uncomfortable

g. Evoked potentials (EPs)
   i. Principle: electrodes are placed on the scalp appropriate to type of evoked response (potential) tested: brain stem auditory evoked response (BAER), visual evoked response (VER), or somatosensory evoked response (SER). As a stimulus is applied (i.e., a clicking noise for BAER, a strobe light or pattern-shift for VER, and electrical stimulation of peripheral nerve for SER), evoked response is amplified, averaged by computer, displayed on the oscilloscope, and

recorded on paper. Evoked potential wave latencies and amplitudes are compared with normal responses and right and left responses in the subject

    ii. Clinical uses

        (a) BAER is useful in determining brain stem function

        (b) VER is a useful index of hemispheric function and in diagnosis of multiple sclerosis

        (c) SER may demonstrate lesions of peripheral pathways, spinal cord, or brain stem

        (d) Multimodal evoked potentials (MEPs) (two or all three methods) may be done to confirm or refute clinical diagnosis

        (e) Useful in determining prognosis in severe head injury

        (f) May be done during intracranial or spine surgery to monitor patients' response to surgical procedure

    iii. Preprocedure and postprocedure care: no specific care needed. Patient's temperature must be above 97°F prior to BAER

4. CBF measurements

  a. Transcranial Doppler study

    i. Principle: An ultrasonic frequency is emitted from probe and is reflected from moving blood cells. The direction and velocity of blood movement alters the frequency of the reflected waves. The difference between the emitted frequency and received frequency is the Doppler shift. Blood moving toward the probe is recorded as positive and away from the probe, negative. If the middle cerebral artery (MCA) velocity is greater than 120 cm/second, the ratio of the MCA to the cervical internal carotid artery (ICA) velocities of greater than 3 is indicative of cerebral vasospasm

    ii. Clinical uses: Measure blood flow velocity and direction in the large intracranial vessels to determine cerebral vasospasm, brain death, stenotic vessels. Detects active emboli

        (a) Advantages

            (1) Noninvasive, portable, relatively inexpensive

            (2) Can be repeated often and safely

            (3) Can be used to monitor changes

        (b) Disadvantages

            (1) Anatomic variations of arteries may make it difficult to distinguish from arterial disease

            (2) Absolute velocities vary with age, hematocrit, $PaCO_2$, cardiac output, and degree of activation of brain tissue supplied by the artery being insonated

            (3) Does not detect bilateral symmetric disease, long regions of vasoconstriction or stenosis, or distal artery disease

    iii. Preprocedure and postprocedure care: no specific care required; no known complications

  b. Xenon (^{133}Xe)

    i. Principle: xenon isotope inhalation technique is a method of monitoring CBF that can be done at the bedside. It is based on the principle that the rate of uptake and clearance of an inert diffusible gas is proportional to CBF. Extracranial collimators measure the washout of inhaled or injected ^{133}Xe, and give accurate data on the regional blood flow. Cannot measure flow to cerebral subcortical areas and may miss focal areas of ischemia near areas of high flow

 ii. Clinical use: valuable in patients with cerebrovascular disorders. Is used to delineate the influence of CBF on outcome from head injury

 iii. Preprocedure and postprocedure care: no specific care. No risks involved in procedure with the exception of radiation exposure

c. Stable xenon CT

 i. Principle: A CT scan is done after inhalation of mixture of O_2 and 30% to 35% xenon, a radiodense, lipid-soluble gas that acts as a contrast agent during the procedure. Arterial concentration can be determined by measuring end-tidal exhaled gases. Provides excellent anatomic resolution of blood flow to the brain, particularly in the deep structures. Immediate results of CBF can be obtained

 ii. Clinical use: beneficial when both CT scan and CBF measurements are needed, as with head trauma patients. Also useful when CBF to specific or discrete areas of the brain needs to be determined

 iii. Preprocedure and postprocedure care: no specific preprocedure care necessary. After the procedure, the patient may experience hypotension, nausea, sedation, or hypoventilation and should be monitored carefully

d. Single photon emission tomography (SPECT)

 i. Principle: uses a rotating gamma camera system to detect disintegration of single photon-emitting radioisotopes, such as ^{99m}technetium, ^{133}xenon, ^{201}thallium, ^{123}iodine, and hexamethyl-propyleneamineoxime (HM-PAO). Because the tracers have a distribution that is dependent on blood flow, it can delineate regions of perfusion defect after insult. However, only ^{133}xenon measures absolute CBF values

 ii. Clinical use: An adjunct measurement or a primary modality if other blood flow techniques are not available in patients who are thought to have regional blood flow changes

 iii. Preprocedure and postprocedure care: no specific care required. The radioisotope may be administered at varying times prior to scanning

e. Positron emission tomography (PET)

 i. Principle: positron-emitting isotopes of carbon, fluorine, nitrogen, or O_2 are administered, and the gamma rays emitted are recorded by detectors placed in pairs around the head

  (a) Provides high-sensitivity, quantitative measurements in a three-dimensional tomographic format

  (b) Can generate images of regional CBF, O_2 metabolism, glucose metabolism, and blood volume

  (c) PET scanning with 18-fluorodeoxyglucose (FDG) measures glucose utilization and can determine the rate of glycolysis in the brain

 ii. Clinical uses

  (a) Permits study of physiologic processes and precise measurement of blood flow and metabolism in discrete areas of the brain

  (b) Is not common in clinical practice; predominantly a research tool

 iii. Preprocedure and postprocedure care: no specific care necessary, although patients undergoing 18-FDG studies should take nothing by mouth (NPO) for at least 4 hours before testing

f. Jugular venous O_2 saturation (SjO_2)

    i. Principle: indirect assessment of CBF and metabolism. Placement of fiberoptic catheter into the jugular bulb allows for continuous recording of jugular venous O_2 saturation and intermittent sampling of venous blood gases. When venous and arterial blood gases are analyzed simultaneously, the values can be used to calculate the arteriovenous O_2 difference and, in conjunction with CBF measurements, determine the cerebral metabolic rate for O_2

    ii. Clinical uses: may be able to detect episodes of cerebral ischemia. Normal SjO_2 is approximately 65%; a saturation below 55% is indicative of global ischemia and warrants treatment

    iii. Preprocedure and postprocedure care: no specific preprocedure care. After insertion, a lateral or slightly oblique cervical radiograph should be obtained to confirm catheter position in the jugular bulb. Because many readings are caused by poor catheter position or calibration, an algorithm for diagnosing the problem should be employed

COMMONLY ENCOUNTERED NURSING DIAGNOSES

. . . .

Alteration in Cerebral Tissue Perfusion Related to Increased Intracranial Pressure

See Increased Intracranial Pressure.

. . . .

Impaired Gas Exchange Related to Altered Oxygen Supply or Oxygen Carrying Capacity

See Chapter 1, The Pulmonary System.

. . . .

Ineffective Breathing Pattern Related to Inadequate Airway from Depressed Level of Consciousness, Intracranial Pathology, or Metabolic Imbalance

1. **Assessment for defining characteristics**
   a. Tachypnea
   b. Shallow, rapid respirations
   c. Deep, labored respirations
   d. $PaCO_2$ greater than 45 mm Hg or less than 30 mm Hg
   e. Altered level of responsiveness
   f. ICP greater than 20 mm Hg
   g. Nasal flaring
   h. Change in alveolar minute ventilation
   i. Arterial pH below 7.35
2. **Expected outcomes**

a. $PaCO_2$ remains between 35 and 45 mm Hg or at ordered level
b. ICP stays below 20 mm Hg
c. Normal acid-base balance is maintained

3. **Nursing interventions**
   a. Monitor pulmonary status as patient's condition warrants
   b. Maintain mechanical ventilation as ordered
   c. Suction as necessary to keep airway patent
   d. Maintain $PaCO_2$ within ordered range
   e. Monitor ICP; maintain below 20 mm Hg
   f. Administer sedation as ordered to maintain adequate ventilation
   g. Monitor neurologic status
   h. Monitor pH, lactate levels

4. **Evaluation of nursing care**
   a. $PaCO_2$ is maintained below 45 mm Hg and as ordered
   b. ICP remains below 20 mm Hg
   c. There is no laboratory evidence of metabolic acidosis

Ineffective Airway Clearance Related to Increased Secretions, Depressed Level of Consciousness

See Chapter 1.

1. **Additional nursing interventions**
   a. Turn the patient every 2 hours, and position to maintain mobility of secretions while keeping the head of the bed at 30° or as ordered. A specialty bed that provides continual rotation of 40° may be helpful
   b. Suction as necessary to maintain patent airway; monitor ICP during suctioning, limit suctioning to 15 seconds, and hyperoxygenate prior to and after suctioning

Potential Fluid Volume Deficit Related to Excessive Loss, Decreased Intake, Diabetes Insipidus, Cerebral Salt Wasting Syndrome

1. **Assessment for defining characteristics**
   a. Oliguria
   b. Weight loss
   c. Altered electrolytes (e.g., sodium >150 mEq/L). Sodium is less than 135 mEq/L in cerebral salt wasting syndrome
   d. Serum osmolality above 310 mOsm/L
   e. Urine specific gravity increased
   f. Low blood pressure
   g. Rapid, thready pulse
   h. Increased temperature
   i. History of osmotic or loop diuretic therapy, fluid restriction, hemorrhage
   j. Low central venous pressure (CVP) or pulmonary artery wedge pressure (PAWP)
   k. Altered coagulation studies
   l. Decreased level of responsiveness
   m. Diabetes insipidus: urine output above 200 ml/hour for 3 consecutive hours, with a specific gravity below 1.005

2. **Expected outcomes**
   a. Patient maintains stable vital signs and neurologic status
   b. Urine output is between 30 ml and 100 ml/hour, with specific gravity 1.005 to 1.020
   c. Electrolytes, osmolality, and clotting profile are within normal limits
3. **Nursing interventions**
   a. Monitor vital signs and neurologic status every hour until stable
   b. Measure, record, and report intake and output every hour
   c. Measure specific gravity every 2 to 4 hours
   d. Administer fluid and blood products as ordered. Record effectiveness
   e. Monitor CVP and PAWP. Report deviations from desired range
   f. Monitor electrolytes, serum osmolality, and clotting profile
   g. Weigh daily
   h. Administer exogenous pitressin as ordered; monitor response
4. **Evaluation of nursing care**
   a. Vital signs and neurologic status are maintained within expected range
   b. Urine output is maintained above 30 ml/hour
   c. Electrolytes, serum osmolality, and clotting profile are maintained in normal range

Fluid Volume Excess Related to Syndrome of Inappropriate ADH

See Chapter 5.

Potential for Infection Related to Invasive Lines, Monitoring and Therapeutic Devices, Traumatic and Surgical Wounds

1. **Assessment for defining characteristics**
   a. Presence of invasive monitoring lines
   b. Presence of traumatic wounds or surgical incision
   c. Leaking of CSF around ICP device
   d. Wet dressings
   e. Drainage devices
   f. Presence of tracheal intubation and humidified ventilation
   g. Drainage of purulent material around catheter insertion sites
   h. Redness or swelling of intravenous site or wound
   i. Fever, tachycardia
   j. Laboratory findings consistent with infection, such as elevated WBCs or ESR
2. **Expected outcomes**
   a. Wound and drainage cultures are free of pathogens
   b. Respiratory secretions remain clear and odorless
   c. Wounds and incisions are clean, pink, and free of purulent drainage
   d. Intravenous lines show no signs of inflammation
   e. ICP device has no drainage; remains free of WBCs
3. **Nursing interventions**
   a. Minimize risk of infection by using good hand-washing technique and wearing gloves

b. Use aseptic technique when handling invasive lines and when setting up monitoring systems

c. Culture drainage and secretions per order or unit protocol

d. Change lines every 72 hours and tubings every 24 hours or per hospital protocol

e. Remove invasive line as soon as clinically possible

f. Rotate IV and ICP sites per hospital protocol

g. Monitor lines and wounds for signs of infection

4. **Evaluation of nursing care**

a. Cultures of drainage and secretions are sterile

b. Wounds heal without signs of infection

c. Insertion sites are free of signs of infection

Potential for Injury Related to Seizure Activity

1. **Assessment for defining characteristics**

a. Grand mal seizure (tonic-clonic seizure)

i. Tonic-clonic symmetric movements involving whole body

ii. No focal onset

iii. Loss of consciousness; no purposeful actions or responses

iv. Profuse salivation during seizure

v. Apnea and cyanosis may develop, clear as seizure terminates

vi. Incontinence is common

vii. Usually lasts 1 to 5 minutes

b. Myoclonic: sudden, brief, muscular contractions that may occur singly or repetitively; usually involves arms

c. Partial seizures

i. Motor: focal motor seizures that are confined to specific body parts but may progress and become generalized; may be associated with an aura—that is, a sensory phenomenon preceding seizure activity

ii. Sensory: somatic sensory seizures that patient describes as numbness or tingling; may generalize. Special sensory seizures may include visual, auditory, or vertiginous symptoms

2. **Expected outcomes**

a. Patient does not experience injuries from seizure activity

b. Patient experiences no toxic effects from anticonvulsants

3. **Nursing interventions**

a. Observe seizure activity; record and report observations

i. Note time and signs of impending attack

ii. Observe parts of body involved, order of involvement, and character of movements

iii. Check for deviation of eyes and nystagmus; note change in pupillary size

iv. Assess respiratory pattern and function

v. Assess patient during postictal phase; note neurologic deficits

b. Prevent injuries during convulsive seizure activity

i. Never force anything into the patient's mouth

ii. Do not attempt to restrain the patient's movements

iii. Remove objects from the vicinity that can cause injury

iv. Pad side rails to protect the patient from trauma during convulsive activity

    c. Monitor and maintain therapeutic plasma levels of anticonvulsant medication. Phenytoin and phenobarbital are the most frequently used drugs in the acute setting

    d. Observe for toxic effects of anticonvulsants

        i. Rash: may be anywhere on body, but usually starts on the arms and chest; the face is involved frequently. If a rash is caused by phenytoin, the drug should be discontinued because of the potential for the development of a severe dematologic reaction (Stevens-Johnson syndrome)

        ii. Nystagmus, ataxia, or dysmetria may indicate excessive serum levels of drug

        iii. Liver function test results may become abnormal with some drugs; if severe, may need to change drugs

    e. Diagnose and treat causative factors

    f. Eliminate precipitating factors, such as electrolyte disorders, particularly sodium

4. Evaluation of nursing care

    a. Absence of injury is related to seizure activity

    b. There is adequate control of seizures

    c. Side effects and toxic effects from anticonvulsants are absent or controlled

. . . .

Impaired Verbal Communication Related to Expressive/Receptive Dysphasia

1. Assessment for defining characteristics

    a. Inability to speak

    b. Inability to name objects

    c. Perseveration

    d. Inability to speak sentences

    e. Inability to understand spoken or written language

    f. Use of inappropriate words

    g. Speech unrelated to environmental stimuli

    h. Incessant verbalization

    i. Unable to follow commands

2. Expected outcomes

    a. Patient's needs are met

    b. Patient uses effective methods of communication

3. Nursing interventions

    a. Assess comprehension and expression of written and spoken language

    b. Explain to the patient and family the extent and pathology of language deficit

    c. Encourage patience when communication difficulties arise

    d. Utilize strengths when communicating (e.g., gestures, yes/no, pointing, pictures, alphabet board)

    e. Speak slowly; use short phrases

    f. Allow time for the patient to respond

    g. Repeat or rephrase questions

    h. Communicate for short periods to avoid tiring and frustrating the patient

    i. Collaborate with a speech therapist for specific interventions

j. Involve the family in developing and utilizing effective communication techniques

4. **Evaluation of nursing care:** Patient is able to communicate, and needs are met

. . . .
.
. **Impaired Physical Mobility Related to Weakness or Paralysis of One or More Body Parts**

1. **Assessment for defining characteristics**
   a. Limited range of motion
   b. Decreased muscle strength, control, mass, endurance
   c. Inability to purposefully move in the environment, including bed mobility, transfer, and ambulation
2. **Expected outcomes**
   a. Full joint range of motion and muscle strength are maintained
   b. Patient exhibits no evidence of complications, such as contractures or skin breakdown
3. **Nursing interventions**
   a. Perform range-of-motion exercises to joints, progress from passive to active as tolerated
   b. Assess motor strength every shift
   c. Encourage independent activity as tolerated
   d. Reposition patient frequently if not on a rotational bed; maintain functional anatomic alignment, protect bony prominences. Use rotational beds in acute stages to protect skin from pressure
   e. Collaborate with physical and occupational therapists in teaching of self–range of motion, splinting devices, transfer techniques
   f. Place items within reach of the unaffected arm
   g. Involve the family in therapy as appropriate
   h. Assess integrity of the skin when turning the patient
   i. Have patient up in chair two to four times per day, as tolerated, per order
4. **Evaluation of nursing care**
   a. Joint mobility is maintained
   b. There is no evidence of skin breakdown
   c. Contractures are absent

. . . .
.
. **Alteration in Thought Processes Related to Confusion, Short-Term Memory Loss, Short Attention Span**

1. **Assessment for defining characteristics**
   a. Disoriented to time, place, person, and environment
   b. Diminished problem-solving abilities
   c. Lack of sequential thought (i.e., patient unable to remember events as they occurred or in the proper time sequence)
   d. Noncompliance to requests or instructions
   e. Inability to complete simple tasks
   f. Attempts to carry out activities beyond capabilities
   g. Patients with right hemisphere lesions often have poor judgment and problem-solving capabilities

2. **Expected outcomes**
   a. Patient carries out ADL with minimal assistance or guidance
   b. Patient is fully oriented
   c. Injury does not occur
3. **Nursing interventions**
   a. Orient to environment frequently
      i. Call the patient by name
      ii. Tell the patient your name
      iii. Provide tools to help maintain orientation (e.g., calendar, clock, newspapers, radio, television)
      iv. Keep patient items in same place
   b. Provide simple instructions frequently; assist and encourage as necessary
   c. Protect the patient from injury (e.g., restraints, side rails, call light, bed near nurses' station)
   d. Teach and involve the family as appropriate
4. **Evaluation of nursing care**
   a. Patient is fully oriented
   b. Injury is absent
   c. Patient carries out simple ADL

Ineffective Individual Coping Related to Situational Crisis, Loss of Control and Independence, Change in Role

1. **Assessment for defining characteristics**
   a. Verbal manipulation
   b. Inappropriate use of defense mechanisms
   c. Inability to meet basic needs
   d. Inability to meet role expectations
   e. General irritability
   f. Verification of situational crisis
2. **Expected outcomes**
   a. Patient becomes involved in planning and participating in care
   b. Patient communicates feelings about present situation
   c. Patient develops positive ways to deal with illness or deficits
3. **Nursing interventions**
   a. If possible, assign a primary nurse to provide continuity and promote development of a relationship
   b. Spend time with the patient; allow the patient to express fears and concerns. Help identify and develop coping strategies
   c. Explain present and future treatment plan
   d. Encourage participation in care, allow choices
   e. Give feedback about progress
   f. Determine the patient's ongoing strengths and values
   g. Include the family in planning and implementation
   h. Involve other health professionals (e.g., psychiatric clinical nurse specialist) as necessary
4. **Evaluation of nursing care**
   a. Patient participates and takes responsibility for aspects of care
   b. Patient verbalizes feelings about the situation
   c. Patient incorporates effective coping behaviors

Ineffective Family Coping Related to Disruption of Usual Family Roles, Burden of Care, Changes in Family Member's Present and Future Functioning

1. **Assessment for defining characteristics**
   a. Family member or members express concern for future care of the patient
   b. Family expresses unrealistic expectations of outcome, such as daily improvement
   c. Family expresses concern about their financial, social, and spiritual future
   d. Family is demanding and manipulative with nursing and medical staff
2. **Expected outcomes**
   a. Family describes impact of the patient's illness on relationships and family functioning
   b. Family develops coping strategies, when applicable, to deal with caring for a chronically ill family member
3. **Nursing interventions**
   a. Facilitate family conferences; help family identify key issues, and select support services as needed
   b. Encourage use of coping behaviors that have worked previously; help develop new coping strategies
   c. Assist family in developing realistic expectations of current and future functioning of the patient while maintaining an optimistic attitude
   d. Allow the family to express feelings of hurt, fear, anger, despair, and guilt
   e. Encourage family members to participate in care when possible
   f. Interpret the patient's behavior to the family, particularly if it is bizarre or combative
   g. Refer to professional counseling after consultation with team
4. **Evaluation of nursing care**
   a. Family expresses concerns and identifies how they will cope
   b. Family demonstrates effective coping and adaptive strategies

PATIENT HEALTH PROBLEMS

Increased Intracranial Pressure

1. **Pathophysiology**
   a. Nondistensible intracranial cavity is filled to capacity with essentially noncompressible contents: CSF, intravascular blood, brain tissue water (interstitial and intracellular fluid)
   b. The *Monro-Kellie hypothesis* states that if volume of one of constituents of intracranial cavity increases, a reciprocal decrease in volume of one or both of the others must occur or an overall increase in ICP will result
   c. Principal spatial buffers that resist increases in ICP are displacement of CSF from cranial vault and compression of low-pressure venous system. Increased CSF absorption may also contribute to spatial compensation
      i. Volume of fluid that can be displaced is finite; an increase in ICP

ultimately occurs if volume of intracranial mass exceeds volume of fluid displaced

   ii. Relationship between intracranial volume and pressure has been plotted and an elastance curve (inverse of compliance) constructed (Fig. 3–25). The flat portion of curve reflects little change in pressure with increases in volume (low elastance or high compliance), and the steep portion of curve reflects large pressure changes with small increases in volume (high elastance or decreased compliance). A patient's response to changes in intracranial volume, therefore, depends, in part, on where patient is on volume/pressure curve. The rate of volume change also influences magnitude of ICP change

  d. CBF varies with changes in cerebral perfusion pressure (CPP) and diameter of cerebrovascular bed

    i. Increased ICP can increase CBF indirectly by producing cortical vascular dilatation and appears to be principal mechanism responsible for maintenance of CBF in face of rising ICP

    ii. When ICP approaches MAP, CPP decreases to the point where autoregulation is impaired and CBF decreases

      (a) When autoregulation is impaired, arterioles passively dilate with increases in arterial blood pressure, causing increased CBF; however, pressure in venous system (capacitance system) also rises, cerebral blood volume (CBV) increases, and ICP rises further

      (b) Resultant high capillary pressure causes oozing of plasma from vessels and petechial hemorrhages

      (c) Eventually, perfusion pressure can no longer be maintained and CBF gradually falls as ICP increases

    iii. Increases in CO_2 tension, and to a lesser extent decreases in O_2 tension, also cause arteriolar dilatation and increases in CBF. Hypoxia and hypercapnia thus lead to intracranial hypertension, especially in patients with unstable intracranial dynamics

  e. Herniation syndromes

    i. *Tentorial (uncal)* herniation: expanding lesions above the tentorium,

Figure 3–25 • Elastance curve showing the region of low intracranial pressure and low elastance (A), low intracranial pressure and high elastance (B), and high intracranial pressure and high elastance (C). Region A describes the state of normal intracranial pressure and a "safe" amount of volume buffering capacity. Region B includes patients with a normal intracranial pressure with a dangerously low amount of volume reserve. Region C is clearly abnormal, and the diagnosis is readily confirmed by the level of intracranial pressure. (From Lee, K. R., and Hoff, J. T.: Intracranial pressure. *In* Youmans, J. R. [ed.]: Neurological Surgery. Philadelphia, W. B. Saunders, 1996.)

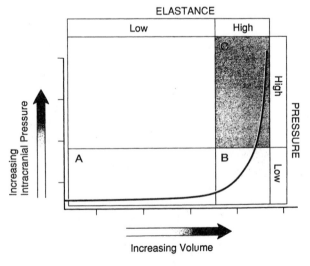

particularly on one side, force the uncus of the temporal lobe over
the medial edge of the tentorium

    ii. *Subfalcine* herniation: unilateral cerebral lesions can cause a shift of
brain tissue from one side to the other, causing the cingulate gyrus
to become distorted under the falx cerebri

    iii. *Tonsillar* (medullary) herniation: displacement of the contents of the
posterior fossa, particularly the tonsils of the cerebellum, through the
foramen magnum causes brain stem distortion and potential
respiratory and vasomotor collapse

    iv. *Central* herniation: midline or bilateral lesions of the cerebrum cause
it to be displaced downward through the tentorial notch causing
pressure on the midbrain. Can progress to tonsillar herniation

  f. A supratentorial lesion that causes tentorial herniation compresses the
ipsilateral oculomotor nerve and impairs its parasympathetic activity,
leading to a larger pupil with a sluggish or absent direct light reflex. In as
many as one third of cases of head injury, the contralateral pupil may
dilate if uncal herniation causes contralateral midbrain compression
against the opposite tentorial edge

  g. Increased ICP can also exert pressure on motor and sensory nerve tracts,
leading to impairment or loss of function usually contralateral to the
compression. Kernohan's notch phenomenon, however, causes ipsilateral
hemiparesis or hemiplegia by compression of the contralateral cerebral
peduncle

  h. Ischemia of vasomotor center in brain stem may trigger Cushing's reflex,
causing rise in systolic pressure, widening pulse pressure, and slowing of
pulse. Respiratory rate and pattern may also change

2. Etiologic or precipitating factors

  a. ICP increases when the volume added to the intracranial cavity exceeds
the compensatory capacity. The rate and extent of the increase in ICP
depends on:

    i. Volume of the mass lesion

    ii. Rate of expansion (i.e., the faster the volume is added, the greater
the rise in ICP)

    iii. Total volume within the intracranial cavity

    iv. Intracranial compliance (elastance) (i.e., the capacity for
compensation)

  b. Increases in brain volume caused by:

    i. Mass lesions: subdural, epidural, or intracerebral hematomas, tumors,
abscesses, or any other space-occupying lesions

    ii. Cytotoxic cerebral edema: intracellular swelling of neurons and glial
cells. Caused by hypoxia or acute hypo-osmolality (water
intoxication). Hypoxia causes anaerobic glycolysis and a decreased
production of ATP. Because there is insufficient ATP to fuel the Na^+-
K^+ pump, Na^+ is no longer pumped out of the cell or K^+ back into
the cell, leading to an accumulation of Na^+ inside the cell. Water
then moves into the cell, causing cellular swelling. Acute hypo-
osmolality causes water to move into the cell via osmosis. Swelling of
the epithelial cells surrounding the capillaries causes vascular
compression and ischemia

    iii. Vasogenic cerebral edema: increase in extracellular fluid space
caused by breakdown of the blood-brain barrier which allows

osmotically active molecules, such as proteins, to leak into the interstitium, drawing water from the vascular system and cells into the interstitium. Caused by most types of cerebral injury or insult including contusions, tumors, or abscesses. Edema is localized around the lesion

c. Cerebrovascular alterations
   i. Venous outflow obstruction
      (a) Rotation, hyperextension, hyperflexion of head, and excessively tight endotracheal or tracheotomy ties all lead to flattening or compression of the jugular veins and inhibit venous return, causing venous engorgement
      (b) Raised intrathoracic and/or intra-abdominal pressures may also impair venous return. Positive end-expiratory pressure, coughing, vomiting, and Valsalva's maneuver may all cause this phenomenon
   ii. Fluctuations in blood pressure or CPP
      (a) Blood pressure that exceeds the limits of autoregulation contributes to increased CBV and cerebral edema
      (b) Autoregulation may be impaired, either globally or regionally, by cerebral injury or insult. CBF to affected area of brain is then dependent on blood pressure (i.e., CBF increases as the blood pressure rises, contributing to cerebral edema and increased ICP). Conversely, as the blood pressure falls, CBF falls and leads to cerebral ischemia
      (c) CPP less than 40 mm Hg exceeds the cerebral vascular capacity for autoregulation; CBF falls, leading to cerebral ischemia
   iii. Vasodilatation
      (a) Hypoventilation causes hypercapnia and vasodilatation, leading to increased CBF and ICP. Abnormal respiratory patterns, obstructed airway, or excess secretions may all cause CO_2 retention
      (b) Hypoxia also causes cerebral vasodilatation, although its effects are not significant until the Pao_2 falls below 60 mm Hg
      (c) Certain anesthetic agents (halothane, ketamine, and nitrous oxide) and drugs (nitroprusside, curare) cause cerebral vasodilatation and lead to increased CBV and increased ICP and thus should be used with caution in the neurosurgical patient

d. Increases in CSF volume (hydrocephalus)
   i. Increased production of CSF is a rare cause of increased CSF volume and is not seen often in clinical practice
   ii. Decreased reabsorption of CSF leading to increased CSF volume is caused in two major ways:
      (a) Obstruction of CSF circulation out of the ventricular system. May be caused by mass lesions in or near ventricles or obstruction of the basal cisterna at the base of the brain
      (b) Impaired reabsorption of CSF from the subarachnoid space into the venous system. May be caused by inflammation of the meninges and obstruction of the arachnoid villa by debris, such as blood cells or bacteria

3. **Nursing assessment data base**
   a. Nursing history

i. Trauma, mass lesion, infectious process, hydrocephalus, or other factors that may lead to raised ICP

ii. ICP monitoring data showing increased ICP

b. Nursing examination of patient

   i. Increased ICP may be present with little or no change in clinical presentation, depending on etiology

   ii. Changes in level of consciousness, motor activity, pupillary size or reflexes, cranial nerve, and vital signs from one assessment to another indicate possible increasing ICP

   iii. Papilledema may be present with longstanding intracranial hypertension

   iv. Other signs and symptoms that indicate a change in patient's neurologic status or increased ICP must be evaluated in light of history and clinical presentation

      (a) Increasing headache

      (b) Blurred vision, diplopia, photophobia

      (c) Seizure activity: may be due to head trauma, anoxia, tumors, or electrolyte disorders in acutely ill patients without history of seizure disorders

      (d) Vomiting: lesions that produce vomiting are those that involve vestibular nuclei, impinge on floor of fourth ventricle, or (less often) produce brain stem compression secondary to increased ICP

      (e) Nuchal rigidity: difficulty or an inability to flex the patient's head and complaints of neck pain indicate irritation of meninges, most commonly due to meningitis or subarachnoid hemorrhage

c. Diagnostic study findings

   i. Lumbar puncture: contraindicated by increased ICP. Reliable measure of ICP only if communication between lumbar subarachnoid space and ventricular system is unobstructed

   ii. ICP monitoring

      (a) Because the brain is deformed and displaced easily by mass lesions, it is thought that persistent differences in pressure do not develop within brain substance, although this remains controversial. There is evidence that there is a pressure differential between the supratentorial and infratentorial regions with lesions of the posterior fossa

         (1) CSF pressure: because CSF is contained within a closed system and pressure is transmitted equally in all directions in fluid, CSF pressure is considered the most accurate indicator of ICP. Choroid plexus pulsations are transmitted to CSF throughout ventricular system and subarachnoid space. The pulsations produce a waveform in the ventricles, although of lower amplitude, with the same characteristics as an arterial waveform. The waveform is further dampened in the subarachnoid space and often resembles a venous waveform

         (2) Intraparenchymal pressure: recent research has demonstrated a linear relationship between intraventricular and intraparenchymal pressure measured with a fiberoptic transducer-tipped probe

(3) Normal ICP is under 10 mm Hg, and pressures between 10 and 20 mm Hg are considered mildly to moderately elevated. Pressures over 20 mm Hg are severely elevated and are usually treated

(b) Indications: patients who benefit from ICP monitoring are those with severe head trauma, known or suspected hydrocephalus, posterior fossa lesions, and subarachnoid hemorrhage. Patients with tumors may benefit from ICP monitoring if the tumor has the potential for obstructing CSF pathways

(c) Techniques

(1) Intraventricular method: A cannula is inserted into the lateral ventricle (usually the anterior horn in nondominant hemisphere) via a twist drill hole through skull. The cannula is connected via a stopcock to fluid-filled pressure tubing to a transducer that is positioned at level of foramen of Monro (the middle of ear may be used as reference). Alternately, a fiberoptic, transducer-tipped catheter may be introduced into the lateral ventricle and connected to a monitor that displays the pressure

a) Advantages: ability to measure CSF pressure directly, drain CSF therapeutically, and withdraw CSF for analysis

b) Disadvantages: risks of infection, inadvertent loss of CSF, and difficulty in placement of cannula if ventricles are small or displaced

(2) Intraparenchymal method: A fiberoptic transducer-tipped probe is placed into the parenchyma of the brain through a twist drill hole in the skull. This is connected to a monitor that provides an analog readout and can be interfaced to the standard pressure monitor to visualize a waveform

a) Advantages: easy to place; not dependent on ventricular size or position

b) Disadvantages: once in place cannot be "re-zeroed" and drift of the transducer can cause erroneous readings. The fiberoptic of the probe is fragile and may break if it is bent when the patient is being transferred or is restless. The probe may become dislodged if the bolt connection is not tight

(3) Subarachnoid method: infrequently used because of many technical difficulties in maintaining the integrity of the system. A hollow bolt is placed into the subarachnoid space through a twist drill hole in the skull. Fluid-filled pressure tubing connects the bolt to the transducer. A fiberoptic transducer-tipped probe may also be placed in the subarachnoid space, although the efficacy depends on the fiberoptic technology used

a) Advantage: its ability to measure CSF pressure directly theoretically increases accuracy of readings

b) Disadvantages:

i) CSF sampling and drainage from this system are not usually possible *ii*) The bolt system needs to be irrigated to keep it patent, and thus the potential for infection is increased

iii) The addition of even a small amount of irrigating solution to the subarachnoid space may increase ICP

iv) Improper placement of either the bolt or the fiberoptic probe results in erroneous measurements

v) The fiberoptic probe cannot be re-zeroed once it is in place

4. Nursing Diagnoses

a. Alterations in cerebral tissue perfusion related to increased ICP

  i. Assessment for defining characteristics

    (a) Changes in level of consciousness, pupillary size and reaction, motor ability, especially abnormal motor responses, and vital signs that may indicate rising ICP

    (b) Rise in ICP to above 20 mm Hg is noted on monitor

    (c) Fall in CPP to below 70 mm Hg as calculated

  ii. Expected outcomes

    (a) ICP remains below 20 mm Hg and CPP remains above 70 mm Hg or as ordered

    (b) Patient experiences no complications as a result of ICP monitoring

  iii. Nursing interventions

    (a) Interventions to maintain ICP monitoring

      (1) For intraventricular and subarachnoid bolt techniques, ensure a closed system to prevent contamination. Because system must be opened to obtain CSF specimens and to zero-balance, take great care to prevent contamination

      (2) Maintain the transducer at the level of the foramen of Monro

      (3) Zero-balance whenever the bed or the patient's position is changed or if erroneous readings are suspected. Keep the transducer and tubing free of air bubbles to avoid dampening of waveform and inaccurate readings

      (4) Report and record changes in waveform, elevations in pressure, and therapy instituted

        a) Normal ventricular pressure is under 10 mm Hg, with pressures between 10 and 20 mm Hg considered mildly to moderately elevated. Pressures above 20 mm Hg are considered severely elevated

        b) Transient increases may occur with suctioning, coughing, Valsalva maneuver, inappropriate positioning of head and neck, or other nursing interventions

        c) Three types of ICP waveforms have been described:

          i) *A waves* (also called *plateau* or *Lundberg waves*): elevations of ICP between 50 and 100 mm Hg, lasting 5 to 20 minutes. May or may not be associated with clinical manifestations of increased ICP. Associated with advanced stages of intracranial hypertension

              ii) *B* and *C waves* are variations in pressure that correspond to respiratory and arterial pressure changes, respectively, but generally are not considered clinically significant

   (b) Interventions to control ICP

      (1) Facilitate venous return

         a) Elevate the head of the bed 15° to 30°, or as ordered

         b) Prevent hyperextension, flexion, or rotation of the head

         c) If the patient has tracheostomy, make sure ties are not too tight. If patient has an endotracheal tube, make sure it is not taped around entire head

      (2) Limit suctioning to 15 seconds to minimize blood gas alterations. Hyperoxygenation before and during suctioning may minimize detrimental effects of suctioning

      (3) Maintain euvolemia and normal electrolytes. Maintain serum osmolality below 310 mOsm/L

      (4) Maintain normothermia (<37.5°C)

      (5) Maintain adequate serum levels of anticonvulsant (usually phenytoin) to prevent seizure activity

      (6) CSF drainage: most effective in reducing ICP if ventricles are of normal size or enlarged

         a) Always drain CSF against a positive pressure to reduce the risk of draining too much CSF or draining it too quickly, leading to the potential for development of intracranial hemorrhage

         b) CSF drainage to control ICP is usually done on an intermittent basis so that monitoring will not be interrupted for prolonged periods. Open the stopcock on the drainage device, and drain CSF until the flow stops, usually 1 to 3 ml, although this is extremely variable, depending on size of the ventricles and degree of brain swelling

         c) If the ventricular catheter is not in optimal position or if the ventricles are small or compressed, CSF drainage may lead to loss of the ICP waveform secondary to collapse of the ventricle around the catheter. The ICP readings under these circumstances may not be accurate and should be interpreted with caution. This can usually be reversed by closing the stopcock to drain and allowing CSF to reaccumulate until an acceptable waveform is established

         d) If the patient has a CSF leak, the ventricular catheter may be left open to drain and closed intermittently (every 30 to 60 minutes) for ICP readings. Draining CSF continually when there is a CSF leak helps the tear in the dura to heal. Drainage of CSF is not always effective in controlling ICP, however, and if the ICP is above 20 mm Hg on intermittent monitoring, increase the frequency of monitoring and employ other interventions

      (7) Hyperventilation causes vasoconstriction and thus reduces

CBF and CBV. Although hyperventilation has been used in the past to control ICP, its use has been found to correlate with poorer short-term outcome in head trauma patients than in patients who were not hyperventilated. Hyperventilation has also been associated with jugular venous desaturation, indicating impaired CBF. Therefore, current recommendations are to maintain a $PaCO_2$ of 30 to 35 mm Hg, if needed, to control intracranial hypertension. Avoid hyperventilation in the first 24 hours after head injury when CBF is low

(8) Sedation with narcotics, benzodiazapines, or propofol often is effective in reducing ICP, particularly in restless or agitated patients. Do not use sedation without ICP monitoring. Morphine is commonly used in repeated bolus doses or as a constant infusion of 2 to 15 mg/hour. If morphine is used over a number of days, taper the dose rather than abruptly discontinuing it

(9) Consider neuromuscular blockade (NMB) with pancuronium, vecuronium, or atracurium or other NMB agents if the ICP remains high (despite CSF drainage and sedation) and if the patient is restless or agitated, has increased muscle tone, or is resisting the ventilator

(10) Mannitol in doses of 0.25 to 1.0 g/kg as a bolus for increases in ICP despite previous therapy is effective in reducing ICP by osmotic diuresis and perhaps by decreasing the viscosity of the blood and improving microcirculation. Mannitol is given as a rapid IV infusion every 4 to 6 hours as needed for ICP above 20 mm Hg. Monitor serum osmolality prior to mannitol administration, and maintain below 310 mOsm/kg. Also monitor renal function if frequent doses of mannitol are given

(11) Maintain CPP above 70 mm Hg with fluid administration, including crystalloids (half normal or normal saline based on serum Na^+ levels) and colloids (blood products as necessary, albumin, or hetastarch). Maintain CVP at 5 to 10 mm Hg or the PAWP between 10 and 14 mm Hg. Vasopressors may be necessary. Dobutamine may be needed if cardiac output is low

(12) Barbiturate therapy is the last step in control of ICP. Pentobarbital is the most common barbiturate used. The mechanism by which barbiturates act to lower the ICP include suppression of metabolism, inhibition of free radical–mediated lipid peroxidation, and alteration of the vascular tone

   a) Criteria: although absolute criteria are lacking, barbiturate therapy is conventionally initiated when the ICP is above 30 mm Hg for more than 30 minutes with a CPP below 70 mm Hg, or an ICP above 40 mm Hg regardless of CPP after maximal therapy to reduce ICP has been employed

   b) Administration: make sure that the patient is euvolemic

and hemodynamically stable before initiating therapy. The loading dose is 10 mg/kg given IV over 30 minutes (slower if blood pressure drops), followed by 5 mg/kg every hour for 3 hours, then 1 to 3 mg/kg/hour maintenance. Vasopressors are usually required to maintain blood pressure and perfusion pressure

    c) Monitoring: initiate pulmonary artery monitoring if it is not already in place. Monitor EEG, and titrate pentobarbital to burst suppression of 8 to 10 seconds of suppression and 1 to 2 seconds of activity

    d) Complications: the potential complications of barbiturate therapy are many and can be severe. Hypotension, pneumonia, hypothermia, and other infections are common

    e) Barbiturates may be discontinued when the ICP has remained under 20 mm Hg for 24 hours or more. Neurologic assessment of the patient is not reliable until the barbiturate levels fall, which sometimes requires 3 or more days

(13) Glucocorticoids are not recommended for reducing ICP or improving outcome in patients with head injury. Glucocorticoids are indicated for patients with other intracranial pathology, most notably intracranial tumors, spinal cord injury tumors, and some infectious processes

· · · · · · · · · ·

Head Trauma

1. **Pathophysiology:** trauma to the head causes both primary injury to the brain (either focal or diffuse) and secondary injuries that result from the cascade of events that the primary injury initiates. Preinjury factors that influence the patient's response to brain injury include those listed in Figure 3–26. Primary injuries are discussed below. The postinjury factors that affect outcome include molecular and biochemical mechanisms, as well as secondary systemic and intracranial insults

   a. Molecular and biochemical mechanisms

     i. Lactate is increased in the brain and CSF after traumatic injury, and this increase correlates with severity of injury

     ii. Release of excitatory amino acids and neurotransmitter substances cause accumulation of intracellular calcium, resulting in neurodegeneration

     iii. Ionic fluxes of calcium, magnesium, and potassium have been implicated in the mechanisms that cause continued cellular damage and death after injury

     iv. Excessive free radicals are produced after brain injury and cause loss of cell membrane integrity, which contributes to neuronal degeneration and cell death

   b. Secondary intracranial insults

     i. Intracranial hypertension correlates with poor outcome

     ii. Brain edema is common after trauma and may be a major factor in increased ICP

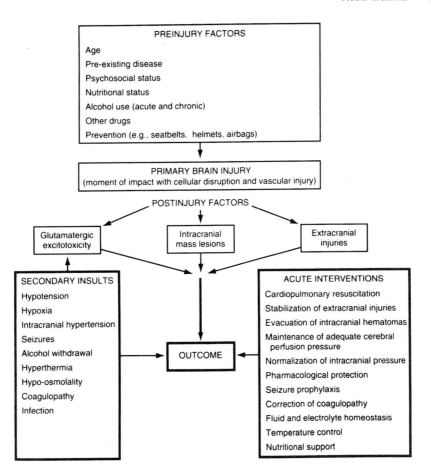

Figure 3-26 • Schematic representation of factors and interventions that influence outcome before and after traumatic brain injury. CPP = cerebral perfusion pressure, ICP = intracranial pressure. (From Kelly, D. F., Nikas, D. L., and Becker, D. P.: Diagnosis and treatment of moderate and severe head injuries in adults. *In* Youmans, J. R. [ed]: Neurological Surgery. Philadelphia, W. B. Saunders, 1996.)

    iii. Seizure activity is deleterious in the early period after injury, as it causes a rapid rise in ICP and increases the metabolic needs of the brain

    iv. Intracranial infections causing meningitis or intracranial abscesses may be caused by a CSF leak, open or penetrating head wounds, or ICP monitoring devices

    v. Cerebral hyperemia contributes to increased ICP

    vi. Brain shift and herniation (see Increased Intracranial Pressure)

  c. Secondary systemic insults (see Fig. 3–26)

    i. Hypotension and hypoxia reduce CPP and oxygenation. The brain is more vulnerable to these insults in the first few hours and days

    ii. Hypoxia is caused by airway obstruction, aspiration, thoracic injury, hypoventilation, or pulmonary shunting

    iii. Hypotension is associated with doubling of mortality rates in patients with severe traumatic brain injury by lowering the CPP, often in the face of already low CBF and high ICP. This may be further complicated by disrupted autoregulation of CBF or vasospasm

iv. Cerebral ischemia may be caused by hypotension, hypoxia, vasospasm, or a combination

v. Hypoventilation causes cerebral vascular vasodilatation and contributes to intracranial hypertension. Hyperventilation below a $PaCO_2$ of 30 mm Hg may compromise CBF by causing vasoconstriction

vi. Hyperthermia increases the metabolic demands of the brain and is associated with a poorer outcome

vii. Both hyperglycemia and hypoglycemia have adverse effects on outcome after brain injury, but exact mechanisms are not understood

viii. Acute hypo-osmolality can lead to cellular swelling

ix. Electrolyte disorders, particularly sodium imbalance, can lead to cellular swelling or dehydration and are often caused by diabetes insipidus, syndrome of inappropriate antidiuretic hormone, or cerebral salt wasting

x. Coagulopathy contributes to intracranial hemorrhage

d. Primary injuries

i. Scalp lacerations: Because of extensive vascularity of scalp and poor contractility of vessels, lacerations can result in significant blood loss that may contribute to hypovolemic shock. In addition, because the venous drainage of the scalp is into the venous sinuses of the brain, a contaminated scalp laceration can lead to infection of the scalp itself, osteomyelitis, or intracranial abscess, particularly if there is an underlying skull fracture

ii. Skull fractures: the amount of brain damage, if any, associated with a skull fracture depends on the degree of inertial loading and direction of the impact as well as deceleration distance and the form of the object hitting the head

(a) Linear skull fracture

(1) Occurs secondary to a force applied over a wide surface area; no displacement of bone

(2) Is a matter of concern if the fracture crosses a major vascular channel, such as the middle meningeal artery, that can cause intracranial bleeding, usually an epidural hematoma

(3) May be open (compound), that is, associated with scalp laceration, which increases the potential for infection

(b) Basilar skull fracture: accounts for about 20% of all skull fractures. Most commonly arises from extension of a vault fracture into the base of the skull but may be caused a direct blow to the skull base

(1) Pneumocephalus (aerocele) occurs in 33% of those with anterior fossa fractures but may not be seen on initial scan. Air-fluid level may be seen on brow-up lateral skull film

(2) CSF leak: Caused by fractures of the frontal or middle basal fossae

a) In 25% of patients with an anterior fossa fracture, a CSF rhinorrhea develops; CSF otorrhea occurs only about 7% of the time and is associated with petrous bone fractures and rupture of the tympanic membrane. If the tympanic membrane is intact, the CSF will seek a course through the eustachian tube into the nasopharynx and will present as CSF rhinorrhea

b) Most leaks occur immediately but may be delayed until resolution of a hematoma or brain swelling or until after surgical repair of fractures

c) Suspected in patients who complain of a salty or sweet taste in the mouth

(3) Meningitis

a) Caused by dural tear with resultant CSF leak

b) Risk is difficult to determine because many cases of dural tearing are undetected

c) May occur weeks or months after injury

d) Need for antibiotics remains controversial. Antibiotics may be indicated if there is a persistent leak for which surgery is contemplated. The most common infecting organism is the pneumococcus

e) A lumbar CSF drain may be used to decrease the flow of CSF to help seal the leak by keeping the CSF pressure in the subarachnoid space low. The drain is usually kept open to drainage so that 10 to 15 ml of CSF is collected every hour

f) Indications for surgery include persistent leak, pneumocephalus, or meningitis in the face of a persistent CSF leak (somewhat controversial)

g) Most CSF leaks heal spontaneously in 5 to 7 days

(4) Cranial nerve injuries: the exact site and orientation of the fracture determine which cranial nerves may be damaged

a) CN I: associated with anterior fossa fractures. Anosmia may be the only symptom of a basilar skull fracture

b) CN V, CN VI, CN VII, CN VIII: associated with petrous bone fractures

c) CN IX, CN X, CN XI, CN XII: may be involved in fractures of the posterior fossa involving the occipital condyle (rare)

(c) Depressed skull fracture

(1) Depression of inner table more than one-half the thickness of the skull caused by falling objects, motor vehicle accidents, or assault. Significant contusion and edema of the scalp occur. If this injury is associated with a laceration, it is classified as an open or compound fracture; without an associated scalp laceration, it is considered a closed or simple fracture. Seventy-five percent or more of depressed fractures are compound fractures. Dural tears and parenchymal injury are seen in a high percentage of patients with compound fractures. Contusions or hematomas of the brain may also occur

(2) Neurologic presentation depends on location and extent of cerebral involvement; focal neurologic deficits may be present

(3) When the venous sinus is involved, potential for bleeding and venous obstruction are the major concerns

        (4) The scalp laceration should be shaved, cleaned, and dressed, and surgery for repair should be carried out within 24 to 48 hours. The bone fragments may be replaced if the wound was clean and surgery is done within 24 to 48 hours. Contaminated bone fragments are removed, and cranioplasty is delayed for 6 to 12 months after initial surgery

        (5) Simple (closed) depressed fractures are usually not elevated except for cosmetic reasons or to treat a progressive focal deficit

        (6) Antibiotic coverage is controversial. Antibiotics should be given if surgery is delayed, if treatment is incomplete (e.g., venous sinus fragment), or if the wound is grossly contaminated

        (7) Early seizures occur in about 10%, late seizures in about 15%. Epileptogenic focus is created at time of injury

  iii. Intracranial hemorrhage

    (a) In about one third of moderately to severely head-injured patients, intracranial hematomas develop

    (b) The clinical presentation of a patient with an intracranial hematomas is consistent with an expanding mass lesion. The clinical course varies, depending on location and rate of accumulation and the presence of other intracranial injuries. It is not possible to differentiate the type of hematoma according to clinical presentation

    (c) Epidural hematoma (EDH): most commonly, arterial bleeding resulting from a fracture over the middle meningeal artery in the temporal area. May also occur in the frontal, occipital, and posterior fossa regions. Hematoma collects above the dura

        (1) Patients (30% to 50%) may have a history of a lucid interval between the time of injury with loss of consciousness and a later deterioration of neurologic status. This phenomenon is not confined to the EDH. Often complains of headache, usually focal. Increasing irritability and agitation should alert the clinician to investigate further

        (2) Because of arterial origin, hematoma can collect rapidly and the patient can deteriorate precipitously

        (3) Posterior fossa EDH may cause nausea, vomiting, headache, stiff neck, and cardiovascular or respiratory instability. Hydrocephalus occurs in about 30% of patients. With these hematomas, there may be delayed onset

    (d) Subdural hematoma (SDH): Hematoma formation below the dura, usually caused by venous bleeding from tearing of the bridging veins. Traditionally, SDH have been categorized into three groups according to timing of presentation:

        (1) Acute: the patient shows immediate signs of deterioration (within 24 hours). Most present in coma or deteriorate within hours of injury. Usually occur as the result of rapid acceleration and deceleration of the head during trauma. Often associated with other intraparenchymal injuries,

which may be a greater factor in determining outcome than the SDH itself. Prognosis is poor

(2) Subacute: symptoms of neurologic deterioration and increased ICP are delayed for 4 to 21 days after injury. Treatment depends on the patient's clinical presentation

(3) Chronic: symptoms do not develop for 3 or more weeks after injury. Usually occur in older patients who suffered seemingly minor head injury or in younger adults who have alcoholic history and brain atrophy. The fluid collection is dark and turbid. Clinical presentation may mimic a variety of other disorders, including dementia and stroke, with vague symptoms such as headache, nausea, vomiting, and gait disturbance. Prognosis is good

(e) Intracerebral hematoma (ICH): Hemorrhage occurs into the parenchyma of the brain; produced by shearing and tensile stresses within the brain tissue that result in rupture of small vessels. Frequently occurs in the white matter of the frontal and temporal regions

(1) A mass lesion of 25 ml or greater generally requires surgical resection

(2) May be single or multiple and are often associated with other intracranial lesions, such as contusions, SDH, and diffuse axonal injury. Often accompany penetrating injuries

(f) Contusions: consist of perivascular hemorrhage around small vessels and necrotic brain. There may be coup and contrecoup contusions (i.e., point of impact injuries and injuries opposite or distant from impact, respectively). Contusions of the frontal and temporal poles of the cerebral hemispheres are common because acceleration and deceleration movements of the cranium and brain cause the brain to move across the bony structures of the base of the skull

(1) Hemorrhagic contusions may coalesce to become an ICH, and may coexist with ICH. May be seen anywhere in the brain; most frequently seen with moderate and severe head injury. Coup and contrecoup areas may be seen. Injury to opposite side of brain may be greater

(2) Deep intracerebral hematomas are often associated with diffuse axonal injury. Development may be delayed for hours to days

(3) Posterior and medial temporal lobe contusions, because of the precarious location near the tentorium, should be removed regardless of the patient's clinical condition

(g) Subarachnoid hemorrhage (SAH): Trauma is the most common cause. May occur with other injuries or as the only evidence of trauma. Results from forces that produce stress sufficient to damage superficial vascular structures in the subarachnoid space. May predispose to cerebral vasospasm, leading to diminished blood supply and ischemic damage

(h) Intraventricular hemorrhage (IVH): bleeding into the ventricles caused by severe brain trauma or gunshot or stab wounds to the brain. Occurs in fewer than 10% of trauma victims but contributes to mortality

iv. Diffuse brain injury (closed head injury)

    (a) Mild concussion represents temporary neurologic dysfunction but is reversible with no persistent sequelae. May be the result of rotational forces on the brain, causing stretching of nerve fibers with subsequent failure of conduction. Repeated mild concussions have cumulative effects. Retrograde amnesia of short duration occurs

    (b) Classic concussion is also reversible and is associated with a brief loss of consciousness with disorientation and retrograde and post-traumatic amnesia. Post-concussion syndrome is common and includes some or all of the following: memory problems, headache, dizziness, information processing problems, visual disturbances, coordination problems, lethargy

    (c) Diffuse axonal injury (DAI), a potentially serious form of closed head injury, is diffuse white matter shearing associated with severe mechanical disruption of axons and neuronal pathways in the hemispheres, diencephalon, and brain stem. As the magnitude of the acceleration forces increases, the tissue stresses extend deeper into the brain and the brain stem. Coma ensues with signs of brain stem and autonomic dysfunction. It is thought that all head trauma involves varying degrees of histopathologic changes consistent with diffuse axonal disruption with a continuum of clinical responses. Severe DAI is associated with 35% or greater mortality; survivors have profound neurologic, psychologic, or personality deficits. Treatment is supportive and preventative, initially focusing on ICP but ultimately focusing on pulmonary and other systemic complications

v. Penetrating injuries

    (a) Gunshot wounds: The most lethal of all injuries to the brain, with a mortality rate above 90% in the United States. Two thirds of victims never reach the hospital

        (1) The pathophysiology of cranial missile injuries is based on three primary events occurring at impact:

            a) Local parenchymal destruction occurs along the bullet track. A temporary cavity forms parallel to the primary track, which may be much larger than the missile diameter, and collapses within milliseconds

            b) A shock wave is then transmitted throughout the intracranial cavity, occurring immediately after impact. With low-velocity insults, which occur with the majority of handgun injuries, local parenchymal damage along the bullet path is the most important factor in determining extent of injury

            c) If the bullet has insufficient energy to exit the skull, it may ricochet off the inner table opposite the entry site, or off a dural barrier such as the falx or tentorium, creating a second and occasionally a third track. The course of such a rebounding bullet is highly variable

        (2) As the impact energy of a missile increases, temporary

cavitation and shock wave effects take on increasing significance in determining the ultimate extent of injury

(3) If vital brain stem structures are transgressed by the projectile, the victim generally dies at that instant. Even without anatomic disruption of vital centers, the shock wave alone may be severe enough to produce transient or permanent medullary failure with cardiopulmonary arrest

(4) Several secondary phenomena further complicate the injury and can lead to death

  a) The pressure wave associated with a bullet entering the skull can cause distant cerebral injuries, such as cerebral contusions and marked rises in ICP, leading to uncal and tonsillar herniation

  b) The mechanism of raised ICP after a cranial gunshot wound in the absence of hematoma formation is not entirely clear. The blast effect may damage cerebral vessels and may impair autoregulation. The blood-brain barrier may be damaged by the shock wave, leading to vasogenic edema. Respiratory arrest may lead to cerebral ischemia, cell death, and cytotoxic edema

(5) Laceration of major cerebral vessels may result in hematoma formation or development of a traumatic aneurysm

(6) Local parenchymal damage causes release of tissue thromboplastin and plasminogen and may result in a consumptive coagulopathy. Multiple indriven bone fragments can create additional areas of brain destruction. Finally, scalp, hair, clothing and other foreign debris may be pulled intracranially by the bullet, providing multiple nidi for infection

(b) Stab wounds: less common than gunshot wounds in the United States, although more common in countries where guns are not as readily accessible. Most stab wounds occur on the left side of the brain because most assailants are right-handed. Although a variety of instruments are used, knives remain the most common weapon

(1) Neurologic symptoms arise from vessel laceration with hematoma formation, laceration of the brain parenchyma, or cranial nerve injury. Dysphasia is also common, given the predominance of left hemisphere injuries

(2) Traumatic aneurysm formation, carotid-cavernous fistula, and arteriovenous fistulas occur in approximately half of all stab wound victims

2. Etiologic or precipitating factors

a. According to epidemiologic data, the number of head-injured patients is estimated at between 200 and 300 per 100,000 population per year, or approximately 500,000 head injuries per year requiring hospitalization

  i. Head injuries account for 30% of trauma patients

  ii. More men than women affected (almost 3:1)

  iii. Younger population (15 to 24 years of age) but also a predominance in the very young and very old

iv. Approximately 10% die before reaching the hospital. Of survivors, about 80% have mild head injuries (GCS = 13–15), 10% have moderate head injuries (GCS = 9–12), and 10% severe head injuries (GCS = 3–8)

b. Causes

  i. Motor vehicle accidents: about 50% of all traumatic brain injuries are caused by motor vehicle crashes involving automobiles, motorcycles, and pedestrians

  ii. Assaults

  iii. Falls

  iv. Domestic accidents

  v. Sports and leisure activities

  vi. Gunshot wounds

  vii. Alcohol use: a compounding factor in up to 75% of head injuries and is a contributing factor in more than half of all fatal motor vehicle crashes in the United States. Alcohol use increases the risk for head injury by impairing gross and fine motor skills, reaction times, and judgment. It also confounds the accuracy of diagnosis by lowering the level of consciousness when the blood alcohol concentration is over 200 mg/dl. Finally, acute alcohol use may adversely affect outcome from head injury

  viii. Other substances: use or abuse of cocaine, amphetamines, narcotics, sedatives, cannabis, and other illicit substances is often associated with head injury

3. **Nursing assessment data base**

a. Nursing history

  i. History of motor vehicle crash or other trauma to the head

  ii. History of alcohol or other substance use or abuse

b. Nursing examination of patient

  i. Severity of head injury is based on the level of consciousness as described by the GCS after initial resuscitation

    (a) Mild head injury (GCS = 13–15):

      (1) A score of 15 is assigned to a patient with a documented head injury but whose neurologic examination has returned to normal

      (2) A patient with a GCS of 14 is usually confused

      (3) A patient with a GCS of 13 is confused and does not open eyes spontaneously

      (4) Patients with a GCS of 13 to 15 usually have a normal CT scan

      (5) Patients with a GCS of 13 and an abnormal CT scan are considered to have a moderate head injury

      (6) Patients with mild head injury may have persistent complaints of neurologic sequelae, such as headaches, visual disturbance, memory problems (particularly short-term memory), short attention span, information processing problems, and dizziness

    (b) Moderate head injury (GCS = 9–12): Most of these patients have an abnormal CT scan. Clinically, the patient is confused, opens the eyes only to commands or painful stimulation, and may follow commands or only localize or withdraw extremities to painful stimulation

    (c) Severe head injury: a post-resuscitation GCS of 3 to 8 or deterioration to a GCS of 8 or less. Patients with severe head injury are usually in a coma, defined as no eye opening, no verbal response, and inability to follow commands

  ii. In addition to the level of consciousness, as described by the GCS, the brain stem reflexes also assist in defining severity of injury. Direct light reflexes may be absent in one or both eyes, with mortality directly related to the degree of impairment. Oculocephalic and oculovestibular reflexes are absent in patients with severe brain injury or brain death

  iii. Scalp lacerations

  iv. Cranial nerve deficits

  v. CSF rhinorrhea or otorrhea

  vi. Hemotympanum and Battle's sign (ecchymosis over mastoid bone) are indications of middle fossa basilar skull fracture; hearing is decreased if CSF is behind tympanic membrane or the tympanic membrane is ruptured. "Raccoon's eyes" (bilateral periorbital edema and ecchymosis) are caused by anterior fossa basilar skull fracture

  vii. Focal neurologic deficits, such as hemiparesis and dysphasia

  viii. Signs of increased ICP in patients with brain swelling or an expanding intracranial lesion

c. Diagnostic study findings

  i. Laboratory: lumbar puncture is contraindicated in the presence of suspected or known intracranial hypertension and adds little to the diagnosis of head injury

  ii. Toxicology: may reveal presence of alcohol or illicit substance

  iii. Radiologic

    (a) CT scan: defines intracranial hematomas, contusions, and occasionally DAI. Shift of the intracranial contents as well as effacement of the ventricles and basilar cisterns is apparent. Edema and brain swelling may be seen, although these are better appreciated 24 hours or more after the insult

      (1) EDH appears lens-shaped

      (2) SDH is crescent-shaped and covers most of the hemisphere

      (3) ICH appears as area of hyperdensity within the parenchyma

      (4) Contusions are heterogeneous areas of hemorrhage and edema

      (5) DAI may be suspected if small hemorrhages in the deep white matter of the brain are seen

    (b) Skull x-rays and bone windows of CT scan: may reveal linear, depressed, basilar skull, or facial-orbital fractures. Basilar skull fractures may not be seen on plain skull radiographs but are usually seen on bone windows of CT scans; diagnosis often made on clinical signs alone. Other radiographic and diagnostic signs of a basilar skull fracture include:

      (1) Air-fluid levels in the sinuses or pneumocephalus are consistent with CSF leaks

      (2) Isotopes injected into the ventricles or via lumbar puncture

help to confirm the diagnosis and may identify the site of a CSF leak

    (3) Facial fractures are often associated with basal skull fractures

  (c) Cervical spine x-rays: always performed in patients with moderate and severe head injury. May reveal fracture or dislocation of spine. Thoracic and lumbar radiographs are indicated in patients involved in a motor vehicle crash or in a fall more than a few feet or patients with localized spine tenderness

  (d) Cerebral angiogram: performed if vascular injury is suspected with gunshot wounds or stab wounds. May also be indicated with severe head injury and suspected vasospasm or infarction

  iv. Transcranial Doppler study: may reveal vasospasm. Incidence varies greatly, with significant vasospasm occurring in severely head-injured patients with SAH most often. Abnormally low-flow velocities are correlated with poor outcome

  v. Although MRI is not usually performed for diagnostic purposes in acute head injury, it does reveal hemorrhage, edema, DAI, and other areas of abnormality

4. Nursing Diagnoses (see Commonly Encountered Nursing Diagnoses)

  a. Potential fluid volume deficit related to blood loss from scalp laceration

  b. Potential for infection related to contaminated scalp laceration

  c. Potential for infection related to CSF leak

    i. Assessment for additional defining characteristics

      (a) Presence of raccoon's eyes or Battle's sign

      (b) CSF rhinorrhea or otorrhea: clear or serous drainage from nose or ear

      (c) Presence of basilar skull fracture or open, depressed skull fracture, particularly involving the frontal or mastoid sinuses

      (d) Evidence of penetrating intracranial injury

      (e) Clinical and laboratory signs of intracranial infection

    ii. Expected outcome: no pathogens will be present in CSF cultures

    iii. Additional nursing interventions

      (a) Monitor for CSF rhinorrhea or otorrhea

      (b) Monitor for signs of intracranial infection, including nuchal rigidity

      (c) When there is a confirmed CSF leak:

        (1) Do not put anything into the patient's nose or ears; this includes tissue, dressings, packing, cotton, suction catheters, nasogastric tubes, oxygen catheter or cannulas

        (2) Instruct the patient not to blow the nose but to allow fluid to flow freely

        (3) Place a dry, sterile dressing loosely over the patient's ear or as a mustache dressing to absorb drainage. Note amount of drainage by charting the type and number of dressings that become saturated over a specified period of time

        (4) Prevent a Valsalva maneuver and vigorous coughing to avert further tearing of the dura and increased CSF flow

        (5) Maintain lumbar drain at ordered level to maintain CSF drainage at 10 to 15 ml/hour or as ordered

      iv. Evaluation of nursing care: no clinical signs of intracranial infection are present

  d. Potential for injury related to cranial defect

      i. Assessment for defining characteristics

        (a) Unprotected brain resulting from skull defect as a result of a depressed skull fracture with surgical repair and removal of bone or craniectomy for other reasons

        (b) Focal neurologic deficit from injury to brain underlying cranial defect

        (c) Seizure activity

      ii. Expected outcome: patient experiences no further brain injury from cranial defect

      iii. Nursing interventions

        (a) Position the patient's head away from the cranial defect. Apply a protective device as indicated

        (b) Assess cranial nerve function; record and report abnormal findings

      iv. Evaluation of nursing care: there is no clinical evidence of brain injury

  e. Potential for injury related to cranial nerve damage from depressed or basilar skull fracture or focal brain injury

      i. Assessment for defining characteristics

        (a) Loss of sensation to one side of the face from a CN V injury

        (b) Loss of movement on one side of the face from a CN VII injury; note whether the patient is unable to close the eye on affected side

        (c) Decreased or loss of hearing from a CN VIII injury on the side of the depressed or basilar skull fracture

        (d) Depressed gag or swallow reflex as the result of CN IX and X injury from posterior fossa fractures or hematomas

      ii. Expected outcome: no further injury to patient as a result of cranial nerve deficits

      iii. Nursing interventions

        (a) Protect the eye on the affected side of CN V or CN VII deficits from corneal abrasion by using eye drops frequently to keep the cornea moist and lubricated; tape the upper eyelid to the cheek with Steri-Strips to keep the eye closed; use a protective eye shield intermittently on alternate eyes

        (b) Teach the patient to chew on the unaffected side when there is a facial palsy from CN VII injury; clean the mouth of food collected on the affected side

        (c) Assess the tongue for injury in patients with CN V or CN VII deficits

        (d) Realize that patients with CN VIII injury cannot hear if you are talking to them on the side of decreased hearing; speak louder or move to the patient's unaffected side. Teach the patient to turn toward the person talking

        (e) Determine the patient's ability to handle secretions. Assess swallowing by having the patient sit upright and giving small amounts of gelatin. If coughing or choking occurs, *do not feed by mouth.* Do not use liquids to assess swallowing

        (f) Consult speech pathologist, occupational therapist, or head and neck surgeon per hospital protocol for a formal swallow evaluation

    iv. Evaluation of nursing care: no injury occurs as a result of cranial nerve deficit

  f. Alteration in cerebral tissue perfusion related to increased ICP (see Increased ICP)

  g. Impaired gas exchange related to altered O_2 supply or O_2-carrying capacity

  h. Ineffective breathing pattern related to inadequate airway from depressed level of consciousness, intracranial pathology, or metabolic imbalance

  i. Ineffective airway clearance related to increased secretions and/or depressed level of consciousness

  j. Potential fluid volume deficit related to excessive loss, decreased intake, diabetes insipidus

  k. Potential fluid volume excess related to high intake for management of cerebral perfusion pressure

    i. Assessment for defining characteristics

        (a) CVP greater than 10 mm Hg

        (b) PAWP greater than 14 mm Hg

        (c) Adventitious breath sounds

        (d) Pulmonary edema on chest radiograph

        (e) Peripheral edema

        (f) Increased ICP

    ii. Expected outcome: pulmonary edema is avoided or treated promptly

    iii. Nursing interventions

        (a) Monitor CVP or PAWP every hour when the patient is receiving large volumes of fluid and is receiving vasopressor therapy

        (b) Auscultate lungs for crackles (rales) every 1 to 2 hours

        (c) Monitor results of chest radiographs for evidence of fluid overload

        (d) Monitor intake and output hourly

        (e) Weigh the patient daily

        (f) Administer diuretics, as ordered, to reduce fluid volume

    iv. Evaluation of nursing care: no clinical evidence of pulmonary edema is present

  l. Potential for infection related to invasive lines

  m. Impaired physical mobility related to spasticity or abnormal flexor or extensor posturing

    i. Assessment for additional defining characteristics

        (a) Increased muscle tone

        (b) Flexor or extensor posturing

        (c) Extreme restlessness, agitation

        (d) Increases in ICP during agitation or abnormal posturing

        (e) Tachycardia, tachypnea, fever

    ii. Expected outcomes

        (a) ICP is maintained below 20 mm Hg

        (b) There is no evidence of skin breakdown or contractures

        (c) There is no injury from agitated responses

    iii. Nursing interventions

        (a) Apply restraining devices as necessary to prevent unintended

extubation, dislodgment of ICP monitoring device, intra-arterial
or intravenous catheters, falls, or other injury. Assess extremities
per unit protocol

(b) Sedate as ordered to control agitation and ICP

(c) Collaborate with physical or occupational therapist in
maintaining range of motion in patients with spasticity or
abnormal posturing

(d) Monitor metabolic responses to increased activity (e.g.,
temperature, respiratory, cardiac, CBF)

   iv. Evaluation of nursing care

(a) Metabolic responses are within desired levels

(b) Musculoskeletal complications are minimal or absent

(c) ICP is controlled below 20 mm Hg; CPP is above 70 mm Hg

(d) There is no skin breakdown from restraining devices

(e) Range of motion of joints is maintained

(f) There is absence of injury from agitated behavior

n. Impaired physical mobility related to weakness or paralysis of one or more
body parts

. . . .

Hydrocephalus

1. **Pathophysiology:** In the adult, hydrocephalus occurs as a complication of
other intracranial pathology. It results when the circulation or reabsorption
of CSF is obstructed by a pathologic process and CSF accumulates in the
ventricles. It is exceedingly rare for increased production of CSF to be the
cause of hydrocephalus

    a. Noncommunicating (obstructive) hydrocephalus is caused by obstruction
    of CSF circulation within the ventricles either by intraventricular masses
    or masses that prevent circulation of CSF to the subarachnoid space. The
    continued production of CSF by the choroid plexus causes the ventricles
    to dilate and compresses surrounding brain tissue

    b. Communicating (nonobstructive) hydrocephalus occurs when CSF is able
    to circulate out of the ventricular system but is not reabsorbed via the
    arachnoid granulations into the venous sinuses at the rate at which it is
    produced

    c. Hydrocephalus may occur acutely within hours or days, subacutely over
    weeks, or chronically over months. The urgency of treatment generally
    correlates directly with the acuity of the development of hydrocephalus
    and the patient's clinical status

2. **Etiologic or precipitating factors**

    a. Tumors or masses in or near the ventricles or basal cisterns or on the
    convexity of the brain that obstruct the subarachnoid space

    b. Cysticercosis, an infectious process caused by a parasite, forms cysts in the
    subarachnoid spaces, basal cisterns, or in the ventricles causing
    obstruction of CSF flow

    c. Subarachnoid hemorrhage, intraventricular hemorrhage, and meningitis
    cause inflammation of the meninges and impede CSF reabsorption by
    obstructing the arachnoid villae

3. **Nursing assessment data base**

    a. Patient history of aforementioned conditions

    b. Nursing examination of patient (see Increased Intracranial Pressure)
       i. Headache, usually bifrontal
      ii. Nausea
     iii. Vomiting, more common in the morning
     iv. Truncal ataxia and a wide-based gait
      v. Visual disturbances, such as loss of acuity, diplopia, or inability to look up, (i.e., the "sunset eyes" syndrome)
     vi. Incontinence
    vii. Lethargy
   viii. Papilledema
    c. Diagnostic study findings
       i. CT scan reveals enlarged ventricles and, specifically, presence of dilated temporal horns of the lateral ventricles and an enlarged, round third ventricle
      ii. CT scan may also show the cause of hydrocephalus
     iii. MRI may be useful in delineating the cause of hydrocephalus
     iv. Lumbar puncture is contraindicated in a patient with hydrocephalus and increased ICP
      v. Angiography is used to evaluate vascular lesions that cause hydrocephalus, such as aneurysms and arteriovenous malformation (AVM)

4. Nursing diagnoses

    a. Alteration in tissue perfusion related to increased intracranial pressure (see Commonly Encountered Nursing Diagnoses)
       i. Potential for complications after shunt placement
         (a) Assessment for defining characteristics
           (1) Overdrainage: can cause headache and collapse of the ventricles, causing the brain to be pulled away from the skull, tearing the small bridging veins, and causing a subdural hematoma. Rarely, an epidural hematoma may form. Signs of increased ICP may occur
           (2) Shunt malfunction: insufficient drainage by the shunt because of mechanical obstruction, causing CSF to accumulate intracranially. Signs of increased ICP occur. Signs of partial obstruction include headache, ataxia, lethargy, visual disturbance, nausea and vomiting, and urinary incontinence
           (3) Shunt infection: usually occurs within the first 2 months after shunt placement (although it may occur later), leading to ventriculitis, meningitis, or cerebral abscess formation. Morbidity is high. Symptoms are nonspecific. There are signs of shunt obstruction as well as signs of infection, such as fever, nuchal rigidity, headache, vomiting, and abdominal discomfort (in patients with ventriculoperitoneal shunts)
         (b) Expected outcomes: shunt complications will be recognized early and care implemented promptly
         (c) Nursing interventions
           (1) Monitor the patient in the immediately postoperative period for signs of hematoma formation (signs of increasing ICP)

   (2) Administer antibiotics as ordered, perioperatively for shunt placement and if shunt infection has been diagnosed

   (3) Monitor CSF laboratory analysis and cultures

   (4) Promptly report change in the patient's neurologic status

   (5) Prepare the patient for emergency CT scan in the event of neurologic deterioration

   (6) Prepare the patient for emergency ventriculostomy. This may be done in the patient with shunt obstruction and is usually done in patients with shunt infection

   (7) Prepare the patient for surgery

  (d) Evaluation of nursing care: patient maintains baseline neurologic status

 b. Impaired verbal communication related to expressive/receptive dysphasia

 c. Ineffective family coping related to change in patient's present and future functioning and burden of care

Brain Tumors

1. **Pathophysiology:** brain tumors act as space-occupying lesions and are life-threatening because they destroy brain tissue and nerve structures and cause increased ICP. Tumors may be spherical, well delineated, and encapsulated or diffuse and infiltrating masses. The tumor may enlarge as a result of cell proliferation, necrosis, edema, or hemorrhage. Tumors cause neurologic symptoms owing to compression, invasion, or destruction of brain tissue. The pathophysiologic complications include cerebral edema, intracranial hypertension, seizures, focal neurologic deficits, hydrocephalus, and hormonal changes. Tumors are classified by histologic features and grade of malignancy (grades I to IV, with IV the most malignant). Prognosis is determined by histologic type, grade of tumor, location and size of tumor, the patient's age, the patient's clinical status prior to surgery, and duration of symptoms

 a. Glioma: nonencapsulated, infiltrates and displaces brain tissue; arises from neuroglial cells; comprises 40% to 50% of intracranial tumors

  i. Astrocytoma: usually grade I to II, but may advance to higher grades (glioblastoma); may occur in brain or spinal cord. The 5-year survival of grades I and II is 50% to 85%

   (a) Anaplastic astrocytoma: if well differentiated and only mildly to moderately anaplastic, 5-year survival rates are 41% to 51%. True anaplastic astrocytomas (grade III) have a 5-year survival of 18% to 48%

   (b) Cerebellar astrocytoma: tend to be lower grade, with a 20% to 50% 5-year survival

   (c) Optic nerve glioma: a slowly growing astrocytoma of the optic nerves and optic chiasm. May affect hypothalamic function and vision. Often cured with surgical excision

  ii. Oligodendroglioma: a rare, slow-growing tumor in adults; arises from oligodendrocytes; occurs in cerebral hemispheres, usually calcified. Survival depends on location and grade of tumor, with 5-year survival of up to 85% in well-differentiated tumors (grade I) and as low as 17% in highly malignant tumors (grade IV)

      iii. Glioblastoma multiforme: constitutes about 50% of primary brain tumors; malignant (grades III and IV), occur throughout cerebral hemispheres, may cross the midline. Grows rapidly, invades tissues, and causes edema and mass effect. Usually is necrotic and poorly differentiated. Survival is less than 10% at 5 years; is usually fatal in 9 to 12 months

      iv. Brain stem glioma: although gliomas may be of variable malignancy, they are often diagnosed on clinical presentation alone because of the difficulty in obtaining tissue by biopsy without causing further damage. Generalized enlargement of the brain stem indicates a poor prognosis, as does higher grade of tumor. Although 3-year survival is reported at 48%, the 5-year survival is less than 20%

      v. Ependymoma: arises from cells lining the ventricles and the central canal. This slow-growing tumor causes obstructive hydrocephalus and cranial nerve or cerebrellar dysfunction

      vi. Medulloblastoma: a highly malignant tumor arising from the cerebellum. Causes obstructive hydrocephalus; is most common in young children or adults. Survival is usually less than 5 years, but prognosis is improved with surgery and chemotherapy

      vii. Pineal region tumor: Of varying histology and malignancy. Pinealocytomas are slow growing, whereas pinealoblastomas are highly malignant. Other tumors of germ cell origin may also occur in this region. Because they are relatively rare and often not diagnosed by biopsy, the prognosis is difficult to determine with certainty

  b. Extra-axial tumor: arises from supporting structures of the central or peripheral nervous system

      i. Meningioma: makes up 15% to 20% of all primary brain tumors. Arises from meningeal tissues. Vascular, firm, encapsulated, slow growing, and benign. The prognosis is good unless size or location makes surgery more difficult. A malignant form of meningioma is relatively rare but is more likely than other tumors of the brain to metastasize to other structures of the craniospinal axis

      ii. Acoustic neuroma (schwannoma): composes 10% of all primary brain tumors. Also called acoustic schwannoma because it arises from Schwann cells of CN VIII. Originates at the junction of the cerebellum and pons. Often affects function of CN VII and VIII and sometimes CN V, CN IX, and CN X. This tumor is slow growing and benign

  c. Developmental tumor

      i. Hemangioblastoma: a slow-growing, vascular tumor that develops from embryonic vascular elements. Is most frequently found in the cerebellum

      ii. Craniopharyngioma: found in suprasellar region, thought to arise from the pituitary hypophysis. Occurs primarily in children and young adults. Benign but recurrence is common

      iii. Chordoma: a slow growing tumor found in both brain and spinal cord. Grows aggressively along the base of the skull from the clivus to the cerebellum. Invades bone. Is difficult to excise completely

  d. Pituitary tumor: makes up 10% to 15% of primary brain tumors. Although this tumor arises from the pituitary gland and is technically an endocrine tumor, because of the intracranial nature of its extension and the close relationship to the hypothalamus and hypothalamic functions, it is considered along with other brain tumors

    i. Nonsecreting tumor (chromophobe adenoma): a space-occupying lesion that produces endocrine dysfunction by compressing the pituitary gland or hypothalamus and producing hypopituitarism. Causes compression of the optic chiasm and visual changes. Represents 90% of all pituitary tumors

    ii. Secreting tumors

       (a) Prolactin-secreting tumor (prolactinoma): produces galactorrhea

       (b) Growth-hormone secreting tumor (eosinophilic pituitary adenoma): giantism occurs if tumor develops in childhood; acromegaly occurs if tumor develops in adulthood

       (c) ACTH-secreting tumor: stimulates production of cortisol from adrenal gland and symptoms of Cushing's syndrome (see Chapter 5)

  e. Metastatic tumor: Most common brain tumor. Metastases originate most commonly from the breast in women and from the lungs in men. Primary cancers of the gastrointestinal and genitourinary tracts may also metastasize. Lesions may be single or multiple or encapsulated or diffuse, and they affect meninges or brain tissue. Neurosurgical operative management depends on the prognosis of the patient from the primary cancer and the number of metastatic lesions. Generally, if there is more than one lesion, intracranial surgery is not performed. Most patients with metastatic disease die from their primary cancer

2. Etiologic or precipitating factors: the causes of tumor growth are not fully understood. Theories include an abnormality in the structure or function of one or more genes, the influence of hormones, an angiogenesis factor (a substance in tumor cells that stimulates capillary growth), chemicals, radiation, viruses, trauma, and diet, and environmental exposure to carcinogens. Metastatic tumors reach the brain by hematogenous spread, usually through the arterial circulation

3. Nursing assessment data base

  a. Nursing history

    i. Subjective findings

       (a) Patient's chief complaint

         (1) Headache: the most common symptom with tumors. May be generalized or localized. Initially worse in the morning, eventually more constant

         (2) Seizures: another very common presenting symptom. May be focal or generalized. An initial seizure occurring in adults is highly suggestive of an intracranial tumor

         (3) Mental changes and drowsiness

       (b) Other symptoms

         (1) Visual changes (caused by papilledema from chronic intracranial hypertension)

         (2) Vomiting: may occur without nausea or abdominal discomfort. Unrelated to meals, more common in morning. Only occasionally is projectile

         (3) Dizziness, instability, vertigo

       (c) Objective findings

(1) Historic symptoms secondary to size and location of tumor (see Nursing examination of patient)

(2) Family history: some tumors have genetic relationship

(3) Social history: Noncontributory

(4) Medication history: current medications

b. Nursing examination of patient: findings are secondary to location of tumor, rate of growth, and degree of invasion of the brain tissue

  i. Frontal lobe tumor

  (a) Inappropriate behavior

  (b) Inattentiveness

  (c) Inability to concentrate

  (d) Loss of self-restraint and social behavior

  (e) Impaired recent memory

  (f) Difficulty with abstraction

  (g) Flat affect, inactivity, apathy

  (h) Expressive aphasia (if lesion is in the dominant hemisphere)

  (i) Motor weakness, usually contralateral hemiparesis

  ii. Parietal lobe tumor

  (a) Hyperesthesia

  (b) Paresthesia: tingling, crawling, burning

  (c) Loss of two-point discrimination

  (d) Astereognosis

  (e) Autotopognosia

  (f) Anosognosia

  (g) Agraphesthesia

  (h) Gerstmann's syndrome:

      (1) Finger agnosia

      (2) Loss of left-right discrimination

      (3) Agraphia

      (4) Acalculia

  (i) Constructional apraxia

  (j) Homonymous hemianopsia

  (k) Unilateral neglect

  iii. Temporal lobe tumor

  (a) Psychomotor seizures

  (b) Homonymous heminopsia

  (c) Homonymous quadranopsia

  (d) Receptive aphasia if lesion is in the dominant hemisphere

  (e) Alterations in hearing

  iv. Occipital lobe tumor

  (a) Contralateral homonymous hemianopsia

  (b) Visual hallucinations

  (c) Seizures with a visual aura

  v. Pituitary and hypothalamic region tumor

  (a) Visual defects

  (b) Hypopituitarism

  (c) Headache

  (d) Cushing's syndrome

  (e) Acromegaly

  (f) Endocrine dysfunction

  (g) Menstrual dysfunction

vi. Ventricular and periventricular tumors
  (a) Hydrocephalus
  (b) Headache
  (c) Change in level of consciousness
vii. Cerebellar tumor
  (a) Ataxia
  (b) Incoordination
  (c) Dysmetria
  (d) Dizziness
  (e) Nystagmus
viii. Brain stem tumor
  (a) Cranial nerve deficits
  (b) Cerebellar dysfunction
  (c) Vomiting
  (d) Obstructive hydrocephalus
c. Diagnostic study findings
  i. Visual field and funduscopic examination: reveals papilledema, visual field defects
  ii. Skull films: may reveal deviation of calcified pineal gland, erosion of bone, calcified areas
  iii. CT scan: without and with contrast enhancement. Reveals size and location of tumor, presence of cerebral edema, hydrocephalus. Confirms presence of calcified areas within tumor
  iv. MRI: reveals size and location of the tumor, vascularity and extent of cerebral edema. Also reveals characteristics of tumor based on different imaging sequences of MRI at different times during the imaging process
  v. Cerebral angiography: reveals vascularity of tumor and vessels that supply it. May also demonstrate displacement and distortion of uninvolved vessels and formation of new vessels
  vi. Endocrine studies: very helpful in pituitary and sometimes hypothalamic tumors. Abnormally high or low values indicate secreting tumor or destruction of secreting cells
  vii. Other tests may be performed for further differentiation of tumor (CBF and radionucleotide studies)

4. **Nursing diagnoses** (see Commonly Encountered Nursing Diagnoses)
  a. Alteration in cerebral perfusion related to increased ICP
  b. Impaired gas exchange related to altered oxygen supply or oxygen-carrying capacity
  c. Impaired breathing pattern related to depressed level of consciousness, intracranial pathology, or metabolic imbalance
  d. Ineffective airway clearance related to increased secretions and depressed level of consciousness
  e. Potential for fluid volume deficit related to excessive loss, decreased intake, or cerebral salt wasting syndrome
  f. Potential for fluid volume excess related to the syndrome of inappropriate ADH secretion (SIADH)
  g. Potential for infection related to invasive lines, monitoring, and therapeutic devices
  h. Impaired verbal communication related to expressive and receptive dysphasia

    i. Impaired physical mobility related to weakness or paralysis of one or more body parts

    j. Alteration in thought processes related to confusion, short-term memory loss, or short attention span

    k. Potential for injury related to seizures

    l. Ineffective individual coping related to situational crisis, loss of control and independence, or change in role

    m. Ineffective family coping related to disruption of usual family roles, burden of care, or changes in family member's present and future functioning

Intracranial Aneurysms

1. **Pathophysiology**
   a. Dilatation of an artery resulting from weakness in media layer and internal elastic laminar layer of the arterial wall. The aneurysm itself is composed mainly of collagen of variable thickness
   b. Ninety-five percent of aneurysms occur close to the circle of Willis at bifurcations of the internal carotid, middle cerebral, and basilar arteries and in relation to the anterior and posterior communicating arteries. They are associated with hypoplasia of vessels, particularly the anterior cerebral arteries (ACAs) and posterior communicating arteries (P-Com). More than 50% of all aneurysms occur on the anterior or posterior communicating arteries; the middle cerebral artery is the next most common location
   c. Most cerebral aneurysms occur in vessels of anterior portion of circle of Willis
   d. About 20% of patients have multiple aneurysms
   e. The overall incidence of aneurysms in the general population is about 1%, and about half of these rupture. The incidence of ruptured aneurysms is close to zero for children and rises in each decade of life
   f. High arterial pressures and continuous arterial pulsations are thought to lead to ballooning of weakened arterial wall
   g. Rupture of aneurysm causes SAH in more than 95% of patients, and about 50% have either ICH or IVH. ICH is most commonly seen with rupture of middle cerebral artery and anterior communicating artery aneurysms
   h. Clot forms in and around the rupture site and may inhibit continuing hemorrhage
   i. ICP rises in proportion to worsening clinical grade and the occurrence of hydrocephalus and vasospasm. CBF also falls, more in patients with vasospasm

2. **Etiologic or precipitating factors**
   a. Hemodynamic factors, arteriosclerosis, and breakdown of the internal elastic membrane contribute to formation and growth of aneurysms
   b. No specific precipitating causes exist for all patients
   c. A familial association is seen in some patients, but the causes are not known
   d. Hypertension is not a major factor in the etiology of aneurysms, but it is a poor prognostic sign if it is present after rupture

e. Fewer than 10% of aneurysms are traumatic, septic, or arteriosclerotic in origin

3. Nursing assessment data base

a. Nursing history
   i. Subjective findings
      (a) Presenting complaint: "Worst headache of my life"
      (b) Nausea, vomiting, dizziness
      (c) Photophobia, painful neck or back
      (d) Brief loss of consciousness
   ii. Objective findings
      (a) Signs of meningeal irritation: nuchal rigidity, headache, photophobia, low back pain
      (b) Altered level of consciousness
      (c) Focal neurologic deficit depends on the location of the aneurysm or ICH
   iii. Family history: no clear genetic or familial link in all cases, but familial aggregations do occur in a minority of patients
   iv. Social history
      (a) Alcohol and illicit drug use (particularly cocaine) have been associated with SAH
      (b) Cigarette smoking or cardiovascular risk factors may increase risk of hemorrhage

b. Nursing examination of patient
   i. Clinical presentation
      (a) Mild to severe headache
      (b) Nausea or vomiting
      (c) Seizures
      (d) Meningismus—nuchal rigidity, headache, photophobia, diplopia, Kernig's or Brudzinski's sign sometimes present
      (e) Neurologic deficit—motor, sensory, speech
      (f) Altered level of consciousness
   ii. Physical examination: neurologic examination reveals varying signs and symptoms, depending on severity and location of hemorrhage. Aneurysms are graded using the Botterell, Hunt and Hess, or World Federation of Neurologic Surgeons scale. In some systems, grade 0 represents an unruptured aneurysm. The following is the Hunt and Hess scale:
      (a) Grade I: alert, no neurologic deficit; minimal headache; slight nuchal rigidity
      (b) Grade II: awake, no neurologic deficit other than a cranial nerve palsy; mild to severe headache; nuchal rigidity; no vasospasm
      (c) Grade III: drowsiness, confusion, mild focal neurologic deficit
      (d) Grade IV: unresponsiveness, hemiplegia; vasospasm may or may not be present
      (e) Grade V: comatose, moribund; extensor posturing; vasospasm likely

c. Diagnostic study findings
   i. Laboratory: lumbar puncture: not performed if signs of increased ICP are present or likely based on CT findings. If bloody CSF is found, one can differentiate it from a traumatic tap by spinning the blood down in a centrifuge and checking the supernatant for

xanthochromia (a yellowish color), indicating hemorrhage occurred at least 4 hours ago and the cells have had time to lyse. Elevated CSF protein and increased WBC and RBC counts are seen. CSF pressure may be elevated

ii. Radiologic
   (a) CT scan, the initial study of choice, reveals ICH, intraventricular blood, amount and distribution of SAH, and hydrocephalus. The degree of SAH and the risk of vasospasm are graded with the Fisher grading scale
      (1) Grade I = no blood seen on CT; low risk of vasospasm
      (2) Grade II = diffuse blood, not dense; moderate risk of vasospasm
      (3) Grade III = dense blood in the fissures and basal cisterns; high risk of vasospasm
      (4) Grade IV = intracerebral or intraventricular clot, diffuse or no blood in basal cisterns; low risk of vasospasm
   (b) If CT or lumbar puncture reveals SAH, a cerebral angiogram is done to illustrate the size, shape, and location of aneurysm and spasm of involved vessels

iii. MRI reveals evidence of hemorrhage and hydrocephalus but is not the study of choice

iv. MRA may noninvasively diagnose aneurysm

v. Transcranial Doppler studies may reveal increased blood flow velocity greater than 120 cm/second indicating vasospasm, with flow velocities above 200 cm/second diagnostic of severe spasm

vi. CBF studies may reveal decreased flow if vasospasm is present or if significant brain damage has occurred as a result of intraparenchymal bleeding or hydrocephalus

4. Nursing diagnoses
   a. Potential for alteration in cerebral tissue perfusion related to rebleeding
      i. Assessment for defining characteristics
         (a) Rebleeding is most common in the first day or two after the initial rupture in patients who have not had their aneurysm clipped surgically; incidence decreases progressively to a rate of 3% per year after the first year in unclipped aneurysms
         (b) A sudden change in the patient's neurologic status is usually indicative of rebleeding although vasospasm or acute hydrocephalus may also be the cause. Increased ICP may also occur with rebleeding
      ii. Expected outcome: signs of rebleeding are recognized and appropriately managed
      iii. Nursing interventions
         (a) Prepare the patient and family for surgery
            (1) Patients with Hunt and Hess grades I, II, or III ruptured aneurysm usually undergo surgical repair of the ruptured aneurysm within 24 hours of the bleeding episode to prevent rebleeding
            (2) If the patient presents days after the initial bleed and has evidence of severe vasospasm on transcranial Doppler studies, surgery may be delayed until vasospasm has resolved

(3) Patients who are a poor neurologic grade (IV or V) despite therapy to control ICP may be treated medically until neurologic status improves

(b) Monitor the patient's neurologic status postoperatively

(c) Maintain blood pressure at ordered levels, being careful to avoid even transient incidents of hypotension

(d) Monitor serum anticonvulsant levels to maintain a seizure-free state

iv. Evaluation of nursing care

(a) Signs of rebleeding are recognized and interventions initiated

(b) Patient and family are prepared for surgery

b. Potential for alteration in cerebral tissue perfusion related to vasospasm

(a) Assessment for defining characteristics

(1) Vasospasm may occur immediately or as long as 3 weeks after SAH; commonly occurs between 3 and 14 days after rupture. The incidence and degree of vasospasm are directly related to the amount of blood in the subarachnoid space

(2) No neurologic symptoms or subtle or dramatic changes in the patient's level of consciousness may occur. Focal deficits may worsen during vasospasm

(3) Decreases in blood pressure may worsen neurologic deficits

(4) Ischemia may occur if vasospasm is severe or if blood pressure drops

(b) Expected outcome: vasospasm is recognized and managed appropriately

(c) Nursing interventions

(1) Use calcium channel blockers to prevent or lessen the neurologic effects of vasospasm. Nimodipine is usually given immediately after SAH is diagnosed at a dose of 60 mg every 4 hours. If it causes hypotension, the dose is reduced to 30 mg every 2 hours

(2) Hypervolemia, hemodilution, hypertension (so-called triple-H therapy) is optimally employed after the aneurysm has been surgically clipped if vasospasm develops. Pulmonary complications may occur; hemodynamic monitoring with a CVP catheter or pulmonary artery catheter in older patients helps guide therapy

(3) Hemodilution and hypervolemia are accomplished with a combination of colloid (usually in the form of 5% albumin, 250 to 500 ml every 6 hours) and crystalloid solutions. The objective is to drop the hematocrit level to about 30% and increase cardiac output to 6.5 to 8 L/min, CVP to 8 to 10 mm Hg, or PAWP to 12 to 16 mm Hg

(4) If these measures are not adequate to increase the blood pressure and CPP to the desired range, vasopressors may be used. Dopamine is often the first drug used. However, at low doses it is a renal stimulant and increased urine output may compromise attempts to increase the circulating volume. Phenylephrine (Neo-Synephrine) or norepinephrine (Levophed) is frequently used.

Dobutamine may be needed to improve cardiac performance. A CPP of greater than 70 mm Hg and a systolic blood pressure of 160 to 180 mm Hg or greater are usually the goal of therapy

    (5) If patient is hypertensive, drugs may be used to control blood pressure only if it reaches dangerously high levels

  (d) Evaluation of nursing care: vasospasm is controlled with triple-H therapy

 c. Potential for alteration in cerebral tissue perfusion related to hydrocephalus

   i. Assessment for defining characteristics

    (a) Acute onset of hydrocephalus leads to a rapid rise in ICP (see Increased Intracranial Pressure). Emergency ventriculostomy is necessary to drain CSF and control ICP

    (b) Occurrence of hydrocephalus may be delayed days or weeks after SAH. The patient will begin to experience symptoms such as drowsiness, ataxia, headache, blurred vision, diplopia, nausea, vomiting, and incontinence

   ii. Expected outcomes: hydrocephalus is recognized early, and intervention is initiated promptly

   iii. Nursing interventions

    (a) Hydrocephalus is initially treated with a ventriculostomy until the ICP is normal and ventricular and subarachnoid spaces are clear of blood. The ventricular size is monitored with serial CT scans. If the patient requires frequent CSF drainage to keep the ICP below 20 mm Hg and the ventricular system is enlarged on CT scan, a ventriculoperitoneal shunt is usually placed

   iv. Evaluation of nursing care: hydrocephalus is recognized and treated

 d. Fluid volume excess related to hypervolemic, hypertensive and hemodilution therapy (see Traumatic Brain Injury, Nursing Diagnoses, Potential fluid volume excess related to high intake for CPP management)

 e. Potential for infection related to invasive lines and monitoring and therapeutic devices

 f. Other nursing diagnoses may apply if patient has neurologic deficits (see Nursing Diagnoses)

Arteriovenous Malformations

1. **Pathophysiology:** abnormal vascular network consisting of one or more direct connections between the arterial inflow and venous outflow without an intervening capillary network, although an abnormal proliferation of capillaries adjacent to the AVM is often seen. AVMs primarily occur in the supratentorial structures and most frequently involve the vessels of the middle cerebral arterial tree, followed by those of the anterior and then posterior circulation. Grossly, AVMs appear as a tangled mass of dilated vessels. The vessels become passively enlarged secondary to high flow volume and increased venous pressure produced by the arteriovenous (A-V) shunt. The arterial walls become thin as a result of collagenous replacement of the normal smooth muscle component of the media. Saccular aneurysms are

found in 10% to 15% of patients with AVMs, most occurring on arteries hemodynamically related to the AVM. Because most AVMs do not become symptomatic until the third decade of life, it is thought that the size of the AVM increases not only by enlargement of the feeding vessels and draining veins but also by recruitment of additional vessels not initially involved in the lesion. Symptoms are caused by the mass effect of the malformation, increased flow recruitment and subsequent "steal" from adjacent brain tissue, and by venous hypertension

2. **Etiologic or precipitating factors:** development of congenital lesions in the fourth to eighth week of embryonic life

3. **Nursing assessment data base**
   a. Nursing history
      i. Hemorrhage: most common presenting symptom in patients with AVMs; leads to headache and decreased level of consciousness. Most hemorrhages occur in the parenchyma, but 5% to 10% may be intraventricular, occasionally subdural or subarachnoid. Smaller AVMs may be more likely to bleed. The morbidity and mortality rates from the AVM hemorrhage are lower than from hypertensive or aneurysmal hemorrhages, probably because most AVMs bleed from the low-pressure venous portion of the lesion and the brain tissue involved is mainly nonfunctional
      ii. Seizures: the second most common presenting symptom; may occur more often in patients with large AVMs
      iii. Other symptoms
         (a) Headache
         (b) Hydrocephalus: an uncommon presenting symptom but may occur as a result of SAH
         (c) Intellectual deterioration may occur in older patients secondary to the mass effect of larger AVM or to "steal phenomenon"
         (d) Many AVMs are found incidentally
   b. Nursing examination of patient
      i. In absence of hemorrhage, clinical symptoms correlate to the site of the lesions
      ii. Signs of cerebral ischemia
      iii. Signs of increased ICP
   c. Diagnostic study findings
      i. Cerebral angiography: the most definitive study. Reveals feeding and draining vessels, size and location of AVMs, ICH, and cerebral vasospasm
      ii. CT: A noncontrast scan may show areas of calcification in and around the AVM. A contrast-enhanced scan often shows large tortuous feeding arteries or draining veins
      iii. MRI: demonstrates location, size, and reduced blood flow to the area around the AVM; cerebral edema
      iv. Lumbar puncture: this study is contraindicated if increased ICP is known or suspected. CSF will be bloody or xanthochromic if SAH has occurred
      v. Functional MRI is helpful in delineating the proximity of the AVM to functional areas of brain

4. **Nursing diagnoses** (see Commonly Encountered Nursing Diagnoses)
   a. Alteration in cerebral tissue perfusion related to increased ICP

b. Potential for injury related to seizures

c. Potential for infection related to invasive lines

d. Other nursing diagnoses may apply if the patient has neurologic deficits

Stroke

1. **Pathophysiology:** Ischemic-hypoxic brain damage results from decreased CBF, either focal or diffuse, which causes hypoxia of cerebral tissues leading to anaerobic glycolysis. Ischemia induces inhibition of synaptic transmission as a result of neurotransmitter depletion caused by inadequate adenosine triphosphate (ATP). May be reversible. Subsequently, structural changes of neuronal membranes occur in which ATP is depleted and intracellular ionic balances cannot be maintained. Cellular swelling and neuronal death follow

   a. Occlusive vascular disease

      i. Thrombosis

         (a) The most common cause of stroke

         (b) Lacunar strokes are small, irregular areas of infarction and necrosis associated with thrombosis of small arteries of the deep white matter of the brain

         (c) Atherosclerosis of large cerebral vessels causes progressive narrowing, leading to progressive levels of deficits. Plaques may embolize to smaller vessels

      ii. Embolus

         (a) May be calcified plaques from extracranial vessels, vegetation from diseased heart valves, fat, air, or tumor fragments. Blood clots from extracranial sources, such as those arising from a diseased heart, are common

         (b) Emboli become lodged at bifurcations of arteries where blood flow is most turbulent. Fragments may become lodged in smaller vessels

   b. Hemorrhage

      i. Accounts for as many as 25% of strokes

      ii. Bleeding into parenchyma of brain causes irritation of and pressure on cerebral tissues and nerves, leading to loss of function and death of neurons

      iii. Hypertensive intracranial hemorrhage usually occurs in the basal ganglia, cerebellum or brain stem but may affect more superficial areas of the cerebrum

2. **Etiologic or precipitating factors**

   a. Thrombosis

      i. Longstanding hypertension

      ii. Diabetes mellitus

      iii. Cardiac disease

      iv. Atherosclerosis

      v. Vascular inflammatory processes

   b. Embolus

      i. Extracranial arterial plaques or clots

      ii. Clots produced by other hematologic conditions, such as polycythemia

      iii. Other substances in the vascular system such as air, fat, and infectious emboli

c. Hemorrhage
  i. Hypertensive vascular disease (most common cause)
  ii. Ruptured intracranial aneurysm, AVM, vascular tumor
  iii. Traumatic intracerebral hemorrhage
  iv. Systemic hemorrhagic disorders and diathesis
3. Nursing assessment data base
  a. Nursing history
    i. Subjective findings
      (a) Decreased neurologic function
      (b) Headache
      (c) Seizure (uncommon)
      (d) Other symptoms: reports of prior neurologic symptoms
    ii. Objective findings
      (a) History of etiologic or precipitating factors
      (b) Transient ischemic attacks (TIA): an ischemic event that results in reversible short-lived (<24 hours but may be only minutes) neurologic deficit, such as loss of vision in one eye (amaurosis fugax), numbness or weakness of a hand or leg, dyarthria, aphasia. Lacunar TIAs generally result in a pure motor or pure sensory deficit lasting more than an hour
      (c) Reversible ischemic neurologic deficit (RIND): a neurologic deficit that lasts more than 24 hours but leaves little or no neurologic deficit
      (d) Family history: vascular or heart disease; diabetes mellitus; hypertension
      (e) Social history
        (1) Cigarette smoking
        (2) Illicit drug use, particularly cocaine
        (3) Heavy alcohol use
        (4) Longstanding stress
        (5) Medication history
          a) Oral contraceptive use, especially in women at risk (e.g., smokes, hypertension, migraines)
          b) All current therapeutic drugs
  b. Nursing examination of patient
    i. Main presenting feature in hemorrhagic or embolic stroke is sudden onset of signs and symptoms
    ii. Clinical presentation varies, depending on the area of the brain involved and extent of injury
    iii. Patients with injury to right cerebral hemisphere may exhibit some or all of the following dysfunctions
      (a) Left homonymous hemianopia: blindness in left half of both visual fields
      (b) Left hemiparesis or hemiplegia
      (c) Sensory agnosia
        (1) *Astereognosis:* inability to recognize objects placed in hand without aid of visual clues
        (2) *Astatoagnosia:* inability to determine position of body parts
        (3) Tactile inattention: lack of attention to simultaneous stimuli

        (4) *Anosognosia:* unawareness of neurologic deficit (e.g., hemiplegia)

        (5) *Constructional apraxia:* patients do not complete the left half of figures they are drawing

        (6) *Dressing apraxia:* inability to dress oneself properly

        (7) Neglect: inattention to objects in the left visual field and to left auditory stimuli

        (8) Deviation of the head and eyes to the right

    iv. Patients with injury to the left cerebral hemisphere may exhibit some or all of the following dysfunctions:

      (a) Right homonymous hemianopia: blindness in the right half of both visual fields

      (b) Right hemiparesis or hemiplegia

      (c) Sensory agnosia

        (1) Astereognosis

        (2) Astatoagnosia

        (3) Finger agnosia: inability to identify the finger touched

        (4) Right-left disorientation

      (d) Aphasia

        (1) Expressive (motor): inability to speak or write language or to name familiar objects

        (2) Receptive (sensory): inability to understand spoken words (auditory aphasia) or written words (visual aphasia–dyslexia)

        (3) Mixed or global: a combination of expressive and receptive language difficulties; if complete, a devastating disability. Most patients suffer incomplete dysfunction, which makes some recovery possible

      (e) Deviation of head and eyes to left

  c. Diagnostic study findings

    i. Laboratory

      (a) CSF: RBCs and increased protein after hemorrhage

      (b) Serum glucose: should be checked to rule out hypoglycemic coma, diabetes mellitus

      (c) Clotting profile: check adequacy of clotting

    ii. Radiologic

      (a) CT scan

        (1) Ischemia and infarctions are revealed as areas of decreased absorption or density; best seen 24 hours or more after occlusive event

        (2) Hemorrhage appears as an area of increased absorption or density and is seen immediately after the event

      (b) Cerebral angiography: may reveal vessels in spasm, aneurysms, AVMs, or vessels displaced or stretched

    iii. Special

      (a) MRI: reveals infarction, hemorrhage, and areas of edema. May reveal causative factor, depending on etiology

      (b) Many direct and indirect noninvasive tests for detecting carotid artery disease are available

      (c) CBF studies

(1) Xenon isotope (^{133}Xe) inhalation technique: may reveal hemispheric or global decrease in CBF

(2) PET: provides quantitative values for CBF, CBV, and brain cell metabolism to define infarction size and location. Expensive, not readily available

4. **Nursing diagnoses** (see Commonly Encountered Nursing Diagnoses)

   a. Potential for injury related to intracranial hemorrhage secondary to thrombolytic therapy (e.g., streptokinase, urokinase, tissue plasminogen activator [tPA])

      i. Assessment for defining characteristics

         (a) Increase in neurologic deficit

         (b) New neurologic deficit

         (c) Decreased level of consciousness

         (d) Increased ICP

         (e) Headache

      ii. Expected outcome: deficit is recognized promptly, and therapy is stopped

      iii. Nursing interventions

         (a) Monitor the patient's neurologic status frequently during thrombolytic therapy

         (b) Stop infusion of the thrombolytic drug promptly if the patient's neurologic condition changes

         (c) Report changes to the physician and prepare the patient for CT scan

      iv. Evaluation of nursing care: the deficit is recognized promptly, and therapy is stopped appropriately

   b. Impaired physical mobility related to hemiparesis or hemiplegia

   c. Unilateral neglect related to cerebral impairment, usually a right hemisphere lesion

      i. Assessment for defining characteristics

         (a) There is consistent inattention to stimuli on affected side

         (b) Patient demonstrates inadequate self-care

         (c) Patient positions self inappropriately on the affected side

         (d) Patient attempts to move or get up without assistance for the affected side

         (e) Patient does not look toward the affected side

         (f) Homonymous hemianopsia is present

         (g) Patient does not recognize affected body parts as part of the body

      ii. Expected outcomes

         (a) Patient demonstrates increased awareness of and attention to affected side

         (b) Patient does not experience injury

      iii. Nursing interventions

         (a) Create a safe environment:

            (1) Orient the patient

            (2) Provide good lighting

            (3) Position the patient's bed and personal objects in the unaffected visual field

            (4) Keep side rails up and the call light within reach, restraining the patient only if necessary

(b) Protect the neglected side during activities

(c) Teach the patient to scan the affected visual field or side

(d) Gradually move objects to the affected side, and encourage the patient to attend to that side

(e) Include the family in interventions

iv. Evaluation of nursing care

(a) Patient attends to and is aware of affected side

(b) There is absence of injury

Meningitis

1. **Pathophysiology**
   a. Although the skull and meninges provide barriers to microbial invasion, once access is gained, the CNS has limited immunologic defenses. This inability to provide a rapid response to infection results in proliferation of bacteria that other organs would resist, and mortality rates from infection are higher than in other body sites. Pathologic organisms gain access to the subarachnoid space and meninges
       i. Via blood stream, sinuses, or middle ear
       ii. Directly through penetrating injuries, ventriculostomy catheters, surgical wound contamination
       iii. Indirectly as result of cerebral abscess or encephalitis
   b. Bacterial exudate forms in the subarachnoid space, and meninges become inflamed. Congestion of tissues and blood vessels leads to cortical irritation; increased ICP may result from hydrocephalus or vasogenic and cytotoxic cerebral edema
   c. Progressive involvement includes:
       i. Vasculitis leading to ischemia or infarction
       ii. Ependymitis or pyocephalus
       iii. Petechial hemorrhage within brain
       iv. Hydrocephalus or subdural hygroma
       v. Cranial nerve neuritis

2. **Etiologic or precipitating factors**
   a. Infecting organisms: organism varies widely, depending on the cause (e.g., traumatic CSF leak, postoperatively, gunshot wound)
       i. Virus: enterovirus, mumps virus, herpesvirus, arbovirus
       ii. Bacteria
           (a) The most common organisms after neurologic surgery are staphylococci, usually *Staphylococcus aureus* but also *S. epidermidis*
           (b) Gram-negative enteric bacilli, including *Escherichia coli, Serratia, Klebsiella, Citrobacter, Proteus, Pseudomonas,* and *Acinetobacter*
           (c) *Neisseria meningitidis* (meningococcal meningitis): one of most contagious
           (d) *Haemophilus influenzae*
           (e) *Streptococcus pneumoniae*
           (f) *Mycobacterium tuberculosis*
   b. Sources of infection
       i. Neurologic surgery: contamination during surgery, local wound infection from irrigation systems or drains
       ii. Penetrating head injury: stab wounds, gunshot wounds, depressed skull fractures

    iii. Basal skull fracture resulting in dural tears with CSF leak

    iv. Otitis media or sinusitis

    v. ICP monitoring devices

    vi. Septicemia, septic emboli

    vii. Dental abscesses or recent dental therapy

3. Nursing assessment data base

  a. Nursing history

    i. Subjective findings

      (a) Headache that has grown progressively worse

      (b) Neck or back pain upon flexion

      (c) Nausea and vomiting

      (d) Photophobia

    ii. Objective findings

      (a) Presence of etiologic or precipitating factors; a highly suspect injury, procedure, or pathologic condition

      (b) Social history: IV drug abuse

      (c) Medications: immunosuppressant drugs, such as steroids

      (d) Seizures

      (e) Irritability, confusion

  b. Nursing examination of patient

    i. Inspection

      (a) Signs of infection

        (1) Fever

        (2) Tachycardia

        (3) Chills

        (4) Skin rash: petechiae or purpura most common in meningococcal meningitis

      (b) Meningeal irritation

        (1) Headache

        (2) Nuchal rigidity: resistance to flexion of neck

        (3) Brudzinski's sign: adduction and flexion of the patient's legs as the examiner flexes the patient's neck

        (4) Kernig's sign: after the examiner adducts the patient's thigh against the abdomen, the examiner's attempts to extend the leg are met with resistance

      (c) Neurologic abnormalities

        (1) Decreased level of consciousness

        (2) Cranial nerve involvement

          a) Optic (CN II): papilledema may be present; blindness can occur

          b) Oculomotor, trochlear, abducens (CN III, CN IV, CN VI): impairment of ocular movement, ptosis and unequal pupils, and diplopia are common findings

          c) Trigeminal (CN V): photophobia

          d) Facial (CN VII): facial paresis

          e) Acoustic (CN VIII): tinnitus, vertigo, deafness

        (3) Focal neurologic signs (hemiparesis, hemiplegia)

        (4) Seizures

      (d) Complications

        (1) Waterhouse-Friderichsen syndrome (adrenal hemorrhage)

with resulting hemorrhage and shock. May be seen in fulminating meningococcal meningitis
(2) Disseminated intravascular coagulation (DIC)
(3) Brain abscess, subdural effusions, encephalitis
(4) Hydrocephalus
(5) Cerebral edema
c. Diagnostic study findings
  i. Laboratory findings
    (a) CSF: results depend on type of organism
      (1) Elevated protein level seen in most cases; higher level in bacterial than in viral meningitis
      (2) Low glucose content seen in most cases of bacterial meningitis; may be normal in viral meningitis
      (3) Purulent, turbid; may be clear with some viruses
      (4) Cells: predominantly polymorphonuclear leukocytes in bacterial form, lymphocytes in viral form
    (b) Cultures: specimens of CSF, blood, drainage from sinuses or wounds are obtained to identify organism. Make sure that specimens are transported to the laboratory immediately as prompt culturing is necessary for certain organisms
    (c) Nasopharyngeal smear: causative bacteria may be present
    (d) Electrolytes: either hyponatremia or hypernatremia may be seen
  ii. Radiologic findings
    (a) CT scan: usually normal in acute uncomplicated meningitis but may show diffuse enhancement in some types or reveal hydrocephalus
    (b) Skull x-rays: infected sinuses may be seen; basilar skull fracture may be evident
  iii. Other diagnostic findings: EEG may show generalized slow-wave activity
4. **Nursing diagnoses** (see Commonly Encountered Nursing Diagnoses)
  a. Alteration in cerebral tissue perfusion related to increased ICP
  b. Potential for injury related to seizures
  c. Fluid volume deficit related to decreased intake, increased output
  d. Alteration in comfort secondary to meningeal irritation
    i. Assessment for defining characteristics
      (a) Complaints of headache, pain in neck or back
      (b) Guarding or protective behavior (e.g., unwillingness to move in bed)
      (c) Narrowed focus: altered time perception, withdrawal from social contact
      (d) Facial mask of pain
      (e) Moaning, crying
      (f) Increased blood pressure, pulse, respiratory rate
    ii. Expected outcomes
      (a) Patient articulates factors that intensify pain and modifies behavior appropriately
      (b) Patient expresses relief from pain
    iii. Nursing interventions
      (a) Assess symptoms of pain, and administer pain medication as ordered. Monitor and record effectiveness and side effects

        (b) Perform comfort measures to promote relaxation

        (c) Plan activities with patient to provide distraction (e.g., radio, visitors, television, or reading if patient is able)

        (d) Explain reasons for pain (e.g., nuchal rigidity) to increase pain tolerance

        (e) Manipulate environment to promote periods of uninterrupted rest (e.g., turning down lights)

        (f) Place the patient in a comfortable position

    iv. Evaluation of nursing care

        (a) Factors that intensify pain diminish

        (b) Relief of pain reported

  e. Hyperthemia related to infectious process

    i. Assessment for defining characteristics

        (a) Fever

        (b) Tachycardia

        (c) Tachypnea

        (d) Warm, flushed skin

        (e) Seizures

    ii. Expected outcomes

        (a) Temperature remains below 100.5°F (38.0°C)

        (b) Fluid intake stays equal to or greater than output

        (c) Patient does not experience seizures

    iii. Nursing interventions

        (a) Administer antibiotic therapy as ordered and at the first suspicion of infection, even before CSF is obtained for analysis

        (b) Monitor temperature every 2 to 4 hours as patient's condition indicates

        (c) Administer antipyretic medications as ordered

        (d) Employ other cooling measures as indicated: remove blankets, use tepid water/alcohol sponge, use a hypothermia blanket

        (e) Monitor systemic responses to fever or infection (e.g., vital signs, respiratory rate, level of consciousness)

        (f) Prevent skin irritation or breakdown if sponge baths or a hypothermia blanket is used

    iv. Evaluation of nursing care

        (a) Temperature is maintained below 100.5°F (38.0°C)

        (b) Fluid intake is adequate

        (c) Seizures are absent

Acute Spinal Cord Injury

1. **Pathophysiology**

  a. Compression, contusion, or transection of the spinal cord can be caused by bony dislocation, fracture fragments, rupture of ligaments, vessels or intravertebral discs, interruption of the blood supply, or overstretching of neural tissue

  b. Subsequent histopathologic changes may be the result of decreased spinal cord blood flow mediated by loss of autoregulation, progressive edema causing small vessel compression, decreased tissue oxygenation, and release of a vasoactive substance, such as dopamine, serotonin, or norepinephrine. Ionic shifts lead to diminished ATP levels and calcium influx into cells, causing further destruction, mediated at least in part by uncoupling of blood flow and oxidative metabolism

2. **Etiologic or precipitating factors**
   a. Most spinal cord injuries are caused by trauma, including motor vehicle accidents, falls, sports injuries (the most common being diving accidents), gunshot wounds, or stab wounds
   b. There are about 8000 to 10,000 new cases of spinal cord injury per year. The cervical spine is most frequently injured in motor vehicle accidents, especially when shoulder and lap restraints are not used
   c. Mechanisms include hyperextension, flexion, vertical compression, and rotational injuries leading to fractures, dislocations, or subluxation of the bony elements and stretching, crushing, or vascular compromise of the spinal cord
   d. Disease processes (e.g., tumors, ruptured AVMs, infectious processes, or hematomas) may also precipitate acute loss of function

3. **Nursing assessment data base**
   a. Nursing history
      i. Trauma resulting in acute decrease or loss of function
      ii. Acute decrease in function secondary to other spinal cord processes without a history of trauma
   b. Nursing examination of patient
      i. Assess any neck pain or tenderness
      ii. Assess motor and sensory function of the corticospinal and spinothalamic tracts and the posterior columns (see Physiologic Anatomy and Nursing Examination of Patient)
      iii. Type and extent of lesion
         (a) Complete transection: total loss of motor and sensory function below the level of the lesion; irreversible
         (b) Incomplete lesion: varying degrees of motor and sensory loss below the level of the lesion; represents sparing of some tracts. Prognosis is much better
            (1) Central cord syndrome: greater motor weakness in upper extremities than in lower, varying sensory loss
            (2) Brown-Séquard syndrome: hemisection of the cord, ipsilateral loss of motor, position and vibratory sense, contralateral loss of pain and temperature perception
            (3) Anterior cord syndrome: complete motor loss and loss of pain and temperature below the level of the lesion, with sparing of proprioception, vibration and touch
            (4) Other incomplete lesions cause patchy motor and sensory loss
      iv. Level of the lesion
         (a) C1–4: quadriplegia with total loss of respiratory function
         (b) C4–5: quadriplegia with possible phrenic nerve involvement caused by edema which results in loss of respiratory function
         (c) C5–6: quadriplegia with gross arm movements, diaphragmatic breathing
         (d) C6–7: quadriplegia with biceps intact, diaphragmatic breathing
         (e) C7–8: quadriplegia with triceps, biceps, and wrist extension intact

but no function of intrinsic hand muscles; diaphragmatic breathing

    (f) T1–L2: paraplegia with varying loss of intercostal and abdominal muscle function

    (g) Below L2: cauda equina injury; mixed picture of motor and sensory loss, bowel and bladder dysfunction

    v. Spinal shock: areflexia with flaccid paralysis immediately or shortly after injury. Is due, in part, to sudden withdrawal of predominantly facilitatory influences from higher centers, persistent inhibition from below the lesion acting on extensor reflexes, and axonal degeneration, particularly of axons severed near the cell body. The intensity of spinal shock is variable, as is the return of reflex function when spinal shock subsides. The spastic paralysis typical of an upper motor neuron lesion is then manifested. Duration varies considerably

  c. Diagnostic study findings

    i. Laboratory findings: CSF analysis may be helpful in pathology other than trauma

    ii. Spinal series is done initially to discern fractures, dislocations, or penetrating injury. All seven cervical vertebrae and the cervicothoracic junction must be visualized

    iii. CT demonstrates the bony pathology exquisitely. Myelography shows impingement of the spinal canal by disc or bony fragments. Three-dimensional reconstruction is possible

    iv. MRI is best at demonstrating soft tissue injury and pathology of the spinal cord; does not elucidate the bony injury

    v. Angiography is done in cases of gunshot and stab wounds to assess for vascular injuries, if chest injury suggests aortic involvement, or in suspected vascular malformations

4. Nursing diagnoses

  a. Potential for recovery related to spinal cord injury

    i. Assessment for defining characteristics: decreased motor or sensory function secondary to trauma to the spinal cord

    ii. Expected outcome: improved sensory or motor function

    iii. Nursing interventions

      (a) Begin methylprednisolone within 8 hours of injury. Loading dose is 30 mg/kg given IVPB over 15 minutes; wait 45 minutes, then begin 5.4 mg/kg/hour for 23 hours

      (b) Assess sensory and motor function for signs of improvement

    iv. Evaluation of nursing care: improved sensory or motor function

  b. Potential for decreased cardiac output related to sympathetic blockade

    i. Assessment for defining characteristics

      (a) Hypotension: neurogenic shock caused by loss of sympathetic tone in spinal cord injury above T5; usually in complete lesions. Vasodilatation, decreased venous return, and hypotension result. May be further complicated by hemorrhage from other injuries

      (b) Bradycardia: caused by sympathetic blockade. May lead to junctional rhythm or ventricular escape. Aggravated by hypothermia and hypoxia

      (c) Vasovagal reflex: bradycardia caused by hypoxia and vagal stimulation induced by suctioning. May lead to cardiac arrest

    ii. Expected outcomes

(a) Systolic blood pressure is maintained at normal levels

(b) Patient experiences no bradycardia or arrest during suctioning or other nursing interventions

iii. Nursing interventions

(a) Hypotension: fluid replacement with colloids and crystalloid is used to maintain normal blood pressure; vasopressors may be required

(b) Bradycardia: treated with atropine if patient is symptomatic or if dysrhythmias occur. Treat complicating factors, such as hypothermia or hypoxia

(c) Vasovagal reflex: Oxygenate before and after suctioning; monitor cardiac rate and rhythm

iv. Evaluation of nursing care

(a) Cardiac output is maintained within normal limits

(b) There is no bradycardia or cardiac arrest from vasovagal reflex

c. Alteration in temperature regulation related to poikilothermism

i. Assessment for defining characteristics

(a) Core temperature drifts toward ambient temperature and patient becomes hypothermic or hyperthermic, depending on the environmental temperature

(b) Results from interruption of sympathetic pathways to temperature-regulating centers in the hypothalamus

ii. Expected outcome: core temperature is maintained above 94°F (34°C)

iii. Nursing interventions

(a) Ensure a cool environment to avoid hyperthermia

(b) Treat with a warming mattress if patient is hypothermic

(c) Monitor temperature every 2 hours until stable, then according to unit protocol

iv. Evaluation of nursing care: core temperature is maintained above 94°F (34°C)

d. Alteration in tissue perfusion related to deep venous thrombosis (DVT)

i. Assessment for defining characteristics

(a) Decreased rate of blood flow and flaccid paralysis contribute to venous stasis in legs and pelvis

(b) The usual clinical signs of tenderness, a positive Homans sign, and swelling of the extremities are often difficult to detect in patients with sensory loss and paralysis and are late signs in the development of DVT

(c) Venography remains the gold standard for diagnosis of DVT

ii. Expected outcomes

(a) Patient does not experience inflammation, redness, or swelling of extremities

(b) There is no clinical evidence of DVT

iii. Nursing interventions

(a) Avoid placing IV catheters in paretic limbs, particularly lower extremities

(b) Frequent range-of-motion exercises may be useful in prevention if used early in the patient's course but should not be performed in suspected or known DVT (may embolize)

(c) Prophylactic anticoagulation with low-dose heparin (e.g., 5000 units subcutaneously every 12 hours) has been recommended. Low-molecular-weight heparin may also be used

(d) Antiembolic stockings and alternating-pressure devices may be effective in conjunction with heparin therapy

(e) Early mobilization of the patient into a chair may also prevent venous stasis

iv. Evaluation of nursing care: absence of venous thrombosis

e. Inadequate gas exchange related to pulmonary embolus (see Chapter 1)

i. Assessment for additional defining characteristics

(a) Because of loss of sensation and decreased respiratory ability secondary to spinal cord injury, the usual subjective symptoms of embolism, such as chest pain, dyspnea, and tachypnea, may not be apparent

(b) Likewise, hemoptysis will not be manifested because of poor coughing ability in patients with cervical lesions

(c) Embolism should be suspected in patients with abrupt changes in oxygenation via pulse oximetry, ABGs, or mental status changes

f. Ineffective breathing pattern related to paralysis of respiratory muscles, ineffective cough

i. Assessment for defining characteristics

(a) Paradoxical breathing: because of paralysis of abdominal and intercostal muscles in patients with cervical cord lesions, as the patient inspires, the accessory muscles are used, the diaphragm moves upward, and the abdomen inverts. The opposite occurs on expiration

(b) Hypoventilation: injury below C4 results in diaphragmatic breathing and decreased tidal volume and vital capacity. Paralysis of abdominal and intercostal muscles leads to ineffective cough and atelectasis. Abdominal distention may further restrict diaphragmatic excursions

(c) Pneumonia: collection of secretions in dependent segments of lung caused by immobility, ineffective cough, and decreased vital capacity. Artificial airways offer easy access for infection. Aspiration is a common complication

ii. Expected outcomes

(a) Adequate ventilation is maintained, as evidenced by ABG analysis

(b) Patient does not experience pneumonia

iii. Nursing interventions

(a) Auscultate for adventitious sounds every 2 hours

(b) Suction as necessary to keep airway clear using sterile technique

(c) Monitor pulmonary function tests (e.g., vital capacity and tidal volume, pulse oximetry, ABGs)

(d) Assist the patient with diaphragmatic coughing

(e) Provide chest physical therapy per unit protocol

(f) Provide incentive spirometry every hour; teach patient and family how to provide

(g) Ensure adequate hydration

(h) Get patient out of bed three to four times per day when the spine is stabilized

(i) Monitor sputum cultures

(j) Provide nasotracheal fiberoptic intubation and mechanical ventilation if the patient experiences atelectasis or pneumonia

    iv. Evaluation of nursing care

      (a) Adequate ventilation is maintained

      (b) Patient does not experience pneumonia

g. Potential for fluid volume deficit related to gastric dilatation or hemorrhage from gastric ulceration or concomitant abdominal trauma

    i. Assessment for defining characteristics

      (a) Gastric dilatation and ileus: can interfere with diaphragmatic functioning, causing hypoventilation and hypoxia. Vomiting and aspiration may occur

        (1) Abdominal distention

        (2) Decreased or absent bowel sounds

        (3) Vomiting

        (4) Coffee-ground gastric aspirate

      (b) Gastric stress ulcer: probably the result of vagal stimulated gastric acid production and/or release of ACTH

        (1) Gastric aspirate and stool guaiac-positive

        (2) Fall in hematocrit

        (3) Decreased blood pressure

      (c) Hemorrhage secondary to abdominal trauma is difficult to diagnose because of loss of usual clinical indicators (e.g., pain). May progress rapidly as a result of loss of sympathetic compensation

        (1) Abdominal distention

        (2) Decreased or absent bowel sounds

        (3) Fall in hematocrit

        (4) Decreased blood pressure

        (5) Decreased CVP or PAWP

        (6) Tachycardia may not be obvious because of sympathetic blockade

        (7) Intraperitoneal lavage may detect the presence of intra-abdominal hemorrhage. Abdominal CT is useful

    ii. Expected outcomes

      (a) Patient does not experience fluid volume deficit from gastric dilatation and ileus or hemorrhage

      (b) Abdominal injury is recognized early

    iii. Nursing interventions

      (a) Inspect the abdomen for distention

      (b) Monitor the amount, quality, and occult blood in gastric aspirate

      (c) Antacids and H_2 antagonists have been recommended in the prevention and treatment of ulcers, although the use of sucralfate may be effective in reducing the incidence of pneumonia from translocation of gastric bacteria in patients who are intubated

      (d) Gastric bleeding has been treated with both warm and cold water lavage. Assess the patient for coagulation defects. Intra-arterial infusion of vasopressin has been used. Gastrectomy may be necessary

      (e) Monitor hematocrit and blood volume. Administer fluid as necessary

        iv. Evaluation of nursing care: hemorrhage is avoided or detected and is treated promptly

    h. Urinary retention related to atonic bladder or areflexia

        i. Assessment for defining characteristics

           (a) Urinary retention: may lead to reflux, stone formation, back pressure, and renal deterioration

           (b) Bladder distention

           (c) No urine output

           (d) Signs of urinary tract infection: cloudy urine, foul odor, sediment, positive urine culture

        ii. Expected outcomes

           (a) Patient maintains adequate urinary elimination

           (b) Maintain sterile urine cultures

        iii. Nursing interventions

           (a) Indwelling urinary catheter necessary during hemodynamic instability; once stable, intermittent catheterization should be initiated

           (b) Monitor output. Intermittent catheterization should be done often enough to keep output at 600 ml each time patient is catheterized

           (c) Monitor urine cultures. Early detection is essential because infection can greatly prolong the period of spinal shock and may lead to sepsis

           (d) Begin teaching patient self-catheterization as soon as feasible

        iv. Evaluation of nursing care

           (a) Urinary elimination is adequate

           (b) There is no urinary tract infection

    i. Potential impairment of skin integrity related to immobilization and paralysis

        i. Assessment for defining characteristics

           (a) Denervated areas break down more quickly and heal more slowly than those with normal nerve supply. Poor circulation may also contribute

           (b) Physical immobility

           (c) Presence of traction

        ii. Expected outcomes: no skin breakdown occurs

        iii. Nursing interventions

           (a) Use kinetic beds, such as the Roto-Rest kinetic table, until the patient's cervical spine is stabilized by surgery or a Halo device placement

           (b) Inspect the skin often, and protect potential vulnerable areas from breakdown, such as bony prominences of the heels, elbows, sacrum, and back of the head

           (c) Once the cervical spine is stable, transfer the patient to a chair three to four times per day

        iv. Evaluation of nursing care: absence of skin breakdown

    j. Impaired physical mobility related to paralysis and spasticity (see Commonly Encountered Nursing Diagnoses)

        i. Assessment for additional defining characteristics

           (a) Muscle atony and wasting: occurs during the flaccid paralysis that characterizes spinal shock

      (b) Contractures may be due to spastic paralysis that occurs as spinal shock dissipates

  k. Disturbance in self-concept related to change in body image, role performance, personal identity (see Chapter 9, Psychosocial Aspects)

    i. Additional nursing interventions

      (a) Encourage participation in care, particularly skin care (cooperating and assisting with turning), urinary tract care (maintaining adequate hydration, learning self-catheterization, if physically possible), and respiratory care (incentive spirometry)

    ii. Evaluation of nursing care

      (a) Adaptation to tetraplegia or paraplegia is a long-term process. Patients will rarely attain significant acceptance while in the acute care setting. While seeming to understand and accept that paralysis may be permanent, almost all patients maintain hope of return of function. As long as this hope does not interfere with the patient's progress toward rehabilitation, do not discourage it

      (b) Patient participates in decisions about various aspects of care

  l. Powerlessness related to total physical dependency (see Chapter 9)

  m. Ineffective individual coping related to situational crisis, loss of control and independence, and change in role

  n. Ineffective family coping related to burden of care and changes in patient's present and future functioning

Status Epilepticus

1. **Pathophysiology**
   a. Tonic-clonic seizures cause a rapid succession of many action potentials in single cells
   b. Heavy metabolic demand is placed on cells, leading to decline of high-energy phosphates (e.g., ATP) and failure of the Na^+-K^+-ATPase pump
   c. Cerebral metabolic rate, O_2 and glucose utilization, and glycolysis increase two to three times normal
   d. CBF increases three to five times normal owing, in part, to increased arterial pressure and cerebrovascular dilation
   e. Cellular swelling may occur with prolonged seizures and may be due to the osmotic effects from uptake of increased amounts of metabolic by-products (e.g., lactate, amino acids, ammonia) and failure of the sodium-potassium pump
   f. Systemic metabolic acidosis contributes to cardiovascular collapse
   g. Hyperthermia occurs as a result of increased metabolic activity
2. **Etiologic or precipitating factors**
   a. Withdrawal from anticonvulsant medications
   b. Acute alcohol withdrawal
   c. Electroshock therapy
   d. CNS infections (e.g., meningitis, encephalitis, abscesses)
   e. Brain tumors, particularly in frontal lobe
   f. Acute withdrawal from chronically used drugs that have sedative or depressant effects
   g. Metabolic disorders (e.g., uremia, hypoglycemia, hyponatremia)
   h. Craniocerebral trauma

     i. Cerebral edema

     j. Cerebrovascular disease

3. Nursing assessment data base

   a. Nursing history

       i. Presence of one or more etiologic or precipitating factors

      ii. Seizure activity that persists

   b. Nursing examination of patient

       i. Absence (petit mal): 200 to 300 absences in 24 hours. Rarely occurs; not life-threatening

      ii. Epilepsia partialis continua: partial or focal seizures that occur regularly or are continuous. Not usually accompanied by loss of consciousness. May generalize—that is, become tonic-clonic seizures

     iii. Tonic-clonic (grand mal); grand mal seizures that recur, with incomplete recovery between seizures. As seizures repeat, the postictal interval becomes progressively shorter. Seizures may become continuous. Life-threatening owing to metabolic and physical exhaustion that occurs

     iv. Electrical status: little or no clinical evidence of seizure activity, although the EEG shows continuous spike discharges

   c. Diagnostic study findings

       i. Laboratory findings

         (a) Electrolyte abnormalities, hypoglycemia, and hypoxemia may precipitate seizure activity or may result from prolonged seizures

         (b) Serum enzymes, particularly CPK, are elevated after seizure activity

         (c) Myoglobinuria is common after prolonged seizures

      ii. Radiologic findings: after seizures are controlled, diagnostic studies may be done to find precipitating or complicating cause

     iii. EEG shows seizure activity

4. Nursing diagnoses (see Commonly Encountered Nursing Diagnoses)

   a. Potential for injury related to metabolic complications of seizure activity

       i. Assessment for additional defining characteristics

         (a) Respiratory and metabolic acidosis

         (b) Hypoxemia

         (c) Hypoglycemia

         (d) Hyperthermia

         (e) Electrolyte imbalances

         (f) Renal impairment secondary to myoglobinuria

      ii. Expected outcomes

         (a) Oxygenation and ventilation are maintained

         (b) Patient experiences no complications of drug therapy

         (c) Seizures are stopped and controlled

     iii. Nursing interventions

         (a) Establish and maintain patent airway and adequate ventilation

            (1) Endotracheal intubation and controlled ventilation with ventilator may be necessary if seizures cannot be controlled rapidly

            (2) Monitor ABGs frequently, and treat respiratory or metabolic acidosis

            (3) Maintain adequate oxygenation; seizure activity increases O_2 consumption

(b) Assess causes or contributing factors
  (1) Analyze blood for glucose, sodium, potassium, calcium, phosphorus, magnesium, and blood urea nitrogen as severe imbalance of any of these may precipitate or perpetuate seizures
  (2) Obtain toxic screen for drugs (e.g., PCP, alcohol, lead)
  (3) Obtain anticonvulsant drug levels (e.g., barbiturate, phenytoin)
  (4) Obtain blood specimens for culture if sepsis is suspected
  (5) CBC with differential may reveal disorders that are associated with seizures (e.g., lead poisoning, sickle cell anemia, leukemia)
(c) Stop seizure activity: the following drugs may be used:
  (1) Lorazepam (Ativan)
    a) Dose: 4 mg IV (0.44 mg/kg); repeat after 15 minutes if seizures persist. Therapeutic plasma levels: 30 to 60 μg/ml
    b) Onset: usually within 15 minutes
    c) Result: respiratory depression may occur but is not seen as frequently as with diazepam
  (2) Diazepam
    a) Dose: 10 to 20 mg IV at 5 mg/minute. Do not dilute. Therapeutic plasma levels: 0.5 μg/ml or greater. Onset of action: almost immediate. Duration of action is 30 to 60 minutes
    b) Result: Respiratory and cardiovascular depression may occur in compromised patients or if diazepam is used with phenobarbital
    c) Mechanism of action: thought to be enhancement of the inhibitory neurotransmitter GABA
  (3) Phenobarbital
    a) Dose: 5 to 8 mg/kg IV at 60 mg/minute. Therapeutic plasma levels: 20 to 40 μg/ml. Onset of action: 5 to 20 minutes. Duration of action: about 24 hours
    b) Result: depression of blood pressure, respiration, and consciousness may occur
    c) Mechanism of action: thought to include increased neuronal threshold to electrical and chemical stimuli, depressed physiologic excitation, enhanced inhibition at the synapse, and reduced calcium uptake by depolarized nerve terminals
  (4) Phenytoin
    a) 12 to 18 mg/kg IV no faster than 50 mg/minute. Therapeutic plasma levels: 10 to 20 μg/ml. Onset of action: 10 to 20 minutes. Duration of action: 24 hours
    b) Administration: IV, as close to infusion site as possible. Line should be flushed with saline or absolute alcohol to preclude precipitation or crystallization with glucose. Because of its basic pH, should not be given intramuscularly
    c) Monitor the electrocardiogram (ECG) continuously for

dysrhythmias or conduction changes. Use with caution in patients with heart block or Stokes-Adams syndrome. Hypotension may occur, particularly if given too fast

    d) Major mechanism of action: decreases intracellular influx of Na^+ and Ca^{2+}, blocking neurotransmitter release

  (5) If seizure activity is not stopped with these medications in the usual doses, high-dose pentobarbital therapy may be employed

    a) Loading doses: 5 to 10 mg/kg over 1 hour; then 5 mg/kg per hour three times

    b) Maintenance: 1 to 3 mg/kg per hour IV piggy back

    c) Monitor EEG continuously

    d) Monitor serum levels

(d) Monitor closely to prevent complications

  (1) Insert a nasogastric tube to gastric suction to prevent vomiting and aspiration

  (2) Establish IV route for medications

  (3) Monitor cardiac rate and rhythm, and arterial blood pressure

  (4) Make cardiovascular drugs readily available

  (5) Assess neurologic status frequently

  (6) Treat hyperthermia with antipyretics and external cooling

(e) Maintain fluid and electrolyte balance

  (1) Maintain accurate intake and output

  (2) Administer glucose solutions IV on the basis of blood glucose levels

  (3) Assess electrolytes, calcium and magnesium levels, and renal and liver function

  (4) Myoglobinuria may result from prolonged seizure activity and can lead to renal failure; treat with fluid and diuretics

(f) Maintain a seizure-free state

  (1) If diazepam is used to stop seizures, anticonvulsant drugs, preferably phenytoin, must be given simultaneously to prevent recurrent seizures

  (2) Phenytoin is often preferred because it does not mask neurologic signs

  (3) Phenobarbital may be used if sedation is not a concern

(g) Investigate and treat underlying pathology

  (1) Signs of head trauma

  (2) Signs of drug abuse (e.g., needle tracks)

  (3) Diagnostic tests for intracranial pathology (e.g., CT scan, angiography)

  (4) Diagnostic tests for conditions that are associated with seizures (e.g., fluid and electrolyte imbalance, white or red blood cell abnormalities)

iv. Evaluation of nursing care

(a) Seizure activity is controlled

(b) There are no complications from the use of anticonvulsant medications

(c) Metabolic responses are controlled

(d) The underlying cause is treated, if possible
  b. Hyperthermia related to seizure activity
       i. Assessment for defining characteristics
          (a) Fever
          (b) Persistent tonic-clonic seizure activity, focal or generalized
          (c) Tachycardia
      ii. Expected outcome: patient's temperature stays below 100°F (38°C)
     iii. Nursing interventions
          (a) Administer antipyretics as ordered
          (b) Give a tepid sponge bath if hyperthermia persists, if temperature is above 103°F, or as ordered
          (c) Stop seizure activity
      iv. Evaluation of nursing care
          (a) Temperature is maintained below 100°F (38°C)
  c. Other nursing diagnoses that may be applicable include (see Commonly Encountered Nursing Diagnoses)
       i. Impaired gas exchange related to altered oxygen supply
      ii. Ineffective breathing pattern related to depressed level of consciousness
     iii. Ineffective airway clearance related to increased secretions and depressed level of consciousness
      iv. Potential fluid volume deficit related to excessive loss and decreased intake

Guillain-Barré Syndrome (Landry–Guillain-Barré–Strohl Syndrome, Polyneuritis, Polyradiculoneuritis, Infectious polyneuritis)

1. **Pathophysiology:** Edema and inflammation of spinal nerve roots, with subsequent demyelination resulting in impaired nerve impulse conduction. Focal perivascular lymphocytic infiltration occurs within nerve roots, peripheral nerves, and CNS. Demyelination classically begins in distal nerves and ascends symmetrically, resulting in ascending paralysis. This process may halt at any point or may progress to quadriplegia and involvement of motor cranial nerves. Remyelination occurs proximally and proceeds distally, with complete recovery in most cases
2. **Etiologic or precipitating factors**
   a. Cause unknown, but probably an autoimmune disease
   b. A viral infection may precede onset of symptoms by 2 to 3 weeks. Vaccinations have been associated with syndrome
   c. Previous surgery and preexisting illnesses (e.g., Hodgkin's disease or systemic lupus erythematosus) have also been associated with syndrome
   d. Many patients have no prior history
3. **Nursing assessment data base**
   a. Nursing history
        i. Subjective findings
           (a) Progressive, ascending weakness; mild to moderate sensory changes, primarily tingling and muscle pain
           (b) Mild shortness of breath in early stages
   b. Nursing examination of patient
        i. Muscle weakness: symmetric involvement (distal muscles most severely affected)

    ii. Cranial nerve involvement: motor cranial nerves may be affected. In order of occurrence:

      (a) Dysphagia (CN IX, CN X)

      (b) Facial weakness (CN VII)

      (c) Extraocular muscle paralysis (CN III, CN IV, CN VI)

      (d) Masseter muscle paralysis (CN V)

      (e) Paralysis of the SCM and trapezius muscles (CN XI)

      (f) Paralysis of the tongue (CN XII)

   iii. Decreased vital capacity due to weakness of respiratory muscles

   iv. Paresthesias, hyperesthesia, hypalgesia

   v. Muscle tenderness

   vi. ANS dysfunction manifested by fluctuation in blood pressure and heart rate

  c. Diagnostic study findings

    i. CSF: elevated protein with normal WBC and RBC counts, referred to as ''albumino-cytologic dissociation'' (a classical finding). Protein level is highest 10 to 20 days after onset

    ii. Electromyography and nerve conduction studies may be abnormal 1 to 2 weeks after onset

4. Nursing diagnoses (see Commonly Encountered Nursing Diagnoses)

  a. Powerlessness related to total physical dependency

  b. Disturbance in self-concept related to change in body image

  c. Alteration in tissue perfusion related to venous thrombosis

  d. Alteration in respiratory function related to paralysis of respiratory muscles, ineffective coughing and deep breathing

  e. Potential for infection secondary to invasive lines

  f. Impaired physical mobility related to paralysis

  g. Ineffective individual coping related to situational crisis, loss of control and independence, change in role

  h. Ineffective family coping related to disruption of usual family roles, burden of care, changes in family member's present and future functioning

  i. Potential autonomic nervous system dysfunction

    i. Assessment for defining characteristics

      (a) Fluctuations in blood pressure: hypertension more common than hypotension

      (b) Alteration in heart rate: may fluctuate widely

      (c) Flushed, warm skin

      (d) Vasovagal reflex

    ii. Expected outcomes

      (a) Patient maintains adequate blood pressure and heart rate

      (b) Patient does not experience complications from vasovagal reflex

   iii. Nursing interventions

      (a) Monitor blood pressure frequently as condition indicates; administer vasoactive drugs as indicated

      (b) Bradycardia: treat with atropine if symptomatic

      (c) Tachycardia: beta blockers may be used

      (d) Vasovagal reflex: oxygenate prior to and after suctioning. Atropine may be necessary

   iv. Evaluation of nursing care

      (a) Blood pressure and heart rate are within normal limits

(b) A vasovagal reflex response is absent
j. Discomfort related to hyperesthesias, paresthesias, or deep muscle aches
   i. Assessment for defining characteristics
      (a) Reports of muscular pain that feels like a "charley horse"
      (b) Hypersensitivity of skin that feels like pins and needles, tingling
      (c) Reports of sharp, shooting sensations like an "electric shock"
      (d) Facial expression of discomfort (if CN VII is not affected)
      (e) Hot flashes caused by ANS dysfunction
   ii. Expected outcome: patient reports relief of discomfort
   iii. Nursing interventions
      (a) Assess symptoms of pain, and administer pain medication as ordered
      (b) Perform comfort measures to promote relaxation
      (c) Plan activities with patient to provide distraction
      (d) Explain reason for discomfort
      (e) Manipulate environment to promote periods of uninterrupted rest
      (f) Position the patient in a comfortable position, reposition often
      (g) Involve the family in pain control measures
      (h) Pain medications may be helpful for muscular pain but are rarely effective in controlling the discomfort of the sharp, shooting pain
   iv. Evaluation of nursing care: patient reports relief of discomfort
k. Inadequate nutrition related to decreased intake (See Chapter 7, The Gastrointestinal System)
   i. Assessment for additional defining characteristics
      (a) Inability to chew (CN V)
      (b) Absent gag reflex, inability to swallow (CN IX and CN X)
      (c) Facial paralysis (CN VII)
      (d) Paralysis of tongue (CN XII)
      (e) Gastric dilatation, ileus
   ii. Expected outcomes
      (a) Aspiration is avoided
      (b) Optimal body weight is maintained
   iii. Nursing interventions
      (a) Weigh the patient daily or per unit protocol
      (b) Monitor intake and output (I & O)
      (c) Administer parenteral nutrition, preferably via gastric route
   iv. Evaluation of nursing care
      (a) There is no aspiration
      (b) Optimal body weight is maintained
l. Potential for complications related to plasmapheresis
   i. Assessment for defining characteristics
      (a) Hypotension
      (b) Hypoprothrombinemia with bleeding
      (c) Cardiac arrhythmias
      (d) Hypocalcemia
   ii. Expected outcome: complications are recognized and treated promptly
   iii. Nursing interventions

(a) Monitor vital signs, particularly blood pressure, and ECG during and after treatments

(b) Monitor electrolyte balance; observe for signs of hypocalcemia

(c) Plasmapheresis: usually done by a specially trained technician

(d) Plasmapheresis may be done every day or every other day for a total of 4 to 6 exchanges

(e) Replace plasma that is removed with saline and 5% albumin or fresh frozen plasma; maintain adequate IV access

    iv. Evaluation of nursing care: complications are recognized and treated promptly

Recovery from General Anesthesia

1. **Pathophysiology**
   a. Recovery from inhaled anesthetics is function of alveolar ventilation, solubility coefficient of agent, and duration of anesthesia
   b. Recovery from narcotic-based anesthesia depends on dose given, postoperative renal function, and urine output
   c. Recovery from neuromuscular blocking agents is influenced by nature of agent given, dose, and renal and hepatic function
2. **Etiologic and/or precipitating factors**: depend on preoperative condition, type of surgery, anesthetic agent used, duration of anesthesia, and intraoperative course
3. **Nursing assessment data base**
   a. Nursing history
      i. Subjective findings: symptoms from previous surgical procedures
      ii. Objective findings
         (a) Presence of etiologic and precipitating factors: dependent on preoperative condition, type of surgery, anesthetic agent used, duration of anesthesia, and intraoperative course
         (b) Family history: malignant hyperthermia
         (c) Social history
            (1) Illicit drug use
            (2) Smoking
         (d) Medication history: current medications, dosage, and frequency
   b. Nursing examination of patient
      i. Inspection
         (a) Cough reflexes from the carina, then the larynx, return first
         (b) Swallow and vomiting reflexes return next with recovery of pharyngeal muscle tone
         (c) Consciousness returns along with diminution of respiratory and cardiovascular depression
      ii. Auscultation
         (a) Breath sounds are diminshed
         (b) Blood pressure may be lowered or fluctuate
   c. Diagnostic study findings
      i. Laboratory findings
         (a) CBC: may reveal inadequate erythrocyte volume or platelets if blood loss was significant
         (b) Electrolytes and chemistries: may reveal imbalances

        (c) ABGs: may reveal hypoxemia, hypoventilation or hyperventilation, metabolic or respiratory acidosis or alkalosis

        (d) Clotting studies: may reveal coagulopathy

    ii. Radiologic findings: chest x-ray may reveal pulmonary edema, pneumothorax, atelectasis, or aspiration pneumonia

4. Nursing diagnoses

  a. Potential for injury related to systemic complications secondary to general anesthesia

    i. Assessment for defining characteristics

      (a) Cardiovascular

        (1) Dysrhythmias and conduction defects cased by hypoxemia, drugs

        (2) Hypotension: may be caused by blood loss, fluid loss, anesthesia, depressant effects of cellular elements, vasodilatation

        (3) Hypertension: caused by pain, hypercapnea, hypoxemia, or fluid overload

      (b) Respiratory

        (1) Hypoxemia: ventilation-perfusion mismatch, shunt, atelectasis

        (2) Hypoventilation or hyperventilation: obtundation, pain

        (3) Pneumothorax

        (4) Pulmonary edema

        (5) Pulmonary embolus

        (6) Aspiration pneumonia

        (7) Atelectasis

      (c) Renal

        (1) Acute tubular necrosis: resulting from excessive circulating hemoglobin or myoglobin

        (2) Prerenal oliguria: resulting from hypovolemia, hypoperfusion

      (d) Bleeding

        (1) Loss of vascular integrity

        (2) DIC

      (e) Nausea and vomiting

      (f) Agitation and pain

      (g) Hypothermia or hyperthermia

      (h) Fluid and electrolyte imbalances

      (i) Persistent neuromuscular blockade

      (j) Anoxic-ischemic brain damage

    ii. Expected outcomes

      (a) Patient recovers completely from anesthetic agents

      (b) There are no systemic complications or sequelae

    iii. Nursing interventions

      (a) Assess physical and psychologic status of patient preoperatively to provide baseline data for postoperative assessment

      (b) The anesthesiologist-surgeon reports the following information to the nurse:

        (1) Patient's name, age, native language

        (2) Surgical procedure, length of surgery, name of surgeon

        (3) Preoperative medications and anesthetic agent used

    (4) Medical history, including medications, allergies, mental status, and communication handicaps

    (5) Intraoperative course, including vital signs, medications, dysrhythmias, and estimated blood loss and replacement

    (6) Monitoring required and problems anticipated from anesthesia or the surgical procedure

(c) The anesthesiologist and nurse carry out the initial assessment on the patient's admission to the recovery room or intensive care unit (ICU)

(d) Because different anesthetic agents have different durations of action, assess the effect of each drug given. Seek factors that may affect reversal of anesthesia (see Etiologic or Precipitating Factors):

    (1) Assess arousability by calling the patient's name

    (2) Assess gag and swallow reflexes

    (3) Assess for reversal of neuromuscular blockade

        a) Ability to sustain head lifting, eye opening, and hand grasp

        b) Ability to extrude tongue for 5 to 10 seconds

        c) Vital capacity of 10 to 15 ml/kg and inspiratory force of -25 cm H_2O

        d) Neostigmine or physostigmine may be given to hasten reversal

    (4) Give naloxone to reverse respiratory depression of opiates; however, its duration may be shorter than that of the narcotic and respiratory depression may reoccur 30 to 60 minutes after naloxone. Maintain observation

        a) Along with reversal of narcotics come pain, coughing, and agitation

        b) Patients who are intubated with respiratory support may be allowed to recover from effects of narcotics without reversal

(e) Continuous monitoring for systemic complications

    (1) Respiratory

        a) Measure of ventilation: vital capacity (VC), tidal volume (VT), minute ventilation (VE), dead space ventilation/tidal volume ratio (VD/VT), inspiratory force

        b) Rate, rhythm, use of accessory muscles

        c) Breath sounds, adventitious sounds

        d) ABGs

    (2) Cardiovascular

        a) ECG: rate, rhythm, conduction

        b) Blood pressure via cuff, Doppler device, or intra-arterial catheter

        c) Hemodynamic integrity: CVP, PAP, PAWP, cardiac output as necessary

        d) Peripheral circulation and pulses

        e) Heart sounds

  (3) CNS

        a) Level of consciousness

        b) Protective reflexes, pupillary reflexes

        c) Motor ability
        d) ICP monitoring as necessary; calculate CPP
        e) Tests for neuromuscular blockade reversal. Note that neuromuscular blockade may be increased by hypothermia, hypermagnesemia, hypocalcemia, inhalation anesthetic agents, almost all antibiotics, furosemide, and renal failure
    (4) Temperature
        a) Hypothermia may be caused by cold environments, obtundation of thermoregulatory centers, and vasodilatation
        b) Hyperthermia may be caused by infection, seizures, or reaction of anesthetic agents—malignant hyperthermia
    (5) Renal
        a) Fluid balance, urine output
        b) Electrolytes
        c) Blood urea nitrogen (BUN), creatinine
    (6) Gastrointestinal
        a) Nausea and vomiting
        b) Aspiration the most common complication
        c) Opiates stimulate vomiting reflex while obtunding protective reflexes
    (7) Pain: control with opiates if severe
        a) Note that opiates may cause nausea if used alone
        b) Monitor the patient for respiratory and cardiovascular depression
        c) Titrate the dose to patient response
        d) Do not give barbiturates and phenothiazine drugs alone (i.e., without an analgesic) in patients who are in pain because they cause increased sensitivity to pain and cause restlessness
        e) Initially, give analgesics intramuscularly or intravenously
  iv. Evaluation of nursing care
    (a) Preoperative status returns after anesthesia
    (b) Systemic complications and sequelae are prevented or treated
b. Potential for hyperthermia related to malignant hyperthermia
  i. Assessment for defining characteristics
    (a) High body temperature (>105.8°F [41°C])
    (b) Marked skeletal rigidity
    (c) Metabolic and respiratory acidosis, frequently with a base deficit of greater than 10 mmol
    (d) Myocardial changes, usually manifested as dysrhythmias
    (e) Marked hyperkalemia
    (f) Muscle breakdown, as manifested by gross increases in serum CPK and myoglobinuria
    (g) Family history of disorder
  ii. Expected outcomes
    (a) Temperature is maintained in the normal range
    (b) Experiences no systemic complications

   iii. Nursing interventions
     (a) Monitor temperature frequently in known or suspected susceptible patients
     (b) Administer dantrolene sodium as ordered, usually 2 to 4 mg/kg IV in fast running IV (pH 9 to 10). May be repeated at 15-minute intervals as necessary, up to 10 mg/kg total
     (c) Monitor electrolytes, particularly calcium and potassium
     (d) Monitor CPK levels
     (e) Monitor urine for signs of myoglobinuria; send specimen for analysis
     (f) Monitor cardiac rate and rhythm
     (g) Monitor ABGs and serum bicarbonate levels
   iv. Evaluation of nursing care
     (a) Malignant hyperthermia is recognized and treated promptly
     (b) No systemic complications occur
  c. Nursing diagnoses that may be applicable should complications develop:
   i. Impaired gas exchange related to altered oxygen supply or oxygen-carrying capacity
   ii. Ineffective breathing pattern related to depressed level of consciousness, intracranial pathology, and metabolic imbalance
   iii. Ineffective airway clearance related to increased secretions and depressed level of consciousness
   iv. Fluid volume deficit related to excessive loss and decreased intake
   v. Fluid volume excess related to excessive intake
   vi. Alteration in comfort or pain related to surgical procedure or wound

Encephalopathy

1. **Pathophysiology**: neurologic degeneration from a direct or indirect effect on the brain caused by one or more of the following pathologic changes: build-up of toxic metabolic products, structural changes in the brain, changes in blood flow to the brain, changes in the electrical activity of the brain, changes in the supply or utilization of neurotransmitter substances, or other cellular changes that alter neurologic functioning
  a. Encephalopathy is not a disease in itself but is a result of other systemic diseases or disorders of the brain. Therefore, hypoxia, metabolic changes, infectious diseases and structural changes can all lead to an encephalopathy
  b. Encephalopathies caused by hydrocephalus, traumatic head injury, brain tumors, meningitis, stroke (one cause of ischemic-hypoxic injury), vascular disorders, and seizures have been discussed earlier
  c. For discussion of the neurologic changes caused by metabolic conditions such as hepatic, renal, or electrolyte dysfunction, refer to Chapters 1, 2, 4, 5, and 7
2. **Etiologic or precipitating factors**
  a. Disorders of any body system can lead to neurologic changes if the disease progresses far enough for long enough
  b. Many of the diseases that lead to encephalopathy are the end stage of that disease (e.g., uremic or hepatic encephalopathy)

3. **Nursing assessment data base**
   a. Nursing history
      i. Subjective findings
         (a) Vary widely from memory problems to behavioral disorders and depressed level of consciousness
         (b) Neurologic changes are consistent with the cause of the encephalopathy
      ii. Objective findings
         (a) Family history: most helpful in degenerative or hereditary disorders that may lead to encephalopathy
         (b) Social history: an example is chronic alcohol abuse, which leads to thiamine deficiency and Wernicke's encephalopathy; may be consistent with precipitating cause of primary disorder
         (c) Medical history: consistent with neurologic changes that correlate with cause of the encephalopathy
   b. Nursing examination of patient: a complete neurologic examination is warranted to delineate the exact neurologic deficits (see Assessment)
   c. Diagnostic study findings (vary, depending on the precipitating cause)
      i. Laboratory findings
      ii. Radiographic findings
      iii. MRI
4. **Nursing diagnoses**: see Commonly Encountered Nursing Diagnoses and sections related to the primary cause of the encephalopathy

References

GENERAL

Martin, N. A. (ed): Neurosurgical intensive care. Neurosurg. Clin. North Am. 5(4):573–849, 1994.

Wilkins, R. H., and Rengachary, S. S. (eds.): Neurosurgery. Vols. 1–3. New York, McGraw Hill, 1996.

Youmans, J. R. (ed): Neurological Surgery. Vols. 1–5. Philadelphia, W. B. Saunders, 1996.

PHYSIOLOGIC ANATOMY

Barr, M. L.: The Human Nervous System: An Anatomical Viewpoint. Philadelphia, JB Lippincott, 1993.

DeGroot, J. L.: Correlative Neuroanatomy. San Mateo, Calif., Appleton & Lange, 1991.

DeMeyer, W. E.: Neuroanatomy. New York, John Wiley & Sons, 1988.

Gilman, S.: Manter and Gatz's Essentials of Neuroanatomy and Neurophysiology. Philadelphia, F. A. Davis, 1992.

Guyton, A. C.: Basic Neuroscience Anatomy and Physiology. Philadelphia, W. B. Saunders, 1991.

Parent, A.: Carpenter's Human Neuroanatomy. Baltimore, Williams & Wilkins, 1996.

NURSING ASSESSMENT DATA BASE AND NURSING DIAGNOSES

DeMeyer, W.: Technique of the Neurological Examination. New York, McGraw-Hill, 1994.

Marshall, L. F., and Marshall, S. B.: Differential diagnosis of altered states of consciousness. *In* Youmans, J. R. (ed.): Neurological Surgery. Vol. 1. Philadelphia, W. B. Saunders, 1996, pp. 61–70.

Miller, D. W., and Hahn, J. F.: General methods of clinical examination. *In* Youmans, J. R. (ed.): Neurological Surgery. Vol. 1. Philadelphia, W. B. Saunders, 1996, pp. 3–43.

Van Hoozen, B. E., Van Hoozen, C. M., and Albertson, T. E.: Pulmonary considerations and complications in the neurosurgical patient. *In* Youmans, J. R. (ed.): Neurological Surgery. Vol. 2. Philadelphia, W. B. Saunders, 1996, pp. 570–645.

Young, B., and Ott, L.: Nutrition and parenteral therapy. *In* Youmans, J. R. (ed.): Neurological Surgery. Vol. 2. Philadelphia, W. B. Saunders, 1996, pp. 646–663.

INCREASED INTRACRANIAL PRESSURE AND HEAD TRAUMA

Alberico, A. M., Ward, J. D., Choi, S. C., et al.: Outcome after severe head injury: Relationship to mass lesions, diffuse injury, and ICP course in pediatric and adult patients. J Neurosurg 67:648–656, 1987.

Chan, K. H., Dearden, N. M., Miller, J. D., et al.: Multimodality monitoring as a guide to treatment of intracranial hypertension after severe brain injury. Neurosurgery 32:547–554, 1993.

Constantini, S., Cotev, S., Rappaport, Z. H., et al.: Intracranial pressure monitoring after elective intracranial surgery. J. Neurosurg. 69:540–544, 1988.

Cooper, P. R. (ed.): Head Injury. Baltimore, Williams & Wilkins, 1993.

Corrigan, J. D., and Mysiw, J.: Agitation following traumatic head injury: Equivocal evidence for a discrete stage of cognitive recovery. Arch. Phys. Med Rehabil. 69:487–492, 1988.

Doberstein, C., and Martin, N. A.: Cerebral blood flow in clinical neurosurgery. In Youmans, J. R. (ed.): Neurological Surgery. Vol. 2. Philadelphia, W. B. Saunders, 1996, pp. 519–569.

Eisenberg, H. M., Frankowski, R. F., Contant, C. F., et al.: High-dose barbiturate control of elevated intracranial pressure in patients with severe head injury. J. Neurosurg. 69:15–23, 1988.

Fortune, J. B., Feustel, P. J., Weigle, C. G. M., et al.: Continuous measurement of jugular venous oxygen saturation in response to transient elevations of blood pressure in head-injured patients. J. Neurosurg. 80:461–468, 1994.

Gennarelli, T. A.: Cerebral concussion and diffuse brain injuries. In Cooper, R. R. (ed.): Head Injury. Baltimore, Williams & Wilkins, 1993, pp. 137–158.

Gentry, L. R., Godersky, J. C., Thompson, B., et al.: Prospective comparative study of intermediate-field MR and CT in the evaluation of closed head trauma. Am. J. Radiol. 150:673–682, 1988.

Gentry, L. R., Godersky, J. C., and Thompson, B.: MR imaging of head trauma: Review of the distribution and radiopathologic features of traumatic lesions. Am. J. Radiol. 150:663–672, 1988.

Grolomund, P., Weber, M., Seiler, R. W., et al.: Time course of cerebral vasospasm after severe head injury. Lancet, May 21, 1988, p. 1173.

Kadowaki, M. H., Watanabe, H., Numoto, M., et al.: Necessity for ICP monitoring to supplement GCS in head trauma cases. Neurochirurgia (Stuttg) 31:39–44, 1988.

Kelly, D. F., Nikas, D. L., Becker, D. P.: Diagnosis and treatment of moderate and severe head injuries in adults. In Youmans, J. R. (ed.): Neurological Surgery. Vol. 3. Philadelphia, W. B. Saunders, 1996, pp. 1618–1718.

Klauber, M. R., Marshall, L. F., Luerssen, T. G., et al.: Determinants of head injury mortality: Importance of the low risk patient. Neurosurgery 24:31–36, 1989.

Lee, K. R., and Hoff, J. T.: Intracranial pressure. In Youmans, J. R. (ed.): Neurological Surgery. Vol. 2. Philadelphia, W. B. Saunders, 1996, pp. 491–518.

Liau, L. M., Bergsneider, M., Becker, D. P.: Pathology and pathophysiology of head injury. In Youmans, J. R. (ed.): Neurological Surgery. Vol. 3. Philadelphia, W. B. Saunders, 1996, pp. 1549–1594.

Nikas, D. L. (ed.): Head trauma: Part 1. The spectrum of critical care. Crit. Care Nurs. Q. 10:(1), 1987.

Nikas, D. L.: Critical aspects of head trauma. Crit. Care Nurs. Q. 10:19–44, 1987.

Nikas, D. L.: Prognostic indicators in patients with severe head injury. Crit. Care Nurs. Q. 10:25–34, 1987.

Nikas, D. L. (ed.): Head Trauma: Part 2. Nursing issues and controversies. Crit. Care Nurs. Q. 10:(3), 1987.

Robertson, C. S., Contant, C. F., Narayan, R. K., et al.: Cerebral blood flow, AVDO$_2$, and neurological outcome in head injured patients. J Neurotrauma 9(Suppl.):349–358, 1992.

Sahquillo-Barris, J., Lamarca-Ciuro, J., Vilalta-Castan, J., et al.: Acute subdural hematoma and diffuse axonal injury after severe head trauma. J. Neurosurg. 68:894–900, 1988.

Sundberg, G., Nordstrom, C. H., Messeter, K., et al.: A comparison of intraparenchymatous and intraventricular pressure recording in clinical practice. J. Neurosurg. 67:841–845, 1987.

Yonas, H: Measurement of cerebral blood flow. In Wilkins, R. H., and Rengachary, S. S. (eds): Neurosurgery. Vol. 2. New York, McGraw-Hill, 1996, pp. 2007–2010.

HYDROCEPHALUS

Black, P. McL.: Hydrocephalus in adults. In Youmans, J. R. (ed.): Neurological Surgery. Vol. 2. Philadelphia, W. B. Saunders, 1996, pp. 927–944.

Milhorat, T. H.: Hydrocephalus: Pathophysiology and clinical features. In Wilkins, R. H., and Rengachary, S. S. (eds.): Neurosurgery. New York, McGraw-Hill, 1996, pp. 3625–3632.

BRAIN TUMORS

Black, P. M.: Meningiomas. Neurosurgery 32:643–657, 1993.

Fuller, G. N., and Burger, P. C.: Classification and biology of brain tumors. In Youmans, J. R. (ed.): Neurological Surgery. Vol. 4. Philadelphia, W. B. Saunders, 1996, pp. 2495–2520.

Fuller, G. N., and Burger, P. C.: Gliomas: Pathology. In Wilkins, R. H., and Rengachary, S. S. (eds.): Neurosurgery. New York, McGraw-Hill, 1996, pp. 735–748.

Galicich, J. H., Arbit, E., Wronski, M.: Metastatic Brain Tumors. In Wilkins, R. H., and Rengachary, S. S. (eds.): Neurosurgery. New York, McGraw-Hill, 1996, pp. 807–822.

Kaye, A. H., and Laws, E. R. (eds.): Brain Tumors. New York, Churchill Livingstone, 1995.

Martuza, R. L.: Neuro-oncology: An overview. In Wilkins, R. H., and Rengachary, S. S. (eds.): Neurosurgery. New York, McGraw-Hill, 1996, pp. 505–510.

McDermott, M. W., and Wilson, C. B.: Meningiomas. In Youmans, J. R. (ed.): Neurological Surgery. Vol. 4. Philadelphia, W. B. Saunders, 1996, pp. 2782–2825.

Morantx, R. A. and Walsh, J. W. (eds.): Brain Tumors: A Comprehensive Text. New York, Marcel Dekker, 1994.

Young, B., and Patchell, R. A.: Brain metastases. In Youmans, J. R. (ed.): Neurological Surgery. Vol. 4. Philadelphia, W. B. Saunders, 1996, pp. 2748–2760.

INTRACRANIAL ANEURYSMS

Black, P. M.: Hydrocephalus and vasospasm after subarachnoid hemorrhage from ruptured intracranial aneurysms. Neurosurgery 18:12–16, 1986.

Friedman, D: Pre- and postoperative management of a patient with a ruptured aneurysm. In Wilkins, R. H. and Rengachary, S. S. (eds.): Neurosurgery. New York, McGraw-Hill, 1996, pp. 2261–2270.

Hijdra, A., Vermeulem, M., van Gijn, J., et al.: Rerupture of intracranial aneurysms: A clinicoanatomic study. J. Neurosurg. 67:29–33, 1987.

MacDonald, R. L., and Weir, B.: Pathophysiology and clinical evaluation of subarachnoid hemorrhage. In Youmans, J. R. (ed.): Neurological Surgery, Vol. 2. Philadelphia, W. B. Saunders, 1996, pp. 1224–1242.

Mayberg, M. R.: Intracranial arterial spasm. In Wilkins, R. H., and Rengachary, S. S. (eds.): Neurosurgery. New York, McGraw-Hill, 1996, pp. 2245–2254.

McKenna, P., Willison, J. R., Phil, B., et al.: Cognitive outcome and quality of life one year after subarachnoid hemorrhage. Neurosurgery 24:361–367, 1989.

Ohman, J., and Heiskanen, O.: Effect of nimodipine on the outcome of patients after aneurysmal subarachnoid hemorrhage and surgery. J. Neurosurg. 69:683–686, 1988.

Shaffrey, M. E., Shaffrey, C. I., Lanzino, G., et al.: Nonoperative treatment of aneurysmal subarachnoid hemorrhage. In Youmans, J. R. (ed.): Neurological Surgery. Vol. 2. Philadelphia, W. B. Saunders, 1996, pp. 1264–1271.

Weir, B., and McDonald, R. L.: Intracranial aneurysms and subarachnoid hemorrhage: An overview. In Wilkins, R. H., and Rengachary, S. S. (eds.): Neurosurgery. New York, McGraw-Hill, 1996, pp. 2191–2214.

ARTERIOVENOUS MALFORMATIONS

Batjer, H. H., Devous, M. D., Seibert, G. B., et al: Intracranial arteriovenous malformation: Relationship between clinical factors and surgical complications. Neurosurgery 24:75–79, 1989.

Camarata, P. J., and Heros, R. C.: Arteriovenous malformations of the brain. In Youmans, J. R. (ed.): Neurological Surgery. Vol. 2. Philadelphia, W. B. Saunders, 1996, pp. 1372–1404.

Garretson, H. D.: Intracranial arteriovenous malformations. In Wilkins, R. H., and Rengachary, S. S. (eds.): Neurosurgery. New York, McGraw-Hill, 1996, pp. 2433–2442.

Solomon, R. A.: Vascular malformations affecting the nervous system. In Rengachary, S. S., and Wilkins, R. H. (eds.): Principles of Neurosurgery. St. Louis, Mosby-Year Book 1994, pp. 12.1–12.15.

Spetzler, R. F., Martin, N. A., Carter, L. P., et al.: Surgical management of large AVMs by staged embolization and operative excision. J. Neurosurg. 67:17–28, 1987.

STROKE

Barnett, N. J. M., Mohr, J. P., Stein, B. M., et al. (eds): Stroke, Pathophysiology, Diagnosis and Management. New York, Churchill Livingstone, 1992.

Bogousslavsky, J., and Caplan, L. (eds): Stroke Syndromes. Cambridge, Cambridge University Press, 1995.

Davis, J. N., and Gerber, O.: Medical management of ischemia cerebral vascular disease. In Wilkins, R. H., and Rengachary, S. S. (eds.): Neurosurgery. New York, McGraw-Hill, 1996, pp. 2131–2135.

Lougheed, M. G.: Brain resuscitation and protection. Med. J. Aust. 148:458–466, 1988.

Mathern, G. W., Martin, N. A., and Becker, D. P.: Cerebral ischemia: Clinical pathophysiology. In Cerra, F. B., and Shoemaker, W. C. (eds.): Critical Care: State of the Art. Fullerton, Calif., Society of Critical Care Medicine, 1987.

Moossy, J.: Pathology of ischemic vascular disease. In Wilkins, R. H., and Rengachary, S. S. (eds.): Neurosurgery. New York, McGraw-Hill, 1996, pp. 1193–1198.

Ratcheson, R. A., Kiefer, S. P., Selman W. R.: Pathology and clinical evaluation of ischemic cerebrovascular disease. In Youmans, J. R. (ed.): Neurological Surgery. Vol. 2. Philadelphia, W. B. Saunders, 1996, pp. 1113–1138.

Tammer, B., Gross, C. E., Kindt, G. W., et al.: Medical management of acute cerebral ischemia. In Youmans, J.

R. (ed.): Neurological Surgery. Vol. 2. Philadelphia, W. B. Saunders, 1996, pp. 1139–1158.

Tu, Y. K., Heros, R. C., Candia, G., et al.: Isovolemic hemodilution in experimental focal cerebral ischemia: Part 1. Effects on hemodynamics, hemorrheology, and intracranial pressure. J. Neurosurg. 69:72–81, 1988.

Tu, Y. K., Heros, R. C., Karacostas, D, et al.: Isovolemic hemodilution in experimental focal cerebral ischemia: Part 2. Effects on regional cerebral blood flow and size of infarction. J. Neurosurg. 69:82–91, 1988.

MENINGITIS

Abolnik, I. Z., Perfect, J. R., Durack, D. T.: Acute bacterial meningitis. In Wilkins, R. H. and Rengachary, S. S. (eds.): Neurosurgery. New York, McGraw-Hill 1996, pp. 3299–3306.

Dempsey, R., Rapp, R. P., Young, B., et al.: Prophylactic parenteral antibiotics in clean neurosurgical procedures: A review. J. Neurosurg. 69:52–57, 1988.

Gormley, W. B., del Busto, R., Saravolatz, L. D., et al.: Cranial and bacterial infections. In Youmans, J. R. (ed.): Neurological Surgery. Vol. 5. Philadelphia, W. B. Saunders, 1996, pp. 3191–3220.

Petrak, R. M., Pottage, J. C., Harris, A. A., et al: Haemophilus influenzae meningitis in the presence of a cerebrospinal fluid shunt. Neurosurgery 18:79–81, 1986.

Ross, D., Rosegay, H., Pons, V.: Differentiation of aseptic and bacterial meningitis in postoperative neurosurgical patients. J. Neurosurg. 69:669–674, 1988.

Sack, T.: Prophylactic antibiotics in traumatic wounds. J. Hosp. Infection 11(Suppl.):251–258, 1988.

SPINAL CORD INJURY

Becker, D. M., Gonzalez, M., Gentilli, A., et al.: Prevention of deep venous thrombosis in patients with acute spinal cord injuries: Use of rotating treatment tables. Neurosurgery 20:675–677, 1987.

Benzel, E. C.: Management of acute spinal cord injury. In Wilkins, R. H., and Rengachary, S. S. (eds.): Neurosurgery. New York, McGraw-Hill, 1996, pp. 2861–2866.

Bracken, M. B., Shepard, M. J., Collins, W. F., et al.: A randomized, controlled trial of methylprednisolone or naloxone in the treatment of acute spinal-cord injury. N. Eng. J. Med. 322:1405–1411, 1990.

Geisler, F. H., Dorsey, F. C., Coleman, W. P.: Recovery of motor function after spinal-cord injury: A randomized, placebo-controlled trial with GM-1 ganglioside. N. Eng. J. Med. 324:1829–1838, 1991.

Hamilton, M. G., Hull, R. D., Pineo, G. F.: Venous thromboembolism in neurosurgery and neurology patients: A review. Neurosurgery 34:280–296, 1994.

Hull, R. D.: Venous thromboembolism in spinal cord injury. Chest 102(Suppl):658–663, 1992.

Levi L, Wolf, A., Belzberg, H: Hemodynamic parameters in patients with acute cervical cord trauma: Description, intervention, and prediction of outcome. Neurosurgery 33:1007–1017, 1993.

Mammen, E. F.: Pathogenesis of venous thrombosis. Chest 102(Suppl.):640–644, 1992.

Marshall, L. F., Knowlton, S., Garfin, S. R., et al: Deterioration following spinal cord injury. J. Neurosurg. 66:400–404, 1987.

McBride D. Q.: Spinal cord injury syndromes. In

Greenberg, J. (ed.): Handbook of Head and Spine Trauma. New York, Marcel Dekker, 1993, pp. 393–412.

McBride D. Q., and Rodts, G. E.: Intensive care of patients with spinal trauma. Neurosurg. Clin. North Am. 5(4):1–12, 1994.

Merli, G. J.: Management of deep vein thrombosis in spinal cord injury. Chest 102:652–657, 1992 suppl.

Nikas, D. L.: Pathophysiology and nursing interventions in acute spinal cord injury. Trauma Q. 4(3):23–44, 1988.

Steudel, W. I., Rosenthal, D., Lorenz, R., et al: Prognosis and treatment of cervical spinal injuries with associated head trauma. Acta Neurochir. Suppl. 43:85–90, 1988.

Tator, C. H.: Pathophysiology and pathology of spinal cord injury. In Wilkins, R. H., and Rengachary, S. S. (eds.): Neurosurgery. New York, McGraw-Hill, 1996, pp. 2847–2860.

Tator, C. H., and Fehlings, M. G.: Review of the secondary injury theory of acute spinal cord trauma with emphasis on vascular mechanisms. J. Neurosurg. 75:15–26, 1991.

Yao, S. T.: Deep vein thrombosis in spinal cord–injured patients: Evaluation and assessment. Chest 102(Suppl.):645–648, 1992.

Young W.: Secondary injury mechanisms in acute spinal cord injury. J Emerg. Med 11:13–22, 1993.

STATUS EPILEPTICUS

Leppik, E.: Status epilepticus. In Wyllie, E. (ed.): The Treatment of Epilepsy. Philadelphia, Lea & Febiger, 1994, pp. 678–685.

Shorvon, S. D.: Status Epilepticus: Its Clinical Feature and Treatment in Children and Adults. Cambridge, England, Cambridge University Press, 1994.

GUILLAIN-BARRÉ SYNDROME

Parry, G. J.: Guillain-Barré Syndrome. New York, Thieme Medical Publishers, 1993.

Ropper, A., Wijdicks, E. F. M., Truax, B. T.: Guillain-Barré Syndrome. Contemporary Neurology Series. Philadelphia, F. A. Davis, 1991.

RECOVERY FROM GENERAL ANESTHESIA

Brown, D.: Neurological complications of anesthesia. In Aminoff, M. J. (ed.): Neurology and General Medicine. New York, Churchill Livingstone, 1995, pp. 895–914.

Drain, C. B.: The Post Anesthesia Care Unit. Philadelphia, W. B. Saunders, 1994.

Frost, E. A. M., Goldiner, P. C.: Postanesthesia Care. Norwalk, Conn., Appleton & Lange, 1990.

Gallagher, T. J. (ed.): Postoperative Care of the Critically Ill Patient. Baltimore, Williams & Wilkins, 1995.

Goldman, D. R., Brown, F. H., Guarnieri, D. M. (eds.): Perioperative Medicine. New York, McGraw-Hill, 1994.

Gronert, G. A., Mott, J., and Lee, J.: Aetiology of malignant hyperthermia. Br. J. Anaesth. 60:253–267, 1988.

Litwack, K. (ed.): Post Anesthesia Nursing. Nurs. Clin. North Am. 28:483–514, 1993.

Rosenberg, H.: Clinical presentation of malignant hyperthermia. Br. J. Anaesth. 60:268–273, 1988.

Vender, J. S., and Spiess, B. D.: Postanesthesia Care. Philadelphia, W. B. Saunders, 1992.

... The Renal System

June L. Stark, R.N., B.S.N., M.Ed.

PHYSIOLOGIC ANATOMY

Process of Urine Formation

This function occurs in the nephron and involves four processes: filtration, reabsorption, secretion, and excretion

1. **Anatomic structures** (Fig. 4–1)
   a. Cortical layer
      i. Outermost layer of the kidney: the metabolically active portion where aerobic metabolism occurs and where ammonia and glucose are formed
      ii. Metabolic needs are more than satisfactorily met by an excessive oxygen supply
   b. Medullary layer
      i. Middle layer of the kidney: region of glycolytic metabolism that supplies energy for active transport
      ii. Region of active metabolism with high oxygen consumption but a limited oxygen supply
      iii. Composed of six to 10 renal pyramids, formed by collecting ducts
      iv. Site of the deepest part of the long loops of Henle in the nephron
   c. Renal sinus, pelvis, and collecting system
      i. Papillae: rounded projections of renal tissues located at the apical ends of renal pyramids positioned with the base facing the cortex and the apices facing the renal pelvis. The apical portion opens into the minor calices
      ii. Corticomedullary junction: point of division between the cortex and the medulla formed by the base of the pyramids
      iii. Renal lobe: composed of a pyramid plus the surrounding cortical tissue
      iv. Calix
         (a) Minor calix wraps around the papilla and collects urine flow from the collecting duct

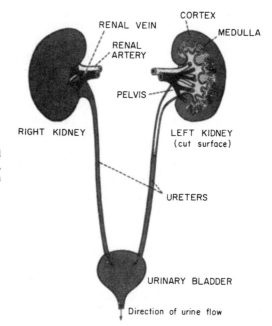

Figure 4–1 • General organizational plan of the urinary system. (From Guyton, A. C.: Textbook of Medical Physiology, 8th ed. Philadelphia, W. B. Saunders, 1996.)

   (b) Major calix channels urine from the renal sinus to the renal pelvis
   (c) Urine flows from the renal pelvis to the ureter
d. Nephron: anatomic microscopic structure (Fig. 4–2)
   i. Structural and functional unit of the kidney
   ii. Approximately 1 million in each kidney
   iii. Compensates for a significant degree of nephron destruction by:
      (a) Filtering a greater solute load

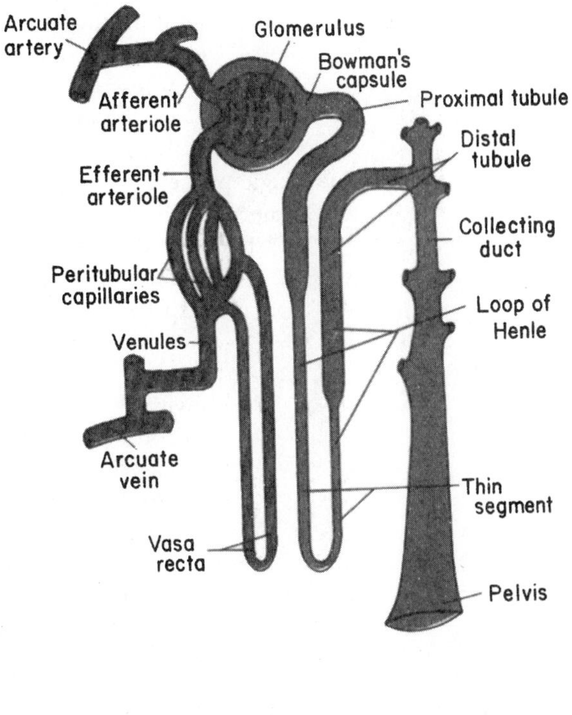

Figure 4–2 • The functional nephron. (From Guyton, A. C.: Textbook of Medical Physiology, 8th ed. Philadelphia, W. B. Saunders, 1996.)

      (b) Hypertrophy of the remaining functional nephrons

    iv. Types of nephrons, based on location and function

      (a) Cortical nephrons are located in the outer region of the cortex and contain short loops of Henle with a low capacity for sodium reabsorption

      (b) Juxtamedullary nephrons are located in the inner cortex adjacent to the medulla. They have long loops of Henle that penetrate deep into the medulla and have a greater capacity for concentration of urine because they are sodium-retaining nephrons

    v. Functional segments of the nephron

      (a) Renal corpuscle

        (1) Bowman's capsule: specialized portion of the proximal tubule that supports the glomerulus

        (2) Glomerulus: capillary bed

          a) Semipermeable membrane, normally permeable to water, electrolytes, nutrients, and wastes; relatively impermeable to large protein molecules, albumin, and erythrocytes

          b) Composed of three cellular layers: endothelial, basement membrane, and epithelial cells contribute to the characteristic semipermeability of this membrane

          c) Characteristics of cellular layers: endothelial cells contain fenestrations 50 to 100 nm wide, favoring the movement of water and solute. Remaining layers are less porous, with openings 1500 nm thick, which may explain the impedance of macromolecules

          d) Electrical potential of the membrane possesses a negative charge, favoring passage of positively charged molecules and impeding negatively charged molecules, such as albumin

      (b) Renal tubules

        (1) Segmentally divided into the proximal convoluted tubule, descending loop of Henle, ascending loop of Henle, distal convoluted tubule, and collecting duct

        (2) Each segment has a specific cellular structure and function

2. Physiologic processes

  a. Glomerular ultrafiltration: first step in the formation of urine

    i. Characteristics of filtrate

      (a) Normal: protein-free, plasma-like substance with a specific gravity of 1.010

      (b) Abnormal: increased permeability of the glomerular membrane allows erythrocytes and protein to be filtered into urine. Specific gravity of urine may artificially increase because of the presence of protein or glucose

      (c) Increased amount of serum osmotic substances (glucose, urea) can result in diuresis

    ii. Filtration is determined by the pressure and presence of a normal semipermeable glomerular membrane

      (a) Glomerular hydrostatic pressure is 50 mm Hg and favors filtration. This capillary hydrostatic pressure reflects cardiac output

      (b) Colloid osmotic pressure of 25 mm Hg and Bowman's capsule pressure of 10 mm Hg oppose hydrostatic pressure and thus oppose filtration

          (1) Colloid osmotic pressure results from oncotic pressure of plasma proteins in the glomerular blood supply

          (2) Bowman's capsule pressure reflects renal interstitial pressure

      (c) Net filtration pressure is derived from the following formula:

Glomerular hydrostatic pressure (facilitates):	+50 mm Hg
Colloid osmotic pressure (opposes):	−25 mm Hg
Bowman's capsule pressure (opposes):	−10 mm Hg
Net pressure favoring filtration:	+15 mm Hg

  iii. Glomerular filtration rate (GFR)

      (a) Clinical assessment tool to determine renal function

      (b) Definition: volume of plasma cleared of a given substance per minute (may be determined by using endogenous creatinine)

      (c) GFR equation

$$GFR = \frac{(Ux \times V)}{Px}$$

where

x = a substance freely filtered through glomerulus and not secreted or reabsorbed by tubules (e.g., creatinine)

P = plasma concentration of x

V = urine flow rate (ml/min)

U = urine concentration of x

      (d) Normal adult GFR is 125 ml/min or 180 L/day

      (e) Normal adult urine volume is 1 to 2 L/day, reflecting greater than 99% reabsorption of filtrate

      (f) Factors affecting GFR

          (1) Changes in glomerular hydrostatic pressure

              a) Secondary to changes in systemic blood pressure

              b) Variation in afferent or efferent arteriolar tone

          (2) Alterations in oncotic pressure

              a) Dehydration

              b) Hypoproteinemia or hyperproteinemia

          (3) Alterations in Bowman's capsule pressure

              a) Urinary tract obstruction

              b) Nephron destruction

              c) Interstitial edema of the kidney

b. Tubular functions of reabsorption, secretion, and excretion comprise the following steps in urine formation (Fig. 4–3)

  i. Conversion of 180 L of plasma filtered per day to 1 to 2 L of excreted urine

  ii. Absorption and secretion by two processes

      (a) Passive mechanisms: solute movement without the expenditure of metabolic energy

          (1) Diffusion: solute following either a concentration or an electrical gradient

              a) A solute moves from a solution of higher concentration through a semipermeable membrane to a solution of lower concentration

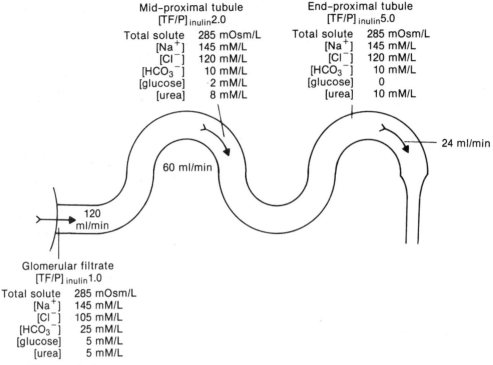

Figure 4–3 • Transport of water and some solutes in the proximal tubule. (From Maude, D. L.: Kidney Physiology and Kidney Disease. Philadelphia, J. B. Lippincott, 1977.)

    b) The electrical gradient causes a solute to passively migrate to the opposite charged compartment (e.g., sodium, a positive ion, migrates to a negatively charged compartment, whereas chloride, a negative ion, moves toward a positively charged compartment)

  (2) Osmosis: water following an osmotic gradient

    a) Water moves from an area of low concentration to an area of higher concentration

    b) An osmotic agent, such as sodium or mannitol, is a particle that is limited to a compartment

  (b) Active mechanisms: ion transport requiring energy (adenosine triphosphate [ATP]) permits ions to move against a concentration gradient

  (c) Maximal tubular transport capacity: active reabsorption mechanisms in the tubule have limited capacity for reabsorption of certain substances. Glucose is a prime example. A plasma glucose level of 375 mg/minute, which is the transport maximum (Tm), reflects no excretion in the urine, whereas a plasma glucose level above 375 mg/minute is reflected by glucose excretion in the urine. The Tm for glucose can vary from one nephron to another; as a result, glucose can sometimes spill into the urine at lower serum levels

 iii. Proximal convoluted tubule

  (a) Reabsorbs 60% to 80% of the filtrate, which remains isotonic to plasma

(b) Major function is active reabsorption of sodium chloride (NaCl) with passive reabsorption of water

(c) Other nutrients reabsorbed are glucose, amino acids, phosphates, uric acid, and potassium

(d) Regulates acid-base balance through reabsorption of the carbonate (HCO_3^-) and secretion of hydrogen ions (H^+)

(e) Secretes organic acids and foreign substances, such as drugs

iv. Loop of Henle

  (a) Variations in length depend on type of nephron

    (1) Juxtamedullary, with long loops

    (2) Cortical, with short loops

  (b) Two distinct segments

    (1) Descending segment, the thin limb, is permeable to water and impermeable to sodium

    (2) Ascending segment, the thick limb, has an active sodium and chloride pump and is impermeable to water

  (c) Major function is concentration or dilution of urine, accomplished by a countercurrent mechanism that maintains hyperosmolar concentration in the interstitium of the renal medulla

v. Distal convoluted tubule

  (a) Receives hyposmotic (or hypotonic) urine from ascending loop of Henle

  (b) Major functions are

    (1) Reabsorption of water, sodium chloride, and sodium bicarbonate

    (2) Secretion of potassium, ammonia, and hydrogen ions

  (c) Water permeability here is controlled by antidiuretic hormone (ADH); sodium reabsorption is determined by aldosterone

vi. Collecting duct

  (a) Receives urine, which is isotonic to plasma, from the distal convoluted and collecting tubules

  (b) Functions with the distal convoluted tubule and is influenced by ADH and aldosterone

  (c) Final adjustments of urine are made in this segment before urine enters the renal pelvis and progresses to the ureter and bladder

c. Aging process: in individuals above age 65 years, renal function is diminished by 10% and may progressively diminish with increasing age

Renal Hemodynamics: Normal Blood Flow Patterns

1. **Renal vasculature**

a. Specialized arrangement of renal blood vessels reflects interdependence of blood supply with kidney function

b. Pathway of blood supply

i. Kidney: aorta→segmented renal arteries→interlobar artery→arcuate artery→interlobular artery→(nephron)→interlobular vein→arcuate vein→interlobar vein→renal vein→inferior vena cava

       ii. Nephron: afferent arteriole→glomerular capillary→efferent arteriole→peritubular capillary→vasa recta adjacent to tubules→interlobular vein→renal vein→inferior vena cava

  c. Juxtaglomerular apparatus: site of renin synthesis

     i. Specialized cells composed of juxtaglomerular cells and macula densa

       (a) Juxtaglomerular cells: smooth muscle cells contain granules of inactive renin

       (b) Macula densa: portion of the distal tubule making contact with afferent arterioles of its respective glomerulus

     ii. Responds to arterial blood pressure in afferent and efferent arterioles and to the sodium content in the distal tubule

2. Renal blood flow (RBF) parameters

  a. Receives 20% to 25% of cardiac output or 1200 ml/minute

  b. Translates into a flow rate of 4 ml/g/minute to the kidney

  c. Oxygen extraction from renal cells is high, but the amount is not significant enough to account for flow rate; rather, the flow is required to support normal renal function

  d. RBF is

     i. Higher in males than females

     ii. Increased with age until maturity and then decreased in the elderly

     iii. Decreased with exercise

     iv. Increased in the supine position

     v. Increased in the afternoon and decreased at night

3. Distribution of RBF

  a. Renal tissue

     i. Cortex: metabolically active region receives most of the blood supply (80%)

     ii. Medulla: site of anaerobic metabolism receives 20% of blood supply

  b. Nephrons receive 600 to 650 ml/minute of renal plasma flow

4. Intrarenal autoregulation: general principles

  a. Mean arterial pressure (MAP) is maintained in a range of 80 to 180 mm Hg to prevent large changes in GFR

  b. Major site of autoregulation is the afferent arteriole

  c. Increase in the renal arterial pressure causes afferent vasoconstriction; decrease causes both afferent and efferent vasoconstriction, producing an increased GFR/RBF ratio

  d. Changes in vascular tone of the efferent arteriole (primarily vasoconstriction) complement efforts to maintain GFR by compensating for reduced blood flow

  e. Autoregulation is essentially absent at an MAP of 70 mm Hg or below

5. Neural control

  a. Route of nerve supply: along renal blood vessels

  b. Renal neurologic intervention is vasoconstrictive

  c. Hypotension decreases systemic arterial pressure, stimulating the carotid sinus and aortic arch baroreceptors to trigger the sympathetic response and the release of circulating epinephrine

  d. The sympathetic response decreases both RBF and GFR by vasoconstricting both afferent and efferent arterioles

  e. Other factors that stimulate an increased sympathetic tone are stress, fear, and exercise

f. The neuronal effect is not the primary factor in autoregulation. A denervated kidney is successfully transplanted and still has the ability to compensate for changes in blood pressure

6. **Hormonal modulation of RBF** (see renal regulation of blood pressure)
   a. Renin-angiotensin system: a mechanism to sustain systemic blood pressure and plasma volume
      i. Responds to a decreased afferent arteriolar pressure by increasing angiotensin II levels
      ii. Angiotension II vasoconstricts renal blood vessels, particularly the efferent artery, which reduces RBF but increases GFR
   b. Renal prostaglandins: modulate the effects of vasoactive substances on the kidney

7. **Pharmacologic effects**
   a. Epinephrine and norepinephrine: cause efferent arterioles to vasoconstrict, leading to a fall in the filtration fraction and a dose-related decrease in RBF
   b. Dopamine: pharmacologic action on RBF is dose-related; causes a vasodilatory effect on renal vasculature in doses between 1 and 4 $\mu g/kg/min$ intravenously (IV) (optimal dose 3 $\mu g/kg/minute$); doses above 10 $\mu g/kg/minute$ cause renal vasoconstriction, decreasing RBF and GFR
   c. Furosemide and mannitol: increase GFR initially by increasing blood flow to the kidney and later by decreasing intratubular pressure

. . . .

Body Water Regulation: Maintenance of Volume and Concentration of Body Water Content via Thirst-Neurohypophyseal-Renal Axis

1. **Thirst:** regulator of water intake
   a. Thirst center is located in the anterior hypothalamus
   b. Neuronal cells of this center are stimulated by intracellular dehydration, causing sensation of thirst
   c. Role is maintenance of satiety state (i.e., drinking exact amount of fluid to return body to normal hydration state)

2. **ADH:** sodium osmoreceptor mechanism for control of extracellular fluid (ECF) osmolality and sodium concentration
   a. ADH is synthesized in the paraventricular and supraoptic nuclei of the hypothalamus. It then travels along axons of the supraopticohypophysial tract to be stored or released from the posterior pituitary. The supraoptic area of the hypothalamus may overlap with the thirst center, thus leading to an integration of the thirst mechanism, osmolality detection, and ADH release
   b. Release of ADH occurs with the following:
      i. An increased serum osmolality stimulates osmoreceptor cells in the hypothalamus. Normal serum osmolality is 285 to 295 mOsm/L. These cells transmit a message along neurohypophysial tracts, stimulating ADH release from the posterior pituitary
      ii. Volume contraction states, leading to reversal in inhibitory effect on ADH release, are controlled by stretch receptors in the left atrium, thus allowing activation of the ADH mechanism
   c. In the presence of ADH, water reabsorption occurs in the distal tubule and collecting ducts, resulting in:
      i. Production of hypertonic urine

      ii. Hypotonic medullary interstitium

      iii. Eventual correction of contracted ECF

   d. Inhibition of ADH secretion occurs when serum osmolality is decreased, as seen during water intoxication

   e. When ADH secretion is inhibited, the distal tubule and collecting duct become relatively impermeable to water

      i. Large volumes of hypotonic filtrate are delivered to the collecting duct, resulting in dilute urine

      ii. Final results are excess water loss in comparison to extracellular solute concentration, returning serum osmolality to normal limits

3. Countercurrent mechanism of the kidney: mechanism for the concentration and dilution of urine; adjusts urine osmolality from 50 to 1200 mOsm/L

   a. Isotonic glomerular filtrate leaves the proximal tubule and enters the loop of Henle at 300 mOsm/L

   b. Descending limb loop of Henle is permeable to water only. This water is gradually drawn into the hypertonic medullary interstitium, resulting in

      i. Gradual increase in osmolality of the glomerular filtrate as it becomes dehydrated; at hairpin turn of the loop, osmolality is dramatically increased by removal of water and sodium chloride pumping action; osmolality can reach 1000 to 1200 mOsm/L

      ii. Medullary interstitium concurrently becomes hypotonic

   c. The thick ascending limb of loop of Henle is permeable to sodium choride and impermeable to water. The medullary interstitium becomes more hypertonic as its sodium concentration is increased by pumping action at the ascending limb

   d. A dilute filtrate reaches the distal tubule

      i. In the absence of ADH, dilute filtrate is excreted unchanged, resulting in dilute urine with water excretion in excess of solute

      ii. In the presence of ADH, water is reabsorbed from dilute filtrate in the collecting duct, resulting in excretion of concentrated urine

Electrolyte Regulation

1. Sodium regulation: normal serum concentration is 136 to 145 mEq/L solute

   a. Sodium is the major extracellular cation and osmotically active solute. Because variation in body sodium can be associated with an exchange of water between intracellular and extracellular compartments, sodium affects ECF volume

   b. Renal reabsorption sites: normal percentages of reabsorbed filtered sodium

      i. Proximal tubule: 65% of filtered sodium

      ii. Loop of Henle: 25% of filtered sodium

      iii. Distal tubule: 6% of filtered sodium

      iv. Collecting duct: 2% to 4% of filtered sodium

   c. Three major factors influence sodium excretion:

      i. GFR

      ii. Aldosterone

      iii. Atrial natriuretic peptides (ANPs): previously called the "third factor." ANPs represent a group of peptides that play a role in regulating and monitoring fluid, electrolyte, and cardiovascular balance

d. Sodium reabsorption increases at renal tubules during the following conditions
 i. Decreased GFR secondary to renal hypoperfusion (e.g., shock): less sodium is delivered to renal tubules, and less is excreted
 ii. Aldosterone secretion
  (a) Aldosterone is a mineralocorticoid secreted from the zona glomerulosa of the adrenal cortex
  (b) Its major effects are to increase renal tubular reabsorption of sodium and to control selective renal excretion of potassium
  (c) Result of aldosterone secretion is an increased quantity of sodium in ECF, which in turn promotes water reabsorption. At the same time, potassium ions are secreted into the distal tubule and collecting duct to be excreted
  (d) Regulating factors for aldosterone secretion are the potassium concentration in ECF, renin-angiotensin-aldosterone mechanism, total amount of body sodium, and adrenocorticotropic hormone (ACTH)
 iii. ANP action: causes a natriuretic, diuretic, and hypotensive effect secondary to its potent vasodilatory properties. The increased urinary excretion of sodium is matched by an accompanying loss of potassium and phosphate. Researchers are examining the potential benefits of ANP's vasodilatory effect on the prevention of acute renal failure (ARF)
e. Sodium reabsorption decreases at renal tubules during the following conditions:
 i. Increased GFR (excess ECF volume): the effect is increased perfusion to kidneys and therefore increased GFR. More sodium is delivered into renal tubules, and more is excreted in the urine
 ii. Inhibition of aldosterone secretion, resulting in renal sodium excretion
 iii. ANP
 iv. Secretion of ADH
 v. Diuretics, especially loop-affecting diuretics

2. **Potassium regulation:** normal serum concentration is 3.5 to 5.5 mEq/L
a. Potassium is the major intracellular cation necessary for maintenance of osmolality and electroneutrality of cells
b. Renal transport sites: potassium is actively reabsorbed in the proximal tubule and actively and passively secreted in the distal tubule to maintain electroneutrality of urine. This electrical gradient is determined primarily by reabsorption of sodium from urine
c. Factors enhancing potassium excretion:
 i. Increase in cellular potassium
  (a) Increase the exchange between sodium and potassium ions. Potassium ions are excreted into urine, and sodium is reabsorbed
  (b) Acute metabolic or respiratory alkalosis results in movement of potassium ions into cells
 ii. High-volume flow rates in the distal portion of the nephron increase the number of available potassium ions and thus increase the excretion of potassium
 iii. Aldosterone, which provides a feedback mechanism for maintenance of ECF potassium, functions as follows:

      (a) Elevation of serum potassium stimulates secretion of aldosterone

      (b) Aldosterone acts on distal nephrons and collecting ducts, enhancing retention of sodium and excretion of potassium

      (c) Excretion of excess potassium eventually returns potassium to a normal level

3. Calcium regulation: normal serum concentration is 8.5 to 10.5 mg/dl

  a. Major functions of calcium ions

    i. Transmission of nerve impulses

    ii. Roles in blood coagulation and activation of clotting mechanism

    iii. Formation of bones and teeth

    iv. Maintenance of cellular permeability

    v. Generation of cardiac action potential and pacemaker function

    vi. Contraction of cardiac and vascular smooth muscle

  b. Renal transport sites: 98% of filtered calcium is reabsorbed

    i. Reabsorptive pathways are similar to those used for sodium transport

    ii. Most active reabsorption occurs in the proximal tubule

    iii. Other sites include the loop (20% to 25%) and the distal tubule (10%)

  c. Factors influencing calcium reabsorption:

    i. Parathyroid hormone (PTH):

      (a) Decrease in serum calcium stimulates secretion of PTH

      (b) PTH stimulates tubular reabsorption of calcium at the distal portion of the nephron, stimulates increased phosphate excretion, and mobilizes calcium and phosphate from bone

    ii. Vitamin D: calcium absorption from the small intestine depends on the presence of activated vitamin D (1,25-dihydroxycholecalciferol)

      (a) Activation process: absorption of ultraviolet light converts 7-dehydrocholesterol in skin to cholecalciferol

        (1) Liver further hydroxylates vitamin D to form 25-hydroxycholecalciferol

        (2) Kidney further hydroxylates to final activated form of vitamin D (1,25-dihydroxycholecalciferol)

      (b) PTH stimulates this activation process

      (c) Reduction in serum calcium levels results in decreased urinary calcium excretion; therefore, activated vitamin D must be available to absorb calcium from the small intestine in order to maintain adequate serum calcium levels

    iii. Corticosteroid effect

      (a) Large doses decrease calcium absorption in intestines

      (b) Suspected of interfacing with activation of vitamin D in liver

    iv. Diuretic effect

      (a) Diuretics can cause sodium and calcium excretion. The ultimate effect of reduced serum calcium concentration is decreased excretion

      (b) Volume loss: decrease in total body fluid volume, leading to diminished GFR and reduced calcium excretion

4. Phosphate: normal serum concentration is 3.0 to 4.5 mg/dl

  a. The phosphate ion is found in large quantities in bone. Phosphates play a significant role in intracellular energy-producing reactions. They may also be connected with deoxyribonucleic acid (DNA), ribonucleic acid (RNA), and genetic code information. Phosphates are used by kidneys to buffer hydrogen ions

b. Renal transport sites: reabsorption of phosphate is an active process that occurs in the proximal tubule and is dependent on the presence of sodium. Factors influencing phosphate excretion include the following:

   i. PTH secretion: inhibits reabsorption of phosphates

   ii. Alterations in GFR

     (a) Increased GFR results in decreased reabsorption of plasma phosphates

     (b) Decreased GFR results in increased reabsorption of plasma phosphates

5. **Magnesium**: normal serum concentration is 1.5 to 2.2 mEq/L

  a. The magnesium ion is the second major intracellular cation and is a significant factor in cellular enzyme systems and biochemical reactions

  b. Magnesium may have a role in the management of myocardial infarction (MI), since magnesium administration decreases the mortality rate in MI by 24% and improves ventricular function by 25%. This benefit may be attributed to magnesium's ability to enhance coronary blood flow, conserve potassium, improve cellular function, and diminish the risk of dysrhythmias

  c. Renal transport site: the reabsorptive process is similar to that for calcium and is linked to sodium reabsorption along renal tubules

  d. Factors influencing reabsorption

   i. Availability of sodium: sodium ion is necessary for reabsorptive process

   ii. Availability of PTH, although this has a minimal effect on magnesium reabsorption

6. **Chloride**: normal serum concentration is 96 to 106 mEq/L

  a. Renal transport sites: reabsorbed with sodium at all sodium absorptive sites in the nephron

  b. Factors influencing excretion

   i. Acidosis: bicarbonate reabsorbed while chloride is excreted to maintain electrochemical balance

   ii. Alkalosis: bicarbonate excreted while chloride is reabsorbed to maintain electrochemical balance

Excretion of Metabolic Waste Products

Excretion plays a primary role in renal function. The kidney excretes more than 200 metabolic waste products. The two products measured for the interpretation of renal function are blood urea nitrogen (BUN) and serum creatinine.

1. **Urea**: a nitrogen waste product of protein metabolism that is filtered and reabsorbed along the entire nephron

  a. Is an unreliable measurement of GFR, since urea excretion is influenced by:

   i. Urine flow (decrease in urine flow rate may allow for reabsorption of urea)

   ii. Extrarenal factors, such as hypoperfusion states

   iii. Catabolic state as seen with fever or infection

   iv. Changes in protein metabolism

   v. Drugs

   vi. Diet

vii. Gastrointestinal bleeding
  b. Elevation in BUN without an associated rise in creatinine (>25:1 ratio) suggests
    i. Volume depletion
    ii. Low renal perfusion pressure
    iii. Increased catabolic process
  c. Elevations of both BUN and creatinine (at a 10:1 ratio) indicate renal disease
2. **Creatinine**: a waste product of muscle metabolism
  a. Amount produced each day is proportional to the body's muscle mass and occurs at a constant rate
  b. The normal kidney excretes creatinine at a rate equal to the kidney's blood flow or GFR
  c. Creatinine is freely filtered
  d. A combination of equal creatinine production and excretion makes it a reliable reflection of kidney function
  e. An elevated serum creatinine level can be directly related to a change or deterioration in kidney function

Renal Regulation of Acid-Base Balance

The kidneys regulate acid-base balance by minimizing wide variations in body fluid balance in conjunction with the retention or excretion of hydrogen ions. Normal acid-base balance is also regulated by the lungs and the body buffers (serum bicarbonate, blood, and plasma proteins).

1. **Bicarbonate** (HCO_3^-) reabsorption
  a. Takes place mostly in the proximal tubule but also in the distal tubule
  b. Occurs with sodium ions
  c. Occurs when filtrate contains more than 28 mEq/L (Tm), as in acidemia and volume contraction (contraction alkalosis)
2. **Hydrogen ion secretion**
  a. Passive secretion occurs in the proximal tubule, and active secretion occurs distally in exchange for sodium ions
  b. Acid is buffered by ammonia (NH_3^+) or phosphate (HPO_4^{-2}) before excretion, providing for hydrogen (H^+) excretion without lowering pH
  c. Is increased during acidemia and decreased during alkalemia
3. **Renal buffers of hydrogen ions**
  a. Buffers that are filtered by the glomerulus
    i. Bicarbonate is completely reabsorbed (up to 28 mEq/L)
    ii. Phosphate (HPO_4^{-2}) is secreted and then reacts with hydrogen
    iii. $H^+ + HPO_4^{-2} = H_2PO_4^{-1}$
  b. Buffers produced by the kidney tubule
    i. Bicarbonate can be synthesized in the distal tubule. The process involves excretion of hydrogen into urine at the same time that bicarbonate is delivered by ECF with sodium. Hydrogen and bicarbonate both come from the distal tubule cell as a result of ionization of carbonic acid (H_2CO_3); thus

$$\overset{CA}{H_2CO_3 \leftrightarrows H^+ + HCO_3^-}$$

      ii. Carbonic acid comes from hydration of carbon dioxide (CO_2) via carbonic anhydrase (CA)

$$\overset{\text{CA}}{H_2O + CO_2 \leftrightharpoons H_2CO_3}$$

      iii. Carbon dioxide is derived from either cellular metabolism or dissolved carbon dioxide in venous blood; thus new bicarbonate can be made in the distal tubule from extraurinary sources

      iv. Complete equation

$$\overset{\text{CA}}{H_2O + CO_2 \leftrightharpoons H_2CO_3 \leftrightharpoons H^+ + HCO_3^-}$$

4. Summary of renal responses to acidemia
    a. Increased hydrogen ion secretion at the distal tubule with an increased excretion of titratable acids (HPO_4^{-2})
    b. All bicarbonate (HCO_3^-) is reabsorbed in the proximal tubule
    c. Production of ammonia to accommodate hydrogen ion excretion

$$NH_3 + H^+ \leftrightharpoons NH_4^+$$

    d. Urinary pH can be as low as 4 because of excretion of a more acid urine in the presence of acidemia

5. Summary of renal responses to alkalemia
    a. Decreased hydrogen ion secretion in the distal tubule
    b. Excess bicarbonate excretion
    c. Decreased production of ammonia
    d. Urine is alkaline, with a pH over 7

Renal Regulation of Blood Pressure

This regulation involves five mechanisms.

1. Maintenance of volume and composition of ECF
    a. Normal plasma volume is essential for control of blood pressure
    b. Alterations in plasma volume eventually affect blood pressure
      i. Reduction of plasma volume lowers arterial blood pressure, leading to compensation by vasoconstriction
      ii. Expansion of plasma volume results in increased cardiac preload, affecting Starling's curve, with an ultimate rise in blood pressure

2. Aldosterone–body sodium balance determines ECF volume: aldosterone preserves sodium balance by stimulating renal tubular reabsorption of this ion, in exchange for primarily potassium excretion

3. Renin-angiotensin-aldosterone system: preserves blood pressure and avoids serious volume reduction
    a. Juxtaglomerular apparatus: contains inactivated renin granules
      i. Factors that trigger juxtaglomerular cells to release renin reflect diminished GFR
        (a) Decreased arterial blood pressure in the afferent and efferent arteriole
        (b) Reduced sodium content or concentration at the distal tubule
        (c) Increased sympathetic stimulation of kidneys
    b. Renin is released from juxtaglomerular cells into the afferent arteriole

    c. On entering circulation:
        i. Renin acts on angiotensinogen to split away the vasoactive peptide, angiotensin I
        ii. Angiotensin I changes to angiotensin II in the presence of angiotensin-converting enzyme (ACE), found primarily in the lung and liver but also in the kidney and all blood vessels
        iii. Angiotensin II is a potent systemic vasoconstrictor
    d. Circulatory effect of angiotensin II on arterial blood pressure
        i. Significant constriction of peripheral arterioles
        ii. Venous constriction, a moderate response resulting in reduction of vascular volume
        iii. Renal arteriolar constriction that results in the renal retention of sodium and water; this expands ECF volume, thus increasing arterial blood pressure
    e. Fluid volume response to angiotensin II restores effective circulating volume by:
        i. Angiotensin II's stimulating the release of aldosterone, which enhances renal sodium reabsorption
        ii. Vasoconstriction, to further decrease GFR, leading to sodium reabsorption
        iii. Stimulation of the thirst mechanism

4. Renal prostaglandins: modulating effect
    a. Major renal prostaglandins (PGs) are PGE_2, PGD_2, and PGI_2: vasodilators. PGA_2 is a vasoconstrictor
    b. Physiologic role: modulation, amplification, and inhibition. Vasoactive substances (angiotensin, norepinephrine, bradykinins) stimulate the synthesis and release of prostaglandins. Prostaglandins modulate action of the vasoactive substances
    c. Prostaglandins cause a diminished arterial blood pressure and an increase in RBF. This is accomplished by arterial vasodilation and inhibition of the distal tubules' response to ADH. The suppressed ADH response leads to sodium and water excretion, which ultimately decreases the effective circulatory volume
    d. Pharmacologic prostaglandin inhibitors are the nonsteroidal anti-inflammatory drugs (NSAIDs)
        i. Salicylic acid
        ii. Ibuprofen (Motrin)
        iii. Indomethacin (Indocin)
        iv. Naproxen (Naprosyn)

5. Kallikrein-kinin system: renal kallikreins are proteases that release kinins and are excreted in the urine. Kinins stimulate both the renin-angiotensin and prostaglandin systems, appearing to link renal hemodynamics and fluid/electrolyte excretion

Red Blood Cell Synthesis and Maturation

1. Erythropoietin secretion: stimulates production of erythrocytes in bone marrow and prolongs life of erythrocytes
2. Mechanism of erythropoietin synthesis and secretion:
    a. Normal kidneys either produce erythropoietin or synthesize an enzyme that catalyzes its formation

b. Stimulus for synthesis is believed to be decreased oxygen delivery to the kidney

3. **Erythropoietin deficiency**: primary cause of anemia seen in chronic renal failure, with bleeding as the second most common cause

NURSING ASSESSMENT DATA BASE

Nursing History

1. **Patient health history**
   a. Previous health problems: indicate the presence of or predisposition to renal disease
      i. Kidney disease
      ii. Urinary tract disease
      iii. Cardiovascular disease
         (a) Hypertension: blood pressure control and treatment may prevent or halt renal damage. Hypertension develops in 70% to 80% of patients with advanced renal failure
         (b) Congestive heart failure (CHF) with diminished renal perfusion
         (c) Atherosclerosis
      iv. Diabetes mellitus: renal disease caused by vascular disease alterations, infection, or neuropathy
      v. Immunologic disorders and allergies
      vi. Pulmonary disease (Goodpasture's syndrome)
      vii. Recent infections (streptococcal infection)
      viii. Recent blood transfusions (history of incompatibility reaction)
      ix. Other: toxemia of pregnancy, renal transplant, anemia, recent surgery, dialysis, drugs and toxins, renal calculi, azotemia, hematuria, and exposure to chemicals or poisons
   b. History of specific signs and symptoms
      i. Signs and symptoms of urinary tract disorders
         (a) Dysuria
         (b) Abnormal appearance of urine
            (1) Hematuria (grossly bloody)
            (2) Pyuria (cloudy)
            (3) Biliuria or bilirubinuria (orange)
            (4) Myoglobinuria (usually clear; Hematest positive on dipstick)
         (c) Frequency, urgency, hesitancy of urination
         (d) Nocturia
         (e) Polydipsia
         (f) Patterns of urine output
            (1) Normal volume: approximately 1500 ml/24 hr
            (2) Oliguria: less than 400 ml/24 hr
            (3) Anuria: no urine output
            (4) Polyuria: excessive urine output exceeding daily fluid intake

(5) Nonoliguria: normal urine volume or excess urine volume in the presence of acute renal failure

(g) Incontinence

(h) Fever

(i) Pain in costovertebral angle, flank, or groin

(j) Weight gain or loss

    (1) Patterns of weight gain

    (2) Patterns of weight loss

    (3) Dry weight: the ideal weight, which minimizes the symptomatology, for a patient with renal failure as achieved by a dialysis treatment

(k) Body image changes associated with uremia or renal disease

    (1) Skin color

    (2) Uremic odor

    (3) Arteriovenous access and Tenckhoff or other catheters

    (4) Edema

    (5) Weight changes

    (6) Donated organ

    (7) Impaired mobility

    (8) Corticosteroid-induced changes: moon face, added fat pads, and facial hair

    (9) Self-perception

        a) Focus of control

        b) Feelings of hopelessness, helplessness, and powerlessness

        c) Disorientation to time, place, or person

        d) Change in problem-solving abilities

2. **Family history**: genetic renal disease can account for approximately 30% of all azotemic patients. Genetically transmitted diseases that can cause or precipitate renal disease include:

  a. Hypertension

  b. Diabetes mellitus

  c. Gout

  d. Malignancy

  e. Polycystic kidney disease and medullary cystic disease

  f. Hereditary nephritis (Alport's syndrome)

  g. Renal calculi

  h. Cardiovascular disease

3. **Social history and habits**

  a. Social history

    i. Psychosocial stressors

      (a) Identify stressors

      (b) Recognize expressions of stress such as denial, anxiety, anger, and noncompliance

      (c) Coping

         (1) Describe methods of coping used in the past

         (2) Assess effectiveness of coping strategies

         (3) Assess for adaptation versus maladaptation

         (4) Signs of maladaptation: chronic depression and expressions of suicide

ii. Role changes: determine impact of role changes on the patient's ability to function
   (a) Role in family: description of family unit structure (hierarchical scheme and roles); determine whether family function is cohesive or dysfunctional
   (b) Identify role changes: often the patient moves from independence reluctantly into an ambivalent role of independence–dependence
   (c) Relation with surrogate dialyzer
   (d) Relation with organ donor
iii. Sexuality
   (a) Activity prior to renal disease
   (b) Renal dysfunction may contribute to sexual dysfunction
   (c) Hemodialysis has been associated with decreased libido, impotence, and infertility
   (d) Assess return of sexual functioning after the transplantation
   (e) Sexual dysfunction may be caused by antihypertensive agents

b. Habits
   i. Dietary habits
      (a) Dietary and fluid restrictions
      (b) Pattern of dietary intake: number of meals and nutritional value of intake
      (c) Tolerance of diet: presence or absence of nausea and vomiting; likes and dislikes
      (d) Fluid and electrolyte imbalances
      (e) Weight loss, increased infection, diminished energy levels, impaired mobilization, and impaired wound healing
      (f) Fatigue
         (1) Changes in energy level at critical periods during the day
         (2) Fatigue with activities of daily living, exercise, and leisure times
      (g) Mobility: extent of stability on ambulation

4. Medication history

a. Nephrotoxic agents: antibiotic therapy (tetracyclines, aminoglycosides, gentamicin, amphotericin B)
b. Diuretics
c. Cardiac glycosides (digoxin)
d. Antihypertensives and antiarrhythmic agents
e. Electrolyte replacement therapy
f. Immunosuppressives
   i. Corticosteroids
   ii. Azathioprine, cyclophosphamide, antithymocyte globulin (ATG), cyclosporine, monoclonal antibody (OKT3), and tacrolimus (FK-506)

Nursing Examination of Patient

1. Inspection

a. Diminished level of consciousness (lethargy, coma)
b. Skin
   i. Abnormal color: grayish tinge from anemia and yellowish tinge if retained carotenoids or urochrome pigments

    ii. Capillary integrity: easily bruised

    iii. Skin turgor

    iv. Purpura lesions: in some forms of renal failure

  c. Eye: cataracts, periorbital edema

  d. Ear: nerve deafness

  e. Edema

    i. Presence and significance depend on amount of water and sodium retained

    ii. Edema of renal failure is often related to hypoalbuminemia

  f. Respiratory rate and pattern: a pattern similar to Kussmaul respirations may be seen

  g. Muscle tremors, weakness, and weight loss seen with uremic syndrome

  h. Tetany (rare)

    i. Result of severe hypocalcemia or very rapid correction of acidosis

    ii. Positive Chvostek's and Trousseau's signs

  i. Asterixis

    i. Indicative of progressive uremic state

    ii. Ask the patient to face the examiner, and raise the upper extremities in a fixed hyperextension position

      (a) Palms of the hands should be visible to the examiner, with fingers separated

      (b) Positive sign occurs within 30 seconds: irregular movements of wrists and flapping movements of fingers

  j. Fatigue levels

  k. Mobility: extent and strength with ambulation

  l. Nutritional status

    i. Measure skinfold thickness of triceps (normal is greater than 25 mm for men, 15 mm for women)

    ii. Anemia: pale skin, weakness, shortness of breath

  m. Arteriovenous access: type, patency, signs of infection

2. Palpation: to determine the size and shape of the kidney and to check for presence of tenderness, cysts, and masses

  a. Right kidney is easier to palpate because its position is lower in the abdomen

  b. Palpate the bladder for the presence of urine and distention

  c. Palpate the flank area to elicit tenderness or pain

  d. Palpate pulses for a baseline reading and to determine abnormalities

3. Percussion

  a. Perform at the costovertebral angles to elicit various degrees of pain and tenderness associated with:

    i. Pyelonephritis

    ii. Calculi

    iii. Renal abscess or tumor

    iv. Glomerulonephritis

    v. Intermittent hydronephrosis

  b. Percuss the abdomen for the presence of ascites

4. Auscultation: listen for aortic and renal artery bruits, heard in the flanks or intercostal regions of the anterior abdomen

. . . .

Diagnostic Studies

1. **Laboratory findings**
   a. Blood
      i. Complete blood cell count: reduced hematocrit and hemoglobin levels may reflect bleeding or a lack of erythropoietin
      ii. Serum creatinine: to determine changes in GFR, with a normal level of 0.6 to 1.2 mg/dl
         (a) A proportional relationship exists between creatinine excretion and production
         (b) A significant elevation in creatinine is compatible with renal disease and can be correlated with the percentage of nephron damage
      iii. BUN
         (a) Normal BUN level: 10 to 20 mg/dl
         (b) Ratio of BUN to serum creatinine above 20:1: suspect extrarenal problem (dehydration, catabolic state). This elevation in both BUN and creatinine results from decreased GFR
         (c) Ratio of 10:1: suspect renal failure
      iv. Serum chemistries (calcium, phosphate, alkaline phosphatase, bilirubin, uric acid, sodium, potassium, chloride, carbon dioxide, magnesium)
      v. Baseline arterial blood gases
      vi. Serum glucose, cholesterol, albumin
      vii. Clotting profile
      viii. Serum osmolality
      ix. Serum protein and albumin
   b. Urine
      i. Visual examination for color and clarity
         (a) Clear and colorless with hyposthenuria
         (b) Cloudy when infection is present
         (c) Foamy when albumin is present
      ii. Osmolality (50 to 1200 mOsm/kg)
      iii. Specific gravity (1.003 to 1.030): wide range of normal; test provides reasonable estimate of urinary osmolality but actually measures density
         (a) Below normal (<1.010): suspect diabetes insipidus, overhydration, or CHF
         (b) Above normal (>1.030): suspect proteinuria, glycosuria, the presence of x-ray contrast media, or severe dehydration
      iv. Creatinine clearance (C_{CR}): 24-hour urine collection
         (a) Purpose
            (1) To determine the presence and progression of renal disease
            (2) To estimate the percentage of functioning nephrons
            (3) To determine specific medication dosages
         (b) In 24 hours, the following occurs:

$$\frac{U_{cr} \times V}{P_{cr}} = C_{cr}$$

where

U_{cr} = amount of urinary creatinine excreted

V = urine volume/minute

P_{cr} = plasma creatinine level

 (c) In average-sized patients, a satisfactory 24-hour collection always has approximately 1 g of creatinine, regardless of the degree of renal function

 v. Culture and sensitivity: check for infection

 vi. pH (normal range 4 to 8)

  (a) Average value is 6

  (b) Alkaline urine is frequently seen with infection. In the absence of infection, consider renal tubular acidosis if both alkaline urine and systemic acidosis are present

 vii. Glucose: appears in urine when the renal threshold for glucose is exceeded

 viii. Acetone: seen in urine during starvation and diabetic ketoacidosis. A false-positive result occurs when the patient is taking salicylates

 ix. Protein

  (a) Expressed qualitatively as 1+ to 4+

  (b) Diagnostic for the presence of glomerular membrane disease such as nephrotic syndrome or for the detection of myeloma proteins causing renal failure

 x. Spot urine electrolytes

  (a) Screening test for tubular function

  (b) Measure sodium, potassium, and chloride concentrations

  (c) Assessment of the kidney's ability to conserve sodium and concentrate urine

 xi. Urinary sediment

  (a) Casts: precipitation of protein within the kidney that takes the shape of the tubule in which it originally was formed

   (1) Hyaline casts: entirely protein; small amounts are normal in urine. If present in large amounts, suspect significant proteinuria such as albumin or myeloma protein

   (2) Erythrocyte casts: diagnostic for active glomerulonephritis or vasculitis

   (3) Leukocyte casts: indicative of an infectious process

   (4) Granular casts: small number, possibly the result of degenerating erythrocyte or leukocyte casts

   (5) Fatty casts: when seen in abundance, consider lipoid nephrosis or nephrotic syndrome

   (6) Renal tubular casts: seen in acute renal failure

  (b) Bacteria: presence determined by Gram's stain

  (c) Erythrocytes: small numbers are normal; in abundance during active glomerulonephritis, interstitial nephritis, malignancies, and infection

  (d) Leukocytes: small numbers are normal; present in infection and interstitial nephritis

  (e) Renal epithelial cells: rarely seen; present in abundance during acute tubular necrosis, nephrotoxic injury, and allergic reaction in the kidney

        (f) Crystals: seen in diseases of stone formation or following certain intoxications

        (g) Eosinophils: when present, indicate allergic reaction in the kidney

    xii. Nucleomatrix test: noninvasive, quantitative, painless examination for transitional cell cancer of the bladder

2. Radiologic findings

   a. Plain abdominal x-ray determines position, shape, and size of the kidney and identifies calcification in the urinary system

   b. Intravenous pyelogram (IVP)

      i. Visualizes the urinary tract for diagnosis of partial obstruction, renovascular hypertension, tumor, cysts, and congenital abnormalities

      ii. Complications include allergic reaction to dye; dehydration

     iii. Is contraindicated in the presence of:

        (a) Poor renal function: can further compromise function because of the dye's dehydrating effect and nephrotoxicity

        (b) Multiple myeloma: IVP dye may precipitate myeloma protein in the kidney

        (c) Pregnancy: avoid abdominal irradiation

        (d) Heart failure: dye has an acute osmotic effect that can further compromise cardiac function by expanding vascular volume

        (e) Diabetes mellitus

        (f) Sickle cell anemia: elevation in renal oncotic pressure from dye can promote sickling and infarction of renal tissue

   c. High-excretion tomography: indicated when kidneys cannot be readily visualized on IVP

   d. Renal scan: determines renal perfusion and function; can provide information about obstructions and renal masses

      i. Radioactive dye is taken up by normal kidney tubule cells. A decrease in uptake indicates hypoperfusion due to any cause

      ii. Commonly used to assess status of renal transplants

   e. Retrograde pyelography: is used to examine upper region of the urinary collecting system

   f. Retrograde urethrography: is used to examine the urethra

   g. Cystoscopy: detects bladder or urethral pathology

   h. Renal arteriography (angiography)

      i. Identifies tumors and differentiates the type of renal or renovascular disease

      ii. Complications

        (a) Dye can be allergenic and cause same complications as IVP dye

        (b) Puncturing of a peripheral artery, with consequent hematoma, embolism, or thrombus formation, is the greatest technical risk

   i. Voiding cystourethrography: identifies abnormalities of the lower urinary tract, urethra, and bladder to determine the presence of reflux and residual urine

   j. Diagnostic ultrasonography

      i. Identifies hydronephrosis

      ii. Differentiates between solid and cystic tumors

     iii. Localizes cysts or fluid collections

    k. Computed tomography (CT): identifies tumors and other pathologic conditions that create variations in body density (e.g., abscess or lymphocele)

    l. Magnetic resonance imaging (MRI)

       i. Better tissue characterization than CT

       ii. Provides direct imaging in several planes for detection of renal cystic disease, inflammatory processes, and renal cell carcinoma

       iii. Identifies morphologic changes in renal transplantation

       iv. Detects alterations in blood flow (i.e., slow or absent flow)

    m. Magnetic resonance urography: a form of magnetic imaging that offers results similar to an IVP, without the use of dye

    n. Chest radiograph: identifies pulmonary edema, cardiomegaly, left ventricular hypertrophy, uremic lung, Goodpasture's disease, and infections

3. Kidney biopsy: the most common invasive diagnostic tool

    a. Indicated for renal disease that cannot be definitely diagnosed by other methods

    b. Determines the cause and extent of lesions; helpful in planning of treatment regimen

    c. Biopsy

       i. Open: for severe anatomic deformities or if a "deep specimen" is needed for diagnosis

       ii. Closed: a simple percutaneous procedure

    d. Contraindications to open biopsy: bleeding tendency, hydronephrosis, hypertension, cystic disease, and neoplasms

COMMONLY ENCOUNTERED NURSING DIAGNOSES

Fluid Volume Excess

A state in which an individual experiences increased fluid retention and edema because of the kidney's inability to excrete excess body water.

1. Assessment for defining characteristics

    a. Intake greater than output

    b. Weight gain

    c. Oliguria or anuria

    d. Elevated blood pressure

    e. Edema: peripheral, anasarca, ascites, periorbital, pulmonary

    f. Neck vein distention; elevated central venous pressure (CVP)

    g. Bounding pulses

    h. Dyspnea, orthopnea

    i. Lung sounds: crackles

    j. Muffled heart sounds

    k. Pulmonary congestion on chest x-ray

    l. Decreased hemoglobin and hematocrit values

    m. Elevated pulmonary artery pressure (PAP) and pulmonary wedge pressure (PAWP)

    n. Low specific gravity (1.015 or less) or dilute urine

    o. Dilutional effect on electrolytes

    p. Anxiety, restlessness

    q. Stupor (seen with water intoxication)

2. **Expected outcomes**

    a. Patient maintains dry weight

    b. CVP, PAP, and PAWP are normal

    c. Patient is free of edema

    d. Breath sounds are clear bilaterally

    e. Intake and output (I&O) are balanced

3. **Nursing interventions**

    a. Identify common causes of fluid excess

        i. Expansion of blood volume secondary to renal sodium retention

        ii. Diminished plasma proteins leading to a decrease in plasma oncotic pressure

        iii. Increased capillary permeability

    b. Document I&O; compare with daily weight. Consider insensible losses: fluid losses via lungs, skin, and bowel (600 to 800 ml/day)

    c. Assess renal function

        i. Urine volume, creatinine clearance, and BUN: creatinine ratio

        ii. Urinalysis

        iii. Urine concentration: specific gravity, osmolality, and spot electrolytes

        iv. A 24-hour urine collection for protein evaluation

    d. Restrict fluids in overhydration associated with impaired renal function, impaired cardiac function, or syndrome of inappropriate ADH (SIADH) secretion

4. **Evaluation of nursing care**

    a. A 24-hour I&O balance is negative or zero

    b. Absence of edema: adventitious breath sounds, hypertension

    c. Compliance with fluid restriction

Fluid Volume Deficit

A state in which an individual experiences vascular, cellular, or intracellular dehydration related to active fluid loss. Volume deficit may occur in the diuretic phase of acute renal failure.

1. **Assessment for defining characteristics**

    a. Weight loss

    b. Output greater than intake

    c. Hypotension

    d. Increased pulse

    e. Poor skin turgor

    f. Dry skin and mucous membranes

    g. Thirst

    h. Decreased CVP

    i. Increased body temperature

    j. Urine output

        i. Polyuric phase: large volume of dilute urine with low specific gravity

        ii. Dehydration with normal renal function: oliguria, concentrated urine with an elevated specific gravity

    k. Weakness

l. Stupor (seen with severe hypovolemia)

2. Expected outcomes
   a. Patient's weight is normal and stable
   b. Fluid balance is maintained
   c. Vital signs and hemodynamic parameters are normal
   d. Urine output is within normal limits

3. Nursing interventions
   a. Identify common causes of fluid deficit
      i. Renal water losses
         (a) Diuretic abuse
         (b) Salt-wasting nephropathies
         (c) Diabetes insipidus (nephrogenic, central)
         (d) Osmotic diuresis (hyperglycemia, urea)
         (e) Postobstruction diuresis
      ii. Gastrointestinal losses
         (a) Diarrhea, vomiting, nasogastric (NG) suction
         (b) Fistula and wound drainage
         (c) Blood losses
      iii. Skin: insensible losses
      iv. Third space phenomena
   b. Document intake and output; compare with daily weight
   c. Assess renal function
      i. Urine volume, creatinine clearance, BUN:creatinine ratio
      ii. Urinalysis
      iii. Urine concentration: specific gravity, urine osmolality, and spot electrolytes
      iv. A 24-hour urine collection for protein evaluation
   d. Administer fluid therapy

4. Evaluation of nursing care
   a. The 24-hour intake and output balance is positive or zero
   b. Patient has stable, normal weight
   c. Vital signs and hemodynamic parameters are normal
   d. Urine volume and specific gravity are normal

Altered Nutrition: Less Than Body Requirements Related to Uremia

Uremic symptoms and strict dietary restrictions often precede this condition.

1. Assessment for defining characteristics: presence of uremic symptoms (see Nursing History earlier)

2. Expected outcomes
   a. Patient's intake meets nutritional requirements
   b. Patient maintains stable baseline weight
   c. Muscle mass is adequate
   d. Serum protein and albumin levels are normal

3. Nursing interventions
   a. Identify causes of inadequate nutritional intake and plan care aimed at etiology
   b. Teach appetite-enhancing measures
      i. Provide oral hygiene prior to meals
      ii. Give small, frequent meals

      iii. Identify food preferences, especially those high in complex carbohydrates and essential amino acids

  c. Teach the essential elements of the renal patient's diet

      i. Essential amino acids and adequate calories

      ii. Adjusted protein and electrolyte intake (sodium and potassium) to avoid uremic symptoms and electrolyte imbalances. Diminished protein intake causes the use of the protein stored in muscles, which leads to body muscle wasting. Providing increased calories can help avoid this situation

      iii. Provide vitamins and iron supplements (folic acid, multivitamins)

  d. Monitor pattern of changes in weight and nutritional intake

  e. Assess for noncompliance with dietary instructions

4. Evaluation of nursing care

  a. There is weight gain with a stabilization pattern

  b. There is an absence of muscle wasting

  c. Serum protein and albumin levels are or approach normal limits

Risk of Alterations in Blood Pressure: Hypertension

In renal failure, the hypertensive state is usually created by the retention of fluid or the stimulation of the renin-angiotensin mechanism. Preexisting hypertension is a common variable.

1. Assessment for defining characteristics

  a. Hypertension: defined as a diastolic pressure above 90 mm Hg and systolic pressure above 140 mm Hg

  b. Headache

  c. Dizziness

  d. Blurred vision

2. Expected outcomes

  a. Diastolic pressure stays below 90 mm Hg, and systolic pressure stays below 140 mm Hg

  b. There is an absence of symptoms associated with hypertension

  c. Patient complies with antihypertensive medication regimen

3. Nursing interventions

  a. Identify causes of hypertension (see Chapter 2)

  b. Collaborate with the health team to control hypertension

      i. Monitor blood pressure frequently

      ii. Restrict salt and water intake

      iii. Avoid drugs that can elevate blood pressure (such as corticosteroids and sympathomimetic-containing antihistamines)

  c. Administer diuretics, as ordered, to treat edema and hypertension

      i. General characteristics of diuretics

        (a) Inhibit the active transport of sodium or chloride, resulting in an increase in urine output

        (b) The diuretic effect reduces effective plasma circulating volume, thereby lowering blood pressure

      ii. Complications

        (a) Volume depletion

        (b) Hypokalemia

        (c) Hyperkalemia (seen with potassium-sparing diuretics)

             (d) Hyperuricemia

             (e) Hyponatremia

             (f) Metabolic alkalosis

             (g) Hypochloremia

             (h) Azotemia

iii. Types of diuretics

    (a) Osmotic diuretic: a nonabsorbable solute (mannitol)

        (1) Exerts an osmotic effect, causing water diuresis in excess of sodium chloride

        (2) Side effects: blurred vision, rhinitis, rebound plasma volume expansion, thirst, urinary retention, and fluid and electrolyte imbalance

    (b) Loop diuretics: the most potent diuretics available (furosemide and ethacrynic acid). The primary site of action is the thick segment of the medullary ascending loop of Henle

        (1) Block the reabsorption of sodium chloride, thus contributing to a large diuresis of isotonic urine. Potassium excretion is also enhanced

        (2) Increase RBF by exerting a vasodilatory effect on renal vasculature

        (3) Side effects: volume depletion, agranulocytosis, thrombocytopenia, transient deafness, abdominal discomfort, hypokalemia, hypochloremic alkalosis, and hyperglycemia

        (4) Prolonged use without electrolyte replacement results in all other electrolyte imbalances

    (c) Thiazides (hydrochlorothiazide)

        (1) Sodium reabsorption is inhibited in the ascending loop of Henle and the beginning portion of the distal tubule

        (2) Increased potassium excretion occurs with a weak carbonic anhydrase inhibitory effect

        (3) Side effects: rashes, leukopenia, thrombocytopenia, hypercalcemia, and acute pancreatitis

    (d) Potassium-sparing diuretics (spironolactone, amiloride hydrochloride, triamterene): aldosterone inhibitors

        (1) Promote sodium secretion into the distal tubule and potassium reabsorption, causing a mild diuresis while protecting the body's potassium level

        (2) Usually selected for patients receiving digoxin and diuretic therapy who cannot tolerate low serum potassium levels or when a mild diuretic effect is desirable

        (3) Side effects: hyperkalemia, hyponatremia, headache, nausea, diarrhea, urticaria, and gynecomastia or menstrual disturbances

    (e) Carbonic anhydrase inhibitors (acetazolamide sodium)

        (1) Inhibit the enzyme carbonic anhydrase

        (2) Increase the excretion of sodium by interfering with sodium bicarbonate reabsorption. Sodium bicarbonate is lost in the urine, creating a hyperchloremic metabolic acidosis

        (3) Are beneficial when an alkaline urine is desirable

(4) Side effects: hyperchloremic acidosis, renal calculi, rash, nausea, vomiting, anorexia, and deteriorating renal function

(f) Other: pharmacologic agents that increase both cardiac output and GFR contribute to diuresis (e.g., xanthines [theophylline, aminophylline] and digoxin)

iv. General nursing considerations in administration of diuretics

(a) Collaborate with the physician to determine the weight and fluid balance desired at the conclusion of diuretic therapy

(b) Observe for fluid, electrolyte, and acid-base disorders

(c) Maintain intake and output records correlated with daily weights

(d) Monitor serum potassium levels, especially if the patient is taking digoxin (hypokalemia increases the risk of digitalis toxicity)

(e) Consider administering potent or high doses of diuretics in the early morning or afternoon unless a Foley catheter is in place

(f) Monitor blood pressure during aggressive diuresis because hypotension can indicate dehydration and impending circulatory collapse

(g) Advise the patient to report the onset of side effects, such as difficulty with hearing

(h) Be aware that a diminished response to diuretics may be related to electrolyte imbalances, particularly hyponatremia, hypochloremia, and hypokalemia

v. Administer antihypertensive agents as ordered

(a) Rationale is to decrease the possibility of complications, such as cerebrovascular accidents and renal failure

(b) General actions

(1) Diminish adrenergic nerve stimulation to the vasculature, thus decreasing peripheral resistance

(2) Vasodilate by relaxing the vascular smooth muscle

(3) Reduce preload caused by vasodilatation

(c) Categories of antihypertensive agents

(1) Central and peripheral antiadrenergics or sympathetic blockers: primary action causes postsynaptic alpha-adrenergic agonist to inhibit or reduce the sympathetic response. Occurs at any of three sites

a) In the central nervous system (clonidine hydrochloride, methyldopa, guanabenz)

b) At the peripheral nerve endings (reserpine, guanethidine monosulfate, guanadrel sulfate, pargyline hydrochloride)

c) At the alpha and beta receptor sites (alpha: prazosin hydrochloride, terazosin hydrochloride, doxazosin mesylate, labetalol; beta: atenolol, betaxolol hydrochloride, carteolol hydrochloride, penbutolol sulfate, bisoprolol, metoprolol tartrate, acebutolol, esmolol hydrochloride, propranolol, nadolol, timolol maleate, pindolol)

d) Primary effect is achieved through reduction of systemic vascular resistance (SVR); beta blockers work by decreasing cardiac output

e) RBF may be reduced, causing stimulation of the renin-angiotensin mechanism

  i) This is counterbalanced by the tendency of the drugs to cause salt and water retention

  ii) This response warrants the use of diuretics in conjunction with sympathetic blockade therapy

(2) Vasodilators: act directly on blood vessel walls to relax smooth muscle. These agents decrease SVR without interfering with the sympathetic response. Arterioles are the site for relaxation

  a) The hypotensive response to these drugs can result in a reflex tachycardia

  b) The renin-angiotensin mechanism is initiated: salt and water are reabsorbed

  c) These responses can be avoided by administering vasodilators in conjunction with a diuretic and a beta-blocker

  d) Examples of vasodilators are captopril, lisinopril, enalapril, minoxidil, diazoxide, pinacidil, hydralazine, and nitroprusside

(3) ACE inhibitors (captopril, enalapril): specifically for the patient with renin-mediated hypertension. These agents inhibit angiotensin-converting enzyme, thus preventing the conversion of angiotensin I to angiotensin II

(d) General nursing considerations in administration of antihypertensive agents

  (1) On admission, obtain baseline blood pressure in lying, sitting, and standing positions and in both arms; record if a difference exists

  (2) Maintain a graphic sheet of blood pressure readings

  (3) Schedule antihypertensive doses at regular intervals over a 24-hour period

  (4) Question holding the dose prior to hemodialysis

  (5) During initiation or adjustment of the antihypertensive agent, obtain blood pressure immediately prior to administering (especially with prazosin hydrochloride [Minipress])

  (6) Routine blood pressure should be obtained within 1 hour of medication administration

  (7) Establish blood pressure parameters for withholding medications

  (8) Observe for symptomatology, relate blood pressure readings, then report

  (9) If postural hypotension occurs, take blood pressure recordings with the patient lying and sitting

  (10) Be aware that antihypertensive drugs may cause changes in libido. This issue should be addressed, and the patient should be directed to counseling

  (11) Monitor the patient's response to antihypertensive therapy

    d. Treat hypotension
       i. Administer fluid challenges with volume expanders (normal saline, albumin, dextran) to increase blood pressure
       ii. If hypotension persists after correcting volume depletion, vasopressors (e.g., dopamine) are indicated
    e. Treat renal hypoperfusion
       i. Restore plasma volume and/or blood pressure in an effort to increase cardiac output. Colloid is the most effective volume expander and consistently increases renal perfusion
       ii. Other agents that may augment RBF are mannitol, dopamine, furosemide, ethacrynic acid, prostaglandin, and bradykinin

4. Evaluation of nursing care
    a. A normal or slightly elevated blood pressure supports renal perfusion
    b. Patient is free of hypertensive symptoms
    c. Patient complies with antihypertensive medication regime

Risk of Acid-Base Imbalances: Metabolic Acidosis

A condition commonly associated with renal failure caused by the inability of the kidney to excrete hydrogen ions

1. Assessment for defining characteristics
    a. The pH value is below 7.35, and the bicarbonate level is below 22 mEq/L
    b. Kussmaul's respirations
    c. Hypotension
    d. Fatigue
    e. Headache
    f. Cardiac dysrhythmias, decreased myocardial contractility
    g. Diminished level of consciousness progressing to coma; seizures
    h. Chronic acidotic conditions result in skeletal system disorders, such as osteitis, fibrosis, and osteomalacia

2. Expected outcomes
    a. The pH stays within a physiologic range
    b. Respiratory and cardiac function stay normal

3. Nursing interventions: identify and treat common causes of metabolic acidosis (see Chapter 1, The Pulmonary System)

4. Evaluation of nursing care
    a. The pH and bicarbonate levels are within normal limits
    b. Symptoms associated with metabolic acidosis are absent

Risk of Anemia

Anemia is related primarily to a lack of erythropoietin secretion by the kidney but can also be caused by actual blood loss (e.g., stress ulcer).

1. Assessment for defining characteristics (see Chapter 6, The Hematologic System)

2. Expected outcome: Patient maintains an asymptomatic level of anemia

3. Nursing interventions
    a. Identify common causes of anemia associated with renal failure
       i. Suppression of erythropoietin
       ii. Actual blood losses
       iii. Uremic syndrome

b. Treat chronic anemia associated with renal failure
   i. Oral iron or iron dextran (Imferon), unless the patient has excess body iron stores
   ii. Folic acid and pyridoxine (vitamin B_6): important, especially in dialysis patients because these are dialyzable vitamins
   iii. Anabolic steroids (e.g., nandrolone decanoate): stimulate erythrocyte formation
   iv. Epoetin alfa (recombinant human erythropoietin): stimulates erythrocyte production and prevents the anemia of chronic renal failure. Effect of the drug on erythrocytes does not begin until 2 to 6 weeks, with peak results in 3 months after administration; as a result, it is not used in acute renal failure

4. **Evaluation of nursing care**
   a. Patient maintains acceptable hematocrit level (usually 20% to 24% with traditional therapy and 30% to 33% with epoetin alfa therapy)
   b. Patient complies with pharmacologic and nutritional supplement therapy

Risk of Uremic Syndrome

The uremic state results from the kidney's inability to excrete toxic waste products. Uremic symptoms occur at BUN levels above 100 mg/dl or at a GFR below 10 to 15 ml/minute.

1. **Assessment for defining characteristics**
   a. Early uremia
      i. Sensorium change (e.g., loss of attention span, lethargy)
      ii. Nausea, vomiting, stomatitis
      iii. Weight loss, muscle wasting
      iv. Skin changes (pruritus, pale yellow tinge, dryness, ecchymoses)
      v. Uremic fetor
      vi. Edema
   b. Progressive uremia
      i. Renal osteodystrophy, soft tissue calcification
      ii. Pericarditis, heart murmurs
      iii. Bleeding secondary to platelet dysfunction
      iv. Gastritis, colitis (rare), constipation
      v. Skin changes (uremic frost is rare)
      vi. Hyperkalemia and hyponatremia
      vii. Carbohydrate intolerance
      viii. Peripheral neuropathy
      ix. Decreased immune response
      x. Pleuritis, pulmonary edema
      xi. Hyperparathyroidism (secondary)
      xii. Increased rate of atherosclerosis
      xiii. Sexual dysfunction and infertility
2. **Expected outcome**: BUN level is maintained below 100 mg/dl or at a level that minimizes uremic symptoms
3. **Nursing interventions**: based on minimizing azotemia and preventing dehydration
   a. Restrict oral protein intake

    b. Remove blood if it is present in the gastrointestinal tract because this is another protein source that can be metabolized to ammonia and urea. These metabolites cannot be handled by diseased kidneys

    c. Consider dialysis to maintain BUN below 100 mg/dl. In each patient, uremic symptoms develop at individual levels of BUN. Establish this value for each patient, and strive to maintain BUN below this level

4. Evaluation of nursing care

    a. BUN is below 100 mg/dl

    b. Patient is free of or has minimized uremic symptoms

Risk of Infection

Infections are the major cause of death in patients with acute renal failure and can seriously compromise the patient with chronic renal failure.

1. Assessment for defining characteristics

    a. Presence of renal disease and uremic symptoms

    b. History of repeated infections

    c. Fever and chills, cough

    d. Wound drainage

    e. Cloudy, concentrated urine

    f. Tachycardia, hypotension, or both

    g. Alterations in skin integrity or wound sites

    h. Increased leukocyte count

2. Expected outcome: patient remains free of infection

3. Nursing interventions

    a. Recognize that patients with renal failure have an impaired immune response secondary to uremic toxins and reduced phagocytosis by the reticuloendothelial system

    b. Implement the following precautions

        i. Obtain a urine specimen for culture on admission: urinary tract infection (UTI) may be asymptomatic

        ii. Prevent introduction of microorganisms

            (a) Avoid indwelling urinary catheters

            (b) Avoid unnecessary invasive monitoring procedures

        iii. Use an aseptic technique for urinary and intravenous catheter care

        iv. Maintain the BUN at 80 to 100 mg/dl or lower to minimize susceptibility to infection

        v. Maintain skin integrity: avoid unnecessary venipuncture

        vi. Maintain adequate nutritional intake (protein, calories)

        vii. Institute positive prevention measures (e.g., pulmonary toilet)

        viii. Prevent cross-contamination between patients

        ix. Use universal precautions

        x. Implement isolation techniques for hepatitis antigen–positive patients receiving hemodialysis

4. Evaluation of nursing care: there is no infection

Risk of Bone Disease: Osteomalacia, Osteitis Fibrosa

Chronic hypocalcemia can precipitate hyperparathyroidism, which leads to the mobilization of calcium from the bone and results in softening of the bone (osteomalacia).

1. **Assessment for defining characteristics**
   a. History of chronic hypocalcemia, hyperparathyroidism, or both
   b. Bone pain, fractures
   c. Activity intolerance
   d. Radiologic examination of the skull, hands, and feet reveals signs of demineralization
2. **Expected outcomes**
   a. Asymptomatic hypocalcemia
   b. There are no fractures or bone pain
   c. Patient maintains ability to ambulate
   d. Patient is compliant with the treatment regimen for hypocalcemia
3. **Nursing interventions**
   a. Monitor serum calcium and phosphorus levels, and avoid hypocalcemia and hyperphosphatemia
   b. Provide pharmacologic therapy to prevent secondary hyperparathyroidism and bone disease
      i. Hyperphosphatemia may be treated by dietary restriction, although the more common therapy is administration of antacids (e.g., calcium carbonate) that bind dietary phosphates in the intestines. These antacids should maintain the plasma phosphorus level below 5 mg/dl. Side effects of these phosphate-binding gels include
         (a) Constipation
         (b) Hypophosphatemia
         (c) Aluminum deposits (if an aluminum hydroxide gel is used) accumulating in fat, the brain, or other body tissues
      ii. Approaches to vitamin D administration
         (a) Administer large dosages of vitamin D tablets (50,000 to 125,000 units/day) to compensate for the vitamin D resistance experienced in renal failure
         (b) Administer dihydrotachysterol (synthetic analog of vitamin D)
         (c) Administer 1,25-vitamin D (the completely activated form) in dosages of 0.24 to 1 mg/day
      iii. Calcium carbonate administration provides a secondary benefit, as a calcium supplement
      iv. Explain the importance of taking calcium carbonate medication, which prevents the development of secondary hyperparathyroidism
      v. Secondary hyperparathyroidism is manifested as hypercalcemia, hyperphosphatemia, and progressive deterioration of the skeletal system. Treatment for uncontrollable hyperparathyroidism is subtotal parathyroidectomy
4. **Evaluation of nursing care**
   a. Serum calcium level is within safe range
   b. Patient is free of pain
   c. Patient complies with medication therapy

. . . .

Altered Metabolism and Excretion of Pharmacologic Agents Related to Renal Failure

A state resulting from the failed kidneys' inability to metabolize or excrete pharmacologic agents.

1. **Assessment for defining characteristics**
   a. Unusual untoward pharmacologic effects
   b. Enhanced sensitivity to drugs
   c. Retention of the active or toxic metabolites of a medication
   d. Increased azotemia caused by an elevation in metabolic wastes from drug usage
2. **Expected outcomes**
   a. Patient tolerates pharmacologic therapy
   b. There are no untoward pharmacologic effects
   c. Prescribed serum drug levels are adequate
3. **Nursing interventions**
   a. Recognize alterations in the body's use of drugs during renal failure
      i. Distribution of drugs in a uremic state
         (a) Decreased stores of body fat affect lipid-soluble drugs
         (b) Low cardiac output states restrict the degree of renal metabolism or excretion of these agents
         (c) Acidemia alters tissue uptake of drugs
         (d) Increased body water has a dilutional effect
         (e) Decreased protein binding causes competition by various drugs for tissue binding sites, leading to a higher concentration of the unbound drugs
      ii. Uremic effects that can alter drug absorption
         (a) Decreased gastrointestinal motility
         (b) Alteration in gastric pH
         (c) Effects of electrolyte imbalances on the gastrointestinal tract
         (d) Inability of the kidney to excrete or metabolize drugs
         (e) Diminished protein binding
   b. Follow general principles for drug administration during renal insufficiency
      i. Reduce drug dosage
      ii. Increase intervals between doses
      iii. Question orders for nephrotoxic agents
      iv. Closely observe the patient to prevent or assess toxicity due to drug accumulation
      v. Report any untoward signs, especially an elevation in serum creatinine, so that the drug can be reconsidered, reduced in dosage, or discontinued
      vi. Monitor serum drug levels, especially in situations requiring a specific drug concentration (e.g., antibiotics, digoxin)
      vii. To ensure a more stable serum concentration, administer initial loading doses of drugs that have a long half-life (e.g., digoxin)
4. **Evaluation of nursing care**
   a. Patient tolerates pharmacologic therapy
   b. There are no untoward drug effects
   c. BUN and serum creatinine levels are stable
   d. Desired serum drug levels

. . . .

Ineffective Patient and Family Coping

Insufficient, ineffective, or compromised support, comfort, assistance, or encouragement, usually by a supportive primary person (family member or close friend).

Patients may need to manage adaptive tasks related to the stress of renal failure on themselves and the family.

1. **Assessment for defining characteristics**
   a. Maladaptive signs of a patient's coping
      i. Verbalization of an inability to cope or inability to ask for help
      ii. Inability to meet role expectations and solve problems
      iii. Diminished social participation
      iv. Destructive behavior toward self or others
      v. Failure to comply with treatment regimen
      vi. Change in usual communication patterns
   b. Maladaptive signs of family coping
      i. Patient communicates concern regarding family's response to his or her renal disease
      ii. Family members demonstrate preoccupation with their own personal reaction: fear, anticipatory grief, guilt, anxiety
      iii. Family has inadequate understanding of the patient's condition, or therapy interferes with effective supportive behaviors
      iv. Family withdraws from communication with the patient
      v. Family demonstrates overprotective or underprotective behaviors

2. **Expected outcomes**
   a. Patient demonstrates increased functional independence
   b. Patient appropriately expresses ideas, feelings, and needs
   c. Patient is compliant with treatment regimen
   d. Patient participates in family activities
   e. Patient participates in dialysis unit's exercise rehabilitation program
   f. Patient resumes employment
   g. Patient receives appropriate support from family
   h. Patient and family adjust to role changes
   i. Patient seeks support system in times of family crisis

3. **Nursing interventions**
   a. Identify common causes of stress in the patient and family
      i. Exacerbations of illness; frequent hospitalizations
      ii. Life-threatening nature of renal disease
      iii. Inability to perform activities of daily living
      iv. Restrictions caused by a shunt, a fistula, or a Tenckhoff catheter; demands of dialysis schedule and other treatments
      v. Reversal in family roles
      vi. Effects on sexual behavior and sexuality
      vii. Question of maintaining or resuming work
      viii. Financial burden of care
   b. Recognize the psychologic consequences of renal disease and its treatment
      i. Denial, depression, and dependency
      ii. Suicide rate with hemodialysis is believed to be 100 times that of the normal population
   c. Assess the patient's ability to cope with the disease (see Chapter 9, Psychosocial Aspects)
   d. Specific nursing interventions directed at supporting adaptation in the patient with renal failure
      i. Teach the patient about the various treatment alternatives and encourage participation in the selection of the treatment method

    ii. Provide support systems
       (a) Visits with successfully adjusted patients
       (b) Support for family members. Patients with supportive families tend to have fewer physical complications, survive longer, and adjust more readily

4. Evaluation of nursing care
  a. Patient demonstrates the following:
    i. Participation in self-care and social and family activities
    ii. Use of adaptive coping mechanisms, such as functional denial
    iii. Increased self-esteem with acceptance of body image changes
    iv. Cooperation with health care personnel
    v. Compliance with the treatment regimen
  b. Family demonstrates the following:
    i. Decreased levels of anxiety
    ii. Adaptive changes in family roles
    iii. Participation in patient care
    iv. Use of support systems

PATIENT HEALTH PROBLEMS

Acute Renal Failure

This syndrome has varying causes and affects approximately 20% of the critically ill. ARF can present as a single disease or as a portion of a more complex syndrome involving multiple organ failure, resulting in an acute deterioration of renal function. Oliguria with ARF is associated with a mortality rate of 50% in the critically ill and a rate of 50% to 70% in trauma or postoperative patients. Nonoliguria with ARF carries a better prognosis and a lower mortality rate of 26%. Because of these high mortality rates, prevention of ARF remains the best intervention.

1. Pathophysiology
  a. Prerenal conditions
    i. Physiologic states lead to diminished renal perfusion without renal tubular damage
    ii. Effects of diminished kidney perfusion
       (a) Decreased renal artery pressure
       (b) Decreased afferent arterial pressure (<100 mm Hg), which diminishes forces favoring filtration
  b. Intrarenal conditions
    i. Cortical involvement of vascular, infectious, or immunologic processes
       (a) Causes renal capillary swelling and cellular proliferation, which eventually decrease GFR
       (b) Edema and cellular debris obstruct glomeruli
       (c) Ultimate result is oliguria
    ii. Medullary involvement occurs after prolonged ischemia/ hypoperfusion or nephrotoxic injury to tubular portion of nephrons (Fig. 4–4)

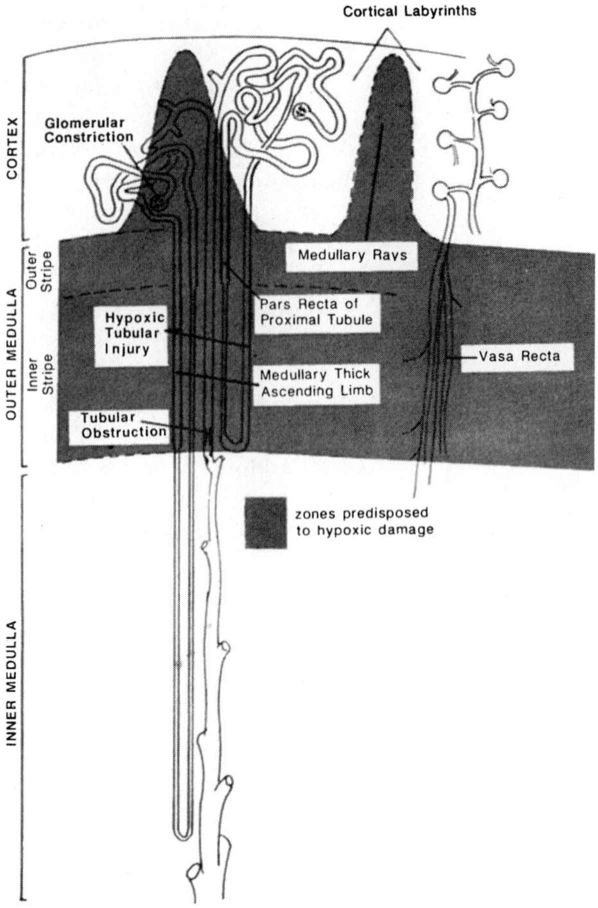

Figure 4–4 • Anatomy of intrarenal zones predisposed to hypoxic injury in acute renal failure. (From Heyman, S. N., Fuch, S., and Brezis, M.: The role of indwelling ischemia in ARF. New Horiz. 3(4):597, 1995.)

(a) Medullary hemodynamics: hypoperfusion states and oxygen insufficiency disrupt the fine balance between limited oxygen supply and high oxygen consumption in the outer medullary region; may contribute to ARF from hypoxic medullary damage
    (1) Conditions predisposing to hypoperfusion
        a) Endotoxin
        b) Rhabdomyolysis
        c) Hypercalcemia
        d) Nonsteroidal anti-inflammatory drugs
        e) Radiologic contrast agents
        f) Antibiotics (i.e., amphotericin, cyclosporine)
    (2) Pharmacologic agents can also alter the hemodynamics of the medullary region, especially if administered in the absence of volume depletion (i.e., furosemide bolus, mannitol, dopamine). Other substances suspected of improving medullary hemodynamics are nitric oxide, which is normally produced by the macula densa to control glomerular blood flow and renin release, and ANP, an endogenous vasodilator

(b) Tubular necrosis produced as localized damage in a patchy pattern. Extent of damage in nephrotoxic, ischemic/hypoperfusion, sepsis-associated, and multiple organ failure (MOF) injury differs

  (1) Nephrotoxic injury affects the epithelial cellular layer, which can regenerate

  (2) Ischemic and hypoperfusion injury alters renal tubular cells, with the damage to the basement membrane. The tubular basement membrane cannot regenerate

   a) Cellular injury may involve several factors: adenosine triphosphate (ATP) depletion, oxygen free radical formation, loss of epithelial cell polarity, and increased calcium levels

   b) ATP depletion: begins 30 seconds after the kidney is hypoperfused. The normal homeostatic benefits of cellular ATP are lost, including preservation of cellular volume, ionic composition, and membrane integrity

   c) Oxygen free radicals: the production of oxygen free radicals is a normal process resulting from oxidative metabolism

     i) Because these substances are highly reactive and volatile, intracellular mechanisms exist (composed of enzyme systems and antioxidants) for the rapid breakdown and destruction of the oxygen free radical in an act of defense

     ii) When left unopposed, as during ischemic events, these radicals disrupt cellular functioning. For example, during ischemia, the renal cell is unstable and unable to protect itself from the oxygen free radicals, resulting in renal cell injury

   d) Loss of epithelial cell polarity: ischemia alters the passage of water, electrolytes, and other charged elements through the tubule's epithelial wall, leading to a concentration defect

   e) Increased calcium levels: ischemic and hypoperfusion states cause a rise in intracellular calcium levels that causes renal vasoconstriction and a decrease in GFR

  (3) Systemic inflammatory response syndrome (SIRS) injury occurs as the result of an extreme and prolonged inflammatory response. The explanation of this response exemplifies the role of the immune system in the pathogenesis of ARF. Endotoxin produces a significant decrease in renal perfusion that is exacerbated by renal vasoactive substances that alter renal cellular metabolism and the localized renal vasoconstriction that contributes to ARF

  (4) Multisystem organ dysfunction syndrome (MODS) is characterized by the rapid, progressive, and sequential deterioration of vital organ functions

   a) It begins a few days after trauma or a prolonged inflammatory event with pulmonary failure, followed by failure of the liver, intestines, and kidneys

        b) The impact on the kidneys involves a combination of the immune response as well as ischemia/hypoperfusion and, possibly, a nephrotoxicity event

        c) All of these factors act on the renal cells, contributing to the formation of acute tubular necrosis (ATN)

(c) Three or four phases of recovery: the classic form of ARF has four phases from onset to oliguria, followed by the diuretic and recovery phases. The nonoliguric form has only three phases from onset to nonoliguria. The nonoliguric phase seems to be synonymous with the diuretic phase, which suggests that nonoliguric ARF reflects less tubular damage

(d) Onset, or initial phase, precedes the actual necrotic injury and correlates with a major alteration in renal hemodynamics

    (1) Associated with a decrease in RBF and GFR

    (2) Most important factor altering RBF is a decrease in cardiac output

    (3) Other mechanisms contributing to the decreased renal perfusion are either an increase in sympathetic activity or an accentuation of the renal vascular resistance

    (4) A consistent increase in cardiac output during this phase produces a consistent increase in RBF and protects the patient from the impending ARF

(e) Oliguric phase reflects four processes:

    (1) Obstruction of tubules by cellular debris, tubular casts, or tissue swelling

    (2) Total reabsorption or back-leak of urine filtration through the damaged tubular epithelium and into circulation

    (3) Tubular cell damage with the development of necrotic, patchy areas. The cell leaks ATP and potassium, edema is present, mitochrondria are altered, and calcium leaks into the cell

    (4) Renal vasoconstriction: continues and may contribute to the decreased GFR

(f) The nonoliguric phase reflects less tubular damage; symptomatology resembles that of the diuretic phase

    (1) Urine output may exceed 1 L/hr

    (2) Solute is present in the urine at approximately 350 mOsm/L

    (3) Creatinine clearance is as high as 15 ml/min, and sodium excretion is low

    (4) Hyperkalemia remains a significant problem

    (5) Duration of this phase is short, reaching the recovery phase in 5 to 8 days

(g) Diuretic phase signifies that tubular function is returning

    (1) Tubular obstruction relieved, but cellular edema remains as scar tissue forms on necrotic areas

    (2) Large daily urine output, sometimes exceeding 3L

    (3) Output due to the osmotic-diuretic effect produced by elevated BUN and impaired ability of tubules to conserve sodium and water

(4) Recovery phase

    a) Occurs after gradual improvement of kidney function extending over a 3- to 12-month period

    b) Residual impairment in GFR may result

c. Postrenal conditions: associated with obstruction of the urinary collecting system

    i. Partial obstructions: can increase renal interstitial pressure, increasing opposing forces of glomerular filtration. End result is diminished urine output

    ii. Complete obstruction: impediment of urine flow accompanies bilateral kidney involvement. The "back-up" pressure of urine compresses the kidneys

2. Etiologic or precipitating factors

a. Prerenal failure

    i. Hypovolemia secondary to hemorrhage, gastrointestinal losses, and third-spacing phenomena, decreasing extracellular fluid (ECF) volume

    ii. Excessive use of diuretics

    iii. Impaired myocardial contractility

    iv. Sepsis, progressing to gram-negative shock with vasodilatation

    v. Increased renal vascular resistance from anesthesia or surgery

    vi. Bilateral renal vascular obstruction caused by embolism or thrombosis

b. Intrarenal failure (cortical involvement)

    i. Acute poststreptococcal glomerulonephritis

    ii. Acute cortical necrosis

    iii. Systemic lupus erythematosus (SLE)

    iv. Goodpasture's syndrome

    v. Bilateral endocarditis

    vi. Pregnancy as seen with abruptio placentae and abortion

    vii. Malignant hypertension

c. Intrarenal failure (medullary involvement): ATN is the most common type of ARF and is the result of nephrotoxic injury, ischemic injury, SIRS, and MODS

    i. Nephrotoxic injury: occurs after exposure to nephrotoxic agents, the effects of which are accentuated by dehydration, creating more extensive tubular damage. Nephrotoxic damage may also compound the clinical picture of renal deterioration associated with sepsis. Examples of nephrotoxic agents:

        (a) Antibiotics: aminoglycosides, tetracyclines, penicillins

        (b) Carbon tetrachloride

        (c) Heavy metals: lead, arsenic, mercury, uranium

        (d) Pesticides and fungicides

        (e) X-ray contrast media

    ii. Ischemic injury: during ischemia, MAP drops below 60 mm Hg for over 40 minutes. Causes include massive hemorrhage, transfusion reaction (tubules are obstructed with hemolyzed erythrocytes), and cardiogenic shock

    iii. SIRS: renal injury can result from endotoxins, an inflammatory or immune response, or renal hypoperfusion

    iv. MODS: triggered by the inflammatory or immune response, leading to the progressive deterioration of organs, with the kidney as a prime target

   d. Postrenal failure: obstructive process can occur anywhere, from the kidney to the urinary meatus

  3. Nursing assessment data base: complete the general assessment for the renal patient (described earlier), and refer to the section for specific elements concerning ARF

   a. Nursing history: establish whether a rapidly reversible form of ARF is present

    i. Subjective findings

     (a) Patient's chief complaint: change in the volume or lack of urine output

     (b) Other symptoms: fatigue, lethargy, weakness

    ii. Objective findings

     (a) Etiologic or precipitating factors: collect data necessary to determine the etiology of the abrupt decrease in renal function, the elevated BUN and creatinine levels, and the decrease in urine volume

      (1) Prerenal conditions: history of any of the conditions described in pathophysiology

      (2) Intrarenal conditions: history of exposure to nephrotoxic agents or drugs, to hypotensive-ischemic catastrophes causing ATN, or to other causes of intrarenal pathology mentioned in the previous section

      (3) Postrenal conditions (bilateral obstruction): history of any of the causes of postrenal pathology mentioned in the previous section

     (b) Family history

      (1) Describes the family unit and impact of ARF

      (2) Describes the perception of the family members' support of the patient

     (c) Social history

      (1) Employment status, including type of work and impact of disease on work performance

      (2) Sexual dysfunction: uremia depresses the libido and sexual function of the patient with ARF, but, because these patients are often hospitalized, this factor may not be an issue until discharge is planned

     (d) Medication history

      (1) Diuretics: check for excessive use

      (2) Antibiotics: check whether patient is taking nephrotoxic antibiotics

      (3) Vasopressors: check whether high dosages are received

   b. Nursing examination of patient: clinical presentation during the first few days of oliguria or nonoliguria is dominated by the primary disease process or underlying illness (see general Nursing Examination of Patient)

    i. Inspection: additional areas to examine

     (a) Neurologic: confusion, lethargy, stupor, and neuromuscular involvement, including twitching and weakness secondary to metabolic acidosis

(b) Cardiovascular: electrocardiogram (ECG) reveals dysrhythmias secondary to electrolyte or cardiac involvement (e.g., heart failure)

(c) Genitourinary: oliguria (<400 ml/24 hr) or nonoliguria

(d) Gastrointestinal: weight loss secondary to anorexia, nausea and vomiting, "coffee ground" emesis, or melena

(e) Integument: dry skin, edema, pallor, bruising, uremic frost, and pruritus

(f) Musculoskeletal: impaired mobility

(g) Other: examine for signs of local infection. Systemic infection may present as shaking chills and fatigue

ii. Palpation

(a) Cardiac: tachycardia, irregular pulse secondary to electrolyte imbalances

(b) Genitourinary: flank pain

iii. Percussion

(a) Bladder: small in oliguria, distended in lower urinary tract obstruction

(b) Abdominal distention: secondary to constipation

iv. Auscultation

(a) Blood pressure may be normal or increased as the disease state progresses

(b) Friction rub may indicate uremic pericarditis

(c) Pulmonary rales (crackles) are associated with pulmonary edema

(d) If patient is on hemodialysis, assess vascular access for patency by checking bruit or thrill

c. Diagnostic study findings

i. Laboratory

(a) Prerenal

(1) Urinary sodium level less than 10 mEq/L

(2) Specific gravity greater than 1.020

(3) Serum BUN to creatinine ratio (>25:1)

(4) Minimal or no proteinuria

(5) Normal urinary sediment

(b) Intrarenal (cortical disease)

(1) Urinary sodium level less than 10 mEq/L

(2) Specific gravity varies

(3) Moderate to heavy proteinuria

(4) Serum BUN and creatinine values elevated but remain in a 10:1 ratio

(5) Hematuria

(6) Urinary sediment with erythrocyte casts and leukocytes

(c) Intrarenal (medullary disease)

(1) Urinary sodium level greater than 20 mEq/L

(2) Specific gravity 1.010

(3) Minimal to moderate proteinuria

(4) Serum BUN and creatinine elevated

(5) Urinary sediment with numerous renal tubular epithelial cells, tubular casts, and a rare erythrocyte

(d) Postrenal
    (1) Serum BUN and creatinine elevated when complete obstruction present
    (2) Bacteriology report significant for a specific organism
(e) Special
    (1) Antistreptolysin-O (ASO) titer: to diagnose recent streptococcal infection, which may cause poststreptococcal glomerulonephritis
    (2) Antiglomerular basement membrane titers: to diagnose Goodpasture's syndrome, a devastating disease of pulmonary hemorrhage and renal failure
    (3) Serum studies for complement components: a fall in complement levels is seen in active complement-mediated glomerulonephritis (e.g., lupus nephritis)
    (4) Serum electrophoresis for immunoglobulin levels: abnormal proteins, as seen in multiple myeloma, can damage kidneys irreversibly
 ii. Radiologic: to rule out obstruction as the cause of oliguria or anuria, since its immediate treatment may reverse symptoms of renal failure

4. Nursing diagnoses
 a. Risk for ARF: prevention of ARF remains the best intervention, with the preservation of renal function as the desired outcome
  i. Assessment for defining characteristics
   (a) Sudden decrease in or cessation of urine output
   (b) Severe dehydration
   (c) Prolonged hypotensive episode
   (d) Presence of septic shock, trauma, or burns
   (e) Presence or suspicion of MODS
  ii. Expected outcomes
   (a) ARF is resolved
   (b) Normal renal function and output are resumed
  iii. Nursing interventions
   (a) Identify patients at high risk for ARF
    (1) Hemodynamically unstable
    (2) Multiple trauma
    (3) Multisystem organ failure
    (4) Intravenous (IV) hemolysis
    (5) Receiving nephrotoxic drugs
    (6) Rhabdomyolysis
    (7) Blood loss or hypotension in surgical patients
   (b) Monitor for prerenal or onset stage of ATN
    (1) Renal hypoperfusion from any cause can diminish GFR as the MAP drops to 70 mm Hg or below
     a) Hypotension: renal autoregulation is essentially absent at a MAP of 70 mm Hg or below
     b) Oliguria (occasionally anuria): urine is dilute, with a urine osmolality similar to plasma osmolality and a urinary sodium of 10 mEq/L or less
     c) Renal vasoconstriction: occurs in response to decreased cardiac output and hypotension as revealed by a decreased urinary output not responding to IV fluid administration or increased serum renin levels

(c) Correct hypotension or renal hypoperfusion by fluid administration or pharmacologic agents: Augmentation of renal blood flow does not protect the tubules from damage but may limit the extent of the damage, creating a nonoliguric ATN

(1) Fluid administration: the best modality for reinstating renal perfusion is to increase cardiac output through the administration of fluids

(2) Pharmacologic intervention: the persistence of renal hypoperfusion despite volume resuscitation warrants additional pharmacologic interventions, including diuretics (e.g., mannitol, furosemide) and vasoactive agents (e.g., dopamine hydrochloride, prostaglandins)

a) Mannitol: exerts a protective effect on the kidney; prevents cellular debris, reducing the chance for tubular obstruction; and augments blood flow

b) Furosemide: acts as both a diuretic and an augmentor of RBF when administered in conjunction with dopamine hydrochloride

i) The diuresis encourages the removal of the sloughed tubular cells, thereby eliminating the tubular obstruction

ii) Administer either an IV bolus or a continuous infusion. The recommended bolus dose is 100 to 200 mg every 6 to 8 hours. The continuous infusion dose generally begins low, approximately 20 to 40 mg/hr; If the patient does not respond, doses can be increased by 20 mg every 2 hours until results are achieved

iii) The maximal dose should not exceed 4 mg/kg/min in order to avoid ototoxicity

c) Dopamine hydrochloride: administered in doses varying from 1 to 3 μg/kg/minute to maintain RBF, increase GFR, and preserve urine output

d) Prostaglandin: an experimental agent

(d) Monitor and report changes in urine output (onset of oliguria, nonoliguria, or anuria)

(e) Obtain urine and blood specimens for laboratory analysis, and interpret results

iv. Evaluation of nursing care

(a) Renal perfusion is improved, and ATN is prevented

(b) Urine output is over 30 ml/hr with normal concentration

(c) Balanced 24-hour total on I&O record coincides with daily weight

b. Urinary elimination, altered patterns: the state in which an individual experiences a disturbance in urine elimination. Oliguria, anuria, and nonoliguria/polyuria are the urinary patterns associated with ARF

i. Assessment for defining characteristics (see Nursing History)

ii. Expected outcomes

(a) Fluid I&O are balanced

(b) Levels of electrolytes are physiologic

(c) Urinary output pattern returns to normal

iii. Nursing interventions
   (a) Monitor and record all I&O
   (b) Assess the character of the urine: color, clarity, concentration, specific gravity, and odor
   (c) Report changes in the volume or character of the urine output; changes may reflect a recovering kidney. Adjust therapeutic regimen to match the stage of renal recovery
   (d) Assess fluid status; monitor for signs of dehydration or volume overload
   (e) Monitor serum electrolytes and assess for the following:
      (1) Oliguria or anuria: expect retention of electrolytes
      (2) Nonoliguria or polyuria: expect either accumulation or uncontrolled loss of electrolytes
iv. Evaluation of nursing care
   (a) Zero fluid balance remains despite the alteration in urine output
   (b) Electrolyte balance is maintained
   (c) Urine volume and concentration are normal
c. Fluid volume excess (see Commonly Encountered Nursing Diagnoses): associated with an oliguric phase of ATN and either an oliguric or anuric pattern of urine output
   i. Additional expected outcomes
      (a) Weight is lost or stable (as appropriate)
      (b) Patient has alert mental status
      (c) Dialysis is effective in treating fluid imbalances
   ii. Additional nursing intervention: implement dialysis for repeated episodes of symptomatic fluid volume excess
d. Fluid volume deficit: a state associated with the diuretic or nonoliguric stage of ARF, caused by the excessive loss of urinary volume without adequate volume replacement (see Commonly Encountered Nursing Diagnoses)
   i. Assessment for additional defining characteristics: presence of diuretic or nonoliguric state
   ii. Additional expected outcome: there is stable weight or weight gain
   iii. Additional evaluation of nursing care
      (a) There is weight gain or stable weight
      (b) Patient has alert mental status
e. Potential for uremic syndrome (see Commonly Encountered Nursing Diagnoses)
   i. Additional expected outcomes
      (a) There are no debilitating symptoms (e.g., nausea, vomiting, fatigue)
      (b) Patient is stable on dialysis
   ii. Additional nursing interventions
      (a) Assess for the presence of uremic symptoms
      (b) Implement conservative measures for controlling BUN
      (c) Initiate dialysis for uncontrollable symptomatic azotemia, acidosis, hypercatabolism, hyperkalemia, and volume overload
      (d) Monitor for indications for hemodialysis, traditionally the first form of dialysis for ARF
         (1) ARF

(2) Chronic renal failure when medications and diet no longer provide effective therapy

(3) Rapid removal of toxic substances from the blood stream (e.g., alcohol, aspirin, barbiturates, some antibiotics, poisons)

(4) Dialysis to keep BUN under 100 mg/dl to improve survival

(5) Uremic pericardial friction rub

(e) Monitor for contraindications for hemodialysis:

    (1) Intolerance to systemic heparinization

    (2) Labile cardiovascular status incompatible with rapid changes in extravascular fluid volume

    (3) Hemodynamic instability

(f) Monitor for indications for peritoneal dialysis: traditionally considered the second dialysis option for ARF upon the contraindications for hemodialysis

    (1) Fluid overload

    (2) Electrolyte or acid-base imbalance

    (3) Acute or chronic renal failure

    (4) Intoxication from dialyzable drugs and poisons

    (5) Peritonitis or pericarditis

    (6) Unavailability of vascular access for hemodialysis

(g) Monitor for contraindications to peritoneal dialysis: bleeding disorder, abdominal adhesions, and recent peritoneal surgery

(h) Monitor for indications and contraindications for the continuous renal replacement therapies (CRRT), which include slow continuous ultrafiltration (SCUF), continuous arteriovenous hemofiltration (CAVH), continuous arteriovenous hemodialysis (or hemodiafiltration) (CAVHD), continuous venovenous hemofiltration (CVVH), and the newest form, continuous venovenous hemodialysis (or hemodiafiltration) (CVVHD). CVVHD involves the use of a hollow-fiber hemofilter capable of rapid fluid removal during hypotensive or low blood flow states. Adaptations in this procedure include the addition of peritoneal dialysis fluid or a blood pump. This form of dialysis is often selected after hemodialysis and peritoneal dialysis have been contraindicated, although the CRRTs have demonstrated a unique benefit in dialysis as well as blood purification in the critically ill. Another practice is the combination of different forms of dialysis (e.g., CAVH and hemodialysis)

    (1) Indications for CAVH and other adaptations of this procedure

        a) Conditions of fluid overload or cardiovascular instability requiring a continuous method of fluid removal or compensation for azotemia

        b) ARF (e.g., ATN)

        c) Diuretic-resistant edema

        d) Acute pulmonary edema

        e) Post cardiac surgery

        f) Recent myocardial infarction

        g) Ascites

        h) Inability to tolerate the cardiovascular impact of rapid fluid losses associated with hemodialysis

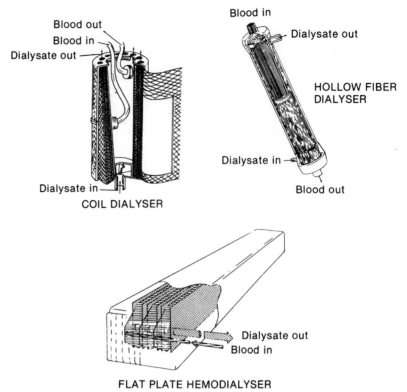

Figure 4–5 • Types of hemodialyzers. (From Levine, D. Z.: Care of the Renal Patient, 3rd ed. Philadelphia, W. B. Saunders, 1997.)

(2) Contraindications to CAVH and other adaptations of this procedure: very few, primarily hematocrit above 45%

(i) Initiate hemodialysis, an extracorporeal technique for removing waste products or toxic substances from the systemic circulation (Fig. 4–5)

(1) Principles of hemodialysis include osmosis (optional), diffusion, and convection/ultrafiltration

a) Osmosis: movement of water across a semipermeable membrane from an area of lesser to greater osmolality

b) Diffusion: movement of molecules from an area of higher to an area of lower concentration

c) Ultrafiltration/convection: movement of particles through a semipermeable membrane by hydrostatic pressure

(2) Anticoagulation

a) Prior to the procedure, heparinization is done to keep blood anticoagulated within the hemodialysis machine (regional heparinization)

b) For patients without complications, 5000 units of heparin is administered to start and 2000 units/hour while the patient is on the machine (general heparinization); the dosage may have to be adjusted to meet the needs of individual patients *c)* Patients should be monitored closely for signs of bleeding

     (3) Shunt care (rarely utilized)

           a) Auscultate for bruit or palpate for thrill to assess shunt patency

           b) Promptly report any suspicion of clotting, color change of blood, separation of serum from erythrocytes, or absence of pulsations in the tubing

           c) Provide adequate hydration to minimize clotting

           d) Change the sterile dressing over the shunt at least daily. Reinforce the dressing as necessary

           e) *Do not* perform venipuncture, give IV therapy, give injections, or take blood pressure with a cuff on the shunt arm

           f) Instruct the patient in care of the shunt site

     (4) Arteriovenous fistula care

           a) *Do not* perform venipuncture, start IV therapy, give injections, or take blood pressure with a cuff on the arm with a fistula

           b) Palpate the thrill or auscultate the bruit to confirm patency

           c) Avoid circumferential dressings and restrictive clothing

           d) Report bleeding, skin discoloration, drainage, or other signs of infection. Obtain drainage for culture

           e) For profuse bleeding, apply a pressure dressing

     (5) Femoral vein catheter care

           a) Palpate peripheral pulses in the cannulated extremity

           b) Observe for bleeding or hematoma formation. Apply a pressure dressing, and notify the physician

           c) Properly position the catheter to avoid dislodgment during the dialysis procedure

           d) If the femoral vein catheter is to be maintained after dialysis, connect it to a pressurized IV flow system. Add to the infusion solution a low dose of heparin, usually 500 units/1000 ml. Maintain a secure aseptic dressing to minimize the risk of infection. Discourage ambulation

           e) On removal of the femoral catheter, apply direct pressure to the puncture site for 5 to 10 minutes or the amount of time necessary to stop bleeding after dialysis (and after its period of heparinization). Complete this procedure with the application of a pressure dressing and a period of bed rest

  (j) Initiate peritoneal dialysis (Fig. 4–6)

     (1) Principles include diffusion and osmosis: Ultrafiltration is possible but is rarely used. To ultrafiltrate on peritoneal dialysis, choose from two methods. One method is to administer a vasopressor in conjunction with the peritoneal dialysis; vasoconstriction of the peritoneal blood vessel creates a vasodynamic hydrostatic pressure favoring the ultrafiltration process. The second method involves

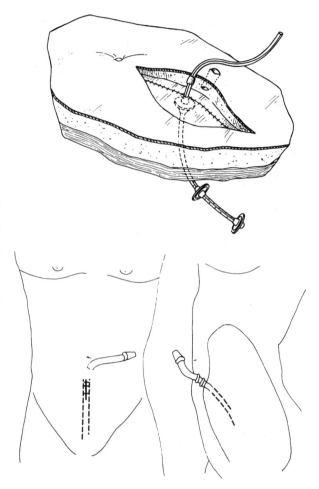

Figure 4–6 • Permanent peritoneal catheter in place, showing its position with respect to the different layers of the abdominal wall *(top)*, the anteroposterior position *(lower left)*, and the catheter angle with respect to abdominal wall *(lower right)*. (From Levine, D. Z.: Care of the Renal Patient, 3rd ed. Philadelphia, W. B. Saunders, 1997.)

skipping the dwell time and simply instilling peritoneal dialysis fluid as fast as possible and draining immediately after. This creates a siphoning effect with a negative pressure promoting water removal. Important nursing tasks include:

a) Explain the procedure to the patient: include the duration, limited mobility, and discomfort
b) Weigh the patient before and after treatment
c) Prepare equipment using an aseptic technique: use an automated peritoneal dialysis machine when available because it provides a closed system, decreasing the risk of infection
d) Prepare the dialysate solution, 1.5%, 2.5%, or 4.25% glucose; select a concentration according to the desired osmotic gradient necessary for water removal
e) Add medications to the dialysate as prescribed
   i) Heparin to prevent clotting in the dialysis catheter
   ii) Potassium chloride: dosage varies according to serum potassium levels and the requirement for digitalization precautions

       iii) Antibiotics for treatment of peritonitis

       iv) Insulin for treatment of hyperglycemia

       v) Lidocaine for control of local discomfort (~50 mg/ 2 L of dialysis fluid)

    f) Patient must void before the procedure to eliminate bladder distention and thus decrease the risk of bladder perforation during trocar or Tenckhoff insertion. If the patient is unable to void, a catheter is necessary

    g) Warm the dialysate solution to body temperature

    h) Assist the physician during trocar insertion

    i) First dialysate solution must be drained immediately to determine whether the catheter is patent; outflow should drain in a steady stream

    j) Allow all other infusions to "pool" or "dwell" in the abdomen (~20 to 45 minutes) for optimal fluid and electrolyte exchange

    k) Drain at the end of the dwell time and observe characteristics of the dialysate outflow

       i) Normal: clear, pale yellow

       ii) Cloudy: infection or peritonitis

       iii) Brownish: bowel perforation

       iv) Amber: bladder perforation

       v) Blood-tinged: a common occurrence in the first to fourth exchange; if bleeding continues, abdominal bleeding or uremic coagulopathy may be present

    l) Obtain a periodic culture specimen and sensitivity of the outflow fluid

    m) Monitor and record the total body I&O; record the positive and negative balance

    n) Monitor vital signs during the outflow phase, including changes in baseline blood pressure, pulse rate, and rhythm indicative of impending shock or overhydration. When using a hypertonic dialysate (4.25%), expect an osmotic effect and monitor glucose levels in all patients, especially in those with diabetes

(k) Initiate CRRTS: SCUF, CAVH, CAVHD, CVVH, or CVVHD

    (1) SCUF/CAVH (Fig. 4–7):

       a) Uses the principle of ultrafiltration, the exchange of primarily plasma water along with particles (e.g., potassium, BUN, creatinine) by convection

       b) Rate of exchange depends on membrane area, fiber diameter, hematocrit, plasma protein concentration, pressure gradient, and blood flow rate

       c) Administration of replacement fluid with CAVH only

    (2) CAVHD: incorporates the use of peritoneal dialysis fluid with ultrafiltration, thus combining the principles of diffusion and convection. The peritoneal dialysis fluid administration is regulated by a volumetric pump at 15 ml/ minute. The dialysis fluid enters the ultrafiltration compartment of the hemofilter and flows in the opposite direction of the blood flow

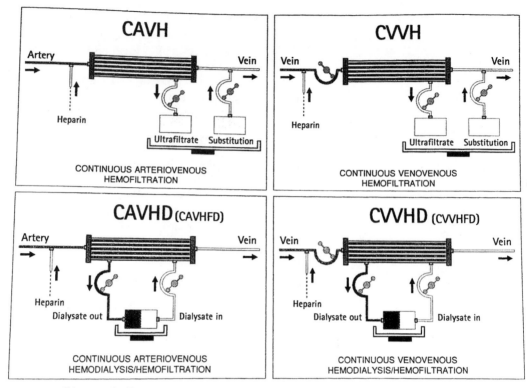

Figure 4–7 • The available continuous renal replacement therapies. CAVH = continuous arteriovenous hemofiltration; CVVH = continuous venovenous hemofiltration; CAVHD (CAVHFD) = continuous arteriovenous hemodialysis/hemodiafiltration (continuous arteriovenous high-flux dialysis); CVVHD (CVVHFD) = continuous venovenous hemodialysis/hemodiafiltration (continuous venovenous high-flux dialysis). (From Ronco, C., Barbacini, S., Digito, A., Zoccali, G.: Achievements and new directions in continuous renal replacement therapies. New Horiz. 3(4):709, 1995.)

    (3) CVVH: an adaptation of the previous principles. A blood pump with a venovenous blood access is used with administration of replacement fluid. Ultrafiltration is the primary principle involved

    (4) CVVHD: use of a blood pump in conjunction with the dialysate flowing countercurrent to the blood, for the ultrafiltration, diffusion, and osmotic dialysis effect

    (5) Overview of method

       a) Prepare the patient: explain the procedure. Obtain baseline serum studies, clotting time, chemistries, ABG studies, and CBC. Administer a loading dose of heparin

       b) Prepare the hemofilter, apply blood pump if initiating CVVH or CVVHD, and connect to the vascular access properly

       c) Attach the peritoneal dialysis fluid infusion if initiating CAVHD

       d) Determine the blood flow through the hemofilter and the resulting ultrafiltration rate, and begin fluid replacement therapy

       e) Monitor fluid replacement according to the patient's condition and desired rate of filtrate output to prevent circulatory collapse

  f) Regulate blood pressure, oncotic pressure, and
   ultrafiltration compartment to optimize the amount of
   filtrate (according to the prescribed dialyzing device)

  g) Maintain accurate hourly total body I & O records

f. Risk of electrolyte imbalances: patient with ARF is at risk for a number of
electrolyte imbalances, varying with the phase of ARF

 i. Assessment for defining characteristics

  (a) Oliguric phase

   (1) Hyperkalemia (see Hyperkalemia, Nursing Examination of
    Patient)

   (2) Hypocalcemia (see Hypocalcemia, Nursing Examination of
    Patient)

   (3) Hyperphosphatemia: defining characteristics are the same
    as for hypocalcemia

  (b) Diuretic or nonoliguric phase

   (1) Hypokalemia: results from the loss of potassium in the
    urine (see Hypokalemia, Nursing Examination of Patient)

   (2) Hyperkalemia: seen in the early period of nonoliguria

   (3) Hypercalcemia: occurs in patients who have experienced
    severe rhabdomyolysis (see Hypercalcemia, Nursing
    Examination of Patient)

   (4) Hypophosphatemia: occurs with large amounts of
    phosphate lost in the urine

 ii. Expected outcomes

  (a) Patient is asymptomatic, or levels of electrolytes are normal

  (b) Patient tolerates therapeutic interventions to correct electrolyte
   imbalances

  (c) Patient is compliant with preventive measures for control of
   electrolyte levels

 iii. Nursing interventions

  (a) Prevent or practice early detection of electrolyte imbalances
   associated with ARF

  (b) Collaborate with the physician to determine specific therapeutic
   interventions for each electrolyte imbalance (see specific
   electrolyte imbalances)

  (c) Monitor serum electrolyte levels to assess the therapeutic
   response

  (d) Initiate dialysis for persistent symptomatic electrolyte imbalances

 iv. Evaluation of nursing care

  (a) Serum electrolyte levels are in a normal or a near-normal or
   acceptable range

  (b) Symptoms associated with electrolyte imbalance are absent

g. Risk of metabolic acidosis: a state created by the kidney's inability to
excrete hydrogen ions (see Commonly Encountered Nursing Diagnoses)

 i. Additional expected outcomes

  (a) The pH is maintained within an asymptomatic range

  (b) Patient tolerates dialysis treatment for correction of metabolic
   acidosis

 ii. Additional nursing interventions

  (a) Collaborate with the physician to establish a desired baseline
   value for pH

      (b) In emergency situations, administer sodium bicarbonate slowly by IV infusion to correct systemic pH; repeated infusions can cause a significant sodium overload that could precipitate pulmonary edema

      (c) Implement dialysis for repeated episodes of symptomatic acidosis

  h. Risk of infection (see Commonly Encountered Nursing Diagnoses)

    i. Assessment for additional defining characteristics: BUN level over 80 to 100 mg/dl coincides with an increased risk of infection

    ii. Additional nursing intervention: monitor for early signs of septic shock (SIRS)

  i. Risk of anemia: the risk of anemia in ARF results from actual bleeding secondary to primary etiology or uremia, a lack of erythropoietin, or the presence of septic shock and SIRS, which is commonly associated with the onset of disseminated intravascular coagulation (see Commonly Encountered Nursing Diagnoses)

    i. Assessment for additional defining characteristics

      (a) Actual bleeding

        (1) Positive guaiac test of nasogastric drainage, vomitus, stool, or other drainage

        (2) Ecchymotic areas

        (3) Hematoma

      (b) Decreased hematocrit and hemoglobin secondary to a lack of erythropoietin: anemia occurring in the absence of any signs of actual bleeding during ARF

    ii. Additional nursing interventions

      (a) Assess for actual bleeding

      (b) Collaborate with the physician to determine the range of hematocrit levels requiring blood transfusions with packed cells

  j. Altered nutrition: less than body requirements (see Commonly Encountered Nursing Diagnoses)

    i. Assessment for additional defining characteristics

      (a) ARF associated with accelerated protein catabolism contributing to a negative nitrogen balance

      (b) Uncontrollable high BUN levels indicative of a hypercatabolic state

      (c) Glucose intolerance due to insulin resistance associated with ARF

      (d) Presence of lipid and fatty acid metabolic disturbance; lipid clearance is reduced by 50%

    ii. Additional nursing interventions

      (a) Assess for the presence of hypercatabolism

        (1) Repeated elevations of BUN over 100 mg/dl despite the use of routine dialysis

        (2) Signs of rapid muscle wasting

      (b) Consider total calories of 30 to 35 kcal/kg/day of carbohydrate and lipid combination with the glucose and triglycerides controlled. Amino acids, both essential and nonessential, are administered at 2 g/kg/day to diminish protein catabolism

      (c) Be aware that hyperalimentation and daily dialysis have been associated with increased survival rates in ARF as well as promoting renal tubular cell regeneration. Hyperalimentation requirements include large amounts (2 g/day) of both essential and nonessential amino acids

(d) IV glucose and lipid solution can also be considered

(e) Administer water-soluble vitamins. Avoid excessive doses of vitamin C (not exceeding 250 mg/day), which may exacerbate ARF. Be cautious with vitamin A administration, since excessive intake in the absence of renal excretion can lead to vitamin A toxicity

(f) Monitor serum protein, albumin, hematocrit, and urea levels in conjunction with daily weights to determine the effectiveness of nutritional therapy

k. Risk of impaired skin integrity: This problem is created in ARF by uremia, malnutrition, and immobility

  i. Assessment for defining characteristics

    (a) Dry skin

    (b) Itching

    (c) Bruising

    (d) Uremic frost

    (e) Infection

    (f) Edema

    (g) Presence of wounds, skin ulcers, or both

    (h) Changes in skin texture and thickness

  ii. Expected outcomes

    (a) Intact skin

    (b) Presence of wound healing

  iii. Nursing interventions

    (a) Initiate a regimen to keep skin clean, dry, and intact to prevent infection

      (1) Bathe the patient's skin daily to remove waste products

      (2) Apply creams or ointments

      (3) Administer medications to relieve itching (e.g., diphenhydramine)

      (4) Use oil in a bath to prevent dryness

      (5) Clean bruises and open areas to prevent infection

      (6) Monitor for the presence of edema

      (7) Help the patient to avoid tight-fitting shoes or clothing that may create pressure points susceptible to breakdown

    (b) Use aseptic technique during wound care

  iv. Evaluation of nursing care

    (a) Skin is dry, clean, and intact

    (b) There is no itching

    (c) There is no infection

    (d) Wounds are healing

l. Sleep pattern disturbance: disruption of sleep time interferes with the healing process and desired life style. During renal failure, this state results from interruptions associated with the intensity of the care, the critical care environment, and the uremic condition. This has been demonstrated in nursing research, which revealed an increase in the number of recalled nightmares the night prior to dialysis at the uremic peak, resulting in a disturbed sleeping pattern

        i. Assessment for defining characteristics
- (a) Frequent interruptions of the patient's sleep cycle for monitoring of health status
- (b) Lack of 90-minute periods of uninterrupted sleep
- (c) Patient's complaint of lack of sleep
- (d) Restless during sleep, with frequent awakening
- (e) Fatigue, irritability, and lethargy related to sleep deficit

      ii. Expected outcomes
- (a) Patient receives three to four 90-minute periods of uninterrupted sleep
- (b) Patient has no symptoms of sleep deprivation

    iii. Nursing interventions
- (a) Obtain a sleep history (i.e., day or night sleeper)
- (b) Organize care to minimize patient interruptions
- (c) Limit noise in the environment
- (d) Provide three to four 90-minute cycles of sleep each 24-hour period

    iv. Evaluation of nursing care
- (a) Patient receives three to four 90-minute cycles of sleep
- (b) Patient is oriented to time, place, person, and surroundings
- (c) Patient verbalizes feeling rested

m. Knowledge deficit related to ARF: the absence or deficiency of information related to aspects of the condition or its treatment; ARF often is associated with a lack of knowledge by both patient and family

        i. Assessment for defining characteristics: the patient lacks understanding of the following:
- (a) Monitoring equipment
- (b) Dietary and fluid restrictions
- (c) Dialysis machine and procedures
- (d) Etiology and course of renal disease
- (e) Prospects for recovery

      ii. Expected outcomes
- (a) Patient verbalizes basic knowledge of ARF and its treatment
- (b) There is enhanced participation in care as a result of better understanding

    iii. Nursing interventions
- (a) Assess the patient's level of readiness to learn
- (b) Assess uremic effects on learning: memory, attention span, and thought processing
- (c) Teach the patient key points about the critical care experience, ARF, and the treatment regimen

    iv. Evaluation of nursing care
- (a) Patient conveys basic knowledge of the disease process and the treatment
- (b) Cooperates with care based on knowledge
- (c) Expresses decreased anxiety related to information needs

n. Altered metabolism/excretion of pharmacologic agents resulting from the acutely failed kidney's inability to metabolize or excrete medications (see Commonly Encountered Nursing Diagnoses)

        i. Additional nursing interventions
- (a) Be aware of nephrotoxic agents usually ordered for ARF
  - (1) Antibiotics: gentamicin, carbenicillin, and amikacin

(2) Diuretics: furosemide in large doses

    (b) Monitor BUN and serum creatinine levels to determine the drug effect on renal function

    (c) Monitor serum drug levels

    (d) Collaborate with the physician to determine the need for modifying the pharmacologic administration

        (1) Reduced drug dosage

        (2) Increased intervals between doses

o. Ineffective patient and family coping: the sudden onset of ARF compounds its psychosocial impact (see Commonly Encountered Nursing Diagnoses)

    i. Additional expected outcomes

       (a) Patient maintains minimal level of anxiety

       (b) Patient cooperates with health care providers

       (c) Patient exhibits trust of health care providers

       (d) Patient uses support systems appropriately

    ii. Additional nursing interventions

       (a) Identify common causes of stress in the patient

          (1) Sudden, unexpected onset of loss of health

          (2) Uncertainty of the future: balance between hope and despair for recovery of renal function

          (3) Body image changes: loss of urine-making ability, arteriovenous or peritoneal access, bruises, and changes in skin color and texture

          (4) Long-term hospitalization, including a stay in the intensive care unit (ICU), removes the patient from home and work

          (5) Fear of loss of life

    iii. Additional evaluation of nursing care

       (a) Patient expresses decreased feelings of anxiety

       (b) Patient participates in care

       (c) Patient demonstrates trust in caregivers

       (d) Patient participates during sessions offering psychosocial support

Chronic Renal Failure

Chronic renal failure (CRF) is a slowly progressive renal disorder culminating in end-stage renal disease (ESRD). The decline in kidney function correlates with the degree of nephron loss.

1. **Pathophysiology:** systemic changes occur when overall renal function is less than 20% to 25% of normal

    a. Bricker's "intact nephron" hypothesis: provides an explanation of the kidney's ability to compensate and preserve homeostasis despite a significant loss (80%) of nephron function. During CRF, injury occurs to the nephrons in a progressive manner. The remaining intact nephrons compensate for the loss of functioning nephrons by cellular hypertrophy, which enables nephrons to accept larger blood volumes for clearances, resulting in the excretion of greater solute levels

    b. Four stages of CRF: each stage correlates with a certain degree of nephron loss

      i. Diminished renal reserve: 50% nephron loss

        (a) Kidney function is mildly reduced, whereas the excretory and regulatory functions are sufficiently maintained to preserve a normal internal environment. The patient usually is problem free

        (b) The serum creatinine value usually doubles; a normal value of 0.6 mg/dl rises to 1.2 mg/dl, which is still within normal limits

     ii. Renal insufficiency: a 75% nephron loss

        (a) Evidence of impaired renal capacity that appears in the form of mild azotemia, slightly impaired urinary concentrating ability, and anemia

        (b) Factors that exacerbate renal disease at this stage by increasing nephron damage are infection, dehydration, drugs, cardiac failure, and instability of primary disease

    iii. ESRD: 90% of nephrons are damaged

        (a) Renal function has deteriorated so that persistent abnormalities exist

        (b) Patient requires artificial support to sustain life (dialysis or transplantation)

    iv. Uremic syndrome

        (a) The body's systemic responses to the build-up of uremic waste products and the results of the failed organ system

        (b) Usually described as the constellation of signs and symptoms demonstrated by renal failure

        (c) Symptoms may be avoided or diminished by the initiation of early dialysis treatment

2. Etiologic or precipitating factors

  a. Tubulointerstitial disease or interstitial nephritis

     i. Chronic pyelonephritis (most common cause)

    ii. Analgesic abuse nephropathy

    iii. Myeloma kidney

    iv. Uric acid renal disease

    v. Hyperkalemic nephropathy

    vi. Cystic disease of the kidney

    vii. Sarcoidosis

    viii. Immunologic mechanisms (transplant rejection, allergic response, hypersensitivity)

    ix. Radiation nephritis

    x. Idiopathic organ nephritis

    xi. Hypokalemic nephropathy

  b. Glomerulonephropathies

     i. Focal glomerulosclerosis (gamma A immunoglobulin [IgA]-type antibody: benign and hereditary nephritis)

    ii. Crescentic glomerulonephritis (rapidly progressing)

    iii. Membranoproliferative glomerulonephritis

    iv. Lipoid nephrosis

    v. Membranous glomerulonephritis

    vi. Chronic glomerulonephritis

    vii. Diabetes mellitus: Kimmelstiel-Wilson syndrome

    viii. Systemic lupus erythematosus

    ix. Goodpasture's syndrome

    x. Polyarteritis nodosa
   xi. Wegener's granulomatosis
  xii. Bacterial endocarditis
 xiii. Henoch-Schönlein purpura

c. Nephrotic syndrome: seen in patients with glomerular or tubular disorders

d. Renal vascular disorders
    i. Systemic vasculitis (i.e., polyarteritis nodosa, hypersensitivity vasculitis)
   ii. Scleroderma
  iii. Coagulopathies
     (a) Hemolytic-uremic syndrome
     (b) Preeclampsia and pregnancy
     (c) Cortical necrosis
   iv. Thromboembolic disease
     (a) Renal vein thrombosis
     (b) Renal atheroembolus
    v. Sickle cell nephropathy
   vi. Hypertensive nephrosclerosis: benign, malignant, or accelerated

e. Renal cancer
    i. Renal cell carcinoma (most common renal neoplasm)
   ii. Secondary neoplasms such as bronchogenic carcinoma and adenocarcinoma of the stomach

3. Nursing assessment data base: complete the general assessment for the renal patient (described earlier), then refer to this section for specific elements concerning CRF

a. Nursing history: determine the stage of CRF and the patient's tolerance of each stage. A history of the patient's experiences with renal replacement therapies is also collected
    i. Subjective findings
     (a) Patient's chief complaints: fatigue and weakness
     (b) Other symptoms: nausea, vomiting, bone pain, chest pain (pleuritic)
   ii. Objective findings
     (a) Etiologic or precipitating factors: consider all possibilities until the reversible disorders have been identified and eliminated
       (1) Past examinations reveal a pattern of deteriorating renal reserve
       (2) Unexplained symptoms
         a) General: fever, lassitude, anorexia, edema, nausea, weakness, anemia, headache, tremors, coma
         b) Specific: hematuria, proteinuria, flank pain
       (3) Pregnancies with recurrent pyelitis, edema, or hypertension
       (4) Deafness (Alport's syndrome)
       (5) Chronic urinary tract or renal infections: dysuria, frequency, polyuria
       (6) Recent respiratory or skin infection (Goodpasture's syndrome or poststreptococcal infections)
       (7) History of etiologic or precipitating factors
         a) Drug sensitivity
         b) Allergies
         c) Extensive vascular disease

           d) Enuresis past age 6 years: suggestive of congenital stricture or neurologic abnormalities of the urinary tract

     (b) Family history

          (1) Genetic predisposition to actual kidney disorder (polycystic disease, Alport's syndrome, cystinuria, Fanconi's syndrome)

          (2) Positive for gout, diabetes mellitus, hypertension, vascular disease, systemic lupus erythematosus, arthritis, or heart disease

          (3) Family unit: impact and past adjustment to CRF

          (4) Role of the family in care (e.g., home dialysis)

     (c) Social history: present employment status and impact of CRF on employment

     (d) Medication history: past as well as present response to current use

          (1) Diuretics

          (2) Antihypertensives

          (3) Immunosuppressives: presence of bone marrow suppression or infection; past episodes of rejection

          (4) Use or abuse of analgesics, phenacetin-containing compounds, and methysergide

     (e) Other

          (1) Uremic symptoms: determine the number and severity

          (2) Sexual dysfunction

          (3) Self-image: alteration may be associated with loss of health, diminished body image, and renal function

          (4) Dietary restrictions: usually 60 g of protein, 2 g of sodium, and 2 g of potassium with fluid restriction. Diet varies according to the individual case and the source of the renal replacement therapy

          (5) Renal replacement therapy: determine the types used

b. Nursing examination of patient: patient may present at any stage of CRF (see Nursing Examination of Patient and same section under Acute Renal Failure)

   i. Inspection

     (a) Neurologic

          (1) Uremic seizures

          (2) Hypocalcemia with associated signs and symptoms such as tetany, seizures, and numbness and tingling in the fingertips, around the oral cavity, in the nose, and in the toes plus possible ECG changes (prolonged ST segment)

          (3) Alterations in mobility, with diminished strength, muscle atrophy, bone pain, and change in gait

          (4) Muscle paralysis secondary to hyperkalemia and muscle wasting secondary to malnutrition, particularly in a protein-deficient diet

     (b) Respiratory: deep, rapid respirations; Kussmaul's respirations

     (c) Cardiovascular

          (1) 12-lead ECG changes consistent with uremic pericarditis

          (2) Dysrhythmias or cardiac arrest associated with electrolyte imbalances

     (d) Genitourinary: normal urine volume to oliguria or anuria

   ii. Palpation

     (a) Pulse: normal to bradycardia or tachycardia secondary to uremic or electrolyte effects

     (b) Genitourinary: palpable masses in both upper quadrants may be indicative of polycystic disease

c. Diagnostic studies

   i. Laboratory findings

     (a) Urinalysis: the following abnormalities may be the first indicators of renal disease:

       (1) Proteinuria: may exceed 3 g/24 hr in patients with glomerulonephropathies and nephrotic syndrome

       (2) Hematuria: gross or microscopic

       (3) Leukocyte casts and pyuria: indicate infection in the urinary tract. Suspect renal disease when pyuria occurs in conjunction with hematuria, casts, and proteinuria

       (4) Eosinophiluria: may occur in allergic interstitial nephritis

       (5) Epithelial cells: renal tubular cells with lipid droplets in the cytoplasm suggest nephrotic syndrome. Large numbers of these cells are present in glomerulonephritis and pyelonephritis

       (6) Casts: provide important diagnostic clues

         a) Erythrocyte casts suggest hematuria of glomerular origin

         b) Leukocyte casts indicate intrarenal inflammation

         c) Mixed leukocyte and erythrocyte casts may be prominent in acute exudative glomerulonephritis

         d) Fatty casts are seen in glomerular diseases in conjunction with moderate to heavy proteinuria

         e) Granular casts are common in many diseases

         f) Waxy and broad casts occur in the last stages of renal failure

       (7) Urine culture can detect the presence of infection

       (8) Urine osmolality varies with the stage of CRF

       (9) Creatinine clearance:

         a) A decrease of 10 to 50 ml/minute or a renal reserve of 25% is associated with the onset of renal insufficiency and its symptoms

         b) A creatinine clearance of 10 to 15 ml/minute is consistent with ESRD

     (b) Serum

       (1) Creatinine: an inverse relationship exists between serum creatinine and GFR versus the stages of CRF

         a) Diminished renal reserve: a 50% nephron loss is reflected by either a normal creatinine level of 1.4 mg/dl or a twice normal creatinine level of 2.8 mg/dl

         b) Renal insufficiency: a 75% nephron loss causes the serum creatinine level to quadruple

         c) ESRD: a 90% nephron loss correlates with a serum creatinine value of 10 mg/dl or greater

         d) Uremic syndrome: a creatinine value of 10 mg/dl or above is maintained by some form of dialysis treatment

        (2) BUN: in CRF, the BUN level correlates well with uremia. Levels above 100 mg/dl are usually associated with uremic symptoms; therefore, BUN can be used to determine the frequency and duration of dialysis requirements

        (3) Uric acid: increased serum levels may suggest gouty nephropathy when there is an elevation out of proportion to the degree of renal failure

        (4) Serum triglycerides: may be elevated

        (5) Glucose tolerance test: determines the presence of carbohydrate intolerance

    ii. Radiologic findings: IVP

      (a) Small kidneys, or one atrophied kidney and one normal-sized kidney, may indicate bilateral disease. Unilateral disease always causes compensatory hypertrophy of the contralateral kidney

      (b) Enlarged kidneys suggest polycystic disease or obstruction

      (c) Scarring and altered calices can suggest chronic pyelonephritis or analgesic nephropathy

    iii. Renal biopsy: is used to establish a diagnosis, determine reversible etiologic mechanisms, and establish appropriate therapy

    iv. Special: baseline motor nerve conduction velocity studies and long bone x-ray films of the skull, hands, and feet determine the development of uremic neuropathy and bone disease

4. Nursing diagnoses (see Commonly Encountered Nursing Diagnoses)

  a. Fluid volume excess: accompanies ESRD with the onset of anuria or oliguria

    i. Assessments for additional defining characteristics

      (a) Noncompliance with fluid restriction between dialysis treatments

      (b) Ineffective dialysis treatments

    ii. Additional expected outcomes

      (a) Normal blood pressure is maintained

      (b) Patient is compliant with fluid restriction

    iii. Additional nursing interventions

      (a) Teach the patient the risks of abusing fluid restriction; encourage compliance

      (b) Obtain daily weight; determine dry weight

      (c) Implement a fluid restriction (amount equals insensible losses)

      (d) Collaborate with the physician to evaluate the effectiveness of dialysis treatments and the need for more aggressive treatment

      (e) Assess for hypertension. Consider the severity of hypertension and the need for blood pressure control by rapid fluid removal via dialysis

      (f) Assess the degree of edema and the impact on skin integrity

  b. Risk of electrolyte imbalance: accompanies the inability to concentrate urine. Any electrolyte is at risk of imbalance during ESRD, but the most common imbalances are hyperkalemia, hypocalcemia, and hyperphosphatemia (see specific imbalances)

  c. Risk of acid-base imbalances: metabolic acidosis

    i. Additional expected outcomes

      (a) There is a symptom-free pH level

      (b) Dialysis is successful in controlling acidosis

  ii. Additional nursing interventions
   (a) Provide dialysis and oral sodium bicarbonate for long-term control
   (b) Be aware of the method by which dialysis controls acidosis
    (1) Acetate or lactate found in a hemodialysis and peritoneal dialysis bath is absorbed into the body. These elements enter the Krebs cycle to be converted to bicarbonate. This conversion process requires the presence of oxygen at the tissue level
    (2) Bicarbonate bath: a specifically adjusted hemodialysis machine that dialyzes with a bath containing bicarbonate. The patient receiving bicarbonate does not have to carry out the metabolic conversion expected with acetate–lactate

d. Risk of anemia
 i. Assessment for additional defining characteristics: the hematocrit value is maintained with the administration of epoetin usually within the range of 32% to 35% in the general hemodialysis population
 ii. Additional nursing interventions
  (a) Assess the degree of anemia
  (b) Determine the baseline hematocrit
  (c) Assess the epoetin alfa dosage on a routine basis
  (d) Epoetin alfa (DNA recombinant-engineered erythropoietin): an effective replacement agent for erythropoietin
   (1) Administration after a 3-month duration results in a near-normal hematocrit (range, 30% to 36%) associated with a mild to moderate improvement in exercise tolerance and work capacity, increased aerobic performance, and improved oxygen transport to tissue
   (2) Cardiac output and ejection fraction also show improvement
   (3) Side effects are minimal: higher hematocrit levels increase blood viscosity, which potentially leads to problems during dialysis treatment, a shortened life of fistula, hypertension, and limited reuse of dialyzers. These effects are minimized when the hematocrit is maintained in the lower ranges of normal

e. Risk of uremic syndrome
 i. Additional expected outcome: patient is able to accomplish activities of daily living
 ii. Additional nursing interventions
  (a) Assess to determine the extent or degree of uremia
   (1) Monitor for cardiovascular involvement secondary to uremia
    a) Uremic pericarditis from the accumulation of uremic toxins. Observe for pericardial friction rub, shortness of breath (relieved by sitting upright and leaning), fever, and ECG changes (ST elevations in the leads reflecting the involved epicardial surface)
    b) Pericardial effusion: look for loss of friction rub; increased severity of chest pain; rapid, thready pulse; increased CVP; and hypotension

    c) Cardiac tamponade: if untreated uremic pericardial effusion; monitor for hypotension, pulsus paradoxus, increased jugular venous pulse (JVP), decreased cardiac output, and distant heart sounds

    d) Pulmonary edema: seen with fluid overload and left ventricular failure (see Chapter 1)

    e) Arteriosclerosis: acceleration of vascular changes associated with aging. It is the second most common cause of death in the hemodialysis population. Organ failure commonly associated with ischemia created by the vascular changes; hypertension

    f) Symptomatic hyperkalemia (see specific section on this disorder)

    g) Hypertension

      i) Hypertensive retinopathy: arteriolar narrowing secondary to vascular changes or spasms

       [a] Grade I: arteriolar narrowing

       [b] Grade II: arteriolar narrowing and arteriovenous nicking

       [c] Grade III: arteriolar narrowing, arteriovenous nicking, and hemorrhages or exudates

       [d] Grade IV: all of the preceding plus papillary edema

      ii) Hypertensive encephalopathy: stupor, confusion, restlessness, nausea and vomiting, and seizures progressing to coma

  (2) Collaborate with the health care team in the treatment of cardiovascular complications

  (3) Monitor manifestations of pulmonary involvement

    a) Pleural effusion

    b) Uremic pneumonitis (uremic lung): associated with fluid overload; in severe cases, mimics the picture of adult respiratory distress syndrome

 (d) Treat pulmonary involvement

    a) Initiate frequent dialysis

    b) Provide antibiotics as necessary

    c) Provide pulmonary toilet

    d) Administer oxygen

    e) Monitor progress with ABG analysis and chest x-rays

  (5) Monitor for manifestations of neurologic involvement

    a) Encephalopathy

    b) Peripheral neuropathy

      i) "Burning" sensation of the feet progressing to paresthesia and intense pain on the dorsal and ventral surfaces of the feet

      ii) Footdrop and diminished muscle strength

      iii) Impaired gait and possibly paralysis

      iv) Slowing of nerve conduction velocity and a segmental demyelination of the nerves

  (6) Minimize alterations in neurologic effects

    a) Orient the patient as necessary

    b) Protect from hyperirritability and seizures

          c) Correct electrolyte imbalances (hypocalcemia)

          d) Reverse the encephalopathy and minimize the peripheral neuropathy by dialysis

  (7) Monitor for manifestations of endocrine and metabolic involvement

          a) Hyperuricemia and gout: accumulation of uric acid

             i) Joint pain and inflammation

             ii) Low-grade fever

             iii) Hypertension

          b) Secondary hyperparathyroidism: combination of hypercalcemia and demineralization of bone with metastatic calcifications

          c) Hyperlipidemia: an increase in type IV lipoprotein is most commonly seen with CRF

          d) Carbohydrate intolerance: manifested as moderate levels of hyperglycemia and elevated insulin levels

          e) Assess for sexual dysfunctions

             i) Amenorrhea or abnormal menstruation

             ii) Impotence

             iii) Infertility

             iv) Decreased libido

             v) Diminished testosterone production and reduced ovulation

  (8) Collaborate with the health care team in the treatment of endocrine-metabolic disorders

          a) Administer allopurinol for gout accompanied by hyperuricemic levels

          b) Adjust dietary intake and administer low-dose corticosteroids to decrease serum lipid levels

          c) Initiate dialysis to partially improve glucose tolerance

          d) Transplant to normalize sexual function; dialysis may provide some improvement

  (9) Manifestations of gastrointestinal involvement

          a) General: anorexia, nausea, vomiting

          b) Uremic bowel: diarrhea or constipation, malabsorption syndrome, weight loss, and fatigue

          c) Peptic ulcer disease: gastric pain and possibly bleeding

          d) Gastrointestinal symptoms: minimize or alleviate with dialysis; administer a protein-restricted diet; administer zinc to improve taste sensation; consider a broad-spectrum antibiotic

          e) Bleeding, gastrointestinal ulceration, or pain: use nonmagnesium-containing antacids

 (10) Monitor for manifestations of hematologic involvement

          a) Anemia

          b) Platelet function abnormality: decrease in platelet adhesiveness, sometimes accompanied by a mild thrombocytopenia

             i) Increased tendency toward bleeding. If bleeding occurs, the hematocrit will fall below 20% for reasons beyond renal failure

        ii) Bruising and purpura

(11) Initiate dialysis to minimize the uremic effect on platelet functions

    a) Iron and folic acid supplements

    b) Testosterone and other androgens that may reverse anemia

(12) Monitor for manifestations of musculoskeletal involvement: osteomalacia (renal rickets)

    a) Hypocalcemia with reciprocal hyperphosphatemia

    b) Bone pain

    c) Impaired growth process

    d) Pathologic fractures

(13) Treat musculoskeletal effects: monitor serum calcium levels and administer calcium tablets and 1,25-dihydroxycholecalciferol (a form of activated vitamin D) in conjunction with phosphate-binding therapy (calcium carbonate)

f. Management of therapeutic regimen, patient, and family: hemodialysis continues to be the standard for treatment of ESRD

  i. Assessment for defining characteristics: patient needs to continue therapy for CRF

  ii. Expected outcomes

    (a) Circulatory access is maintained

    (b) Patient has hemodialysis treatment, usually three times a week (3 to 5 hours for each treatment)

    (c) Patient complies with rigid diet and fluid restrictions

    (d) Patient has home hemodialysis

      (1) Proper environment is available: adequate space, plumbing, and hygiene

      (2) Patient demonstrates signs of compliance and adaptation to the disease process

      (3) Patient demonstrates ability to physically tolerate dialysis procedure

      (4) There is evidence of established family support system or acceptance of a surrogate dialyzer

      (5) Patient demonstrates ability to learn technical and aseptic skills

    (e) Patient undergoes chronic peritoneal dialysis: follows same principles and procedures as acute peritoneal dialysis; differences relate to the patient's expectations and the use of an automated peritoneal dialysis machine

      (1) Patient's expectations for peritoneal dialysis

        a) Maintenance of Tenckhoff catheter

        b) Use of aseptic technique throughout the procedure

        c) Able to obtain treatment three to four times a week for 10 hours each treatment

        d) Adheres to dietary and fluid restrictions

      (2) Expectations for home peritoneal dialysis

        a) Proper environment: treatment requires space and storage area for equipment *b)* Psychologic stability: not as necessary for home peritoneal dialysis because rapid fluid shifts and dramatic cardiovascular effects are not associated with this treatment

        c) Family support systems: helpful but not essential because most patients use dialysis at night, and the family routine may not be disrupted

        d) Cognitive ability: less technological skill is required, but aseptic technique is essential

    (f) Patient demonstrates ability to perform continuous ambulatory peritoneal dialysis (CAPD)

        (1) Patient recognizes that exchanges are made 24 hours a day, 7 days a week. Frequency of exchanges can vary. Each exchange is for 6 to 8 hours during the day and 8 to 12 hours at night

        (2) Patient completes a rigorous training program

        (3) Patient demonstrates proper care of the Tenckhoff catheter

        (4) Patient adheres to the treatment schedule

        (5) Patient stores the dialysis equipment appropriately

        (6) Patient demonstrates measures to avoid complications, including peritonitis, back strain, visceral herniation, obesity, and fluid excess

  iii. Nursing interventions

    (a) Provide patient and family teaching to ensure the capability of continuing the therapeutic regimens

    (b) Provide patient and family teaching to avoid the development of complications from CRF or its treatment

    (c) Collaborate with the multidisciplinary team and home care services to provide continuity of care

  iv. Evaluation of nursing care: patient meets all expected outcomes for the therapeutic regimen ordered

g. Management of the therapeutic regimen related to renal transplantation: promotes primary disease management by minimizing complications, slowing the progression of the primary disease process, and decreasing the mortality rate

  i. Assessment for defining characteristics

    (a) Recipient selection criteria: begins with the presence of irreversible ESRD

        (1) Age: up to 70 years

        (2) Preexisting antibodies (to donor kidney)

        (3) No medical or surgical contraindications

        (4) Functioning bladder or urinary tract

        (5) No psychosis, severe personality disorder, or history of noncompliance

    (b) "Last resort" alternative: patient may be accepted based on the inability to participate in other treatment alternatives. This may be due to a lack of vascular access or physical tolerance of the procedure

    (c) Tissue typing compatibility

        (1) ABO blood typing: to determine blood type compatibility between donor and recipient

(2) HLA typing: serologic testing for specification of the HLA-A, -B, and -C locus antigen plus lymphocyte-defined typing of the D locus

(3) Mixed lymphocyte culture (MLC): reveals the degree of difference between the D loci of the donor and the recipient

(4) Cross-match for preformed antibody (microlymphocytotoxicity cross-match): presence of preformed antibodies significantly decreases the viability of any graft

(d) Immunocompetent cells: two kinds of lymphocytes are involved in the rejection processes:

(1) B lymphocytes: for humoral immunity and antibody-producing cells; responsible for hyperacute rejection and partially involved in acute and chronic rejection

(2) T lymphocytes: cell-mediated immunity involved in acute and chronic rejection. Three types: effectors, helpers, and suppressors

(e) Presence of rejection: types of rejection

(1) Hyperacute: irreversible process; occurs within minutes or hours of surgery

(2) Accelerated: occurs from the second to fifth day in the immediate postoperative period; physiologically is similar to hyperacute rejection. It is rarely reversible, involving both humoral and cellular immunity

(3) Acute: often reversible with high doses of antirejection medication

a) Occurs most frequently 2 weeks after transplantation but can be seen from the first week postoperatively up to 1 year

b) T cells or cellular immunity is the primary mechanism

c) Antigen leaves the graft and enters the serum, where it is recognized and incorporated into macrophage RNA. With reexposure to antigen, macrophage releases RNA-antigen complexes into the serum, where plasma lymphocytes manufacture specific antibody. The plasma lymphocytes then travel to the kidney for the immunologic attack

(4) Chronic: cannot be reversed; ultimately leads to organ failure

a) Occurs at 1 to 5 years after transplantation

b) B-cell or humoral response to antibody

c) A slow, chronic immunologic response, with gradual deterioration of renal tissue

d) Response involves primarily the glomerular basement membrane and endothelial layer of the blood vessels

ii. Expected outcomes

(a) Renal transplantation is successful in restoring normal renal function

(b) Patient recovers satisfactorily from transplant surgery without complications

        (c) Patient demonstrates ability for self-care and follow-up care
following transplant surgery

    iii. Nursing interventions

        (a) Instruct the patient and family about transplantation as a
treatment alternative, including:

            (1) Survival rates: patient selection criteria; treatment
expectations, such as antirejection medications; frequent
clinic visits the first year; and dietary limitations

            (2) Benefits: replacement of renal function, alleviation of most
pathophysiologic effects of uremia, and return to many
normal life activities

            (3) Complications, including rejection; immunosuppressive
effects: increased susceptibility to infections, risk of
malignancies, esophagitis, peptic ulcer, and acute
pancreatitis; and surgical complications

        (b) Provide preoperative teaching

            (1) Report to the hospital on request

            (2) Expected preoperative work-up

            (3) Description of the surgical procedure

                a) The kidney is transplanted into the iliac fossa

                b) Revascularization is usually accomplished by
anastomosing the renal artery to the hypogastric artery
and the renal vein to the external iliac vein (Fig. 4–8)

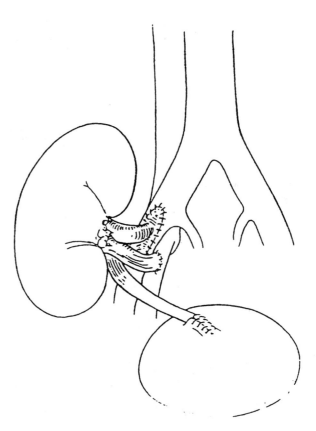

Figure 4–8 • The standard anastomosis. The donor renal artery is shown anastomosed end-to-end on a Carrel aortic patch to the recipient external iliac artery. The donor renal vein is anastomosed to the recipient external iliac vein. The donor ureter is anastomosed to the recipient bladder with an antireflux technique. (From Danovitch, G. M. [ed.]: The Handbook of Kidney Transplantation. Boston, Little, Brown & Co., 1992, p. 138. With permission of Lippincott Publishers.)

        c) The ureter is anastomosed to the recipient's ureter at the pelvis of the kidney (ureteropelvic anastomosis), or the donor's ureter can be implanted into the host's bladder (ureteroneocystostomy)

    (4) Immediate postoperative recovery period care

  (c) Provide postoperative teaching

    (1) How to obtain and record daily I&O, temperature, blood pressure, and weight records

    (2) Antirejection medication and side effects

    (3) Need to communicate signs and symptoms of rejection

        a) Fever

        b) Pain, tenderness, redness, and swelling at the site of the graft

        c) Weight gain

        d) Decreased urine output

        e) Hypertension

    (4) Activity limitations in first 3 months:

        a) Avoidance of lifting or strenuous exercise

        b) Avoidance of crowds

    (5) Need to report signs and symptoms of infection

    (6) Knowledge of diet

    (7) Schedule of clinic visits

  (d) Administer antirejection medications as ordered:

    (1) Corticosteroids to suppress the production of cytotoxic T cells and prevent the production of interleukin-2, which initiates the immunologic response

    (2) Azathioprine (Imuran): begin dosing at 2 to 3 mg/kg/day and decrease gradually to 1 mg/kg/day to prevent or deter acute rejection episodes

    (3) Cyclosporine: to inhibit T-cell proliferation

    (4) Antilymphocyte globulin (ALG): to deplete circulating T cells and suppress cell-mediated immunity allograft responses. Toxicity: agranulocytosis and hemolytic response and predisposition to infection

    (5) Monoclonal antibody (OKT3): administered over 14 days to suppress or inactivate one of two antigen-recognition sites on T cells (T2 or T3)

    (6) Cyclophosphamide (Cytoxan): used when azathioprine is contraindicated: to diminish the production of antibodies and initiate the destruction of circulating lymphocytes

    (7) FK-506: newest agent approved for liver transplants, approved with some exceptions for renal transplants; actions similar to those of cyclosporine

  iv. Evaluation of nursing care

    (a) Patient verbalizes an understanding of the renal transplantation preparation, surgical procedure, and postoperative regimen

    (b) Patient demonstrates an ability to participate in recovery and home care following surgical procedures

    (c) Family members actively participate in the patient's care

h. Alteration in nutrition: less than body requirements

i. Knowledge deficit: CRF, dialysis, and transplant procedures: the absence or deficiency of cognitive information related to a topic; a state created from the complexities of CRF, demanding a wide range of patient and family teaching sessions to produce a knowledgeable patient

    i. Assessment for defining characteristics

      (a) Patient verbalizes a lack of knowledge concerning the disease process or treatment

      (b) Patient is noncompliant with the treatments or medications

      (c) Patient lacks participation in self-care activities

    ii. Expected outcomes

      (a) Patient has increased knowledge of CRF, the treatment, and the medications

      (b) Patient complies with treatment expectations

      (c) Patient participates in care

    iii. Nursing interventions

      (a) Assess knowledge level related to CRF, its treatment, and medications

      (b) Assess uremic effect on learning

        (1) Decreased attention span

        (2) Diminished memory

        (3) Alteration in thought processes

      (c) Develop a teaching plan including reinforcement

      (d) Instruct the patient about all aspects of CRF

        (1) Normal renal function and renal disease state

        (2) Fluid management

        (3) Dietary management

        (4) Medications (action, dosage, times)

        (5) Avoidance of infection

        (6) Rest periods to minimize fatigue

        (7) Skin care

        (8) Treatment alternatives; after the patient and the family acquire knowledge of the benefits and disadvantages of each treatment, support the family's decision

      (e) Instruct the patient and family about dialysis

        (1) Dynamics of hemodialysis or peritoneal dialysis

        (2) Special diet and fluid allowances

        (3) Care of dialysis access

        (4) Need for weight control

        (5) Signs and symptoms of complications such as an electrolyte imbalance

    iv. Evaluation of nursing care: patient is able to describe preoperative and postoperative care

j. Body image disturbance: a disruption in the way one perceives one's body image; results from the effects of uremia, dependency on treatments, and primary illness other than renal disease (see Chapter 9)

k. Sexual dysfunction: a state in which an individual experiences a change in sexual function that is viewed as unsatisfying, unrewarding, or inadequate; a result of uremia and its treatments

    i. Assessment for defining characteristics

      (a) Decreased libido

      (b) Impotence

      (c) Amenorrhea

      (d) Infertility

(e) Verbalization of problem

(f) Actual or perceived limitation imposed by renal disease

(g) Altered relationships with significant others

(h) Change of interest in self and others

  ii. Expected outcomes

(a) Level of sexual functioning is satisfactory

(b) Loss of reproductive functioning is resolved

  iii. Nursing interventions

(a) Obtain a sexual history

(b) Advise the patient of methods to optimize sexuality, promote personal respect between partners, and encourage the recognition of individual needs for love and tenderness

(c) Consider methods that may improve sexual functioning

(d) Allow the patient to verbalize, providing emotional support for the patient and sexual partner

  iv. Evaluation of nursing care

(a) Verbalizes achievement of a satisfactory level of sexual functioning

(b) Verbalizes acceptance of loss of reproductive functioning

Electrolyte Imbalances—Potassium Imbalance: Hyperkalemia

The serum potassium level in hyperkalemia is above 5.5 mEq/L

1. **Pathophysiology**

a. Inability of kidney tubules to excrete potassium ion owing to tubular damage, salt depletion, and increased potassium load from injured tissues

b. Decreased renal perfusion diminishes potassium excretion as a result of a limited amount of sodium available for exchange with potassium (e.g., in cardiac failure)

2. **Etiologic or precipitating factors**

a. Acute and chronic renal failure

b. Increased cellular destruction with potassium release as occurs in burns, trauma, crash injuries, severe catabolism, acute acidosis, intravascular hemolysis, and rhabdomyolysis

c. Excessive administration and ingestion of potassium chloride

d. Adrenal cortical insufficiency: hypoaldosteronism

e. Low cardiac output or sodium depletion

f. Acidosis: precipitates the movement of intracellular potassium to the extracellular space

3. **Nursing assessment data base**

a. Nursing history: it is difficult to obtain specific information leading to the detection of electrolyte imbalances. Suspect imbalances in the presence of renal and endocrine disease, in association with a history of excessive loss of body fluid (e.g., vomiting, diarrhea), and in some special situations with drug intoxication (indiscriminate use of electrolyte replacement, hormonal therapy, and vitamins)

  i. Subjective findings

(a) Patient's chief complaints: lethargy and weakness

(b) Other symptoms: nausea, abdominal cramps, diarrhea, small urine volumes, or the absence of urine output

ii. Objective findings
   (a) Etiologic or precipitating factors (see preceding)
   (b) Medication history
      (1) Potassium chloride supplements to correct potassium losses caused by diuretic therapy
      (2) Kayexalate, a sodium-exchange resin administered as a conservative measure for potassium removal
b. Nursing examination of patient: all electrolyte imbalances generally present as evidence of abnormal neuromuscular function such as irritability, hyporeflexia or hyperreflexia, seizures, weakness, and cardiac dysrhythmias
   i. Inspection
      (a) Neurologic: apathy and confusion
      (b) Respiratory: deep rapid respirations when hyperkalemia is accompanied by acidosis or shallow respirations as a result of muscle paralysis
      (c) Cardiovascular: dysrhythmias on ECG
      (d) Genitourinary: oliguria
      (e) Gastrointestinal: abdominal cramping
      (f) Musculoskeletal
         (1) Irritability to flaccid paralysis and numbness of extremities
         (2) Fatigue, diminished exercise tolerance
         (3) Mobility: diminished due to paralysis
   ii. Auscultation: hyperactive bowel sounds, tachycardia, bradycardia
c. Diagnostic study findings
   i. Serum potassium levels exceed 5.5 mEq/L
   ii. ECG: progressive changes reveal peaked and elevated T waves→ widened QRS→prolonged PR interval→flattened or absent P wave and ST segment depression→asystole

4. Nursing diagnoses
a. Risk of electrolyte excess: hyperkalemia
   i. Assessment for defining characteristics (see Nursing assessment data base)
      (a) Myocardial manifestations of hyperkalemia
         (1) Myocardial depressant effect on conduction and contractility
         (2) Progressive ECG changes associated with bradycardia and hypotension
         (3) Disappearance of P wave progressing to idioventricular rhythm and asystole
   ii. Expected outcomes
      (a) Serum potassium level stays within normal limits
      (b) Cardiac function is within normal limits
   iii. Nursing interventions
      (a) Initiate cardiac monitoring: observe for changes in heart rate and rhythm
      (b) In emergency situations (i.e., if serum potassium level > 6.5 mEq/L or ECG change indicates severe hyperkalemia), administer:
         (1) Glucose, insulin, and sodium bicarbonate IV to temporarily drive potassium into cells

         a) Essential to follow up with other measures, such as sodium polystyrene sulfonate (Kayexalate) and sorbitol administration or dialysis for permanent removal of potassium

         b) If refractory hyperkalemia occurs, dialysis is indicated

      (2) Calcium chloride or calcium gluconate intravenously to stimulate cardiac contractility: contraindicated in patients taking digoxin

   (c) Administer Kayexalate (a cation-exchange resin) and sorbitol (a nonabsorbuble sugar) to reverse hyperkalemia

      (1) Kayexalate: sodium is "exchanged" 1:1 for a potassium ion in the bowel cell wall; therefore, assess the amount of sodium as well as potassium loss

      (2) Sorbitol: induces an osmotic diarrhea that contributes to potassium loss from the bowel

      (3) Routes of administration: oral or by enema. For rectal administration, Kayexalate solution is retained for at least 30 minutes for maximal effect. In both cases, ensure that the Kayexalate and sorbitol mixture is expelled, especially postoperatively, because retained Kayexalate can cause bowel obstruction and perforation

   (d) Monitor serum potassium levels at frequent intervals

   (e) Teach the patient about the need to remain compliant with potassium restrictions

  iv. Evaluation of nursing care

   (a) Serum potassium level below 5.5 mEq/L or in an asymptomatic range

   (b) Absence of cardiac complications of hyperkalemia

Electrolyte Imbalances—Potassium Imbalance: Hypokalemia

The serum potassium level in hypokalemia is below 3.5 mEq/L.

1. **Pathophysiology**
   a. Potassium loss exceeding intake
   b. Alkalosis: stimulates the secretion of potassium in the distal tubule
   c. Intracellular shifting of potassium

2. **Etiologic or precipitating factors**
   a. Alkalosis
   b. Abnormal gastrointestinal losses: nasogastric suction and drainage
   c. Liver disease
   d. Diuretic therapy
   e. Renal tubular acidosis
   f. Increased adrenal corticosteroid secretion or corticosteroid therapy
   g. Laxative abuse or diarrhea
   h. Starvation
   i. Prolonged episode of vomiting
   j. Bartter's syndrome: hypokalemia, hyponatremia, hypomagnesemia, metabolic alkalosis, and hyperreninemia

3. **Nursing assessment data base**
   a. Nursing history: see Hyperkalemia for a detection of electrolyte imbalance
      i. Subjective findings
         (a) Patient's chief complaints: feeling drowsy, weakness with muscle tenderness
         (b) Other symptoms: nausea, vomiting, and constipation
      ii. Objective findings
         (a) Additional etiologic or precipitating factors (see preceding)
            (1) Dietary indiscretion: either prolonged dieting without adequate potassium intake or starvation
            (2) Hyperalimentation without adequate potassium replacement
         (b) Medication history
            (1) Potassium chloride supplements prescribed but not taken
            (2) Diuretics—prescribed to treat hypervolemia or renal failure may cause potassium loss
   b. Nursing examination of patient
      i. Inspection
         (a) Neurologic
            (1) Drowsiness to coma, malaise, and confusion
            (2) Muscle cramping (commonly in calf muscle)
            (3) Muscular weakness progressing to paralysis
         (b) Respiratory: shallow respirations secondary to muscle weakness
         (c) Cardiovascular: dysrhythmias on ECG
         (d) Genitourinary: polyuria
         (e) Gastrointestinal: vomiting
      ii. Palpation: diminished pulses
      iii. Auscultation
         (a) Heart sounds: irregular rhythm secondary to dysrhythmias; possible enhanced digitalis effect
         (b) Bowel sounds: diminished secondary to paralytic ileus
         (c) Blood pressure: hypotension
   c. Diagnostic study findings
      i. Serum potassium levels below 3.5 mEq/L
      ii. ECG: depressed ST segments, flat or inverted T wave, presence of U wave, and ventricular dysrhythmias
4. **Nursing diagnoses**
   a. Risk of electrolyte deficit: hypokalemia
      i. Assessment for defining characteristics (see Nursing Assessment Data Base)
         (a) Additional manifestations of hypokalemia
            (1) Dizziness
            (2) Abdominal distention
            (3) Polyuria (impaired concentrating ability) and polydipsia
         (b) Myocardial manifestations of hypokalemia
            (1) General: increased myocardial excitability or irritability
            (2) Associated dysrhythmias: premature atrial complex (PAC), premature ventricular contraction (PVC), sinus bradycardia, paroxysmal atrial tachycardia, atrioventricular (AV) blocks, AV dissociation, junctional dysrhythmias, and ventricular tachycardia
            (3) Increased incidence of ectopy with digoxin administration

ii. Expected outcomes
  (a) Serum potassium level remains above 3.5 mEq/L or within asymptomatic range
  (b) Cardiac function is within normal limits
iii. Nursing interventions
  (a) Provide cardiac monitoring: observe for ECG changes and presence of dysrhythmias
  (b) Monitor serum potassium levels
  (c) Record the amount of urine output and other drainage (gastric aspirate, diarrhea) to aid in calculating total body potassium balance
  (d) Recognize and treat signs of alkalosis
  (e) Administer oral potassium supplements when indicated: dilute to prevent gastrointestinal irritation and to facilitate absorption
  (f) Never give IV potassium chloride rapidly: large concentrations can precipitate hyperkalemia, producing a necrotic effect on the vessel wall and possibly inducing ventricular fibrillation
  (g) Determine whether the patient is receiving digitalis or diuretics: correct potassium losses, since these can precipitate digitalis toxicity and decrease the effectiveness of most diuretics
  (h) Emergency treatment
    (1) Slowly administer IV potassium chloride while the patient is monitored with an ECG for dysrhythmias
    (2) Monitor for signs and symptoms of hyperkalemia
    (3) Maintain a record of serum potassium levels to assess the adequacy of replacement therapy
  (i) Follow-up: if the patient is receiving digitalis and diuretics, consider potassium chloride supplements or potassium-sparing diuretics
iv. Evaluation of nursing care
  (a) Asymptomatic serum potassium levels are above 3.5 mEq/L
  (b) There are no cardiac complications of hypokalemia

Electrolyte Imbalances—Sodium Imbalance: Hypernatremia

The serum sodium level in hypernatremia is above 145 mEq/L.

1. **Pathophysiology**
   a. Increased ECF volume: sodium and water retention
   b. Less total body water in relation to the quantity of body sodium, with increased amounts of water loss in comparison to the amount of sodium loss

2. **Etiologic or precipitating factors**
   a. Normal kidneys: lack of ADH or neurohypophyseal insufficiency (e.g., diabetes insipidus, water loss in excess of salt)
      i. Potassium depletion: causes a concentrating defect in the kidney, leading to polyuria
      ii. Hypercalcemia: polyuria and dehydration
      iii. Drugs (e.g., osmotic diuretics or sodium bicarbonate, or sodium choride solution); also mineralocorticoids, laxatives, and antacids
      iv. Excessive adrenocortical secretion
      v. Loss of the thirst mechanism (e.g., in a comatose patient)

      vi. Uncontrolled diabetes mellitus with osmotic diuresis secondary to hyperglycemia

    b. Abnormal renal function: inability of renal tubules to respond to ADH (nephrogenic diabetes insipidus, decrease in GFR, causing stimulation of aldosterone release)

3. Nursing assessment data base

    a. Nursing history (see Hyperkalemia)

      i. Subjective findings

        (a) Patient's chief complaint

          (1) Complaints associated with "edematous states" and hypoproteinemia: excessive weight gain and possibly shortness of breath

          (2) Complaints associated with "dehydration states" (sodium retention, water loss): extreme thirst, febrile conditions, decreased urine output, and dry mucous membranes

        (b) Other signs and symptoms: muscle weakness and a change in volume of urine output

      ii. Objective findings

        (a) Etiologic or precipitating factors

          (1) Presence of hyperadrenocortical secretion

          (2) Absence of the thirst mechanism (patients older than age 65 or comatose)

          (3) Diabetes mellitus

          (4) Hypercalcemia

          (5) Episodes of dehydration

          (6) Episodes of overhydration

          (7) Renal tubule disease

          (8) Established history of dietary abuse, noncompliance with fluid and sodium restriction, or episodes of large water volume loss without an equal sodium loss

        (b) Medication history

          (1) Laxatives and antacids: contain high sodium content (e.g., sodium bicarbonate)

          (2) Diuretics: promote a greater loss of water than sodium

          (3) Corticosteroids: conserve sodium and waste potassium

        (c) Other

          (1) Dietary restrictions: diet and fluid restrictions with modifications of sodium

          (2) Renal replacement therapy: dialysis

    b. Nursing examination of patient

      i. Inspection

        (a) Neurologic: restlessness, irritability, lethargy, confusion to coma, twitching, and seizures

        (b) Respiratory: labored breathing associated with pulmonary edema (dyspnea)

        (c) Genitourinary

          (1) Oliguria or anuria with dehydration

          (2) Polyuria with osmotic diuresis

         (d) Gastrointestinal: anorexia

        (e) Integument: dry, flushed skin; dry mucous membranes; edematous tongue; pitting edema

(f) Musculoskeletal: muscle weakness
ii. Palpation: thready, weak pulse with increased ECF, and tachycardia with decreased ECF
iii. Auscultation: hypertension with increased ECF and hypotension with decreased ECF
c. Diagnostic studies: laboratory evaluation
  i. Serum sodium level above 145 mEq/L and elevated hematocrit
  ii. Serum osmolality greater than 295 mOsm/L
  iii. Urine specific gravity greater than 1.030
  iv. Urine osmolality 800 to 1400 mOsm/L
  v. Urine sodium greater than 40 mEq/L when hypernatremia is due to sodium excess and normal to low sodium value during a water deficit

4. Nursing diagnoses
a. Risk of electrolyte excess: hypernatremia
  i. Assessment for defining characteristics
    (a) Manifestations of hypernatremia (see Nursing assessment data base)
    (b) Manifestations of dehydration (water loss only)
      (1) Warm, flushed, dry skin and mucous membranes with poor skin turgor
      (2) Initial elevated body temperature
      (3) Hypotension with or without postural changes
      (4) Initial tachycardia, progressing to bradycardia
      (5) Thirst
  ii. Expected outcomes
    (a) Sodium in a normal range or in a high, asymptomatic range
    (b) Normal fluid status
  iii. Nursing interventions
    (a) Monitor for complications of hypernatremia
      (1) If the ECF volume (increased sodium and water) is increased, edematous states lead to hypertension, high cardiac output, and pulmonary congestion
      (2) If sodium retention occurs in the presence of water loss, severe dehydration leads to hypotension, increased serum osmolality, shock, and respiratory arrest
      (3) General: neuromuscular involvement can lead to coma, seizures, and death
    (b) For hypernatremia caused by excessive water losses
      (1) Attempt to lower the plasma sodium level by water replacement
      (2) Administer water in excess of sodium if the patient requires volume (5% dextrose in water [D5W] or one-half normal saline or both)
      (3) Monitor serum sodium levels, serum osmolality, and urine osmolality
      (4) Assess the hydration status: too rapid a correction can lead to acute pulmonary edema
        a) Maintain intake and output records
        b) Monitor body weight
      (5) Perform neurologic assessments and correlate with serum sodium levels

        (c) For hypernatremia with normal hydration status and sodium retention

            (1) Determine precipitating factors and treat as ordered

            (2) Correct gradually by encouraging sodium losses via diuretics or by administering fluids

            (3) Be aware that too rapid a correction of sodium levels can cause cerebral edema

            (4) Monitor serum and urine sodium levels and osmolality levels

            (5) Assess neurologic status

     iv. Evaluation of nursing care

        (a) Sodium level is asymptomatic

        (b) Serum osmolality is 280 to 295 mOsm/L

        (c) Urine osmolality is within a normal range

        (d) Hydration status is normal

Electrolyte Imbalances—Sodium Imbalance: Hyponatremia

The serum sodium level in hyponatremia is below 136 mEq/L.

1. Pathophysiology

    a. Excess of water relative to the amount of sodium in the body, producing a dilutional effect on the sodium concentration

    b. Salt (NaCl) loss in excess of water loss

2. Etiologic or precipitating factors

    a. Water excess: excessive water intake without salt; SIADH secretion

    b. Sodium depletion

      i. Diuretics

      ii. Diarrhea

     iii. Nasogastric suction

     iv. Abnormal losses via diaphoresis

      v. Salt-losing renal diseases: interstitial nephritis

     vi. Hyperglycemia (glucose-induced diuresis)

    vii. Bartter's syndrome (hyponatremia, hypokalemia, hypomagnesemia, metabolic alkalosis, and hyperreninemia)

    c. Congestive heart failure and cirrhosis of the liver

      i. Decreased cardiac output increases water retention by the kidneys

      ii. Kidneys may retain larger amounts of water

3. Nursing assessment data base

    a. Nursing history

      i. Subjective findings

        (a) Patient's chief complaints

          (1) Complaints associated with dehydration: thirst and muscle weakness

          (2) Complaints associated with overhydration: edema and muscle weakness

        (b) Other signs and symptoms

          (1) Increased or decreased urine output

          (2) Limitations of accomplishing activities of daily living, exercise, and ambulation

     ii. Objective findings

        (a) Etiologic or precipitating factors

           (1) Hypoactive adrenal gland

           (2) Renal tubular disease (sodium-wasting nephritis)

           (3) Aggressive diuretic therapy

           (4) Prolonged episodes of vomiting or diarrhea

           (5) History of dietary abuse, noncompliance with fluid and sodium intake requirements, or episodes of both water and sodium loss

        (b) Medication history

           (1) Diuretics: cause loss of sodium and water

           (2) Laxatives: cause sodium loss via the stool

      (c) Other: renal replacement therapy (dialysis)

   b. Nursing examination of patient

     i. Inspection

        (a) Neurologic: malaise, confusion to coma, seizures, headache

        (b) Respiratory: dyspnea with pulmonary edema

        (c) Genitourinary: normal urine output to polyuria

        (d) Gastrointestinal: abdominal cramps

        (e) Integument: poor skin turgor

     ii. Palpation: rapid pulse with water overload

     iii. Auscultation

        (a) Increased or decreased CVP

        (b) Blood pressure: may range from hypotension to normal to hypertension

        (c) Crackles with fluid overload

   c. Diagnostic study findings: laboratory

     i. Serum sodium level below 136 mEq/L and decreased hematocrit caused by water excess

     ii. Urine volume and specific gravity can be normal

     iii. Urine sodium less than 20 mEq/L if it is due to a sodium deficit and normal to elevated if it is due to water excess

4. Nursing diagnoses

   a. Risk of electrolyte deficit: hyponatremia

     i. Assessment for defining characteristics

        (a) Manifestations of hyponatremia (see preceding)

           (1) Malaise, confusion to coma

           (2) Headache

           (3) Muscular weakness

           (4) Weight loss

           (5) Poor skin turgor

           (6) Decreased CVP

           (7) Abdominal cramps, nausea

           (8) Urinary sodium under 20 mEq/L

           (9) Permanent neurologic changes; can occur with a serum sodium level below 110 mEq/L

        (b) Manifestations of water intoxication

           (1) Headache

           (2) Confusion to delirium, seizures

           (3) Weight gain

           (4) Good skin turgor

           (5) Decreased hematocrit, BUN

    (6) Increased CVP; elevated JVP

    (7) Serum osmolality below 280 mOsm/L

    (8) Normal or increased urinary sodium above 25 mEq/L

    (9) Increased risk of pulmonary edema

  ii. Expected outcomes

   (a) Serum sodium level is within normal limits or at an asymptomatic level

   (b) Normal fluid status is maintained

  iii. Nursing interventions

   (a) For sodium and water losses

    (1) Administer a diet high in sodium with adequate fluid intake

    (2) Anticipate fluid replacement with normal or hypertonic saline. Watch carefully for pulmonary edema

    (3) Obtain serum sodium and urine sodium and osmolality concentrations to determine the effectiveness of therapy

    (4) Monitor neurologic signs

    (5) Discontinue diuretic agents if they are implicated in the etiology

    (6) Maintain I&O records

   (b) For water intoxication

    (1) Restrict fluid intake (a restriction of 500 ml/day may be appropriate)

    (2) Administer diuretics if ordered

    (3) Monitor serum sodium levels to determine whether sodium replacement is indicated as normal fluid status is restored

    (4) Monitor neurologic status

    (5) Do not give hypertonic saline in SIADH secretion. Saline does not correct the basic cause and may precipitate CHF

    (6) In SIADH secretion, restrict all water intake because decreased sodium is a result of an inability to excrete water normally

  iv. Evaluation of nursing care

   (a) Asymptomatic sodium levels

   (b) Urinary sodium above 30 to 40 mEq/L

   (c) Normal hydration status

Electrolyte Imbalances—Calcium Imbalance: Hypercalcemia

The serum calcium level in hypercalcemia is above 10.5 mg/dl.

1. **Pathophysiology**
   a. Increased mobilization of calcium from bone occurs in primary hyperparathyroidism, immobilization, and thyrotoxicosis
   b. Increased intestinal reabsorption of calcium may occur with large dietary intake or excessive administration of vitamin D
   c. Altered renal tubular reabsorption of calcium occurs
2. **Etiologic or precipitating factors**
   a. Primary hyperparathyroidism causes increased tubular reabsorption of calcium

b. Metastatic carcinoma with ''osteolytic lesions'' and multiple myeloma; hypercalcemia is the result of lesions releasing calcium into plasma
c. Hypophosphatemia
d. Immobilization: prolonged bed rest causes calcium to be mobilized from bones, teeth, and intestines
e. Alkalosis: increases calcium binding to protein; decreases serum calcium levels
f. Thyrotoxicosis
g. Excessive doses of vitamin D increase reabsorption of calcium from the intestine
h. Drugs: thiazide diuretic therapy inhibits calcium excretion
i. Renal tubular acidosis

3. **Nursing assessment data base**
   a. Nursing history
      i. Subjective findings
         (a) Patient's chief complaints: lethargy and muscle weakness
         (b) Other signs and symptoms
             (1) Anorexia, nausea, and vomiting
             (2) Increased fatigue
             (3) Increased urine output
             (4) Constipation
      ii. Objective findings
         (a) Etiologic or precipitating factors: presence of those identified previously
         (b) Medication history
             (1) Vitamin D (excessive intake)
             (2) Calcium supplements (excessive intake)
             (3) Thiazide diuretics
   b. Nursing examination of patient
      i. Inspection
         (a) Neurologic: lethargy, confusion, coma, and subtle personality changes
         (b) Cardiovascular: if the patient is taking digitalis, hypercalcemia may enhance digitalis effects, which can contribute to dysrhythmias or cardiac arrest
         (c) Genitourinary: polyuria, flank and thigh pain associated with renal calculi
         (d) Gastrointestinal: nausea, vomiting, and inadequate peristalsis related to the hypotonicity of smooth muscle of the bowel, leading to constipation
         (e) Musculoskeletal: hypotonicity and weakness of muscles, pathologic fractures, and metastatic calcifications
         (f) Other: observe for metastatic calcifications, usually calcium crystals deposited in the cornea and visible by slit-lamp examination. If these changes are extensive, they will be visible to the naked eye as band keratopathy (semilunar whitish bands, beginning as ''parentheses'' at the lateral margins of the cornea and extending in a band across the cornea)
   c. Diagnostic studies
      i. Laboratory
         (a) Serum calcium level above 10.5 mg/dl

       (b) Sulkowitch's urine test for calcium
- ii. Radiologic
  - (a) Renal calculi
  - (b) Calcium deposits visible on bone films
  - (c) Nephrocalcinosis: calcium deposits in renal parenchyma
- iii. Special: ECG reveals shortening of the ST segment

4. Nursing diagnoses
- a. Risk of electrolyte excess: hypercalcemia
  - i. Assessment for defining characteristics (see preceding)
    - (a) Additional manifestations of hypercalcemia
      - (1) Headache
      - (2) Abdominal pain
      - (3) Hypertension (occurs in 33% of all cases)
      - (4) Deep bone pain
      - (5) Polydipsia secondary to polyuria
    - (b) Myocardial manifestations of hypercalcemia: ECG changes reveal shortened ST segment and AV blocks that may progress to cardiac arrest
  - ii. Expected outcomes
    - (a) Calcium stays within normal limits or in an asymptomatic range
    - (b) Cardiac function is normal
  - iii. Nursing interventions
    - (a) Provide cardiac monitoring
    - (b) If administering digitalis, do so cautiously. Hypercalcemia enhances the action of digitalis, and toxicity can result
    - (c) Monitor I&O record and status of renal function
    - (d) Anticipate the use of therapies to reduce serum calcium level
      - (1) Normal saline infusion and diuretics reduce calcium absorption
      - (2) Corticosteroids decrease gastrointestinal absorption of calcium
      - (3) Mithramycin therapy stimulates bone uptake of calcium
      - (4) Oral phosphate binds calcium
    - (e) Monitor serum calcium levels to determine the effectiveness of interventions
  - iv. Evaluation of nursing care
    - (a) Asymptomatic calcium level
    - (b) Normal neuromuscular and cardiac function

Electrolyte Imbalances—Calcium Imbalance: Hypocalcemia

The serum calcium level in hypocalcemia is below 8.5 mg/dl.
1. Pathophysiology
- a. Excessive gastrointestinal losses of calcium secondary to diarrhea, diuretics, and increased levels of lipoproteins
- b. Malabsorption syndromes, such as vitamin D deficiency and hypoparathyroidism

2. Etiologic or precipitating factors

   a. Hypoparathyroidism
- i. Surgical ablation of parathyroids
- ii. Parathyroid adenoma
- iii. Idiopathic
- iv. Depletion of magnesium: needed for effective action of PTH

   b. CRF
- i. Hyperphosphatemia: potentiates peripheral deposition of calcium
- ii. Vitamin D resistance: inability to absorb calcium from the intestine; vitamin D mediated

   c. Vitamin D deficiency secondary to CRF, hepatic failure, and rickets: "active" vitamin D is necessary for calcium absorption

   d. Chronic malabsorption syndrome resulting from:
- i. Magnesium depletion
- ii. Gastrectomy
- iii. High-fat diet: fat impairs calcium absorption
- iv. Small bowel disorder: inability to absorb vitamin D

   e. Increased thyrocalcitonin: stimulates osteoblasts to prevent calcium entry into serum

   f. Malignancy
- i. Osteoblastic metastasis: calcium is consumed for abnormal bone synthesis
- ii. Medullary carcinoma of thyroid: abnormal secretion of thyrocalcitonin

   g. Acute pancreatitis: precipitation of calcium in an inflamed pancreas and intra-abdominal lipids

   h. Hyperphosphatemia: calcium and phosphate bind together and precipitate in tissues
- i. Cytotoxic drugs (cytolysis of bone)
- ii. Increased oral intake of phosphates
- iii. CRF (decreased excretion of phosphate)

3. Nursing assessment data base

   a. Nursing history
- i. Subjective findings
  - (a) Patient's chief complaints: muscle and abdominal cramps
  - (b) Other symptoms
    - (1) Bone pain
    - (2) Lethargy
    - (3) Constipation
    - (4) Nausea and vomiting
    - (5) Functional and physical limitations (ambulation and exercise)
- ii. Objective findings
  - (a) Etiologic or precipitating factors
    - (1) Presence of CRF
    - (2) Starvation or history of dietary abuse
    - (3) Malabsorption syndrome
    - (4) Noncompliance with phosphate binders
    - (5) Carcinoma with metastasis
    - (6) Acute pancreatitis
    - (7) Massive infection of subcutaneous tissue

(b) Medication history
    (1) Phosphate binders–gels administered in renal failure to bind phosphate in the gut, leaving calcium free to be absorbed
    (2) Vitamin D supplements: promote calcium absorption
    (3) Calcium supplements
    (4) Diuretics: promote renal loss of calcium
(c) Other: renal replacement therapy

b. Nursing examination of patient
  i. Inspection
    (a) Neurologic: lethargy, muscle tremors, and cramps may accompany minor reductions in calcium level
    (b) Respiratory: labored and shallow breathing, wheezes, and bronchospasm if the respiratory musculature is involved Neuromuscular irritability can cause airway obstruction and bronchial spasm
    (c) Cardiovascular: dysrhythmias
    (d) Genitourinary: oliguria or anuria secondary to obstruction by renal calculi
    (e) Gastrointestinal: distended abdomen secondary to constipation or diarrhea
    (f) Musculoskeletal: tetany and generalized tonic-clonic seizures develop with severe reductions
    (g) Other: bruising or bleeding. Bleeding can occur secondary to changes in the clotting mechanism because calcium is necessary for normal clotting
  ii. Palpation
    (a) Chvostek's sign: tap a finger on the supramandibular portion of the parotid gland and observe twitches in the upper lip on side of stimulation. This muscle spasm indicates a positive test
    (b) Pulses: irregular secondary to dysrhythmias
  iii. Auscultation
    (a) Bowel sounds: absent secondary to paralytic ileus
    (b) Trousseau's sign: apply a blood pressure cuff to the upper arm and inflate
      (1) If carpopedal spasm results, the test is positive
      (2) If no spasm appears in 3 minutes, the test is negative
      (3) Remove the cuff and tell the patient to hyperventilate (30 times/min)
      (4) Respiratory alkalosis that develops can also produce a carpopedal spasm (a positive result if it occurs)

c. Diagnostic studies: serum calcium level below 8.5 mg/dl

4. Nursing diagnoses
a. Risk of electrolyte deficit: hypocalcemia
  i. Assessment for additional defining characteristics (see Nursing examination of patient)
    (a) Manifestations of hypocalcemia
      (1) Tetany: early signs include numbness and tingling of the extremities and around the oral cavity
      (2) Laryngeal stridor: may predispose to respiratory arrest
      (3) Increased incidence of fractures
      (4) Decreased cardiac output predisposing to cardiac arrest

(b) Myocardial manifestations of hypocalcemia
    (1) ECG changes: prolonged ST segment and QT interval
    (2) Impaired myocardial contractility: may lead to hypotension, heart failure, and cardiac arrest

ii. Expected outcomes
    (a) Serum calcium level is within normal limits, and patient is asymptomatic
    (b) There is no evidence of complications from hypocalcemia

iii. Nursing interventions
    (a) Provide cardiac monitoring
    (b) Administer 10% calcium gluconate or calcium chloride slowly IV (1 ml/minute) for emergency interventions: monitor for decreased cardiac output, enhanced digitalis effects, and dysrhythmias
    (c) Chronic hypocalcemia necessitates daily oral doses of calcium, usually administered in the range of 1.5 to 3 g/day
    (d) Administer vitamin D supplements, if ordered
    (e) With phosphate deficiency, replace phosphates before administering calcium. Hyperphosphatemia usually accompanies this imbalance
    (f) Monitor serum calcium and phosphate levels
    (g) Implement seizure precautions; provide a quiet environment
    (h) Monitor respiratory status; bronchospasm may precipitate respiratory arrest
    (i) Teach patients warning signs of tetany or seizures, and instruct them to report the immediate onset of these symptoms
    (j) Monitor the therapeutic effectiveness via Chvostek's and Trousseau's signs plus ECG

iv. Evaluation of nursing care
    (a) Patient is asymptomatic, and calcium level is within normal limits
    (b) There is no neuromuscular or cardiac involvement

Electrolyte Imbalances—Phosphate Imbalance: Hyperphosphatemia

The serum phosphate level in hyperphosphatemia is above 4.5 mg/dl.

1. Pathophysiology
    a. Inability to excrete phosphate via the kidney because of a decrease in GFR to one tenth of normal or because of renal failure
    b. Excessive intake due to dietary or cathartic abuse and drugs (cytotoxic agents)

2. Etiologic or precipitating factors
    a. Acute or chronic renal failure (inability to excrete phosphate)
    b. Hypoparathyroidism: PTH causes hypophosphatemia and lowers body phosphate
    c. Cathartic abuse or phosphate-containing laxatives or enemas
    d. Cytotoxic agents for neoplasms: serum phosphate increases as a result of cytolysis
    e. Overadministration of IV or oral phosphates

3. **Nursing assessment data base**
    a. Nursing history
        i. Subjective findings
            (a) Patient's chief complaint: muscle cramping
            (b) Other symptoms: seizures, joint pain
        ii. Objective findings
            (a) Etiologic or precipitating factors
                (1) Renal failure
                (2) Vague neurologic complaints
                (3) Seizures of unknown origin
                (4) Metastatic calcifications
                (5) Hypocalcemia
                (6) Noncompliance with the use of phosphate-binding gel
            (b) Medication history: the following are prescribed for hyperphosphatemia:
                (1) Phosphate-binding gels: promote binding of phosphate in the intestines and prevent phosphate absorption
                (2) Calcium supplement: if hypocalcemia is present
            (c) Other renal replacement therapy
    b. Nursing examination of patient: presents with vague symptomatology similar to hypocalcemia
        i. Inspection
            (a) Neurologic: seizures caused by a chronic phosphate elevation that can depress calcium levels, precipitating the seizure
            (b) Musculoskeletal: joint pain secondary to the precipitation of calcium and/or phosphate in soft tissue and joints
    c. Diagnostic study findings
        i. Laboratory: serum phosphate greater than 4.5 mg/dl
        ii. Special: ECG changes comparable with those seen in hypocalcemia
4. **Nursing diagnoses**
    a. Risk of electrolyte excess: hyperphosphatemia
        i. Assessment for defining characteristics: synonymous with assessment parameters provided for hypocalcemia. A natural inverse relationship exists between these two ions, so that hyperphosphatemia leads to a reciprocal hypocalcemia
        ii. Expected outcomes
            (a) Phosphate level stays within normal limits or within a safe asymptomatic range
            (b) There are no episodes of tetany or seizures
        iii. Nursing interventions
            (a) Administer aluminum hydroxide gels to bind phosphate in the intestines, limiting its absorption and thus reducing serum phosphate levels
            (b) Teach the patient the purpose of gels (they are easy to confuse with antacids because of the similarity in drug preparation)
            (c) Monitor serum phosphate and calcium levels to determine the effectiveness of therapy
            (d) Implement dialysis for the rapid correction of hyperphosphatemia if necessary
            (e) Administer acetazolamide to increase urinary phosphate excretion via a normal kidney
        iv. Evaluation of nursing care

(a) Serum phosphate level is within normal limits

(b) There is no neuromuscular symptomatology

. . . .

Electrolyte Imbalances—Phosphate Imbalance: Hypophosphatemia

The serum phosphate level in hypophosphatemia is below 3.0 mg/L.

1. **Pathophysiology**
   a. Increased cell uptake to form sugar phosphates: occurs during hyperventilation or glucose administration
   b. Decreased phosphate absorption from the bowel
   c. Renal phosphate wasting (loss of proximal tubular function): seen in Fanconi's syndrome and vitamin D–resistant rickets

2. **Etiologic or precipitating factors**
   a. Inadequate phosphate intake (seen in chronic alcoholism)
   b. Chronic phosphate depletion: occurs in osteomalacia and rickets
   c. Long-term hyperalimentation lacking in phosphates. Glucose phosphorylation uses phosphate and can lead to phosphate depletion if no replacement is available
   d. Hyperparathyroidism: causes renal phosphaturia
   e. Malabsorption syndrome
   f. Abuse or overadministration of phosphate-binding gels
   g. Fanconi's syndrome: loss of phosphates in urine, leading to osteomalacia (adults)

3. **Nursing assessment data base**
   a. Nursing history
      i. Subjective findings
         (a) Patient's chief complaints: vague, including muscle weakness, muscle wasting, and fatigue
         (b) Other symptoms: confusion, lack of appetite, changes in weight, and impaired ambulation
      ii. Objective findings
         (a) Etiologic or precipitating factors
            (1) Presence of metabolic acidosis
            (2) Alcohol abuse without adequate nutritional intake
            (3) Starvation
            (4) Renal failure
            (5) Malabsorption syndrome
         (b) Medication history
            (1) Phosphate binders: overuse
            (2) Diuretics: prolonged use may (rarely) lead to phosphate depletion
         (c) Other: renal replacement therapy
   b. Nursing examination of patient
      i. Inspection
         (a) Neurologic: confusion, malaise
         (b) Respiratory: dyspnea secondary to hypoxia resulting from a deficit in the erythrocyte phosphate content necessary for 2,3-diphosphoglycerate (2,3-DPG). Shortness of breath can also be the result of cardiac failure
         (c) Genitourinary: decreased urine output secondary to cardiac failure

(d) Integument: cool skin secondary to decreased cardiac output. Myocardial contractility diminishes because of inadequate intracellular phosphates

(e) Musculoskeletal: muscle weakness and wasting

   (1) Symptoms result from acute depletion of intracellular phosphate, which leads to a diffuse muscle-wasting necrosis called rhabdomyolysis

   (2) Skeletal changes occur with long-standing hypophosphatemia, which results from excessive losses of external phosphate

ii. Palpation: tachycardia secondary to a decrease in cardiac output

iii. Auscultation

   (a) Hypotension

   (b) Crackles secondary to cardiac failure

c. Diagnostic study findings

   i. Laboratory: serum phosphate level below 3.0 mg/dl, low serum alkaline pyrophosphate level, and high serum pyrophosphate level

   ii. Hypercalcemia and hypercalciuria: indicators of acute phosphate depletion in hyperparathyroidism; PTH increases serum calcium by taking it from bone and decreases serum phosphate by excreting it into urine

   iii. Radiologic: skeletal abnormalities resembling osteomalacia (i.e., pseudofractures characterized by thickened periosteum and new bone formation over what appears to be an incomplete fracture)

4. Nursing diagnoses

a. Risk of electrolyte deficit: hypophosphatemia

   i. Assessment for defining characteristics (see preceding)

      (a) Manifestations of hypophosphatemia

         (1) Anorexia

         (2) Malaise

         (3) Muscle wasting and weakness

         (4) Hemolysis and hypoxia

      (b) Manifestations of hypercalcemia: hypophosphatemia creates a reciprocal hypercalcemia

   ii. Expected outcomes

      (a) Asymptomatic serum phosphate level

      (b) No neuromuscular signs of hypophosphatemia

   iii. Nursing interventions

      (a) Treat primary cause of hypophosphatemia

      (b) Replace phosphates intravenously, then orally

      (c) Discontinue phosphate-binding gels

      (d) Monitor phosphate and calcium levels

   iv. Evaluation of nursing care

      (a) Asymptomatic phosphate level

      (b) Absence of neuromuscular involvement

Electrolyte Imbalances—Magnesium Imbalance: Hypermagnesemia

The serum level in hypermagnesemia is above 2.5 mEq/L.

1. **Pathophysiology**
   a. Decreased excretion secondary to renal failure
   b. Increased magnesium intake
   c. Acidosis
2. **Etiologic or precipitating factors**
   a. Renal failure
   b. Adrenal insufficiency
   c. Excessive intake or administration of magnesium-containing antacid gels or laxatives
   d. Acidotic states (e.g., diabetic ketoacidosis)
3. **Nursing assessment data base**
   a. Nursing history
      i. Subjective findings: patient's chief complaints are muscle weakness and fatigue
      ii. Objective findings
         (a) Etiologic or precipitating factors
            (1) Renal failure
            (2) Laxative or antacid abuse
            (3) Adrenal insufficiency
            (4) Diabetes mellitus
            (5) Acidosis
         (b) Medication history
            (1) Laxatives: milk of magnesia or others containing magnesium
            (2) Antacids: containing magnesium hydroxide
   b. Nursing examination of patient
      i. Inspection
         (a) Neurologic: lethargy to coma
         (b) Respiratory: depressed respirations to apnea
         (c) Cardiovascular: bradycardia
         (d) Musculoskeletal: muscle weakness, loss of deep tendon reflexes, and seizures
      ii. Auscultation: hypotension secondary to depressed myocardial contractility can progress to cardiac arrest
   c. Diagnostic study findings
      i. Laboratory serum magnesium level over 2.5 mEq/L
      ii. ECG: peaked T wave similar to that in hyperkalemia
4. **Nursing diagnoses**
   a. Risk of electrolyte excess: hypermagnesemia
      i. Assessment for defining characteristics (see earlier)
         (a) Sudden onset of vague neuromuscular symptomatology (lethargy, confusion, coma, seizures)
         (b) Depressed respiratory rate
         (c) Cardiac involvement: bradycardia, peaked T wave, and signs of depressed myocardial contractility
      ii. Expected outcomes
         (a) Serum magnesium level returns to within normal limits
         (b) There is no neuromuscular or cardiac involvement
      iii. Nursing interventions
         (a) Determine the primary cause of hypermagnesemia and intervene
         (b) Consider dialysis if excesses are due to renal failure

(c) Teach the patient to avoid medications containing magnesium

(d) Observe for respiratory distress and support the patient symptomatically while decreasing the magnesium level.

(e) If renal function is normal, administer diuretics or saline-induced diuresis to encourage magnesium loss. During the period of diuresis, maintain I&O record to prevent dehydration, which may exacerbate symptoms

(f) Monitor ECG and neurologic signs

(g) Monitor serum magnesium levels

(h) Consider calcium gluconate administration to minimize symptoms of increased magnesium

    iv. Evaluation of nursing care

(a) Magnesium levels are asymptomatic

(b) There are no neuromuscular or cardiac complications

Electrolyte Imbalances—Magnesium Imbalance: Hypomagnesemia

The serum level in hypomagnesemia is below 1.5 mEq/L.

1. Pathophysiology

    a. Decreased intake of magnesium

    b. Diminished intestinal reabsorption

    c. Excess losses in urine, a wound, or extracellular drainage

    d. Alkalosis (in some instances)

    e. Excessive adrenal corticoid secretions

2. Etiologic or precipitating factors

    a. Starvation and malabsorption syndrome

    b. Bartter's syndrome

    c. Prolonged hyperalimentation without adequate magnesium replacement

    d. Excessive diuretic therapy

    e. Toxemia of pregnancy

    f. Excessive fistula or gastrointestinal losses containing magnesium (e.g., severe diarrhea, nasogastric suction without replacement)

    g. Chronic alcoholism

    h. Alkalotic states (in some instances)

    i. Excessive corticosteroid administration

    j. Hypocalcemia

    k. Hypoparathyroidism

    l. Hyperaldosteronism

    m. Hyperthyroidism

    n. Acute and chronic pancreatitis

    o. Cisplatin treatment for cancer

3. Nursing assessment data base

    a. Nursing history

        i. Subjective findings

(a) Patient's chief complaints: muscle weakness or tremors

(b) Other symptoms: anorexia, nausea, and dizziness

        ii. Objective findings

(a) Etiologic or precipitating factors (see earlier)

         (b) Medication history

            (1) Diuretics

            (2) Corticosteroids with an aldosterone component may precipitate hypomagnesemia

        (c) Other: renal replacement therapy

    b. Nursing examination of patient

      i. Inspection

        (a) Neurologic: lethargy, confusion, and coma

        (b) Cardiovascular: dysrhythmias

        (c) Musculoskeletal: hyperirritability, tremors, facial twitching, and seizures

      ii. Palpation

        (a) Pulse: irregular secondary to dysrhythmias or enhanced digitalis effect

        (b) Positive Chvostek's sign

      iii. Auscultation

        (a) Blood pressure: normal to decreased

        (b) Positive Trousseau's sign

    c. Diagnostic study findings

      i. Laboratory: serum magnesium levels below 1.5 mEq/L

      ii. ECG: flat or inverted T waves, possible ST segment depression, and prolonged QT interval

4. Nursing diagnoses

    a. Risk of electrolyte deficit: hypomagnesemia

      i. Assessment for defining characteristics

        (a) Vague neurologic symptoms that may have sudden onset without obvious explanations, such as confusion, coma, tremors to tetany, ataxia, psychosis, and seizures

        (b) Anorexia and nausea

        (c) Dizziness

        (d) Muscle weakness

      ii. Expected outcomes

        (a) Serum magnesium level returns to normal, especially in acute myocardial infarction

        (b) Absence of neuromuscular symptoms

      iii. Nursing interventions

        (a) Administer magnesium sulfate 50% IM or IV. In acute myocardial infarction, the infusion rates and amount of IV magnesium dosing vary from 33 mmol to 91.6 mmol

        (b) Consider the administration of calcium gluconate when replacing large boluses of magnesium. Calcium retards the effects of sudden reversal to hypermagnesemia

        (c) If hypokalemia occurs simultaneously with hypomagnesemia, correct the magnesium deficit first

        (d) Be aware that hypomagnesemia enhances digitalis, causing digitalis toxicity

        (e) Correct alkalosis

        (f) Establish seizure precautions

        (g) Monitor serum magnesium levels

        (h) Monitor ECG changes

        (i) Consider dietary replacement (seafood, green vegetables, whole grains, and nuts)

iv. Evaluation of nursing care
  (a) Level of magnesium is asymptomatic
  (b) There are no neuromuscular symptoms

Renal Trauma

This problem occurs most often in men between the ages of 20 and 40 years.

1. **Pathophysiology:** renal trauma may result from the combination of an applied force and the hydrostatic pressure generated within this liquid-containing organ, the kidney. Following are the results of renal tissue trauma:
   a. Disruption of the renal system caused by:
      i. Nonpenetrating injuries (blunt trauma): 80% to 90% of all renal injuries
      ii. Penetrating injuries: 10% to 20% of all renal injuries
   b. Classifications of renal injury according to severity
      i. Contusions: constitute approximately 85% of all renal injuries (e.g., subcapsular hematomas, minor cortical lacerations). The renal collecting system is not involved
      ii. Lacerations: deep renal parenchyma injury (10% of all renal injuries). Damage can involve the renal collecting system
      iii. Fractures: extensive lacerations at various sites in the renal parenchyma, with collecting system damage
      iv. Vascular or pedicle injuries: renal arterial intima tears or vessel disruptions. Renal arterial tears cause blood collections between the intima and the intact media, usually leading to thrombosis, sometimes of the entire vessel's length
2. **Etiologic or precipitating factors**
   a. Nonpenetrating renal injuries
      i. Vehicular accident (e.g., impact with dashboard, steering wheel)
      ii. Impact to the abdomen or flank after an assault or a sports injury
      iii. Sudden deceleration or acceleration accidents (e.g., pedestrian-vehicular accident or falls from significant heights). These accidents typically precipitate vascular injuries
   b. Penetrating renal injuries: associated with a high incidence of intraperitoneal visceral injury, hemorrhage, fistulas, and infections
      i. Gunshot wounds
      ii. Stab wounds
      iii. Vehicular crashes
      iv. Industrial accidents
      v. Other sources of trauma
3. **Nursing assessment data base**
   a. Nursing history (acute event)
      i. Subjective findings
         (a) Patient's chief complaint: pain in the flank or an upper quadrant of the abdomen
      ii. Objective findings
         (a) Etiologic or precipitating factors: history of a traumatic incident
         (b) Family history
            (1) Description of the family unit
            (2) Adequacy as a support system

(c) Social history: alcohol or drug abuse

(d) Medication history: medications taken by the patient prior to trauma

b. Nursing examination of patient

i. Inspection

(a) Abdomen: observe the abdomen and flanks for symmetry

(b) Genitourinary

(1) Observe the external genitalia, perineum, and urethral meatus for blood or ecchymosis

(2) Inspect for type of trauma to provide indicators of renal injury

a) High-velocity trauma: contributes to secondary renal necrosis, fistula, hemorrhage, and infection. Significant renal trauma with hemorrhage may require nephrectomy

b) Low-velocity trauma: associated with a low incidence of complications

c) Nonpenetrating injury: should be suspected on a description of the abdomen, back, or lower chest as the site of trauma

(3) Monitor signs and symptoms of blunt or penetrating wound in the region of the kidneys indicating renal injury. Note that injuries from blunt trauma may initially lack a typical clinical picture of renal trauma

a) Costovertebral angle pain

b) Renal colic: from clots obstructing the collecting system

c) Hematoma over the posterior aspect of the 11th or 12th rib or in the flank area (absence of hematoma does not rule out renal injury in 24% of all cases)

d) Flank mass

e) Hematuria, gross or microscopic: a common sign suggesting renal injury; however, a correlation does not exist between the degree of hematuria and the extent of the injury

f) Fractured ribs overlying the kidney

g) Ecchymosis at the site of entrance wounds in the lateral abdomen and the flank

h) Tenderness in the flank or an upper quadrant of the abdomen; crepitation or contusion in the flank

i) Retroperitoneal bleeding

ii. Palpation

(a) Palpate the suprapubic areas and the flanks for tenderness, masses, or the presence of rib fractures

(b) Palpate the pelvis for fractures

iii. Percussion: to determine the presence of a collection of fluid or solid material

iv. Auscultation: blood pressure is normal to decreased secondary to blood loss or a response to trauma

v. Other: examine other organ systems for injuries concomitant with renal injury (60% to 80% incidence), such as the liver, colon, lung, spleen, small bowel, stomach, pancreas, duodenum, and diaphragm

c. Diagnostic studies
   i. Laboratory
      (a) Serum
         (1) BUN and creatinine: an elevation of BUN indicates a catabolic process in the trauma victim or a hypovolemic state. An elevation of both BUN and creatinine levels indicates significant renal injury
         (2) Hematocrit and hemoglobin: a decrease indicates hemorrhage; origin must be determined
         (3) Electrolytes: a variety of results may occur. Potassium level usually is elevated secondary to leakage from cells because of trauma, acidosis, or catabolism. Other values usually reflect a decrease if the actual loss has occurred through a wound or fistula drainage
      (b) Urine
         (1) Volume: may be diminished if significant renal damage or obstruction or hypovolemia is present
         (2) Urinalysis: erythrocytes and protein may be present, but renal trauma can still exist without this response
         (3) Hematuria: gross or microscopic
   ii. Radiologic examination
      (a) Plain film of the abdomen
         (1) Rib fractures over the kidney
         (2) Obliteration of a renal or psoas shadow
         (3) Displacement of the bowel
      (b) High-dose infusion pyelogram: to establish the status of the uninvolved kidney as well as the traumatized organ. Results suggestive of renal injury are:
         (1) Delayed excretion of dye
         (2) Renal outline enlargement
         (3) Diminished concentration of contrast media level in renal parenchyma: outlines the collecting system and ureters
         (4) If the patient is in shock, a radiologic examination should include only the first two studies
      (c) Tomography: particularly helpful when a nonpenetrating injury is suspected. Establishes an 80% to 95% accuracy for the location and extent of renal parenchymal damage. To perform this examination, the patient must maintain a systolic blood pressure above 90 mm Hg
      (d) Ultrasonography: has a minimal value in interpreting a nonpenetrating injury. The study can determine renal parenchymal injury and locate a hematoma
      (e) Renal scan: determines the status of renal blood flow and the presence of parenchymal injury
      (f) Retrograde pyelography: provides minimal information and can contaminate the traumatized victim
      (g) Renal angiography: a more precise examination tool when an injury is not clearly defined by other radiologic studies. Is indicated in cases of continuous bleeding that impairs visualization or causes extravasation of contrast medium

(h) Computed tomography (CT): provides an exact means for determining the extent of an injury

(i) Surgical exploration: is usually indicated for all hematomas. If exploration reveals a major laceration, then repair can occur immediately

4. Nursing diagnoses

a. Decreased tissue perfusion related to fluid volume deficit and hemorrhage

   i. Assessment for defining characteristics

    (a) Hypotension

    (b) Cool, clammy skin

    (c) Tachycardia, dysrhythmias

    (d) Decreased hematocrit and hemoglobin

    (e) Shortness of breath, Kussmaul respirations

    (f) Evidence of frank bleeding may occur, such as an enlarged abdomen

    (g) Restlessness, confusion, lassitude, feelings of impending doom

    (h) Hematuria: gross or microscopic

  ii. Expected outcomes

    (a) Hemodynamic stability is maintained

    (b) Fluid and blood volume are adequately replaced

 iii. Nursing interventions

    (a) Monitor for systemic complications of renal trauma

      (1) Ileus

      (2) Hemorrhage or rebleeding

      (3) Extravasation of urine

      (4) Sepsis

      (5) Shock

      (6) Impairment or loss of renal function

      (7) Fistula formation

      (8) Perinephric or renal abscess

      (9) Late complications: hypertension, hydronephrosis, chronic pyelonephritis, calculus formation, and intrarenal calcification

    (b) Initial period

      (1) Maintain patent airway

      (2) Provide adequate oxygenation

      (3) Control hemorrhage

      (4) Type and cross-match blood

      (5) Establish multiple IV lines in major vessels with at least one central line

      (6) Reestablish normal fluid and blood volume

      (7) Obtain frequent vital signs

      (8) Obtain laboratory data: serum electrolytes, BUN, creatinine, amylase, ABG, CBC

    (c) After minor injury

      (1) Maintain bed rest

      (2) Monitor hematocrit and hemoglobin levels

      (3) Monitor the presence of hematuria

      (4) Obtain vital signs and report any sudden changes

      (5) Provide analgesics

        (6) Administer broad-spectrum antibiotics as prescribed

        (7) Begin ambulation once urine clears of gross hematuria

        (8) Be aware that renal tissue heals from a minor injury within 4 to 6 weeks

    (d) After major injury

        (1) Administer fluids as warranted

        (2) Maintain I&O record

        (3) Provide analgesics

        (4) Provide preventive pulmonary maintenance therapies

        (5) Administer broad-spectrum antibiotics as prescribed; renal parenchyma is susceptible to infection secondary to hematuria, ischemia, and urinary extravasation

        (6) Obtain urine for culture and analysis

        (7) Obtain hematocrit, hemoglobin, electrolytes, BUN, and creatinine values

        (8) Monitor vital signs; hypertension may be a sign of constricting parenchymal fibrosis

        (9) Maintain patency of Penrose drain (usually placed in the renal fossa to extrude liquefying hematoma)

       (10) Monitor the presence of hematuria

       (11) Provide adequate nutrition

       (12) Ambulate on the first postoperative day

  iv. Evaluation of nursing care

    (a) Stable vital signs; acceptable ABG values

    (b) Homeostatic fluid, electrolyte, and protein status

    (c) Injuries managed to prevent complications and promote healing

b. Risk of extravasation of urine related to renal trauma

  i. Assessment for defining characteristics

    (a) Midline bulging: from an overdistended bladder

    (b) Lower quadrant distention: indicative of fluid collection

    (c) Lower abdominal pain or mass: resulting from a bladder rupture and the presence of extravasated urine

    (d) Fluid collection on sides of abdomen or thighs

    (e) Abdominal palpation reveals pain, possibly indicative of peritonitis secondary to urine extravasation

    (f) Severe abdominal pain and rebound tenderness that may reflect severe, advancing peritonitis

    (g) Presence of hematuria (not always present): microscopic or gross

    (h) Anuria (rare)

    (i) Indications for surgery

        (1) Shattered kidney: nephrectomy is indicated

        (2) Vascular injuries

        (3) Deep renal lacerations (controversial)

        (4) Pulsatile hematoma

        (5) Urinary extravasation

        (6) Expanding hematoma

        (7) Necrotic renal parenchyma

        (8) Continually decreasing hematocrit

  ii. Expected outcomes

    (a) Renal and genitourinary integrity is restored

    (b) Infection is prevented

(c) Follow-up care of the renal system is obtained

iii. Nursing interventions

(a) Assess the presence and extent of renal and urinary tract trauma

(b) Obtain a urine sample on admission to the emergency department

(c) Be aware that an inability to void warrants catheterization. When a catheter cannot be passed because of increased resistance, a radiologic examination of the urinary tract is indicated. Catheters should never be forced because obstruction suggests trauma or hematoma

(d) Blood passage through a catheter necessitates removal of the catheter. Urology consultation must immediately follow

(e) Assess urine for hematuria, commonly associated with a ruptured bladder

(f) Observe for signs of extravasated urine (see preceding assessment for defining characteristics)

(g) Note that extravasated urine contributes to infection (i.e., peritonitis) in the trauma victim. Monitor temperature closely

(h) Provide adequate fluid replacement to sustain urine output. Hypotension or hypovolemia contributes to oliguria or anuria, but these two urinary output patterns may also result from renal trauma. Massive muscle breakdown secondary to trauma may contribute to rhabdomyolysis, which may cause renal tubular blockage

(i) Prepare the patient for surgery if indicated

(j) Maintain the patency of the catheter; constant irrigation may be prescribed

(k) Provide effective pain management

(l) Provide aseptic wound care

iv. Evaluation of nursing care

(a) Renal function remains intact

(b) Urinary collecting tract remains patent

(c) There is no infection

(d) Wound heals

References

PHYSIOLOGIC ANATOMY

Barchman, M. J., and Bernard, D. B.: Clinical and laboratory evaluation of altered renal function. *In* Krane, R. J., Siroky, M. B., and Fitzpatrick, J. M. (eds.): Clinical Urology. Philadelphia, J. B. Lippincott, 1994.

Brenner, B. M.: The Kidney, 4th ed. Philadelphia, W. B. Saunders, 1991.

Gilbert, B. R., Leslie, B. R., and Vaughan, E. D.: Normal Renal Physiology. *In* Walsh, P. C., Retik, A. B., Stamey, T. A., and Vaughan, E. D. (eds.): Campbell's Urology. Philadelphia, W. B. Saunders, 1992, pp. 70–90.

Hunter, S.: When your patient needs a contrast dye injection. Nursing 26(1):32c–32d, 1996.

Knox, D. M., and Martof, M. T.: Effects of drug therapy on renal function of healthy older adults. J. Gerontol. Nurs. 4(2):35–40, 1995.

Kruse, J. A.: Acid-base interpretations. *In* Prough, D. S., and Traystman, R. J. (eds.): Critical Care: State of the Art. Anaheim, Calif., Society of Critical Care Medicine. 14:275–298, 1993.

Radke, K. J.: The aging kidney: Structure, function, and nursing implications. ANNA J. 21(4):181–193, 1994.

Stark, J.: Interpreting BUN and creatinine levels. Nursing 24:58–61, 1994.

Stark, J.: The renal system. *In* Alspach J. G. (ed.): Core Curriculum for Critical Care Nursing, 4th ed. Philadelphia, W. B. Saunders, 1991.

NURSING ASSESSMENT DATA BASE/ COMMONLY ENCOUNTERED NURSING DIAGNOSES

Brasfield, K.: Renal and fluids clinical assessment. *In* Thelan, L. A., Davie, J. K., and Urden, L. D. (eds.):

Textbook of Critical Care Nursing: Diagnosis and Management. St. Louis, Mosby-Year Book, 1990, pp. 622–626.

Espinel, C. H.: Diagnosis of acute and chronic renal failure. Clin. Lab. Med. 13(1):89–102, 1993.

Gokal, R.: Quality of life in patients undergoing renal replacement therapy. Kidney Int. Suppl. 40:S23–S27, 1993.

Killington, A.: Psychosocial impact of renal disease. Br. J. Nurs. 2(18):905–908, 1993.

Kim, M. J., McFarland, G. K., and McLane, A. M.: Pocket Guide to Nursing Diagnosis, 6th ed. St. Louis, Mosby-Year Book, 1995.

Meyer, K. B.: The outcomes of ESRD and its treatment. Adv. Ren. Replace. Ther. 2(2):101–111, 1995.

Pfettscher, S. A.: Assessment of the learner: Physiological readiness. Adv. Ren. Replace. Ther. 2(3):191–198, 1995.

Porter, G. A.: Assessing the outcome of rehabilitation in patients with end-stage renal disease. Am. J. Kidney Dis. 24 (Suppl.):S22–S27, 1994.

Seidel, H. M., Ball, J. W., and Dains, J. E.: Physical Examination, 2nd ed. St. Louis, Mosby-Year Book, 1991, pp. 403–456.

Szczepanik, M. E.: Assessment and selection considerations: ESRD patient and family education materials and media. Adv. Ren. Replace. Ther. 2(3):207–216, 1995.

Wilson, R. F.: Critical Care Manual, 2nd ed. Philadelphia, F. A. Davis, 1992, pp. 565–751.

ACUTE RENAL FAILURE

Ardaillou, R., Dussaule, J. C., Michael, D., et al.: Renal effects of atrial natriuretic factor and control of its secretion in various diseases. Adv. Nephrol. 19:145–186, 1990.

Ash, S. R., and Bever, S. L.: Peritoneal dialysis for ARF: The safe, effective and low cost modality. Adv. Ren. Replace. Ther. 2(2):160–163, 1995.

Baer, C. L.: Acute renal failure: Recognizing and reversing its deadly course. Nursing 20:34–39, 1990.

Baer, C. L., and Lancester, L. E.: Acute renal failure. Crit. Care Nurs. Q. 14(4):1–21, 1992.

Baud, L., and Ardaillou, R.: Reactive oxygen species: Production and role in the kidney. Am. J. Physiol. 251:F765–F776, 1986.

Bellomo, R., and Ronco, C.: Adequacy of dialysis in ARF of the critically ill: The case for continuous therapies. Int. J. Artif. Organs 19(2):129–142, 1996.

Bellomo, R., and Mehta, R.: Acute renal replacement in the intensive care unit: Now and tomorrow. New Horiz. 3(4):760–767, 1995.

Berstein, A. D., and Hold, A. W.: Vasoactive drugs and the importance of renal perfusion pressure. New Horiz. 3(4):650–661, 1995.

Bohler, J.: Treatment of ARF in ICU patients. Int. J. Artif. Organs 19(2):108–110, 1996.

Bosworth, C.: SCUF/CAVH/CAVHD: Critical differences. Crit. Care Nurs. Q. 14(4):45–55, 1992.

Brady, H. R., and Singer, G. G.: Acute renal failure. Lancet 346:1533–1540, 1995.

Breslow, M. J.: Hemodynamic changes in sepsis: Pathophysiology and treatment. A critical care medicine review. In Prough, D. S., and Traystman, R. J. (eds.): Critical Care: State of the Art. Anaheim, Calif., Society of Critical Care Medicine. 14:299–320, 1993.

Brivet, F. G., Kleinknecht, D. J., and Loirat, P.: Acute renal failure in ICU: Causes, outcomes and prognostic factors of hospital mortality. A prospective, multicenter study. Crit. Care Med. 24(2):192–198, 1996.

Dolleris, P. M.: Diuretic and vasopressor usage in acute renal failure: A synopsis. Crit. Care Nurs. Q. 14(4):28–31, 1992.

Douglas, S.: Acute tubular necrosis. AACN Clin. Issues Crit. Care Nurs. 9(3):688–697, 1992.

Eliahou, H. E., Marcusohn, G., and Knecht, A.: A multiple system organ failure is gradually replacing isolated ATN in severe trauma. In Timio M., and Wizman, V. (eds.): Cardionephrology. Milan, Italy, Wichtig Editore, 1991.

Fry, D. E., Pearlstein, L., and Fulton, R. L.: Multiple system organ failure: The role of uncontrolled infection. Arch. Surg. 151:136–140; 1980.

Gaudio, K. M., Stromski, M., Thulu, G., Ardito, T., Kashgarian, M., and Siegel, N. S.: Post-ischemic hemodynamics and recovery of renal adenosine triphosphate. Am. J. Physiol. 251:F603–F609, 1986.

Golper, T. A., and Price, J.: Continuous venovenous hemofiltration for acute renal failure in the ICU setting. ASAIO J. 40(4):936–939, 1994.

Guerriero, W. G.: Initial assessment of medical management of patients with urologic trauma. Probl. Urology 2:269–278, 1988.

Hagland, M.: Making sense of continuous renal replacement therapy. Nurs. Times 90(40):37–39, 1994.

Heyman, S. N., Fuchs, S., and Brezis, M.: The role of indwelling ischemia in ARF. New Horiz. 3(4):597–605, 1995.

Higley, R. R.: Continuous arteriovenous hemofiltration: A case study. Crit. Care Nurse 16(5):37–43, 1996.

Hulman, P., and Wolfson, M.: The patient with acute renal failure. Hosp. Med. 29(7):82–95, 1994.

Ito, S., Carretero, O. A., and Ale, K: Nitric oxide in the regulation of renal blood flow. New Horiz. 3(4):615–623, 1995.

Johnson, J. P., and Rokawh, M. D.: Sepsis or ischemia in experimental ARF: What have we learned? New Horiz. 3(4):608–614, 1995.

Kelleher, R. M.: Dialysis in the surgical intensive care patient: A case study. Crit. Care Nurs. Q. 14(4):72–77, 1992.

Kellerman, P. S., and Molitoris, B. A.: Pathogenetic mechanisms of ischemic acute renal failure. In Jacobson, H. R., Striler, G. E., and Klahr, S. (eds.): The Principles and Practices of Nephrology. Philadelphia, B. C. Decker, 1992.

Kierdorf, H. P.: The nutritional management of ARF in the intensive care unit. New Horiz. 3(4):689–707, 1995.

Kierdorf, H., and Sieberth, H. G.: Continuous treatment modalities in ARF. Nephrol. Dial. Transplant. 10(11):2001–2003, 1995.

Kirby, S., and Davenport, A.: Haemofiltration/dialysis treatment in patients with acute renal failure. Care Crit. Ill. 12(2):154–158, 1996.

Knaus, W. A., Draper, E. A., and Wagner, D. P.: Prognosis in acute organ system failure. Ann. Surg. 202:685–693, 1985.

Krane, N. K.: A systemic approach to azotemia. J. Am. Acad. Phys. Assist. AAPA. 3(7):529–533, 1990.

Levy, E. M., Viscoli, C. M., and Horwitz, R. I.: The effect of ARF on mortality: A cohort analysis. J.A.M.A. 275(9):1489–1494, 1996.

Martin, S. J., and Danziger, L. H.: Continuous infusion of loop diuretics in the critically-ill: A review of the literature. Crit. Care Med. 22(8):1323–1329, 1994.

Mehler, P. S., Schrier, R. W., and Anderson, R. J.: Clinical presentation and prognosis of acute renal failure. In:

Jacobson, H. R., Striker, G. E., and Klahr, S. (eds.): The Principles and Practice of Nephrology. Philadelphia, B. C. Decker, 1992.

Peschman, P.: Acute hemodialysis: Issues in the critically-ill. AACN Clin. Issues Crit. Care Nurs. 3(3):545–557, 1992.

Pinson, J. M.: Preventing complications in the CAVH patient. Dimens. Crit. Care Nurs. 11(5):242–248, 1992.

Ronco, C., and Bellmo, R.: Basic mechanisms and definitions for CRRT. Int. J. Artif. Organs 19(2):95–99, 1996.

Schetz, M., Ferdinande, P., and Vanden Berghe, G.: Pharmacokinetics of continuous renal replacement therapy. Intensive Care Med. 21(7):612–620, 1995.

Stark, J.: Acute tubular necrosis: Differences between oliguria and nonoliguria in acute renal failure. Crit. Care Q. 14(4):22–27, 1992.

Stark, J.: Dialysis options in the critically ill patient: Hemodialysis, peritoneal, and continuous renal replacement therapy in acute renal failure. Crit. Care Nurs. Q. 14(4):40–44, 1992.

Stark, J.: Dialysis choices: Turning the tide in acute renal failure. Nursing 27(2):41–48, 1997.

Strohschein, B. L., Caruso, D. M., and Greene, K. A.: Continuous venovenous hemofiltration. Am. J. Crit. Care 3(2):92–99, 1994.

Valle, B. K., Valle, G. A., and Lemburg, L.: Volume control: A reliable option in the management of "refractory" congestive heart failure. Am. J. Crit. Care 4(20):169–173, 1995.

Weinman, M.: Natriuretic peptides and acute renal failure. New Horiz. 3(4):624–633, 1995.

CHRONIC RENAL FAILURE

Acchiaedo, S. R.: Uremia and adequate dialysis treatment. Semin. Nephrol. 14(3):274–281, 1994.

Annis, C., Ransdell, R., and Annis, C.: Patient education: A continuing repetitive process. ANNA J. 23(2):217–221, 1996.

Bhatla, B., Khanna, R., and Twardowski, Z. J.: Peritoneal access. J. Postgrad. Med. 40(3):170–178, 1994.

Buckalew, V. M.: Pathophysiology of progressive renal failure. South. Med. J. 87(10):1028–1033, 1994.

Brown, T. E., and Carter, B. E.: Hypertension and end stage renal disease. Ann. Pharmacother. 28(3):359–366, 1994.

de Zeeuw, D., Apperloo, A. J., and de Jong, P.: Management of CRF. Curr. Opin. Nephrol. Hypertens. 1(1):116–123, 1992.

Dunn, S. A.: How to care for the dialysis patient. Am. J. Nurs. 93(6):26–34, 1993.

Felsenfeld, A. J., and Llach, F.: Parathyroid gland function in chronic renal failure. Kidney Int. 43(4):771–789, 1993.

Green, I.: Laboratory tests in ESRD patients undergoing dialysis. Health Technol. Assess. 2:1–12, 1994.

Hayslip, D. M., and Suttle, C. D.: Pre-ESRD patient education: A review of the literature. Adv. Ren. Replace. Ther. 2(3):217–226, 1995.

Levin, N. W.: Adequacy of dialysis. Am J. Kidney Dis. 24(2):308–315, 1994.

Lowrie, E. G.: Chronic dialysis treatment: Clinical outcomes and related processes of care. Am. J. Kidney Dis. 24(2):255–266, 1996.

Mason, N. A.: Drug-nutrient interactions in renal failure. J. Ren. Nutr. 5(4):214–220, 1995.

McCormick, T. R.: Ethical issues in caring for patients with renal failure. ANNA J. 20(5):549–555, 1993.

Nolph, K. D.: Peritoneal dialysis update 1994. J. Postgrad. Med. 40(3):151–157, 1994.

Olsen, J.: Clinical Pharmacology Made Ridiculously Simple. Miami, Med Master, Inc., 1994.

Packer, K. P.: Dream content and subjective sleep quality in stable patients on chronic dialysis. ANNA J. 23(2):201–211, 1996.

Paganini, E. P.: In search of an optimal hematocrit level in dialysis patients: Rehabilitation and quality of life implications. Am. J. Kidney Dis. 24(Suppl. 1):S10–S16, 1996.

Price, C. A.: Issues related to the care of the critically ill patient with end stage renal failure. AACN Clin. Issues Crit. Care Nurs. 3(3):585–596, 1992.

Stark, J.: Renal management. Crit. Care Nurs. Clin. North Am. 2(1):53–138, 1990.

Steinman, T. I.: Kidney protection: how to prevent or delay CRF. Geriatrics 51(8):28–35, 1996.

Summerton, H.: End stage of renal failure: The challenge to the nurse. Nurs. Times 91(6):27–29, 1995.

Wagner, C. D.: Family needs of chronic hemodialysis patients: A comparison of perception of nurses and families. ANNA J. 23(1):19–26, 1996.

Wilson, B. M.: Promoting compliance: The patient-provider partnership. Adv. Ren. Replace. Ther. 2(3):199–206, 1995.

RENAL TRANSPLANT

Barry, J. M.: Renal transplant. In Walsh, P. C., Retick, A. B., Staney, T. A., and Vaughan, E. D. (eds.): Campbell's Urology. Philadelphia, W. B. Saunders, 1992, pp. 1501–2518.

Barry, J. M.: Renal transplant. In Krane, R. J., Siroky, M. B., and Fitzpatrick, J. M. (eds.): Clinical Urology. Philadelphia, J. B. Lippincott, 1994.

Coolican, M. B., Stark, J., Doka, K. J., and Coor, C. A.: Education about death, dying, and bereavement in nursing programs. Nurse Educ. 6(3):591–598, 1994.

McKay, D. B., Milford, E. L., and Sayegh, M. H.: Clinical aspects of renal transplantation. In Brenner, B. M. (ed.): The Kidney, 5th ed. Philadelphia, W. B. Saunders, 1996, pp. 2602–2652.

Stark, J., Boller, J., and Morse, M.: The nurse moderator role in making the critical difference. Crit. Care Nurs. Clin. North Am. 6(3):587–590, 1994.

Stark, J., Wikoren, B., and Martone, L.: Partners in organ donation: Piloting a successful nurse requestor program. Crit. Care Nurs. Clin. North Am. 6(3):591–598, 1994.

ELECTROLYTE IMBALANCES

Abraham, W. T., and Schroer, R. W.: Body fluid volume regulation in health and disease. Adv. Intern. Med. 39:23–47, 1994.

Allon, M.: Hyperkalemia in end-stage disease: Mechanisms and management. J. Am. Soc. Nephrol. 6(4):1134–1142, 1995.

Braxmeyer, D. L., and Keyes, J. L.: The pathophysiology of potassium balance. Crit. Care Nurse 16(5):59–71, 1996.

Chenevey, B.: Overview of fluids and electrolytes. Nurs. Clin. North Am. 22(4):749–759, 1987.

Devecchi, A. F.: Adequacy of fluid/sodium balance and

blood pressure control. Perit. Dial. Int. 14(Suppl. 3):S110–S116, 1994.

Eckart, J., and Neeser, G.: Management of fluid balance. Int. J. Artif. Organs 19(2):106–107, 1996.

Goldsmith, W. K., Auden, J., and Chernow, B.: Magnesium and calcium: Two keys to unlocking the dilemmas of cardiovascular diseases. *In* Prough, D. S., and Traystman, R. J. (eds.): Critical Care: State of the Art. Anaheim, Calif., Society of Critical Care Medicine. 14:169–206, 1993.

Halperin, M. L.: Fluid, Electrolyte, and Acid-Base Physiology: A Problem-Based Approach, 2nd ed. Philadelphia, W. B. Saunders, 1994.

Hutchison, A. J., and Gokal, R.: Adequacy of calcium and phosphate balance in peritoneal dialysis. Perit. Dial. Int. 14(Suppl. 3):S117–S122, 1994.

Innerarity, S. A.: Hyperkalemic emergencies. Crit. Care Nurs. Q. 14(4):32–39, 1992.

Innerarity, S. A., and Stark, J. L.: Fluid and Electrolytes, 3rd ed. Springhouse, Pa., Springhouse, 1997.

Kupin, W. L., and Narins, R. G.: The hyperkalemia of renal failure: Pathophysiology, diagnosis, and therapy. Contrib. Nephrol. 102(1):1–22, 1993.

Leunissen, K. M.: Fluid status in hemodialysed patients. Nephrol. Dial. Transplant. 10(2):153–155, 1995.

Nora, N. A., and Singer, I.: Interpretation of hypercalcemia in a patient with end-stage renal disease. Arch. Intern. Med. 152(6):1321–1322, 1992.

Schrier, R. W.: Renal and Electrolyte Disorders, 4th ed. Boston, Little, Brown & Co., 1992.

Sciarini, P., and Dungan, J. M.: A holistic approach for management of fluid volume excess in hemodialysis patients. ANNA J. 23(3):299–305, 1996.

Torralbo, A., Portoles, J., Perez, A. J., and Barrientos, A.: Hypomagnesemic hypocalcemia in chronic renal failure. Am. J. Kidney Dis. 21(2):167–171, 1993.

Toto, K. H.: Regulation of plasma osmolality: The thirst and vasopressin. Crit. Care Nurs. Clin. North Am. 6(4):661–674, 1994.

Winchester, J. F., Rotellar, C., Goggins, M., Robino, D., Rakowski, T. A., and Argy, W. P.: Calcium and phosphate balance in dialysis patients. Kidney Int. Suppl. 41:5174–5178, 1993.

Zeidel, M. L., Strange, K., Emma, F., and Harris, H. W.: Mechanism and regulation of water transport in the kidney. Semin. Nephrol. 13(2):155–167, 1993.

RENAL TRAUMA

Better, O. S.: Preventing acute renal failure in trauma victims. Physician Assist. 16(8):41–44, 1992.

Carpinito, G. A.: Lower urinary tract trauma. *In* Krane, R. J., Siroky, M. B., and Fitzpatrick, J. M. (eds.): Clinical Urology. Philadelphia, J. B. Lippincott, 1994.

Dixon, D. M., Carroll, P. R., and McAvinch, J. W.: The Management of Renal and Ureteral Trauma. *In* Krane, R. M., Siroky, M. B., and Fitzpatrick, J. M. (eds.): Clinical Urology. Philadelphia, J. B. Lippincott, 1994.

Lazar, L.: Conservative treatment of an injured hydronephrotic kidney: The role of percutaneous nephrostomy. J. Trauma. 40(2):304–305, 1996.

Peters, P. C., and Sagalowsky, A. I.: Genitourinary trauma. *In* Walsh, P. C., Retick, A. B., Stamey, T. A., and Vaughan, E. D. (eds.): Campbell's Urology. Philadelphia, W. B. Saunders, 1992, pp. 1571–1594.

Schmidlin, F. R., Schmid, P., and Kurtyka, T.: Force transmission and stress distribution in a computer-simulated model of the kidney: An analysis of the injury mechanisms in renal trauma. Trauma 40(5):791–795, 1996.

Stamatos, C. A., and Reed, E.: Nutritional needs of trauma patients: Challenges, barriers, and solutions. Crit. Care Clin. North Am. 6(3):501–514, 1994.

Stark, J.: Acute renal failure in trauma: Current perspectives in multiple systems organ failure. Crit. Care Nurs. Q. 16(4):49–60, 1994.

VonRueden, K. T., and Dunham, C. M.: Sequelae of massive fluid resuscitation in trauma patients. Crit. Care Clin. North Amer. 6(3):463–472, 1994.

chapter

● **5**

································

⁞

⁞... The Endocrine System

Kim Litwack, Ph.D., R.N., CPAN, CAPA, FAAN

PHYSIOLOGIC ANATOMY

················
⁞
⁞ **Foundational Concepts**

1. **Definition of a hormone**
   a. Molecules are synthesized and secreted by specialized cells and released into the blood, exerting biochemical effects on target cells away from the site of origin
   b. Hormones control metabolism, transport of substances across cell membranes, fluid and electrolyte balance, growth and development, adaptation, and reproduction
2. **Chemically categorized by physiologic action**
   a. Peptide or protein hormones: vasopressin (antidiuretic hormone [ADH]) thyrotropin-releasing hormone (TRH), insulin, growth hormone (GH [somatotropin]), follicle-stimulating hormone (FSH), luteinizing hormone (LH), corticotropin (adrenocorticotropic hormone [ACTH]), calcitonin
   b. Steroids: aldosterone, cortisol, estradiol, progesterone, testosterone
   c. Amines and amino acid derivatives: norepinephrine, epinephrine, triiodothyronine (T_3), thyroxine (T_4)
3. **Hormone receptors**
   a. Specificity of hormone action is determined by the presence of a specific hormone receptor on or in the target cell
   b. Receptors distinguish hormones from each other and translate the hormonal signal into a cellular response
   c. The hormone-receptor complex initiates intracellular events that lead to the biologic effects of the hormone acting on the target cell
4. **Mechanisms of hormone action**
   a. Activation of cyclic adenosine monophosphate (cAMP), thyrotropin (thyroid-stimulating hormone [TSH]), ACTH, parathyroid hormone (PTH), and ADH
   b. Activation of genes: steroid hormones and gonadal hormones
5. **Feedback control of hormone production** (Fig. 5–1)
   a. Feedback control can be positive (low hormone levels stimulating the

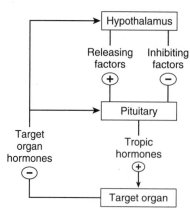

Figure 5-1 • Regulatory feedback loops of the hypo-thalamic-pituitary-target organ axis. (From Wilson, J., and Foster, D.: Williams Textbook of Endocrinology, 7th ed. Philadelphia, W. B. Saunders, 1985.)

release of its controlling hormone) or negative (high hormone levels inhibiting the release of its controlling hormone)
   b. Feedback control systems allow self-regulation and prevent hormonal overproduction

Pituitary Gland

1. **Location**: base of skull in sphenoid bone. Connected to hypothalamus by the pituitary stalk, which links the nervous and endocrine systems
2. **Composition**
   a. Anterior lobe (adenohypophysis: 75% of gland): hormones controlled by hypothalamic releasing or inhibiting hormones in response to stimuli received in the central nervous system
   b. Posterior lobe (neurohypophysis: 25% of gland)
      i. Hormones are controlled by nerve fibers originating in hypothalamus and terminating in posterior pituitary gland
      ii. Hormones are synthesized in hypothalamus, stored in posterior pituitary, and released after activation of the cell bodies in the nerve tract
3. **Anterior pituitary hormones**
   a. GH
      i. Regulation of secretion
         (a) Stimulation: growth hormone–releasing hormone (GRH) in response to physical and/or emotional stress, starvation, hypoglycemia, other protein-depleted states
         (b) Inhibition: somatostatin from hypothalamus, postprandial hyperglycemia, and pharmacologic doses of corticosteroids
      ii. Physiologic activity
         (a) Increases rate of protein synthesis
         (b) Increases lipolysis
         (c) Decreases protein catabolism
         (d) Decreases carbohydrate use
         (e) Stimulates bone and cartilage growth
         (f) Works with insulin, thyroid hormone, and sex steroids to promote growth
      iii. Disorders resulting from dysfunction

(a) Excess: gigantism (prepubertal), acromegaly (postpubertal)

(b) Deficiency: dwarfism (prepubertal)

b. ACTH

   i. Regulation of secretion

      (a) Stimulation: corticotropin-releasing hormone (CRH) in response to physical and/or emotional stress, trauma, hypoglycemia, hypoxia, surgery, decreased plasma cortisol levels

      (b) Inhibition: increased plasma cortisol levels exert negative feedback on CRH and ACTH. Stress can overcome this negative feedback

   ii. Physiologic activity: production and release of adrenocortical hormones (glucocorticoids, adrenal androgens, and mineralocorticoids)

   iii. Disorders resulting from dysfunction

      (a) Excess: Cushing's disease

      (b) Deficiency: adrenal insufficiency (chronic), addisonian crisis (acute)

c. TSH

   i. Regulation of secretion

      (a) Stimulation: TRH in response to concentration of thyroid hormone

      (b) Inhibition: somatostatin from hypothalamus, increased thyroid hormone levels

   ii. Physiologic activity

      (a) Increases synthesis of thyroid hormone

      (b) Releases stored thyroid hormone

      (c) Stimulates iodide uptake into thyroid cells

      (d) Increases size, number, and secretory activities of thyroid cells

   iii. Disorders resulting from dysfunction: see Thyroid Gland section

d. Other anterior pituitary hormones under hypothalamic control

   i. LH

   ii. FSH

   iii. Prolactin

4. Posterior pituitary hormones

a. ADH

   i. Regulation of secretion

      (a) Stimulation: increase in plasma osmolality, hypoxia, reduction in blood volume or blood pressure

      (b) Inhibition: a decrease in plasma osmolality

   ii. Physiologic activity

      (a) Increases water permeability in renal collecting duct epithelial cells, thereby controlling extracellular fluid osmolality

      (b) In pharmacologic amounts, constricts arterioles to increase blood pressure

   iii. Disorders resulting from dysfunction

      (a) Excess: syndrome of inappropriate ADH (SIADH) secretion

      (b) Deficiency: diabetes insipidus

b. Oxytocin

   i. Dilatation of cervix, vagina, lower segment of the uterus, and nipple stimulation, causes reflex release of oxytocin

ii. Oxytocin stimulates uterine contractions and milk ejection during lactation

Thyroid Gland

1. **Location**: immediately below larynx laterally and anterior to the trachea
2. **Composition**: two lobes connected by an isthmus
   a. Follicular cells produce T_3 and T_4
   b. Parafollicular cells (C cells): produce thyrocalcitonin
3. **Regulation of secretion** (thyroid hormone)
   a. Stimulation: TSH stimulates thyroid hormone release, which is regulated by TRH from the hypothalamus. Decreased levels of thyroid hormone stimulate TSH and TRH
   b. Inhibition: elevated thyroid hormone levels inhibit TSH and TRH
4. **Physiologic activity**
   a. Increases metabolic activity of cells, resulting in increased oxygen consumption, increased rate of chemical reactions, and heat production
   b. Stimulates carbohydrate, fat, and protein metabolism
   c. Works with insulin, GH, and sex steroids to promote growth
   d. Critical in fetal neural and skeletal system development: intrauterine hypothyroidism causes cretinism
   e. Positive chronotropic and inotropic effects on the heart
   f. Required for normal hypoxic and hypercapneic drive in respiratory centers
   g. Increases erythropoiesis
   h. Increases metabolism and clearance of steroid hormone and insulin
5. **Disorders resulting from dysfunction**
   a. Thyroid enlargement (goiter)
   b. Excess: hyperthyroidism (chronic), thyroid storm (acute)
   c. Deficiency: hypothyroidism (chronic), myxedema coma (acute)
   d. Complications of hyperthyroidism: Graves' disease
6. **Thyrocalcitonin** (calcitonin)
   a. Regulation of secretion
      i. Stimulation: increase in calcium levels
      ii. Inhibition: decrease in calcium levels
   b. Physiologic activity
      i. Decreases blood calcium by inhibiting calcium mobilization from bone and decreasing calcium resorption in kidney
      ii. Decreases phosphate levels by inhibiting bone remodeling and by increasing phosphate loss in urine
   c. Disorders resulting from dysfunction are usually not significant because calcitonin is a relatively weak hypocalcemic agent in humans
   d. Used as a pharmacologic agent to control hypercalcemia of malignancy

Parathyroid Glands

1. **Location**: four glands on posterior surface of thyroid gland
2. **Composition**: chief cells release PTH
3. **Regulation of secretion**
   a. Stimulation: decrease in serum calcium

b. Inhibition: increase in serum calcium and in vitamin D metabolites, hypermagnesemia, and hypomagnesemia

4. **Physiologic activity**
   a. Kidney
      i. Increases renal tubular reabsorption of calcium and magnesium
      ii. Decreases renal tubular reabsorption of phosphate and bicarbonate
      iii. Stimulates formation of active form of vitamin D
   b. Gastrointestinal tract: increases calcium absorption
   c. Bone: larger amounts increase calcium reabsorption

5. **Disorders resulting from dysfunction**
   a. Excess: hypercalcemia results from hyperparathyroidism
   b. Deficiency: hypocalcemia results from hypoparathyroidism

Adrenal Glands

1. **Location**: retroperitoneal, superior to kidney
2. **Composition**: two separate endocrine tissues that produce distinct hormones
   a. Cortex (90% of gland) produces aldosterone, glucocorticoids, and adrenal androgens
   b. Medulla (10% of gland) produces catecholamines
3. **Cortical hormones**
   a. Glucocorticoids (cortisol is major hormone)
      i. Regulation of secretion
         (a) Stimulation: ACTH
         (b) Inhibition: cortisol exerts negative feedback on the anterior pituitary and hypothalamus
      ii. Physiologic activity
         (a) Carbohydrate metabolism
            (1) Increases gluconeogenesis
            (2) Decreases glucose uptake in muscle and adipose tissue (insulin-antagonistic effect)
         (b) Protein metabolism
            (1) Decreases protein stores and protein synthesis in all cells except liver
            (2) Increases protein catabolism
            (3) Promotes gluconeogenesis
         (c) Promotes lipolysis
         (d) Increases tissue responsiveness to other hormones, such as glucagon and catecholamines
         (e) Anti-inflammatory effects
            (1) Decreased migration of inflammatory cells to sites of injury
            (2) Inhibition of production and/or activity of vasoactive substances
            (3) Prevention of immune response to tissue antigens released by injury
      iii. Disorders resulting from dysfunction
         (a) Excess: Cushing's syndrome
         (b) Deficiency: Addison's disease (chronic), adrenal crisis (acute)
   b. Mineralocorticoids (aldosterone is major hormone)
      i. Regulation of secretion

TABLE 5–1. Adrenergic Responses of Selected Organs

Organ	Receptor Type	Effect
Heart		
SA node	β_1	Inotropic ($\uparrow$ rate)
AV node	β_1	$\uparrow$ Automaticity and conduction speed
Ventricle	β_1	$\uparrow$ Automaticity, conduction speed, and contractility
Arterioles	α	Vasoconstriction
	β_2	Vasodilation
Kidney	β	$\uparrow$ Renin release
Lung: bronchial muscle	β_2	Relaxation (dilatation)
Liver	α, β	$\uparrow$ Glycogenolysis
Pancreas	α	$\downarrow$ Insulin and glucagon release
	β	$\uparrow$ Insulin and glucagon release
Uterus	α	Contraction
	β_2	Relaxation

      (a) Stimulation: renin-angiotensin system as well as hyponatremia, hyperkalemia, and ACTH

      (b) Inhibition: hypokalemia, sodium loading, and increased plasma volume

    ii. Physiologic activity

      (a) Increases sodium reabsorption, indirectly increasing extracellular fluid volume

      (b) Increases potassium excretion

    iii. Disorders resulting from dysfunction

      (a) Excess: primary aldosteronism, characterized by potassium depletion, extracellular fluid volume expansion, and hypertension

      (b) Deficiency: Addison's disease (chronic), adrenal crisis (acute)

      (c) Adrenal androgens: not of significance in critical care

4. Medullary hormones: epinephrine and norepinephrine

    a. Regulation of secretion: stimulation from fear, anxiety, pain, trauma, fluid loss, hemorrhage, extremes in temperature, surgery, hypoxia, hypoglycemia, hypotension

    b. Physiologic activity (Table 5–1)

      i. Fight or flight (stress) response

      ii. Critical in the recovery from insulin-induced hypoglycemia

      iii. Major insulin antagonists

    c. Disorders resulting from dysfunction

      i. Excess: pheochromocytoma. Tumor produces epinephrine and/or norepinephrine, causing hypertension

      ii. Deficiency: persons with an intact sympathetic nervous system manifest no clinically significant disability

Pancreas

1. Location: lies transversely behind the peritoneum and stomach

2. **Composition**: exocrine and endocrine components. Endocrine functions originate from islet cells, which constitute less than 2% of the total pancreatic volume; 65% of the islet cells are beta cells, which produce insulin. Glucagon is produced by the alpha cells; somatostatin and gastrin are produced from the delta cells

3. **Insulin**
   a. Regulation of secretion
      i. Stimulation: increases in blood glucose, gastrin, secretin, cholecystokinin, gastrointestinal hormones, and beta-adrenergic stimulation
      ii. Inhibition: alpha-adrenergic effects of somatostatin, catecholamines, and drugs, including diazoxide, phenytoin, and vinblastine
   b. Physiologic activity
      i. Carbohydrate metabolism
         (a) Increases glucose transport across cell membrane in muscle and fat
         (b) Increases glycogenesis
         (c) Inhibits gluconeogenesis
      ii. Protein metabolism
         (a) Increases amino acid transport across cell membrane
         (b) Increases protein synthesis
         (c) Decreases protein catabolism
      iii. Fat metabolism
         (a) Increases triglyceride synthesis
         (b) Increases fatty acid transport across cell membrane
         (c) Inhibits lipolysis
      iv. Works with thyroid hormone, the sex steroids, and GH to promote growth
   c. Disorders resulting from dysfunction
      i. Excess: hypoglycemia
      ii. Deficiency: diabetes mellitus (type I, insulin dependent)

4. **Glucagon**
   a. Regulation of secretion
      i. Stimulation: hypoglycemia, catecholamines, gastrointestinal hormones, and glucocorticoids
      ii. Inhibition: hyperglycemia and somatostatin
   b. Physiologic activity
      i. Increases blood glucose via glycogenolysis and gluconeogenesis
      ii. Increases lipolysis
      iii. Increases amino acid transport to liver and conversion of amino acids to glucose precursors
      iv. Is a major insulin-antagonistic hormone
      v. Critical hormone in the recovery of insulin-induced hypoglycemia
   c. Deficient glucagon production is thought to play a role in defective glucose counterregulation in insulin-induced hypoglycemia in type I diabetes mellitus
   d. Available as a pharmacologic agent to correct insulin-induced hypoglycemia

5. **Somatostatin**
   a. Present in islet cells, hypothalamus, and gastrointestinal tract

  b. Physiologic activity: inhibits secretion of insulin, glucagon, GH, TSH, and gastrointestinal hormones (gastrin, secretin)

Gonadal Hormones (Testosterone, Estrogen, Progesterone)

Not of significance in critical care

NURSING ASSESSMENT DATA BASE

Nursing History

1. **Patient health history**
   a. Presence of pathophysiologic processes that can result in endocrine dysfunction
      i. Trauma, vascular interruption
      ii. Surgical infection
      iii. Infection, inflammation
      iv. Autoimmune processes
      v. Neoplasms and the chemotherapeutic agents and radiotherapy to treat the neoplasms
      vi. Infiltrative disorders
      vii. Acquired immunodeficiency syndrome (AIDS)
   b. Presence of preexisting chronic endocrine disorder (diagnosed or undiagnosed)
   c. Poor compliance with pharmacologic therapy for a preexisting endocrine disorder
   d. Presence of an unrelated critical illness in a patient with a preexisting chronic endocrine disorder
2. **Indicators of altered health patterns**
   a. Cognitive and perceptual
      i. Personality changes, lethargy, emotional lability, attention span deficit, memory impairment
      ii. Visual disturbances
      iii. Changes in level of consciousness
      iv. Depression, paranoia, delusions, delirium
      v. Verbalizations that indicate lack of knowledge or misconceptions regarding self-care management
   b. Nutrition and metabolism
      i. Change in weight
      ii. Nausea, anorexia, vomiting
      iii. Polydipsia
      iv. Temperature intolerances
      v. Edema
   c. Elimination
      i. Diarrhea or constipation
      ii. Polyuria, anuria, oliguria, nocturia
      iii. Excessive perspiration

    d. Activity and exercise
      i. Fatigue, weakness
      ii. Impairment in activities of daily living
    e. Sleep and rest: restlessness, inadequate sleep
    f. Sexual
      i. Menstrual irregularities
      ii. Impotence
      iii. Decreased libido
      iv. Infertility
    g. Roles and relationships
      i. Discord in previously stable relationships
      ii. Physical and emotional inability to engage in usual role activity
    h. Coping and stress tolerance
      i. Inability to cope
      ii. Past or present psychiatric history
    i. Health perception and health management: evidence of noncompliance

3. Family history: endocrine disorders in other family members

4. Social history
    a. Elderly persons may be at special risk for development of an endocrine crisis because of changes associated with aging and decreased thirst mechanism
    b. Economically disadvantaged persons may be at risk for development of an endocrine crisis because many of the regimens for treating chronic endocrine disorders are costly and necessitate regular medical follow-up
    c. Teenagers with poor compliance, particularly diabetic patients, are at increased risk of crisis

5. Medication history
    a. Use of pharmacologic agents to treat chronic endocrine disorders
    b. Use of pharmacologic agents that may stimulate or inhibit hormone release, or interfere with hormone action at target tissue
    c. Exposure to radiographic contrast dyes

Nursing Examination of Patient

1. Inspection
    a. General appearance
      i. Stature
      ii. Fat distribution in relation to gender and maturational level
      iii. Mobility, tremor, hyperkinesis
      iv. Scars, especially in the neck area
      v. Hair distribution and texture in relation to gender and maturational level
      vi. Edema
      vii. Goiter
      viii. Seizure activity
      ix. Presence of medical alert identification
    b. Face
      i. Shape
      ii. Hydration status of oral cavity
      iii. Periorbital edema

      iv. Eyelid lag, eyelid retraction, stare

      v. Conjunctival irritation, dry eyes

      vi. Protruding or sunken eyeballs

  c. Skin

      i. Color, unusual pigmentation

      ii. Texture, temperature

      iii. Turgor, moisture

      iv. Evidence of bruising, striae, thinning, edema

2. Palpation: enlarged or nodular thyroid gland

3. Percussion: abnormal deep tendon reflexes

4. Auscultation

  a. Neck: bruits over thyroid gland

  b. Heart: distant heart sounds, third heart sound

  c. Blood pressure: hypotension, hypertension

  d. Heart rate and rhythm disturbances

  e. Altered respiratory pattern

  f. Hypoactive bowel sounds

  g. Evidence of pleural or pericardial effusions

5. Additional findings: hypothermia or hyperthermia

Diagnostic Studies in the Critically Ill Patient

1. Laboratory: blood and urine

  a. Electrolytes

  b. Glucose, ketoacids, blood urea nitrogen, cholesterol, creatinine, serum creatine phosphokinase

  c. Plasma osmolality, hematocrit, white blood cell count with differential

  d. Arterial blood gases (ABGs)

  e. Specific hormone assays

  f. Urine specific gravity, osmolality, pH

2. Radiologic (to identify precipitating factor)

  a. X-ray (skull, chest, abdomen)

  b. Scans (thyroid, pancreas)

  c. Computed axial tomography

  d. Magnetic resonance imaging

  e. Arteriography

  f. Bone mineral densitometry

3. Electrocardiographic (ECG)

4. Visual field testing

COMMONLY ENCOUNTERED NURSING DIAGNOSES

Fluid Volume Deficit (Actual or Potential)

1. Assessment for defining characteristics

  a. Dry skin and mucous membranes

  b. Decreased skin turgor

    c. Hypotension, orthostasis, tachycardia

    d. Hypernatremia

    e. Weight loss

    f. Polyuria

    g. Insufficient oral fluid intake

    h. Negative balance of intake and output

2. **Expected outcome**: patient is able to achieve and maintain fluid and electrolyte balance

3. **Nursing interventions**

    a. Monitor hydration status

    b. Monitor electrolyte status

    c. Use flow sheet to document trends in intake, output, vital signs, central venous pressure (CVP), urine specific gravity, peripheral perfusion, body weight, laboratory, and other hemodynamic parameters

    d. Administer prescribed fluid and electrolyte therapy

    e. Administer prescribed hormone replacement

    f. Provide skin and oral care

    g. See disorder-specific information for diabetes insipidus, diabetic ketoacidosis, and acute adrenal insufficiency

4. **Evaluation of nursing care**

    a. Laboratory parameters are within physiologic range

    b. No signs or symptoms of dehydration (see defining characteristics)

Fluid Volume Excess (Actual or Potential)

1. **Assessment for defining characteristics**

    a. Intake greater than output

    b. Weight gain

    c. Third heart sound

    d. Evidence of pulmonary congestion and dyspnea

    e. Deterioration in mental status

    f. Hemodilution

    g. Abnormal electrolyte values

    h. Edema

2. **Expected outcome**: patient is able to achieve and maintain fluid and electrolyte balance

3. **Nursing interventions**

    a. Monitor hydration status

    b. Monitor electrolyte status

    c. Use flowsheet to document trends in intake, output, vital signs, CVP, urine specific gravity, body weight, neurologic status, laboratory, and other hemodynamic parameters

    d. Identify patients at risk for fluid overload. Closely monitor fluid replacement rates in these patients, and restrict fluids if necessary

    e. Assess pulmonary status

    f. Administer prescribed diuretic agents

    g. See interventions for myxedema coma and SIADH secretion

4. **Evaluation of nursing care**

    a. Laboratory parameters are within physiologic range

    b. Hemodynamic parameters are within patient's normal range

c. Intake approximates output
d. No dependent or pulmonary edema

Altered Nutrition, Less Than Body Requirements

1. **Assessment for defining characteristics**
   a. Weight loss of 10% to 20%
   b. Ketosis
   c. Generalized fatigue and muscle weakness
   d. Decreased serum albumin
2. **Expected outcomes**
   a. Body weight stabilizes
   b. Patient is able to achieve and maintain normal carbohydrate, fat, and protein metabolism
   c. No evidence of ketosis
3. **Nursing interventions**
   a. Provide sufficient calories and vitamins
   b. Administer hormone replacement or antihormone therapy
   c. Obtain daily weight
   d. See specific discussions for hyperthyroid crisis and diabetic ketoacidosis
4. **Evaluation of nursing care**
   a. Positive nitrogen balance is maintained
   b. Body weight returns to normal range for patient

Knowledge Deficit

1. **Assessment for defining characteristics**
   a. Verbalizes lack of knowledge or skill related to condition and/or self-care
   b. Follow-through of instructions is inaccurate
   c. Statements indicate misconceptions
   d. Patient requests information
2. **Expected outcomes**
   a. Patient and family (including significant others) are able to verbalize self-care knowledge and demonstrate skills necessary to implement prescribed regimen
   b. Patient and family are able to verbalize knowledge of self-care practices necessary to prevent recurring endocrine crises
   c. Patient and family are able to state the importance of compliance with medications and life style changes (e.g., diet)
3. **Nursing interventions**
   a. Assess patient and family's knowledge of the health disorder and the required self-care
   b. Initiate self-care education for patient and family, to continue after discharge from intensive care unit (ICU)
   c. See interventions for specific patient health problems
4. **Evaluation of nursing care**: patient and family demonstrate knowledge of condition and self-care requirements

Altered Health Maintenance Related to the Need for Hormonal Replacement and Regulation

1. **Assessment for defining characteristics**
   a. Lack of knowledge about basic health practices
   b. Lack of behaviors adaptive to environmental changes
   c. Reported or observed inability to take responsibility for meeting basic health practices
   d. Lack of health-seeking behavior
   e. Expressed interest in improving health behaviors
2. **Expected outcome**: patient is able to identify, manage, and/or seek help to maintain health
3. **Nursing interventions**
   a. Assist patient in identifying needs relating to maintaining hormonal control
   b. Provide opportunity for discussion of health alteration and related self-care needs
   c. Assist patient in understanding how choice of health care practices will affect hormonal control
   d. Help patient to identify risk factors for poor control
   e. Teach patient about importance and use of hormonal replacement medications
   f. Reinforce patient's contact with appropriate resources and educators upon discharge from ICU
   g. Provide patient with positive feedback on behaviors that are effective in maintaining control

PATIENT HEALTH PROBLEMS

Diabetes Insipidus

1. **Pathophysiology**: occurs when any organic lesion of the hypothalamus or posterior pituitary interferes with ADH synthesis and transport or release. Deficiency results in an inability to conserve water
2. **Etiologic or precipitating factors**
   a. Central/neurogenic diabetes insipidus (ADH-sensitive)
      i. Familial, idiopathic
      ii. Traumatic: head injury
      iii. Craniopharyngioma, pituitary tumor
      iv. Infections: meningitis, encephalitis
      v. Vascular: aneurysm
      vi. Infiltrative disorders (histiocytosis X, sarcoidosis)
   b. Nephrogenic diabetes insipidus (ADH-insensitive)
      i. Renal: polycystic kidneys, pyelonephritis
      ii. Multisystem disorders: multiple myeloma, sarcoidosis, sickle cell disease
      iii. Familial

    c. Pharmacologic agents: ethanol, lithium, and phenytoin inhibit ADH secretion and action

    d. Insufficient exogenous ADH in the person with diabetes insipidus

3. Nursing assessment data base

    a. Nursing history

       i. Subjective findings

         (a) Polydipsia

         (b) Fatigue

       ii. Objective findings

         (a) Patient health history: presence of precipitating factor

         (b) Social history: identification of patient with impaired thirst mechanism or who is confused, incapacitated, or unable to secure fluids

         (c) Medication history: use of medications that impair ADH release or action

    b. Nursing examination of patient

       i. Inspection

         (a) Decreased skin turgor

         (b) Dry mucous membranes

         (c) Polyuria (5 to 20 L/24 hours)

       ii. Auscultation: tachycardia; hypotension if the patient has become dehydrated

    c. Diagnostic study findings

       i. Plasma osmolality elevated ($>$295 mOsm/kg), urine osmolality decreased ($<$500 mOsm/kg; can be as low as 30 mOsm/kg)

       ii. Hypernatremia

      iii. Low urine specific gravity (1.001 to 1.005)

      iv. Water deprivation test: with adequate stimulus for ADH release (simple dehydration), kidneys cannot concentrate urine. Differentiates psychogenic polydipsia from diabetes insipidus

       v. ADH test: to demonstrate that kidneys can concentrate urine with exogenous ADH. Differentiates nephrogenic from central diabetes insipidus

      vi. Low plasma ADH levels in patients with central diabetes insipidus

4. Nursing diagnoses

    a. Actual or potential fluid volume deficit related to inability to conserve water

       i. See Commonly Encountered Nursing Diagnoses section

       ii. Additional nursing interventions

         (a) Administer hormonal replacement (central diabetes insipidus)

           (1) Aqueous pitressin (intravenous [IV] or subcutaneous)

           (2) Lysine vasopressin (nasal)

           (3) Desmopressin acetate (DDAVP)

         (b) Administer pharmacologic agents (nephrogenic diabetes insipidus)

           (1) Chlorpropamide: stimulates ADH release and augments renal tubular response to ADH

           (2) Thiazide diuretics and sodium restriction: mild sodium depletion and reduced solute load will enhance water reabsorption

         (c) Document intake and output, body weight, urine specific gravity, plasma, and urine osmolality. With neurosurgery patients, record for 7 to 10 days postoperatively because diabetes insipidus can be triphasic in nature (manifests, then appears to resolve, only to reappear and be permanent)

    (d) Assist with water deprivation and ADH tests

    (e) Explain diagnostic procedures to patient and family

  iii. Evaluation of nursing care

    (a) Vital signs and other hemodynamic parameters are within patient's normal range

    (b) Intake approximates output

    (c) Laboratory parameters (plasma and urine osmolality, electrolytes, urine specific gravity) are within normal limits

    (d) Patient is alert and oriented

    (e) Mucous membranes are moist

    (f) Skin is warm and dry with good turgor

b. Potential knowledge deficit regarding self-care management of permanent diabetes insipidus

  i. Assessment for defining characteristics

    (a) Patient has newly diagnosed diabetes insipidus

    (b) Patient has not taken medication as prescribed at home

    (c) Patient is unable to state signs and symptoms that necessiate physician notification

  ii. Expected outcome: patient and family are able to state regimen for managing diabetes insipidus

  iii. Nursing interventions

    (a) Initiate medication instruction

    (b) Instruct patient and family to notify physician of edema, weight gain, polydipsia, or polyuria

  iv. Evaluation of nursing care

    (a) Patient and family are able to state purpose, name, dose, and schedule of medication and importance of compliance

    (b) Patient is able to accurately administer medication

    (c) Patient and family are able to identify changes in fluid balance that warrant notifying physician

SIADH Secretion

1. **Pathophysiology:** syndrome characterized by plasma hypotonicity and hyponatremia that results from aberrant secretion of ADH that in turn results from failure of the negative feedback system. Dysfunction results in water intoxication

2. **Etiologic or precipitating factors**

a. Central nervous system disorders

  i. Traumatic: skull fracture, subdural hematoma, subarachnoid hemorrhage, cerebral contusion

  ii. Neoplasms

  iii. Infection: meningitis, encephalitis, brain abscess, Guillain-Barré syndrome, AIDS

  iv. Vascular: aneurysm, cerebral vascular accident

b. Stimulation of ADH release via hypoxia and/or decreased left atrial filling pressure

      i. Pulmonary infections
      ii. Asthma
      iii. Congestive heart failure
      iv. Positive pressure ventilation
   c. Pharmacologic agents: either increase ADH secretion or potentiate its action
      i. Cancer chemotherapy: cyclophosphamide, vincristine
      ii. Chlorpropamide, acetaminophen, amitriptyline, thiazide diuretics, carbamazepine, pentamidine
   d. Excessive exogenous ADH therapy
   e. Ectopic ADH production associated with bronchogenic, prostatic, or pancreatic cancers and with leukemia

3. Nursing assessment data base
   a. Nursing history
      i. Subjective findings
         (a) Headache, lethargy
         (b) Nausea
      ii. Objective findings: in patient health history, presence of a precipitating factor
   b. Nursing examination of patient
      i. Inspection
         (a) Muscle twitching or seizure activity
         (b) Vomiting
         (c) Confusion, impaired memory
      ii. Percussion: delayed deep tendon reflexes
   c. Diagnostic study findings
      i. Hyponatremia
      ii. Decreased plasma osmolality
      iii. Elevated urine sodium and osmolality
      iv. Elevated plasma ADH levels
      v. Inability to excrete water load

4. Nursing diagnoses
   a. Fluid volume excess related to inability to excrete water (see Commonly Encountered Nursing Diagnoses section)
      i. Assessment for defining characteristics
         (a) Hyponatremia with hypo-osmolality
         (b) Elevated urine osmolality
         (c) Weight gain
         (d) Neurologic changes
      ii. Expected outcome: fluid balance is restored to normal
      iii. Nursing interventions
         (a) Recognize subtle signs indicative of water intoxication: decreased level of consciousness, headache, fatigue, weakness
         (b) Manage fluid therapy
             (1) Fluid restriction and replacement may be based on urine output plus insensible losses
            (2) Use of hypertonic sodium chloride infusion in patients with severe hyponatremia and/or seizure activity is controversial. May precipitate heart failure, fluid overload, and cerebral osmotic demyelination syndrome

        (3) Diuretics: decrease the effectiveness of ADH. Can cause significant electrolyte imbalance

        (4) Monitor IV infusion rate and urine output in patients at risk

    (c) Monitor electrolytes and replace as required

    (d) Document intake and output, body weight, urine specific gravity, hydration, cardiovascular, and neurologic assessments

    (e) Assist with diagnostic studies and explain procedures to patient and family

    (f) Administer therapy aimed at precipitating factors

  iv. Evaluation of nursing care

    (a) Intake approximates output

    (b) Laboratory parameters (plasma and urine osmolality, serum sodium) are within normal limits

    (c) Patient's body weight returns to normal

    (d) Patient is alert and oriented

b. Potential for injury related to impaired cognitive state and physical inactivity

  i. Assessment for defining characteristics

    (a) Confusion, impaired memory, lethargy

    (b) Restlessness, fatigue, weakness

    (c) Imposed physical inactivity

    (d) Unfamiliar environment and personnel

  ii. Expected outcome: remains free from personal injury

  iii. Nursing interventions

    (a) Institute seizure precautions

    (b) Reorient the confused patient

    (c) Prevent complications of immobility

  iv. Evaluation of nursing care: patient is free from personal injury

Thyrotoxicosis (Thyroid Storm)

1. **Pathophysiology:** life-threatening augmentation of the signs and symptoms of hyperthyroidism. Manifested by severe tachycardia, heart failure, shock, hyperthermia (up to 105.3°F [40°C]), restlessness, agitation, abdominal pain, nausea, vomiting, and coma. Rare, because most hyperthyroid patients are well controlled by antithyroid drug therapy

2. **Etiologic or precipitating factors**
   a. Surgical procedures or trauma of any kind
   b. Infection
   c. Poor compliance with antithyroid therapy (rare)
   d. Other: diabetic ketoacidosis, trauma, eclampsia

3. **Nursing assessment data base**
   a. Nursing history
     i. Subjective findings
       (a) Confusion, agitation, overt psychosis
       (b) Weakness, fatigue, tremor
       (c) Nausea, abdominal pain
       (d) Heat intolerance
     ii. Objective findings
       (a) Patient health history: diagnosis is confirmed in the presence of

high fever and altered mental status in a severely ill hyperthyroid patient
- (b) Social and family history: in view of acute nature of disease, not applicable at this time
- (c) Medication history
  - (1) Past or present use of methimazole or propylthiouracil, with disruption of established medication regimen
  - (2) Use of antiarrhythmic agents
- b. Nursing examination of patient
  - i. Inspection
    - (a) Warm, moist, flushed, soft skin
    - (b) Hyperkinesis and tremor
    - (c) Eyelid lag, retracted eyelids, stare, exophthalmos, irritated eyes
    - (d) Alopecia
    - (e) Coma
  - ii. Palpation
    - (a) Goiter: diffuse or multinodular, nontender
    - (b) Hepatomegaly
    - (c) Hyperthermia (105°F [40°C])
  - iii. Percussion: hyperreflexia
  - iv. Auscultation
    - (a) Audible bruits over thyroid gland
    - (b) Tachycardia, irregular pulse
    - (c) Hypotension and shock (late sign)
    - (d) Third heart sound
    - (e) Adventitious breath sounds caused by pulmonary edema
- c. Diagnostic study findings
  - i. Elevated total and free T_3 and T_4 and reduced TSH
  - ii. Elevated hepatic aminotransferases; hyperbilirubinemia common
  - iii. Elevated alkaline phosphatase

4. Nursing diagnoses
- a. Hyperthermia related to accelerated metabolic state secondary to thyroid hormone excess
  - i. Assessment for defining characteristics
    - (a) Hyperthermia (100° to 106°F [38° to 41°C])
    - (b) Flushed, warm, diaphoretic skin
    - (c) Tachypnea
    - (d) Tachycardia, atrial fibrillation
    - (e) Delirium
  - ii. Expected outcome: body temperature is restored to normal
  - iii. Nursing interventions
    - (a) Pharmacologic management
      - (1) Propylthiouracil, carbimazole, and methimazole
      - (2) Ipodate sodium
      - (3) Beta-adrenergic blocking agents (propranolol is drug of choice)
    - (b) Thermoregulation
      - (1) Institute cooling measures, but avoid causing patient to shiver
      - (2) Measure body temperature every hour or continuously

(3) Supply sufficient fluids and electrolytes to replace losses from diaphoresis

(4) Provide comfort measures appropriate to the febrile patient

(5) Administer antibiotics if precipitator is infectious

(6) Administer antipyretics as ordered. Do not use salicylates: they inhibit T_4 and T_3 binding and therefore increase free T_4 and T_3

iv. Evaluation of nursing care: body temperature within normal range

b. Potential for decreased cardiac output related to excessive demands on cardiovascular system resulting from hyperthermia and increased sensitivity of cardiac catecholamine receptors

  i. Assessment for defining characteristics

   (a) Dysrhythmias, tachycardia

   (b) Hypotension and shock

   (c) Congestive heart failure

  ii. Expected outcome: acceptable cardiac output is restored and maintained

  iii. Nursing interventions

   (a) Administer beta-adrenergic blocking agents

   (b) Perform frequent cardiovascular, respiratory, and neurologic assessments

   (c) Identify patients at risk for cardiovascular collapse (elderly patients; patients with preexisting coronary heart disease; those with known cardiac risk factors)

   (d) Record intake and output

   (e) Closely regulate fluid replacement

   (f) Interventions for hyperthermia will also diminish the demands on the cardiovascular system

  iv. Evaluation of nursing care

   (a) Hemodynamic parameters and urine output are within normal limits

   (b) Patient is alert and oriented

   (c) Patient is able to tolerate brief periods of physical activity without exhaustion

c. Altered nutrition, less than body requirements, related to hypermetabolism and inadequate diet

  i. Assessment for defining characteristics

   (a) Weight loss

   (b) Inadequate food intake

   (c) Muscle weakness

   (d) Abdominal pain, nausea, vomiting, diarrhea

  ii. Expected outcomes

   (a) Stabilization of body weight

   (b) Positive nitrogen balance

  iii. Nursing interventions

   (a) Administer IV fluids, electrolytes, B-complex vitamins, and glucose

   (b) Provide assistance with eating

   (c) Obtain daily weights

   (d) Institute calorie count to quantify nutritional adequacy

   (e) Consult dietician to provide meals that are generous in calories, protein, and appeal

   (f) Consider nutritional support if patient is unwilling or unable to eat

   (g) Note glucose levels: hyperglycemia may result from decreased peripheral and hepatic insulin sensitivity

  iv. Evaluation of nursing care

   (a) Patient's body weight stabilizes

   (b) Calorie count reveals that nutritional intake is adequate for current metabolic needs

 d. Potential for injury related to impaired cognitive state (see this nursing diagnosis for SIADH)

  i. Additional nursing interventions

   (a) Provide interventions to prevent injury

   (b) Ensure safe environment

   (c) Monitor patient's judgment, decision-making abilities, and attention span

   (d) Provide eye protection for the patient with exophthalmos (eye drops, artificial tears, eye patches)

   (e) Assist patient in activities of daily living

   (f) Reorient patient as to time, place, person, and circumstance

  ii. Evaluation of nursing care: patient is free from injury

 e. Knowledge deficit regarding hyperthyroidism and its management

  i. Assessment for defining characteristics

   (a) Patient and family request information regarding disease management

   (b) Poor compliance with previous instructions

  ii. Expected outcome: patient and family are able to state regimen for managing hyperthyroid state

  iii. Nursing interventions

   (a) Explain symptoms and treatment of hyperthyroidism

   (b) Outline current medication therapy (purpose, name, dose, schedule)

   (c) Encourage continued medical follow-up for definitive treatment (radioiodine therapy or surgery)

  iv. Evaluation of nursing care

   (a) Patient and family are able to state the importance of medical follow-up for hyperthyroidism

   (b) Patient and family are able to state specifics of medication regimen and importance of compliance

Myxedema Coma

1. **Pathophysiology:** life-threatening emergency resulting from extreme hypothyroidism. Often occurs in presence of concurrent illness, but may manifest as initial finding in hypothyroidism

2. **Etiologic or precipitating factors**

 a. Decompensation of a preexisting hypothyroid state after infection, trauma, exposure to cold, administration of tranquilizers, barbiturates, and narcotics or other physical stress. Preexisting hypothyroidism may result from:

    i. Thyroidectomy

    ii. Destruction of thyroid gland after radioactive iodine therapy for hyperthyroidism

    iii. Chronic thyroiditis

    iv. Hashimoto's thyroiditis (autoimmune thyroiditis)

    v. Dysfunction within the hypothalamic-pituitary axis (hypophysectomy, pituitary irradiation, pituitary infarction)

  b. Insufficient provision of exogenous thyroid hormone (hypothyroid patient who discontinues replacement therapy, critically ill patient who has preexisting hypothyroidism but does not receive continued replacement therapy while hospitalized)

3. Nursing assessment data base

  a. Nursing history

    i. Subjective findings: Compromised mental status makes subjective assessment difficult

    ii. Objective findings

      (a) Patient health history: presence of a precipitating factor

      (b) Family history of Graves' disease, Hashimoto's thyroiditis, or type I diabetes mellitus

      (c) Social history: Family reports subtle change in patient's behavior (e.g., memory impairment or confusion)

      (d) Medication history

        (1) Past or present use of levothyroxine or desiccated thyroid; disruption of an established medication regimen

        (2) Lithium carbonate: blocks thyroid hormone synthesis and release and can cause hypothyroidism

  b. Nursing examination of patient

    i. Inspection

      (a) Nonpitting edema: cool, rough, dry skin

      (b) Enlarged tongue

      (c) Loss of eyebrows and scalp hair

    ii. Palpation: Goiter may not be palpable because of atrophy, prior radiation, or prior surgery

    iii. Percussion: Delayed deep tendon reflexes

    iv. Auscultation

      (a) Slow, shallow respiration

      (b) Bradycardia

      (c) Blood pressure inconclusive

    v. Other clinical measurements

      (a) Hypothermia ($91°$ to $95°F$ [$32°$ to $35°C$])

      (b) Exaggerated response to sedatives

  c. Diagnostic study findings

    i. Hyponatremia

    ii. Respiratory acidosis, hypoxemia

    iii. Hypoglycemia

    iv. Enlarged cardiac outline, pleural and pericardial effusions on x-ray

    v. ECG: sinus bradycardia, T-wave depression, ST changes, prolonged RT and QT intervals

    vi. Low T_4, T_3 resin uptake, increased TSH

       vii. High cholesterol, hyperlipoproteinemia

      viii. Because of potential for concurrent adrenal insufficiency, rapid ACTH stimulation test should be performed in patients with myxedema

4. Nursing diagnoses

  a. Hypothermia related to deficient thermogenesis secondary to decreased metabolic rate associated with profound hypothyroidism

    i. Assessment for defining characteristics

      (a) Body temperature below 94°F (34.4°C)

      (b) Decreased level of consciousness

      (c) Bradycardia

      (d) Marked peripheral vasoconstriction

    ii. Expected outcome: body temperature is restored to normal

    iii. Nursing interventions

      (a) Administer thyroid hormone replacement

      (b) Implement gradual rewarming

      (c) Monitor temperature every 1 hour or continuously

      (d) Assess vital signs, hemodynamic parameters, neurologic status, and peripheral perfusion

      (e) Because of greatly decreased metabolic rate, drug turnover and degradation will be delayed

      (f) Administer glucocorticoids as ordered. Thyroid replacement may aggravate preexisting adrenal insufficiency

      (g) Take measures to prevent infection. Patient's response to infection will not include fever

    iv. Evaluation of nursing care: body temperature is restored to normal

  b. Ineffective breathing pattern related to reduced central ventilatory drive and respiratory muscle weakness

    i. Assessment for defining characteristics

      (a) Hypercapnia and hypoxemia

      (b) Depressed level of consciousness

    ii. Expected outcome: hypoxemia is resolved or is improved with oxygen supplementation or mechanical ventilatory support

    iii. Nursing interventions

      (a) Administer thyroid hormone replacement. Decreased ventilatory response may be secondary to hypothermia. T_4 assists with thermogenesis and thus can help improve ventilatory drive

      (b) Assess respiratory, cardiac, and neurologic status

      (c) Initiate endotracheal intubation and mechanical ventilation for hypercapneic respiratory failure

      (d) Avoid pharmacologic agents that depress the ventilatory drive

      (e) Monitor blood gas values

      (f) Administer oxygen, encourage deep breathing, assist with repositioning, remove secretions as necessary

      (g) Ensure adequate nutritional intake (oral, enteral, or parenteral) to prevent further respiratory muscle weakness

      (h) Implement measures to prevent infection. Hypothyroid patients are susceptible to bacterial infections

    iv. Evaluation of nursing care: blood gas values are within acceptable limits for patient

c. Knowledge deficit regarding hypothyroidism and its management
    i. Assessment for defining characteristics
        (a) Patient and family request information regarding management of hypothyroidism
        (b) Patient's preadmission behavior suggests poor compliance or understanding
    ii. Expected outcome: patient and family are able to state regimen for managing hypothyroidism
    iii. Nursing interventions
        (a) Explain symptoms and treatment of hypothyroidism and importance of compliance
        (b) Outline current medication schedule (purpose, name, dose, schedule)
    iv. Evaluation of nursing care: patient and family are able to state the medication regimen and importance of compliance

Hypoparathyroidism and Hyperparathyroidism

1. **Pathophysiology:** parathyroid gland dysfunction or production of a tumor-derived PTH-related peptide is associated with disturbances in calcium and phosphorus balance and bone metabolism. See Chapter 4, The Renal System, for further discussion of pathophysiology of calcium-phosphorus imbalances
2. **Etiologic or precipitating factors**
    a. Hyperparathyroidism
        i. Primary hyperparathyroidism: increased secretion of PTH resulting from benign neoplasm or adenoma (80% of cases)
        ii. Secondary hyperparathyroidism is a compensatory response to hypocalcemia caused by chronic renal failure, osteomalacia, or intestinal malabsorption syndromes
    b. Humoral hypercalcemia of malignancy: squamous cell carcinomas of lung, head, and neck: hypernephroma; ovarian cancers secrete a PTH-like peptide
    c. Hypoparathyroidism: inadequate PTH with hypocalcemia
        i. Congenital absence of parathyroid glands
        ii. Surgical removal or damage to the parathyroid gland (thyroidectomy, radical neck surgery)
        iii. Autoimmune
        iv. Hypomagnesemia: interferes with PTH secretion
3. **Nursing assessment data base** See Chapter 4. Diagnostic study findings include laboratory measurements of intact PTH, vitamin D levels, total and ionic calcium, phosphorus, magnesium, and urinary cAMP
4. **Nursing diagnoses**
    a. Hypercalcemia: see Chapter 4. Interventions include hydration and possible administration of loop diuretics. Treatment for humoral hypercalcemia of malignancy may include calcitonin, glucocorticoids, diphosphonates, or plicamycin (mithramycin)
    b. Hypocalcemia: see Chapter 4. Interventions include administration of calcium, vitamin D, and magnesium

Acute Adrenal Insufficiency (Addisonian Crisis)

1. **Pathophysiology:** deficiency of cortisol production with electrolyte and fluid abnormalities that result in life-threatening cardiovascular collapse
2. **Etiologic or precipitating factors**
   a. Acute injury to or infection of adrenal glands
   b. Patient with chronic adrenal insufficiency who has a critical illness
   c. Abrupt cessation of corticosteroid therapy
3. **Nursing assessment data base**
   a. Nursing history
      i. Subjective findings
         (a) Acute adrenal crisis produces cardiovascular collapse. Examiner will be unable to collect subjective data
         (b) Patient may complain of nausea and abdominal pain
      ii. Objective findings
         (a) Patient health history: presence of a precipitating factor
         (b) Medication history
            (1) Current or past corticosteroid use of 20 mg of hydrocortisone or its equivalent for longer than 7 to 10 days has the potential for suppressing the hypothalamic-pituitary-adrenal axis. Recovery may take 2 to 12 months or longer
            (2) Adrenal hemorrhage may occur with anticoagulant therapy
            (3) Ketoconazole and etomidate can interfere with steroid biosynthesis
            (4) Rifampin increases metabolic clearance rate of corticosteroids
   b. Nursing examination of patient
      i. Inspection
         (a) Confusion, altered mental status
         (b) Vomiting
         (c) Petechiae
         (d) Hyperpigmentation (chronic insufficiency)
      ii. Auscultation
         (a) Tachycardia
         (b) Severe hypotension, vascular collapse
      iii. Other clinical measurements: fever
   c. Diagnostic study findings
      i. Hyponatremia
      ii. Hyperkalemia
      iii. Azotemia
      iv. Hypoglycemia (more severe in children than in adults)
      v. Hypercalcemia
      vi. Eosinophilia
      vii. ACTH stimulation test will confirm diagnosis
4. **Nursing diagnoses**
   a. Fluid volume deficit related to ACTH deficiency
      i. See Commonly Encountered Nursing Diagnoses section
      ii. Additional nursing interventions
         (a) Rapid administration of IV fluids and electrolytes (usually 0.9% normal saline)

   (b) Hormonal replacement
       (1) Glucocorticoid (hydrocortisone)
       (2) Mineralocorticoid (fludrocortisone)
   (c) Monitor fluid balance, body weight
   (d) Monitor heart rate and rhythm
   iii. Evaluation of nursing care
       (a) Vital signs and other hemodynamic parameters are within patient's normal range
       (b) Electrolytes and fluid balance parameters are within normal limits
 b. Potential knowledge deficit regarding long-term steroid management
   i. Assessment for defining characteristics
       (a) Patient and family request information regarding corticosteroid use
       (b) Patient's preadmission behavior suggests poor compliance or understanding
   ii. Expected outcome: patient and family are able to state self-care actions necessary when taking corticosteroids
   iii. Nursing interventions
       (a) Initiate medication instruction
       (b) Instruct patient and family in importance of compliance and gradual corticosteroid tapering (if appropriate)
   iv. Evaluation of nursing care: patient and family are able to state purpose, name, dose, and schedule of steroid regimen and importance of compliance

Diabetic Ketoacidosis (DKA)

1. **Pathophysiology:** DKA is the most serious metabolic complication of insulin-dependent diabetes mellitus. DKA is a state of insulin deficiency combined with insulin-antagonistic hormones (glucagon, cortisol, catecholamines, and GH). Result is altered metabolism of carbohydrate, fat, and protein (Fig. 5–2) and hyperglycemia
   a. Decreased insulin in combination with gluconeogenesis and increased insulin resistance results in exaggerated hepatic glucose production
   b. Ketosis and metabolic acidosis resulting from increased synthesis of ketones and lactic acidosis

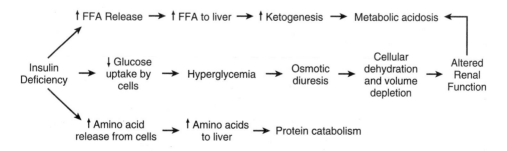

Figure 5–2 • Metabolic consequences of insulin deficiency. FFA = free fatty acid. (From Skillman, T.: Diabetic ketoacidosis. Heart Lung 7:596, 1978.)

    c. Fluid and electrolyte imbalance: osmotic diuresis caused by glycosuria. Accompanied by loss of sodium, potassium, and chloride

    d. Altered mental status results from hyperosmolality, cellular dehydration, acidosis, and possible impaired oxygen dissociation as glycosylated hemoglobin binds oxygen more tightly

2. Etiologic or precipitating factors

    a. Diagnosed diabetes mellitus

        i. Insufficient exogenous insulin: dose missed or insufficient for needs

        ii. Infection or trauma in a diabetic patient

    b. Undiagnosed diabetes mellitus

3. Nursing assessment data base

    a. Nursing history

        i. Subjective findings

           (a) Blurred vision

           (b) Nausea, abdominal cramping, polyphagia

           (c) Polydipsia, polyuria

           (d) Fatigue, weakness, weight loss

           (e) Muscle cramps

        ii. Objective findings

           (a) Presence of a precipitating factor

           (b) Family history of endocrine disorders

           (c) Social history

               (1) Family reports poor compliance with established diabetes self-care regimen

               (2) One third of patients admitted for DKA have associated educational deficits or psychosocial distress

               (3) Teenagers with poor compliance

           (d) Medication history

               (1) Use of insulin or a continuous infusion device in which flow rate has been disrupted

               (2) Thiazide diuretics, diazoxide, and phenytoin decrease insulin release

               (3) Glucocorticoids increase gluconeogenesis

    b. Nursing examination of patient

        i. Inspection

           (a) Diminished level of consciousness

           (b) Polyuria and polydipsia

           (c) Vomiting, anorexia

           (d) Decreased skin turgor, dry mucous membranes

           (e) Acetone odor to breath (ketosis)

        ii. Auscultation

           (a) Tachycardia

           (b) Orthostatic hypotension

           (c) Tachypnea, Kussmaul respiration

        iii. Palpation: abdominal tenderness

    c. Diagnostic study findings

        i. Elevated plasma and urine glucose levels (plasma glucose, 500 to 800 mg/dl)

        ii. Metabolic acidosis

        iii. Positive serum and urine ketoacids

        iv. Azotemia

  v. Mild hyponatremia

  vi. ECG may reflect hypokalemia, although serum potassium may be normal or excessive

  vii. Hypocalcemia in 30% of patients

  viii. Hyperosmolality

4. Nursing diagnoses

 a. Fluid volume deficit related to osmotic diuresis induced by hyperglycemia. Deficit worsened by vomiting and/or inadequate oral intake

  i. See Commonly Encountered Nursing Diagnoses section

  ii. Additional nursing interventions

   (a) Administer intravenous fluids and electrolytes as ordered, via an infusion pump. Begin fluid therapy with 0.9% NaCl solution. When plasma glucose level reaches 250 to 300 mg/dl, add 5% dextrose solution to NaCl to prevent hypoglycemia

   (b) Intake and output

   (c) Assess vital signs, other hemodynamic parameters, and neurologic status

   (d) Obtain body weight

   (e) Maintain skin integrity

   (f) Encourage oral fluids as tolerated

   (g) Inform physician of signs of cardiovascular compromise

   (h) Decline in neurologic status may signal development of cerebral edema

   (i) Assess for evidence of fluid overload

   (j) Maintain flow sheet of laboratory and hemodynamic parameters

  iii. Evaluation of nursing care

   (a) Vital signs and other hemodynamic parameters are within acceptable range for patient

   (b) Laboratory parameters are within normal limits

   (c) Fluid balance is restored

 b. Altered nutrition, less than body requirements, related to catabolic effects of insulin deficiency and stress hormone excess

  i. Assessment for defining characteristics

   (a) Loss of weight despite polyphagia

   (b) Ketosis

   (c) Fatigue, weakness

   (d) Hyperglycemia, glucosuria

  ii. Expected outcome: normal metabolism of carbohydrate, fat, and protein is restored

  iii. Nursing interventions

   (a) Administer rapid-acting, IV regular insulin (bolus followed by continuous infusion)

   (b) Switch to subcutaneous insulin 1 to 2 hours before stopping the continuous insulin infusion, to prevent the recurrence of ketosis and accelerated hyperglycemia

   (c) Hourly serum glucose monitoring

   (d) Measure urine ketones

   (e) Offer foods and fluids as tolerated

   (f) Obtain weight daily

   (g) Administer antibiotics if precipitator is an infectious process

  iv. Evaluation of nursing care

(a) Blood glucose decreases 100 mg/dl/hour
(b) Blood glucose stabilizes at 150 to 200 mg/dl
(c) Persistent ketosis is absent
(d) Patient is able to tolerate oral feedings
(e) Body weight is stabilized

c. Acid-base imbalances are caused by ketosis that is secondary to insulin deficiency and stress hormone excess
   i. Assessment for defining characteristics
     (a) Acetone odor to breath
     (b) Tachypnea, Kussmaul respiration
     (c) Positive findings for serum and urine ketones
     (d) Metabolic acidosis
     (e) Increased anion gap
     (f) Depressed level of consciousness
   ii. Expected outcome: acid-base balance is restored
  iii. Nursing interventions
     (a) Assess ABG, respiratory and neurologic status
     (b) Administer intravenous fluids and insulin as primary therapies for correction of acidosis
     (c) Sodium bicarbonate is rarely required unless pH is less than 7.0; is used with goal of myocardial and cerebral protection
     (d) Measure urine ketones
     (e) Monitor for hypokalemia while acidosis and volume deficits are being corrected
     (f) Note and promptly report laboratory and/or clinical evidence of increasing acidosis
   iv. Evaluation of nursing care
     (a) Acid-base and potassium levels are within normal limits
     (b) Anion gap is normal
     (c) No acetone odor is detected on breath

d. Potential hypoglycemia related to insulin therapy and a decrease in circulating insulin-antagonistic hormones
   i. Assessment for defining characteristics
     (a) Blood glucose less than 50 mg/dl
     (b) Signs and symptoms of hypoglycemia, as discussed in Hypoglycemic Episode section
   ii. Expected outcome: blood glucose is maintained between 80 and 120 mg/dl
  iii. Nursing interventions
     (a) Assess for the signs and symptoms of hypoglycemia
     (b) If diabetes is established, secure information regarding past experiences with hypoglycemia
     (c) Instruct patient and family in the signs and symptoms of hypoglycemia
     (d) Plan interventions for prevention of hypoglycemia, because hypoglycemia can precipitate dysrhythmias and extend infarcts
       (1) Monitor the trend of laboratory data, especially blood glucose levels
       (2) Keep physician informed of trends evidenced in clinical and laboratory data
       (3) Add 5% dextrose to 0.9% sodium chloride (NaCl) when

serum glucose is 250 to 300 mg/dl. Insulin infusion may be decreased or stopped at this point

   (e) If hypoglycemia occurs, patient will require administration of a rapid-acting carbohydrate; administer IV or orally if patient's consciousness is not depressed

   (f) Perform bedside blood glucose measurement any time hypoglycemia is suspected

   (g) After treatment of a suspected hypoglycemic episode, monitor patient's response to the carbohydrate source provided

  iv. Evaluation of nursing care

   (a) Blood glucose level is between 80 and 100 mg/dl

   (b) Patient evidences no signs or symptoms of hypoglycemia

   (c) Patient and family are able to state symptoms of hypoglycemia

e. Potential knowledge deficit regarding home management of hyperglycemia

  i. Assessment for defining characteristics

   (a) Patient is unable to state appropriate sick day management

   (b) Patient discontinued insulin and/or home monitoring before admission

   (c) Patient delayed notifying health care team about deteriorating condition

   (d) Patient has newly diagnosed type I diabetes mellitus

   (e) Patient unable to state troubleshooting guidelines in the event of sustained unexplainable hyperglycemia while using continuous subcutaneous insulin-infusion device

  ii. Expected outcome: patient and family are able to state self-management knowledge and skills necessary to prevent recurrence of DKA

  iii. Nursing interventions

   (a) If diabetes is established, identify precipitating factors by securing and documenting data regarding

    (1) Home medication regimen

    (2) Presence of infections or illness

    (3) Presence of emotional stressors

    (4) Past history of hyperglycemic crisis

    (5) Results of recent home glucose and ketone testing before admission

    (6) Evidence of insulin infusion device malfunction (if used)

   (b) If precipitating factors point to a deficit in self-care knowledge or skill or to noncompliance with the self-care regimen, refer patient to diabetes educator upon transfer from ICU

   (c) Instruct patient and family in causes, symptoms, and treatment of hyperglycemia and hypoglycemia

  iv. Evaluation of nursing care

   (a) Patient and family are able to identify causes and symptoms of hyperglycemia and hypoglycemia

   (b) Patient and family are able to state the impact of infection and other stressors on blood glucose levels

   (c) Patient and family are able to state the importance of continuing the prescribed insulin regimen

Hyperglycemic, Hyperosmolar Nonketotic Coma (Hyperglycemic, Nonacidotic Diabetic Coma)

1. **Pathophysiology:** life-threatening hyperglycemic emergency accompanied by hyperosmolality, severe dehydration, and alterations in neurologic status without ketosis. Pathophysiologic processes (Fig. 5–3) include
   a. Relative insulin deficiency that impairs glucose transport across the cell membrane. Insulin present may be sufficient to inhibit lipolysis or ketogenesis in the liver but not to control hyperglycemia
   b. Hyperosmolality resulting from hyperglycemia and hypernatremia may impair insulin secretion, promote insulin resistance, and inhibit free fatty acid release from adipose tissue
   c. Fluid shifts from intracellular to extracellular space to offset hyperosmolality
   d. Osmotic diuresis caused by hyperglycemia results in extracellular fluid volume depletion
   e. Severe electrolyte losses (sodium, chloride, phosphate, magnesium, potassium) occur with osmotic diuresis
   f. Volume depletion compromises glomerular filtration, diminishing urinary escape of glucose
   g. Coma results from cellular dehydration caused by hyperosmolality

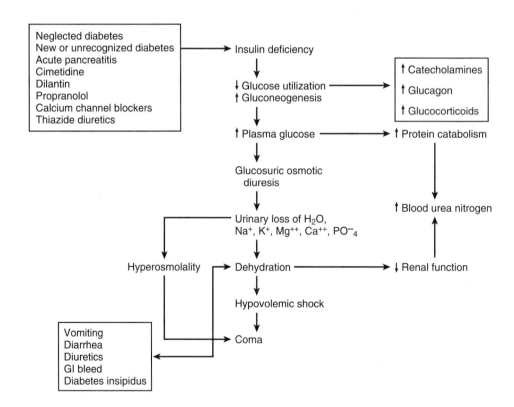

Figure 5–3 • Pathogenesis of hyperglycemic, hyperosmolar nonketotic coma. GI = gastrointestinal. (From Matz, R.: Hyperglycemic hyperosmolar nonacidotic coma: Not a rare event. Clin. Diabetes 6:31, 1988. With permission of the American Diabetes Association, Inc.)

2. Etiologic or precipitating factors
  a. Inadequate insulin secretion and/or action (newly diagnosed type II, non–insulin-dependent diabetes)
  b. Majority of patients are elderly and severely dehydrated
  c. Concomitant illnesses that increase glucose production or contribute to dehydration, including sepsis, pancreatitis, stroke, uremia, burns, myocardial infarction, and gastrointestinal hemorrhage

3. Nursing assessment data base
  a. Nursing history
    i. Subjective findings
      (a) Lethargy, fatigue
      (b) Polydipsia, polyuria, polyphagia
    ii. Objective findings
      (a) Patient health history: presence of a precipitating factor
      (b) Family history of type II diabetes
      (c) Social history
        (1) Family gives a history of a protracted, gradual deterioration in the person's physical and mental condition
        (2) Patient at risk includes persons who cannot gain ready access to fluids or who cannot recognize or express their need for fluids
      (d) Medication history
        (1) Use of insulin or oral hypoglycemic agent, disruption of established medication regimen
        (2) Use of medications known to elevate glucose levels and/or resist insulin action, including thiazide diuretics, phenytoin, sympathomimetics
        (3) Preadmission medications that suggest cardiovascular or renal disease, because crisis is more common in late middle age and in elderly people with preexisting renal or cardiovascular disease
  b. Nursing examination of patient
    i. Inspection
      (a) Flushed skin and dry mucous membranes
      (b) Coma
    ii. Auscultation
      (a) Tachycardia
      (b) Hypotension
      (c) Shallow, rapid respirations
  c. Diagnostic study findings
    i. Severely elevated glucose levels ($>$1000 mg/dl)
    ii. No ketosis
    iii. Electrolyte levels vary with state of hydration; often severely depleted as a result of osmotic diuresis. Hypokalemia necessitates potassium replacement
    iv. Plasma hyperosmolality ($>$330 mOsm/kg)
    v. Acidosis, if present, usually caused by lactic acid or renal dysfunction

4. Nursing diagnoses
  a. Fluid volume deficit: refer to coverage in DKA section. Fluid deficits are usually greater than with ketoacidosis and are commonly corrected with rapidly administered 0.9% NaCl. Because many of these patients are

elderly or have underlying heart disease, central venous catheters or pulmonary artery catheters may be placed to assess for heart failure
   b. Altered nutrition, less than body requirements. Refer to coverage in DKA section. IV route for insulin administration is preferred because of poor peripheral perfusion in these severely dehydrated patients
   c. Potential hypoglycemia: refer to coverage in DKA section
   d. Potential for impaired peripheral tissue perfusion related to dehydration, hyperviscosity, increased platelet activity
      i. Assessment for defining characteristics
         (a) Cool, pale extremities
         (b) Hypotension
         (c) Diminished peripheral pulses
      ii. Expected outcomes
         (a) Color, temperature, and pulse quality are normal and equal bilaterally
         (b) Negative Homans' sign
      iii. Nursing interventions
         (a) Assess and document the status of the circulation in extremities, including color, temperature, and quality of bilateral peripheral pulses
         (b) Assess and report signs and symptoms indicative of thrombus formation, such as positive Homans' sign, localized redness, swelling, tenderness, or increased warmth
         (c) Perform active or passive range-of-motion exercises
         (d) Avoid constricting garments or positions that may impede circulation
         (e) Provide foot care, including inspection and prevention of foot injury
      iv. Evaluation of nursing care: patient exhibits no signs of impaired peripheral perfusion
   e. Potential for ineffective family coping related to gravity of illness and/or inadequate knowledge regarding illness and treatment
      i. Assessment for defining characteristics
         (a) Family describes preoccupation with personal reaction to situation (fear, anticipatory grief, guilt, anxiety)
         (b) Family requests information regarding illness and its treatment
      ii. Expected outcomes
         (a) Family is able to verbalize feelings and concerns
         (b) Family is able to use health care providers for information and support
      iii. Nursing interventions
         (a) Elicit concerns of family
         (b) Explain basic rationale for treatment
         (c) Explain the precipitating factors and the circumstances surrounding admission to the hospital
         (d) Keep family informed of patient status
         (e) Discuss usual reactions to acute illness, such as guilt, anxiety, grief
      iv. Evaluation of nursing care: family exhibits coping behaviors appropriate for patient's condition and treatment

. . . .

Hypoglycemic Episode

1. **Pathophysiology:** decrease in serum glucose level to 50 mg/dl or below. Glucose production (feeding and/or liver gluconeogenesis) lags behind glucose use. May be caused by decreased insulin resistance, decreased clearance of insulin or oral hypoglycemia agents or drug interactions
2. **Etiologic or precipitating factors**
   a. Insulin therapy
      i. Insulin dose greater than body's current needs
      ii. Sudden rotation of sites from hypertrophied area to one with unimpaired absorption
   b. Sulfonylurea (oral hypoglycemic) therapy
   c. Insufficient caloric consumption
      i. Meal or snack missed or delayed
      ii. Intake decreased because of nausea, vomiting, anorexia
      iii. Enteral tube feedings interrupted
   d. Strenous physical exercise that is uncompensated by an increase in food intake or a decrease in insulin dose
   e. Potentiation of hypoglycemic medications
      i. Renal and hepatic insufficiency
      ii. Medications that potentiate the action of sulfonylureas (phenylbutazone, large doses of salicylates, sulfonamides)
   f. Excessive alcohol intake, which inhibits gluconeogenesis
   g. Decreased requirements for exogenous insulin resulting from
      i. Recovery from physiologic stress, which decreases the levels of insulin-antagonistic hormones, thus decreasing the need for insulin
      ii. Weight loss, which decreases insulin resistance
      iii. Immediate postpartum period: sudden reduction in anti-insulin effects of placental hormones
      iv. Decrease in steroid dose
   h. Pentamidine used to treat *Pneumocystis carinii* infection is associated with pancreatic islet cell necrosis with resultant acute increase in insulin release
   i. Other health problems
      i. Adrenal insufficiency and hypopituitarism
      ii. Severe liver disease
      iii. Pancreatic islet cell tumor
3. **Nursing assessment data base**
   a. Nursing history
      i. Subjective findings
         (a) Headache, fatigue
         (b) Irritability
         (c) Hunger
      ii. Objective findings
         (a) Presence of a precipitating factor
         (b) Medication history
            (1) Regular insulin can be associated with a rapid fall in glucose levels and may prompt more adrenomedullary symptoms. Intermediate acting insulins or continuous insulin infusion devices may prompt a more gradual drop in plasma glucose, thus producing central nervous system symptoms (neuroglycopenia)

(2) Patients taking beta-adrenergic blocking agents (e.g., propranolol) may not exhibit adrenomedullary symptoms. Beta-adrenergic blocking agents can also impair recovery from hypoglycemia by inhibiting glycogenolysis

b. Nursing examination of patient

  i. Inspection

    (a) Pale skin

    (b) Tremors

    (c) Altered responsiveness or coma

    (d) Medical alert identification indicating diabetes mellitus

  ii. Palpation

    (a) Cool, clammy skin

    (b) Tachycardia and tachydysrhythmias

c. Diagnostic study findings: serum glucose level less than 50 mg/dl

4. Nursing diagnoses

a. Actual or potential hypoglycemia related to disparity between available fuel (glucose) and circulating insulin levels

  i. Assessment for defining characteristics

    (a) See subjective and objective findings

    (b) See physical and diagnostic findings

  ii. Expected outcome: plasma and capillary glucose levels are restored and remain within normal range

  iii. Nursing interventions

    (a) Identify patients at risk for hypoglycemia

    (b) If diabetes is established, secure information regarding past experience with hypoglycemia

    (c) Determine serum glucose level in any patient exhibiting symptoms

    (d) Administer oral or IV glucose if hypoglycemia occurs

    (e) Inform physician of episode

    (f) Observe patient closely until he or she is completely recovered

    (g) Remeasure glucose 20 to 30 minutes after treatment. Treat again if necessary

    (h) Assess cardiovascular and neurologic systems during and after the episode. Hypoglycemia has the potential for causing dysrhythmias and extending infarcts

    (i) Reevaluate current fluid and nutritional status to prevent recurrence

    (j) Instruct patient who is receiving insulin or oral hypoglycemic agents about the signs and symptoms of hypoglycemia and the need to report these promptly to the nurse

    (k) Maintain flow sheet documenting food intake, glucose levels, and diabetes-related medications

  iv. Evaluation of nursing care

    (a) Serum glucose level is within normal range

    (b) No signs or symptoms of hypoglycemia

b. Potential knowledge deficit regarding hypoglycemia management and prevention

  i. Assessment for defining characteristics

    (a) Patient and family request information regarding causes, symptoms, treatment, and prevention of hypoglycemia

(b) Precipitating event for hypoglycemic episode suggests that patient and family have inadequate knowledge of hypoglycemia and its management

ii. Expected outcome: patient and family are able to state causes, symptoms, treatment, and prevention of hypoglycemia

iii. Nursing interventions

(a) Instruct patient and family in causes, symptoms, treatment, and prevention of hypoglycemia

(b) If patient was admitted with a severe hypoglycemic episode, secure data regarding possible precipitating factors and most effective treatment

(c) If precipitating factors point to knowledge or skill deficit or to noncompliance, refer patient to diabetes educator

(d) Reinforce the importance of performing home blood glucose monitoring and when to notify physician

iv. Evaluation of nursing care

(a) Patient and family are able to identify causes, symptoms, and management of hypoglycemia

(b) Patient and family are able to perform home blood glucose monitoring

References

PHYSIOLOGIC ANATOMY

Bongard, F., and Sue, D.: Current Critical Care Diagnosis and Treatment. Norwalk, Conn., Appleton & Lange, 1994.

Genuth, S.: The endocrine system. *In* Berne, R., and Levy, M. (eds): Physiology, 3rd ed. St. Louis, Mosby-Year Book, 1993, pp. 478–578.

Goldman, D.: Surgery in patients with endocrine dysfunction. Med. Clin. North Am. 71:499–509, 1987.

Greenspan, F.: Basic and Clinical Endocrinology, 3rd ed. Norwalk, Conn., Appleton & Lange, 1991.

Wall, R.: Anesthetic challenges in the patient with endocrine disease. ASA Refresher Course Lectures (143:1–7). Chicago, American Society of Anesthesiologists, 1993.

NURSING ASSESSMENT DATA BASE

Dirksen, S., Lewis, S., and Collier, I.: Clinical Companion to Medical-Surgical Nursing. St. Louis, Mosby-Year Book, 1996.

COMMONLY ENCOUNTERED NURSING DIAGNOSES

Kim, M. J., McFarland, G., and McLane, A.: Pocket Guide to Nursing Diagnoses, 6th ed. St. Louis, Mosby-Year Book, 1995.

DIABETES INSIPIDUS, SIADH

Lindeman, C.: S.I.A.D.H.: Is your patient at risk? Nursing 22:60–68, 1992.

Moses, A., and Streeten, D.: Disorders of the neurohypophysis. *In* Isselbacher, K. (ed.): Harrison's Principles of Internal Medicine, 13th ed. New York, McGraw-Hill, 1994, pp. 1682–1691.

Smith-Rooker, J. L., Garrett, A., and Hodges, L. C.: Case management of the patient with pituitary tumor. MED-SURG Nurs. 2:265–274, 1993.

ACUTE ADRENAL INSUFFICIENCY

Epstein, C.: Adrenocortical insufficiency in the critically ill patient. AACN Clin. Issues Crit. Care Nurs. 3:705–718, 1992.

Gill, J.: Primary hyperaldosteronism. Endocrinologist 1:365–374, 1991.

Wall, R.: Anesthetic management of pheochromocytoma. Prog. Anesthesiol. 5:342–354, 1991.

THYROTOXICOSIS, MYXEDEMA COMA

Coffland, F.: Thyroid-induced cardiac disorders. Crit. Care Nurs. 25:81–97, 1993.

Federman, D.: Hyperthyroidism in the geriatric population. Hosp. Pract. 26:61–70, 1991.

Miller, M.: Disorders of the thyroid. *In* Brocklehurst, J., Tallis, R., and Fillit, H. (eds.): Textbook of Geriatric Medicine, 4th ed. Edinburgh, Churchill Livingstone, 1992, pp. 85–97.

Spittle, L.: Diagnoses in opposition: Thyroid storm and myxedema coma. AACN Clin. Issues Crit. Care Nurse 3:300–307, 1992.

DIABETIC KETOACIDOSIS, HHNK, HYPOGLYCEMIA

Diabetes update '93. Nursing 23:59–64, 1993.

Gusek, A.: 10 commonly asked questions about diabetes. Am. J. Nurs. 94:19–22, 1994.

Hirsch, I., and McGill, J.: Role of insulin in management of surgical patients with diabetes mellitus. Diabetes Care 13:980–985, 1990.

Nathan, D.: Long-term complications of diabetes mellitus. N. Engl. J. Med. 328:1676–1680, 1993.

Peragallo-Dittko, V.: A core curriculum for diabetes education, 2nd ed. Chicago, American Association of Diabetes Educators, 1993.

Reising, D.: Acute hypoglycemia. Nursing 25:41–49, 1995.

Roizen, M.: Perioperative management of the diabetic patient. ASA Refresher Course Lectures (164:1–5). Chicago, American Society of Anesthesiologists, 1993.

Wilson, B.: What nurses don't know about managing NIDDM. MEDSURG Nurs. 3:152–161, 1994.

HYPOPARATHYROIDISM AND HYPERPARATHYROIDISM

Fitzpatrick, L., and Bilezikian, J.: Primary hyperparathyroidism. *In* Becker, K. (ed): Principles and Practice of Endocrinology and Metabolism. Philadelphia, J.B. Lippincott, 1990, pp. 319–352.

chapter

Hematologic and Immunologic Systems

Stacey Young-McCaughan, R.N., Ph.D.(C), OCN®,
Lieutenant Colonel, U.S. Army Nurse Corps, and
Bonnie Mowinski Jennings, R.N., D.N.Sc., FAAN, Colonel,
U.S. Army Nurse Corps

PHYSIOLOGIC ANATOMY

Hematologic System

1. **Anatomic structures**
    a. Bone marrow
        i. Bone marrow is the spongy center of the bones where the hematologic and immunologic cell lines originate and mature before being released into the circulation
        ii. Bone marrow is present throughout the bones of the body, although the majority of the cells are produced in the vertebrae, ribs, skull, pelvis, and proximal epiphyses of the femur and humerus
    b. Liver
        i. The liver is located in the upper right quadrant of the abdomen in the peritoneal space below the diaphragm and under the rib cage. The liver receives 24% of the cardiac output—approximately 1500 ml of blood flow each minute—via the hepatic artery and portal vein
        ii. The liver has many diverse functions. As part of the hematologic system, the liver synthesizes various plasma proteins, including clotting factors and albumin. In addition, the liver clears damaged and nonfunctioning red blood cells (RBCs), or erythrocytes, from circulation
2. **Components**
    a. Pluripotent stem cell
        i. The pluripotent stem cell is a self-renewing cell from which all the differentiated bone marrow cell lines derive

ii. Various developmental cell lineages can be identified in the bone marrow before the mature cells are released into the circulation (Fig. 6–1)

b. Red blood cells

i. RBCs are biconcave disc-shaped cells enveloped with a tough, flexible membrane

ii. Erythropoiesis, or the production of RBCs, occurs in the bone marrow, where the pluripotent stem cell gives rise to the erythrocyte lineage, as shown in Figure 6–1. Erythropoiesis is regulated by the glycoprotein erythropoietin, which is produced primarily by the kidneys. In response to decreased oxygen levels in the blood, the kidney produces more erythropoietin, which acts on the bone marrow to increase and accelerate erythropoiesis. Iron, cobalamin (vitamin B$_{12}$), and folic acid are all needed for RBC production

iii. RBCs have a life span of approximately 120 days, at the end of which they are filtered out of circulation by the spleen and liver. Iron released from the heme is transported by transferrin back to the bone marrow, where it is recycled to make new RBCs. The porphyrin ring of the heme is reduced to bilirubin and eliminated as bile through the intestine

iv. Genetically determined antigens are located on the RBC cell membrane. The major antigens are named A and B. On the basis of the presence or absence of these two antigens, four major blood groups are defined (Table 6–1). Persons without antigen will form a naturally occurring antibody against the absent antigen shortly after birth. Rh is another type of RBC antigen that is different from A and B antigens. Persons without the Rh antigen (known as *Rh-negative*

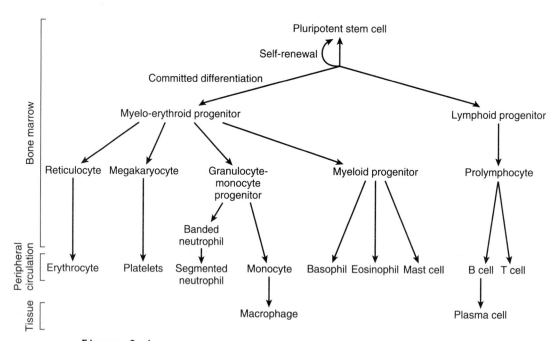

Figure 6–1 • Maturation of cells constituting the hematologic and immunologic systems. (Data from Appelbaum, 1993; Parslow, 1994; and Workman, 1995.)

TABLE 6–1. Red Blood Cell (RBC) Antigen Groups

Characteristic	O*	A	B	AB†
Genotype	OO	AA or AO	BB or BO	AB
Antigen A present	No	Yes	No	Yes
Antigen B present	No	No	Yes	Yes
Antibody against A	Yes	No	Yes	No
Antibody against B	Yes	Yes	No	No

* Type O blood is considered the universal donor blood because no major blood group antigens are present on the RBCs and so the blood can be transfused to any patient in an emergency.
† A person with type AB blood is considered the universal recipient because no natural antibodies are present and a person with this blood type can receive blood from any donor in an emergency.

persons) form antibody against Rh only when exposed to Rh-positive blood. Rh-negative persons can be exposed to the Rh antigen if they receive Rh-positive blood through transfusion. An Rh-negative woman can be exposed to the Rh antigen if she delivers an Rh-positive baby

   c. Platelets (thrombocytes)
      i. Platelets are non-nucleated cell fragments of megakaryocytes produced in the bone marrow (see Fig. 6–1)
      ii. Platelets activate the blood clotting system by going to sites of blood vessel or tissue injury, forming a platelet plug, and releasing cytokines that recruit more platelets and the clotting factors to the injury site
      iii. The life span of a platelet is approximately 10 days
   d. Clotting factors are proteins and other substances, numbered I to XIII, that form a fibrin matrix at sites of blood vessel or tissue injury. Factors commonly referred to include
      i. Factor I, also known as *fibrinogen*
      ii. Factor II, also known as *prothrombin*
      iii. Factor III, also known as *tissue thromboplastin* or *tissue factor*
      iv. Factor IV, also known as *calcium*
      v. Factor VIII, also known as *antihemophilic factor*
   e. Plasma is the straw-colored fluid that carries the blood components through the circulatory system and is made up primarily of water, proteins (albumin, globulins, and fibrinogen), small amounts of nutrients, electrolytes, hormones, enzymes, and metabolites. Serum is plasma without clotting factors

3. Functions
   a. Oxygenation
      i. The RBCs transport oxygen from the lungs to the tissues and carry carbon dioxide from the tissues to the lungs for excretion. Hemoglobin in the RBCs combines easily with both oxygen and carbon dioxide
      ii. The affinity of hemoglobin for oxygen and the mechanism of how oxygen is bound to hemoglobin in the lungs and released in the tissues is best described by the oxyhemoglobin dissociation curve (see Chapter 1, The Pulmonary System)
   b. Hemostasis
      i. Vascular constriction

    ii. Platelet plug
      (a) Injury to a blood vessel causes platelets to adhere to the exposed surfaces
      (b) Platelets then degranulate, releasing serotonin, von Willebrand factor, adenosine diphosphate (ADP), fibrinogen, and thromboxane from cell vesicles into the surrounding environment constricting the blood vessel, to minimize blood loss, and recruiting more platelets and clotting factors to the area. The coagulation cascade is initiated through mechanisms dependent on phospholipids in the platelet membrane
      (c) The platelets form an initial, unstable plug
   iii. Coagulation
      (a) At the same time the platelet plug is forming, the coagulation cascade is initiated
      (b) Two primary mechanisms activate the coagulation cascade (Fig. 6–2)
        (1) The extrinsic pathway is activated after tissue trauma when factor III released from the damaged tissues comes in contact with factor VII (proconvertin) circulating in the blood
        (2) The intrinsic pathway is activated after endothelial damage when factor XII (Hageman factor) circulating in the blood comes in contact with collagen

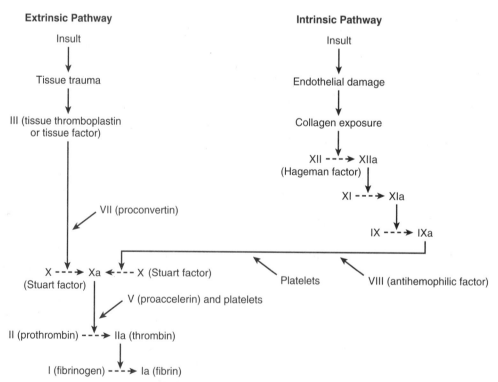

Figure 6–2 • Intrinsic and extrinsic coagulation cascades. (Modified from Secor, V. H.: Mediators of coagulation and inflammation: Relationship and clinical significance. Crit. Care Nurs. Clin. North Am. 5[3]:411–433, 1993.)

       (c) At each step in the cascade, an inactive proenzyme is converted to an active enzyme by proteolytic cleavage. Calcium, coenzymes, or phospholipids are required for some of the reactions to proceed

       (d) The last step of the cascade is the conversion of factor I (fibrinogen) to factor Ia (fibrin), forming a stable fibrin clot

    iv. Limiting and focusing hemostasis to sites of blood vessel damage

       (a) Platelet aggregation and the coagulation cascade are normally initiated only when blood comes in contact with nonvascular tissues, thereby localizing hemostasis to sites of injury

       (b) As the clot extends to areas where the blood vessel is intact, antithrombin III, a plasma protein normally circulating in the blood, inactivates thrombin. Heparin greatly improves the activity of antithrombin III

       (c) The fibrin clot is eventually removed by an enzyme called *plasmin.* Damaged endothelial cells secrete a protein that converts the inactive form of plasmin, plasminogen, to its active form so that degradation of the fibrin clot can begin. Like antithrombin III, plasminogen normally circulates freely in the blood. As the fibrin clot is degraded, fibrin split products can be detected in the blood

Immunologic System

1. Anatomic structures

  a. Bone marrow (see preceding description)

  b. Thymus

    i. The thymus is a bi-lobed lymphoid organ located in the mediastinum below the thyroid. Early in life, lymphocytes released from the bone marrow migrate to the thymus, where they mature into T cells before being released into the circulation

    ii. During fetal development and throughout the first 2 years of life, the thymus grows rapidly. After puberty the thymus slowly involutes as the circulating, long-lived T-cell population is maximized

  c. The lymph system is a separate vessel system that collects plasma and leukocytes that are not returned to the circulatory system from the tissue capillary beds. This lymph fluid is filtered and returned to the circulatory system, thereby maintaining appropriate tissue fluid pressures and preventing edema. Lymph fluid is propelled along the system by normal contraction of skeletal muscles

    i. Lymph fluid is a pale yellow liquid made up of plasma, leukocytes, enzymes, and antibodies; it lacks clotting factors and thus coagulates very slowly

    ii. Lymphatic capillaries and vessels are a network of open-ended tubes with one-way valves that collect lymph fluid from the tissues and eventually return it to the venous system via both the right lymphatic duct, which drains into the right subclavian vein, and the thoracic duct, which drains into the left subclavian vein

    iii. Lymph nodes are small, flat, bean-shaped patches of tissue located along the length of the lymphatic system that filter microorganisms from the lymph fluid before it is returned to the blood stream

(a) Lymph nodes can become swollen with white blood cells (WBCs), or leukocytes, that are responding to invading microorganisms if an infectious process is occurring in the area drained by the lymph node

(b) Lymph nodes can also become swollen with metastatic cancer cells that have migrated away from the primary site and become trapped in the network of the lymph node

d. The spleen is a lymphoid organ located in the upper left quadrant of the abdomen that clears damaged or nonfunctioning RBCs and filters antigens from the blood for evaluation by lymphocytes

2. **Components**

a. Pluripotent stem cell (see earlier description)

b. WBCs circulate throughout the body, detecting and destroying bacteria, viruses, fungi, parasites, and other proteins identified as foreign to the body. The pluripotent stem cell gives rise to all WBC lineages. The different WBCs mature primarily in the bone marrow before being released into circulation (see Fig. 6–1). The average life span of a WBC in circulation is 12 hours

i. Granulocytes or myeloid series of leukocytes

(a) Neutrophils

(1) Because these cells are segmented polymorphonuclear neutrophils, they are also known as "segs," "PMNs," "polys," or "neuts." Because these cells are also granulocytes, they are also known as "grans"

(2) Neutrophils are the most numerous of the WBCs. They are efficient phagocytic cells that are able to migrate through endothelial cells to sites of microbial invasion

(3) Neutrophils are often destroyed during phagocytosis. Pus is the accumulation of cellular debris from the destruction of microorganisms and neutrophils at the site of infection

(b) Monocytes and macrophages

(1) Monocytes are released from the bone marrow into the peripheral circulation where they mature. When they enter the tissue, they become highly efficient phagocytic macrophages

(2) Some macrophages move throughout the body, whereas others stay in one particular tissue and are named according to where they reside. For example, Kupffer cells are liver macrophages, Langerhans cells are skin macrophages, alveolar macrophages are lung macrophages, mesangial cells are kidney macrophages, and microglial cells are central nervous system macrophages

(3) Unlike neutrophils, which are often destroyed during phagocytosis, macrophages can phagocytose many foreign antigens, surviving months to years

(c) Eosinophils are motile, phagocytic cells that combat multicellular parasitic infections. They are also associated with allergic reactions and other inflammatory processes

(d) Basophils

(1) Basophils are nonphagocytic cells that attract immunoglobulin E (IgE) antibodies to their cell membranes. When the IgE binds antigen, the basophils

   release histamine, triggering a massive inflammatory
   response

   (2) Basophils are involved in various inflammatory conditions.
   Their exact role in immunity has yet to be determined

(e) Mast cells

   (1) Mast cells, like basophils, attract IgE antibodies to their cell
   membranes. Also, like basophils, mast cells release histamine
   when the IgE binds antigen, triggering a massive
   inflammatory response

   (2) Mast cells and basophils differentiate along separate
   pathways. Basophils circulate in the blood and survive only
   days, whereas mast cells are located in the tissue and live
   weeks or months

   (3) IgE-mediated mast cell degranulation is responsible for type
   I hypersensitivity reactions

ii. Lymphocytes or lymphoid series of leukocytes

(a) B cells, or B lymphocytes

   (1) B cells manufacture and express antigen-binding proteins
   called *immunoglobulins* on their cell membrane

   (2) When the B cell immunoglobulin binds a particular antigen,
   the cell is stimulated to differentiate into two separate cells
   called *plasma cells* and *memory B cells*

      a) Plasma cells are antibody factories that immediately
      produce and secrete large amounts of antibody to bind
      to the antigen

      b) Memory B cells go into a resting state but can be quickly
      reactivated to produce plasma cells and antibody if
      exposed to the same antigen in the future

   (3) Antibodies are secreted protein immunoglobulins that can
   bind to more of the same antigen. There are four major
   types of antibodies

      a) Immunoglobulin M (IgM) is the first immunoglobulin to
      be secreted during the primary immune response to an
      antigen

      b) Immunoglobulin G (IgG) is secreted during the
      secondary immune response and is more specific to a
      particular antigen

      c) Immunoglobulin A (IgA) is present in secretions such as
      mucus and breast milk

      d) IgE attaches to the cell membranes of basophils and mast
      cells. When IgE binds to antigen, it triggers the cell to
      release histamine

(b) T cells or T lymphocytes

   (1) T cells mature in the thymus and recognize antigen in
   association with cell membrane proteins. The cell
   membrane proteins are known as *major histocompatibility
   complexes* (MHC). There are two classes of MHC proteins (I
   and II) that work with different T cells as part of the
   immune system. Class I MHC are found on all cells, whereas
   Class II MHC are found on B cells and macrophages

       (2) T helper (T_H) cells, also called *CD4 cells* because they display the membrane glycoprotein antigen CD4, recognize class II MHC molecules on the cell surface of B cells and macrophages. In response to recognition of a foreign antigen–MHC II complex, T_H cells secrete hormones, called *cytokines,* that activate other components of the immune system (see also Acquired Immunity)

       (3) T cytotoxic (T_C) cells, also called *CD8 cells* because they display the membrane glycoprotein CD8, recognize class I MHC molecules on the surface of cells. In response to recognition of a foreign antigen–MCH I complex, T_C cells secrete cytotoxic substances that directly destroy the cell (see also Acquired Immunity)

    (c) Natural killer (NK) cells are a type of null cell (neither T nor B) lymphocyte. NK cells do not express antigen-binding receptors but do have cytotoxic capabilities against bacteria-infected and virus-infected cells as well as against tumor cells

  c. Complement is a group of more than 20 serum proteins, named C1 to C9, that act through an enzymatic cascade against invading pathogens. These proteins act sequentially and in concert to lyse microorganisms and/or infected cells

  d. Cytokines are protein hormones secreted by cells to signal other cells. Examples of cytokines include interferon, interleukin, tumor necrosis factor (TNF), granulocyte-macrophage colony-stimulating factor (GM-CSF), granulocyte colony-stimulating factor (G-CSF), erythropoietin, and thrombopoietin

  e. Eicosanoids are a type of fatty acid that regulate a variety of physiologic processes, some of which are listed in Table 6–2. Eicosanoids are short-lived compounds that signal cells in a local area. Many commonly prescribed drugs inhibit eicosanoid production but, in the process, affect other physiologic processes dependent on eicosanoid regulation. Figure 6–3 shows how steroids and nonsteroidal anti-inflammatory drugs (NSAIDs) act to disrupt eicosanoid production

TABLE 6–2. Functions of Eicosanoids

Prostaglandins

  Cardiovascular: vasodilation
  Gastrointestinal: maintenance of mucosal barrier
  Endocrine: temperature elevation
  Genitourinary: uterine contraction
  Hematologic: antiplatelet aggregation
  Immunologic: inflammatory response

Thromboxanes

  Cardiovascular: vasoconstriction
  Hematologic: platelet aggregation

Leukotrienes

  Pulmonary: bronchial smooth muscle contraction
  Immunologic: leukocyte activation

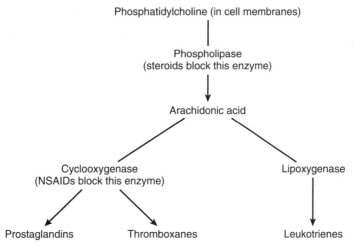

Figure 6-3 • Eicosanoid production. NSAID = nonsteroidal anti-inflammatory drug.

3. **Functions**
   a. Innate immunity
      i. Anatomic and physiologic barriers
         (a) Mechanical barrier of the skin and mucosa
         (b) Acid pH of the skin and in the stomach
         (c) Flushing or mechanical removal of pathogens (e.g., bladder emptying, gastrointestinal motility, coughing and sneezing, ciliary activity)
         (d) Mucous secretions (e.g., saliva, tears) that contain enzymes and IgA
      ii. Inflammation
         (a) The hallmarks of inflammation are rubor (erythema), tumor (edema), calor (heat), and dolor (pain) that occur as a result of
            (1) Vasodilation of the capillary bed in the affected area
            (2) Increased capillary permeability, allowing fluid and immune competent cells into the area
            (3) An influx of phagocytic cells to attack microorganisms
         (b) The eicosanoids thromboxane and leukotriene are potent mediators of inflammation that increase the migration of inflammatory cells to the area and increase capillary permeability
      iii. Phagocytosis
         (a) Neutrophils and macrophages are capable of ingesting and digesting antigens such as microorganisms, dead cells, and cellular debris
         (b) Inside the phagocytic cell, lysozymes break down antigens, recycling usable products and displaying antigenic protein pieces on their class II MHC for evaluation by T cells
      iv. Complement pathway
         (a) The complement pathway can be triggered either by antigen-antibody complexes or by components of the infectious agents themselves
         (b) The complement pathway acts against invading pathogens by inducing inflammation, attracting neutrophils and monocytes, promoting phagocytosis, and building a membrane attack

complex (MAC) which makes a hole in the microorganism's cell membrane, thereby killing it

b. Acquired immunity

  i. Antibody-mediated immunity is aimed primarily at extracellular microorganisms and is also responsible for immediate hypersensitivity reactions

   (a) Immunoglobulins on B cells bind antigen on the cell surface. The B cells internally process the antigen-antibody complex, re-displaying the antigen on the B cell's surface on a Class II MHC

   (b) A T_H CD4 cell then binds the antigen displayed on the Class II MHC of the B cell and, recognizing it as foreign, secretes cytokines that stimulate the B cell to both secrete IgM and differentiate into antibody-secreting plasma cells and memory B cells

   (c) When antibody binds to an antigen, it does not actually destroy the antigen, but it facilitates its neutralization, elimination, or destruction in the following ways:

    (1) Neutralization or binding the antigen so that the function of the antigen is disrupted until the antigen can be phagocytized

    (2) Opsonization or coating the invading microorganism so that it can be easily recognized as foreign and phagocytized

    (3) Activation of complement, which lyses the invader's cell membrane

  ii. Cell-mediated immunity is aimed primarily at intracellular microorganisms, viruses, and cancer and is also responsible for delayed hypersensitivity reactions and transplanted tissue rejection. When T_C CD8 cells recognize foreign antigen on a cell's surface on class I MHC, the T_C cell secretes cytotoxic substances that destroy the foreign cell. This is particularly important in eliminating virus-infected cells, tumor cells, and cells of a transplanted tissue graft

c. Tolerance

  i. In addition to recognizing foreign antigens and initiating an immunologic response, the immune system must also be able to recognize its own proteins and not mount an immune response against self

  ii. This process of self-recognition occurs as part of normal neonatal growth and development

  iii. Autoimmune diseases occur when there is a breakdown of tolerance in which the immune system identifies its own proteins as foreign and inappropriately mounts a response to destroy these self proteins

  iv. Examples of autoimmune diseases include systemic lupus erythematosus, rheumatoid arthritis, acute rheumatic fever, Graves' disease, Hashimoto's thyroiditis, and type I diabetes mellitus

d. Hypersensitivity reactions

  i. Hypersensitivity reactions, or allergies, are exaggerated immune responses that can be uncomfortable and potentially harmful to the patient

  ii. There are four types of hypersensitivity reactions, classified according to the time between exposure and reaction, immune mechanism involved, and site of reaction

(a) *Type I* immediate hypersensitivity reactions are mediated by IgE reacting to common allergens such as dust, pollen, animal dander, insect stings, some foods, and various drugs. These reactions can be local, resulting in local swelling and discomfort, or systemic, resulting in anaphylaxis and possibly in death if not recognized and treated promptly

(b) *Type II* immediate hypersensitivity reactions are mediated by antibody and complement. These reactions can occur with a mismatched blood transfusion or as a response to various drugs

(c) *Type III* immediate hypersensitivity reactions result in tissue damage caused by precipitation of antigen-antibody immune complexes. These reactions can occur with serum sickness or as a response to various drugs

(d) *Type IV* delayed hypersensitivity reactions result from migration of immune cells to the site of exposure days after the exposure to the antigen. These reactions can occur with contact dermatitis, measles rash, or tuberculin skin testing or as a response to various drugs. Transplanted graft rejection is a type IV hypersensitivity reaction

iii. Hypersensitivity reactions to drugs, or drug allergies, are one of many possible adverse drug reactions. Drug-induced hypersensitivity reactions can be any of the four types of hypersensitivity

NURSING ASSESSMENT DATA BASE

. . . .
.
: Nursing History

1. **Client health history**
   a. Many times in the process of seeking medical attention for some other reason, a hematologic or immunologic problem is identified
   b. Past medical history indicating a potential or existing hematologic or immunologic problem would include
      i. Recent, recurrent, or chronic infections
      ii. Cancer or prior treatment for cancer
      iii. Human immunodeficiency virus (HIV)
      iv. Liver disorders
      v. Kidney disorders
      vi. Malabsorption disorders
      vii. Any prolonged bleeding or delayed healing with prior surgeries and/or dental extractions
      viii. History of having blood transfused
      ix. History of splenectomy
      x. Placement of prosthetic heart valves
      xi. Placement of an indwelling venous access device indicating the patient needed long term venous access
   c. Review of systems with patient and/or family for signs and symptoms
      i. General: fatigue, weakness, lethargy, malaise, fever, chills, night

   sweats, dyspnea, restlessness, apprehension, pain, altered mental status, vertigo, dizziness, confusion

  ii. Skin: pruritus, change in skin color, rash, unusual bruising, ulcers or other lesions

  iii. Head and neck: headache, change in vision, sinus pain, epistaxis, gingival bleeding, sore throat, pain with swallowing, enlarged lymph nodes

  iv. Respiratory: cough, hemoptysis, dyspnea, orthopnea

  v. Cardiovascular: palpitations, dizziness with position changes

  vi. Gastrointestinal: change in eating habits, anorexia, abdominal fullness, nausea, vomiting, hematemesis, change in bowel habits, hematochezia, melena, pain with defecation, change in weight

  vii. Genitourinary: hematuria, pain with urination, menorrhagia, enlarged inguinal lymph nodes

  viii. Musculoskeletal: swelling of joints, tenderness or pain in bones or joints

  ix. Endocrine: heat or cold intolerance

2. **Family history** indicating a potential hematologic or immunologic problem: hemophilia, sickle cell anemia, cancer, or death at a young age for reasons other than trauma

3. **Social history and habits** that may assist with the diagnosis and treatment of the underlying condition include

 a. Any unusual or excessive exposure to chemicals (e.g., gasoline, benzene, solvents, glues, paints, varnishes) or radiation (e.g., x-rays) at work or in pursuing a hobby

 b. Any unusual dietary preferences, pica

 c. Excessive alcohol consumption

 d. Sexual preference, number of partners, history of sexually transmitted diseases, current contraceptive method, use of safe sex practices

 e. Intravenous drug use

4. **Medication history**

 a. Current medications or a recent change in medication may suggest an underlying hematologic or immunologic problem. Always ask about over-the-counter medication use, because many of these contain aspirin or NSAIDs

 b. Many medications used to treat nonhematologic and nonimmunologic problems can have effects on the hematologic and immunologic systems. Examples of these drugs include

  i. Analgesics and anti-inflammatory drugs

   (a) Aspirin and aspirin-containing drugs, such as

    (1) Oxycodone and aspirin (Percodan)

    (2) Bismuth subsalicylate (Pepto-Bismol)

   (b) NSAIDs, such as

    (1) Ibuprofen (Motrin)

    (2) Indomethacin (Indocin)

    (3) Ketoprofen (Orudis)

    (4) Ketorolac (Toradol)

    (5) Sulindac (Clinoril)

   (c) Steroids, such as

    (1) Dexamethasone (Decadron)

    (2) Prednisone

   ii. Antibiotics, such as
     (a) Chloramphenicol (Chloromycetin)
     (b) Isoniazid (INH)
     (c) Para-aminosalicylic acid (PAS)
     (d) Penicillin
     (e) Streptomycin
     (f) Trimethoprim-sulfamethoxazole (Bactrim, Septra)
     (g) Zidovudine (AZT)
  iii. Anticoagulants, such as
     (a) Heparin
     (b) Warfarin (Coumadin)
  iv. Anticonvulsants, such as
     (a) Carbamazepine (Tegretol)
     (b) Phenytoin (Dilantin)
   v. Antidiabetic agents, such as chlorpropamide
  vi. Antineoplastic chemotherapy agents, such as
     (a) Cyclophosphamide (Cytoxan)
     (b) Cytosine arabinoside (ara-C)
     (c) Daunorubicin (daunomycin)
     (d) Doxorubicin (Adriamycin)
     (e) Etoposide (VP-16)
     (f) Hydroxyurea (Hydrea)
     (g) Methotrexate
     (h) Nitrogen mustard
     (i) Paclitaxel (Taxol)
     (j) Vinblastine (Velban)
  vii. Antipsychotic, such as clozapine (Clozaril)
 viii. Antirheumatic agents, such as
     (a) Gold
     (b) Methotrexate
  ix. Cardiovascular agents, such as
     (a) Digoxin
     (b) Methyldopa (Aldomet)
     (c) Procainamide (Pronestyl)
     (d) Quinidine sulfate
   x. Diuretics, such as chlorothiazide (Diuril)
  xi. Hormones, such as
     (a) Estrogens
     (b) Androgens
  xii. Immunosuppressives, such as
     (a) Azathioprine (Imuran)
     (b) Cyclophosphamide (Cytoxan)
     (c) Cyclosporine
     (d) Methotrexate
     (e) Vincristine (Oncovin)
 xiii. Oral contraceptives

Nursing Examination of Patient

1. **Inspection**
  a. Temperature: exceeds 101°F (38.3°C)

b. Skin: pallor, jaundice, flushing, rash, petechiae, purpura, ecchymoses, hematomas, urticaria, integrity
c. Head and neck: integrity of mucosal membranes, tongue appearance (e.g., smooth, coated), conjunctival bleeding
d. Chest: shortness of breath, hemoptysis
e. Abdomen: vomiting, hematemesis, hematuria, diarrhea, melena
f. Musculoskeletal: swelling of joints

2. **Palpation and percussion**
   a. Skin: warm to touch
   b. Neck: enlarged lymph nodes
   c. Abdomen: hepatomegaly, splenomegaly, enlarged lymph nodes in the axilla or groin
   d. Musculoskeletal: pain with palpation

3. **Auscultation**
   a. Tachycardia
   b. Hypotension
   c. Orthostatic changes (pulse increases 20 beats and blood pressure decreases 20 points when patient moves from lying to sitting or standing)
   d. Tachypnea
   e. Crackles, rhonchi
   f. Decreased breath sounds

Diagnostic Studies

1. **Laboratory** (see Table 6–3 for normal values)
   a. Blood
      i. Complete blood count (CBC) with differential
         (a) The total WBC count measures the total number of WBCs found in 1 µl of blood
         (b) The differential measures the contribution that each type of WBC (neutrophils, monocytes, basophils, eosinophils, and lymphocytes) makes to the total WBC count.
            (1) A "shift to the right" on a CBC indicates that only a small percentage of the WBCs are neutrophils. The lower the neutrophil count, the greater the patient's risk of infection. To calculate the absolute neutrophil count (ANC), multiply the percentage of neutrophils indicated on the differential of the CBC by the total number of WBCs. See Figure 6–4 for a sample calculation
            (2) A "shift to the left" on a CBC indicates that a large percentage of the WBCs are neutrophils. This usually implies that the bone marrow has been stimulated to produce more neutrophils to fight a severe infection
         (c) The RBC count is a measure of the total number of RBCs found in 1 mm³ of blood
         (d) The hemoglobin count (Hb) is a measure of the amount of hemoglobin in 1 dl of blood and is an indicator of the blood's oxygen-carrying capacity

TABLE 6–3. Normal Laboratory Blood Values*

White blood cell count (WBC): 5000–10,000/μl
White blood cell count differential
   Neutrophils: 50%–62% of total WBC
   Bands: 3%–6% of total WBC
   Monocytes: 3%–7% of total WBC
   Basophils: 0%–1% of total WBC
   Eosinophils: 0%–3% of total WBC
   Lymphocytes: 25%–40% of total WBC
Red blood cell count (RBC)
   Men: 4.5–5.5 × 10^6/L
   Women: 4.0–5.0 × 10^6/L
Hemoblogin (Hb)
   Men: 14.0 to 17.4 g/dl
   Women: 12.0–16.0 g/dl
Hematocrit (HCT)
   Men: 42% to 52%
   Women: 36%–48%
Mean corpuscular volume (MCV): 84–96 fl
Mean corpuscular hemoglobin concentration (MCHC): 32–36 g/dl
Mean corpuscular hemoglobin (MCH): 28–34 pg
Platelets: 140,000–440,000/mm³ (can be annotated 140K–440K)
Reticulocyte count
   Men: 0.5%–1.5% of total RBC
   Women: 0.5%–2.5% of total RBC
Erythrocyte sedimentation rate (ESR)
   Men: 0–15 mm/hour
   Women: 0–20 mm/hour
Serum iron
   Men: 75–175 μg/dl
   Women: 65–165 μg/dl
Total iron-binding capacity (TIBC): 240–450 μg/dl
Ferritin
   Men 18–270 μg/L
   Women 18–160 μg/L
Bleeding time: 3–10 minutes†
Thrombin time (TT): 7–12 seconds†
Prothrombin time (PT): 11–13 seconds†
Partial thromboplastin time (PTT): 30–45 seconds†
International Normalized Ratio (INR): 0.9–1.1
Fibrin split products (FSPs): negative at 1:4 dilution
D-dimers: <250 mg/ml
Fibrinogen (factor I): 200–400 mg/dl
Serum bilirubin
   Total bilirubin: 0.2–1.0 mg/dl or 3.4–17.1 μmol/L
   Direct: 0.0–0.2 mg/dl or 0.0–3.4 μmol/L
   Indirect: 0.2–0.8 mg/dl or 3.4–13.68 μmol/L
Coombs' antiglobulin test
   Direct: negative for antibody on RBC
   Indirect: negative for antibody in serum
T cell counts
   Total T cells: 812–2318 cells/μl
   T_H cells (CD4 cells): 589–1505 cells/μl
   T_S cells: 325–997 cells/μl
   T_H/T_S ratio: >1.0

* Be sure to check your institution's normal values.
† Normal values depend on the measurement method.
Data from Fischbach, F. T.: A Manual of Laboratory and Diagnostic Tests, 5th ed. Philadelphia, J. B. Lippincott, 1996.

CBC Report	
6.5	WBC $\times$ 10^3
4.51	RBC $\times$ 10^6
14.0	HGB g/dl
40.8	HCT %
90.5	MCV fl
30.9	MCH pg
34.2	MCHC g/dl
333	PLT $\times$ 10^3

Automated Differential

35.0	LYMPH %
10.3	MONO %
46.3	NEUT %
7.3	EOS %
1.0	BASO %

Manual Differential

SEGMENTED NEUTROPHILS %	49
BANDED NEUTROPHILS %	1
LYMPHOCYTES %	32
MONOCYTES %	8
EOSINOPHILS %	9
BASOPHILS %	1

Figure 6–4 • Calculating the absolute neutrophil count from the complete blood count (CBC) report. HCT = hematocrit; HGB = hemoglobin; MCH = mean corpuscular hemoglobin; MCHC = mean corpuscular hemoglobin concentration; MCV = mean corpuscular volume; PLT = platelets; RBC = red blood cell; WBC = white blood cell.

To calculate the absolute neutrophil count (ANC), use the *manual differential* because it is more accurate. Multiply the percent of segmented neutrophils (49% in this example) and the percent of banded neutrophils (1% in this example) by the total number of WBCs (6500 in this example). Banded neutrophils are included in the calculations of the ANC because they are developmentally nearly mature neutrophils and can function as mature neutrophils (see Fig. 6–1). If a manual differential has not been done, the automated differential can be used; if the total WBC count is >10,000/μl or <3000/μl, a manual differential should be requested.

Generic Calculation:
(% neutrophils + % bands) (WBC) = ANC
Calculations for this example:
(.49 + .01) (6500) = 3250

(e) The hematocrit (HCT) is the percentage of RBCs in a volume of whole blood

(f) The mean corpuscular volume (MCV) is the average size (volume) of RBCs

(g) The mean corpuscular hemoglobin concentration (MCHC) is the average concentration of hemoglobin in the RBCs

(h) The mean corpuscular hemoglobin (MCH) is the average amount of hemoglobin per RBC

(i) The platelet count is the total number of platelets per 1 mm^3 of blood

ii. The reticulocyte count measures the number or percent of immature RBCs in the peripheral circulation

iii. The erythrocyte sedimentation rate (ESR, or sed rate) measures the rate at which RBCs settle out of anticoagulated blood in 1 hour. The ESR can be elevated in inflammatory conditions or anemia. Rather than as a diagnostic test, ESR is best used to assess response to treatment

iv. Serum iron level is a measure of the amount of iron in serum

v. The total iron-binding capacity (TIBC) reflects the body's ability to transport available iron

vi. Ferritin is a rough measure of the body's iron stores and is a good indicator of the body's iron storage status

vii. Bleeding time refers to the primary phase of hemostasis: how long it takes platelets to adhere to the broken blood vessel and form the platelet plug. Bleeding time is a rough gauge of platelet function

viii. Thrombin time (TT) measures the time it takes thrombin (factor IIa) to convert fibrinogen (factor I) to fibrin (factor Ia). It is markedly prolonged by the presence of any heparin

ix. Prothrombin time (PT) measures clotting ability of the extrinsic coagulation cascade (factor VII) and the common pathway (factor X [Stuart factor], factor V [proaccelerin], factor II [prothrombin], and factor I [fibrinogen]). The PT is used to monitor warfarin (Coumadin) therapy

x. Partial thromboplastin time (PTT) is a more sensitive measure of the clotting ability and a test of the common pathway (factor X [Stuart factor], factor V [proaccelerin], factor II [prothrombin], and factor I [fibrinogen]). The PTT is used to monitor heparin therapy

xi. The International Normalized Ratio (INR) is a comparative rating of PT ratios in which the measured PT is adjusted by the International Reference Thromboplastin. It is a more uniform way of monitoring warfarin therapy

xii. Fibrin split products are measures of the levels of fibrin degradation products

xiii. D-dimers also reflect levels of fibrin degradation products but are a more specific test for disseminated intravascular coagulation (DIC) because they are specific for fibrinolysis

xiv. Fibrinogen measures the blood level of fibrinogen (factor I)

xv. Serum bilirubin, resulting from the breakdown of hemoglobin in the RBCs, reflects the various amounts of bilirubin in the blood

    (a) Conjugated or direct bilirubin circulates freely in the blood until it is cleared by the liver and excreted in bile. An increase in conjugated bilirubin is indicative of a dysfunction or blockage of the liver

    (b) Unconjugated or indirect bilirubin is protein bound. An increase in unconjugated bilirubin often is evidence of increased RBC destruction

    (c) Total bilirubin is a measure of both conjugated and unconjugated bilirubin

xvi. Serum protein electrophoresis (SPEP) determines the levels of serum proteins in blood, particularly levels of immunoglobulins

xvii. Coombs' test

    (a) The direct Coombs test detects the presence of antibody on the RBC membrane

    (b) The indirect Coombs test detects antibody in the serum

xviii. T-cell counts reflect the levels of T cells in the blood

xix. HIV antibody tests include the enzyme-linked immunosorbent assay (ELISA) and the Western blot. Both of these tests are used to detect the presence of antibody to HIV. The Western blot is a more specific and sensitive test

xx. Blood and tissue typing

    (a) Blood typing detects ABO and Rh antigens present on RBCs and is necessary for compatibility testing before blood product transfusions

    (b) A more specific blood typing test detects human leukocyte antigens (HLAs) and is necessary for compatibility testing before some types of tissue transplantation (e.g., bone marrow transplantation)

xxi. Blood cultures detect and identify microorganisms in the blood

b. Sputum cultures detect and identify microorganisms in the sputum

  c. Urine tests

    i. Urinalysis can detect gross amounts of blood or protein in the urine

    ii. Urine cultures detect and identify microorganisms in the urine

    iii. Urine protein electrophoresis (UPEP) determines the levels of proteins excreted in the urine, particularly levels of immunoglobulins

  d. Stool Hemoccult detects microscopic amounts of blood in the stool

2. Noninvasive methods: Radiologic

  a. Spleen ultrasonography is used to estimate the size of the spleen

  b. In a liver-spleen scan, a radioactive tracer is used to evaluate the size as well as the function of the liver and spleen

  c. In a gallium scan, a radioactive tracer is used to detect the presence of malignant tissue, particularly malignant lymphoid tissues

  d. In a lymphangiogram (LAG), contrast dye is used to radiologically visualize the lymph system, particularly the size and architecture of lymph nodes

3. Invasive methods

  a. Biopsies

    i. A bone marrow biopsy includes aspiration of bone marrow fluid and removal of a needle core biopsy sample of the bone marrow tissue for pathologic examination

    ii. In a lymph node biopsy, one or more lymph nodes are removed for pathologic examination

  b. Skin tests can serve as a barometer of immune functioning, pointing out hyposensitivities or hypersensitivities to a particular antigen. Examples of allergens used in skin testing include allergenic extracts (e.g., dust, pollen, animal dander); purified protein derivative (PPD) for tuberculin skin tests; mumps virus; *Candida albicans;* and skin fungi

COMMONLY ENCOUNTERED NURSING DIAGNOSES

Altered Protection (Risk for Infection) Related to Disease or Treatment

1. Assessment for defining characteristics

  a. Reports of fever, chills, night sweats, sore throat, cough, malaise, pain with swallowing, pain with urination, pain with defecation, diarrhea, reddened areas, sore areas, swollen areas (these symptoms may not be present if patient is neutropenic and unable to mount a WBC response)

  b. Flushing, lethargy; skin warm to touch

  c. Abnormal vital signs: temperature exceeding 101°F (38.3°C); hypotension; tachycardia

  d. WBC count is less than 1500/μl, ANC is less than 500/μl (see Fig. 6–4)

2. Expected outcomes

  a. Vital signs are within normal limits for the patient

  b. The patient has no signs or symptoms of active infection

  c. The WBC count is maintained within an acceptable range

  d. The patient and family verbalize an understanding of underlying pathology and infection prevention

3. **Nursing interventions** (see Table 6–4)
4. **Evaluation of nursing care**
    a. The patient is afebrile
    b. The patient has no signs or symptoms of active infection
    c. The patient can maintain an ANC exceeding 1000/μl
    d. The patient and family can describe how to reduce the patient's risk of infection

Altered Protection (Risk for Hemorrhage) Related to Disease and/or Treatment

1. **Assessment for defining characteristics**
    a. Reports of unusual bruising, prolonged bleeding, hematemesis, hemoptysis, hematochezia, melena, hematuria, menorrhagia
    b. Petechiae, purpura, ecchymoses, hematomas, gingival bleeding, conjunctival bleeding
    c. Platelet count is less than 50,000/mm^3; PT and PTT are prolonged
2. **Expected outcomes**
    a. The patient is without evidence of spontaneous bleeding
    b. The patient is able to maintain platelet counts and levels of clotting factors within an acceptable range
    c. The patient and family verbalize an understanding of underlying pathology and bleeding precautions
3. **Nursing interventions** (see Table 6–5)
4. **Evaluation of nursing care**
    a. The patient shows no evidence of spontaneous bleeding
    b. The patient can maintain a platelet count of more than 50,000/mm^3 and PT and PTT times are within prescribed ranges as determined by the patient's therapy and care provider
    c. The patient and family can describe how to reduce the patient's risk of bleeding

Potential Fluid Volume Deficit Related to Fever, Vomiting, Diarrhea, Hemorrhage, or Shock

1. **Assessment for defining characteristics**
    a. Reports of thirst, sweating, vomiting, polyuria, diarrhea, lightheadedness
    b. Pallor, mucosal dryness, loss of skin turgor, decreased venous filling
    c. Abnormal vital signs: fever, tachycardia, hypotension, changes in orthostatic vital signs
    d. Decreased urine output and concentrated urine with specific gravity exceeding 1.020
    e. Altered mental status
2. **Expected outcomes**
    a. Vital signs are within normal limits for the patient
    b. The patient maintains an adequate urine output
3. **Nursing interventions**
    a. Administer intravenous fluids and blood products as prescribed
        i. Transfuse blood products (Table 6–6)

TABLE 6–4. Nursing Actions for the Patient Who Is Neutropenic: Compromised Host Precautions

1. The patient should have a private room. It does not have to be an isolation room. The door may be left open. A "Compromised Host Precaution" sign should be posted on the door.

2. All persons entering the patient's room must wash their hands before touching the patient for any reason. This is the most important way to prevent infection. The patient and family should be encouraged to remind all staff and visitors to wash their hands before touching the patient.

3. Administer hematopoietic growth factors as prescribed. Hematopoietic growth factors, also called colony-stimulating factors (CSFs), are cytokines that stimulate production of various blood cell components. Because hematopoietic growth factors take several days to increase white blood cell counts, they are best used in anticipation of neutropenia (e.g., immediately after cytotoxic chemotherapy).

4. Monitor vital signs every 2 to 4 hours. Notify physician immediately for temperature exceeding 101°F (38.3°C) to consider the need for an infectious fever work-up and initiating or changing antibiotics. An infectious fever work-up usually includes two sets of blood cultures, a chest radiograph, sputum culture, urine culture, wound culture, and other cultures for suspected sites of infection. For patients with an indwelling venous access device (VAD), one set of cultures is usually drawn from the VAD and one set is drawn from a peripheral site. To assist with the localization of the infection, mark the culture bottles clearly with regard to where the specimen was obtained. The offending organism is more likely to grow in blood cultures if cultures are drawn as the patient's temperature is rising than after the patient's temperature has peaked.

5. Invasive procedures should be kept to a minimum. Invasive devices such as catheters and tubes should be removed as soon as the patient's medical condition permits.

6. Careful attention to aseptic technique must be observed, especially for performing phlebotomy, handling intravenous lines, or performing other invasive procedures.

7. Designate a particular stethoscope and thermometer to be used exclusively in caring for the patient.

8. Masks are not required; they are actually discouraged. Staff with upper respiratory tract or other infections should not care for the patient.

9. Clean table tops, equipment, and room floor frequently with hospital-approved disinfectant, clean cloths, and clean mops.

10. The patient should be taught to wash his or her hands before and after eating, using the toilet, and performing any self-care procedure. If possible, the patient should shower every day. Liquid soap instead of bar soap should be used.

11. Encourage the patient to cough and deep breathe every 4 hours. Mobility should be encouraged. Smoking should be discouraged.

12. Only canned or cooked foods should be served. Raw fruits, raw vegetables, and milk products are not served because of the risk of bacteria (e.g., *Escherichia coli, Pseudomonas aeruginosa*, and *Klebsiella* species) on or in these food items. The patient should be encouraged to choose appropriate foods from the menu. The diet roster should be annotated "Compromised Host Precautions" so that the nutrition care staff can verify that appropriate choices are being made.

13. Tests, scans, and appointments away from the patient's room should be coordinated in advance to eliminate or minimize waiting time in common waiting areas.

14. The patient should wear a clean mask when outside the room, especially in heavily traveled public areas such as corridors, elevators, and waiting rooms. The mask may be removed when the patient is in less public areas. A new mask should be used for each trip out of the room.

15. Some hospitals allow flowers and plants in the patient's room; however, they should not be handled by the patient because of the possibility of *E. coli* contamination of the water and dirt.

16. No humidifiers with standing water should be used in the patient's room. If a wall humidifier is needed, the water should be changed every day.

17. Teach the patient and family about underlying pathophysiologic processes that put the patient at risk for infection and about precautions to minimize the risk of infection.

Data from Dean, Haeuber, and Rivera, 1996; Fischer, Knobf, and Durivage (1993); and Young-McCaughan (1995).

TABLE 6–5. Nursing Actions for the Patient Who Is at Risk for Hemorrhage

1. Administer blood product transfusions as prescribed. If a platelet transfusion is to be given in preparation for a procedure, it is best to give the transfusion immediately before the procedure so that the greatest number of platelets will be available to stop bleeding caused by the procedure.
   a. See Table 6–6 (Blood Products that Can Be Transfused).
   b. See Table 6–7 (Considerations in Administering Blood Products).
   c. See Table 6–8 (Types of Blood Transfusion Reactions).

2. Minimize the number of invasive procedures done to the patient that might result in prolonged bleeding.
   a. Draw as much blood for laboratory work as possible with one venipuncture.
   b. Avoid prolonged tourniquet use.
   c. Apply direct pressure for 5 to 10 minutes after all invasive procedures such as venipuncture or bone marrow biopsies.
   d. Avoid intramuscular injections.

3. Implement measures to avoid damage to the rectal mucosa that might cause bleeding:
   a. Avoid taking the patient's temperature rectally.
   b. Avoid administering suppositories.
   c. Avoid administering enemas.
   d. Prevent constipation by increasing fiber in the diet or administering stool softeners as ordered.

4. When measuring blood pressure, inflate the cuff only until the pulse is obliterated, to prevent petechiae along the arm. Set automated sphygmomanometers to the lowest appropriate pressure.

5. Instruct patient to use a soft-bristle toothbrush. If the patient is experiencing oral bleeding, toothettes or mouth rinses can be used to maintain oral hygiene.

6. Instruct the patient to use an electric razor, not a straight-edged razor, to shave.

7. As much as possible, avoid the use of drugs that interfere with platelet function, such as aspirin, aspirin-containing drugs (e.g., bismuth subsalicylate [Pepto-Bismol], oxycodone [Percodan]), and nonsteroidal anti-inflammatory drugs (NSAIDs).

8. Teach the patient and family about underlying pathophysiologic processes that put the patient at risk for hemorrhage and about precautions to minimize their risk of bleeding.

Adapted with permission from Young-McCaughan, S.: Hematologic and lymphatic disorders. *In* Linton, A. D., Matteson, M. A., and Maebius, M. K. (eds.): Introductory Nursing Care of Adults. Philadelphia, W. B. Saunders, 1995.

      ii. Keep special considerations related to blood product administration in mind (Tables 6–7 and 6–8)
  b. Treat underlying condition as prescribed
  c. Encourage oral fluid intake as patient's condition allows
  d. Monitor fluid balance with intake and output recordings and daily weights
4. **Evaluation of nursing care**
  a. Patient maintains vital signs within normal limits. When patient moves from lying to sitting or standing, the pulse and blood pressure do not change more than 20 points
  b. Patient's urine output exceeds 30 ml/hour
  c. The patient's 24-hour intake and output are approximately equal
  d. The patient's weight is stable

TABLE 6-6. Blood Products That Can Be Transfused

Blood Component	Indications	Usual Amount in One Unit	Recommended Infusion Rate	Special Considerations
Packed red blood cells (PRBC)	Symptoms caused by a low HCT or Hb, such as shortness of breath, tachycardia, decreased blood pressure, chest pain, lightheadedness, fatigue	250–300 ml/unit	2–4 hours/unit	Can expect the Hb to rise approximately 1 g/dl/unit and HCT to rise 3% per unit If >10 units of PRBC are administered over a short time, FFP may be needed to correct dilutional coagulopathies RBCs are preserved in citrate; if multiple units of RBCs are administered over a short time, the citrate can bind with the patient's calcium, decreasing serum calcium levels
Platelets	Bleeding from thrombocytopenia	60 ml/pack; usually four to six packs are pooled for a platelet transfusion	As quickly as the patient can tolerate	Platelet count can be expected to increase 12,000/m^3 for each multiple donor pack of platelets
Fresh frozen plasma (FFP)	Clotting deficiencies, hemophilia, rapid reversal of warfarin (Coumadin) effects, massive RBC transfusions	200–280 ml/unit	10 ml/minute	FFP contains all clotting factors except platelets
Cryoprecipitate	Hemophilia A, DIC	10 ml/bag; usually 10 bags are pooled for a transfusion	10 ml/minute	Cryoprecipitate contains factors I (fibrinogen) and VIII
Albumin	Shock, burns, cerebral edema	25 g repeated every 15–30 minutes as needed but not to exceed 250 g/48 hours	As quickly as the patient can tolerate	No need for blood typing or crossing; solution is hyperosmolar
Intravenous immunoglobulin (IVIG)	Idiopathic thrombocytopenic purpura (ITP), bone marrow transplant (BMT), acquired immunodeficiency syndrome (AIDS), severe combined immunodeficiency disease (SCID)	100–2000 mg/kg usually reconstituted in 1 L of D5W	Administer slowly for the first 15–30 minutes; if the patient's vital signs are stable, the infusion rate can be increased 1 mg/kg/hour every 15 minutes up to a maximum of 5 mg/kg/hour	No need for blood typing or crossing; hang with D5W, not normal saline (as normally recommended with blood products)

Data from the American Red Cross (1992); Coffland and Shelton (1993); and Timmerman (1993).
HCT = hematocrit; Hb = hemoglobin count; RBC = red blood cell; DIC = disseminated intravascular coagulation; D5W = 5% dextrose in water.

TABLE 6–7. Considerations in Administering Blood Products

Irradiated Blood Products

Irradiating blood products with 1500–2500 cGy kills 85%–90% of the lymphocytes and thus reduces the incidence of cytomegalovirus (CMV) infection, alloimmunization of the patient to future blood transfusions, and transfusion-associated graft-versus-host disease (GVHD). All patients who are or may in the future be candidates for bone marrow transplantation should receive irradiated and/or filtered blood products. Irradiated blood products must be specifically ordered from the blood bank. Irradiating blood products at these doses does not affect red blood cells, platelets, or granulocytes.

CMV-Negative Blood Products

CMV infection is commonly observed and nonlethal in immunocompetent persons. More than 80% of the population are exposed to CMV early in life and undergo seroconversion. For patients who need a bone marrow transplant but who have never been exposed to the virus, a CMV infection during transplantation could be life-threatening. To prevent unnecessary exposure to the virus, CMV-negative patients who may be bone marrow transplant candidates should receive only CMV-negative cellular blood products. CMV-negative blood products must be specifically ordered from the blood bank.

Alloimmunization

After repeated blood product transfusions, a patient exhibits large numbers of antibodies to a wide variety of distinct blood cell antigens. As a result, the transfused cells are destroyed and patient's blood counts do not improve with transfusion. Red blood cell transfusions contain only one person's blood in a unit; however, platelet transfusions normally contain many persons' platelets for transfusion and thus expose the patient to a greater number of antigens. When a patient becomes alloimmunized to platelets, *single-donor* platelets can be ordered. Single-donor platelets are plasmapheresed from only one donor, thus exposing the patient to fewer new antigens. Eventually the patient will become alloimmunized even to single-donor platelets.

Premedication for Blood Products

Premedication with acetaminophen (Tylenol) and/or diphenhydramine (Benadryl) can help alleviate the symptoms of a febrile blood transfusion reaction, in which the recipient's antibodies react to the donor leukocytes.

Intravenous Fluids

Hang blood products only with normal saline, to prevent hemolysis of the cells. The only exception to this is intravenous immunoglobulin, which is hung with 5% dextrose in water.

Filtering Blood Products

Standard blood filters trap clots that are 170–260 μm in size or larger. Smaller microaggregate filters can trap nonviable leukocytes, platelets, and fibrin strands that are 20–40 μm in size or larger. With leukocyte removal filters, leukocytes adhere to a filter media. These filters are rated on the efficiency of leukocyte removal, not size. Different filters are designed to be used with specific blood products. Some institutions use filters to remove white blood cells in lieu of giving CMV-negative blood products, especially when CMV-negative cellular blood products are not readily available.

Data from Greenbaum (1991), Higgins (1996), and Timmerman (1993).

• •

Potential for Impaired Gas Exchange Related to Anemia, Hemoglobin Abnormalities, Blood Loss, or Disease

1. Assessment for defining characteristics

a. Dyspnea

TABLE 6–8. Types of Blood Transfusion Reactions

Reaction	Mechanism	Symptoms	Occurrence	Treatment
Hemolytic	Type II antigen-complement reaction to transfusion of ABO-incompatible blood	Fever, chills, nausea, dyspnea, chest pain, back pain, hypotension	Shortly after the transfusion starts	Stop the transfusion Notify the physician immediately Be prepared to provide supportive therapy to maintain hemodynamic status and renal perfusion
Anaphylactic	Type I hypersensitivity reaction to plasma proteins	Urticaria, wheezing, dyspnea, hypotension	Within 30 minutes of the start of the transfusion	Stop the transfusion Notify the physician immediately Be prepared to administer epinephrine and steroids
Febrile	Recipient's antibodies react to donor leukocytes	Fever, chills	Within 30–90 minutes of the start of the transfusion	Stop the transfusion Notify the physician immediately
Circulatory overload	Patient's cardiovascular system is unable to manage the additional fluid load	Cough, frothy sputum, cyanosis, decreased blood pressure	Any time during the transfusion and up to several hours afterwards	Stop the transfusion Call for help Be prepared to administer oxygen and/or furosemide (Lasix)

Data from the American Red Cross (1992); Coffland and Shelton (1993); and Jeter and Spivey (1995).

    b. Pallor, cyanosis

    c. Abnormal vital signs: tachycardia, tachypnea

    d. Hb is less than 7 g/dl, HCT is less than 21 g/dl

    e. PaO$_2$ is less than 80 mm Hg when patient is breathing room air

    f. Altered mental status, particularly confusion

2. Expected outcomes

    a. Vital signs are within normal limits for patient

    b. Patient can maintain the Hb and HCT within acceptable ranges

    c. PaO$_2$ returns to normal range without supplemental oxygen

3. Nursing interventions: see Table 6–9

4. Evaluation of nursing care

    a. Patient's respiratory rate is less than 20/minute

    b. Patient's Hb exceeds 10 g/dl and HCT exceeds 30 g/dl

    c. Patient's PaO$_2$ is less than 98 mm Hg when breathing room air

· ·

Potential for Activity Intolerance Related to Disease or Treatment

1. Assessment for defining characteristics

    a. Reports of fatigue, weakness, malaise, inability to sleep, inability to concentrate

    b. Changes in vital signs with activity: increased heart rate, decreased blood pressure, increased respiratory rate

    c. Inability to perform activities of daily living without assistance

2. Expected outcomes

    a. Vital signs are within normal limits for the patient

    b. The patient can accomplish activities of daily living without tachycardia or hypotension

    c. The patient expresses a reduction in fatigue

3. Nursing interventions

    a. Plan care to allow for periods of uninterrupted rest

    b. Assist patient with activities of daily living as needed

    c. Monitor vital signs as an indication of activity tolerance

4. Evaluation of nursing care

TABLE 6–9. Nursing Actions for the Patient Who Is Anemic, Has Hemoglobin Abnormalities, or Has Suffered Blood Loss

---

1. Administer oxygen as prescribed
2. Administer blood products as prescribed
    a. See Table 6–6 (Blood Products That Can Be Transfused)
    b. See Table 6–7 (Considerations in Administering Blood Products)
    c. See Table 6–8 (Types of Blood Transfusion Reactions)
3. Administer the hematopoietic growth factor erythropoietin as prescribed
4. Allow for rest between periods of activity, because the anemic patient can tire easily
5. Elevate the patient's head on pillows during episodes of shortness of breath
6. Provide extra blankets if the patient feels too cool
7. Teach the patient and family about underlying pathophysiology and how to manage the symptoms of anemia

---

Adapted with permission from Young-McCaughan, S.: Hematologic and lymphatic disorders. *In* Linton, A. D., Matteson, M. A., and Maebius, M. K. (eds.): Introductory Nursing Care of Adults. Philadelphia, W. B. Saunders, 1995.

a. Patient's pulse increases no more than 20 beats with nonaerobic activity and returns to baseline within 5 minutes of stopping the activity

b. The patient states that the level of fatigue with activities of daily living is manageable

Potential for Pain Related to Disease or Treatment

See Chapter 9, Psychosocial Aspects.

Potential for Fear or Anxiety Related to Disease or Treatment

See Chapter 9.

Potential for Altered Family Processes

See Chapter 9.

PATIENT HEALTH PROBLEMS

Anemia

1. **Pathophysiology**
   a. Anemia is a reduction in the number of RBCs, the quantity of hemoglobin, or the volume of RBCs. Because the main function of RBCs is oxygenation, anemia results in varying degrees of hypoxia
   b. The body compensates for anemia in the following ways:
       i. Increased cardiac output and respiratory rate
       ii. Redistribution of blood to sustain blood supply to the brain and heart by reducing blood supply to the skin, gut, and kidneys
       iii. Increased production of erythropoietin by the kidney to stimulate erythropoiesis
   c. Acute blood loss, such as with arterial rupture, dramatically changes the body's hemodynamic status, necessitating emergency intervention. Chronic blood loss occurring over weeks or months, such as with slow gastrointestinal bleeding or menorrhagia, allows the body time to compensate; the symptoms of chronic blood loss may be more insidious. Although patients with chronic anemia are not usually admitted to the critical care setting, chronic anemia can complicate other medical conditions that do necessitate treatment in a critical care setting
2. **Etiologic or precipitating factors**
   a. Inadequate RBC production
       i. Aplastic anemia
       ii. Chronic inflammatory diseases (e.g., rheumatoid arthritis, chronic osteomyelitis)
       iii. End-stage renal disease

iv. Bone marrow infiltration with malignant cells

v. Current treatment or recent history of treatment with antineoplastic chemotherapy

vi. Any history of radiation therapy to bones where blood cells are made (i.e., vertebrae, ribs, skull, pelvis, femur, or humerus)

vii. Bone marrow transplantation

viii. Dietary deficiencies, particularly in iron, cobalamin (B_{12}), or folate

ix. Drug-induced (e.g., zidovudine)

b. Increased RBC destruction

i. Immune-mediated

(a) Autoimmune hemolytic anemia

(b) Cytotoxic hypersensitivity reaction (e.g., drug-induced)

ii. RBC membrane defects (e.g., hereditary spherocytosis)

iii. Hemoglobin defects (e.g., sickle cell anemia, thalassemia)

iv. Mechanical (e.g., trauma from prosthetic heart valves)

c. Major blood loss

3. **Nursing assessment data base**

a. Nursing history

i. Subjective: fatigue; dyspnea, especially with exertion; altered mental status (e.g., dizziness, especially when changing position from lying down to sitting or standing; inability to concentrate; confusion)

ii. Objective: palpitations

b. Nursing examination of patient

i. Inspection: pallor, possibly jaundice, shortness of breath

ii. Palpation and percussion

(a) Bone pain possible if bone marrow is infiltrated with malignant cells

(b) Hepatosplenomegaly possible with liver disease, some types of malignant disease; the liver and spleen can be tender with palpation and percussion

iii. Auscultation: tachycardia, hypotension, orthostatic changes in vital signs

c. Diagnostic study findings

i. Laboratory

(a) Blood

(1) Hb less than 7 g/dl, HCT less than 21 g/dl

(2) Other findings vary with the cause of anemia and can include increased reticulocyte count, decreased serum iron level, increased or decreased TIBC, decreased ferritin level, increased indirect bilirubin level, positive result of Coombs' test

(b) Urine: can be positive for blood

(c) Stool: can be positive for blood

(d) Tissue: a bone marrow biopsy may be obtained to evaluate bone marrow production of RBCs or the presence of bone marrow infiltration with malignant cells

ii. Radiologic: a gastrointestinal series may be obtained to detect the source of bleeding

iii. Endoscopy: to detect the source of bleeding

4. **Nursing diagnoses** (see Commonly Encountered Nursing Diagnoses section)

a. Potential for impaired gas exchange related to disease

b. Potential fluid volume deficit related to hemorrhage
c. Potential for activity intolerance related to disease or treatment
d. Potential for pain related to disease or treatment (see Chapter 9)
e. Potential for fear or anxiety related to disease or treatment (see Chapter 9)
f. Potential for altered family processes (see Chapter 9)

. . . .

Disseminated Intravascular Coagulation

1. **Pathophysiology**
   a. DIC is a hypercoagulable state that occurs when the normal coagulation cascade is over-stimulated, which results in simultaneous thrombosis and hemorrhage
   b. DIC is always secondary to another pathologic process. Coagulation takes place normally, but it occurs at so many sites in the body that the normal inhibitory mechanisms are overwhelmed. Eventually all available platelets and clotting factors are depleted, and systemic uncontrolled hemorrhage results
2. **Etiologic or precipitating factors**
   a. Overwhelming sepsis
   b. Shock
   c. Major trauma, crush injuries, burns
   d. Malignancy
   e. Acute tumor lysis syndrome (see the Leukemia section)
   f. Obstetric complications, such as abruptio placentae or fetal demise
3. **Nursing assessment data base**
   a. The diagnosis of DIC is based on a constellation of findings, including the sudden onset of a bleeding disorder without a prior history of bleeding or blood coagulation abnormalities
   b. Nursing history
      i. Subjective: reports of spontaneous bleeding for no obvious reason
      ii. Objective: a preceding or concurrent pathologic process that is known to precipitate DIC
   c. Nursing examination of patient
      i. Inspection: petechiae; purpura; ecchymoses; hematomas; epistaxis; conjunctival bleeding; spontaneous and/or uncontrollable hemorrhage from multiple unrelated sites, such as sites of venipuncture, tubes, drains, lines, incisions, and wounds
      ii. Palpation, percussion, and auscultation: findings are usually noncontributory except to identify the underlying pathologic process
   d. Diagnostic study findings
      i. Laboratory: prolonged PT, decreased fibrinogen, increased fibrin split products, increased D-dimers, and prolonged TT
      ii. Radiologic: findings are usually noncontributory except to identify the underlying pathologic process
4. **Nursing diagnoses** (see Commonly Encountered Nursing Diagnoses section)
   a. Altered protection (risk for hemorrhage) related to disease or treatment; additional nursing considerations include assisting with the diagnosis and treatment of the underlying condition that precipitated the DIC
   b. Potential fluid volume deficit related to hemorrhage; additional nursing considerations include the following:

      i. Blood component replacement therapy is often prescribed. However, blood component replacement therapy is controversial, inasmuch as some providers believe that additional platelets and clotting factors perpetuate the abnormal DIC feedback loop

     ii. Some providers prescribe heparin to interrupt the DIC cycle. Heparin inhibits the conversion of prothrombin to thrombin, thus slowing the coagulation cycle and allowing the body to replenish platelets and clotting factors. However, heparin therapy is also controversial, inasmuch as some providers believe that it exacerbates clinical bleeding

  c. Potential for impaired gas exchange related to disease

  d. Potential for fear or anxiety related to disease or treatment (see Chapter 9)

  e. Potential for altered family processes (see Chapter 9)

Thrombocytopenia

1. Pathophysiology

  a. The number of platelets available to assist with coagulation is inadequate, which puts the patient at increased risk of hemorrhage

  b. In various hematologic malignancies such as leukemia and lymphoma, the cancerous cells crowd out normal cell lines in the bone marrow, resulting in thrombocytopenia, as well as neutropenia and anemia. Treatment includes treating the underlying malignancy with antineoplastic chemotherapy, which can itself also cause pancytopenia

  c. Treatment of either solid tumor or hematologic malignances with antineoplastic chemotherapy is a major cause of thrombocytopenia. Chemotherapy indiscriminately targets rapidly dividing cells in the bone marrow, including megakaryocytes. Thrombocytopenia can be expected to appear 10 to 14 days after treatment; it lasts until the bone marrow is able to replenish its megakaryocyte pool

  d. Various antibody-mediated autoimmune disorders can result in thrombocytopenia when IgG is erroneously directed against the patient's own platelets

2. Etiologic or precipitating factors

  a. Decreased platelet production

      i. Bone marrow infiltration with malignant cells (e.g., leukemia, multiple myeloma, malignant metastases)

     ii. Current treatment or recent history of treatment with antineoplastic chemotherapy

    iii. Any history of radiation therapy to bones in which blood cells are made

    iv. Bone marrow aplasia

  b. Increased platelet destruction

      i. DIC (see Disseminated Intravascular Coagulation section)

     ii. Antibody-mediated

       (a) Immune thrombocytopenic purpura (ITP)

         (1) Agents known to induce ITP include sulfonamides, thiazide diuretics, chlorpropamide, quinidine, and gold

         (2) Patients with HIV infection are at increased risk for development of ITP

          (b) Heparin-induced thrombocytopenia and thrombosis

          (c) Alloimmunization after multiple platelet transfusions (see Table 6–7)

       iii. Thrombotic thrombocytopenic purpura (TTP) or hemolytic uremic syndrome (HUS) (see Hypercoagulable Disorders section)

       iv. Sepsis

   c. Sequestration of platelets in spleen (e.g., with liver disease and portal hypertension)

   d. With massive transfusions of RBCs over a short period of time, a dilutional thrombocytopenia can occur

3. Nursing assessment data base

   a. Nursing history

       i. Subjective: unexplained bleeding

       ii. Objective: petechial rash

   b. Nursing examination of patient

       i. Inspection: pallor; petechiae; purpura; ecchymoses; oozing of blood from venipuncture sites; conjunctival bleeding; bleeding from the oropharynx, gastrointestinal tract, or genitourinary tract

       ii. Palpation and percussion: splenomegaly may be present

       iii. Auscultation: findings are noncontributory

   c. Diagnostic study findings

       i. Laboratory

          (a) Blood

             (1) Platelets are less than $50,000/mm^3$

             (2) Both Hb and HCT are usually decreased as a result of blood loss

          (b) Urine: can be positive for blood

          (c) Stool: can be positive for blood

          (d) Tissue: bone marrow biopsy to determine whether adequate platelets are being made in the bone marrow

       ii. Radiologic: spleen ultrasonography or liver-spleen scan to determine size of spleen

4. Nursing diagnoses (see Commonly Encountered Nursing Diagnoses section)

   a. Altered protection (risk for hemorrhage) related to disease or treatment; additional nursing considerations for patients with ITP:

       i. ITP in children usually appears after a viral infection and spontaneously resolves in 90% of cases. Adult ITP is not as well understood. Only 10% to 20% of adult patients have a spontaneous remission, and so adults are much more likely to need treatment

       ii. Treatment for ITP can include steroids, intravenous immunoglobulin (IVIG), splenectomy, and immunosuppressive therapy

       iii. In approximately 75% of adult patients with ITP, platelets will be sequestered in the spleen, and so splenectomy is done to remove this storehouse, thereby increasing the circulating blood levels of platelets

       iv. Immunosuppressive therapy with cytotoxic drugs (e.g., vincristine or cyclophosphamide) can be used in patients who do not respond to splenectomy

       v. Platelet transfusions are *not* indicated because the underlying problem is platelet consumption, not platelet production. If platelets are transfused, they are immediately destroyed

b. Potential fluid volume deficit related to hemorrhage

c. Potential for fear or anxiety related to disease or treatment (see Chapter 9)

d. Potential for altered family processes (see Chapter 9)

. . . .

Hypercoagulable Disorders

1. **Pathophysiology**

   a. Hypercoagulable disorders occur when the normal mechanisms of hemostasis involving platelets and clotting factors are disrupted, resulting in uncontrolled or inappropriate clotting. Paradoxically, a secondary bleeding disorder develops in many of these patients when their reservoirs of platelets and clotting factors are depleted

   b. Venous thromboses result from activation of the coagulation cascade caused by venous stasis, ischemia, or infarction. Arterial emboli result when a venous thrombus breaks away from its site of origin and migrates into the arterial vascular system. Pulmonary embolus, myocardial infarction, and thrombotic cerebrovascular accidents can be caused by arterial emboli. Patients are often admitted to critical care units for hemodynamic and neurologic support, as well as for thrombolytic therapy with streptokinase, urokinase, or tissue plasminogen activator (t-PA). Anticoagulation therapy puts these patients at risk for bleeding, although they have an underlying hypercoagulable disorder (see Chapters 2, The Cardiovascular System, and 3, The Neurologic System)

   c. TTP appears to be an exaggerated immunologic response to vessel injury that results in extensive thrombus formation and decreased blood flow to the affected site. These patients are critically ill; fever, thrombocytopenia, hemolytic anemia, renal impairment, and neurologic symptoms develop. HUS appears to be a variant of TTP that is seen more commonly in children. Patients with HUS tend to have more severe renal impairment, but fewer neurologic signs and symptoms, than do patients with TTP

   d. DIC is another hypercoagulable disorder (see Disseminated Intravascular Coagulation section)

2. **Etiologic or precipitating factors**

   a. Changes in blood flow (e.g., deep vein thrombosis)

   b. Changes in circulating blood coagulation factors (e.g., TTP)

   c. Changes in the vessel wall

3. **Nursing assessment data base**

   a. Nursing history

      i. Subjective: unexplained bleeding and other symptoms may be present, depending on the organ system involved

      ii. Objective: sudden painful swelling of one extremity and other signs may be present, depending on the organ system involved

   b. Nursing examination of patient

      i. Inspection: temperature exceeding 101°F (38.3°C), petechiae, purpura, ecchymoses, hematomas

      ii. Palpation and percussion: circumference of one extremity is different from that of the other; tenderness or pain with palpation

      iii. Auscultation: changes in vital signs may be present, depending on the organ system involved; with an arterial thrombosis, decreased blood flow in one extremity may be detected with Doppler ultrasonography

c. Diagnostic study findings
i. Laboratory
(a) With venous stasis, laboratory values may be normal until anticoagulation therapy begins
(b) With TTP, RBCs are decreased; reticulocytes, bilirubin level, and lactate dehydrogenase level are increased; and fragmented RBCs are seen on peripheral smear
ii. Radiologic: angiography or venography can indicate vessel blockage

4. **Nursing diagnoses** (see Commonly Encountered Nursing Diagnoses section)
a. Altered protection (risk for hemorrhage) related to disease or treatment; additional nursing considerations:
i. For patients with venous thromboses: treatment of these patients includes anticoagulation with intravenous heparin, switching to oral warfarin (Coumadin) before discharge from the hospital
ii. For patients with arterial thromboses receiving a thrombolytic agent: see Chapter 2
iii. For patients with TTP: the main treatment is plasmapheresis with administration of fresh frozen plasma to replace the clotting factors removed with pheresis. Plasmapheresis is usually done daily or every other day for several weeks until the patient's hematologic parameters stabilize. Other treatments include steroids, antiplatelet agents (e.g., aspirin or dipyridamole [Persantine]), and splenectomy
(a) Plasmapheresis presumably removes the immunologic agent that triggered the TTP. The patient's blood is centrifuged in a pheresis machine that separates the blood components so that the plasma can be selectively removed. The patient's own WBCs, RBCs, and platelets are reinfused during the treatment. Critically ill patients can become hemodynamically unstable during this procedure, requiring close monitoring and timely interventions to maintain cardiac output and blood pressure
(b) Platelet transfusions are usually contraindicated because they may contribute to the ongoing thrombotic process. Heparin is not used in the treatment of TTP because it does not affect platelet aggregation
b. Potential fluid volume deficit related to fever, hemorrhage, or shock
c. Potential for fear or anxiety related to disease or treatment (see Chapter 9)
d. Potential for altered family processes (see Chapter 9)

: Neutropenia

1. **Pathophysiology**
a. Occurs when the total number of neutrophils is abnormally low, putting the patient at increased risk of infection. The longer the patient is neutropenic, the greater the chance of infection. Patients are often admitted to critical care units with a diagnosis such as sepsis or acute leukemia that is complicated by neutropenia
b. The most common sites of infection seen in neutropenic patients are the

lung (pneumonia), blood (septicemia), skin, urinary tract, and gastrointestinal tract (mucositis, esophagitis, perirectal lesions). The major infectious gram-negative bacilli include *Klebsiella pneumoniae* and *Escherichia coli*. The major infectious gram positive cocci include *Staphylococcus aureus*, *Enterococcus*, and *Staphylococcus epidermidis*. Because affected patients do not have adequate numbers of WBCs to mount an immunologic response, the classical signs of infection may be absent. Fever may be the only sign of infection
   c. See also Chapter 8, Septic Shock section
2. **Etiologic or precipitating factors**
   a. Decreased neutrophil production
      i. Bone marrow infiltration with malignant cells
      ii. Recent history of antineoplastic chemotherapy, especially if high-dose chemotherapy was administered as part of bone marrow transplantation
      iii. Any history of radiation therapy to bones in which blood cells are made
      iv. Drug-induced (e.g., zidovudine, clozapine)
      v. Autoimmune (e.g., systemic lupus erythematosus, rheumatoid arthritis)
   b. Increased neutrophil use: overwhelming sepsis
3. **Nursing assessment data base**
   a. Nursing history
      i. Subjective: malaise, fever, chills, night sweats, rash, sore throat, dyspnea, abdominal pain, diarrhea, sinus pain, headache, confusion, pain with swallowing, pain with urination, pain with defecation
      ii. Objective: cough, diarrhea
   b. Nursing examination of patient
      i. Inspection: temperature exceeding 101°F (38.3°C), loss of integrity of skin and mucous membranes (especially at intravenous and central venous catheter sites), shortness of breath
      ii. Palpation and percussion: pain, lymphadenopathy
      iii. Auscultation: tachycardia, hypotension, crackles, rhonchi
   c. Diagnostic study findings
      i. Laboratory
         (a) ANC less than 500/μL (see Fig. 6–4)
         (b) Possibly a bone marrow biopsy, depending on the clinical situation
      ii. Radiologic: findings are usually noncontributory to the diagnosis of neutropenia, but studies may be indicated to identify the source of infection secondary to neutropenia
4. **Nursing diagnoses** (see Commonly Encountered Nursing Diagnoses section)
   a. Altered protection (risk for infection) related to disease or treatment; additional nursing considerations:
      i. Broad-spectrum antibiotics are prescribed for neutropenic fevers even without a documented source of infection
      ii. Fungal infections, particularly with *Candida albicans* or *Aspergillus*, should be suspected if fever persists beyond 5 days of treatment with broad-spectrum antibiotics
      iii. Infections with herpes simplex virus, cytomegalovirus, varicella zoster virus, or other viruses are also possible

iv. The goal of antibiotic therapy is to support the patient until his or her own WBCs are available to fight the infection

b. Potential for fear or anxiety related to disease or treatment (see Chapter 9)

c. Potential for altered family processes (see Chapter 9)

Acute Leukemia

1. Pathophysiology

a. Leukemia is a cancer of the WBCs. There are many different types of leukemia, each based on which WBC lineage is affected and how quickly the leukemic clone multiplies. Acute nonlymphocytic leukemia (ANLL), also called acute myelogenous leukemia (AML), is cancer of the granulocyte cell line (see Fig. 6–1) affecting primarily adults. Acute lymphocytic leukemia (ALL) is a cancer of the lymphocyte cell line (see Fig. 6–1) affecting primarily children. The leukemic cells themselves are nonfunctional. They crowd out the normal bone marrow cells, thereby inducing pancytopenia, manifested as anemia, neutropenia, and thrombocytopenia

b. Patients with leukemia are usually treated on oncology wards, but two complications of leukemia, overwhelming sepsis and acute tumor lysis syndrome, bring patients to critical care units for hemodynamic support and close observation

   i. Overwhelming sepsis can occur in leukemic patients because they do not have enough functional WBCs to mount an immunologic response to even common pathogens. Infection is the most common cause of morbidity and mortality in this patient population. (See patient health problems in the Neutropenia section and in Chapter 8, Septic Shock section)

   ii. Acute tumor lysis syndrome can occur when a large number of tumor cells are rapidly destroyed by chemotherapy, which results in potentially life-threatening electrolyte changes. Acute tumor lysis syndrome occurs with malignancies such as leukemia and lymphoma, in which tumor cells are rapidly dividing, creating a large tumor burden before the disease is diagnosed. Because of their high growth fraction, theses tumors are exquisitely sensitive to chemotherapy. The first doses of chemotherapy cause large numbers of tumor cells to be lysed, releasing their cellular contents into the blood stream. The four hallmarks of acute tumor lysis syndrome resulting from massive tumor lysis are hyperuricemia, hyperkalemia, hyperphosphatemia, and hypocalcemia. Acute renal failure can occur with acute tumor lysis syndrome if uric acid crystallizes in the distal tubules and collecting ducts of the kidney

2. Etiologic or precipitating factors

a. Largely unknown, probably multifactorial

b. Excessive radiation exposure

c. Previous exposure to certain chemicals (e.g., benzene)

d. Previous exposure to certain drugs (e.g., alkylating chemotherapy agents)

e. Chromosomal abnormalities (e.g., as in Down's syndrome)

3. Nursing assessment data base

a. Nursing history
   i. Subjective: fatigue, malaise, bone pain, headache, reports of fever, chills, night sweats
   ii. Objective: pallor, petechial rash, easy bruising, weight loss
b. Nursing examination of patient
   i. Inspection: temperature exceeding 101°F (38.3°C), flushing, lethargy, petechiae, purpura, ecchymosis, hematomas
   ii. Palpation and percussion: possible lymphadenopathy, possible hepatomegaly, possible splenomegaly
   iii. Auscultation: tachycardia, hypotension
c. Diagnostic study findings: Laboratory
   i. Very high or very low total WBC count with primarily immature blast cells seen on the differential
   ii. Low RBC and platelet counts are usually also seen because these cell lines are crowded out of bone marrow by leukemic cells
   iii. In acute tumor lysis syndrome, uric acid levels exceed 7.2 mg/dl, potassium levels exceed 5.3 mg/dl, PO_4 exceeds 4.5 mg/dl, and Ca^{2+} is less than 8.6 mg/dl
   iv. A bone marrow biopsy is usually done to help with the diagnosis and guide treatment
4. **Nursing diagnoses** (see Commonly Encountered Nursing Diagnoses section)
   a. Altered protection (risk for infection) related to disease or treatment; additional nursing considerations for the patient with acute leukemia include:
      i. The acute leukemias are initially treated with high-dose chemotherapy, called *induction therapy,* to induce bone marrow hypoplasia, and allow normal cells to repopulate the bone marrow. In general, patients are hospitalized 2 to 3 weeks. If they remain hemodynamically stable and not infected, they are discharged from the hospital and monitored as outpatients until normal bone marrow function returns (i.e., they can make adequate amounts of RBCs, WBCs, and platelets)
      ii. After induction therapy, patients with ANLL are hospitalized for the same high doses of chemotherapy, called *intensification and consolidation therapies,* two to four more times over the ensuing 2 to 4 months; active treatment is then finished
      iii. Bone marrow transplantation is one form of intensification therapy (see Bone Marrow Transplantation and Peripheral Blood Stem Cell Transplantation section)
      iv. After induction therapy, patients with ALL are treated with lower doses of chemotherapy, called *maintenance therapy,* as outpatients for 1 to 3 years
   b. Altered protection (risk for hemorrhage) related to disease or treatment
   c. Potential for electrolyte imbalances (hyperkalemia, hyperphosphatemia, hypocalcemia) related to acute tumor lysis syndrome (see Chapter 4, The Renal System); additional nursing considerations for the patient at risk for acute tumor lysis syndrome include:
      i. In anticipation of the possibility of acute tumor lysis syndrome, medical management should include aggressive intravenous hydration, alkalinization of the urine, and allopurinol administration before chemotherapy is initiated

     ii. After chemotherapy is started, blood electrolytes should be monitored frequently and adjustments to the plan of care rapidly implemented as indicated. Hemodialysis may be necessary to prevent acute tumor lysis syndrome even with aggressive management

     iii. For patients with WBC counts exceeding 100,000/µl, leukapheresis may be done to remove the leukemic WBCs from circulation before initiating chemotherapy. This reduces the risk of acute tumor lysis syndrome

  d. Potential fluid volume deficit related to fever, hemorrhage, or shock

  e. Potential for pain related to disease or treatment (see Chapter 9)

  f. Potential for fear or anxiety related to disease or treatment (see Chapter 9)

  g. Potential for altered family processes (see Chapter 9)

Bone Marrow Transplantation and Peripheral Blood Stem Cell Transplantation

1. **Pathophysiology**

  a. Bone marrow transplantation (BMT) and peripheral blood stem cell transplantation (PBSCT) are procedures to reconstitute the hematologic and immunologic systems after patients with malignancies receive doses of chemotherapy and radiation therapy high enough to permanently kill the bone marrow. BMT is also used in patients with aplastic anemia, in an attempt to repopulate the marrow. Harvested marrow or peripheral stem cells are infused into the patient intravenously. Through their innate homing mechanism, the cells travel to the bone marrow and reestablish normal hematopoiesis

  b. Types of transplants

     i. In allogeneic BMT, bone marrow from an HLA-matched donor is used. Overall, there is a 25% chance that a sibling of a patient needing a BMT will be an HLA match. The chances of finding an HLA-matched, unrelated donor (MUD), for a so-called MUD allogeneic transplant, are much smaller

     ii. In autologous BMT, or bone marrow rescues, bone marrow from the patient is harvested and preserved before chemotherapy is initiated; the rescued bone marrow is infused after treatment. Using the patient's own bone marrow eliminates the risk of rejection and graft-versus-host disease (GVHD); however, the risk of cancer recurrence is higher. This type of BMT is the best option for patients with a solid tumor who require high doses of chemotherapy and radiation therapy but who have healthy bone marrow that can be harvested before treatment and returned after therapy. Patients with hematologic malignancies can have their bone marrow harvested during remission, purged of malignant cells, and then returned after high-dose therapy

     iii. In PBSCT, the patient's bone marrow is stimulated with colony-stimulating factors, and then the patient's peripheral stem cells are harvested through repeated phereses. After chemotherapy and radiation therapy treatment, the patient's stem cells are reinfused, as in BMT. As with autologous BMT, the risks of rejection and GVHD are eliminated. In addition, stem cells re-engraft more quickly than bone marrow, reducing the length of neutropenia and risk of infection. Often, PBSCT is performed concurrently with autologous BMT

c. Major complications of BMT and PBSCT

    i. Infection is an omnipresent concern in the care of patients undergoing BMT (see Neutropenia section). After transplantation, although WBC and neutrophil counts approach normal levels, the patient's cellular immune function can be compromised for more than a year

    ii. Thrombocytopenia can be profound and prolonged in the patient undergoing BMT or PBSCT because of the high doses of chemotherapy and radiation therapy (see Thrombocytopenia section)

    iii. Renal insufficiency can occur as a result of inadequate blood flow to and through the kidneys, damage to the kidneys (by aminoglycosides, amphotericin B, cisplatin chemotherapy, cyclosporine, radiation therapy, and acute tumor lysis syndrome), and obstruction of kidney outflow from tumor masses

    iv. Hepatic veno-occlusive disease (VOD) occurs as a result of high-dose chemotherapy and radiation therapy, which damage the liver hepatocytes and venules. Blood flow in and out of the liver is obstructed, resulting in ischemia, ascites, and increasing serum bilirubin levels. The kidney reabsorbs sodium and water that tend to move into interstitial and peritoneal spaces, further contributing to ascites. Complications of VOD include decreased tissue perfusion, electrolyte abnormalities, and coagulopathies. VOD can occur in 10% to 50% of patients undergoing BMT and is fatal in 50% of the patients in whom it develops

    v. GVHD occurs when T lymphocytes in the transplanted tissue recognize the recipient's tissue as foreign; these grafted T lymphocytes attack the host. GVHD can be either acute, occurring within 100 days of transplantation, or chronic, occurring after 100 days. Some form of GVHD develops in 40% to 50% of patients receiving allogeneic BMT, and between 30% and 60% of the patients with GVHD die from the disease or infectious complications. The transplanted tissue T lymphocytes attack primarily the epithelial cells of the skin, gastrointestinal tract, biliary ducts, and lymphoid system, resulting in a maculopapular erythematous rash; large amounts of green, watery, heme-negative diarrhea; and elevated bilirubin and liver enzyme levels

2. Etiologic or precipitating factors (i.e., indications for BMT or PBSCT)

a. Doses of chemotherapy and radiation used to treat a malignancy that are toxic to bone marrow

b. Genetic defect (e.g., severe combined immunodeficiency disease)

c. Aplastic syndromes (e.g., aplastic anemia, agranulocytosis)

3. Nursing assessment data base during transplantation

a. Nursing history

    i. Subjective: malaise; fatigue; weakness; lethargy; chills; night sweats; sore throat; dyspnea; sinus pain; headache; confusion; pain with swallowing, urination, or defecation

      ii. Objective: petechial rash; cough; diarrhea

  b. Nursing examination of patient

      i. Inspection: temperature exceeding 101°F (38.3°C), pallor, jaundice, petechiae, rash, weight changes, shortness of breath, loss of integrity of skin and mucous membranes, diarrhea, bleeding from oropharynx, bleeding from gastrointestinal tract, bleeding from genitourinary tract

      ii. Palpation and percussion: hepatomegaly

      iii. Auscultation: tachycardia, hypotension, crackles, rhonchi, hyperactive bowel sounds

  c. Diagnostic study findings

      i. Laboratory

        (a) Expect WBC, HCT, Hb, and platelets all to be low

        (b) With renal insufficiency, increased creatinine and electrolyte abnormalities

        (c) With VOD, increased bilirubin, increased liver enzymes, prolonged PT, and prolonged PTT

        (d) Definitive diagnosis of VOD and/or GVHD often requires a tissue biopsy; however, biopsy is often contraindicated because of coagulopathies

      ii. Radiologic: specific to complication being investigated

4. Nursing diagnoses (see Commonly Encountered Nursing Diagnoses section)

  a. Altered protection (risk for infection) related to disease or treatment; additional nursing considerations for the patient undergoing BMT or PBSCT:

      i. Prophylactic use of the antifungal drug fluconazole decreases the incidence of *Candida albicans* infection in BMT patients. Prophylactic treatment with acyclovir can decrease the incidence of reactivation of herpes simplex virus and cytomegalovirus in seropositive patients undergoing BMT

      ii. For the patient with GVHD, treatment includes immunosuppressive drug therapy to suppress the transplanted T lymphocytes (with antithymocyte globulin or murine monoclonal antibody to CD3), cyclosporine, low-dose methotrexate, and hemodynamic support (see also Transplant Rejection section)

  b. Altered protection (risk for hemorrhage) related to disease or treatment

  c. Potential fluid volume deficit related to fever, vomiting, diarrhea, hemorrhage, or shock; additional nursing considerations for the patient with VOD:

      i. Intravenous fluid infusions, diuretics, blood cell replacement, and drug dosages must all be meticulously managed

      ii. Both heparin and recombinant human t-PA have been used with some success to prevent and remove fibrin and clots in the liver

  d. Potential for acute renal insufficiency and failure related to disease or treatment (see Chapter 4)

  e. Potential for activity intolerance related to disease or treatment

  f. Potential for pain related to disease or treatment (see Chapter 9)

  g. Potential for fear or anxiety related to disease or treatment (see Chapter 9)

  h. Potential for altered family processes (see Chapter 9)

Transplant Rejection

1. **Pathophysiology**
   a. When tissue from one person is transplanted into another person, the immune system of the recipient can recognize the transplanted tissue, or allograft, as foreign. Rejections occur through various mechanisms:
      i. T_C lymphocytes can directly attack the allograft, resulting in acute transplant rejection, occurring within hours of the transplantation
      ii. B lymphocytes can make antibodies against the allograft; these activate the complement pathways and attract platelets. Fibrin accumulates on the transplanted tissue, causing ischemia. In this way the allograft is slowly rejected over many months to years
   b. HLA matching of donor to recipient before transplantation is an attempt to choose a donor whose antigens match the recipient's as closely as possible so that the recipient's immune system is not triggered to attack the allograft after the transplantation procedure
   c. Various combinations of drugs are also given to suppress the recipient's immune system and minimize the immune response to the allograft. However, these drugs also suppress the patient's ability to fight bacteria, viruses, fungi, and parasites, putting the patient at increased risk for infection. Combinations of steroids (which inhibit the inflammatory response by inhibiting the production of prostaglandins) and azathioprine (which inhibits B-cell and T-cell proliferation) are commonly used to chronically suppress the immune system after organ transplantation. Several newer drugs target the T cells, preserving B cell function and thus more of the patient's immune function. Examples of these drugs are cyclosporine, FK506 (Tacrolimus), anti-lymphocyte globulin (ALG), anti-thymocyte globulin (ATG), and murine monoclonal antibody to CD3 (OKT3)
   d. Allogeneic BMT is fundamentally different from solid organ transplantation. In allogeneic BMT, the immune system itself is being transplanted into a new host. Therefore, it may attack any tissue in the new host, resulting in GVHD (see Bone Marrow Transplantation and Peripheral Blood Stem Cell Transplantation section). Because GVHD is usually a limited (albeit serious) problem, the majority of patients undergoing an allogeneic BMT can eventually discontinue immunosuppressive therapy. For patients receiving a solid organ transplantation, the host's own immune system attacks the donated organ, and so recipients must receive lifelong immunosuppressive therapy
2. **Etiologic or precipitating factors:** activation of the immune response against transplanted tissue
3. **Nursing assessment data base**
   a. Nursing history
      i. Subjective: malaise, poor appetite, myalgia, tenderness of allograft
      ii. Objective: swelling of allograft
   b. Nursing examination of patient
      i. Inspection: temperature exceeding 101°F (38.3°C)
      ii. Palpation and percussion: swelling and tenderness of allograft
      iii. Auscultation: findings are usually noncontributory
   c. Diagnostic study findings are specific to the organ transplanted

4. **Nursing diagnoses** (see Commonly Encountered Nursing Diagnoses section)
   a. Altered protection (risk for infection) related to disease or treatment
   b. Potential for fear or anxiety related to disease or treatment (see Chapter 9)
   c. Potential for altered family processes (see Chapter 9)

Immunosuppression

1. **Pathophysiology**
   a. Immunosuppression occurs when some defect in the immunologic system puts the patient at increased risk for infection. The longer the patient is immunosuppressed, the greater the risk of infection. Neutropenia is one form of immunosuppression (see Neutropenia section). Although there are primary forms of immune dysfunction, patients are more often admitted to critical care units with immunosuppression as a complication to an underlying disease
   b. Various drugs prescribed to suppress one part of the immune system have untoward effects on other parts of the hematologic and immunologic systems
      i. Both the NSAIDs and steroids inhibit portions of the pathway that synthesizes prostaglandins, thromboxanes, and leukotrienes, which are responsible for many normal hematologic and immunologic processes (see Fig. 6–3). These agents may also mask the usual signs and symptoms of infection such as fever
      ii. After organ transplantation, various immunosuppressive drugs are used to suppress the immune system and prevent transplant rejection. These drugs act primarily on B cells and T cells and suppress not only the immunologic response to the allograft but also the patient's ability to fight bacteria, viruses, fungi, and parasites. Commonly used immunosuppressive drugs in transplant patients are described in the Transplant Rejection section
2. **Etiologic or precipitating factors**
   a. Drug-induced
      i. Steroids
      ii. Azathioprine (Imuran)
      iii. Cyclosporine
      iv. History of antineoplastic chemotherapy especially high dose as is administered for BMT
   b. Genetic (e.g., severe combined immunodeficiency disease)
   c. Decreased neutrophil production (see Neutropenia section)
   d. HIV infection (see HIV Infection section)
3. **Nursing assessment data base**
   a. Nursing history
      i. Subjective: malaise, chills, night sweats, sore throat, dyspnea, sinus pain, headache, confusion, pain with swallowing, pain with urination, pain with defecation
      ii. Objective: cough, diarrhea
   b. Nursing examination of patient
      i. Inspection: temperature exceeding 101°F (38.3°C), shortness of breath, loss of integrity of skin and mucous membranes (especially intravenous and central venous catheter sites)

        ii. Palpation and percussion: lymphadenopathy

       iii. Auscultation: tachycardia, hypotension, crackles, rhonchi

  c. Diagnostic study findings: Laboratory cultures positive for unusual or opportunistic organisms (e.g., *Pneumocystis carinii*)

4. Nursing diagnoses (see Commonly Encountered Nursing Diagnoses section)

  a. Altered protection (risk for infection) related to disease or treatment; additional nursing considerations for the immunosuppressed patient:

        i. Antibiotics are used to prevent infection as well as to treat documented infections

       ii. If immunosuppression is secondary to a drug intervention (e.g., NSAIDs, steroids, cyclosporine), the drug dose may have to be decreased despite the risk of a recurrence or flare-up of the underlying disease that the immunosuppressive drug was being used to treat

  b. Potential for fear or anxiety related to disease or treatment (see Chapter 9)

  c. Potential for altered family processes (see Chapter 9)

HIV Infection

1. Pathophysiology

  a. HIV type 1, previously known as human T lymphocyte virus-3 (HTLV-3), is a retrovirus that infects cells expressing CD4 on their cell membranes, primarily T_H lymphocytes and macrophages. The HIV copies its RNA into the host cell's DNA and then remains quiescent until the host cell is activated to mount an immunologic response. Activation of the host CD4 cells also initiates replication and production of the HIV RNA, which is released into the circulation. This newly made HIV then infects other cells expressing CD4

  b. Disease course

        i. The initial stage of HIV infection lasts 4 to 8 weeks. High levels of virus are in the blood. The patient experiences generalized flu-like symptoms

       ii. The virus then enters a latent stage in which it is inactive in infected, resting CD4 cells, replicating only when the host cell is activated for an immune response. Levels of virus are high in the lymph nodes, where CD4 cells reside, but low in the blood. T_C cells, which express CD8 and so are not infected by HIV, and B cells attempt to destroy the CD4 cells harboring the virus. However, the T_C cells and B cells are crippled without adequate T_H support. This latent stage lasts on the average between 2 and 12 years, during which time the patient is asymptomatic. During this time, the number of CD4 cells declines

       iii. During the third stage of HIV infection, the patient begins to experience opportunistic infections. Levels of CD4 cells are usually below 500/mm^3 and declining, whereas levels of virus in the blood are increasing. This stage can last 2 to 3 years

       iv. Once the CD4 cell levels drop below 200/mm^3, the patient is considered to have acquired immunodeficiency syndrome (AIDS). Virus levels in the blood are high. This stage ends in death, usually within 1 year

    c. Complications of HIV infection

        i. Opportunistic fungal, parasitic, or viral infections: oral candidiasis, *P. carinii* pneumonia, recurrent herpes simplex, cytomegalovirus retinitis, *Cryptosporidium* enteritis, *Cryptococcus neoformans* meningitis, toxoplasmosis

        ii. Secondary cancers: Kaposi's sarcoma, non-Hodgkin's lymphoma, anal cancer, cervical cancer

        iii. Wasting syndrome

        iv. Dementia

    d. More than two thirds of HIV-infected patients cared for in critical care units are admitted because of respiratory failure, predominantly caused by *P. carinii*

2. Etiologic or precipitating factors: HIV is transmitted via intimate sexual contact, contaminated needles, or contaminated blood products; from mother to fetus; and from mother to breast-feeding infant

3. Nursing assessment data base

    a. Nursing history

        i. Subjective: fatigue, night sweats, sore throat, dyspnea, pain, history of frequent infections, social history of intravenous drug abuse with shared needles, history of unprotected sexual contact with persons possibly infected with HIV, history of blood transfusion

        ii. Objective: weight loss, diarrhea

    b. Nursing examination of patient

        i. Inspection: temperature exceeding 101°F (38.3°C), shortness of breath, loss of integrity of skin and mucous membranes, possibly cachexia

        ii. Palpation and percussion: possibly lymphadenopathy

        iii. Auscultation: tachycardia, hypotension, crackles, rhonchi

    c. Diagnostic study findings

        i. Laboratory

            (a) Western blot result is positive for HIV (note: the ELISA is a less expensive screening test for HIV antibody. If the ELISA result is positive, a Western blot should be performed to confirm the results because false-positive results do occur with ELISA)

            (b) CD4 lymphocyte counts are less than $500/mm^3$

            (c) Nonreactive skin panel

            (d) Infection with unusual or opportunistic organisms (e.g., *P. carinii*)

        ii. Radiologic: infiltrates on chest radiograph

4. Nursing diagnoses (see Commonly Encountered Nursing Diagnoses section)

    a. Altered protection (risk for infection) related to disease or treatment; additional nursing considerations for the patient with HIV: treatment of HIV infection can include

        i. Anti-retroviral therapy with zidovudine (AZT, Retrovir), didanosine (ddI, Videx), zalcitabine (ddC, Hivid), or stavudine (d4T, Zerit)

        ii. Prophylactic antibiotic therapy with trimethoprim-sulfamethoxazole (Bactrim, TMP-SMX, Septra), aerosolized pentamidine (Pentam), and/or other agents

        iii. Anti-retroviral agents with HIV-1 protease inhibitors such as saquinavir (Invirase), indinavir (Crixivan), nelfinavir (Viracept), and/or ritonavir (Norvir)

b. Anticipatory grieving (see Chapter 9)

c. Potential for activity intolerance related to disease or treatment

d. Potential for pain related to disease or treatment (see Chapter 9)

e. Potential for altered family processes (see Chapter 9)

f. Potential for fear or anxiety related to disease or treatment (see Chapter 9)

Anaphylactic Type I Hypersensitivity Reactions

1. **Pathophysiology**
   a. After a first, sensitizing exposure to a specific allergen, such as an insect sting, in which abnormally large amounts of IgE antibodies are made, subsequent exposures to the same allergen trigger an exaggerated antibody reaction. When the patient comes in contact with the antigen a second time, IgE triggers the release of histamine, heparin, and other cytokines from mast cells, causing bronchiole constriction, peripheral vasoconstriction, and increased vascular permeability, quickly progressing to airway obstruction, pulmonary edema, peripheral edema, hypovolemia, hypotension, shock, and circulatory collapse
   b. Prompt diagnosis and treatment of anaphylaxis with epinephrine, antihistamines, steroids, and hemodynamic support is of paramount importance
2. **Etiologic or precipitating factors**
   a. Drugs (e.g., penicillin, local anesthetics, vaccines, contrast dye)
   b. Insect stings
   c. Foods (e.g., shellfish, milk, eggs, fish, wheat)
3. **Nursing assessment data base**
   a. Nursing history
      i. Subjective: apprehension, dyspnea
      ii. Objective: restlessness
   b. Nursing examination of patient
      i. Inspection: urticaria, facial edema, tachypnea, stridor, cyanosis
      ii. Auscultation: tachycardia, hypotension, wheezing
   c. Diagnostic study findings: usually noncontributory to diagnosis of anaphylaxis
4. **Nursing diagnoses** (see Commonly Encountered Nursing Diagnoses section)
   a. Potential for impaired gas exchange related to disease
   b. Potential for fluid volume deficit related to shock
   c. Potential for fear or anxiety related to disease or treatment (see Chapter 9)

References

PHYSIOLOGIC ANATOMY

Abbas, A. K., Lichtman, A. H., and Pober, J. S.: Cellular and Molecular Immunology. Philadelphia, W. B. Saunders, 1994.

Huddleston, V. B.: The inflammatory/immune response: Implications for the critically ill. *In* Huddleston, V. B. (ed.): Multisystem Organ Failure: Pathophysiology and Clinical Implications. St. Louis, Mosby-Year Book, 1992, pp. 16–36.

Huddleston, V. B.: Inflammatory mediators and multisystem organ failure. *In* Huddleston, V. B. (ed.): Multisystem Organ Failure: Pathophysiology and Clinical Implications. St. Louis, Mosby-Year Book, 1992.

Janeway, C. A., Jr., and Travers, P.: Immunobiology. New York, Garland Publishing, 1994.

Kuby, J. (ed.): Immunology, 2nd ed. New York, W. H. Freeman, 1994.

Parslow, T. G.: The phagocytes: Neutrophils and macrophages. *In* Stites, D. P., Terr, A. I., and Parslow, T. G. (eds.): Basic and Clinical Immunology, 8th ed. Norwalk, Conn., Appleton & Lange, 1994, pp. 9–21.

Secor, V. H.: Mediators of coagulation and inflammation: Relationship and clinical significance. Crit. Care Nurs. Clin. North Am. 5:411–433, 1993.

Secor, V. H.: The inflammatory/immune response in critical illness: Role of the systemic inflammatory response syndrome. Crit. Care Nurs. Clin. North Am. 6:251–264, 1994.

Stites, D. P., Terr, A. I., and Parslow, T. G. (eds.): Basic and Clinical Immunology, 8th ed. Norwalk, Conn., Appleton & Lange, 1994.

Workman, M. L.: Essential concepts of inflammation and immunity. Crit. Care Nurs. Clin. North Am. 7:601–615, 1995.

NURSING ASSESSMENT DATA BASE

Fischbach, F. T.: A Manual of Laboratory and Diagnostic Tests, 5th ed. Philadelphia, J. B. Lippincott, 1996.

Fischer, D. S., Knobf, M. T., and Durivage, H. J.: Cancer Chemotherapy Handbook, 5th ed. St. Louis, Mosby-Year Book, 1997.

Shannon, M. T., Wilson, B. A., and Stang, C. L.: Govoni and Hayes Drugs and Nursing Implications, 7th ed. Norwalk, Conn., Appleton & Lange, 1992.

COMMONLY ENCOUNTERED NURSING DIAGNOSES

American Red Cross: Circular of information for the use of human blood and blood components. AABB OP1594/ARC 1751, 1995.

Anderson, K. C., and Braine, H. G.: Specialized cell component therapy. Semin. Oncol. Nurs. 6:140–149, 1990.

Coffland, F. I., and Shelton, D. M.: Blood component replacement therapy. Crit. Care Nurs. Clin. North Am. 5:543–556, 1993.

Dean, G. E., Haeuber, D., and Rivera, L. M.: Infection. *In* McCorkle, R., Grant, M., Frank-Stromborg, M., and Baird, S. B. (eds.): Cancer Nursing: A Comprehensive Textbook (2nd ed.): Philadelphia, W. B. Saunders, 1996, pp. 963–978.

Erickson, J. M.: Blood support for the myelosuppressed patient. Semin. Oncol. Nurs. 6:61–66, 1990.

Fuller, A. K.: Platelet transfusion therapy for thrombocytopenia. Semin. Oncol. Nurs. 6:123–128, 1990.

Greenbaum, B. H.: Transfusion-associated graft-versus-host disease: Historical perspectives, incidence, and current use of irradiated blood products. J. Clin. Oncol. 9:1889–1902, 1991.

Higgins, V. L.: Leukocyte-reduced blood components: Patient benefits and practical applications. Oncol. Nurs. Forum 23, 659–667, 1996.

Jeter, E. K., and Spivey, M. A.: Noninfectious complications of blood transfusion. Hematol. Oncol. Clin. North Am. 9:187–204, 1995.

Kefer, C. A., Godwin, J., and Jassak, P. E.: Blood component therapy. *In* McCorkle, R., Grant, M., Frank-Stromborg, M., and Baird, S. B. (eds.): Cancer Nursing: A Comprehensive Textbook (2nd ed.). Philadelphia, W. B. Saunders, 1996, pp. 485–503.

McNally, J. C., Somerville, E. T., Miaskowski, C., and Rostad, M. (eds.): Guidelines for Oncology Nursing Practice, 2nd ed. Philadelphia, W. B. Saunders, 1991.

Phillips, G. R., Kauder, D. R., and Schwab, C. W.: Massive blood loss in trauma patients: The benefits and dangers of transfusion therapy. Postgrad. Med. 95(4):61–72, 1994.

Snyder, E. L., and Mechanic, S. A.: Transfusion therapy. *In* DeVita, V. T., Hellman, S., and Rosenberg, S. A. (eds.): Cancer: Principles and Practice of Oncology (5th ed.). Philadelphia, J. B. Lippincott, 1997, pp. 2607–2620.

Spector, D.: Transfusion-associated graft-versus-host disease: An overview and two case reports. Oncol. Nurs. Forum 22:97–101, 1995.

Timmerman, P. R.: Intravenous immunoglobulin in oncology nursing practice. Oncol. Nurs. Forum 20:69–75, 1993.

Young-McCaughan, S.: Hematologic and lymphatic disorders. *In* Linton, A. D., Matteson, M. A., and Maebius, M. K. (eds.): Introductory Nursing Care of Adults. Philadelphia, W. B. Saunders, 1995, pp. 509–536.

    See also: Bociek and Armitage, 1996; Fischbach, 1996; Fischer, Knobf, and Durivage, 1997; Vose and Armitage, 1995.

PATIENT HEALTH PROBLEMS

Anemia

Erickson, J. M.: Anemia. Semin. Oncol. Nurs. 12:2–14, 1996.

    See also Coffland and Shelton, 1993; Fischer, Knobf, and Durivage, 1997; Haeuber and Spross, 1991; Higgins, 1996.

Disseminated Intravascular Coagulation

Bell, T. N.: Disseminated intravascular coagulation: Clinical complexities of aberrant coagulation. Crit. Care Nurs. Clin. North Am. 5:389–410, 1993.

Bell, T. N.: Coagulation and disseminated intravascular coagulation. *In* Huddleston, V. B. (ed.): Multisystem Organ Failure: Pathophysiology and Clinical Implications. St. Louis, Mosby-Year Book, 1992, pp. 57–81.

Bick, R. L.: Disseminated intravascular coagulation: Objective criteria for diagnosis and management. Med. Clin. North Am. 78:511–543, 1994.

Thrombocytopenia

Ellenberger, B. J., Haas, L., and Cundiff, L.: Thrombotic thrombocytopenia purpura: Nursing during the acute phase. Dimen. Crit. Care Nurs. 12(2):58–65, 1993.

Lapka, D. M. V., Wild, L. D., and Barbour, L. A.: Heparin-induced thrombocytopenia and thrombosis: A case study and clinical overview. Oncol. Nurs. Forum 21:871–876, 1994.

Neumann, M., and Urizar, R.: Hemolytic uremic syndrome: Current pathophysiology and management. AANA J. 21(2):137–143, 1994.

Rintels, P. B., Kenney, R. M., and Crowley, J. P.: Therapeutic support of the patient with thrombocytopenia. Hematol. Oncol. Clin. North Am. 8:1131–1157, 1994.

Rutherford, C. J., and Frenkel, E. P.: Thrombocytopenia: Issues in diagnosis and therapy. Med. Clin. North Am. 78:555–575, 1994.

Shuey, K. M.: Platelet-associated bleeding disorders. Semin. Oncol. Nurs. 12:15–27, 1996.

Wells, J. V., and Isbister, J. P.: Hematologic diseases. *In* Stites, D. P., Terr, A. I., and Parslow, T. G. (eds.): Basic and Clinical Immunology, 8th ed. Norwalk, Conn., Appleton & Lange, 1994, pp. 425–441.
   See also Fischer, Knobf, and Durivage, 1997; Haeuber and Spross, 1991.

Hypercoagulable Disorders

Bick, R. L.: Hypercoagulability and thrombosis. Med. Clin. North Am. 78:635–665, 1994.

Ellenberger, B. J., Haas, L., and Cundiff, L.: Thrombotic thrombocytopenic purpura: Nursing during the acute phase. Dimen. Crit. Care Nurs. 12(2):58–65, 1993.

Neutropenia

Alvir, J. M., Lieberman, J. A., Safferman, A. Z., et al.: Clozapine-induced agranulocytosis: Incidence and risk factors in the United States. N. Engl. J. Med. 329:162–167, 1993.

American Society of Clinical Oncology.: American Society of Clinical Oncology recommendations for the use of hematopoietic colony-stimulating factors: Evidence-based, clinical practice guidelines. J. Clin. Oncol. 12:2471–2508, 1994.

American Society of Clinical Oncology.: Update of recommendations for the use of hematopoietic colony-stimulating factors: Evidence-based clinical practice guidelines. J. Clin. Oncol. 14:1957–1960, 1996.

Appelbaum, F. R.: The application of hematopoietic colony stimulating factors (CSFs) in cancer management. *In* Hubbard, S. M., Greene, P. E., and Knobf, M. T. (eds.): Current Issues in Cancer Nursing Practice Updates. Philadelphia, J. B. Lippincott, 1993, pp. 1–13.

Bociek, R. G., and Armitage, J. O.: Hematopoietic growth factors. CA Cancer J. Clin. 46:165–184, 1996.

Brandt, B.: Nursing protocol for the patient with neutropenia. Oncol. Nurs. Forum 17(1, Suppl.):9–15, 1990.

Freifeld, A. G., Walsh, T. J., and Pizzo, P. A.: Infections in the cancer patient. *In* DeVita, V. T., Hellman, S., and Rosenberg, S. A. (eds.): Cancer: Principles and Practice of Oncology, 5th ed. Philadelphia, J. B. Lippincott, 1997, pp. 2659–2704.

Glaspy, J. A., and Ambersley, J. M.: The promise of colony-stimulating factors in clinical practice. Oncol. Nurs. Forum 17(1, Suppl.):20–24, 1990.

Griffin, J. D.: Hematopoietic growth factors. *In* DeVita, V. T., Hellman, S., and Rosenberg, S. A. (eds.): Cancer: Principles and Practice of Oncology, 5th ed. Philadelphia, J. B. Lippincott, 1997, pp. 2639–2657.

Lee, J. W., and Pizzo, P. A.: Management of the cancer patient with fever and prolonged neutropenia. Hematol. Oncol. Clin. North Am. 7:937–960, 1993.

Oniboni, A. C.: Infection in the neutropenic patient. Semin. Oncol. Nurs. 6:50–60, 1990.

Pizzo, P. A.: Management of fever in patients with cancer and treatment-induced neutropenia. Drug Ther. 328:1323–1332, 1993.

Vose, J. M., and Armitage, J. O.: Clinical applications of hematopoietic growth factors. J Clin Oncol. 13:1023–1035, 1995.
   See also Fischer, Knobf, and Durivage, 1997; Haeuber and Spross, 1991; Wade, 1993.

Acute Leukemia

Callaghan, M. E.: Leukemia. *In* McCorkle, R., Grant, M., Frank-Stromborg, M., and Baird, S. B. (eds.): Cancer

Nursing: A Comprehensive Textbook (2nd ed.). Philadelphia, W. B. Saunders, 1996, pp. 752–772.

Foon, K. A., and Casciato, D. A.: Acute leukemia. *In* Casciato, D. A., and Lowitz, B. B. (eds.): Manual of Clinical Oncology, 3rd ed. Boston, Little, Brown & Co., 1995, pp. 431–445.

Lawrence, J.: Critical care issues in the patient with hematologic malignancy. Semin. Oncol. Nurs. 10:198–207, 1994.

Scheinberg, D. A., Maslak, P., and Weiss, M.: Acute leukemias. *In* DeVita, V. T., Hellman, S., and Rosenberg, S. A. (eds.): Cancer: Principles and Practice of Oncology, 5th ed. Philadelphia, J. B. Lippincott, 1997, pp. 2293–2321.

Stucky, L. A.: Acute tumor lysis syndrome: Assessment and nursing implications. Oncol. Nurs. Forum 20:49–59, 1993.

Wade, J. C.: Management of infection in patients with acute leukemia. Hematol. Oncol. Clin. North Am. 7:293–315, 1993.

Warrell, R. P.: Metabolic emergencies. *In* DeVita, V. T., Hellman, S., and Rosenberg, S. A. (eds.): Cancer: Principles and Practice of Oncology, 5th ed. Philadelphia, J. B. Lippincott, 1997, pp. 2486–2500.

Yeager, K. A., and Miaskowski, C.: Advances in understanding the mechanisms and management of acute myelogenous leukemia. Oncol. Nurs. Forum 21:541–548, 1994.
   See also Vose and Armitage, 1995.

Bone Marrow Transplantation and Peripheral Blood Stem Cell Transplantation

Appelbaum, F. R.: The use of bone marrow and peripheral blood stem cell transplantation in the treatment of cancer. CA Cancer J. Clin. 46:142–164, 1996.

Bearman, S. I., Anderson, G. L., Mori, M., et al.: Venoocclusive disease of the liver: Development of a model for predicting fatal outcome after marrow transplantation. J. Clin. Oncol. 11:1729–1736, 1993.

Buchsel, P. C., and Kapustay, P. M.: Peripheral stem cell transplantation. *In* Hubbard, S. M., Goodman, M., and Knobf, M. T. (eds.): Oncology Nursing: Patient Treatment and Support. J. B. Lippincott, Philadelphia, 1995, pp. 1–14.

Ford, R. C., McDonald, J., Mitchell-Supplee, K. J., and Jagels, B. A.: Marrow transplant and peripheral blood stem cell transplantation. *In* McCorkle, R., Grant, M., Frank-Stromborg, M., and Baird, S. B. (eds.): Cancer Nursing: A Comprehensive Textbook (2nd ed.). Philadelphia, W. B. Saunders, 1996, pp. 504–530.

Hooper, P. J., and Santas, E. J.: Peripheral blood stem cell transplantation. Oncol. Nurs. Forum 20:1215–1223, 1993.

Jassak, P. F., and Riley, M. B.: Autologous stem cell transplant: An overview. Cancer Pract. 2:141–145, 1994.

Lin, E. M., Tierney, D. K., and Stadtmauer, E. A.: Autologous bone marrow transplantation: A review of the principles and complications. Cancer Nurs. 16:204–213, 1993.

McDonald, G. B., Hinds, M. S., Fisher, L. D., et al.: Veno-occlusive disease of the liver and multiorgan failure after bone marrow transplantation: A cohort study of 355 patients. Ann. Intern. Med. 118:255–267, 1993.

Rowe, J. M., Ciobanu, N., Ascensao, J., et al.: Recommended guidelines for the management of autologous and allogeneic bone marrow transplantation: A report for the Eastern Cooperative Oncology Group (ECOG). Ann. Intern. Med. 120:143–158, 1994.

Whedon, M. B. (ed.). Bone Marrow Transplantation: Principles, Practice, and Nursing Insights. Boston, Jones & Bartlett, 1991.

Wujcik, D., Ballard, B., and Camp-Sorrell, D.: Selected complications of allogeneic bone marrow transplantation. Semin. Oncol. Nurs. 10:28–41, 1994.

See also Spector, 1995, and Timmerman, 1993.

Transplant Rejection

Garovoy, M. R., Stock, P., Bumgardner, G., et al.: Clinical transplantation. *In* Stites, D. P., Terr, A. I., and Parslow, T. G. (eds.): Basic and Clinical Immunology, 8th ed. Norwalk, Conn., Appleton & Lange, 1994, pp. 744–764.

See also Wahrenberger, 1995.

Immunosuppression

Wahrenberger, A.: Pharmacologic immunosuppression: Cure or curse? Crit. Care Nurs. Q. 17(4):27–36, 1995.

Lake, K. D., and Kilkenny, J. M.: The pharmacokinetics and pharmacodynamics of immunosuppressive agents. Crit. Care Nurs. Clin. North Am. 4:205–221, 1992.

HIV Infection

Goldschmidt, R. H., and Dong, B. J. Current report—HIV treatment of AIDS and HIV-related conditions—1995. J. Am. Board Fam. Pract. 8:139–162, 1995.

Goldschmidt, R. H., Dong, B. J., and Legg, J. J.: Current report—HIV antiretroviral strategies revisited. J. Am. Board Fam. Pract. 8:62–69, 1995.

Henry, S. B., and Holzemer, W. L.: Critical care management of the patient with HIV infection who has *Pneumocystis carinii* pneumonia. Heart Lung 21:243–249, 1992.

Libman, H.: Pathogenesis, natural history, and classification of HIV infection. Prim. Care 19(3):1–17, 1992.

Wachter, R. M., Luce, J. M., and Hopewell, P. C.: Critical care of patients with AIDS. J.A.M.A. 267:541–547, 1992.

Anaphylactic Type I Hypersensitivity Reactions

Fisher, M.: Treatment of acute anaphylaxis. B.M.J. 311:731–733, 1995.

c h a p t e r

7

... The Gastrointestinal System

Susan L. Smith, R.N., Ph.D.

PHYSIOLOGIC ANATOMY

Upper Gastrointestinal (GI) System (Fig. 7–1)

1. **Oral cavity**
   a. Prepares food for absorption by ingestion, mastication, salivation, and the initial stage of swallowing
   b. Approximately 1000 to 1500 ml/day of saliva are secreted by the submandibular, parotid, and sublingual salivary glands
   c. Stimulation is via the autonomic nervous system (ANS)
2. **Pharynx**
   a. Divisions of the pharynx: nasopharynx, oropharynx, laryngeal pharynx
   b. Closes and seals off trachea as food moves into the esophagus
   c. Swallowing receptors are stimulated when food moves toward the back of the mouth
   d. The motor impulses from the swallowing center during the pharyngeal stage of swallowing are transmitted via cranial nerves V, IX, X, and XII
3. **Esophagus**
   a. Lies posterior to the trachea and the heart and shares a common fibroelastic membrane with the posterior portion of the trachea
   b. Attaches to the stomach below the level of the diaphragm
   c. Sphincters: hypopharyngeal (proximal), gastroesophageal (distal)
   d. Blood supply
      i. Arterial supply: left gastric artery
      ii. Venous drainage
         (a) Splanchnic bed drains entire GI tract
         (b) Gastric vein drains stomach and esophagus
         (c) Direct drainage into azygous and hemiazygous veins of the mediastinum

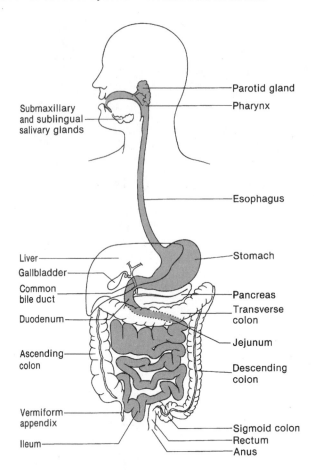

Figure 7–1 • Digestive tract of the human being. (From Westfall, U. E., and Heitkemper, M.: Gastrointestinal physiology. *In* Clochesy, J. M., Breu, C., Cardin, S., et al. [eds.]: Critical Care Nursing, 2nd ed. Philadelphia, W. B. Saunders, 1996, p. 979.)

4. Stomach

    a. Layers of the stomach wall (Fig. 7–2)

        i. Mucosa: receives majority of blood supply

            (a) Epithelium: contains the gastric, cardiac, and pyloric glands

            (b) Lamina propria: contains lymphocytes; site of gut immunologic responsiveness

            (c) Muscularis mucosa: contains thin smooth muscle layer

        ii. Submucosa: contains loose, connective tissue and elastic fibers, blood vessels, and lymphatic vessels

        iii. Muscularis: muscle layer that folds the mucosa into rugae (mucosal folds) at the inner lining of the stomach

        iv. Serosa

    b. Sphincters are responsible for controlling the rate of food passage: cardiac sphincter (proximal), pyloric sphincter (distal)

    c. Secretion of gastric enzymes: necessary for digestion

        i. Cardiac glands: secrete mucus, which is a lubricant and a mucosal barrier from acids

        ii. Fundic glands

            (a) Chief cells: secrete pepsinogen, which, in its activated form (pepsin), digests proteins; optimal pH for pepsin activity is 1.2 to 2.4

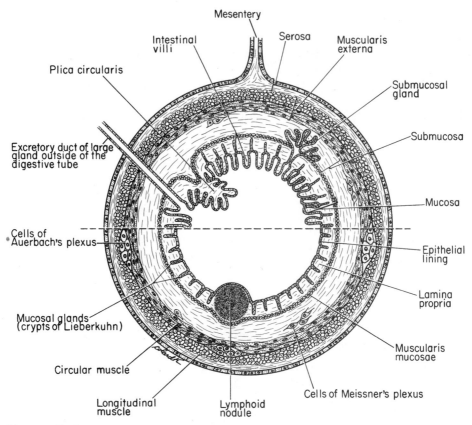

Figure 7–2 • Layers of the intestinal wall. Histologic organization of the digestive tract—the stomach through the large intestine. (From Bloom, W., and Fawcett, D. W.: A Textbook of Histology, 10th ed. Philadelphia, W. B. Saunders, 1975, p. 599.)

   (b) Parietal cells secrete
      (1) Hydrochloric acid, which lowers pH and kills bacteria
      (2) Intrinsic factor, a glycoprotein necessary for vitamin B_{12} absorption
   d. Gastric hormones
      i. Gastrin: secreted in response to distention of the antrum or fundus
         (a) Stimulates secretion of hydrochloric acid by the parietal cells
         (b) Stimulates secretion of pepsin by chief cells
         (c) Increases gastric blood flow, promotes stomach emptying
         (d) Stimulates mucosal cell replication
      ii. Histamine: secreted by mast cells in response to presence of food
         (a) Stimulates gastric acid and pepsin secretion
         (b) Causes contraction of gallbladder, relaxation of sphincter of Oddi
         (c) Increases GI motility
   e. Blood supply
      i. Arterial supply (celiac plexus)
         (a) Right gastric artery
         (b) Left gastric artery
         (c) Gastroduodenal artery into right gastroepiploic artery
         (d) Splenic artery into left gastroepiploic artery

      ii. Venous drainage

        (a) Splanchnic bed drains entire GI tract

        (b) Gastric vein drains stomach and esophagus

  f. Innervation

    i. Intrinsic (enteric) system: independent of central nervous system (CNS) control, contains two networks

      (a) Myenteric (Auerbach's) plexus: influences muscle tone, contractions, velocity, and excitation of the stomach

      (b) Submucosal (Meissner's) plexus: influences secretions of the stomach

    ii. Extrinsic system: via the CNS, parasympathetic, and sympathetic systems

      (a) Parasympathetic: fibers arise from the medulla and spinal segments (i.e., vagus nerves)

        (1) Enhances most GI functions by secretion of acetylcholine

        (2) Increases glandular secretion and muscle tone; decreases sphincter tone

      (b) Sympathetic: motor and sensory fibers arise from the thoracic and lumbar segments; distribution is via sympathetic ganglia (i.e., celiac plexus)

        (1) Fibers run alongside blood vessels and secrete norepinephrine

        (2) System inhibits GI activity

  g. Gastric secretion: approximately 1500 to 3000 ml is secreted daily and mixes with food entering the stomach

  h. Phases of gastric secretion

    i. Cephalic: fibers of the vagus nerve stimulate the stomach to secrete gastrin (from the antrum) and hydrochloric acid

    ii. Gastric: vasovagal reflexes stimulate parasympathetic system to increase the secretion of gastrin

  i. Gastric emptying is proportional to the volume of material in the stomach

  j. Factors that accelerate gastric emptying: large volume of liquids; anger; insulin

  k. Factors that inhibit gastric emptying: fat (most potent stimulus of inhibition), protein, starch, sadness, duodenal hormones

  l. Vomiting: coordinated by the vomiting center in the medulla

    i. Stimuli that induce vomiting: tactile stimulation to the back of the throat, increased intracranial pressure, intense pain, dizziness, anxiety

    ii. ANS discharge may precede vomiting: sweating, increased heart rate, increased salivation, nausea

Lower Gastrointestinal System

1. Small intestine extends from the pylorus to the ileocecal valve (duodenum, jejunum, ileum): primary function is absorption of nutrients

  a. Layers of the intestinal wall (see Fig. 7–2)

    i. Mucosa: innermost layer, receives majority of blood supply, predominant site of nutrient absorption

      (a) Epithelium: covered with villi that contain glands, crypts of Lieberkühn

      (b) Lamina propria: contains lymphocytes; site of gut immunologic responsiveness

      (c) Muscularis mucosa: contains thin smooth muscle layer

    ii. Submucosa: contains loose, connective tissue and elastic fibers, blood vessels, lymphatic vessels, and nerves

    iii. Muscularis: muscle layer

      (a) Function is involuntary motility

      (b) Peristalsis: propulsive movements that move the intestinal contents toward the anus

    iv. Serosa: outermost layer, protects and suspends intestine within the abdominal cavity

b. Blood supply

    i. Arterial supply: derived from the celiac artery and the superior (jejunum, ileum, cecum) mesenteric arteries

    ii. Venous drainage: splanchnic bed drains entire GI tract

      (a) Superior mesenteric vein: drains the small intestine and the ascending and transverse colon

      (b) Inferior mesenteric vein: drains the sigmoid colon and rectum

c. Innervation: same as for stomach

d. Small intestinal digestive enzymes: not secreted, but integral components of the mucosa

    i. Up to 3000 ml/day of digestive enzymes (e.g., lipase, amylase, maltase, and lactase)

    ii. pH is approximately 7.0

e. Intestinal hormones

    i. Secretin: secreted in response to acidic gastric juice from the stomach and to alcohol ingestion

      (a) Augments the action of cholecystokinin (CCK)

      (b) Stimulates release of pancreatic bicarbonate and secretion of water

      (c) Mildly inhibits motility of most of GI tract

    ii. CCK: secreted in response to the presence of fat, protein, and acidic contents in the intestine

      (a) Increases contractility of the gallbladder

      (b) Moderately inhibits stomach motility

      (c) Stimulates secretion of pancreatic digestive enzymes, bicarbonate, and insulin

    iii. Gastric inhibitory peptide (GIP): secreted in response to presence of carbohydrates and fat in intestine: inhibits gastric acid secretion and motility

    iv. Vasoactive intestinal peptide: secreted throughout the gut in response to acidic gastric juice in the duodenum

      (a) Main effects are similar to those of secretin

      (b) Stimulates the secretion of intestinal juices to decrease the acidity of chyme

      (c) Inhibits gastric secretion

    v. Somatostatin: secreted throughout the intestine in response to vagal stimulation, ingestion of food, and release of CCK, GIP, glucagon, and secretin

      (a) Inhibits secretion of saliva, gastric acid, pepsin, intrinsic factor, and pancreatic enzymes

      (b) Inhibits gastric motility, gallbladder contraction, intestinal motility, and blood flow to liver and intestine

(c) Inhibits secretion of insulin and growth hormone
vi. Serotonin: secreted throughout the intestine in response to vagal stimulation, increased luminal pressure, and presence of acid or fat in duodenum; inhibits gastric acid secretion and mucin production
f. Functions
    i. Basic absorption: almost all absorption occurs in the small intestine via four mechanisms: active transport, passive diffusion, facilitated diffusion, non-ionic transport
    ii. Vitamins are absorbed primarily in the intestine, except for vitamin B_{12}, which is absorbed in the terminal ileum; most vitamins are absorbed by passive diffusion, except for the fat-soluble vitamins that require bile salts for absorption
    iii. Water absorption: approximately 8 L of water per day is absorbed by the small intestine
    iv. Electrolyte absorption: most occurs in the proximal small intestine
    v. Iron absorption: absorbed in the ferrous form in the duodenum
        (a) Facilitated by ascorbic acid
        (b) Increases in states of iron deficiency
    vi. Carbohydrate absorption: complex carbohydrates are broken down into monosaccharides or basic sugars (fructose, glucose, galactose) by specific enzymes (e.g., amylase, maltase)
    vii. Protein absorption: protein is broken down into amino acids and small peptides
    viii. Essential amino acids: lysine, phenylalanine, isoleucine, valine, methionine, leucine, threonine, and tryptophan
    ix. Fat absorption

2. Colorectum extends from terminal ileum at the ileocecal valve to rectum
a. Divisions of the colorectum
    i. Cecum: a cul-de-sac to which the appendix is attached
    ii. Ascending colon
    iii. Transverse colon
        (a) Hepatic flexure
        (b) Splenic flexure
    iv. Descending colon
    v. Sigmoid colon
    vi. Rectum: from sigmoid colon to anus
b. Layers of the intestinal wall (see Fig. 7–2)
    i. Mucosa: innermost layer, receives majority of blood supply
        (a) Crypts covered by epithelial cells that produce mucus
        (b) Mucosa contains lymphoid cells
    ii. Submucosa: contains most of nerves
    iii. Muscularis: muscle layer divided into longitudinal bands
        (a) Function is involuntary motility
        (b) Peristalsis: propulsive movements that push the GI contents toward the anus
    iv. Serosa: outermost layer, protects and suspends intestine within the abdominal cavity
c. Blood supply (Fig. 7–3)
    i. Arterial supply
        (a) Superior mesenteric artery: ascending colon and part of transverse colon

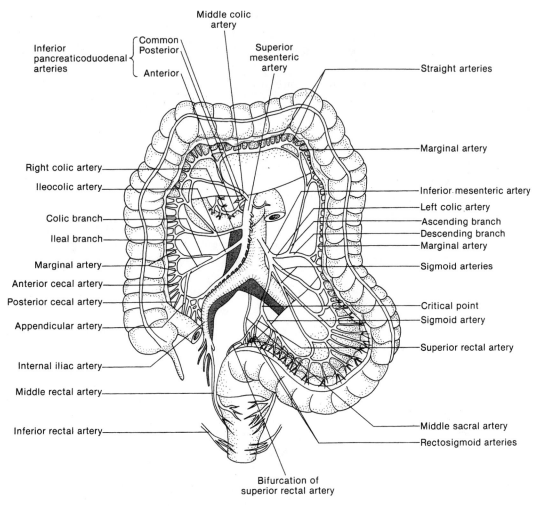

Figure 7–3 • Arterial and venous blood supplies to primary and accessory organs of the alimentary canal. (From Ruppert, S. D., and Englert, D. M.: Patients with gastrointestinal bleeding. *In* Clochesy, J. M., Breu, C., Cardin, S., et al. [eds.]: Critical Care Nursing, 2nd ed. Philadelphia, W. B. Saunders, 1996, p. 1028.)

      (b) Inferior mesenteric artery: transverse colon, sigmoid colon, and upper rectum

      (c) Hypogastric arteries give rise to the middle and inferior rectal and hemorrhoidal arteries

   ii. Venous drainage

      (a) Splanchnic bed drains entire GI tract

      (b) Superior mesenteric vein: ascending colon and part of transverse colon

      (c) Inferior mesenteric vein: transverse colon, sigmoid colon, and rectum

  d. Innervation: same as for the stomach and small intestine

  e. Factors that enhance motility

    i. Bacterial enterotoxins

    ii. Viral infections of the gut

    iii. Regional enteritis

       iv. Ulcerative colitis

       v. Increased bile salts

       vi. Osmotic overload

       vii. Laxatives

  f. Factors that inhibit motility

       i. Low-bulk diet

       ii. Parenteral nutrition

       iii. Bed rest

       iv. Dehydration

       v. Ileus

       vi. Fasting

       vii. Drugs (e.g., morphine SO_4)

  g. Colonic functions

       i. Absorption of approximately 1000 ml/day of water and electrolytes

       ii. Cellulose is broken down by enteric bacteria

       iii. Vitamins (folic acid, vitamin K, riboflavin, nicotinic acid) are synthesized by enteric bacteria

       iv. Fecal elimination: distention of the rectal wall initiates the defecation reflex

Gut Defenses

Mechanisms that exist within the GI tract to protect the integrity of the gut

1. **Mucosal barrier:** physical and chemical barriers that protect the wall of the gut from harmful substances

  a. Epithelial cells: tight junctions between cells make them relatively impervious to large molecules, and rapid proliferation of cells minimizes adherence of flora

  b. Mucus-bicarbonate barrier: forms a layer of alkalinity between the epithelium and luminal acids

2. **Motility:** prevents bacteria in distal small intestine from migrating proximally into sterile parts of GI system

  a. Stomach

       i. Expulsion of toxic substances as a result of stimulation of vomiting center in medulla

       ii. Barrier against reflux of duodenal contents back into stomach

  b. Colon: moves pathogens and potential carcinogens out of body

3. **Gut immunity:** necessary because gut is reservoir of potentially pathogenic bacteria

  a. Gut-associated lymphoid tissue (GALT) in submucosa (lamina propria or Peyer's patches) of GI tract

       i. B lymphocytes that bear surface immunoglobulin A (IgA) or synthesize IgA: secretory IgA prevents bacteria from binding to mucous cells

       ii. Macrophages in the lamina propria

  b. Glutamine is primary fuel of the gut and maintains the gut mucosal barrier

4. **Gastric acid:** intragastric pH below 4.0 is essential

  a. Protects stomach from ingested bacteria and other harmful substances

  b. Prevents bacteria from entering intestine

5. **Commensal bacteria:** natural gut flora are stable and protective in healthy person by competing with pathogenic species for nutrients and attachment sites, and produce inhibitory substances against pathogenic species
   a. Stomach, duodenum, and jejunum are sterile
   b. Ileum contains aerobic and anaerobic bacteria: dietary intake is a major factor in determining intestinal flora
   c. Large intestine contains large numbers of aerobic and anaerobic bacteria, and smaller numbers of yeast and fungi
6. **Impaired gut barrier function** facilitates bacterial translocation, the egress of bacteria and/or their toxins across the mucosal barrier and into the lymphatic vessels and portal circulation

. . . .
Accessory Organs of Digestion (Fig. 7–4)

1. **Liver**
   a. Anatomy: largest solid organ located primarily in the right upper quadrant, but left lobe extends across the midline into the left upper quadrant
      i. Right lobe: anterior and posterior segments
      ii. Left lobe: medial and lateral segments

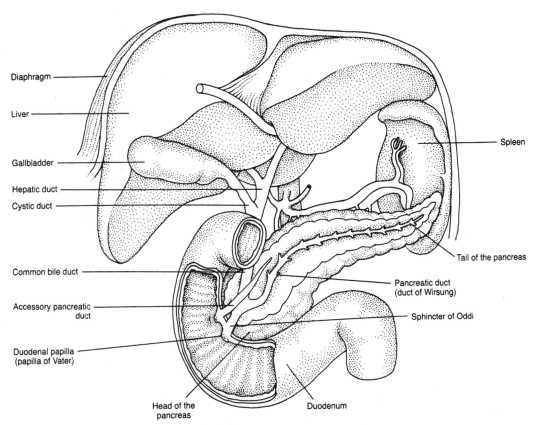

F i g u r e 7 – 4 • Anatomy of the liver and biliary tract. (From Westfall, U. E., and Heitkemper, M.: Gastrointestinal physiology. *In* Clochesy, J. M., Breu, C., Cardin, S., et al. [eds.]: Critical Care Nursing, 2nd ed. Philadelphia, W. B. Saunders, 1996, p. 992.)

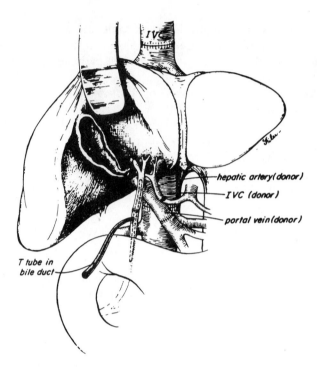

Figure 7–5 • Portal venous circulation. IVC = inferior vena cava. (From Sher, L., and Makowka, L.: The present status of liver transplantation. New Developments in Medicine 4:5–17, 1989. Reprinted with permission of Matthew Bender & Co., Inc.)

    iii. Caudate lobe

    iv. Each segment can be further divided into eight subsegments; important primarily for purposes of surgical resection for hepatic tumors or trauma

    v. Functional unit called *lobule* or *acinus*

  b. Blood supply (Fig. 7–5): the vascular system of the liver is unique in that the blood supply to the liver is via a vein *and* an artery

    i. Portal vein and hepatic artery enter liver at the porta hepatis or hilum

    ii. 25% of cardiac output flows through the liver per minute. Of the blood flow to the liver,

      (a) 75% is supplied by the portal vein

      (b) 25% is supplied by the hepatic artery

    iii. Blood flow to the liver is filtered through hepatic sinusoids that contain macrophages (Kupffer cells) for removing debris and foreign organisms

    iv. Venous drainage

      (a) Begins in central veins in the center of the lobules; central veins empty into hepatic veins

      (b) Hepatic veins: empty into the inferior vena cava

  c. Biliary duct system for draining bile

    i. Begins at the sinusoidal level as bile canaliculi

    ii. These branch, becoming larger and larger to form the right and left hepatic ducts

    iii. Hepatic ducts come together at the porta hepatis to form the common hepatic duct, which becomes the common bile duct after the cystic duct junction

d. Portal triad: branch of portal vein, branch of hepatic artery, and bile duct that flow contiguously throughout the liver

e. Physiology: the liver performs more than 400 functions; some of the more important ones are listed as follows:

    i. Maintains normal serum glucose levels; primary organ of nutrient metabolism: carbohydrate synthesis, metabolism, and transport

        (a) Glycogen storage: approximately 900 kcal of glycogen reserves are stored in the adult liver

        (b) Glycogenesis: conversion of excess carbohydrates to glycogen for storage in liver as metabolic reserve

        (c) Glycogenolysis: conversion of large stores of glycogen in muscles and liver to glucose

        (d) Gluconeogenesis: manufacture of glucose from noncarbohydrate substrate (fat, fatty acids, glycerol, amino acids)

    ii. Plays role in protein synthesis, metabolism, and transport

        (a) Production of plasma proteins (albumin, pre-albumin, transferrin, clotting factors, haptoglobin, ceruloplasmin, alpha$_1$-antitrypsin, complement, alpha-fetoprotein)

        (b) Deamination: metabolism of amino acids

        (c) Transamination: conversion of amino acids to ammonia, conversion of ammonia to urea for urinary excretion

    iii. Plays role in fat and lipid synthesis, metabolism, and transport

        (a) Principal site of synthesis and degradation of lipids (cholesterol, phospholipids, lipoprotein): produces approximately 1000 mg of cholesterol per day

        (b) Exogenous lipoprotein metabolism

        (c) Endogenous lipoprotein metabolism: major lipoprotein synthesized by liver is very-low-density lipoprotein (VLDL); one third of VLDL remnants converted to low-density lipoprotein (LDL)

            (1) Direct removal of VLDL remnants

            (2) Removal of 75% of LDL remnants by LDL receptors in liver

        (d) Conversion of excess carbohydrate to triglyceride, which is stored as adipose tissue

        (e) Conversion of triglyceride to glycerol and fatty acids for energy

        (f) Storage of triglyceride and fat-soluble vitamins (A, D, E, and K)

    iv. Detoxifies and eliminates drugs, hormones, and toxic substances

    v. Produces and secretes 600 to 1000 ml/day of bile

    vi. Stores vitamin B$_{12}$, copper, and iron

    vii. Filters blood via Kupffer cells (macrophages) that reside in the liver sinusoids

2. **Gallbladder:** sac-like organ attached to inferior surface of liver that serves as a reservoir for bile

a. Holds and concentrates approximately 50 ml of bile

b. Cystic duct attaches gallbladder to the common bile duct

c. Common bile duct terminates as the sphincter of Oddi in the duodenum

d. Presence of CCK in blood (in response to chyme in the duodenum): facilitates delivery of bile to duodenum

    i. Contraction of gallbladder

    ii. Relaxation of the sphincter of Oddi

e. Bile is composed of water, bile salts, and bile pigments

  i. Bile salts are responsible for absorption and emulsification of fat and fat-soluble vitamins

  ii. Bile pigments: high in cholesterol and phospholipids, give feces brown color

    (a) Bilirubin is the major bile pigment; is a breakdown product of hemoglobin metabolism from senescent red blood cells

    (b) Serum bilirubin

      (1) Total: indirect bilirubin plus direct bilirubin; when total bilirubin is elevated and cause is unknown, indirect and direct bilirubin fractions can be measured

      (2) Indirect (unconjugated): bilirubin bound to albumin before it binds to glucuronic acid; fat soluble

      (3) Causes of elevation of indirect bilirubin concentration in serum:

        a) Any hemolytic process (e.g., ABO mismatch in blood transfusion, beta-hemolytic streptococcal infection)

        b) Diffuse hepatocellular necrosis

      (4) Direct (conjugated): bilirubin bound to glucuronic acid, water soluble; concentration elevates with biliary tract obstruction (except cystic duct), diffuse biliary tract damage, acute cellular rejection after liver transplantation

      (5) Causes of elevation of direct bilirubin concentration in serum

        a) Bile duct obstruction (e.g., stones, tumor, biliary stricture after liver transplantation)

        b) Cholecystitis

        c) Necrosis of bile duct (e.g., hepatic artery thrombosis)

        d) Autoimmune diseases of biliary stasis (e.g., primary biliary cirrhosis, primary sclerosing cholangitis)

f. Blood supply

  i. Arterial supply: hepatic artery, cystic artery

  ii. Venous drainage: cystic vein

g. Innervation: splanchnic nerve, right branch of vagus nerve

3. **Pancreas:** retroperitoneal gland

  a. Head lies in the C-shaped curve of the duodenum

  b. Body extends horizontally behind stomach

  c. Tail is contiguous with the spleen

  d. Duct of Wirsung: main pancreatic duct whose terminal end, the sphincter of Oddi, empties into the duodenum; shares sphincter of Oddi with the common bile duct

  e. Duct of Santorini: accessory pancreatic duct (not present in all persons), opens into duodenum proximal to the duct of Wirsung

  f. Pancreatic secretions: 1500 to 2000 ml/day, pH of 8.3

    i. Secretion of pancreatic enzymes is induced by parasympathetic (vagal) stimulation

    ii. Food in the intestine stimulates secretion of

      (a) Secretin: results in copious secretion of pancreatic fluid

      (b) CCK: results in secretion of enzymes

  g. Exocrine pancreas (acinar cells): secretes bicarbonate, water, sodium, potassium, and the digestive enzymes

i. Trypsin: digestion of proteins
ii. Amylase: digestion of starches
iii. Lipase: digestion of fats
h. Endocrine pancreas: islets of Langerhans (alpha, beta, delta, and polypeptide cells)
   i. Alpha cells secrete glucagon, which is responsible for glycogenolysis and gluconeogenesis
   ii. Beta cells secrete insulin, which facilitates the use of glucose by tissues
   iii. Delta cells secrete somatostatin, which is responsible for inhibiting secretion of insulin, glucagon, and growth hormone
   iv. Polypeptide cells: associated with hypermotility of GI tract and diarrhea

NURSING ASSESSMENT DATA BASE

Nursing History

1. **Patient health history**
   a. Previous surgery or illness
   b. Abdominal or flank pain: location, duration, character, severity, alleviating and aggravating factors
   c. Oral health status: teeth, gums, tongue, pharnyx
   d. Fecal elimination: diarrhea or constipation, color of stools, presence of blood (black, maroon, or bright red). Clay-colored stool: absence of bile pigment as a result of biliary obstruction or advanced cirrhosis
   e. Urinary elimination: color of urine. Dark (tea-colored) urine: acute hepatocellular necrosis or severe biliary obstruction
   f. Nausea or vomiting: duration, alleviating and aggravating factors, description of vomitus, presence of blood
   g. Heartburn (dyspepsia, reflux): duration, alleviating and aggravating factors
   h. Fatigue, weakness
   i. Easy bruising or bleeding
   j. Food allergies
   k. Fever, night sweats
   l. Nutritional status
      i. Appetite
      ii. Difficulty eating or swallowing
      iii. Eating disorders
         (a) Bulimia
         (b) Anorexia
         (c) Obesity
      iv. Food allergies, intolerances (e.g., lactase deficiency causes lactose intolerance)
      v. Muscle wasting, atrophy
         (a) Wasting of the muscle over the temporal bones in the face

(b) Wasting of the thenar muscle (thenar eminence of thumb)

vi. Predisposing or iatrogenic factors that interfere with adequate nutrition

  (a) Nausea, vomiting

  (b) Pain: oral, abdominal, general

  (c) Ileus

  (1) Functional ileus

  (2) Paralytic ileus

  (3) Mechanical ileus: obstruction (tumor, foreign body, fecal impaction, adhesions)

  (d) Alteration in absorption, use, or storage of nutrients

  (e) Debilitation, fatigue, malaise

  (f) Altered mental status

  (g) Endotracheal intubation

  (h) Poor oral health status

  (i) Surgical loss of part of GI tract

  (j) Chemotherapy; antibiotics; drugs causing anorexia

vii. Increased risk of protein-energy malnutrition

  (a) Overweight: at least 20% over ideal body weight

  (b) Underweight: at least 10% under ideal body weight

  (c) Weight change, unintentional: more than 10% change in normal body weight in preceding 6 months

  (d) Congenital conditions, inborn errors of metabolism

  (e) Increased metabolic needs: fever, infection, hyperthyroidism, burns, recent surgery or soft tissue trauma, skeletal trauma, psychologic stress

  (f) Increased nutrient losses: draining fistulas or abscesses, open wounds, effusions, chronic blood loss, chronic renal dialysis, burns

  (g) Disease of the GI tract: malabsorption, pancreatic insufficiency, severe diarrhea, GI fistula, cirrhosis

  (h) Surgery of the GI tract: stomach or small bowel resection, intestinal bypass

  (i) Catabolic medications or therapies: corticosteroid therapy, immunosuppressive agents, radiation, chemotherapy

viii. Delayed hypersensitivity skin test response for anergy (lack of immune responsiveness)

2. Family history

  a. Carcinoma

  b. Liver disease

  c. Pancreatitis

  d. Diabetes mellitus

  e. Peptic ulcer disease

  f. Anemia

  g. Inflammatory bowel disease: Crohn's disease, ulcerative colitis

  h. Tuberculosis

  i. Obesity

3. Social history

  a. Alcohol, tobacco, and/or other drug abuse

  b. Travel to foreign country where hepatitis is endemic: sub-Sahara region

    c. Sexual promiscuity (homosexual, heterosexual, bisexual): viral hepatitis B and C infection is sexually transmitted

    d. Stress profile: personality type

4. Medication history

    a. Antacids

    b. Carafate

    c. Histamine blockers

    d. Anticholinergics

    e. Laxatives, cathartics

    f. Antidiarrheals

    g. Antiemetics

    h. Diet or weight loss pills

    i. Corticosteroids, other immunosuppressants

    j. Antibiotics

    k. Tranquilizers, sedatives, anxiolytics

    l. Barbiturates

    m. Antihypertensives, diuretics

    n. Analgesics

        i. Salicylates and derivatives

        ii. Acetaminophen (more than 200 preparations contain acetaminophen)

        iii. Nonsteroidal anti-inflammatory drugs (NSAIDs)

        iv. Narcotics

    o. Anticoagulants

Nursing Examination of Patient

1. Anatomic landmarks: used to locate and describe normal anatomic structures and abnormal findings of tenderness or pain and presence of masses

    a. Subcostal margins

    b. Costovertebral angle

    c. Abdominal quadrants (Fig. 7–6), midline of abdomen

    d. Umbilicus

    e. Rectus abdominus muscle

    f. Symphysis pubis

    g. Flanks

2. Inspection

    a. Physical signs of altered nutritional status: cachexia, obesity

    b. Oral cavity: gingivitis, lesions (e.g., herpes simplex, *Candida albicans*, leukoplakia), ability to swallow

    c. Symmetry, size, and contour of abdomen

    d. Condition of umbilicus

    e. Masses, pulsations

    f. Hernias, striae, scars, wounds, stomas, fistulas, tubes, drains

    g. Spider angiomas: found above umbilicus on anterior thorax, head, and neck

    h. Caput medusa: dilated abdominal veins (collateral vessels that come to skin surface) seen in patients with portal hypertension

    i. Jaundice: evident in skin and sclera

    j. Bruises, ecchymoses, hematomas

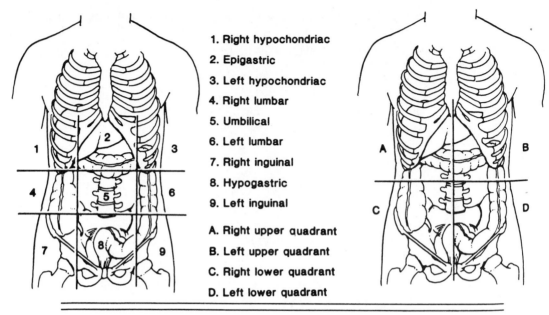

1. Right hypochondriac
2. Epigastric
3. Left hypochondriac
4. Right lumbar
5. Umbilical
6. Left lumbar
7. Right inguinal
8. Hypogastric
9. Left inguinal

A. Right upper quadrant
B. Left upper quadrant
C. Right lower quadrant
D. Left lower quadrant

Figure 7–6 • Regions and quadrants of the abdomen. (From Wright, J. E., and Shelton, B. K.: Desk Reference for Critical Care Nursing. Boston, Jones & Bartlett, 1993, p. 854.)

3. **Auscultation:** done in all quadrants before percussion and palpation to note location and characteristics of bowel and other sounds
    a. Normal bowel sounds: low-pitched, continuous gurgles heard in abdominal quadrants
    b. Abnormal bowel sounds
        i. Factors related to hypoactive sounds
            (a) Peritonitis
            (b) Paralytic ileus
            (c) Inflammation
            (d) Gastric or intra-abdominal bleeding
            (e) Pneumonia
            (f) Mechanical obstruction
        ii. Factors related to hyperactive sounds
            (a) Hyperkalemia
            (b) Gastroenteritis
            (c) Esophageal bleeding
            (d) Diarrhea
            (e) Mechanical obstruction
    c. Abdominal girth
    d. Bruit: denotes partial aortic occlusion
        i. Aortic bruit can be heard 2 to 3 cm above the umbilicus in the epigastric area
        ii. Renal artery bruit can be heard to left and/or right of midline in the epigastric areas
        iii. Iliac artery bruit can be heard in the left and/or right inguinal areas
    e. Venous hum that can be heard over the liver denotes liver disease
    f. Splenic friction rub that can be heard over the spleen denotes inflammation or infarction of the spleen

g. Hepatic friction rub that can be heard over the liver denotes liver tumor

4. Percussion

a. To determine the sizes of the liver and spleen

   i. Liver size can be estimated by percussing from right clavicle straight down the right midclavicular line (MCL) to detect changes in percussion tones

     (a) Over lung tissue, the percussion tone is resonant

     (b) At level of fifth intercostal space, the percussion tone becomes dull, denoting the upper edge of the liver

     (c) Over the bowel, the percussion tone is tympanic, denoting the lower edge of the liver

     (d) The distance between the upper and lower edges of the liver at the MCL is normally about 12 cm

   ii. The spleen can be percussed (dull tones) only if grossly enlarged at the left MCL below the left costal margin

b. To determine the presence of masses

c. To determine abnormal fluid and air collections

5. Palpation

a. Done to elicit tenderness or pain

   i. Visceral pain: dull, poorly localized (e.g., bowel obstruction)

   ii. Somatic pain: sharp, well localized (e.g., late appendicitis, capsular stretching of the swollen liver)

   iii. Rebound tenderness: occurs when palpation is suddenly withdrawn; associated with peritonitis

   iv. Contralateral pain: pain on opposite side of palpation (e.g., early appendicitis)

   v. Referred pain: pain in area distant from source (e.g., left shoulder pain referred from spleen)

   vi. Murphy's sign: severe right upper quadrant pain elicited on deep palpation under right costal margin, exacerbated by deep inspiration, associated with cholecystitis

b. Determine the presence and characteristics of masses

c. Determine tone (relaxed, tense, rigid) of abdominal wall

d. Determine enlarged liver size: palpation of the liver is performed at patient's right side

   i. By supporting the right flank area with the left hand and sliding the fingertips of the right hand under the right costal margin, using firm pressure

   ii. The fingertips are advanced as the patient inhales deeply and the liver edge moves 1 to 3 cm downward

   iii. Fingertips are held steady as the patient exhales and inhales again, and the smooth (normal) edge of the liver may be felt moving past the fingertips

   iv. The liver is not normally palpated more than 1 to 2 cm below right costal margin

Diagnostic Studies

1. Laboratory findings

a. Complete blood count (CBC)

b. White blood cell (WBC) count with differential, platelet count
c. Serum electrolytes, glucose, blood urea nitrogen (BUN)
d. Serum calcium, magnesium
e. Ammonia
f. Cholesterol
g. Serum alanine aminotransferase (ALT; formerly serum glutamate pyruvate transaminase [SGPT]), aspartate aminotransferase (AST; formerly serum glutamic-oxaloacetic transaminase [SGOT]), alkaline phosphatase, lactate dehydrogenase (LDH), gamma-glutamyl transferase (GGT)
h. Serum bilirubin: total, indirect, direct
i. Serum amylase, lipase, cholinesterase
j. Prothrombin time (PT), factor V, factor VII
k. Alpha fetoprotein
l. Blood cultures
m. Urine: amylase, lipase, bilirubin
n. Nutritional parameters
    i. Serum albumin
    ii. Total iron binding capacity
    iii. Serum transferrin, pre-albumin, retinol-binding protein
    iv. Lymphocyte count
    v. WBC count
    vi. Total lymphocyte count
    vii. CBC
    viii. 24-hour urine urea nitrogen
    ix. 24-hour urine creatinine
o. Stool: occult blood, fat, protein, ova and parasites, cultures

2. **Radiologic studies**
a. Abdominal flat-plate x-ray: to visualize the position, size, and structure of abdominal contents, truncal skeleton, and soft tissues of abdominal wall
b. Upper GI series: to visualize position, contours, and size of the entire upper GI tract (especially stomach and duodenum); to detect ulcers, tumors, strictures, and obstructions; and to evaluate melena, hematemesis, or heme-positive nasogastric drainage. Barium swallow: to look at swallowing, motility, and emptying in esophagus
c. Small bowel follow-through: to visualize the small bowel from the ligament of Treitz to the ileocecal valve to detect ulcers, tumors, diverticuli, polyps, and inflammatory bowel disease
d. Lower GI series (barium enema): to visualize position, contours, and size of the entire lower GI tract; to detect ulcers, tumors, strictures, obstructions, polyps, inflammatory bowel disease, and diverticuli; and to evaluate melena after inconclusive upper GI series
e. Cholangiogram: intravenous, percutaneous transhepatic, or T-tube–facilitated study of the biliary ducts
f. Arteriogram: radiologic dye study of any GI branch of the aorta, to evaluate bleeding
g. Splenoportogram: splenic pulp injection resulting in visualization of the portal and splenic veins to evaluate patency of the portal vein and direction of portal venous flow (prograde or retrograde)
h. Nonfluoroscopic abdominal imaging studies
    i. Ultrasonography of abdomen: to visualize the gallbladder, liver, pancreas, and spleen; to determine etiology of masses (cysts,

abscesses, tumors) and presence of foreign bodies (gallstones); and to determine blood flow and vessel patency

    ii. Computed tomography (CT) scan of the abdomen: to visualize gallbladder, liver, pancreas, spleen, extrahepatic bile ducts, and portal vein; and to determine presence of vascular problems, infection, tumors, and pancreatic pseudocyst

    iii. Magnetic resonance imaging (MRI): same applications as CT scan; can also detect blood flow and vessel patency

i. Other studies

    i. Esophagogastroduodenoscopy (EGD) or upper endoscopy: visualization and photography of the esophagus, stomach, and proximal duodenum by means of an endoscope

      (a) To detect obstruction, strictures, ulcers, or tumors

      (b) To evaluate melena, hematemesis, heme-positive nasogastric drainage, dysphagia, odynophagia, dyspepsia, nausea, vomiting, or unexplained abdominal pain

      (c) To perform biopsy, brush cytology studies, and cultures; to place stents; to remove foreign bodies; to place feeding tubes; or to control bleeding

    ii. Colonoscopy: visualization and photography of the colon from the rectum to the ileocecal valve by means of a colonoscope

      (a) To detect polyps, strictures, obstruction, tumors, or inflammatory disease

      (b) To evaluate lower GI bleeding, unexplained chronic abdominal pain, unexplained iron-deficiency anemia

      (c) To perform biopsy, brush cytology studies, polypectomy, and cultures; to remove foreign bodies; and to control bleeding

    iii. Proctosigmoidoscopy (rigid): visualization and photography of the rectum and distal sigmoid colon by means of a rigid proctoscope, to evaluate lower GI bleeding

    iv. Flexible sigmoidoscopy: visualization and photography of the rectum, sigmoid colon, and descending colon up to 65 cm by means of a flexible sigmoidoscope or colonoscope

      (a) To detect inflammatory disease, tumors, obstruction, strictures, and polyps

      (b) To evaluate unexplained chronic diarrhea or pain, lower GI bleeding

      (c) To perform biopsy, brush cytology studies, polypectomy, and cultures; to remove foreign bodies; and to control bleeding

    v. Endoscopic retrograde cholangiopancreatogram (ERCP): visualization and photography of the biliary and/or pancreatic ducts by means of a flexible (fiber-optic) endoscope

      (a) To detect tumors, bile duct stones, pancreatitis, and obstruction

      (b) To evaluate jaundice, elevated liver enzyme levels, and chronic unexplained abdominal pain

      (c) To perform biopsy, brush cytology studies, and cultures; to place stents; or to remove stones

    vi. Biopsy: needle or forceps aspiration of tissue from the esophagus, stomach, duodenum, colon, rectum, or liver for histologic analysis

    vii. Abdominal paracentesis: withdrawal of peritoneal fluid for diagnostic purposes by means of a large-bore needle or syringe

viii. Peritoneoscopy (laparoscopy): examination of the structures and organs within the abdominal cavity by means of a laparoscope

ix. Gastric lavage: insertion of a gastric tube through the nose or mouth to examine secretions for occult blood or pH

x. Schilling's test: vitamin B_{12} absorption test to determine whether vitamin B_{12} absorption is defective and, if so, whether the etiology is intrinsic factor deficiency. Intravenous (IV) unlabeled and radioactive-labeled vitamin B_{12} and intrinsic factor are administered and measured through urinary excretion

COMMONLY ENCOUNTERED NURSING DIAGNOSES

Altered Nutrition

Less than body requirements; related to nausea, vomiting, inadequate dietary intake, altered absorption, increased metabolic needs, diarrhea, ileus, gastric distress

1. **Assessment for defining characteristics**
   a. *Less than ideal weight:* unintentional loss of more than 10% of body weight over 6 weeks
   b. *Starvation:* the process that produces malnutrition as a result of dietary intake that fails to meet the normal or increased metabolic demands of the body
      i. Metabolic responses to *early* starvation
         (a) Decreased metabolic rate
         (b) Decreased temperature
         (c) Decreased serum glucose
         (d) Increased serum levels of catecholamines, glucagon, and cortisol
         (e) Increased serum lactate
         (f) Increased urinary nitrogen excretion, diuresis
         (g) Muscle atrophy and weight loss as results of water and protein loss
      ii. Metabolic responses to *prolonged* starvation
         (a) Increase in metabolic rate, followed by a decrease
         (b) Increase in temperature, followed by a decrease
         (c) Increased or normal serum levels of catecholamines, glucagon, and cortisol
         (d) Increased serum level of lactate
         (e) Increase in urinary nitrogen excretion, followed by a decrease
         (f) Temporary decrease in muscle wasting and weight loss
         (g) Conservation of body fluids, shift of fluids to interstitial spaces (third spacing)
   c. *Malnutrition:* the state that occurs when dietary intake of essential nutrients and calories is insufficient to meet the metabolic demands of the body for a prolonged period of time
      i. Acute malnutrition (kwashiorkor, a maladaptive hypermetabolic state): no wasting, minimal weight loss, visceral protein depletion

(decreased serum albumin, pre-albumin, transferrin), decreased total lymphocyte count

  ii. Protein-energy malnutrition (chronic malnutrition or marasmus, an adaptive hypometabolic state): gradual wasting, cachexia, anorexia, visceral protein preservation (normal serum albumin, pre-albumin, transferrin), decreased total lymphocyte count, decreased BUN

  iii. Negative nitrogen balance: metabolic state in which nitrogen is being lost more rapidly than it can be supplied (protein depletion)

    (a) Body weight at least 10% below ideal weight

    (b) Unintentional weight loss of more than 10% in preceding 6 months

    (c) Cachexia: decreased muscle mass, loss of subcutaneous fat

    (d) Weakness, fatigue

    (e) Apathy, lethargy

    (f) Peripheral edema, ascites

    (g) Oral cavity changes: sore inflamed buccal cavity; redness and swelling of mouth or lips, especially at corners (cheilosis); hyperemic tongue with hypertrophic or atrophic papillae; poor dentition (missing teeth, caries); spongy and receding gums, bleeding gums; halitosis

    (h) Anemia

    (i) Poor wound healing

    (j) Infection, sepsis

    (k) Respiratory failure

    (l) Fatty liver

  iv. Related factors

    (a) Disrupted digestion: patient cannot or will not eat (see Assessment of Nutritional Status section, discussion of factors that interfere with adequate nutrition)

    (b) Increased metabolic needs: patient cannot or will not eat enough

      (1) Increased nutrient losses (e.g., caused by GI fistulas or large wounds)

      (2) Disease or surgery of the GI tract

      (3) Catabolic medications or therapies

      (4) Multisystem organ failure

2. Expected outcomes

a. Meeting of minimum nutrient and caloric needs of the body

b. Prevention of starvation and malnutrition: minimizing of negative nitrogen balance

c. Enhancement of immune response

d. Maintenance of electrolyte and acid-base equilibrium

3. Nursing interventions

a. Record weight

b. Measure intake and output

c. Assess bowel sounds

d. Perform oral hygiene as indicated

e. Assess for increased energy requirements

  i. Surgery

  ii. Trauma, burns

  iii. Infection

       iv. Any other cause of increased metabolic needs

f. In collaboration with nutritional support and/or dietetic services, assess need for nutritional support

     i. Decreased nutritional intake (predisposing or iatrogenic)

     ii. Markedly increased tissue destruction

     iii. Malabsorption

     iv. Decreased use and storage of nutrients

     v. Increased excretion of nutrients

     vi. Markedly increased nutritional requirements

     vii. Dysphagia related to mechanical obstruction (tumor) or neurologic disorder (cerebrovascular accident [CVA])

        (a) Patients are asymptomatic until tumor becomes surgically unresectable

        (b) Symptoms: dysphagia, pain, hoarseness, regurgitation, eructation, hiccups, malaise, weight loss, dehydration, halitosis

     viii. Risk of aspiration

     ix. Comprehensive nutritional assessment

        (a) Visceral protein measurements: serum albumin, pre-albumin, transferrin, retinol-binding protein

        (b) Tests of immunocompetence: total lymphocyte count, cell-mediated immunity (delayed hypersensitivity skin test)

        (c) Nitrogen balance study: 24-hour urine collection to monitor nitrogen losses

        (d) Determination of caloric needs

        (e) Determination of protein needs

g. Administer enteral and/or parenteral nutritional support as ordered

     i. Type of support is influenced by medical diagnosis, treatment, and condition of patient

     ii. Enteral nutritional alimentation: administration of nutritional substances via the GI tract in quantities sufficient to provide caloric needs and positive nitrogen balance in patients with extensive needs for extended periods of time

        (a) The preferred method of feeding: more physiologic, less expensive, entailing fewer complications

        (b) A functional GI tract is required

        (c) Temporary (nasoenteral) feeding tubes: nasogastic, nasoduodenal, nasojejunal

        (d) Long-term feeding tubes

            (1) Gastrostomy: indicated when enteral feeding is expected to continue for more than 3 months

            (2) Jejunal: indicated in patients with upper GI tract obstruction or in those at increased risk of aspiration

                a) Jejunostomy feeding tubes: placed fluoroscopically, endoscopically, or surgically

                b) Needle catheter jejunostomy tube (used for a period of less than 6 weeks): placed at time of GI surgery

        (e) Polymeric formulas: require functional digestive system

            (1) Contain complex carbohydrates, fats, proteins, vitamins, minerals, trace elements, water

            (2) Available in specific caloric densities (1.0, 1.5, and 2.0 kcal/ml)

(3) Numerous specialized products that differ in the amount and type of carbohydrates, proteins, fats, and electrolyte content are available

(f) Predigested or elemental formulas: indicated when feeding is delivered into the intestine at a point (distal jejunum) distal to presence of digestive enzymes; increased osmolality associated with diarrhea

(1) Short bowel syndrome after massive intestinal resection

(2) Diseased mucosa (e.g., Crohn's disease)

(3) Intestinal mucosal atrophy resulting from prolonged NPO status

(4) Exocrine insufficiency (e.g., pancreatitis)

iii. Parenteral nutritional alimentation: intravenous administration of a hypertonic mixture of glucose, amino acids, vitamins, and trace elements sufficient to provide caloric needs and positive nitrogen balance in patients with extensive needs for extended periods of time; may also include fat emulsions

(a) Indicated when the GI tract is nonfunctional, inaccessible, or incapable of adequately digesting and absorbing nutrients

(b) Peripheral alimentation: solutions contain a final dextrose concentration of up to 10% and approximately 45-g equivalents of amino acids; used to maintain *nonstressed* patients who cannot tolerate oral intake for 5 to 7 days

(1) Not usually adequate to meet the critically ill patient's needs

(2) May be used as an adjunct to enteral nutritional support

(c) Central venous alimentation: solutions contain a final dextrose concentration of up to 35% and approximately 8.5-g equivalents of amino acids; used to maintain *stressed* patients who need greater caloric support to maintain positive nitrogen balance and increased use of proteins for tissue growth

(1) Easily modified to meet changing caloric, protein, and metabolic needs

(2) Large amount of calories can be delivered in small volumes

iv. Fat emulsions (intralipid solutions): administered to provide essential fatty acids and prevent essential fatty acid deficiency

(a) Should provide one third of caloric needs

(b) Decrease carbohydrate load to liver to prevent fatty liver

(c) Decreases CO_2 production

h. Maintain patency of enteral feeding tube if used

i. Leaking at exit site

ii. Tube migration

iii. Tube obstruction

i. Monitor patient's physiologic response and tolerance to the enteral feeding regimen

i. Electrolyte imbalances

ii. Dehydration

iii. Hyperglycemia, hypoglycemia

iv. Infection

v. Delayed gastric emptying

      vi. Vomiting

      vii. Aspiration

      viii. Diarrhea, constipation

    j. Care for skin at exit sites of feeding tubes

    k. Maintain integrity of central venous access for parenteral nutrition if used; check for

      i. Occlusion of catheter

      ii. Catheter perforation of vessel

    l. Assess for complications related to insertion of catheter

      i. Pneumothorax, hydrothorax, hemothorax

      ii. Hemomediastinum, hydromediastinum

      iii. Air, catheter embolus

      iv. Arterial puncture

      v. Brachial plexus injury

      vi. Sepsis

    m. Assess for tolerance and complications of parenteral nutritional alimentation

      i. Mucosal atrophy and decreased motility may facilitate proximal migration of bacteria into sterile areas (bacterial translocation)

      ii. Catheter-related infection, sepsis

      iii. Prerenal azotemia

      iv. Hepatic dysfunction, encephalopathy

      v. Hyperglycemia, hypoglycemia

      vi. Hyperkalemia, hypokalemia

      vii. Hypomagnesemia, hypophosphatemia

      viii. Acid-base disturbances

      ix. Fatty acid, trace element, or vitamin deficiency

      x. Complications related to fat emulsion

        (a) Idiosyncratic reaction characterized by fever, respiratory distress, and cardiac arrest (rare)

        (b) Hyperlipidemia

4. Evaluation of nursing care: maintenance of bodily nutrient stores

    a. Preservation of lean body mass

      i. Body weight at least 80% of ideal weight for height and frame size

      ii. Serum albumin level greater than 3.5 mg/dl

      iii. Serum transferrin level greater than 200 mg/dl

    b. Positive nitrogen balance: metabolic state in which the supply of nitrogen to the body exceeds the loss of nitrogen from the body

    c. Maintenance of oral health

Altered Oral Mucous Membrane

Related to malnutrition, dehydration, presence of endotracheal and/or nasogastric tube, bleeding, opportunistic infection, trauma, surgery

1. Assessment for defining characteristics

    a. Mild stomatitis or mucositis

      i. Pale, dry oral mucosa

      ii. Red, engorged uvula

      iii. Dry tongue with raised papillae

      iv. Dry lips

   v. Increased salivation

  b. Moderate stomatitis or mucositis, xerostomia

    i. Red, dry, and wrinkled oral mucosa

    ii. Swollen tongue with inflamed papillae and white coating

    iii. Inflamed mucocutaneous junctions

    iv. Decreased salivation

    v. Blisters on oral mucosa

    vi. Alteration in taste

  c. Severe stomatitis or mucositis, xerostomia

    i. Intense inflammation of the oral mucosa and tongue

    ii. Dry, cracked, swollen lips

    iii. Thick saliva

    iv. Painful, bleeding ulcers

    v. Infection (e.g., *Streptococcus, Candida albicans*)

    vi. Alteration in taste

  d. Discomfort during swallowing (dysphagia)

  e. Gingivitis, dental caries, halitosis

  f. Related factors

    i. Ineffective (in frequency and adequacy) oral hygiene

    ii. Inadequate nutrient intake

    iii. Nondetergent diet (i.e., diet limited to liquids, soft foods)

    iv. Inadequate hydration: NPO for more than 24 hours

    v. Coagulopathy

    vi. Altered immune mechanisms

    vii. Concurrent antibiotic therapy: loss of normal flora, resulting in bacterial and/or fungal overgrowth

    viii. Drugs that decrease salivation: reserpine, chlorpromazine, cholinergic blocking agents, belladonna, antihistamines

    ix. Corticosteroids, chemotherapy

    x. Presence of endotracheal tube, nasogastric tube, and/or other large-bore GI tubes (e.g., Sengstaken-Blakemore tube, Minnesota tube)

    xi. Oxygen therapy

    xii. Tachypnea or mouth breathing

    xiii. Certain disease states: cancer, diabetes, renal insufficiency or failure, cirrhosis

    xiv. Radiation therapy to head and neck

2. Expected outcomes

  a. Lips and oral mucosa are smooth, pink, moist, and intact

  b. Teeth and oral cavity are clean and moist

  c. Patient reports oral comfort when swallowing and talking

3. Nursing interventions

  a. Thoroughly assess the oral cavity (Table 7–1) and establish an individualized oral care and hygiene regimen

  b. Assess potential for trauma from endotracheal, nasogastric, and/or other GI tube

  c. Use interventions to promote comfort, prevent or minimize infection and bleeding, maintain optimal nutritional status

    i. Brush teeth before meals if possible to stimulate appetite and within 30 minutes after meals

    ii. Remove and brush dentures within 30 minutes after meals, then soak in 1.5% hydrogen peroxide solution for at least 30 minutes

TABLE 7–1. A Guide to Physical Assessment of the Oral Cavity

Category	Rating 1	2	3	4
Lips	Smooth, soft, pink, moist, and intact	Slightly dry, wrinkled, reddened areas	Dry, rough, swollen, inflammatory line of demarcation	Very dry, inflamed, cracked, blistered, ulcerated and bleeding (see Fig. 8–27A, B)
Tongue	Smooth, firm, pink, moist, and intact	Papilli prominent, particularly at base; dry; pink with reddened areas	Raised, red papilli all over tongue, giving peppered appearance (very dry and swollen), coating at base	Very dry, thick, grooved, and coated; tip very red and demarcated, sides blistered (see Fig. 8–28A, B)
Oral mucosa	Smooth, pink, moist, and intact	Pale, slightly dry, reddened areas or white pustules	Red, dry, inflamed, edematous, ulcerated	Very red, shiny, edematous with blisters and/or ulcerations
Teeth; dentures	Shiny, no debris; well fitting	Slightly dull with slight debris; slightly loose	Dull with debris on half of visible enamel; loose with areas of irritation	Very dull, covered with debris; unable to wear dentures because of irritation
Saliva	Thin, watery, sufficient quantity	Increase in amount	Saliva scanty, mouth dry	Saliva thick, ropy, viscid or mucid

Oral Dysfunction Score

Range: 5–20   Mild dysfunction: 6–10   Moderate dysfunction: 11–15   Severe dysfunction: 16–20

Adapted from Beck, S.: Oral Exam Guide in "Impact of Teaching a Systematic Protocol for Oral Care on Stomatitis." Cancer Nursing 2:192, 1979.

       iii. Floss teeth daily if possible

       iv. Clean tongue and oral mucosa

       v. Apply water-soluble lubricant frequently to lips and mucosa

4. Evaluation of nursing care

  a. A functional oral cavity

  b. Symptomatic relief of dryness and discomfort

. . . .

Risk for Fluid Volume Deficit

Related to GI fluid loss, third spacing, hemorrhage, sepsis

1. Assessment for defining characteristics (in addition to general defining characteristics of hypovolemia)

  a. Related to hypovolemia caused by sepsis or third-space fluid shifts

     i. Anxiety, altered mental status

     ii. Thirst

     iii. Poor skin turgor

     iv. Tachypnea, dyspnea

     v. Cyanosis, hypoxemia

     vi. Tachycardia

     vii. Decreased pulse pressure, cardiac output/index

     viii. Decreased filling pressures (central venous pressure [CVP], pulmonary capillary wedge pressure [PCWP])

     ix. Orthostatic hypotension (early sign)

     x. Hypotension (late sign)

     xi. Oliguria, anuria

     xii. Elevated urine specific gravity

     xiii. Elevated BUN, creatinine level

     xiv. Hyperosmolarity, hypernatremia

  b. Related to GI blood loss

     i. Hematemesis (emesis of blood that is bright red or resembles coffee grounds)

     ii. Melena (dark blood loss from rectum), hematochezia (bright red blood loss from rectum)

     iii. Bloody drainage

     iv. Cyanosis

     v. Decreased hemoglobin, hematocrit, platelet count

     vi. Prolonged PT

     vii. Decreased fibrinogen

     viii. Elevated BUN

  c. Related to massive blood replacement

     i. Hypothermia

     ii. Hyperkalemia, hypocalcemia

     iii. Metabolic acidosis

     iv. Coagulopathy

  d. Related to sepsis

     i. Increased cardiac output and cardiac index (CI); decreased systemic vascular resistance (SVR)

     ii. Fever

     iii. Signs and symptoms of hypovolemia listed earlier

     iv. Hyperglycemia (early sign)

      v. Metabolic acidosis: increased serum lactate

      vi. Ileus

    e. Related factors

      i. GI bleeding

      ii. Ascites

      iii. Septicemia

      iv. Peritonitis

      v. Pancreatitis

      vi. Malnutrition with hypoalbuminemia

      vii. Excessive GI fluid losses: vomiting, diarrhea, gastric secretions

2. Expected outcome: adequate circulating plasma volume, as evidenced by vital signs, serum electrolytes and lactate level, urine output, filling pressures of heart, and oxygen delivery within normal ranges

3. Nursing interventions

    a. Assess cardiovascular and hemodynamic status

    b. Monitor intake and output for excessive GI losses

    c. Monitor serum electrolytes, lactate level

    d. Assess skin turgor and mucous membranes

    e. Maintain adequate circulating plasma volume

      i. Replace fluid volume losses as ordered

      ii. Maintain hemoglobin greater than 10 g

      iii. Maintain adequate coagulation

        (a) PT less than 16 seconds

        (b) Partial thromboplastin time (PTT) less than 40 seconds

        (c) Platelet count greater than $75,000/cm^3$

        (d) Fibrinogen level greater than 125 mg/dl

      iv. Control bleeding as appropriate and to the extent possible

      v. Administer medications (e.g., inotropes, vasopressors) to support vital signs

      vi. Institute measures to control bleeding as ordered

4. Evaluation of nursing care

    a. Vital signs and hemodynamic parameters within normal ranges

    b. Serum electrolytes and lactate level within normal range

    c. Hemostasis, normal coagulation profile

    d. Fluid intake and losses in balance

Pain (Acute)

Related to infectious conditions, cancer, surgery, trauma, and disruption of mucosal barrier of GI tract; see Chapter 9, Psychosocial Aspects; Commonly Encountered Nursing Diagnoses section, pain subsection.

PATIENT HEALTH PROBLEMS

Acute Pancreatitis

1. Pathophysiology

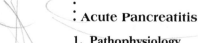

a. Classification of pancreatitis
    i. Acute pancreatitis: pancreatic function returns to normal after resolution of a single episode
    ii. Recurrent acute pancreatitis: more than one episode with pancreatic function returning to normal between episodes; no permanent pancreatic damage
    iii. Recurrent chronic pancreatitis: progressive destruction of the acinar cells as a result of persistent inflammation; patient may experience some pain-free periods
    iv. Chronic pancreatitis: progressive destruction and fibrosis of the acinar cells; patient usually experiences persistent pain
b. Diffuse inflammation, destruction, and autodigestion of the pancreas, all resulting from premature activation of exocrine enzymes (dyschylia) within and around the pancreas
    i. Normal flow of pancreatic enzymes is blocked, causing stagnation and premature activation, resulting in dyschylia (digestion of tissue and fat in and around the pancreas)
       (a) Obstruction of pancreatic duct
       (b) Disruption of pancreatic duct
       (c) Destruction of pancreatic duct
    ii. Pancreatic enzyme inhibitors are inactivated
    iii. Pancreatic and peripancreatic edema with loss of up to 6 L of fluid into interstitial spaces. Mild, interstitial form of pancreatitis can be fatal in elderly patients for this reason
    iv. Release and activation of inflammatory mediators (cytokines), including complement, kinins, histamine, prostaglandin, clotting factors, results in systemic inflammatory response syndrome (SIRS): results in increased vascular permeability, vasodilation, vascular stasis, microthrombosis
c. Forms of acute pancreatitis
    i. Mild, edematous form (interstitial pancreatitis): accounts for 95% of cases; mortality rate, 5%
       (a) Edematous pancreas with minimal or no necrotic damage
       (b) Hypovolemia can occur as a result of massive third spacing of fluids
    ii. Severe, hemorrhagic form (necrotizing pancreatitis): accounts for 5% of cases; mortality rate, 50%
       (a) Extensive peripancreatic tissue necrosis of fat in omentum and retroperitoneum
       (b) Hemorrhage caused by tissue necrosis or erosion of pseudocyst into vascular structure
       (c) SIRS and sepsis
       (d) Multiple organ dysfunction syndrome (MODS) (see Chapter 8, Multisystem; Patient Health Problems section)
          (1) Adult respiratory distress syndrome (ARDS), respiratory failure
          (2) Acute renal tubular necrosis, acute renal failure
          (3) Disseminated intravascular coagulation (DIC)
          (4) Cardiogenic shock: release of myocardial depressant factor
          (5) Hypovolemic shock
          (6) Acute liver failure

2. Etiologic or precipitating factors
  a. Obstruction of pancreatic ducts
    i. Gallstones (biliary, pancreatic)
    ii. Tumor
    iii. Inflammation, infection
    iv. Edema
  b. Alcoholism
  c. Complication of abdominal surgery or diagnostic procedure (e.g., ERCP)
  d. Abdominal trauma: blunt or penetrating
  e. Drug toxicity: cyclosporine, corticosteroids, azathioprine, thiazides, sulfonamides, tetracycline, estrogens
  f. Familial hyperlipidemia
  g. Chronic hyperparathyroidism, hypercalcemia
  h. Infection: *Mycoplasma, streptococcus, salmonella,* paramyxovirus (mumps), cytomegalovirus, Echovirus, Epstein-Barr virus, coxsackievirus, viral hepatitis
  i. Shock

3. Nursing assessment data base
  a. Nursing history
    i. Subjective findings: from mild, almost asymptomatic case to fulminant condition of massive pancreatic necrosis
      (a) Abdominal pain universally manifested
        (1) Epigastric pain that is knife-like and twisting in nature; begins suddenly and reaches apex quickly
        (2) Pain may radiate to all abdominal quadrants and lumbar area
        (3) Differential diagnosis: rule out perforated viscus, leaking abdominal aortic aneurysm, acute mesenteric ischemia
      (b) Visceral pain
        (1) Initial pain caused by capsular distention and release of kinins
        (2) Diffuse, not well localized
        (3) Patient doubled over, with facial expression of pain
      (c) Somatic pain: extrapancreatic involvement (peritoneal, retroperitoneal)
        (1) Sharp, well localized
        (2) Accompanied by nausea, vomiting, rigid abdomen, rebound tenderness
        (3) Standard doses of analgesics may be ineffective for pain relief
    ii. Past medical history
      (a) History of alcoholism
      (b) History of biliary or pancreatic stones
      (c) Family history of pancreatitis
      (d) Family history of hyperlipidemia
      (e) History of bacterial infection such as mumps or scarlet fever
      (f) Drug use: cyclosporine, corticosteroids, azathioprine, thiazides, sulfonamides, tetracycline, estrogens
    iii. Objective findings
      (a) Low-grade fever
      (b) Diaphoresis

(c) Anorexia

(d) Diarrhea

(e) Dehydration

b. Nursing examination of patient

i. Inspection

(a) Patient is doubled over in pain with facial expression of pain

(b) Patient is restless, agitated, apprehensive

(c) Abdomen is distended

(d) Jaundice

(e) Urine is dark, foamy

(f) Steatorrhea: bulky, pale, foul-smelling stools

(g) Extravasation of hemorrhage into tissues in severe, hemorrhagic pancreatitis

(1) Halstead's sign: marbled appearance of abdomen

(2) Cullen's sign: bluish discoloration of the periumbilical area

(3) Turner's sign: bluish discoloration of flanks

(h) Peritoneal lavage reveals blood in peritoneal cavity ("beef broth" tap)

ii. Auscultation: ileus; hypoactive or absent bowel sounds

iii. Percussion: dull percussion tones over the pancreas

iv. Palpation

(a) Abdominal distention, guarding, rigidity

(b) Rebound tenderness

(c) Localized mass (e.g., pancreatic pseudocyst)

c. Diagnostic studies

i. Laboratory findings

(a) Elevated serum amylase level that peaks between 4 and 24 hours after onset and returns to normal within 4 days: degree of elevation does not necessarily correlate with severity of illness. Not a sensitive test unless done early after onset of signs and symptoms

(b) Elevated serum lipase level: stays elevated longer than does serum amylase level

(c) Elevated urine amylase and lipase levels: in patients with good renal function, these are better indexes of pancreatic damage than are serum levels

(d) Decreased serum ionized calcium level (less than 2.0 mg/dl): calcium binds to areas of fat necrosis

(e) Intermittent elevated serum glucose level: indicates beta-cell involvement

(f) Elevated WBC

(g) Others, less diagnostic

(1) Elevated serum bilirubin level

(2) Elevated serum AST, ALT, LDH, alkaline phosphatase

(3) Elevated or decreased hematocrit

(4) Elevated triglyceride level

ii. Radiologic findings: on abdominal plain film; presence of dilated duodenum (sentinel loop) or transverse colon

iii. Other diagnostic findings

(a) Ultrasonography: evidence of diffuse pancreatic enlargement, pseudocyst, or abscess

(b) CT scan: evidence of pancreatic inflammation, pseudocyst, abscess, obstruction of pancreatic duct, peripancreatic and retroperitoneal necrosis

(c) ERCP: evidence of biliary or pancreatic stones. Early ERCP with sphincterotomy and stone extraction may ameliorate the course of biliary pancreatitis

4. **Nursing diagnoses** (see Commonly Encountered Nursing Diagnoses section)
   a. Pain (see Chapter 9, Commonly Encountered Nursing Diagnoses section, pain subsection)
       i. Assessment for additional defining characteristics (see subjective findings from nursing history)
       ii. Expected outcome: patient verbalizes some pain relief
       iii. Additional nursing interventions
           (a) Administer narcotic analgesic as ordered
               (1) The narcotic analgesic of choice is meperidine (Demerol)
               (2) Large doses of narcotic analgesics may be necessary to comfort patient
           (b) Analgesics may be ineffective, so individualized comfort measures are indicated; administer histamine receptor blocker as ordered to increase gastric pH, decrease secretion of enzymes, and decrease pain
       iv. Evaluation of nursing care: patient mentions being comfortable
   b. Risk for fluid volume deficit, related to third-space fluid loss and/or hemorrhage
   c. Gas exchange impaired, related to pulmonary capillary endothelial damage from phospholipase A, resulting in acute respiratory distress syndrome (see Chapter 1, The Pulmonary System; Patient Health Problems section, Adult Respiratory Distress Syndrome subsection)
   d. Nutrition altered, less than body requirements, related to major tissue destruction, hypermetabolic state
   e. Infection, related to peritonitis, abdominal abscess (see Chapter 6, Hematologic and Immunologic Systems; Commonly Encountered Nursing Diagnoses section, infection subsection)

GI Bleeding

1. **Peptic ulcer disease**
   a. Pathophysiology
       i. Ulcerations that occur in the portion of the GI tract exposed to acid-pepsin secretion
       ii. Reflects either an imbalance between acid and pepsin production or loss of protection of the affected mucosa from digestive enzymes
       iii. *Helicobacter pylori*, a bacterium, probably contributes to the development of peptic ulcers; high incidence of colonization with *H. pylori* found in people with peptic ulcers
       iv. Pharmacologic agents may play a role
           (a) Caffeine, alcohol
           (b) Salicylates, indomethacin, phenylbutazone, NSAIDs
           (c) Corticosteroids, antineoplastic agents

b. Etiologic or precipitating factors
   i. Three to four times more common among men
   ii. Gastric ulcers associated with decreased tissue resistance
     (a) Affects older adults
     (b) Associated with malignancy; leads to nonhealing ulcer in stomach
   iii. Duodenal ulcers associated with increased hydrochloric acid level
     (a) Constitute 80% of peptic ulcers
     (b) Most frequent sites are the pylorus and first portion of duodenum (bulb)
     (c) Can occur at any age, are common among young adults
     (d) Common among persons with type A blood
   iv. Cigarette smoking
   v. Familial tendency
c. Nursing assessment data base
   i. Nursing history
     (a) Subjective findings
       (1) Age, gender
       (2) Epigastric pain with bleeding
         a) Heartburn
         b) In patients with duodenal ulcers, pain is relieved by food
         c) Pain stops when bleeding begins
       (3) Nausea, vomiting
     (b) Objective findings: depend on volume of blood loss, rate of bleeding, associated disease, and cardiovascular status
       (1) Bleeding
         a) Hematemesis (blood is bright red or resembles coffee grounds)
         b) Melena
       (2) History of smoking
       (3) History of use of pharmacologic agents listed earlier
       (4) Family history of peptic ulcer disease
       (5) Fever
   ii. Nursing examination of patient
     (a) Inspection
       (1) Weight loss
       (2) Bleeding
       (3) Skin pallor
     (b) Palpation: abdominal tenderness, guarding
     (c) Auscultation
       (1) Hyperactive bowel sounds
       (2) Orthostatic hypotension
       (3) Narrow pulse pressure
   iii. Diagnostic study findings
     (a) Laboratory findings
       (1) Decreased hemoglobin, hematocrit; true extent of blood loss may not be immediately apparent
       (2) Guaiac testing of nasogastric drainage and stool for occult blood
       (3) Colonization by *H. pylori*

(b) Radiologic findings
  (1) Free air under diaphragm with perforated, bleeding ulcers on upright chest x-ray or upright and lateral abdominal x-rays
  (2) Upper GI series to localize ulcer
  (3) Selective mesenteric angiography to localize site of bleeding when endoscopy cannot be performed
(c) Other diagnostic findings
  (1) Nasogastric intubation to obtain gastric aspirate
  (2) Upper GI endoscopy reveals location of ulcer, rules out other causes of bleeding
  (3) Biopsy to rule out carcinoma
  (4) Electrocardiogram (ECG) in elderly patients and those with history of heart disease and anemia
d. Nursing diagnoses
  i. Risk for fluid volume deficit, related to hemorrhage (see Commonly Encountered Nursing Diagnoses section)
  ii. Pain (acute), related to disruption of mucosal barrier of GI tract (see Chapter 9, Commonly Encountered Nursing Diagnoses section, pain subsection)

2. **Variceal bleeding:** 50% of deaths in patients with cirrhosis are caused by variceal bleeding
  a. Pathophysiology
    i. Portal hypertension: increased hydrostatic pressure (greater than 10 mm Hg) within the portal venous system, caused by disruption of normal liver lobular structure, which impedes blood flow (25% of cardiac output per minute) into, through, or out of the liver. Bleeding occurs when the portosystemic gradient is greater than 12 mm Hg
    ii. Formation of collateral portacaval vessels (between the portal venous system and the venae cavae) or varices in the esophagus, duodenum, stomach, peritoneum, retroperitoneum, rectum (Fig. 7–7); purpose is to maintain venous return to the right side of the heart
      (a) Dilated, convoluted veins under increased pressure; vulnerable to spontaneous rupture
      (b) As portal pressure increases, backward venous congestion occurs; this involves the splenic vein and the spleen as a major target organ (splenomegaly) of portal hypertension
    iii. Disease states associated with varices
      (a) Portal vein thrombosis
      (b) Splenic vein thrombosis
      (c) Cirrhosis: multiple causes
      (d) Budd-Chiari syndrome
  b. Etiologic or precipitating factors
    i. Etiologies of portal hypertension
      (a) Prehepatic (presinusoidal) factors: portal vein thrombosis (e.g., umbilical vein catheterization in infancy or hypercoagulable state)
      (b) Intrahepatic (sinusoidal) factors: postnecrotic cirrhosis (e.g., chronic active hepatitis and cirrhosis)

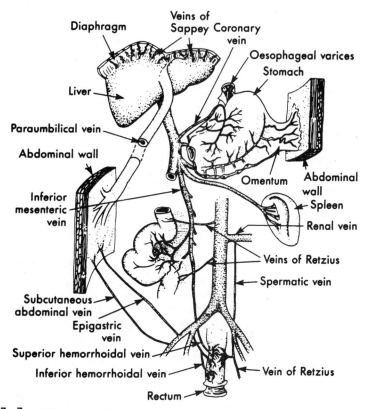

Figure 7-7 • Collateral circulation in the liver. (From Krumberger, J. M.: Gastrointestinal disorders. *In* Kinney, M. R., Packa, D. R., and Dunbar, S. B. [eds.]: AACN's Clinical Reference for Critical-Care Nursing. St. Louis, Mosby–Year Book, 1993, p. 1149.)

      (c) Posthepatic (postsinusoidal) factors: hepatic vein thrombosis (e.g., Budd-Chiari syndrome), veno-occlusive disease after bone marrow transplantation

    ii. Rupture of varices is most often spontaneous

  c. Nursing assessment data base

    i. Nursing history

      (a) Subjective findings: variceal bleeding

        (1) Sudden onset of vomiting: coffee-ground vomitus or bright red blood

        (2) Fatigue

        (3) Anxiety, fear

      (b) Objective findings

        (1) History of liver disease

        (2) Possible history of prior variceal bleeding

        (3) Coagulopathy

          a) Prolonged PT

          b) Decreased platelets

        (4) Hyperdynamic circulation: increased cardiac output, decreased SVR, systolic ejection murmur

        (5) Decreased pulse pressure

        (6) Orthostatic hypotension

        (7) Lethargy, malaise

        (8) Mental status may be altered as a result of encephalopathy

(9) Malnutrition, vitamin deficiencies
ii. Nursing examination of patient
    (a) Inspection
        (1) Visible stigmata of liver disease
            a) Jaundice may be present, but not seen in advanced stage of cirrhosis except in cholestatic liver disease (e.g., primary biliary cirrhosis, primary sclerosing cholangitis)
            b) Ascites
            c) Cachexia
            d) Hematomas, ecchymoses
            e) Spider angiomas
            f) Clubbing of fingers, palmar erythema may be present
            g) Testicular atrophy, gynecomastia in males
            h) Striae
        (2) Pale skin and/or mucous membranes
        (3) Obvious bleeding
    (b) Palpation
        (1) Spleen or liver may be palpably enlarged
        (2) Fluid wave may be palpable, indicating ascites
    (c) Percussion: no notable findings
    (d) Auscultation
        (1) Hyperdynamic circulation: increased heart rate, systolic ejection murmur
        (2) Breath sounds may be decreased as a result of pleural effusions
iii. Diagnostic study findings: the differential diagnosis for variceal bleeding is complex and includes peptic ulcer disease, gastritis, Mallory-Weiss tear of esophagus, Boerhaave's syndrome
    (a) Laboratory findings
        (1) ALT, AST: may be elevated
        (2) Alkaline phosphatase: may be elevated
        (3) GGT: may be elevated
        (4) Bilirubin: may be elevated
        (5) PT: prolonged
        (6) Platelet count: may be decreased
        (7) Hemoglobin, hematocrit: decreased
    (b) Radiologic findings: no specific notable findings
        (1) Doppler ultrasonography: to evaluate patency and flow in portal vein and hepatic veins
        (2) Superior mesenteric artery (SMA) arteriogram: to measure hepatic vein pressure gradient and to image the portal and hepatic venous systems
        (3) CT scan: to document cirrhosis and rule out hepatoma
    (c) Other diagnostic findings: upper GI endoscopy to grade and classify esophageal, gastric, and/or duodenal varices according to size, location, and risk factors
d. Nursing diagnoses (see Commonly Encountered Nursing Diagnoses section)
    i. Risk for fluid volume deficit, related to third-space fluid loss and/or hemorrhage

(a) Assessment for additional defining characteristics: hematemesis

(b) Expected outcome: hemostasis

(c) Additional nursing interventions

 (1) Assess vital signs, hemodynamic status

 (2) Administer fluids and blood products as ordered

  a) Fresh frozen plasma

  b) Clotting factors

  c) Packed red blood cells

  d) Platelets

 (3) Protect airway from aspiration: early endotracheal intubation if bleeding is massive or if patient is hemodynamically unstable or combative

 (4) Prepare patient and assist with endoscopy, injection sclerotherapy, or band ligation of varices

 (5) Prepare patient for transjugular intrahepatic portasystemic shunt (TIPS)

  a) Indicated for acute bleeding not controlled by sclerotherapy or band ligation or for intractable ascites in patients awaiting liver transplantation

  b) Rebleeding rate: 20% during first year

 (6) Administer vasopressin (Pitressin) as ordered

 (7) Administer balloon tamponade to varices via Sengstaken-Blakemore or Minnesota tube

 (8) Prepare patient for surgical shunt procedure (e.g., distal splenorenal shunt) if indicated. Bleeding is controlled in 90% of cases

 (9) Prepare patient for liver transplantation evaluation if indicated

 (10) Prepare patient for surgical devascularization of varices when bleeding is uncontrolled and patient is not a candidate for surgical shunt or liver transplantation

 (11) Frequent oral hygiene

(d) Evaluation of nursing care

 (1) Circulating plasma volume is adequate

 (2) Blood pressure for perfusion pressures is adequate

 (3) Airway is patent; patient does not aspirate blood into lungs

ii. Altered protection (risk for infection), related to altered reticuloendothelial system in liver, malnutrition, ascites (see Chapter 6, Commonly Encountered Nursing Diagnoses section, infection subsection)

3. Carcinoma of the GI tract

a. Gastric neoplasms

i. Pathophysiology

 (a) Benign neoplasms: most common is primary carcinoma beginning in mucosal glands

 (b) Malignant neoplasms

 (c) Begin as atrophic gastritis and progresses to gastric carcinoma, most often in distal stomach at lesser curvature

ii. Etiologic or precipitating factors

 (a) Incidence greater in countries farthest from equator

 (b) Incidence greater in persons of lower socioeconomic status

(c) Incidence greatest in men aged 50 to 70 years

   iii. Nursing assessment data base

      (a) Nursing history

         (1) Subjective findings

            a) Vague epigastric discomfort

            b) Indigestion, belching

            c) Vomiting

            d) Early satiety

            e) Postprandial fullness

            f) Weakness

            g) Weight loss

            h) Type A blood

            i) Prior distal gastrectomy for peptic ulcer disease

         (2) Objective findings

            a) Atrophic gastritis

            b) Blood in stool

            c) Frank bleeding

            d) Pernicious anemia

            e) Hypochlorhydria, achlorhydria

      (b) Nursing examination of patient: no specific findings

      (c) Diagnostic study findings

         (1) Laboratory

            a) Decreased hemoglobin

            b) Positive stool guaiac test

         (2) Radiologic: upper GI radiologic studies reveal "linitis plastica" (leather bottle stomach)

         (3) Other diagnostic tests

            a) Upper GI endoscopy for biopsy and cytology

            b) Histopathologic classification of tumor

            c) Tumor staging

      (d) Nursing diagnoses

         (1) Anemia (see Chapter 6, Commonly Encountered Nursing Diagnoses section, anemia subsection)

         (2) Pain (see Chapter 9, Commonly Encountered Nursing Diagnoses section, pain subsection)

b. Neoplasms of the esophagus

   i. Pathophysiology: most common type is squamous cell carcinoma

   ii. Etiologic or precipitating factors

      (a) Predominates in black males, age 70 to 80

      (b) Achalasia

      (c) Caustic esophageal injury

      (d) Barrett's mucosa

   iii. Nursing assessment data base

      (a) Nursing history

         (1) Subjective findings

            a) Dysphagia: initially with bulky foods, then with soft foods, and eventually with liquids

            b) Vomiting

            c) Reflux

            d) Pain on swallowing

        (2) Objective findings
           a) Weight loss
           b) Aspiration pneumonitis
     (b) Nursing examination of patient: no specific findings
     (c) Diagnostic study findings
        (1) Radiologic: x-ray reveals irregular, ragged mucosal pattern with luminal narrowing
        (2) Other diagnostic tests
           a) Esophagoscopy for visualization, biopsy, and cytology study
           b) Histopathologic classification of tumor
           c) Tumor staging
   iv. Nursing diagnoses
     (a) Anemia (see Chapter 6, Commonly Encountered Nursing Diagnoses section, anemia subsection)
     (b) Pain (see Chapter 9, Commonly Encountered Nursing Diagnoses section, pain subsection)
c. Neoplasms of the colon and rectum
   i. Pathophysiology
     (a) Adenocarcinoma is the most common tumor
     (b) Right colon lesions are polypoid lesions
     (c) Left colon tumors spread, ulcerate, and erode blood vessels
        (1) Obstruction is common
        (2) Associated with liver metastases
     (d) Rectal lesions
        (1) Rectal bleeding
        (2) Local spread to prostate and vagina
        (3) Associated with systemic metastases
   ii. Etiologic or precipitating factors
     (a) Colorectal polyps are associated with colorectal neoplasms
     (b) Metastatic neoplasm in other organ
   iii. Nursing assessment data base
     (a) Nursing history
        (1) Subjective findings
           a) History of familial polyposis, inflammatory bowel disease, familial cancer syndrome, or adenomatous polyposis
           b) Change in bowel habits
               i) Change in size of stool: smaller in diameter
               ii) Difficulty defecating
               iii) Paradoxical diarrhea
           c) Pain: ill defined in right colon neoplasms, colicky in left colon neoplasms, steady and gnawing in rectal neoplasms
           d) Weakness only in right colon neoplasms
        (2) Objective findings: depends on site of neoplasms
           a) Neoplasms of the left colon are accompanied by abdominal distention, pain, vomiting, constipation, cramps, and bright red blood in stool
           b) Right colon neoplasms are accompanied by pain, palpable mass in right lower quadrant, anemia, and brick-red blood in stool

                c) Proximal colon neoplasms are accompanied by pernicious anemia

                d) Rectal neoplasms are accompanied by bright red blood coating the stool

           (b) Nursing examination of patient: no specific findings

           (c) Diagnostic study findings

              (1) Laboratory findings

                a) Decreased hemoglobin

                b) Positive stool guaiac test

              (2) Radiologic findings

                a) Lower GI series (barium enema); see Nursing Examination of Patient, Diagnostic Studies, Radiologic Studies subsection

              (3) Other diagnostic findings

                a) Digital rectal examination yields positive findings for blood

                b) Stool guaiac results positive for blood

                c) Sigmoidoscopy positive for blood, and biopsy done during sigmoidoscopy positive for carcinoma

                d) Histopathologic classification of tumor

                e) Tumor staging

        iv. Nursing diagnoses

          (a) Anemia (see Chapter 6, Commonly Encountered Nursing Diagnoses section, anemia subsection)

          (b) Pain (see Chapter 9, Commonly Encountered Nursing Diagnoses section, pain subsection)

    d. Other neoplasms

      i. Neoplasms of the liver

      ii. Neoplasms of the pancreas

      iii. Neoplasms of the hepatobiliary tract

4. Other upper GI causes of bleeding

    a. Mallory-Weiss tears at gastroesophageal junction

    b. Esophagitis

    c. Stress ulcers: gastric, duodenal

      i. Extremely common in critically ill patients

      ii. Associated with sepsis, shock, burns, trauma, acute head injuries, renal failure, hepatic failure, ARDS, mechanical ventilation, and major operative procedures

      iii. Characterized by mucosal ischemia leading to alterations that result in loss of protective functions

    d. Erosive gastritis, duodenitis

5. Other lower GI causes of bleeding

    a. Crohn's disease, ileitis

    b. Ulcerative colitis

    c. Colitis resulting from ischemia, radiation, chemotherapy

    d. Meckel's diverticulum

    e. Intestinal polyps

    f. Angiodysplasia (arteriovenous malformation of mucosa)

    g. Hemorrhoids

: **Hepatitis**

1. **Pathophysiology**
   a. The essential lesion is an acute inflammation of the entire liver, characterized by centrilobular necrosis and infiltration of the portal tracts by leukocytes
   b. A multisystem infection involving many organs: regional lymphadenopathy, splenomegaly, ulceration of the GI tract, acute pancreatitis, myocarditis, serum sickness, vasculitis, and nephritis
2. **Etiologic or precipitating factors**
   a. Causes may be viral, drug-related, or autoimmune
   b. Multiple viruses cause hepatitis in humans
      i. *Hepatitis A* virus infection (formerly called *infectious hepatitis*)
         (a) RNA virus
         (b) Occurs sporadically or endemically
         (c) Fecal-oral transmission
         (d) Often misdiagnosed as acute gastroenteritis
         (e) Usually self-limiting; symptoms are worse in adults
      ii. *Hepatitis B* virus infection (formerly called *serum hepatitis*)
         (a) DNA virus
         (b) Transmitted in blood and all concentrated body fluids
            (1) 100 million to one billion viral particles per milliliter of blood
            (2) Mother-to-neonate transmission
            (3) Promiscuous homosexual and heterosexual transmission
            (4) Parenteral transmission
               a) Intravenous drug abuse
               b) Transfusion of blood or blood products
            (5) Transmission via contaminated equipment
         (c) More common among homosexuals; among persons with Down's syndrome, hemophilia, renal failure on hemodialysis, or liver disease; and among health care workers
         (d) Associated with delta virus (hepatitis D, an RNA virus), a small RNA particle that is unable to replicate on its own but is capable of infection when activated by presence of hepatitis B virus
            (1) Always occurs as a co-infection with hepatitis B
            (2) Occurs as a super-infection with chronic active hepatitis B infection
      iii. *Hepatitis C* virus infection (formerly called *non-A, non-B hepatitis*)
         (a) RNA virus
         (b) Accounts for more than 90% of post-transfusion hepatitis: chronicity more likely if transfusion-related
         (c) 50% of cases have no known cause
         (d) More common among homosexuals; among persons with hemophilia, renal failure on hemodialysis, or liver disease; and among health care workers
      iv. *Hepatitis E* virus infection (formerly called *epidemic non-A, non-B hepatitis*)
         (a) RNA virus
         (b) Epidemiology and clinical course similar to those of hepatitis A virus infection; enteric transmission

        (c) Most prevalent among young adults

     v. Other: hepatitis non-A, non-B, non-C; hepatitis F; hepatitis G; all viruses in the herpesvirus family (herpes simplex, cytomegalovirus, Epstein-Barr virus, varicella zoster virus)

  c. Can manifest as an acute, acute fulminant, chronic persistent, or chronic active process

     i. Acute hepatitis: acute onset of viral infection, usually self-limiting

     ii. Acute fulminant hepatitis

     iii. Asymptomatic carrier state

        (a) Hepatitis antigen persists in serum for at least 6 months

        (b) Infected person is unable to clear hepatitis antigen from serum because of ineffective cellular immunity

        (c) Carrier is able to transmit hepatitis to others

        (d) Carrier suffers no liver damage

        (e) This form of transmission is the most common

     iv. Chronic persistent hepatitis

        (a) Hepatitis antigen persists in serum for at least 6 months

        (b) Chronic inflammation of the liver persists for at least 6 months

        (c) Infected individual is unable to clear hepatitis antigen from serum because of ineffective cellular immunity

     v. Chronic active hepatitis

        (a) Viral replication persists in the liver

        (b) Liver damage is progressive

        (c) This form is more common among persons with asymptomatic or mild, anicteric cases

        (d) Develops into cirrhosis

        (e) Is associated with primary hepatocellular carcinoma

3. Nursing assessment data base (note: clinical manifestation spans spectrum from asymptomatic and anicteric case to fatal coma; this section addresses only acute viral hepatitis)

  a. Nursing history

     i. Subjective findings

        (a) Mild anicteric (not jaundiced) case: asymptomatic except for flulike symptoms

        (b) Icteric case

           (1) A prodromal period associated with not feeling well: malaise, fatigue

           (2) Symptoms subside with onset of jaundice

           (3) Among smokers and drinkers, loss of desire to smoke or drink

     ii. Objective findings

        (a) History of cultural practices involving body mutilation and/or exposure to others' body fluids

        (b) Recent foreign travel to endemic areas

        (c) Intimate contacts with jaundiced persons

        (d) Promiscuous heterosexual, homosexual, or bisexual practices

        (e) History of intravenous drug abuse

        (f) History of blood transfusions

        (g) Recent dental procedure

        (h) Dark urine, followed by lightening of the urine

        (i) Nausea, vomiting

        (j) Diarrhea

        (k) Fever

   b. Nursing examination of patient

      i. Inspection

        (a) Tattoos

        (b) Jaundice lasting 1 to 4 weeks

      ii. Percussion: enlarged liver

      iii. Palpation

        (a) Tender enlargement of liver

        (b) Tender enlargement of spleen

   c. Diagnostic study findings: laboratory

      i. Increased WBC count

      ii. Increased serum bilirubin; indirect fraction more elevated

      iii. Increased ALT, AST, alkaline phosphatase, GGT

      iv. Hepatitis serology testing (Table 7–2)

4. Nursing diagnoses

   a. Fatigue related to decreased metabolic energy production, altered nutritional status

      i. Assessment for defining characteristics

        (a) Decreased capacity for physical activity

        (b) Impaired ability to concentrate

        (c) Lethargy, excessive drowsiness

        (d) Decreased appetite

        (e) Decreased sense of well-being

        (f) Nonspecific discomfort

      ii. Expected outcome: patient verbalizes feeling well-rested

      iii. Nursing interventions

        (a) Maintain patient on bed rest until symptoms disappear

        (b) Encourage low-fat, high-carbohydrate diet

      iv. Evaluation of nursing care

        (a) Physical energy and activity are restored

        (b) Mental energy and activity are restored

   b. Nutrition altered, less than body requirements, related to major tissue destruction, hypermetabolic state (see Commonly Encountered Nursing Diagnoses section)

Acute (Fulminant) Liver Failure

1. Pathophysiology

   a. A clinical syndrome characterized by sudden and severe impairment of liver function; occurs in persons with previously normal liver function

   b. Massive hepatocellular necrosis

   c. Hepatic encephalopathy develops within 8 weeks of onset of signs and symptoms

   d. Prognosis is very poor

      i. Liver transplantation is the only definitive treatment

      ii. With the exception of acute fulminant liver failure caused by acetaminophen toxicity, the chance of mortality is nearly 100% without liver transplantation

TABLE 7–2. Nomenclature of Serologic Testing for Viral Hepatitis

Serologic Test	Description and Purpose
Hepatitis A Virus (HAV)	
Anti-HAV (total)	Antibody to HAV; detectable at onset of disease before jaundice; presence in serum confers lifelong immunity
IgM	Rises early during infection (detectable at 4–6 weeks after exposure and within 1 week after signs and symptoms develop); indicates acute infection; persists for approximately 6 months
IgG	Rises slowly during infection (detectable at 8–12 weeks after exposure and persists for life)
Hepatitis B Virus (HBV)	
HBsAg	HBV *surface* antigen; most important and commonly used marker for HBV infection; detectable within 30 days of exposure and persists up to 3 months after jaundice unless a carrier state develops, in which case it will persist longer; presence in serum (seropositivity) indicates that disease is infectious
HBcAg	HBV *core* antigen; not detectable in serum, detectable only in hepatocytes
HBeAg	HBV *e* antigen; found only in sera positive for HBsAG; presence in serum (seropositivity) indicates high titer of HBV (extensive viral replication) and increased infectiousness (ongoing viral replication); detectable 4–6 weeks after exposure
Anti-HBs	Antibody to HBsAg; presence in serum (seropositivity) indicates HBV immunity due to HBV infection or vaccination; detectable 4–8 weeks after HBsAg disappears
Anti-HBc (total)	Antibody to HBcAg; detectable 6–14 weeks after exposure during what is referred to as the "window phase" (after HBsAg disappears but before HBsAb appears); persists for life; high titers may indicate persistent infection (carrier state)
IgM	Rises early in infection; if persistent, may indicate chronic infection
IgG	Rises slowly during infection; persists for life
HBeAb	Antibody to HBeAg
HBV-DNA	HBV-DNA detected by process of nucleic acid hybridization
PCR for HBV-DNA	Polymerase chain reaction (PCR) for HBV-DNA; test detects polymerase-containing virions; PCR process amplifies DNA in blood so that it is easily detected; very sensitive test
Hepatitis D Virus (HDV; Delta Hepatitis Virus)	
HDAg (total)	Antigen to HDV; detectable only concurrently with HBV infection
IgM	Rises early in infection; if persistent, may indicate chronic infection
IgG	Rises slowly during infection; persists for life
Anti-HDV	Antibody to HDV; detectable only concurrently with HBV infection
HDV-RNA	HDV-RNA detected by process of nucleic acid hybridization
Hepatitis C Virus (HCV)	
Anti-HCV	Antibody to HCV; presence (seropositivity) in serum is diagnostic for chronic infection only; absence (seronegativity) does not exclude the diagnosis of HCV infection; may see false-positive results
HCV-RNA	HCV-RNA is detected by process of nucleic acid hybridization; presence of HCV-RNA in serum is diagnostic of viremia in acute or chronic HCV hepatitis; the HCV-RNA test is also used to monitor response to interferon-alpha therapy

TABLE 7–2. Nomenclature of Serologic Testing for Viral Hepatitis *Continued*

Serologic Test	Description and Purpose
Hepatitis C Virus (HCV)	
PCR for HCV-RNA	PCR for HCV-RNA; test detects polymerase-containing virions; PCR process amplifies RNA in blood so that it is easily detected; very sensitive test
bDNA	Quantitative test of HCV-RNA for determining amount of virus; research assay not yet licensed by FDA
Hepatitis E Virus (HEV)	
PCR for HEV-RNA	PCR for HEV-RNA; test detects polymerase-containing virions; PCR process amplifies RNA in blood so that it is easily detected; very sensitive test
Serologic Criteria for Diagnosing Acute Hepatitis A Virus Infection	
HAVAb-IgM positive	
Serologic Criteria for Diagnosing Acute Hepatitis B Virus Infection	
HBsAg positive *or*	
HBsAb positive *or*	
HBcAb-IgM positive *or*	
HBV-DNA positive *or*	
PCR for HBV-DNA	
Serologic Criteria for Diagnosing Acute Hepatitis C Virus Infection	
HCVAb positive *or*	
Anti-HCV *or*	
HCV-RNA positive *or*	
Quantitative HCV RNA-bDNA positive *or*	
PCR for HCV-RNA	

From Smith, S. L.: Patients with liver dysfunction. *In* Clochesy, J. M., Breu, C., Cardin, S., et al. (eds.): Critical Care Nursing, 2nd ed. Philadelphia, W. B. Saunders, 1996, p. 1060.
   IgM = immunoglobulin M; IgG = immunoglobulin G; FDA = U.S. Food and Drug Administration.

2. **Etiologic or precipitating factors**
   a. Viral hepatitis: most common cause
   b. Acetaminophen toxicity: intentional (acute) and unintentional (chronic). Acute fulminant hepatic failure caused by acetaminophen toxicity has a better prognosis than that resulting from other causes
   c. Hepatotoxic drugs or substances
   d. Mushroom poisoning (e.g., *Amanita phalloides, A. verna,* and *A. venosa; Galerina autumnaas, G. marginata,* and *G. venedata; Gyromitra* species)
   e. Viral infections: herpesvirus family
   f. Acute Wilson's disease, acute Budd-Chiari syndrome
   g. Veno-occlusive disease and graft-versus-host disease after bone marrow transplantation
   h. Reye's syndrome
3. **Nursing assessment data base**
   a. Nursing history
      i. Subjective findings: prodromal symptoms (vague, flu-like symptoms)
      ii. Objective findings
         (a) History of exposure to viral hepatitis infection, hepatotoxic drugs or agents, poisonous mushrooms
         (b) Recent bone marrow transplantation

        (c) Rapidly progressive liver failure and multisystem organ failure
           (1) Hepatic encephalopathy: rapid progression to hepatic coma
           (2) Intracranial hypertension
           (3) Profound coagulopathy
           (4) Hyperventilation, respiratory alkalosis
           (5) Profound hypoglycemia
           (6) Hepatorenal syndrome
           (7) Sepsis, metabolic acidosis
           (8) Hyperdynamic circulation
           (9) Eventual cardiovascular collapse
          (10) Fever

b. Nursing examination of patient
  i. Inspection
    (a) Jaundice
    (b) Deterioration of mental status and level of consciousness; progression from fully alert state to deep coma can occur in just a few days
  ii. Auscultation: systolic ejection murmur
  iii. Percussion
    (a) Liver is enlarged during acute inflammatory stage
    (b) Liver becomes atrophied as hepatocellular necrosis progresses
  iv. Palpation
    (a) Liver becomes enlarged, tender during acute inflammatory stage
    (b) Liver becomes nonpalpable as hepatocellular necrosis progresses

c. Diagnostic study findings
  i. Laboratory findings
    (a) Increased AST, ALT, alkaline phosphatase, GGT. Severe elevations followed by progression back to normal may be misinterpreted as improvement in patient's status but are not favorable signs; indicate near-complete hepatocellular necrosis
    (b) Increased serum bilirubin
    (c) Prolonged PT
    (d) Factors V and VII levels less than 20% of normal
    (e) Decreased serum glucose
    (f) Increased serum creatinine, BUN
    (g) Increased serum lactate
    (h) Increased serum ammonia
    (i) Positive serologic findings for hepatitis
    (j) Increased WBC count
    (k) Decreased hemoglobin, hematocrit
    (l) Positive cultures of body fluids
    (m) Positive urine toxicology screen
  ii. Radiologic findings
    (a) Bilateral infiltrates on chest x-ray
    (b) Evidence of aspiration pneumonitis
  iii. Other diagnostic findings
    (a) Increased intracranial pressure (ICP), increased mean arterial pressure (MAP), normal cerebral perfusion pressure (CPP) (*early* signs)
    (b) Increased ICP, normal or decreased MAP, decreased CPP (*late* signs)

(c) CT scan of head normal until very *late* in process; rule out intracerebral hemorrhage

(d) Cerebral perfusion scan may show decreased or absence of flow *late* in process; done before liver transplantation to rule out brain death

(e) Positive stool guaiac test result

4. Nursing diagnoses

i. Altered cerebral tissue perfusion, related to acute hepatocellular necrosis

(a) Assessment for defining characteristics

    (1) Assess grade of hepatic encephalopathy (Table 7–3)

    (2) Assess baseline organ system functions: cardiovascular, renal, pulmonary, hematologic

    (3) Assess infectious disease status

(b) Expected outcome: the integrity of the patient's brain will be protected until liver transplantation can be performed

(c) Nursing interventions

    (1) Stabilization of patient is dependent on initial assessment of multiple organ systems

    (2) Elective endotracheal intubation may be necessary before patient progresses to full hepatic coma

    (3) Administer fresh frozen plasma and other blood products as ordered to optimize coagulation status

    (4) Assist with insertion of ICP monitoring device: continuous monitoring of ICP and CPP

    (5) Institute measures to maintain CPP (see Chapter 3, The Neurologic System; Patient Health Problems section, increased intracranial pressure subsection)

        a) Decrease elevated ICP

        b) Maintain normal or elevated MAP

    (6) Administer antibiotics as ordered

    (7) Initiate barbiturate or sedative coma as ordered, to decrease cerebral metabolism

    (8) Administer mannitol as ordered, to decrease ICP

    (9) Institute measures to maintain normothermia

    (10) Administer hypertonic glucose as ordered, to maintain serum glucose greater than 70 mg/dl

    (11) Prepare patient and family for prospect of liver transplantation

(d) Evaluation of nursing care

    (1) Hemostasis is maintained

    (2) Airway is protected

    (3) Tissue perfusion to vital organs is maintained at optimal level; CPP is maintained at greater than 50 mm Hg

ii. At risk for altered tissue perfusion (cerebral, cardiopulmonary, renal, GI, peripheral), related to postoperative complications of liver transplantation

(a) Assessment for defining characteristics

    (1) Hypothermia

TABLE 7–3. Clinical Assessment of Hepatic Encephalopathy

	Grade I	Grade II	Grade III	Grade IV
Level of consciousness	Awake	Decreased, but opens eyes spontaneously	Patient sleeps but is arousable to verbal and painful stimuli; does not open eyes spontaneously	Comatose; no response to pain
Orientation	Total orientation with progression to confusion; then disorientation to time and place	Disoriented to time and place; severe confusion	Complete disorientation when aroused	Comatose
Intellectual functions	Mental clouding; slowness in answering questions; impaired handwriting; subtle changes in intellectual function; psychometric test scores decrease	Amnesia for past events; psychometric test scores decrease	Inability to make computations	Comatose
Behavior	Forgetful, restless, irritable, untidy, apathetic, disobedient	Decreased inhibitions, lethargic	Bizarre behavior (unprovoked rage)	Comatose
Mood	Euphoria, depression, crying	Apathetic, paranoid	Apathy increases	Comatose
Neuromuscular	Muscular incoordination, tremors, yawning, insomnia	Hypoactive reflexes, asterixis, ataxia, slurred speech	Cannot cooperate; nystagmus and Babinski sign; clonus, decortication, decerebration, rigidity, seizures	Seizures; rigidity decreases to flaccidity; dilated pupils
Electroencephalography	Mild to moderate abnormalities	Moderate to severe abnormalities	Severe abnormalities	Severe abnormalities

From: Smith, S. L.: Patients with liver dysfunction. *In* Clochesy, J. M., Breu, C., Cardin, S., et al. (eds.): Critical Care Nursing, 2nd ed. Philadelphia, W. B. Saunders, 1996, p. 1058.

      (2) Nonfunction of transplanted liver (graft) as a result of ischemia, preservation injury, procurement injury, hepatic artery thrombosis

         a) Absence of bile production

         b) Hypoglycemia

         c) Coagulopathy

         d) Sustained increase in serum lactate

      (3) Cardiovascular instability

         a) Hypovolemia

         b) Hypertension

         c) Vasodilation during warming phase of hypothermia

      (4) Pulmonary compromise

         a) Atelectasis

         b) Pleural effusions

         c) Paresis of right hemidiaphragm

         d) Failure to wean, because of poor nutritional status

         e) Unresolved intrapulmonary shunting, hepatopulmonary syndrome

      (5) Renal compromise

         a) Acute tubular necrosis (ATN) related to immunosuppressant drug (e.g., cyclosporine, tacrolimus) toxicity

         b) Unresolved hepatorenal syndrome

      (6) Hematologic abnormalities

         a) Unresolved coagulopathy

         b) Dilutional coagulopathy caused by massive blood replacement

         c) Nonfunction of liver graft

      (7) GI function or endocrine disturbances

         a) Paralytic ileus

         b) Peptic ulcer disease

         c) Biliary tract complications

         d) Hyperglycemia

      (8) Infection

         a) Early: bacterial; caused by technical surgical error; complication of general surgery

         b) Late: opportunistic as a result of immunocompromise

      (9) Acute cellular rejection: elevations in serum AST, ALT, alkaline phosphatase, GGT, bilirubin

  (b) Expected outcomes

      (1) Alterations in tissue perfusion will be recognized in a timely manner

      (2) Expected complications of liver transplantation will be stabilized and resolved without further problems

      (3) See discussion of impaired physical mobility, related to general anesthesia, abdominal surgery in Patient Health Problems section, Acute Abdomen subsection

  (c) Nursing interventions

      (1) Assess for expected side effects

      (2) Institute warming measures for hypothermic patient, monitor for associated hemodynamic changes

(3) Administer IV fluids, electrolytes, and blood products as ordered
(4) Administer antihypertensives and diuretics as ordered
(5) Administer hypertonic glucose and insulin as ordered
(6) Administer anti-infective agents as ordered
(7) Administer immunosuppressant agents as ordered
(8) See discussion of impaired physical mobility, related to general anesthesia, abdominal surgery in Patient Health Problems section, Acute Abdomen subsection

(d) Evaluation of nursing care
(1) See discussion of impaired physical mobility, related to general anesthesia, abdominal surgery in Patient Health Problems section, Acute Abdomen subsection
(2) Patient's hemodynamic parameters are maintained within normal limits
(3) Patient's fluid status and electrolyte status are balanced
(4) Liver graft function is stable

Chronic Liver Failure: Decompensated Cirrhosis

1. **Pathophysiology**
   a. Cirrhosis is a chronic and usually a slowly progressive disease of the liver involving diffuse formation of connective tissue (fibrosis) and nodular regeneration of the liver after necrosis and chronic inflammation of the liver. Changes are irreversible
   b. Cirrhosis can be stable without evidence of serious signs or symptoms for many years, but at some point the decreased functional liver mass becomes incompatible with homeostasis and/or the complications of portal hypertension become life-threatening, at which time the body can no longer elicit compensatory physiologic mechanisms
   c. Portal hypertension: increased hydrostatic pressure (greater than 10 mm Hg) within the portal venous system as a result of disruption of normal liver lobular structure that impedes blood flow (25% of cardiac output per minute) into, through, or out of the liver
      i. Pathophysiologic consequences of portal hypertension
         (a) Formation of collateral portacaval (between the portal venous system and the venae cavae) vessels (varices) in the esophagus, duodenum, stomach, peritoneum, retroperitoneum, and rectum; purpose is to maintain venous return to the right side of the heart (see Patient Health Problems section, GI Bleeding, Variceal Bleeding subsection)
         (b) Splenomegaly: increased size and congestion of the spleen as a result of portal hypertension, with backward venous congestion via the splenic vein of the spleen
            (1) Pancytopenia
               a) Anemia
               b) Leukopenia
               c) Thrombocytopenia
            (2) Spleen pain

(c) Ascites: abnormal accumulation of lymph fluid that has escaped the lymphatic vessels and enters the peritoneal cavity; caused by transudation of fluid from peritoneal surface as a result of increased hydrostatic pressure and decreased oncotic pressure in the portal venous system
  (1) Results from disorder in renal function caused by rise in sinusoidal pressure, excess hepatic lymph, and hypoalbuminemia
    a) Hepatic lymph production increases by approximately 60% for every 1–mm Hg increase in intrahepatic pressure
    b) Survival rate is 40% at 2 years after onset
  (2) Decreased circulating plasma volume
  (3) Secondary aldosteronism
  (4) Compression of inferior vena cava and obstruction of venous return
  (5) Pleural effusions
  (6) Decreased ventilation-perfusion ($\dot{V}/\dot{Q}$) ratio
  (7) Subacute bacterial peritonitis
  (8) Fatigue
  (9) Alteration in balance, gait, mobility
  (10) Alterations in body image
  (11) Alteration in disposition of water-soluble drugs
  (12) Refractory ascites: ascites that is unresponsive to therapies such as salt restriction and diuretics
    a) Potassium-sparing diuretics used to block proximal and distal tubular reabsorption
    b) Necessitates frequent large-volume paracentesis (LVP): removal of large volume of ascites to provide symptomatic relief
    c) Necessitates TIPS if refractory to LVP
    d) Peritoneovenous shunt (LeVeen or Denver shunt) used rarely
    e) Precipitated by worsening liver disease, increased sodium intake, use of NSAIDs (renal function in liver disease dependent on prostaglandins, which are blocked by NSAIDs)
    f) Associated with hepatorenal syndrome
(d) Abnormal renal function in cirrhosis
  (1) Decreased glomerular filtration rate
  (2) Renal vasoconstriction
  (3) Decreased renal blood flow
  (4) Increased sodium reabsorption
  (5) Increased levels of renin and aldosterone
(e) Hepatorenal syndrome: a "functional" form of acute renal failure that occurs in patients with advanced end-stage liver disease and is caused by decreased circulating plasma volume and the release of mediators of vasoconstriction that cause diversion of renal blood flow
  (1) Oliguria in the presence of normovolemia and azotemia
  (2) Highly concentrated urine that is sodium free (urine sodium concentration less than 10 mEq/L)

(3) Patient is severely hyperdynamic; cardiac output as high as 25 L/minute
(4) Precipitating factors
  a) Refractory ascites
  b) Excessive diuresis
  c) Hemorrhage
  d) Infection
(5) Reversible if liver function restored, such as after liver transplantation
(f) Pulmonary alterations
  (1) Pleural effusions
  (2) Intrapulmonary shunts
  (3) Hepatopulmonary syndrome: pulmonary capillary vasodilation and intrapulmonary shunts
(g) Hepatic encephalopathy: neuropsychiatric dysfunction caused by altered ammonia and amino acid metabolism; characterized by a deterioration in intellectual function, personal behavior, and level of consciousness
  (1) Liver unable to synthesize urea from the by-products of protein (endogenous and exogenous) metabolism; establishment of an alternate circulating pathway for toxic substances that cross the blood-brain barrier
    a) Increase in blood levels of aromatic amino acids inhibits neurotransmission and favors sedation
    b) Decrease in blood levels of branched-chain amino acids inhibits neurotransmission and favors sedation
  (2) Grades: I to IV (see Table 7–3)
  (3) Precipitating factors
    a) Worsening liver function
    b) Excessive diuresis
    c) Azotemia
    d) Infection
    e) Hyperaldosteronism: hypokalemia and metabolic alkalosis
    f) Constipation
    g) GI bleeding
    h) Too much dietary protein
    i) Hypoxia
    j) Sedatives
(h) Coagulopathy: alteration in hemostasis resulting from loss of ability of liver to synthesize clotting factors
  (1) Thrombocytopenia secondary to splenomegaly
2. Etiologic or precipitating factors
  a. Alcoholism: most common cause of liver disease in United States. Laënnec's cirrhosis: development of cirrhosis preceded by reversible stage of alcoholic hepatitis
  b. Postnecrotic cirrhosis
    i. Viral hepatitis (chronic active hepatitis B, C, F, or G): postnecrotic cirrhosis
    ii. Drug or toxin induced
    iii. Autoimmune hepatitis

    c. Autoimmune diseases of biliary stasis (primary biliary cirrhosis, sclerosing cholangitis)

    d. Inborn errors of liver metabolism (Wilson's disease [copper metabolism], hemochromatosis [iron metabolism], alpha$_1$-antitrypsin deficiency)

    e. Fatty liver

        i. Protein calorie malnutrition

        ii. Diabetes mellitus

        iii. Chronic corticosteroid use

        iv. Jejunoileal bypass

        v. Short bowel syndrome

    f. Hepatic vein thrombosis (Budd-Chiari syndrome)

    g. Right-sided heart failure: cardiac cirrhosis

3. Nursing assessment data base

    a. Nursing history

        i. Subjective findings

            (a) Fatigue

            (b) Alteration in sleep pattern: insomnia, day/night reversal

            (c) Pruritis

        ii. Objective findings

            (a) Past medical and surgical history

                (1) Medications: prescription and over-the-counter drugs

                (2) Autoimmune diseases

                (3) Blood transfusions

                (4) Spontaneous fractures

                (5) Abdominal pain

                (6) Surgery, anesthesia history

                (7) Family history

            (b) Malnutrition, vitamin deficiencies

            (c) Anemia

            (d) Clay-colored stools

            (e) Fetor hepaticus: musty, sweet breath indicative of encephalopathy

            (f) Altered mental status

            (g) History: substance abuse: alcohol, analgesics, narcotics

            (h) History: possible exposure to hepatitis (blood transfusion, sexual promiscuity, IV drug abuse, tattoos, body piercing, foreign travel)

    b. Nursing examination of patient

        i. Inspection

            (a) Visible stigmata of liver disease

                (1) Possible jaundice

                (2) Abdomen distention with ascites

                (3) Cachexia

                (4) Hematomas, ecchymoses

                (5) Spider angiomas

                (6) Possible clubbing of fingers, palmar erythema

                    a) Shortness of breath

                    b) Cyanosis

                (7) Testicular atrophy, gynecomastia in males

                (8) Striae

            (b) Poor oral health status

(c) Umbilical hernia, caput medusae

(d) Asterixis

ii. Auscultation

(a) Hyperdynamic circulation: increased heart rate, systolic ejection murmur

(b) Breath sounds may be decreased because of pleural effusions

iii. Percussion: possible palpable fluid wave (shifting dullness) indicating ascites; not a sensitive test

iv. Palpation

(a) Enlarged spleen may be palpable

(b) Nodular lower edge

c. Diagnostic studies

i. Laboratory findings: dependent on etiology and stage of disease

(a) ALT, AST, alkaline phosphatase, GGT: not usually elevated in advanced cirrhosis

(b) Bilirubin: not usually elevated in advanced cirrhosis except in diseases of biliary stasis

(c) PT: prolonged; the most sensitive index of liver function in a readily available laboratory test

(d) Platelet count: may be decreased due to splenomegaly

(e) Ammonia: may be elevated. Not a sensitive test: the degree of encephalopathy does not correlate with the degree of elevation of serum ammonia

(f) Hemoglobin, hematocrit, BUN, creatinine, serum sodium: decreased

(g) Hepatitis serologic findings: variable

(h) Ascitic fluid: WBC, culture

(1) WBC greater than 250 polymorphonuclear neutrophil leukocytes/mm^3

(2) *Escherichia coli* and *Klebsiella* species most common organisms

ii. Radiologic findings

(a) Cholangiogram

(b) Endoscopic retrograde cholangiopancreatogram (ERCP)

(c) Abdominal ultrasonography for presence of small amounts of ascites

(d) CT scan: liver volume decreased, spleen volume increased

iii. Other diagnostic findings

(a) Upper GI endoscopy reveals esophageal, gastric, and/or duodenal varices

(b) Abdominal paracentesis for presence of ascites and testing fluid for infection

(c) Liver biopsy: cirrhosis

(d) Electroencephalogram (EEG): may show generalized slowing with hepatic encephalopathy

4. Nursing diagnoses

a. Risk for fluid volume deficit, related to third-space fluid loss and/or hemorrhage (see Commonly Encountered Nursing Diagnoses section)

b. Nutrition altered, less than body requirements, related to major tissue destruction, hypermetabolic state (see Commonly Encountered Nursing Diagnoses section)

c. Altered thought processes, related to hepatic encephalopathy
   i. Assessment for defining characteristics
      (a) Assess for grade of encephalopathy (I to IV) (see Table 7–3)
      (b) Assess for precipitating factors
      (c) Serum ammonia level: does not necessarily correlate with level of encephalopathy
         (1) Very sensitive laboratory test: must be on ice and processed immediately
         (2) Tolerance to high ammonia levels varies widely among individuals
   ii. Expected outcomes
      (a) Progression of encephalopathy is halted, level of encephalopathy is decreased
      (b) Patient is protected from self-injury
   iii. Nursing interventions
      (a) Assess grade of encephalopathy frequently
      (b) Assess for precipitating factors
      (c) Assess potential for self-harm; provide a safe environment
      (d) Maintain patent airway
      (e) Administer medications to cleanse gut and decrease serum ammonia as ordered
         (1) Neomycin: nonabsorbable antibiotic effective against ureolytic organisms
            a) Short-term treatment to induce regular bowel movements
            b) Nephrotoxic, ototoxic
         (2) Lactulose: saline laxative converted in the gut to lactic and acetic acid
            a) Decreases fecal pH and inhibits growth of ammonia-forming bacteria
            b) Promotes diffusion of ammonia from the systemic circulation into the intestine
            c) Causes abdominal cramping, gas, and diarrhea
      (f) Cleanse intestine with enemas as ordered
      (g) Avoid administration of analgesics, sedatives, hypnotics, tranquilizers
   iv. Evaluation of nursing care
      (a) Serum ammonia level is decreased
      (b) Patient does not inflict self-injury
      (c) Patient does not aspirate GI contents into lungs
d. Altered tissue perfusion (cerebral, cardiopulmonary, renal, GI, peripheral), at risk, related to postoperative complications of liver transplantation (see Patient Health Problems section, Acute Hepatic Failure subsection, nursing diagnoses)

Acute Abdomen

A condition associated with the sudden onset of abdominal pain, usually necessitating emergency surgical intervention

1. **Pathophysiology**
   a. Many conditions can cause an acute abdomen; the differential diagnosis is complex
   b. Associated with inflammation of peritoneal cavity and often contamination
2. **Etiologic or precipitating factors:** infection, surgical complication, blunt or penetrating abdominal trauma, ischemia, erosion of mucosal barrier; may be grouped as follows:
   a. Perforated viscus (esophagus, stomach, gallbladder, bile duct, bowel, appendix, diverticulum)
      i. Erosion (e.g., peptic ulcer disease, ischemia)
      ii. Rupture (e.g., ectopic pregnancy, colonic diverticulitis)
      iii. Technical error during abdominal surgery
      iv. Foreign body
      v. Abdominal trauma
      vi. Infection (e.g., cytomegalovirus infection)
   b. Perforated or ruptured blood vessel
      i. Peptic ulcer disease
      ii. Abdominal aortic aneurysm
      iii. Tumor
      iv. Abdominal trauma
   c. Ruptured viscus
      i. Bowel
      ii. Liver fracture
      iii. Pancreas fracture
      iv. Pancreatic pseudocyst
      v. Ectopic pregnancy
   d. Bowel ischemia: intestinal infarction; ischemic and necrotic tissue damage to the intestinal mesentery
      i. Low cardiac output states: cardiac failure
      ii. Hypovolemia
      iii. Occlusion of mesenteric vessels: thromboses, DIC, strangulation
      iv. Constriction of mesenteric vessels
         (a) Sympathetic nervous system stimulation: alpha agonists (e.g., high-dose dopamine, norepinephrine, ephedrine)
         (b) Vasopressin
   e. Bowel obstruction: blockage of the intestine. Classification of bowel obstruction:
      i. Onset: acute, chronic
      ii. Extent: partial, complete
      iii. Location
         (a) Intrinsic: originates within lumen of intestine
         (b) Extrinsic: originates outside lumen of intestine
      iv. Effects on intestine
         (a) Simple: does not occlude blood supply
         (b) Strangulated: occludes blood supply
         (c) Closed loop: obstruction at each end of an intestinal segment
      v. Causal factors
         (a) Mechanical
            (1) Intraluminal obstruction
               a) Gallstones

       b) Fecal impactions

       c) Polypoid tumors

       d) Intussusception

       e) Foreign bodies

    (2) Lesions of the intestine

       a) Tumors

       b) Congenital disorders: Meckel's diverticulum

       c) Inflammatory bowel disease (IBD): diverticulitis, ulcerative colitis, Crohn's disease

       d) Strictures: IBD, radiation

    (3) External lesions

       a) Adhesions: the holding together by scar tissue of two parts that are normally separated; caused by surgery, trauma, or inflammation; the most common cause of bowel obstruction

       b) Tumors

       c) Anomalous vessels

       d) Abscesses, hematomas

       e) Volvulus (torsion)

       f) Hernia

  (b) Paralytic or functional

    (1) Neuromuscular defects

    (2) Megacolon

    (3) Mesenteric vascular occlusion

    (4) Paralytic ileus: peritonitis, sepsis, electrolyte imbalances (hypokalemia, hypocalcemia, hypomagnesemia), surgical or traumatic manipulation of the intestine

f. Infection

  i. Abdominal abscess

  ii. Peritonitis

  iii. Diverticulitis

g. Bowel sloughing: graft-versus-host disease after organ transplantation

h. Multisystem organ failure: intestinal ischemia

3. Nursing assessment data base

a. Nursing history

  i. Subjective findings

    (a) Persistent, severe abdominal pain

    (b) Referred pain

    (c) Nausea, vomiting

    (d) Anorexia

    (e) Generalized weakness

  ii. Objective findings

    (a) History of peptic ulcer disease

    (b) Evidence of abdominal trauma

    (c) History of motor vehicle crash

    (d) Previous abdominal surgery

    (e) History of splanchnic ischemic period

      (1) Cardiac failure

      (2) Hypovolemia, hypotension

    (f) Current pregnancy

b. Nursing examination of patient

      i. Inspection
- (a) Abdominal distention
- (b) Visible peristalsis
- (c) Guarding of abdomen
- (d) Evidence of blunt or penetrating trauma: wound, bleeding, hematoma, foreign body
- (e) Fever
- (f) Rapid, shallow respirations
- (g) Pallor
- (h) Tachypnea
- (i) Dehydration

     ii. Auscultation
- (a) Hyperactive bowel sounds (early); loud, high-pitched tinkling sounds
- (b) Absent bowel sounds (late)
- (c) Abdominal bruit
- (d) Tachycardia
- (e) Decreased breath sounds
- (f) Hypotension (late)

    iii. Percussion: hyperresonance

    iv. Palpation
- (a) Tightness, rigidity of abdomen
- (b) Rebound tenderness

c. Diagnostic studies: differential diagnosis is complex

      i. Laboratory findings
- (a) Elevated WBC with shift to the left: elevated segmented neutrophil and basophil counts, increased bands (immature neutrophils)
- (b) Elevated alkaline phosphatase
- (c) Findings consistent with diagnosis of pancreatitis; elevated serum amylase, lipase
- (d) Findings consistent with hemorrhage
- (e) Arterial blood gases: metabolic acidosis
- (f) Blood and body fluid cultures positive for infectious organisms

     ii. Radiologic findings
- (a) Abdominal flat plate x-ray: alteration in position, size, or structure of abdominal contents; free air in the abdomen
- (b) Cholangiogram: cholangitis
- (c) ERCP: biliary or pancreatic stones, obstruction of ducts
- (d) Arteriogram: bleeding, infarction
- (e) Abdominal CT scan: vascular problems, infection, masses, or pancreatic pseudocyst
- (f) MRI of the abdomen: same as CT scan

    iii. Other diagnostic studies
- (a) Abdominal ultrasonography: masses (cysts, abscesses, tumors), foreign bodies (gallstones), infarction
- (b) EGD: bleeding from peptic ulcer, esophageal tear
- (c) Colonoscopy: lower GI ulceration, perforation, bleeding, abscess, ischemia
- (d) Flexible sigmoidoscopy: lower GI ulceration, perforation, bleeding, abscess, ischemia

        (e) Abdominal paracentesis: blood, bile, pus, urine, or feces in abdominal cavity

        (f) Peritoneoscopy (laparoscopy): bleeding, perforation, rupture, abscess, ischemia

4. Nursing diagnoses

  a. Altered intestinal tissue perfusion, caused by intestinal infarction

    i. Assessment for defining characteristics

      (a) Acute occlusive mesenteric ischemia: caused by thrombosis or embolism, usually in the superior mesenteric artery (atherosclerosis, dissecting aortic aneurysm, systemic vasculitis)

        (1) Intense spasm with severe colicky periumbilical pain

        (2) Constant generalized abdominal pain with rebound tenderness as ischemia progresses

        (3) Hyperactive bowel sounds (early)

        (4) Paralytic ileus

        (5) Abdominal distention

        (6) Vomiting

        (7) Bloody, foul-smelling diarrhea

        (8) Fever, chills, leukocytosis

        (9) Enteric organisms on blood culture

        (10) Septicemic shock (late): hypotension, pallor, metabolic acidosis

        (11) Decreased breath sounds

        (12) High gastric secretion output

        (13) Free air in the intestine on abdominal x-ray (flat plate and upright)

        (14) Increased serum amylase

        (15) Associated with intestinal obstruction caused by compromised intestinal function

        (16) Associated with intestinal perforation caused by intestinal obstruction and intraluminal pressure exceeding surrounding abdominal pressure

        (17) Hypovolemia resulting from third-space fluid loss from intestine

      (b) Chronic occlusive mesenteric ischemia: caused by atherosclerosis, mostly in elderly

        (1) Intermittent ischemic symptoms: intestinal angina (mid-abdominal pain after eating)

        (2) Fear of eating, followed by weight loss and malnutrition

      (c) Nonocclusive mesenteric ischemia: resulting from low blood flow without occlusion: associated with severe hypoxemia

    ii. Expected outcome: patient recovers without complications after surgical removal of necrotic intestine

    iii. Nursing interventions

      (a) Monitor vital signs, hemodynamic parameters

      (b) Assess for development of obstruction and/or perforation of intestine

      (c) Assess bowel sounds

      (d) Keep patient NPO

      (e) Maintain patent nasogastric or duodenal tube

      (f) Administer IV fluids as ordered

      (g) Administer antibiotics (coverage for gram-negative anaerobes) as ordered

      (h) Administer analgesics as ordered

      (i) Administer low-dose dopamine as ordered, to increase splanchnic blood flow

      (j) Administer nitroglycerin as ordered, to decrease abdominal pain

      (k) Administer parenteral nutritional support as ordered

      (l) Treat fever as ordered

      (m) Prepare patient for abdominal surgery; educate patient and family about abdominal surgery

    iv. Evaluation of nursing care

      (a) Patient is comfortable after surgery

      (b) Patient has adequate circulating plasma volume

      (c) Patient or family can state importance of pulmonary hygiene after surgery

b. Potential for impaired gas exchange, related to general anesthesia, abdominal surgery, decreased mobility

    i. Assessment for defining characteristics

      (a) Altered level of consciousness

      (b) Endotracheal intubation, mechanical ventilation

        (1) Impairment of upper and lower respiratory tract immune defense mechanisms

        (2) At risk for pulmonary complications

          a) Airway obstruction

          b) Hypoventilation, atelectasis

          c) Pneumonia

          d) Aspiration

          e) Pulmonary embolism

      (c) Abdominal surgical incisions

        (1) Pain

        (2) Reluctance to breathe deeply or cough

        (3) At risk for wound infection

          a) Wound dehiscence

          b) Evisceration of intestine

        (4) Presence of tubes or drains

      (d) Paralytic ileus

        (1) General anesthesia

        (2) Surgical manipulation of intestine

        (3) Electrolyte imbalances

      (e) Urinary bladder catheterization; at risk for urinary tract infection

    ii. Expected outcomes

      (a) Absence of pulmonary complications

      (b) Absence of infection

    iii. Nursing interventions

      (a) Institute pulmonary hygiene measures

        (1) Assess breath sounds

        (2) Assist patient with coughing and deep breathing

        (3) Turn patient from side to side frequently

      (b) Institute measures to wean patient from mechanical ventilation as ordered. Assess pulmonary function and arterial blood gases

   (c) Have patient ambulate as soon as tolerated

   (d) Institute pain management measures; administer analgesics as ordered

   (e) Maintain patent nasogastric tube until ileus resolves. Assess bowel sounds

   (f) Maintain incisional site or wound care as ordered. Assess surgical incision site or wound for signs of infection

     (1) Tenderness along incision site or wound

     (2) Reddened area around incision site or wound

     (3) Abnormal drainage (color, odor, consistency, purulence) from incision site or wound or associated tubes or drains

   (g) Administer fluid and electrolytes as ordered

  iv. Evaluation of nursing care

   (a) Patient is weaned from mechanical ventilation in a timely manner

   (b) Patient ambulates in a timely manner

   (c) Patient's surgical incision site or wound heals without complications

 c. Risk for fluid volume deficit, related to third-space fluid loss, bowel obstruction, or hemorrhage (see Commonly Encountered Nursing Diagnoses section)

 d. Altered nutrition, less than body requirements, related to major tissue destruction, hypermetabolic state (see Commonly Encountered Nursing Diagnoses section)

 e. Infection, related to peritonitis, abdominal abscess (see Chapter 6, Commonly Encountered Nursing Diagnoses section, altered protection subsection, risk for infection)

Abdominal Trauma

1. Pathophysiology

 a. Injuries occurring from the nipple line to mid-thigh are considered abdominal trauma

 b. Often involves injury to multiple organs

 c. Types of injury

  i. Blood vessel injury

  ii. Laceration of abdominal organ

  iii. Contusion of abdominal organ

  iv. Crush injury with tissue damage and hemorrhage

2. Etiologic or precipitating factors

 a. Penetrating abdominal trauma

  i. Knife (stab) wounds

  ii. Other sharp objects: ice pick, metal objects, wooden objects

  iii. Impalement on sharp object

  iv. Gunshot: visceral injury possible even when bullet does not penetrate abdomen; caused by blast effect; caliber of bullet important

  v. Lower chest wounds can also produce intra-abdominal visceral injury

 b. Blunt abdominal trauma

  i. Moving vehicular crashes: most common cause

   (a) Not wearing seatbelt

(b) Seatbelt-related injuries

(c) Steering wheel injury

(d) Acceleration-deceleration injuries in passengers and pedestrians

(e) Being thrown from vehicle

   ii. Falls

  iii. Physical violence: punch, kick, use of blunt object, rape

  iv. Sports injuries

   v. Crush injuries

  c. Abdominal trauma may be part of a multiple trauma situation

3. Nursing assessment data base

  a. Nursing history

    i. Subjective findings: abdominal pain, tenderness

   ii. Objective findings: vary with etiology and the organs affected

(a) History of blunt or abdominal penetrating trauma

(b) History of multiple traumatic injuries

(c) History of lower chest injury

(d) History of moving vehicular crash

(e) History of alcohol or drug use

  b. Nursing examination of patient

    i. Inspection

(a) Increased abdominal girth

(b) Halstead's sign: marbled appearance of abdomen

(c) Cullen's sign: bluish discoloration of the periumbilical area

(d) Turner's sign: bluish discoloration of flanks

(e) Coopernail sign: bruising of the scrotum or labia

(f) Peritoneal lavage: reveals blood in peritoneal cavity ("beef broth" tap), urine, bile, or feces

(g) Entrance and exit wounds

(h) Impalement of foreign object

(i) Skin pallor

(j) Respiratory difficulty

   ii. Auscultation

(a) Diminished or absent breath sounds

(b) Abdominal bruit

(c) Orthostatic hypotension

(d) Decreased pulse pressure

  iii. Percussion

(a) Dullness, indicating fluid in abdomen

(b) Hyperresonance, indicating a perforated viscus

  iv. Palpation

(a) Abdominal tenderness, pain with guarding

(b) Rebound tenderness

(c) Diminished or absent femoral pulses

  c. Diagnostic study findings

    i. Laboratory findings

(a) Decreased hemoglobin, hematocrit

(b) Increased serum amylase

(c) Increased WBC count

(d) Hematuria

(e) High alcohol blood level

(f) Positive urine toxicology screen

          (g) Stool guaiac test result positive for occult blood
      ii. Radiologic findings
          (a) Abdominal x-ray: loss of psoas shadow, indicating retroperitoneal bleeding, free air in abdomen, location of bullet
          (b) Chest x-ray: fractured ribs
          (c) Arteriogram: may show vascular injuries
          (d) Liver and spleen scan
          (e) Intravenous pyelogram if blood in urine
          (f) Abdominal or pelvic CT scan: hematoperitoneum, retroperitoneal hematoma, liver or spleen fracture, ruptured viscus
      iii. Other diagnostic findings: rectal examination may show presence of blood
  4. Nursing diagnoses
    a. Risk for fluid volume deficit, related to hemorrhage, sepsis (see Commonly Encountered Nursing Diagnoses section)
    b. Nutrition altered, less than body requirements, related to major tissue destruction, hypermetabolic state (see Commonly Encountered Nursing Diagnoses section)
    c. Infection, related to peritonitis, abdominal abscess (see Chapter 6, Commonly Encountered Nursing Diagnoses section, Altered Protection subsection, risk for infection)
    d. Pain (acute), related to surgery, trauma (see Chapter 9, Commonly Encountered Nursing Diagnoses section, pain subsection)

Inflammatory Bowel Disease

1. **Crohn's disease** (regional enteritis, granulomatous colitis, granulomatous ileitis, transmural disease)
    a. Pathophysiology
      i. Recurrent, chronic inflammation of the entire intestinal wall
          (a) Can involve one or more areas of any portion of the GI tract from the mouth to the anus
             (1) Ascending and transverse colon most common sites
             (2) Intermittent (''skip'') lesions common in large or small intestine
          (b) Inflammation begins in the intestinal mucosa and spreads inward and outward to involve the mucosa and serosa
          (c) Bowel becomes congested, thickened, and rigid, with adhesions
          (d) Edema and thickening of the muscularis mucosa may narrow the lumen of the involved colon
          (e) Anal and perianal fistulas and abscesses
          (f) Ulcerations produce fissures that extend inflammation into the lymphoid tissue: granulomatous lesions
          (g) Development of colon cancer is rare
      ii. Associated with multiple systemic manifestations
          (a) Acute manifestations
             (1) Toxic megacolon
             (2) GI hemorrhage
             (3) Perforation of the ileum

(4) Bowel obstruction: increased motility of intestine proximal to obstruction; watery stools; abdominal distention. Stagnation of intestinal contents: bacterial proliferation, alteration of pH, decreased reabsorption of bile

(b) Chronic manifestations

(1) Rheumatoid arthritis

(2) Iritis, scleritis

(3) Sclerosing cholangitis

(4) Urinary tract calculi, obstruction

(5) Iron-deficiency anemia

b. Etiologic or precipitating factors

i. Exact etiology unknown; possible causes include bacterial, viral, allergic, autoimmune, and hereditary factors

ii. Prevalence equal in men and women; most common age at onset is 10 to 30 years

iii. Autoimmune disorders common

iv. Familial predisposition

v. Increased suppressor T-cell activity

vi. Alterations in IgA production

c. Nursing assessment data base

i. Nursing history

(a) Subjective findings

(1) Crampy abdominal pain most often associated with eating. Initially: constant right-sided pain mimics appendicitis

(2) Watery diarrhea

(3) Meals omitted to avoid pain

(b) Objective findings

(1) Weight loss

(2) Malnutrition

(3) Vitamin B_{12} deficiency in Crohn's disease and ulcerative colitis involving the ileum

(4) Steatorrhea

(5) Disease recurs after surgical intervention

ii. Nursing examination of patient

(a) Inspection

(1) Cachexia

(2) Watery stool

(3) Anal excoriation

(4) Malaise

(5) Pallor

(b) Auscultation

(1) Hyperperistalsis

(2) Decreased breath sounds as a result of pain

(c) Percussion: hypertympanic bowel

(d) Palpation

(1) Abdominal tenderness, pain

(2) Abdominal mass common

iii. Diagnostic study findings

(a) Laboratory findings

(1) Decreased hemoglobin, hematocrit

(2) Increased WBC count

(3) Increased alkaline phosphatase

(4) Decreased serum potassium

(5) Decreased serum albumin

(6) Occult blood in stool

(b) Radiologic findings: "string sign" (irregular narrowing of distal ileum) on abdominal x-ray

(c) Other diagnostic findings

(1) Sigmoidoscopy: inflammation of the intestinal mucosa and surrounding musculature, as well as associated findings outlined earlier

    a) Longitudinal and transverse ulcers (cobblestoning)

    b) Stenosis of intestinal lumen

(2) Colonoscopy: to determine extent of disease found on sigmoidoscopy

(3) Rectal biopsy: inflammation of the intestinal mucosa and surrounding musculature, as well as associated findings outlined earlier

d. Nursing diagnoses: At risk for infection, related to alteration in mucosal protection of GI tract

  i. Assessment for defining characteristics

(a) Fever

(b) Cachexia

(c) Malaise

(d) Increased heart rate

(e) Watery, foul-smelling diarrhea

(f) Pus in stool

(g) Blood cultures positive for enteric organisms

  ii. Expected outcomes

(a) Patient will be normothermic

(b) Blood cultures will be negative

(c) Patient will verbalize symptomatic relief from abdominal pain

(d) Patient will verbalize symptomatic relief from diarrhea

  iii. Nursing interventions

(a) Administer analgesics and corticosteroids for symptomatic relief of abdominal pain as ordered

(b) Administer antidiarrheal agents as ordered

(c) Administer antibiotics as ordered

(d) Administer iron, vitamin B_{12}, and folic acid as ordered, for treatment of anemia

(e) Administer parenteral nutritional support as ordered, to rest intestine and replete nutritional deficits

(f) Prepare patient for surgery if necessary

(g) Assess patient's needs for postoperative rehabilitation program if ostomy surgery is indicated

  iv. Evaluation of nursing care

(a) Temperature maintained below 99°F

(b) Negative blood cultures

(c) Absence of pus in stool

(d) Symptoms from diarrhea are minimized

(e) Abdominal pain is minimized

2. Ulcerative colitis
   a. Pathophysiology
      i. Idiopathic inflammation involving the mucosa of the colon
         (a) Uniform inflammation of the mucosal lining of the colon and rectum, no "skip" lesions
         (b) Inflammation begins at the base of the crypt of Lieberkühn; small erosions form and coalesce into ulcers, followed by abscess formation, necrosis, and ragged ulcerations of the mucosa
         (c) Begins in the rectum and progresses proximally in the colon
         (d) Toxic megacolon is associated with fulminant disease: loss of contractility and massive dilatation of the large colon
      ii. Friable colon
      iii. Risk of colon cancer increases significantly after 10 years of ulcerative colitis
   b. Etiologic or precipitating factors
      i. Etiology unknown: genetic, infectious, and immunologic factors suspected
      ii. Autoimmune disorders common
      iii. Prevalence greater among women; most common age at onset is 10 to 40 years
      iv. Prevalence greater among patients of Jewish descent
   c. Nursing assessment data base
      i. Nursing history
         (a) Subjective findings
            (1) Bloody, purulent, watery diarrhea: up to 30 stools per day
            (2) Sensation of rectal urgency
            (3) Crampy pain
         (b) Objective findings
            (1) Bright red blood in stool
            (2) Pus in stool
            (3) Orthostasis
            (4) Abdominal pain
            (5) Weight loss
            (6) Vomiting
            (7) Fever
            (8) Dehydration
            (9) Extracolonic manifestations
               a) Arthritis
               b) Iritis
               c) Skin lesions
               d) Hepatic dysfunction
               e) Anemia
      ii. Nursing examination of patient
         (a) Inspection
            (1) Bloody diarrhea
            (2) Cachexia
            (3) Malaise
            (4) Pallor
            (5) Decreased skin turgor
         (b) Auscultation
            (1) Hyperperistalsis
            (2) Decreased breath sounds as a result of pain

(3) Increased heart rate

(c) Percussion: hypertympanic bowel

(d) Palpation: abdominal tenderness, pain

iii. Diagnostic study findings

(a) Laboratory findings

(1) Decreased hemoglobin, hematocrit

(2) Increased WBC count

(3) Increased alkaline phosphatase

(4) Decreased serum potassium

(5) Decreased serum albumin

(6) Occult blood in stool

(b) Radiologic findings: abdominal x-ray

(1) Crypt abscess, mucosal ulcerations

(2) Dilated loops of bowel

(c) Other diagnostic findings, proctosigmoidoscopy: diffuse erythema, mucosal inflammation, and loss of vascular network

(1) Mucosal bleeding induced by gentle touch

(2) Ulcers

(3) Pseudopolyps

d. Nursing diagnoses

i. At risk for infection, related to alteration in mucosal protection of GI tract (see Crohn's Disease section)

ii. Altered nutrition, less than body requirements, related to major tissue destruction, hypermetabolic state (see Commonly Encountered Nursing Diagnoses section)

References

PHYSIOLOGIC ANATOMY

Huether, S. E.: Structure and function of the digestive tract. *In* McCance, K. L., and Huether, S. E. (eds.): Pathophysiology. The Biologic Basis for Disease in Adults and Children. St. Louis, Mosby–Year Book, 1990.

Huether, S. E., McCance, K. L., and Tarmina, M. S.: Alterations of digestive function. *In* McCance, K. L., and Huether, S. E. (eds.): Pathophysiology. The Biologic Basis for Disease in Adults and Children. St. Louis, Mosby–Year Book, 1990.

Krumberger, J. M.: Gastrointestinal anatomy and physiology. *In* Kinney, M. R., Packa, D. R., and Dunbar, S. B. (eds.): AACN's Clinical Reference for Critical-Care Nursing. St. Louis, Mosby–Year Book, 1993.

Westfall, U. E., and Heitkemper, M.: Gastrointestinal physiology. *In* Clochesy, J. M., Breu, C., Cardin, S., et al. (eds.): Critical Care Nursing, 2nd ed. Philadelphia, W. B. Saunders, 1996.

NURSING ASSESSMENT DATA BASE

Gibson, R. S.: Principles of Nutritional Assessment. New York, Oxford University Press, 1990.

Johnson, D. A., and Cattau, E. L.: Pharmacologic approach to gastrointestinal disease in critical illness. *In* Chernow, B. (ed.): Essentials of Critical Care Pharmacology. Baltimore, Williams & Wilkins, 1990.

Krumberger, J. M.: Gastrointestinal data acquisition. *In*

Kinney, M. R., Packa, D. R., and Dunbar, S. B. (eds.): AACN's Clinical Reference for Critical-Care Nursing. St. Louis, Mosby–Year Book, 1993.

Quinn, A.: Special procedures used in the diagnosis and treatment of gastrointestinal problems. *In* Boggs, R. L., and Woolridge-King, M. (eds.): AACN Procedure Manual for Critical Care. Philadelphia, W. B. Saunders, 1993.

Ross, L. H., and Grant, J. P.: Parenteral nutrition. *In* Chernow, B. (ed.): Essentials of Critical Care Pharmacology. Baltimore, Williams & Wilkins, 1990.

Shuster, M. H.: Nutrition in the critically ill. *In* Clochesy, J. M., Breu, C., Cardin, S., et al. (eds.): Critical Care Nursing, 2nd ed. Philadelphia, W. B. Saunders, 1996.

COMMONLY ENCOUNTERED NURSING DIAGNOSES

Gibson, R. S.: Principles of Nutritional Assessment. New York, Oxford University Press, 1990.

Hathaway, R. G.: Nursing Care of the Critically Ill Surgical Patient. Rockville, Md., Aspen Publications, 1988.

Kim, M. J., McFarland, G., and McLane, A. M. (eds.): Pocket Guide to Nursing Diagnoses, 6th ed. St. Louis, Mosby–Year Book, 1995.

Ross, L. H., and Grant, J. P.: Parenteral nutrition. *In* Chernow, B. (ed.): Essentials of Critical Care Pharmacology. Baltimore, Williams & Wilkins, 1990.

Shuster, M. H.: Nutrition in the critically ill. *In* Clochesy, J. M., Breu, C., Cardin, S., et al. (eds.): Critical Care Nursing, 2nd ed. Philadelphia, W. B. Saunders, 1996.

PATIENT HEALTH PROBLEMS

D'Amico, G., Pagliaro, L., and Bosch, J.: Treatment of portal hypertension: A meta-analysis review. Hepatology 22:332–354, 1995.

Hathaway, R. G.: Nursing Care of the Critically Ill Surgical Patient. Rockville, Md., Aspen Publications, 1988.

Hennessy, K.: Patients with acute pancreatitis. *In* Clochesy, J. M., Breu, C., Cardin, S., et al. (eds.): Critical Care Nursing, 2nd ed. Philadelphia, W. B. Saunders, 1996.

Hoofnagle, J. H., Carithers, R. L., Shapiro, C., and Ascher, N.: Fulminant hepatic failure: Summary of a workshop. Hepatology 21:240–252, 1995.

Johnson, D. A., and Cattau, E. L.: Pharmacologic approach to gastrointestinal disease in critical illness. *In* Chernow, B. (ed.): Essentials of Critical Care Pharmacology. Baltimore, Williams & Wilkins, 1990.

Krumberger, J. M.: Gastrointestinal disorders. *In* Kinney, M. R., Packa, D. R., and Dunbar, S. B. (eds.): AACN's Clinical Reference for Critical-Care Nursing. St. Louis, Mosby–Year Book, 1993.

Lohrman, J. M.: Hepatic dysfunction and Kupffer cell activity. *In* Huddleston, V. B. (ed.): Multisystem Organ Failure. Pathophysiology and Clinical Implications. St. Louis, Mosby–Year Book, 1992.

Murphy, G. P., Lawrence, W., and Lenhard, R. E.: American Cancer Society Textbook of Clinical Oncology, 2nd ed. Atlanta, American Cancer Society, 1995.

O'Neill, P. L.: Gastrointestinal system: Target organ and source. *In* Huddleston, V. B. (ed.): Multisystem Organ Failure. Pathophysiology and Clinical Implications. St. Louis, Mosby–Year Book, 1992.

Quinn, A.: Management of gastrointestinal disorders. *In* Boggs, R. L., and Woolridge-King, M. (eds.): AACN Procedure Manual for Critical Care. Philadelphia, W. B. Saunders, 1993.

Ross, L. H., and Grant, J. P.: Parenteral nutrition. *In* Chernow, B. (ed.): Essentials of Critical Care Pharmacology. Baltimore, Williams & Wilkins, 1990.

Ruppert, S. D., and Englert, D. M.: Patients with gastrointestinal bleeding. *In* Clochesy, J. M., Breu, C., Cardin, S., et al. (eds.): Critical Care Nursing, 2nd ed. Philadelphia, W. B. Saunders, 1996.

Schiffman, M. L., Jeffers, L., Hoofnagle, J. H., and Tralka, T. S.: The role of transjugular intrahepatic portal systemic shunt for treatment of portal hypertension and its complications: A conference sponsored by the National Digestive Diseases Advisory Board. Hepatology 22:1591–1597, 1995.

Shuster, M. H.: Nutrition in the critically ill. *In* Clochesy, J. M., Breu, C., Cardin, S., et al. (eds.): Critical Care Nursing, 2nd ed. Philadelphia, W. B. Saunders, 1996.

Smith, S. L.: Patients with liver dysfunction. *In* Clochesy, J. M., Breu, C., Cardin, S., et al. (eds.): Critical Care Nursing, 2nd ed. Philadelphia, W. B. Saunders, 1996.

Smith, S. L., and Butler, R. W.: Acute Pancreatitis. Aliso Viejo, Calif., AACN, 1993.

Smith, S. L., and Ciferni, M.: Liver transplantation. *In* Smith, S. L. (ed.): Tissue and Organ Transplantation: Implications for Professional Nursing Practice. St. Louis, Mosby–Year Book, 1990.

Smith, S. L., and Ciferni, M.: Liver transplantation for acute hepatic failure: A review of clinical experience and management. Am. J. Crit. Care 2:137–144, 1992.

Smith, S. L., and Ciferni, M. L.: Liver transplantation. Crit. Care Nurs. Clin. North Am. 4:131–148, 1992.

8

:... Multisystem

Marilyn Sawyer Sommers, R.N., Ph.D., CCRN

PATIENT HEALTH PROBLEMS

Systemic Inflammatory Response Syndrome and Septic Shock

1. **Pathophysiology**
   a. Overview and definitions: definitions developed by a consensus conference and reported in Bone and colleagues (1992)
      i. *Systemic inflammatory response syndrome (SIRS):* systemic inflammatory response to a variety of severe clinical insults, such as pancreatitis, ischemia or reperfusion, multiple trauma and tissue injury, hemorrhagic shock, and immune-mediated organ injury
         (a) Response is manifested by two or more of the following conditions:
             (1) Temperature above 38°C or below 36°C
             (2) Heart rate above 90 beats/minute
             (3) Respiratory rate above 20 breaths/minute or PaCO$_2$ below 32 mm Hg
             (4) White blood cell (WBC) count above 12,000/mm^3 or below 4000/mm^3 or above 10% immature (band) forms
         (b) The condition is called SIRS because, in addition to infectious insults, other conditions (Fig. 8–1) also cause a systemic inflammatory response without infection
      ii. *Infection:* microbial phenomenon characterized by an inflammatory response to the presence of microorganisms or the invasion of normally sterile host tissue by organisms
      iii. *Bacteremia:* presence of viable bacteria in blood
      iv. *Sepsis:* systemic response to infection, manifested by two or more of four conditions that define SIRS (see preceding)
      v. *Severe sepsis:* sepsis associated with organ dysfunction, hypoperfusion, or hypotension. Hypoperfusion and perfusion abnormalities may include, but are not limited to, lactic acidosis, oliguria, and acute alterations in mental status

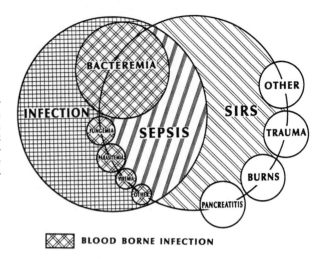

Figure 8–1 • Interrelationship between systemic inflammatory response syndrome (SIRS), sepsis, and infection. (From Bone, R. C., Balk, R. A., Cerra, F. B., et al.: Definitions for sepsis and organ failure and guidelines for the use of innovative therapies in sepsis. Chest 101:1645, 1992.)

vi. *Septic shock:* sepsis-induced state with hypotension despite adequate fluid resuscitation along with the presence of perfusion abnormalities that may include, but are not limited to, lactic acidosis, oliguria, and acute alterations in mental status. Patients receiving inotropic or vasopressor agents may not be hypotensive at the time that perfusion abnormalities are measured

vii. *Multiple organ dysfunction syndrome (MODS):* presence of progressive physiologic dysfunction in two or more organ systems after an acute threat to systemic homeostasis

b. Epidemiology

i. Sepsis is the 13th leading cause of death in the United States

(a) Sepsis is the leading cause of death in non-coronary intensive care units

(b) Bacteremia develops in approximately 500,000 people annually

(c) Sepsis develops in more than 400,000 people annually

(d) Septic shock develops in approximately 100,000 people annually

ii. Mortality rates: approximately 70,000 people die each year of either septic shock or bacteremia

(a) Gram-negative sepsis carries a mortality rate 20% to 50%

(b) Septic shock carries a mortality rate 40% to 60%

(c) Approximately 50,0000 people die of septic shock annually

(d) Approximately 20,000 people die of sepsis without septic shock annually

iii. Health care costs of sepsis are estimated at $5 billion to $10 billion annually

c. Cellular pathophysiology

i. Most episodes of septic shock in adults are thought to be caused by gram-negative bacteria. Septic shock associated with viral infections and gram-positive bacteria may also have mediators in common with the gram-negative bacterial cascade of events

ii. Mediators involved in the massive inflammatory reaction known as SIRS may lead to multiple organ dysfunction and are similar to those released in septic shock

iii. When phagocytic cells destroy bacteria, a cascade of events follows.

All gram-negative bacteria have a common group of molecules in the outer membrane, referred to as lipopolysaccharide (LPS) or endotoxin

   (a) LPS is composed of lipid A and a polysaccharide core linked to an "O-polysaccharide" side chain of repeating sugars
      (1) Lipid A and the polysaccharide core are identical or nearly identical in most gram-negative bacteria
      (2) O-polysaccharide varies for each specific gram-negative organism
   (b) LPS (in particular, lipid A) interacts with the body's immune system to produce a septic state
   (c) LPS binds to a circulating LPS-binding protein (LBP) to form a complex
      (1) Complex can then bind to receptors found on mononuclear leukocytes (mononcytes and macrophages)
      (2) Binding triggers causes the production of mediators known as *cytokines* (soluble molecules released from cells of the immune system whose function is to signal to other cells) (Table 8–1)

iv. Consequences of cytokine production
   (a) Systemic vasodilation with decreased afterload and hypotension
   (b) Increased capillary permeability with decreased preload, third spacing, and interstitial edema
   (c) Relative hypovolemia
   (d) Decreased tissue oxygen extraction
   (e) Platelet aggregation, fibrin deposits, and activation of a clotting cascade, leading to microcirculatory coagulation and tissue hypoxia
   (f) Multiple organ dysfunction

v. Cytokine regulation
   (a) Cytokine production and an inflammatory process are normally strongly repressed by regulatory mechanisms
   (b) Septic shock develops when homeostasis is disrupted and is associated with an overproduction of cytokines

vi. Cytokine cascade: triggering actions of LPS are not fully understood, but bacterial products stimulate production of cytokines by macrophages and monocytes
   (a) Cytokine release begins with tumor necrosis factor-alpha (TNF-α) followed by interleukin (IL)-1 and IL-6
   (b) TNF-α and IL-1 cause a variety of physiologic effects; interferon gamma, released from natural killer cells in response to TNF and bacterial products, amplifies functions of IL-1 and TNF
      (1) Increased temperature set-point, causes fever or may cause hypothermia
      (2) Decreased systemic vascular resistance, increased capillary permeability
      (3) Increased release of leukocytes from bone marrow
   (c) IL-6 is released from T cells and monocytes after tissue injury and may inhibit the release of other cytokines (TNF-α, IL-1)
   (d) Effects of cytokines are mediated at target tissues by nitric oxide,

Text continued on page 722

TABLE 8–1. Cellular Response to Cytokine and Mediator Release in Systemic Inflammatory Response Syndrome

Cytokine/Mediator/Precursor	Release	Cellular Response
Arachidonic Acid Metabolites Arachidonic acid is one of the nutritional essential fatty acids of the body; present in the cell membrane; accounts for 5% to 15% of fatty acids in phospholipids	Arachidonic acid gives rise to mediators during interactions with three enzymes: cyclooxygenase and peroxidase (cyclooxygenase pathway) and lipoxygenase (lipoxygenase pathway) Arachidonic acid gives rise to eicosanoids (physiologically active compounds known as prostaglandins, thromboxanes, and leukotrienes)	See prostaglandins, thromboxanes, and leukotrienes
Bradykinin Vasoactive peptide generated by the kinin system	Bacterial product TNF-α and IL-1 activate Hageman factor, which stimulates release	Vasodilation, hypotension Increased vessel permeability
Histamine Vasoactive amine released from mast cells and basophil granules	C5a of complement cascade binds to mast cells and triggers release	Increased vessel permeability Vasodilation Hypotension
Interleukins Group of molecules involved in signaling between immune system cells	***IL-1*** Bacterial products stimulate release of IL-1 from macrophages, monocytes, lymphocytes, neutrophils, and endothelial cells Similar to TNF-α; related in response; has a synergistic effect Increases in concentration as a "second wave" to TNF-α	Cytokine production (TNF-α, IL-6, IL-8, PAF, leukotrienes, thromboxane, prostaglandins, and itself) Activation of T and B cells, natural killer cells, neutrophils Vasodilation, hypotension Increased vessel permeability Fever, sleep, anorexia Myocardial depression, hypercoagulability, and ACTH release
	IL-6 Released early in sepsis in the presence of bacterial products, TNF-α, and IL-1 Produced by monocytes, macrophages, lymphocytes, and endothelial cells	Fever Cortisol production Decreased IL-1 and TNF-α production Activation of T and B cells Hepatic synthesis of acute-phase proteins

TABLE 8–1. Cellular Response to Cytokine and Mediator Release in Systemic Inflammatory Response Syndrome *Continued*

Cytokine/Mediator/Precursor	Release	Cellular Response
IL-8 (neutrophil-activating factor)	C5a, bacterial products, IL-1, and TNF-α are potent stimulators Produced by macrophages, monocytes, lymphocytes, and endothelial cells	Attraction of PMNs to participate in inflammatory response; stimulation of PMNs to have oxidative burst, degranulation, and release of proteases Tissue damage, cell aggregation Increased vessel permeability
Interferon-γ Molecules involved in signaling among cells of immune system	Released from natural killer cells and T cells in response to TNF-α and IL-1	Enhanced release and amplified actions of TNF-α and IL-1 Increased number of TNF-α receptors on macrophages, making them more sensitive to TNF-α effects Antiviral effect
Leukotrienes Metabolites of arachidonic acid produced in lipoxygenase pathway	PLA$_2$ enzymes, found in most cells, are secreted during shock and in response to TNF-α IL-1, IL-8, complement PLA$_2$ triggers the release of fatty acids, such as arachidonic acid, from many body cells, which triggers leukotriene production Leukotrienes produced from neutrophils, monocytes, and eosinophils in response to PAF, TNF-α, and IL-1	Tissue inflammation Vessel damage Increased permeability of vessels Accumulation of PMNs Vascular and airway construction Vasodilation
MCP-1 Molecules involved in signaling between cells of immune system	Bacterial products, activated complement, and cytokines activate PMNs, monocytes, and endothelial cells to produce MCP-1	Chemotactic agent attracting monocytes and macrophages Oxidative burst from cells increasing metabolism Degranulation Release of proteases with vessel damage and increased vessel permeability
Myocardial Depressant Factors Circulating molecules that may lead to development of myocardial dysfunction	Circulating factors from uncertain origin (specific factors have not been isolated)	Decreased myocardial contractility Decreased ejection fraction Ventricular dilation

Table continued on following page

TABLE 8–1. Cellular Response to Cytokine and Mediator Release in Systemic Inflammatory Response Syndrome *Continued*

Cytokine/Mediator/Precursor	Release	Cellular Response
Nitric Oxide Molecule synthesized by NOS thought to be endothelium-derived relaxant factor	Normally continuously produced by the endothelium; regulates leukocyte adhesion; affects adhesion of platelets and monocytes Released from many body cells in response to LPS, cytokines, and activated mediators Two forms of NOS: inducible form (iNOS), whose production is stimulated by LPS and cytokines; constitutive NOS (cNOS), normally produced in vascular endothelium	Smooth muscle relaxation, vasodilation, hypotension (*Note:* iNOS has a greater potential to produce pathologic hypotension than cNOS does) May depress myocardial function Increased capillary permeability May block platelet aggregation and adhesion
PAF Phospholipid produced by a variety of cells, including endothelium, basophils, and leukocytes	PLA_2 enzymes, found in most cells, are secreted during shock and in response to LPS, TNF-α, IL-1, IL-8, complement, and other cytokines PLA_2 triggers the release of lipid mediators, including PAF, from many body cells	Activation of neutrophils and endothelium; amplification of SIRS Tissue inflammation; may be neurotoxic, GI tract ulceration; vessel damage Increased permeability of vessels; decreased myocardial contractility; vasodilation; hypotension Platelet aggregation; WBC activation
Prostaglandins Metabolites of arachidonic acid produced in cyclooxygenase pathway; 20 carbon unsaturated fatty acids synthesized by most organs of the body	PLA_2 enzymes, found in most cells, are secreted during shock and in response to LPS, TNF-α, IL-1, PAF, complement, thrombin, and other cytokines; PLA_2 causes release of arachidonic acid from the cell membrane and production of prostaglandins Two main types: PGE_2 and PGI_2; prostacyclin	Vasodilation and increased blood flow Fever, immune modulation, lymphocyte inhibitor PGD_2 is produced by mast cells and leads to vasodilation; bronchial constriction PGI_2 inhibits platelet aggregation
Serotonin Monoamine present in platelets and GI tract	Complement C5a stimulates production	Vasodilation; hypotension Increased vessel permeability

TABLE 8–1. Cellular Response to Cytokine and Mediator Release in Systemic Inflammatory Response Syndrome *Continued*

Cytokine/Mediator/Precursor	Release	Cellular Response
Thromboxane A$_2$ Metabolites of arachidonic acid produced in cyclooxygenase pathway	PLA$_2$ enzymes, found in most cells, are secreted during shock and in response to LPS, TNF-α, IL-1, PAF, complement, and thrombin; PLA$_2$ causes release of arachidonic acid from cell membrane and production of thromboxane A$_2$ Synthesized by platelets	Inflammation Platelet aggregation; PMN adherence Increased vascular permeability Vasoconstriction
TNF-α Polypeptide secretory product of monocyte-macrophage system	Released from mononuclear phagocytes in response to LPS Plasma levels rise immediately after administration of endotoxin; levels reach peak before fever, WBCs, or stress hormone levels increase	Increased formation of oxygen radicals; injury to lungs, GI tract, kidney Increased cytokine production (IL-1, IL-6, IL-8, PAF); mediates and replicates all effects of LPS; stimulates arachidonic acid metabolism and production of leukotrienes, thromboxane, prostaglandins, and further production of TNF-α Initial hyperglycemia followed by hypoglycemia; hypotension, metabolic acidosis, coagulopathy Fever, increased oxygen consumption, sleep, anorexia Increased capillary permeability, vasodilation, microvascular constriction Activation of coagulation cascade Activation of NOS to produce NO TNF-β also produced with similar effects

ACTH = adrenocorticotropic hormone; GI = gastrointestinal; IFN = interferon; IL = interleukin; LPS = lipopolysaccharide (endotoxin); MCP-1 = monocyte chemoattractant protein 1; NO = nitric oxide; NOS = nitric oxide synthase; PAF = platelet activating factor; PG = prostaglandin; PLA$_2$ = phospholipase A$_2$; PMNs = polymorphonuclear cells; SIRS = systemic inflammatory response syndrome; TNF = tumor necrosis factor; WBC = white blood cell.

arachidonic acid metabolites (prostaglandins, eicosanoids, platelet-activating factor [PAF]), and lipoxygenase derivatives

(e) TNF-α and IL-1 stimulate production of other cytokines, which leads to a cascade effect with complex amplification and modulation (upregulation and downregulation)

(1) IL-8 induces chemotaxis of activated polymorphonuclear leukocytes and acts as an inflammatory mediator, leading to tissue damage

(2) TNF and IL-1 activate the coagulation cascade

  a) Bacterial products, TNF, and IL-1 induce intravascular coagulation and fibrin deposits

  b) Thromboplastin (factor III) and factor VIII activate the extrinsic coagulation pathway

  c) Factor XII (Hageman factor) activates the intrinsic coagulation pathway

(3) TNF and IL-1 activate the complement (C) cascade by factor XII and bacterial products

  a) C5a component (one of more than 20 proteins involved in the C cascade) is a vasoactive anaphylatoxin that binds to macrophages and monocytes

  b) Complement C stimulates an oxidative burst

  c) Complement C causes the release of oxygen radicals and proteases that damage cells, particularly type II pneumonocytes in lungs

  d) Complement C enhances adherence to endothelium with degranulation (emptying out granules with digestive substances) and aggregation (clumping), leading to microvasculature damage

  e) C5a binds to mast cells, basophils, and platelets to cause the release of histamine, serotonin, prostaglandins, and leukotrienes, resulting in vessel dilation, increased blood flow, increased capillary permeability, and increased plasma leakage

  f) C5a leads to the release of more TNF-α, IL-1, and IL-8

(4) TNF and IL-1 activate the kinin cascade with the production of bradykinin

  a) Potent vasodilator

  b) Increased vascular permeability

d. Role of microbial translocation: controversial theory in humans; describes the passage of microbes or microbial products such as LPS across an injured intestinal mucosal wall from the gut lumen to outside the gut lumen; may be a major contributor to the development of the septic cascade

  i. Common enteric organisms: *Enterococcus, Escherichia coli, Clostridium perfringens, Enterobacter cloacae*

  ii. Conditions that are thought to increase gut permeability and microbial translocation

    (a) Mucosal ischemia and mucosal hypoperfusion caused by shock or mesenteric vasoconstriction from intense sympathetic nervous system stimulation

    (b) Immunoglobulin A (IgA) deficit associated with total parenteral nutrition, thermal injury, glucocorticoid administration, and endotoxin release

(c) Glutamine and fiber deficiencies

(d) Alteration of normal flora

iii. Conditions that contribute to microbial translocation include obstructive jaundice, burns, endotoxemia, hemorrhage, immunosuppression, malnutrition, ischemia, reperfusion injury, total parenteral nutrition, and antibiotic therapy

2. **Etiologic or precipitating factors**

a. Gram-negative organisms account for approximately half of all cases of septic shock and most cases of septic shock in adults

i. Most common sites of origin of bacteremia and sepsis

(a) Urinary tract

(b) Gastrointestinal tract

(c) Respiratory tract

(d) Skin and wounds

ii. Most common organisms in hospitalized patients: gram-negative aerobes

(a) *E. coli*

(b) *Klebsiella* and *Enterobacter* species

(c) *Pseudomonas aeruginosa*

iii. Other gram-negative aerobes: *Serratia marcescens* and *Proteus mirabilis*

b. Other organisms

i. Infections with gram-positive organism are becoming increasingly more common because these organisms are associated with the use of intravenous (IV) catheters and invasive devices. Most common aerobic organisms:

(a) *Staphylococcus aureus* and *Staphylococcus epidermidis*

(b) *Streptococcus viridans* and *Streptococcus pneumoniae*

(c) *Streptococcus defectivus* and *Streptococcus adjacens* (also known as nutritionally variant streptococci)

(d) *Pneumococcus*

(e) *Enterococcus faecalis*

ii. Others

(a) Viruses, protozoa, parasites

(b) Fungi, such as *Candida albicans*

(c) Anaerobic organisms: *Clostridium, Bacteroides fragilis*

c. Predisposing factors for development of bacteremia or sepsis

i. Extremes of age: very old and very young

ii. Granulocytopenia

iii. Prior antibiotic therapy

iv. Severe burn injury, recent trauma, recent surgical procedures, and invasive procedures

v. Functional asplenia

vi. Immunosuppression: infection with human immunodeficiency virus (HIV), chemotherapy, corticosteroids, and bone marrow suppression

vii. Malnutrition and total parenteral nutrition

viii. Alcohol use and abuse; other drugs of abuse

ix. Prolonged intensive care unit stay

(a) Endotracheal intubation longer than 48 hours (aspiration of pharyngeal secretions, contaminated respiratory equipment)

        (b) Ventilator-associated pneumonia

           (1) Most important cause of infections acquired in intensive care units (ICUs)

           (2) Leading cause of death from nosocomial infections

3. Nursing assessment data base

  a. Nursing history

    i. Patient health history

      (a) Significant past medical and surgical history, with a review of all major systems and the identification of recent invasive procedures

        (1) History of chronic disease (diabetes mellitus, alcoholism, and liver, heart, and renal failure) places patients at risk

        (2) Acute illnesses: traumatic injury, burns, cholelithiasis, intestinal obstruction, pancreatitis, appendicitis, peritonitis, and diverticulitis

        (3) Wounds

      (b) Medications, especially those with immunosuppressive properties (chemotherapy, corticosteroids) and antibiotics

      (c) Nutrition history, with a special focus on malnutrition and alcohol use

      (d) Social history: significant others, ability of patient and significant others to manage stress, financial obligations of patient and significant others, and parenting responsibilities of patient

    ii. Family health history: chronic disease or infections

  b. Nursing examination of patient

    i. Vital signs

      (a) Core temperature: above 38°C or below 36°C

      (b) Heart rate above 90 beats/minute

      (c) Respiratory rate: above 20 breaths/minute

      (d) Blood pressure: below 90 mm Hg systolic or:

        (1) Fall in systolic blood pressure of more than 40 mm Hg

        (2) Diastolic blood pressure below 70 mm Hg

      (e) Hemodynamic variables

        (1) Cardiac output/index: usually elevated; above 7 L/minute and 4 L/minute/m², may be low in elderly patients or those with underlying cardiac disorders

        (2) Systemic vascular resistance: below 900 dynes/second/cm^{-5}

        (3) Pulmonary artery wedge pressure (PAWP): normal to low; below 6 mm Hg

        (4) Oxygen delivery and consumption: variable but often decreased as septic shock progresses; oxygen extraction (normally 20% to 25%) below 20% of oxygen delivery

          a) Experts suggest that designations of ''warm shock'' and ''cold shock'' be abandoned and the extent of tissue perfusion be used to determine extent of shock

          b) If derived hemodynamic variables (such as oxygen delivery and consumption) are not available, lactate levels or base deficit can be used (see Diagnostic study findings)

    ii. Inspection: clinical presentation may vary, depending on the patient's underlying health and organ function

       (a) Acute distress with anxiety, restlessness, confusion, and
           disorientation progressing to unresponsiveness
       (b) Flushed, warm, dry skin or pale, cold, mottled skin (particularly
           the elderly); shaking chills and shivering in some patients
       (c) Tachypnea and dyspnea
       (d) Decreased urinary output; interstitial edema
   iii. Palpation
       (a) Tachycardia with rapid, weak, and thready peripheral pulses;
           initially, pulses may be bounding and rapid with a hyperdynamic
           state
       (b) Warm skin (older patients may not present with hyperthermia
           but instead may have cool skin)
   iv. Percussion: dullness over areas of atelectasis
    v. Auscultation
       (a) Pulmonary crackles from interstitial pulmonary edema; wheezing
           without a history of bronchospastic airway disease
       (b) Hypotension; narrowed or widened pulse pressure
c. Diagnostic study findings
    i. Arterial blood gases (ABGs)
       (a) Respiratory alkalosis with $PaCO_2$ below 32 mm Hg attempting to
           compensate for metabolic acidosis, with pH below 7.35 and
           decreased bicarbonate level
       (b) Late: respiratory acidosis with $PaCO_2$ above 45 mm Hg
       (c) Progressive intrapulmonary shunt, with an increasing fraction of
           inspired oxygen needed to maintain PaO_2 and SaO_2 above 92%
   ii. Mixed venous blood gases, arterial lactate level, and base deficit
       (a) Increasing hemoglobin saturation of mixed venous blood ($S\bar{v}O_2$)
           above 80% as tissues are unable to extract oxygen that is
           delivered to them
       (b) Increasing arterial lactate level (>2 mEq/L) as cells use
           anaerobic rather than aerobic pathways for metabolism
       (c) Base deficit more negative than -5
  iii. Complete blood count (CBC) and differential: either increased
       (>12,000/mm³) or decreased (<4000/mm³) or above 10% immature
       (band) forms
   iv. Serum glucose levels: elevated from stress response
    v. Blood cultures and antibiotic sensitivities
       (a) Identify causative organisms; positive blood cultures occur in
           only 50% of septic patients for uncertain reasons (bacteremia
           may be intermittent)
       (b) Urine, sputum, and wound cultures to correlate with blood
           cultures
   vi. Elevated blood urea nitrogen (BUN) and creatinine
  vii. Coagulation studies: may show elevations in prothrombin and partial
       thromboplastin time; decreased fibrinogen level and increased fibrin
       split products
 viii. Decreased platelet levels
   ix. Elevated serum enzymes, indicating liver or cardiac impairment
4. Nursing diagnoses
   a. Altered tissue perfusion (renal, cerebral, cardiopulmonary,

gastrointestinal, peripheral) related to hypovolemia from maldistribution of perfusion

   i. Assessment for defining characteristics

     (a) Hyperdynamic state with increased cardiac output and index is the usual presentation

     (b) Increased arterial lactate levels

     (c) $S\bar{v}O_2$ above 80%; oxygen extraction ratio below 20%

     (d) Decreased urine output

     (e) Decreased gastric mucosal pH showing cellular acidosis

     (f) Diminished bowel sounds or paralytic ileus

     (g) Decreased systemic vascular resistance and hypotension (systolic blood pressure below 90 mm Hg)

     (h) Changes in sensorium (restlessness, anxiety, and disorientation progressing to unresponsiveness)

   ii. Expected outcomes

     (a) Oxygen delivery and oxygen consumption are normal or supranormal

     (b) $S\bar{v}O_2$ is 65% to 75%, and the oxygen extraction ratio is improved (>20%)

     (c) Arterial lactate levels are normal

     (d) Urine output is 1 ml/kg/hour

     (e) Systolic blood pressure is above 90 mm Hg and normal systemic vascular resistance

     (f) Bowel sounds are active, and there is no abdominal distention

     (g) Sensorium is clear, with the patient oriented to time, place, and person

   iii. Nursing interventions

     (a) Monitor hemodynamic parameters and mixed venous oxygen saturation along with derived parameters, such as systemic vascular resistance, oxygen delivery, and oxygen consumption

     (b) Be prepared to administer fluid resuscitation

       (1) Possible suggested end point is a pulmonary artery wedge pressure of 12 mm Hg but varies, depending on the patient's underlying condition

       (2) Type of fluid (colloid versus crystalloid) is controversial; may need blood transfusion if hemoglobin count is low

       (3) See nursing interventions for hypovolemic shock

     (c) Be prepared to administer vasoactive medications as needed if fluid resuscitation fails to maintain blood pressure and organ perfusion

       (1) Dopamine (DA) is the most commonly used initial catecholamine

         a) Often in low doses (1 to 5 μg/kg/minute) for positive inotropic effects and ability to improve renal and splanchnic blood flow

         b) May be used in higher doses (5 to 15 μg/kg/minute) to support blood pressure

       (2) Dobutamine may be used for inotropic effects for myocardial depression but is used with caution in hypotensive patients (or use with α-adrenergic stimulants) because it reduces systemic vascular resistance

(3) Norepinephrine (NE) use is increasing in patients with septic shock who do not respond to fluid resuscitation
    a) Studies indicate that renal function in patients with sepsis receiving NE alone or in combination with DA does not worsen
    b) Some experts recommend NE for hypotension and low-dose DA to increase renal and splanchnic blood flow; others recommend a combination of DA and NE for blood pressure maintenance

(4) Epinephrine increases myocardial oxygen consumption, but some experts recommend it to manage low oxygen delivery and consumption in younger patients

(d) Monitor for symptoms of diminished visceral perfusion
  (1) Decreased or absent bowel sounds
  (2) Elevated serum amylase level
  (3) Decreased platelet count

(e) Avoid Trendelenburg's position, which impairs gas exchange and may decrease cerebral perfusion

(f) Maximize oxygen delivery and utilization; minimize oxygen demand
  (1) Control hyperthermia
    a) Use tepid baths or a cooling blanket
    b) Prevent chills and shivering
    c) Remove extra blankets
    d) Use antipyretic agents other than aspirin to reduce fever
  (2) Reduce the work of breathing as appropriate with mechanical ventilation; work with physicians to sedate and paralyze the patient, as needed, to maintain adequate ventilation and gas exchange
  (3) Limit patient activity; maintain a restful environment; provide periods of uninterrupted rest; maintain family visitations as appropriate
  (4) Manage pain, anxiety, and restlessness with medications and nursing interventions

(g) Administer medications, if appropriate, to modify mediators (Table 8–2)

iv. Evaluation of nursing care
  (a) Hemodynamic parameters and vital signs are within normal limits
  (b) S$\bar{v}$O$_2$ is 65% to 75%; the oxygen extraction ratio is 20% to 25%
  (c) Arterial lactate level and base deficit are normal
  (d) Peripheral pulses are present and equal bilaterally
  (e) Urine output is at least 1 ml/kg/hour
  (f) Sensorium is clear

b. Infection and inflammation related to inadequate primary defenses (broken skin, traumatized tissues), inadequate secondary defenses (immunosuppression), invasive procedures, or malnutrition
  i. Assessment for defining characteristics (see definition of SIRS)
  ii. Expected outcomes
    (a) WBC count is 4000 to 12,000/mm^3
    (b) Temperature is 30° to 38°C

TABLE 8–2. Medications Used in Attempts to Modify Cytokines: Possible Future Direction*

Medication	Rationale
Antibody to tumor necrosis factor (TNF)-α	To bind TNF and decrease cytokine production (particularly the interleukins)
Anti-endotoxin (lipopolysaccharide) antibody	To bind endotoxin and render it ineffective
Antioxidants (vitamin E; N-acetylcysteine)	To block cellular damage from oxygen radicals
Colony-stimulating factors	To increase synthesis and function of white blood cells in response to infection
L-N-monomethyl arginine and aminoguanidine	To inhibit synthesis of nitric oxide through the use of an inducible nitric oxide synthase (iNOS) inhibitor
Nonsteroidal anti-inflammatory drugs (ibuprofen)	To block arachidonic acid metabolism and stabilize the cell membrane
Pentoxifylline	To decrease neutrophil adhesion and TNF levels
Naloxone (Narcan)	To block opioid receptors and receptors that mediate vasodilation

*Much is unknown about the need to modify cytokines, although current investigators are considering the usefulness of these medications in septic shock in humans and animals. Many remain investigational.

     (c) Heart rate is 60 to 100 beats/minute
     (d) Respiratory rate 12 to 20 breaths/minute
   iii. Nursing interventions (see Commonly Encountered Nursing Diagnoses: Hematologic System)
     (a) Additional nursing interventions
       (1) Corticosteroid therapy is not recommended; two meta-analyses published in 1995 (Cronin and colleagues, Lefering and Neugebauer) indicate no beneficial effect in patients with septic shock
       (2) Administer antibiotics on time
       (3) Monitor antibiotic levels, particularly aminoglycoside levels, for renal and ototoxic effects
       (4) Monitor for reactions to antibiotics
         a) Superinfection: infection with organisms such as *C. albicans* is usually controlled by normal body flora
         b) Allergy: rash and anaphylactic shock
         c) Resistance: reemergence of symptoms of fever, purulence, and increased WBC count
       (5) Monitor compliance with unit infection control protocols, as recommended by the Centers for Disease Control and Prevention (CDC)
         a) Hand washing
         b) Dressing change
         c) Wound isolation
         d) Catheter and tubing changes
       (6) Provide oral care frequently

(7) Assist with treatments to limit the nidus of infection
  a) Removal of necrotic tissue
  b) Debridement of burned tissue
  c) Drainage of abscesses
(8) Limit tissue damage and inflammation by prompt stabilization of fractures

  iv. Evaluation of nursing care
  (a) No clinical manifestations of SIRS
  (b) Negative cultures and sensitivities

c. Impaired gas exchange related to alveolar capillary changes (see Chapter 1, The Pulmonary System)

d. Ineffective thermoregulation related to the body's response to infection
  i. Assessment for defining characteristics
    (a) Core temperature below 36°C or above 38°C
    (b) Flushed, warm skin or pale, cool skin
    (c) Increased or decreased metabolic rate
  ii. Expected outcomes
    (a) Core temperature is between 36° and 38°C
    (b) Skin is warm and dry
  iii. Nursing interventions
    (a) Monitor core temperature hourly
      (1) Pulmonary artery (PA) thermistor is the instrument of choice
      (2) If no PA catheter, use a rectal, urinary bladder, esophageal, or tympanic route
    (b) After the source of increased or decreased temperature is identified, maintain normothermia by the use of antipyretic medication as prescribed; avoid aspirin products
    (c) Use tepid baths or a cooling blanket to reduce hyperthermia
      (1) Monitor core temperature at all times to reduce the risk of hypothermia
      (2) Do not decrease temperature too rapidly, because it may lead to shaking chills
      (3) Reposition frequently, and check for tissue breakdown if a cooling blanket is used
    (d) Use warming blankets and a warmed ambient temperature to manage hypothermia
  iv. Evaluation of nursing care: normothermia is achieved

e. Altered nutrition, less than body requirements, related to increased metabolic rate and decreased intake of nutrients
  i. Assessment for defining characteristics
    (a) Increased body temperature
    (b) Loss of body weight
    (c) Increased body metabolism
  ii. Expected outcomes
    (a) Stable body weight is appropriate for gender and body frame
    (b) Nitrogen balance is positive
    (c) Muscle mass is adequate
  iii. Nursing interventions (see Chapter 7, The Gastrointestinal System)
    (a) Initiate enteral feedings as early as possible to limit microbial translocation

(b) Establish caloric requirements based on body size and degree of hypermetabolism; 20 to 25 kcal/kg/day is average

(c) Maintain glucose in a normal range because hyperglycemia (> 200 mg/dl) is associated with poor prognosis

iv. Evaluation of nursing care

(a) Serum albumin level is above 3.5 g/dl

(b) Body weight is within 2 kg of normal

(c) There is no evidence of electrolyte or vitamin imbalances

Multiple Organ Dysfunction Syndrome

1. Pathophysiology

a. Definition developed by a consensus conference and reported in Bone and colleagues (1992): (MODS) is the presence of altered organ function in an acutely ill patient such that homeostasis cannot be maintained without intervention. Other terms used:

   i. Multiple system organ failure (MSOF)

   ii. Multisystem failure (MSF)

b. History of organ failure

   i. Single organ failure

      (a) World War I: profound hypotension with injury led to cardiovascular failure and shock. Results:

         (1) Recognition of the need for aggressive volume replacement in hemorrhagic shock

         (2) Storage of plasma and whole blood by blood banks to be used in volume resuscitation

      (b) World War II and Korean War: resuscitation of war casualties to a preselected blood pressure led to patients surviving an initial insult, only to die from renal failure

         (1) Blood pressure end point was not sufficient; rather, volume loading with salt solutions was needed in addition to blood

         (2) Concept of "third space" evolved

         (3) When urine output became the monitor for adequacy of shock resuscitation, the frequency of renal failure was reduced

      (c) Viet Nam Conflict: pulmonary failure ("shock lung") became a limiting organ system

         (1) Pulmonary failure was attributed to shock and overaggressive fluid resuscitation

         (2) Result: development of high technology pulmonary support

   ii. Advanced technology led to the ability to support patients during critical illness; consequence of that support is the emergence of MODS

c. Epidemiology

   i. MODS develops during 15% of all ICU admissions

   ii. MODS after multiple trauma occurs in 20% to 47% of patients

      (a) Infection is the leading cause of MODS after trauma

      (b) Early, inadequate resuscitation accounts for 50% of MODS

   iii. MODS is responsible for up to 80% of all ICU deaths

      iv. Mortality rates have remained stable at approximately 70% to 80% for the past 20 years in spite of advancements in critical care practice

      v. Death rates increase as a function of the number of organs involved

        (a) When two organ systems are involved, mortality rates are approximately 50% to 60%

        (b) When four organ systems are involved, mortality rates reach 100%

      vi. MODS results in ICU costs of more than $100,000 per patient and approximately $500,000 per survivor

    d. Sequence of organ failure: patients do not necessarily follow the prototype pattern; depends on the reserve of each organ system

      i. Precipitating event: day 1

      ii. Pulmonary failure: day 2 to 3

      iii. Hepatic failure: day 6 to 7

      iv. Stress-induced bleeding: day 10

      v. Renal failure: day 12 to 14

    e. Theories of pathogenesis: all or some of the following hypotheses may exist simultaneously (Fig. 8–2):

      i. "First-hit" model versus "second-hit" model (Fig. 8–3)

        (a) First hit (one-hit): massive tissue injury and shock combine to produce intense SIRS (see Septic Shock) that results in early MODS

        (b) Second hit (two-hits): initial assault and resuscitation followed by secondary but altered SIRS reaction

          (1) Less severely injured patients enter a less intense state of SIRS but are vulnerable to secondary inflammation that amplifies SIRS

          (2) Complications: increasing organ failure, secondary infection, or repeated surgery

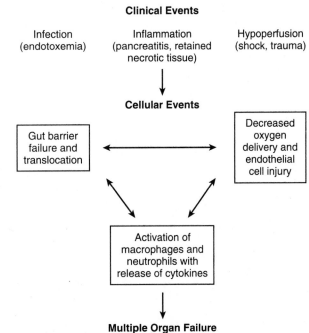

Figure 8–2 • Clinical and cellular events leading to the development of multiple organ dysfunction syndrome (MODS). (From Livingston, D. H., and Deitch, E. A.: Multiple organ failure: A common problem in surgical intensive care unit patterns. Ann. Med. 27:14, 1995.)

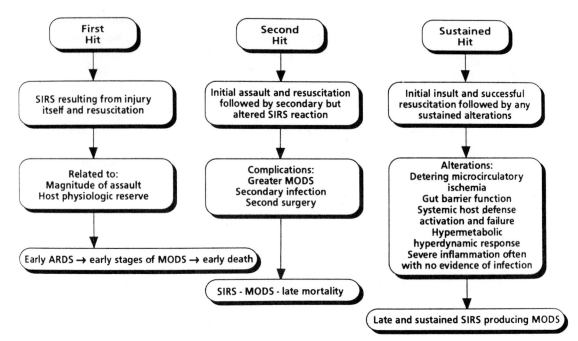

Figure 8–3 • First, second, and sustained hits that can occur with systemic inflammatory response syndrome (SIRS). ARDS = adult respiratory distress syndrome; MODS = multiple organ dysfunction syndrome. (From Bone, R. C.: Toward a theory regarding the pathogenesis of the systemic inflammatory response syndrome: What we do and do not know about cytokine regulation. Crit. Care Med. 24:167, 1996.)

    (c) "Sustained hit": initial insult and successful resuscitation followed by sustained alterations, resulting in late and sustained SIRS producing MODS

  ii. Macrophage/cytokine hypothesis: excessive or prolonged stimulation of macrophages and neutrophils leads to the production of cytokines (see Septic Shock) and other products, which results in harmful cellular and systemic effects

    (a) Cytokines: IL-1, IL-6, IL-8, TNF, and interferon-γ

    (b) A site of infection is not necessary for the development of MODS; up to 30% of patients who die of MODS have no infection

  iii. Microcirculatory hypothesis: failure of oxygen delivery to keep up with oxygen consumption results in tissue ischemia and organ dysfunction

    (a) Ischemia leads to damage of vascular endothelium

    (b) Endothelial cell surface adhesion molecules and interaction between endothelium and cytokines leads to tissue injury

    (c) Tissue injury from ischemia–reperfusion occurs because of oxygen radical formation

    (d) Decreased ability of red blood cells (RBCs) to deform themselves because of peroxidation of lipid membranes leads to the inability of RBCs to move through the circulation

  iv. Gut hypothesis: gut acts as a reservoir for bacteria and endotoxin, which causes and perpetuates the development of MODS (see microbial translocation in SIRS)

   f. Definitions (Hazinski and colleagues, 1993) for organ failure: clinical criteria whose signs are consistent with organ system dysfunction or failure in the absence of other attributable causes

      i. Pulmonary failure: acute respiratory distress syndrome (ARDS)

         (a) Unexplained hypoxemia with suspected sepsis

$$(Pao_2 / FIo_2 < 175\text{--}250 \text{ mm Hg})$$

         (b) Bilateral pulmonary infiltrates on a frontal chest radiograph along with PAWP below 18 mm Hg

         (c) Deterioration of ABG parameters from the baseline

      ii. Hepatobiliary

         (a) Elevation in liver function enzymes twice normal

         (b) Serum bilirubin above 2 mg/dl

      iii. Gastrointestinal

         (a) Paralytic ileus

         (b) Gastrointestinal bleeding

      iv. Renal (not prerenal)

         (a) Oliguria with urine output below .5 ml/kg/hour

         (b) Increase in serum creatinine above normal with urine sodium below 40 mmol/L in patients with normal baseline renal function

         (c) Rise in serum creatinine by 2 mg/dl in patients with chronic renal failure

      v. Central nervous system

         (a) Glasgow Come Scale score below 15 when previously normal or decreased by 1

         (b) Acute change in mental status (confusion, agitation, lethargy)

      vi. Coagulation

         (a) Confirmatory test for disseminated intravascular coagulation (DIC): fibrin degradation products above 1:40 or D-dimers above 2

         (b) Thrombocytopenia or a fall in the platelet count by 25%

         (c) Elevated prothrombin time and partial thromboplastin time

         (d) Clinical evidence of bleeding

  g. MODS scoring: Marshall and associates (1995) developed a scoring system for MODS with physiologic measures of dysfunction in six organ systems; MODS score correlated with risk of mortality (Table 8–3)

      i. Score of 9 to 12: mortality rate 25%

      ii. Score of 13 to 16: mortality rate 50%

      iii. Score of 17 to 20: mortality rate 75%

2. Etiologic or precipitating factors

  a. Predisposition

      i. Chronic diseases and preexisting organ dysfunction: diabetes mellitus, angina pectoris, myocardial infarction, heart failure, chronic obstructive pulmonary disease, acute and chronic renal failure, liver failure, pancreatitis, and HIV infection

      ii. Immunosuppressive therapy: use of corticosteroids or drugs with immunosuppressive properties

      iii. Extremes of age: very old and very young

      iv. Malnutrition, alcohol use, and alcoholism

      v. Cancer

TABLE 8–3. Multiple Organ Dysfunction Score

Organ System	Score				
	0	1	2	3	4
Respiratory (Po/FIO$_2$ ratio)*	>300	266–300	151–225	76–150	≤75
Renal (serum creatinine)†	≤100	101–200	201–350	351–500	>500
Hepatic (serum bilirubin)‡	≤20	21–60	61–120	121–240	>240
Cardiovascular (PAR)§	≤10.0	10.1–15.0	15.1–20.0	20.1–30.0	>30.0
Hematologic (platelet count)‖	>120	81–120	51–80	21–50	≤20
Neurologic (Glasgow Coma Scale)¶	15	13–14	10–12	7–9	≤6

From Marshall, J. C., Cook, D. J., Christou, N. V., et al.: Multiple organ dysfunction score: A reliable descriptor of a complex clinical outcome. Crit. Care Med. 23:1646, 1995.

*The Po$_2$/FIO$_2$ ratio is calculated without reference to the use or mode of mechanical ventilation and without reference to the use or level of positive end-expiratory pressure.

†The serum creatinine concentration is measured in μmol/L without reference to the use of dialysis.

‡The serum bilirubin concentration is measured in μmol/L.

§The pressure-adjusted heart rate PAR is calculated as the product of the heart rate (HR) multiplied by the ratio of the right atrial (central venous) pressure (RAP) to the mean aterial pressure (MAP):

$$PAR = HR \times RAP/mean\ BP$$

‖The platelet count is measured in platelets/mL 10^{-3}.

¶The Glasgow Coma Scale score is preferably calculated by the patient's nurse and is scored conservatively. For the patient receiving sedation or muscle relaxants, normal function is assumed unless there is evidence of intrinsically altered mentation.

      vi. Severe trauma: extensive tissue damage; presence of necrotic tissue; persistent inflammation; hemodynamic instability, inadequate tissue perfusion, and acidosis; hemorrhagic shock and multiple transfusions; burns; inadequate fluid resuscitation; and infection (*Note:* MODS is rarely associated with infection in trauma patients despite a high rate of SIRS)

     vii. Sepsis

   b. Etiology (see SIRS)

      i. SIRS can be initiated by infectious or noninfectious causes

     ii. Normal integrated inflammatory immune response continues unchecked, releasing cellular mediators that cause organ dysfunction

    iii. Clinical and cellular events leading to MODS

       (a) Inflammation: pancreatitis and retained necrotic tissue

       (b) Hypoperfusion: shock and trauma

       (c) Infection: endotoxemia

3. Nursing assessment data base

   a. Nursing history

      i. Past medical and surgical history, with special emphasis on sepsis, shock, trauma, recent surgical procedures, recent infections, and preexisting organ compromise

     ii. Medication history, with particular attention to drugs that cause immunosuppression

       (a) Corticosteroids

       (b) Immunosuppressive drugs following organ transplantation

       (c) Antibiotic use

    iii. Nutritional status of patient (including dietary intake, alcohol use, use of enteral or parenteral nutrition, and normal body weight)

    iv. Social history (see SIRS)

b. Nursing examination of patient
   i. Vital signs (see defintion of SIRS). Note that vital signs vary, depending on the nature of the underlying disorder and the organ systems involved
   ii. Assessment findings depend on the organ system involved
     (a) Pulmonary failure (ARDS) (see Chapter 1)
     (b) Hepatobiliary failure (see Chapter 7)
     (c) Gastrointestinal failure
       (1) Paralytic ileus: abdominal distention, absent bowel sounds, nausea, and vomiting
       (2) Gastrointestinal bleeding (see Chapter 7)
     (d) Intrarenal acute renal failure (see Chapter 4, The Renal System)
     (e) Central nervous system (CNS) failure
       (1) Acute change in mental status (confusion, agitation, lethargy)
       (2) Glasgow Coma Scale score below 15 when previously normal or decreased by 1
     (f) DIC (see Chapter 6, The Hematologic System)
   iii. Inspection: varies across the continuum of organ failure
     (a) Clinical presentation may vary, depending on patient's underlying health, degree of organ dysfunction, number of organs involved, and progression of time
     (b) Acute distress with anxiety, restlessness, confusion, irritability, and disorientation progressing to unresponsiveness and prostration
     (c) Tachypnea, increased work of breathing, intercostal retractions, nasal flaring, and dyspnea
     (d) Tachycardia; cardiac dysrhythmias
     (e) Decreased urinary output despite adequate intake
     (f) Interstitial edema
     (g) Bleeding from orifices, old puncture wounds, and mucous membranes; bruising
     (h) Asterixis (late); jaundiced skin
   iv. Palpation: varies across the continuum of organ failure
     (a) Vocal fremitus: increased because of increased density from pulmonary edema
     (b) Reduced lung expansion
     (c) Rapid, weak, and thready peripheral pulses
     (d) Distended abdomen; enlarged liver
   v. Percussion: varies across the continuum of organ failure
     (a) Dullness over areas of atelectasis, consolidation, and pulmonary edema
     (b) Enlarged liver
   vi. Auscultation: varies across the continuum of organ failure
     (a) Pulmonary crackles from interstitial pulmonary edema; wheezing without a history of bronchospastic airway disease; bronchovesicular breath sounds as consolidation worsens
     (b) Narrowed pulse pressure and variable blood pressure
     (c) Absent bowel sounds
     (d) Pericardial friction rub (late)
c. Diagnostic study findings: same as for SIRS and septic shock

4. Nursing diagnoses

a. Impaired gas exchange related to alveolar-capillary membrane changes (see Chapter 1)

b. Ineffective airway clearance related to secretions, obstruction, and a decreased level of consciousness (see Chapter 1)

c. Ineffective breathing pattern related to the inflammatory process, decreased lung expansion, decreased lung compliance, and tracheobronchial obstruction (see Chapter 1)

d. Altered tissue perfusion (renal, cerebral, cardiopulmonary, gastrointestinal, peripheral) related to hypovolemia from maldistribution (see Septic Shock) or bleeding (see Chapter 6)

e. Risk for alterations in tissue perfusion (peripheral) related to coagulation problems and fluid shifts (see Chapter 7)

f. Risk for infection related to inadequate primary defenses (broken skin, traumatized tissues), inadequate secondary defenses (immunosuppression), invasive procedures, or malnutrition (see Septic Shock)

g. Risk for ineffective thermoregulation related to the body's response to infection or trauma (see Septic Shock)

h. Altered nutrition, less than body requirements, related to an increased metabolic rate and a decreased intake of nutrients (see Septic Shock)

i. Altered urinary elimination related to decreased renal tissue perfusion and cellular injury (see Chapter 4)

j. Impaired skin integrity related to poor nutrition and an increased deposition of wastes in the skin (see Chapter 7)

k. Risk for self-concept, disturbance in the body image related to powerlessness, and changes in the body appearance during a critical illness (see Chapter 9, Psychosocial Aspects)

l. Risk for altered family process related to a situational crisis of a critical illness (see Chapter 9)

m. Risk for fear related to separation from a support system, sensory impairment, and environmental stimuli during a critical illness (see Chapter 9)

Multisystem Trauma

1. Pathophysiology

a. Definitions

i. Injury: physical harm or damage to the body resulting from an exchange, usually acute, of mechanical, chemical, thermal, or other environmental energy that exceeds the body's tolerance

ii. Unintentional injury: accidental harm or damage to the body resulting from sudden, unplanned traumatic events such as motor vehicle crashes, burns, drowning, poisons, falls, explosions, electrical accidents, and accidental firearm injuries

iii. Intentional injury: harm or damage to the body resulting from planned, premeditated harm or damage to the body, for example, assaults (beatings, gunshot wounds, stab wounds), homicides, and suicides

b. Epidemiology

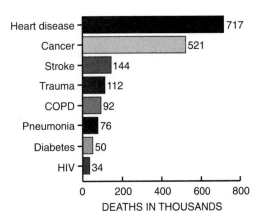

Figure 8–4 • Leading causes of death among United States residents of all ages. COPD = chronic obstructive pulmonary disease; HIV = human immunodeficiency virus. (Data from National Safety Council: Accident Facts. Itasca, Ill., National Safety Council, 1995.)

 i. Injury remains the leading cause of death in people from age 1 to 37 years

 ii. Injury is the fourth leading cause of death for all ages, following heart disease, cancer, and stroke (Fig. 8–4)

 iii. Deaths in 1994 from unintentional injury were approximately 92,000 (Table 8–4)

 iv. Total cost of unintentional injuries in 1994 was estimated at $440.9 billion, including the cost of health care and loss of future economic productivity by injured victims

 v. Approximately 55,000 intentional deaths (particularly suicides and homicides) occur each year; the number of homicides is on the rise in many states

c. Physiologic response to injury

 i. Stress response: initiated by injured tissue, acute blood loss, shock, hypoxia, acidosis, and hypothermia as well as feelings of pain and fear

  (a) Sympathetic nervous system (SNS): afferent nerve signals reach the brain following the presentation of stimuli. Stimulation of splanchnic nerves occurs, leading to the release of epinephrine, norephinephrine, cortisol, and growth hormone into the circulation

TABLE 8–4. Deaths Caused by Unintentional Injury in 1994

Classification	No. of Deaths	Change from 1993
Total unintentional deaths	92,000	+1%
Motor vehicle crashes	43,000	+2%
Falls	13,300	−3%
Poisoning (solids, liquids)	8,000	+11%
Fires	4,200	+5%
Drowning	4,000	−11%
Suffocation	3,000	−6%
Firearms	1,500	0%
Poisoning (gas, vapors)	700	0%
Other	14,500	−1%

Data from the National Safety Council: Accident Facts. Itasca, Ill., National Safety Council, 1995.

          (1) Increase in heart rate and contractility, vasoconstriction, and blood pressure

          (2) Increase in minute ventilation

          (3) Prolonged and excessive stimulation leads to severe and uneven arteriolar vasoconstriction, reduced microcirculatory blood flow, and impaired delivery of oxygen and nutrients to tissues

             a) In the absence of hypovolemia, redistribution of intravascular volume from venous capacitance vessels leads to increased central blood volume and increased intraluminal capillary pressure

             b) Loss of intravascular volume due to increased capillary permeability leads to intravascular hypovolemia, hypoperfusion, and edema formation

          (4) Following restoration of the fluid balance, the body develops a hyperdynamic state to compensate for oxygen debt

             a) Phase lasts 48 to 72 hours and decreases in 7 to 10 days

             b) Inability to achieve and maintain a hyperdynamic state (high cardiac index, oxygen delivery, oxygen consumption) is associated with higher mortality rates

    (b) Hypothalamic-pituitary-adrenal secretions: adrenal secretion of corticosteroids is regulated by both hypothalamus and pituitary gland

          (1) Stimuli: fear, pain, hypotension, hypovolemia, and tissue injury

          (2) Effects of corticosteroid secretion: sodium retention, insulin resistance, hyperglycemia, gluconeogenesis, lipolysis, protein catabolism, and enhancement of the catabolic effects of TNF-α, IL-1, and IL-6

    (c) Antidiuretic hormone (ADH) release: loss of blood volume is sensed by atrial receptors, and hypotension is sensed by pressure receptors in the carotid sinus, aortic arch, and pulmonary artery

          (1) Receptors communicate with neurons in the hypothalamus, which synapse with cells in the posterior pituitary gland

          (2) Posterior pituitary gland releases ADH, which leads to vasoconstriction and water retention

    (d) Renin-angiotensin release: renin is released from juxtaglomerular cells when renal blood flow is diminished or when stimulated by the sympathetic nervous system. Renin catalyzes a reaction that leads to vasoconstriction, aldosterone stimulation, and decreased sodium and water excretion

    (e) Endogenous opioids: released from the pituitary gland as part of an initial stress response to decrease pain, inhibit feedback of pituitary activation, decrease adrenocorticotropic hormone (ACTH) release, and increase insulin release; may decrease immune reponse

    (f) Coagulopathy: from excessive bleeding, massive blood transfusions, and hypothermia

    (g) Locally produced mediators

          (1) Endothelial disruption leads to activation of Hageman factor (factor XII), which leads to activation of other systems

        a) Coagulation cascade, leading to clotting and fibrinolysis

        b) Complement cascade, initiating inflammation and increased capillary permeability

        c) Kinin and plasmin systems

    (2) Activation of arachidonic acid metabolism that leads to activation of other mediators

        a) Prostaglandins: vasoconstriction and platelet aggregation

        b) Leukotrienes: mediator of vascular tone and inflammation

        c) Platelet activation factor (PAF): stimulator of platelet and neutrophil activation, leading to microvascular thrombosis at the site of injury

        d) Activation of cytokine cascades: TNF-α, IL-1, IL-6, and IL-8

    (3) Oxygen radicals: released from ischemic tissues on reperfusion and activated by localized circulating immune effector cells, which leads to further tissue injury

  ii. Psychologic response (varies with circumstances): fear, withdrawal, anger, hostility, anxiety, depression, regression, intrusion or avoidance, and hyperarousal

  iii. Metabolic derangements

    (a) Edema: prolonged trauma and stress leads to a flux of sodium and water from the intravascular space into the interstitial space, leading to intravascular fluid volume deficit and interstitial edema; increased capillary permeability from circulating mediators increases edema

    (b) Increased cardiac output: heart rate and contractility increase as a result of the stress response; when bleeding is controlled and the fluid volume is replaced, hyperdynamic circulation occurs

    (c) Impaired oxygen transport: altered microcirculation due to vasoconstriction at the tissue level leads to decreased tissue perfusion

    (d) Hypermetabolism: oxygen consumption increases to supranormal levels 10% to 25% above the baseline. Extent depends on the severity of injury

    (e) Altered protein metabolism: total body catabolism is increased, particularly within skeletal muscles, resulting in a loss of lean body mass. Hepatic synthesis of proteins increases. Growth hormone induces potent anabolic effects to incorporate amino acids into proteins

    (f) Altered glucose metabolism: glucose increases because of stress hormones; insulin resistance occurs; glucogen stores are converted to glucose

    (g) Altered fat metabolism: lipids in the form of stored fuel are broken down into fatty acids for energy

    (h) Leukocytosis: increased number of granulocytes, which occurs even without infection; increased degranulation

2. Etiologic or precipitating factors

  a. Factors associated with trauma

    i. Physical

      (a) Age: very old and very young are at risk

    (1) Patients above 75 years of age fare worse with trauma than younger patients

     a) Injury is more severe because of increased body fragility, blunted compensatory mechanisms, and the presence of underlying organ dysfunction, with decreased organ reserve

     b) Risk for trauma is higher because of poor vision, weak lower extremities, unsteady gait, or impaired balance

    (2) Very young (<age 5 years) have higher mortality rates than children aged 6 to 14 years

   (b) Gender: more males are injured than females; in 1994, 67% of unintentional injuries occured in males, 33% in females; risk from trauma is 2.5 times higher in males than females

    (1) Pregnancy affects injury severity and outcome

    (2) Females are more at risk than males for domestic violence

   (c) Ethnicity

    (1) Teenaged African American males are 10-fold more likely to die as a result of homicide than European American males of the same age

    (2) Native Americans have the highest rate of unintentional injury; Asian Americans have the lowest

   (d) Type of injury: blunt versus penetrating

   (e) Preinjury health status: preexisting organ dysfunction or conditions, such as diabetes mellitus, chronic obstructive lung disease, atherosclerotic heart disease, hypertension, and cystic kidney disease increase susceptibility for injury and impair the response to injury

  ii. Environmental factors: speed limits, legal drinking age, mandatory helmet laws, availability of guns, living near water, living in cold climates

   (a) Unintentional injury rates are highest in rural areas

   (b) Intentional injury rates are highest in urban areas

  iii. Socioeconomic factors: working in a high-risk occupation (construction work, heavy industry), living in a high crime area, living in a poorly maintained home, and belonging to a gang

  iv. Personality and psychologic factors: risk-taking behaviors, antisocial behavior, mental illness, depression, poor judgment, and previous head injury

  v. Alcohol and other drugs: approximately half of all trauma patients have an alcohol or substance use history; alcohol and other drugs place the patient at risk for injury

   (a) Decreased level of alertness; impaired motor function, coordination, and balance; increased reaction time

   (b) Impaired judgment, perception, and cognitive ability; increased risk-taking behavior and feeling of invulnerability among adolescents; increased violent behavior; reduced inhibitions

   (c) Increased physiologic fragility; injury may be severer, recovery may be slower

  vi. Temporal

   (a) Time of day: death rate from motor vehicle crashes highest between 10 PM and 4 AM

    (b) Day of week

       (1) Weekends are the most common for deaths from motor vehicle crashes, pedestrian accidents, drowning, and homicides

       (2) Suicide rate is highest on Mondays

       (3) Occupational injury is highest on Mondays and Fridays

b. Mechanisms of injury

   i. Blunt injury: trauma that occurs without communication to the outside environment; common causes are motor vehicle crashes and falls; caused by a combination of forces:

    (a) Acceleration: change in the rate of velocity or speed of a moving body; as velocity increases, so does tissue damage

    (b) Deceleration: decrease in the volocity of a moving object; acceleration-deceleration injuries are a common cause of blunt injury

    (c) Shearing: structures slip relative to each other because of forces across a plane

    (d) Crushing and compression: squeezing, stretching, or inward pressure; hollow organs (stomach, bowel, urinary bladder) are less likely to rupture (except in a seat belt injury) compared with solid organs (liver, spleen), which are less compressible

   ii. Penetrating injury: trauma that occurs from the motion of foreign objects that enter into tissue, causing direct damage from entry or indirect damage because of tissue deformation associated with energy transference into surrounding tissues

    (a) Gunshot wounds

       (1) Energy of a missile is dissipated into tissues. When it enters the body, it creates a temporary cavity that distorts, stretches, and compresses surrounding tissues (Fig. 8–5)

       (2) Blast effect (muzzle blast): cavity from a gunshot wound produces damage to structures not in the direct path of a missile

       (3) High-velocity missiles cause extensive cavitation and significant tissue destruction; low-velocity missiles have limited cavitation potential with less tissue destruction

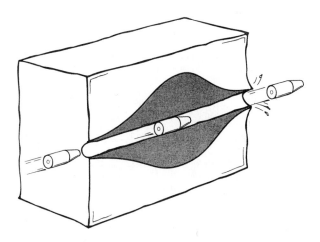

Figure 8–5 • Formation of temporary (gray region) and permanent cavity (white region) during injury from a bullet. The temporary cavity is a localized area of blunt trauma; the permanent cavity occurs with crushing, stretching, and breaking the elastic bonds of tissue along the wound tract of the bullet. (From Hinkle, J., and Betz, S.: Gunshot injuries. AACN Clin. Issues 6:178, 1995. Illustration by Jef Dirig.)

(4) Extent of the injury proportional to the amount of kinetic energy lost by a missile:

$$K = \frac{mass \times (V1^2 - V2^2)}{2}$$

where K = kinetic energy, V1 = impact velocity, and V2 = remaining velocity

(5) Tissue yaw: amount of tumbling and movement of the nose of the missile; the more yaw, the more damage (Fig. 8–6)

(b) Stab wounds: follow a more predictable pattern than gunshot wounds and involve less tissue destruction unless vital organs or vessels are lacerated

(c) Impalement: usually a low-velocity injury that occurs with motor vehicle crashes, with falls, and after being hit with falling or flying objects

(d) Avulsion and degloving: tearing away of tissue, resulting in full-thickness skin loss; caused when skin is sliced by a sharp object or when a person is thrown from a moving vehicle

3. Nursing assessment data base

a. Nursing history

i. Source: patient, family, partner, significant other, prehospital personnel, or bystander

ii. Mechanism of injury

(a) Motor vehicle crashes

(1) Restrained, unrestrained, or airbag; helmet use (motorcycle)

(2) Driver or passenger; location in a vehicle; ejection from a vehicle

(3) Type of vehicle; speed of a vehicle

(4) Direction and force of a collision

(b) Falls

(1) Setting and context: slipping on ice, falling from a balcony during a party

(2) Angle and height of a fall: risk for serious injury is increased at a height above 10 feet; type of impact surface; landing position

Figure 8–6 • Tumbling is the action of forward rotation around the center of mass, similar to a somersault action. Yawing is the deviation or deflection of a bullet's nose in the longitudinal axis from a straight line. The more tumbling and yawing, the more tissue destruction. (From Hinkle, J., and Betz, S.: Gunshot injuries. AACN Clin. Issues 6:179, 1995. Illustration by Jef Dirig.)

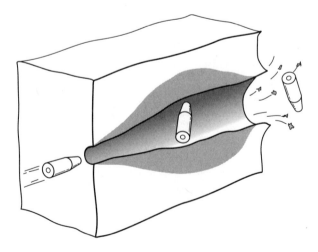

     (c) Gunshot wound

        (1) Type of weapon (handgun, shotgun); caliber of the weapon

        (2) Velocity of the bullet; range at which the weapon was fired; position of the assailant

        (3) Intentional or unintentional

        (4) If self-inflicted, hand dominance

        (5) Estimated depth of penetration; entry site; angle of entry, exit site; angle of exit

     (d) Stab wound

        (1) Type of weapon; size and length of blade

        (2) Intentional or unintentional

        (3) If self-inflicted, hand dominance

        (4) Estimated depth of penetration; entry site; angle of entry

  iii. Description of event

     (a) Location and time

     (2) People involved and their disposition

     (c) Context: during an argument, while at a party, during work, or while driving home

  iv. Alcohol and substance use involvement

   v. Past health history: AMPLE

     (a) *A:* allergies

     (b) *M:* medications

        (1) Prescription and over-the-counter drugs

        (2) Tetanus immunization

     (c) *P:* past illnesses (medical and surgical)

     (d) *L:* last meal (time, quantity, type)

     (e) *E:* events preceding the injury

  vi. Social

     (a) Partner, spouse, housemates, roommates, significant others, contact person, dependents, children, parents, and guardians

     (b) Education; occupation; financial considerations, ability to maintain income, insurance coverage

     (c) Religion

 vii. Other

     (a) Height, weight

     (b) Last menstrual period, potential for pregnancy

b. Nursing examination of patient

   i. Primary survey: rapid assessment (30 seconds to 2 minutes) that simultaneously identifies and manages life-threatening injuries: ABCDE

     (a) *A:* airway; maintain a patent airway. *Note:* stabilizing the cervical spine (cervical collar, sandbags, manual stabilization, taping) is mandatory during airway assessments and interventions

        (1) Assessment: airway is open

           a) Patient speaks or makes appropriate sounds

           b) No foreign material visible in the mouth

           c) Look, listen, and feel for exhaled breath

        (2) If the airway is obstructed, expect some of the following signs:

           a) Inability to speak or make sounds

           b) Substernal and intercostal retractions

            c) No air exchange

            d) Stridor (inspiratory, expiratory)

            e) Nasal flaring (children, infants)

            f) Restlessness and confusion, progressing rapidly to unresponsiveness

        (3) Emergency interventions during the primary survey. *Note:* maintain alignment of the cervical spine

            a) Chin lift or jaw thrust

            b) Suction

            c) Artificial airway: orotracheal or nasotracheal intubation preferred

            d) Cricothyroidotomy: when other means of airway maintenance are not possible or are contraindicated

    (b) *B:* breathing; maintain adequate breathing

        (1) Assessment: spontaneous, regular respirations at least 10 breaths/minute with equal, bilateral chest expansion and audible breath sounds

        (2) If breathing is compromised, expect:

            a) Respiratory rate below 10 or above 29 breaths per minute (adults)

            b) Difficult or labored breathing; intercostal or substernal retractions

            c) Decreased or absent breath sounds

            d) Asymmetric or paradoxical chest expansion

            e) Changes in color (pallor, duskiness, cyanosis)

            f) Tracheal deviation

            g) Restlessness, confusion, anxiety, and disorientation, progressing to unresponsiveness

        (3) Emergency interventions during the primary survey

            a) Manual resuscitator bag with bag-valve-mask and oxygen therapy

            b) Other options as needed in emergencies

               i) Needle or tube thoracostomy

              ii) Cover sucking chest wounds with three-sided occlusive dressing

             iii) Intubation and mechanical ventilation

    (c) *C:* circulation; maintain adequate circulation. *Note:* in early circulatory compromise, few clinical signs may occur

        (1) Assessment: easily palpable carotid pulse, with 50 to 120 beats/minute; patient is awake and answering questions appropriately; capillary refill in less than 2 seconds; no external, uncontrolled bleeding

        (2) If circulation is compromised (late), expect:

            a) Decreased level of consciousness

            b) Cold, damp skin; delayed (>3 seconds) capillary refill

            c) Absent, weak, thready, and rapid (>120 beats/minute) or slow (<50 beats/minute) pulse

            d) Overt or covert uncontrolled bleeding

            e) Hypotension (systolic blood pressure <90 mm Hg), a late sign, generally occurs with a loss of more than 30% of circulating vascular volume

         i) If a radial pulse is present, blood pressure is
            approximately 80 mm Hg

         ii) If a femoral pulse is present, blood pressure is
            approximately 70 mm Hg

         iii) If a carotid pulse is present, blood pressure is
            approximately 60 mm Hg

(3) Emergency interventions during the primary survey

    a) Control of external hemorrhage with direct pressure or pneumatic antishock garment; this is a controversial measure, but it may decrease hemorrhage with lower-extremity or pelvic fracture

    b) Parenteral fluid resuscitation with crystalloid or blood products (after two 2-liter fluid boluses)

    c) Autotransfusion

    d) Vasoactive medications only after fluid deficit is managed

(d) *D:* disability; monitor the level of consciousness

    (1) Assessment: level of alertness, ability to speak or vocalize, response to pain, pupillary response, and gross motor response

    (2) If mental status is compromised, expect:

        a) Decreased alertness; unresponsiveness to verbal and tactile stimulation

        b) Unequal pupils in size or responsiveness; fixed and dilated pupils

        c) Ipsilateral or bilateral deficits in motor response; extremity rigidity

    (3) Emergency interventions during the primary survey

        a) Maintain and protect the airway; maintain breathing and circulation

        b) Emergency measures to control increased intracranial pressure (see Chapter 3, The Neurologic System)

        c) Protect the patient from self-harm

(e) *E:* exposure; completely undress the patient to perform a thorough visual examination

    (1) Entry wounds that appear "minor" may be associated with extensive internal injury

    (2) Until the cervical spine is found to be free of injury, log roll the patient carefully onto the side to maintain spinal alignment

    (3) Cover the patient as soon as possible to prevent hypothermia and institute rewarming measures (see Hypothermia)

ii. Secondary survey: complete head-to-toe physical examination begun as soon as the primary survey and emergency, life-saving interventions are accomplished. *Note:* ongoing trauma resuscitation continues during the secondary survey as needed

iii. Tertiary survey: complete, head-to-toe reexamination of the patient immediately before ambulation or after the patient regains consciousness to identify missed injuries, often occurs days after initial injury and resuscitation

iv. Vital signs: widely variable because of catecholamine response, severity of injury, and medication administration; serial vital signs are essential to detect changes in condition

   (a) Respiratory rate
      (1) Ideal: 12 to 20 breaths/minute
      (2) Typical following trauma: tachypnea; absence of tachypnea following major trauma suggests CNS injury or signficant substance use (alcohol, opioids, and others)
   (b) Heart rate
      (1) Ideal: 60 to 100 beats/minute
      (2) Typical following trauma: tachycardia
         a) Beta blockers may decrease heart rate responsiveness to trauma
         b) Some patients maintain normal heart rates in spite of large amounts of blood loss (particularly during pregnancy)
         c) Some patients with blunt cardiac trauma may have decreased or irregular heart rates because of cardiac dysrhythmias
         d) Well-conditioned athletes have slow heart rates
   (c) Blood pressure
      (1) Ideal: systolic pressure above 90 mm Hg
      (2) Typical following trauma: variable, depending on blood loss and age
         a) Young adults tend to remain normotensive until major blood loss occurs
         b) Older adults may have more limited compensatory mechanisms and may be less able to tolerate volume deficits
         c) Alcohol intoxication may lead to hypotension or hypertension
   (d) Temperature
      (1) Ideal: core temperature above 37°C
      (2) Typical following trauma: decreased core temperature (35° to 37°C) is most common, but hypothermia (<35°C) may occur (see Hypothermia)

 v. Inspection
   (a) Abrasions, ecchymoses, swelling, and skin lacerations may indicate involvement of underlying structures or mechanism of injury. *Note:* absence of external injury does not rule out the possibility of severe underlying injury
   (b) Unusual drainage may indicate injury to internal structures
      (1) Otorrhea, rhinorrhea, and blood from the nose or ears may indicate a basilar skull fracture
      (2) Blood at the urinary meatus may indicate a lower urinary tract injury or a pelvic fracture
   (c) Inspect for protruding bone fragments or viscera
   (d) Note a deformity or dislocation of extremities
   (c) Locate entry and exit wounds of penetrating injuries. Do *not* remove impaled objects until a surgeon is present and ready for the operative procedure, or the injury may be worsened

      vi. Auscultation of the heart and lungs for adventitious sounds and the gastrointestinal tract for hypoactivity or hyperactivity

     vii. Palpation: abnormal findings

        (a) Skull depressions and deformities; facial deformity

        (b) Deformity or abnormal movement of the bony thorax; presence of subcutaneous emphysema

        (c) Abdominal guarding, tenderness, and rigidity

        (d) Pelvic fractures: compress iliac crests toward the midline and rock pelvis back and forth

        (e) Deformities and point tenderness of the extremities and the spine

        (f) Absence of peripheral pulses

    viii. Percussion: note dullness over blood-filled collections or internal hematomas

c. Diagnostic study findings

       i. CBC: reflects amount of blood lost but may take 2 hours to reflect the hematocrit drop with slow bleeding

        (a) Marked drop in hemoglobin and hematocrit after fluid resuscitation with crystalloids due to dilution and mobilization of fluid during the recovery phase

        (b) Leukocytosis with a "shift to the left," reflecting the release of immature cells in response to either trauma or infection

        (c) Platelets: need to be replaced to stem additional bleeding if below 50,000 mm^3

      ii. Blood type and cross-match: to determine the presence of antigens to ensure compatible blood transfusions

     iii. Blood chemistry: to determine *glucose* (usually elevated from stress response and decreased peripheral utilization of insulin), *magnesium* (may be decreased from loss in urine), and *ionized calcium* (often decreased because of citrate used in blood transfusions)

        (a) Baseline levels of BUN, creatinine, and liver function tests to determine the response to injury

        (b) Baseline electrolytes

     iv. Arterial lactate levels: to determine the adequacy of tissue oxygen extraction and to warn of impending organ failure

      v. Arterial and venous blood gases: to determine the adequacy of ventilation, oxygen delivery, and oxygen consumption

        (a) Acidosis may be seen if tissue perfusion deficits exist; hypoxemia may be seen if hypoventilation exists

        (b) Arterial oxygenation may be monitored noninvasively with pulse oximetry

        (c) Base deficit may occur because of perfusion deficits and metabolic acidosis

     vi. Urine and blood toxicology

        (a) Blood alcohol concentration: legal intoxication in most states is 100 mg/dl

        (b) Routine urine toxicology screens for commonly abused substances in a community

     vii. Urinalysis: to determine the presence of blood, bacteria, ketones, glucose, myoglobin, and bilirubin

    viii. Other blood studies: amylase and coagulation studies

        ix. Peritoneal lavage (controversial): often used to determine extent of an abdominal injury or bleeding, particularly in unstable patients with blunt trauma when a solid or hollow organ injury is suspected

        x. Pregnancy test: performed on girls (12–17 years of age) and women of childbearing age; if the patient is verbal, consider the need for a test based on sexual history

        xi. X-rays: are used to locate fractures, abnormal air or fluid collections, and foreign objects such as bullets

           (a) Indicate position of major organs

           (b) In multiple trauma, views of the cervical spine, chest, abdomen, pelvis, and extremities necessary

        xii. Computed tomography (CT): detects the presence of soft tissue injury, hematomas, fractures, and tissue swelling

        xiii. For renal or lower urinary tract injury: intravenous pyelogram (IVP), cystogram, and retrograde urethrogram

        xiv. Other: magnetic resonance imaging (MRI), angiography, ultrasonography, echocardiography, electrocardiogram

4. Nursing diagnoses

  a. Ineffective airway clearance related to tracheobronchial obstruction or trauma (see Chapter 1)

    i. Additional nursing inteventions

      (a) Maintain cervical spine alignment during airway management until cervical spine injury is ruled out

      (b) Do not use the nasotracheal route for intubation if the patient has facial or basilar skull fractures (possible penetration of cribriform plate and latrogenic brain injury)

      (c) Suspect airway compromise in intoxicated patients

  b. Ineffective breathing pattern related to pain, musculoskeletal impairment, decreased lung expansion, or tracheobronchial obstruction (see Chapter 1)

  c. Fluid volume deficit related to active blood loss and decreased circulating volume from fluid shifts (see Chapter 2, the Cardiovascular System)

    i. Additional nursing interventions

      (a) Warm all fluids to body temperature, if possible, to prevent hypothermia

      (b) Use short, large-bore peripheral IV catheters or large-bore trauma catheters at multiple sites for rapid volume resuscitation

        (1) Avoid stopcocks, which slow infusion

        (2) Avoid long lengths of tubing, which increase resistance to flow

      (c) Administer pressurized fluids rapidly by rapid volume infuser or through use of a pressure bag

      (d) Monitor for hypocalcemia and coagulopathy if multiple blood transfusions are needed

  d. Hypothermia related to exposure to cold (see Hypothermia)

  e. Risk for infection related to inadequate primary defenses (broken skin, traumatized tissue) and invasive procedures (see Chapter 6)

  f. Risk for altered peripheral, renal, cardiopulmonary, and cerebral tissue perfusion related to interrupted blood flow from deep vein thromboses and emboli (see Chapters 1 to 4)

  g. Altered nutrition, less than body requirements, related to increased metabolic rate and decreased intake of nutrients (see Septic Shock and Gastrointestinal System)

h. Pain related to physical injury (see Chapter 9)

i. Risk for post-trauma response related to assault or accident

    i. Assessment for defining characteristics: reexperiencing a traumatic event, psychic or emotional numbness, difficulty in interpersonal relationships, or substance use

    ii. Expected outcomes

        (a) Patient verbalizes appropriate coping behaviors

        (b) Patient does not abuse alcohol or other substances

        (c) Patient resumes daily activities to his or her maximum capability

    iii. Nursing interventions

        (a) Discuss the patient's memories of the traumatic event and the emotional response

        (b) Be honest about the level of recovery to baseline status

        (c) Refer the patient appropriately if ineffective coping or substance abuse is demonstrated

    iv. Evaluation of nursing care

        (a) Patient verbalizes coping skills

        (b) Patient resumes activities after rehabilitation appropriate for level of functioning

Burns

1. **Pathophysiology**

    a. Definitions

        i. Burn: tissue injury due to coagulation of cellular proteins as a result of heat produced from thermal, chemical, electrical, or radiation energy; degree of coagulation depends on:

        (a) Temperature of the injuring agent

        (b) Duration of exposure to the injuring agent

        (c) Area exposed to the injuring agent

        ii. Extent of thermal injury: total surface area of the injured tissue (Fig. 8–7)

        iii. Depth of thermal injury: extent of injury down through layers (thicknesses) of skin (Figs. 8–8 and 8–9)

        (a) Zone of hyperemia

            (1) Outer zone of minimal injury; heals rapidly

            (2) Tissue is red (hyperemic) but blanches and refills with pressure

            (3) No cell death

        (b) Zone of stasis

            (1) Middle zone of injury whose cells can either recover or become necrotic over the initial 24 hours following injury

            (2) Tissue is red but does not blanch with pressure

        (c) Zone of coagulation

            (1) Area of injury where the temperature reaches at least 45°C

            (2) Protein coagulation and cell death

            (3) Tissue is black, gray, khaki, to white and does not blanch with pressure

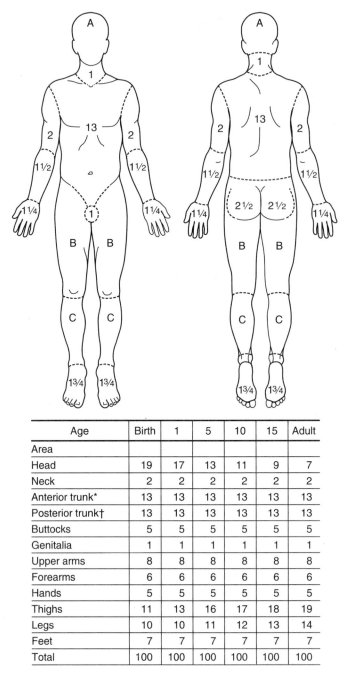

Age	Birth	1	5	10	15	Adult
Area						
Head	19	17	13	11	9	7
Neck	2	2	2	2	2	2
Anterior trunk*	13	13	13	13	13	13
Posterior trunk†	13	13	13	13	13	13
Buttocks	5	5	5	5	5	5
Genitalia	1	1	1	1	1	1
Upper arms	8	8	8	8	8	8
Forearms	6	6	6	6	6	6
Hands	5	5	5	5	5	5
Thighs	11	13	16	17	18	19
Legs	10	10	11	12	13	14
Feet	7	7	7	7	7	7
Total	100	100	100	100	100	100

* Without neck or genitalia.
† Without neck or buttocks.

Figure 8–7 • Lund and Broder chart used for estimating burn size. Numbers are the percentage of body surface area. A = ½ of head; B = ½ of one thigh; C = ½ of one leg. (Redrawn from Lund, C. C., and Browder, N. C.: The estimation of areas of burns. Surg. Gynecol. Obstet. 79:353, 1944.)

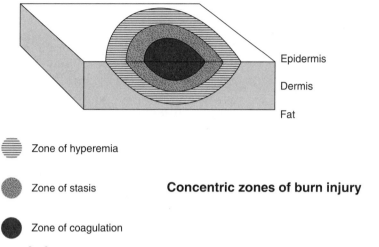

Epidermis

Dermis

Fat

Zone of hyperemia

Zone of stasis   **Concentric zones of burn injury**

Zone of coagulation

Figure 8–8 • Concentric zones of hyperemia, stasis, and coagulation within a burn.

b. Epidemiology
    i. Third leading cause of death for unintentional injury in the United States
    ii. Approximately 2 to 2.5 million Americans experience burns serious enough to require medical care each year
    iii. Approximately 70,000 people require hospitalization each year
    iv. Approximately 12,000 people die each year from burns
    v. Population that composes two thirds of burn fatalities is at the edges of the life span
        (a) Children (mostly preschool): higher mortality rates than adults
        (b) Older adults: aging process makes them less able to respond to conventional therapy. Underlying organ dysfunction leads to a diminished compensatory response to burn injury
c. Cellular pathophysiology: cellular injury occurs when tissues are exposed

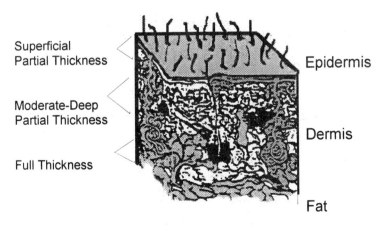

Superficial
Partial Thickness

Epidermis

Moderate-Deep
Partial Thickness

Dermis

Full Thickness

Fat

Burn Depth

Figure 8–9 • Cross-section of human skin demonstrating burn classification by depth.

to an energy source (thermal, chemical, electrical, radiation); responses are both local and systemic

   i. Local response: coagulation of cellular proteins, leading to irreversible cell injury with local production of complement, histamine, and oxygen free radicals

     (a) Complement (particularly C5a) activation and histamine release lead to increased vascular permeability

       (1) C5a attracts neutrophils to the area

       (2) Neutrophil activation leads to a respiratory burst with increased metabolism and production of oxygen free radicals

     (b) Production of oxygen free radicals (by-products formed during oxidative processes; independent molecules with positive or negative charges) such as superoxide or hydroxyl; produce tissue injury

       (1) Attach to electrons from cell lipids and proteins to alter the integrity of the cell membrane and endothelium of microvascular circulation, leading to edema formation

        a) Pulmonary vascular injury, pulmonary interstitial edema, and intra-alveolar hemorrhage

        b) RBC lysis and intravascular hemolysis

       (2) Alter the structure of deoxyribonucleic acid (DNA) and prevent the repair of the genetic code; may lead to total cell destruction

  ii. Systemic response: initiation of SIRS with the release of mediators (see Septic Shock; Table 8–1 for a list of mediators and cytokines)

     (a) Burn injury causes release of vasoactive substances, such as histamine, prostaglandins, interleukins, and arachidonic acid metabolites

     (b) Some experts suggest that bacterial translocation occurs (see Septic Shock)

     (c) Stress hormone production: release of cortisol, glucagon, and epinephrine

 iii. Consequences of local and systemic responses

     (a) Fluid shift from blood into interstitial and intracellular spaces because of increased vascular permeability

       (1) Systemic response occurs when the burn covers 20% or more of the total body surface area

       (2) Sodium-rich fluid and plasma proteins are lost into the interstitium

        a) Decreased capillary oncotic pressure

        b) Increased interstitial oncotic pressure

       (3) May cause increased tissue pressure, leading to compartment syndrome

       (4) May lead to hemoconcentration, increased hematocrit, and increased blood viscosity

     (b) Decreased intravascular volume; decreased blood flow to skin, kidneys, and the gastrointestinal tract

       (1) Compensatory increase in systemic vascular resistance

       (2) Decreased cardiac output

       (3) Further decrease in organ perfusion

        (c) Uncorrected response

          (1) Hypovolemic shock

          (2) Metabolic acidosis from anaerobic metabolism

          (3) Hyperkalemia from cellular lysis and as a complication of metabolic acidosis

       (d) Burn hypermetabolism: increased oxygen consumption, negative nitrogen and potassium balance, excessive muscle wasting, glucose intolerance, hyperinsulinemia, insulin resistance, sodium retention, and peripheral leukocytosis

       (e) Specific organ system changes other than skin

          (1) Immune system: SIRS

          (2) Cardiovascular

             a) Initial: tachycardia, increased blood pressure, decreased cardiac output, and hypovolemia

             b) After 24 hours: increased cardiac output from hypermetabolism

          (3) Pulmonary

             a) Pulmonary hypertension; vascular and perivascular inflammation

             b) Microvascular leak with interstitial pulmonary edema (acute respiratory distress syndrome) and ventilation-perfusion mismatch

             c) Changes with smoke inhalation (Table 8–5)

          (4) Renal

             a) Decreased renal perfusion and ischemic injury

             b) Myoglobinuria from muscle damage, leading to obstructed renal tubules

  d. Classification of burn injury

    i. American Burn Association (Table 8–6)

    ii. Classification by depth

       (a) Superficial partial-thickness (formerly first-degree) burns

          (1) Skin layer: epidermal

          (2) Appearance: pink to red without blistering but there may be slight edema; blanching with pressure

          (3) Discomfort: uncomfortable to touch, but discomfort decreases as burn heals; itching

          (4) Healing: 3 to 5 days without scarring

       (b) Moderate partial-thickness (formerly second-degree) burns

          (1) Skin layer: superficial dermal

          (2) Appearance: red or mottled and pink with blistering; skin moist and weeping; blanching with pressure

          (3) Discomfort: very painful

          (4) Healing: less than 3 weeks

       (c) Deep partial-thickness (formerly second-degree) burns

          (1) Skin layer: deep dermal

          (2) Appearance: pink to pale ivory; wound may be dry with blisters or bullae; no blanching with pressure

          (3) Discomfort: pain response varies from severe to minimal

          (4) Healing: usually 3 to 6 weeks

TABLE 8–5. Chemical, Inhalation, and Electrical Injury

Type/Severity	Description	Reaction	Findings	Management
Chemical Severity of injury depends on: 1. Strength or concentration of chemical 2. Length of contact 3. Quantity of chemical 4. Extent of tissue penetration 5. Mode of chemical's action	Tissue injury and destruction from necrotizing substances 1. *Strong acids* (desiccants): sulfuric and muriatic acid 2. *Corrosives*: phenol, lye, white phosphorus 3. *Oxidizing agents*: chromic acid, potassium permanganate 4. *Vesicants*: dimethyl sulfoxide, chemical warfare agents (gases) 5. *Protoplasmic poisons*: formic acid, tannic acid, hydrochloric acid	Cellular dehydration Denaturation Oxidation Chemical coagulation of protein Precipitation of chemical compounds in cell Protoplasmic poisoning	Burning Discoloration Tissue degeneration; injury to skin and underlying structures continues until chemical is removed or inactivated Localized pain and edema Systemic effects depend on substance	Remove chemical from body contact; brush off chemical powders Flush chemical from wound with large amounts of saline or water for at least 15 minutes; flush eyes for 30 minutes Remove all clothing and discard Do not rub skin; blot or brush off with a washcloth Cover all burned areas with damp sterile dressings until appropriate burn care is instituted
Inhalation Inhaling hot air, steam, or noxious chemicals, which cause damage to respiratory tract	Carbon monoxide inhalation	Carbon monoxide is produced by incomplete burning of materials; displaces oxygen from hemoglobin because hemoglobin has 200 times higher an affinity for carbon monoxide than oxygen	Cherry-red skin color Hypoxia leading to anoxia Elevated carboxyhemoglobin (COHb) level. Normal: 5% for nonsmokers and less than 10% for smokers Exposure levels of COHb 30% to 40% or more COHb cause significant neurologic effects (syncope, severe headache, visual disturbances)	Warmed, humidified 100% oxygen Determine COHb level Bronchodilators Postural drainage Intubation and mechanical ventilation as appropriate Hyperbaric oxygenation if COHb above 25% (accelerates dissociation of COHb from hemoglobin)
	Inhalation above glottis: hot air, steam, smoke (injury usually thermally produced)	Mucosal burns of oropharynx and larynx Injury and swelling	Redness, blistering, edema Risk for upper airway obstruction	Remove patient from smoky or toxic environment Maintain patent airway

	Pathophysiology	Clinical manifestations	Nursing interventions
Inhalation below glottis (injury usually chemically versus thermally produced)	Exposure to toxic fumes or smoke leads to acute respiratory distress syndrome (ARDS) Toxins damage type II pneumocytes and decrease surfactant production Epithelial sloughing with bronchitis occurs 6 to 72 hours after burn injury	Facial burns, singed hair, circumoral or neck burns Sooty or gray mucus Smoky breath Hoarseness or stridor, dyspnea Respiratory distress Dyspnea Decreased lung compliance Sever hypoxemia Ventilation, perfusion imbalances	Provide humidified oxygen Elevate head of bed See ARDS
Electrical Injury caused by intense heat generated from electrical current or lightning Severity of injury depends on: 1. *Amperage:* amount of resistance applied to voltage 2. *Voltage:* measure of force of the flow of current 3. *Type of current:* alternating or direct 4. *Duration of contact:* longer contact causes more injury 5. *Surface area of contact:* larger surface area causes greater injury 6. *Tissue resistance:* high resistance (skin, bone, fat) versus low resistance (blood vessels, nerves, organs) 7. *Current's course in body*	Coagulation necrosis Direct damage to nerves and vessels Tissue anoxia and cell death Asphyxiation caused by tetany of muscles of respiration or respiratory arrest Long bone or vertebral fractures from tetanic contractons of muscles Muscle destruction	White, charred skin; leathery skin Odor of burned skin Decreased or absent pain Cardiac dysrhythmias (ventricular fibrillation, asystole) Entrance and exit wounds with degree of damage greater than is visible Contraction of skeletal muscles Changes in vision, seizure activity, paralysis	Patient should be removed by trained personnel Turn off electrical source Initiate basic life support to maintain airway, breathing, and circulation Administer humidified oxygen Monitor cardiac rhythm Cover entry and exit wounds with damp sterile dressings

TABLE 8–6. American Burn Association Burn Classification

Degree of Injury	Partial Thickness		Full Thickness		Considerations
	Adults	*Children*	*Adults*	*Children*	
Minor	<15%	<10%	<2%	<2%	Does not include special area burns, such as eyes, ears, face, hands, feet, or perineum Does not include people at high risk (extremes of age, people with inhalation injury or electrical injury, people with complex injuries, people with chronic illnesses) Can be treated as an outpatient
Moderate	15%–25%	10%–20%	2%–10%	<5%	Excludes special area burns as above Excludes poor-risk patients as above Can be treated as an outpatient or inpatient, depending on severity and location
Major	>25%	>20%	>10%	>5%	Includes special area burns as above Includes poor-risk patients as above Should be treated at specialized burn unit or burn center

Data from Johnson, J.: Burns. *In* Swearingen, P., and Keen, J. (eds.): Manual of Critical Care Nursing. St. Louis, Mosby–Year Book, 1995; Sadowski, D.: Care of the child with burns. *In* Hazinski, M. F. (ed.): Nursing Care of the Critically Ill Child, 2nd ed. St. Louis, Mosby–Year Book, 1992; Sadowski, D.: Burns. *In* Sommers, M. S., and Johnson, S. (eds.): Davis's Manual of Nursing Therapeutics for Diseases and Disorders (Philadelphia, F. A. Davis, 1997; and Wong, D. L.: Nursing Care of Infants and Children. St. Louis, Mosby–Year Book, 1995.

    (d) Full-thickness (formerly third-degree) burns
        (1) Skin layer: injury extends beneath the dermal layer to fat, muscle, and bone
        (2) Appearance: white, red, to brown or black; no blistering; with or without thrombosed vessels; dry, leathery, and hard; depressed if the underlying muscle is damaged
        (3) Discomfort: pain to superficial pinprick is absent, but deep aching pain occurs
        (4) Healing: more than 1 month, with grafting required

2. Etiologic or precipitating factors
  a. Factors associated with burns
    i. Physical
      (a) Age: incidence highest in very old patients and in children younger than 2 years of age; children 2 to 5 years of age are also at risk
        (1) Older patients (>65 years of age) may have poor vision, risk of overmedicating, or poor living conditions

(2) Very young patients (<5 years of age) lack an understanding of the consequences of their behavior, such as playing with fire or matches

(b) Type of burn: thermal, electrical, chemical, radiation

(c) Preburn health status: preexisting organ dysfunction or conditions, such as diabetes mellitus, chronic obstructive lung disease, heart failure, and hypertension impair compensatory responses to burns

ii. Environmental factors

(a) Presence of fire escapes, smoke alarms, sprinkler systems, firewalls, fire extinguishers

(b) Compliance with federal regulations on combustible and flammable products (nightclothes, plastic in airplanes)

iii. Socioeconomic factors

(a) Working in a high-risk occupation: firefighters, construction workers, roofers, chemical workers, paving contractors, electricians or electrical line workers

(b) Living in a poorly maintained home

(c) Living in areas where arson is a problem

iv. Personality and psychologic factors: risk-taking behaviors, antisocial behavior, mental illness, depression, poor judgment, inadequate child care, geriatric abuse or neglect

(a) Burns are sometimes associated with physical abuse (cigarette burns)

(b) Burns may occur when young children are inadequately supervised

(1) Playing with matches or lighters

(2) Fireworks

(3) Kitchen accidents: boiling water, stoves

(4) Bathroom accidents: hot water in a bathtub

(c) Burn may be a suicide gesture or attempt

v. Alcohol and other drugs of use (see Multisystem Trauma): people who use alcohol often smoke; intoxication increases the risk for burns

vi. Temporal

(a) Most deaths from house fires occur during winter

(b) Injuries from fireworks and barbecue grills occur during summer

b. Causes

i. Thermal: contact with flames or hot objects

(a) House fires are responsible for 75% of all burn deaths, but most of those are due to smoke inhalation or carbon monoxide poisoning

(1) Causes of houses fires: cigarette smoking, malfunctioning heaters, propane tank, electrical wiring

(2) Only 5% of all burn victims have a thermal injury from house fires

(b) Clothing ignition: contact with flames

(1) Responsible for 5% of all burn deaths (up to 75% in elderly population)

(2) Second leading cause of hospitalization, but rates are decreasing because of nonflammable clothing legislation

    ii. Scalds: contact with hot liquids or steam

      (a) Responsible for 3% of all burn deaths and 30% of burn hospital admissions

      (b) Usually caused by hot liquids or steam, hot water in bathtubs and showers, and hot coffee spilled

      (c) Children under age 4 most often affected

      (d) Elderly are susceptible because of fragile, thin skin

   iii. Chemical: contact with caustic or toxic chemicals, leading to tissue coagulation of protein, precipitation of chemical compounds in cells, cellular dehydration, and protoplasmic poisoning

      (a) Home: cleaning agents

      (b) Industry: explosions and contact with chemicals

      (c) Chemical agents

        (1) Oxidizing agents: cause tissue oxidation; potassium permanganate

        (2) Corrosives: cause tissue denaturation (loss of normal properties of cellular proteins); phenol, lye, and white phosphorus

        (3) Desiccants: cause severe cellular dehydration; sulfuric acid

        (4) Vesicants: cause blisters; dimethyl sulfoxide and poisonous gases used in warfare

        (5) Protoplasmic poisons: cause cellular coagulation; acetic acid, tannic acid, and oxalic acid

   iv. Electrical: contact with an electrical current or flash caused by electrical arcing

      (a) Approximately 1000 deaths per year

      (b) Most common in summer: lightning; electrocution in homes, on farms, or in industrial locations

      (c) Household appliances: hair dryers and wall sockets

      (d) Industrial: electrical transmission lines

      (e) Toddlers at risk for biting on electrical cords or putting objects into electrical outlets

   v. Radiation: exposure to ionizing radiation (alpha and beta particles, gamma rays, x-rays) resulting from inadvertent exposure or a catastrophic disaster or accident

      (a) Long-term biologic effect, resulting in chronic health concerns

      (b) Intracellular destruction of DNA, loss of genetic information

      (c) Acute injury similar to early symptoms of thermal injury (pain, swelling, redness, tissue ischemia); several weeks may pass before symptoms appear

3. Nursing assessment data base

  a. Nursing history

    i. Complete description of burn injury

      (a) Time: delay of treatment may result in a minor or moderate burn becoming a major injury

      (b) Location: closed-space injuries are related to smoke inhalation

      (c) Context or situation: falling asleep while smoking; being burned at work; pulling boiling water off a stove

      (d) Burning agent, temperature of agent, and length of exposure

      (e) Actions of witnesses

ii. Suspicion of physical abuse: if abuse is suspected, obtain in-depth information. Factors that raise suspicion:

    (a) Delay in seeking treatment

    (b) Burns not consistent with the reported history

    (c) Bruising at different stages of healing

    (d) Report of the burn differs among household members

    (e) History of previous injury

iii. Past medical and surgical health history, with particular emphasis on organ malfunction: heart failure, hypertension, chronic obstructive pulmonary disease (COPD), diabetes mellitus, and renal failure

iv. Substance use and abuse: detailed history of smoking, alcohol, and other drugs of abuse

v. Family and social history: household members and relationships; household and child care responsibilities; occupation, education, and job status; financial situation and insurance coverage; religion

vi. Allergies, current medications

b. Nursing examination of patient

  i. Primary survey: rapid assessment (30 seconds to 2 minutes) that simultaneously identifies and manages life-threatening injuries

    (a) ABCDE (see Multisystem Trauma for assessments and interventions): *a*irway, *b*reathing, *c*irculation, *d*isability, and *e*xposure

    (b) Interventions that should take place with exposure

      (1) Remove burning clothing to stop further injury, and inspect all skin surfaces

      (2) Remove smoldering clothing by soaking clothes in a saline solution beforehand

      (3) Cover the patient to prevent heat loss

  ii. Secondary survey: a head-to-toe physical assessment is begun as soon as the primary survey and emergency, life-saving interventions are completed. *Note:* ongoing resuscitation continues during the secondary survey as needed

    (a) Note the odor of the smoke (suspect inhalation injury)

    (b) Other findings that increase the suspicion of smoke inhalation: burns of the intraoral cavity, hoarseness, expiratory wheezes, singed nasal hair, circumoral burns, and blackened carbonaceous sputum

    (c) Assess for accompanying traumatic injuries, such as fractures, internal hemorrhage, and head injury

iii. Vital signs: widely variable because of the catecholamine stress response, burn severity, and medication therapy

    (a) Serial vital signs: essential to monitor the response to burns and to interventions

    (b) Respiratory rate

      (1) Ideal: 12 to 20 breaths/minute

      (2) Typical following major burns: tachypnea

      (3) Absence of tachypnea following a major burn indicates CNS suppression (alcohol or other drugs of abuse) or injury, airway obstruction, and restricted chest excursion from injured skin

        a) Monitor for edema of the neck and airway

        b) Monitor for circumferential eschar formation around the neck or chest

        c) Monitor for signs of obstruction: stridor, hoarseness, restlessness, behavior changes, and decreased level of consciousness

(c) Heart rate

  (1) Ideal: 60 to 100 beats/minute

  (2) Typical following burn: tachycardia

    a) Well-conditioned athletes have slow heart rates

    b) Electrical burns may lead to dysrhythmias (ventricular fibrillation, asystole)

    c) Patient may have decreased or absent peripheral pulses or delayed capillary refill

(d) Blood pressure

  (1) Ideal: systolic pressure above 90 mm Hg

  (2) Typical following burns: variable, depending on fluid loss and the patient's age but often hypotension

  (3) Young adults may maintain blood pressure in spite of significant fluid losses

  (4) Older adults have less compensatory mechanisms and less tolerance for fluid deficits

  (5) Alcohol intoxication may lead to either hypotension or hypertension

(e) Temperature

  (1) Ideal: core temperature above 37°C

  (2) Typical following burns: decreased core temperature of 35° to 37°C because of exposure or loss of heat from open wounds

  (3) Hyperthermia may develop because of increased tissue metabolism and infection

(f) Hemodynamics and urinary output: usually a PA catheter is not used during initial burn resuscitation; urine output is more commonly used to determine the success of fluid resuscitation; the PA catheter is used after 72 hours for cardiopulmonary instability

  (1) Ideal: urine output above 1 ml/kg/hour

  (2) Typical following burns: decreased urine output

iv. Inspection of burn: see classification by depth

(a) Location: hands, face, eyes, ears, feet, and genitalia increase severity

(b) Appearance: color, consistency, and changes in vessels

(c) Depth: severity depends on the intensity and duration of the exposure

(d) Extent: percent of the body surface area involved; severity depends on intensity and duration of exposure

(e) Considerations

  (1) Check for entry and exit sites for electrical burns. There may be small entry and exit sites but large areas of injury lying underneath the skin (''iceberg effect''). Internal damage may not be evident for hours or days

  (2) Monitor for increased swelling and edema, which may lead

        to airway obstruction or *compartment syndrome* (increased pressure within an anatomic compartment that compromises the perfusion, viability, and function of associated tissues)

        (3) Depth and severity of a burn may not be evident until several days after the initial injury

   v. Palpation, percussion, and auscultation of body systems to monitor for multisystem effects of an injury and inflammatory response (see MODS and Multisystem Trauma)

c. Diagnostic study findings

   i. ABGs

      (a) Respiratory alkalosis with $PaCO_2$ above 32 mm Hg may occur early because of tachypnea

      (b) Metabolic acidosis with pH above 7.34 occurs after major burns

        (1) The pH usually returns to normal with correction of fluid deficit and correction of low cardiac output states

        (2) Base deficit is typical

      (c) Metabolic acidosis also occurs with topical mafenide acetate (Sulfamylon) application over a large burn

      (d) In severe burns and inhalation injuries, progressively increasing the fraction of inspired oxygen is needed to maintain PaO_2 and SaO_2

   ii. Carboxyhemoglobin (COHb) level: more than 10% is diagnostic of carbon monoxide poisoning (see Table 8–5). Absence of positive COHb does not rule out inhalation injury

   iii. CBC and differential

      (a) The post-burn period is associated with leukocytosis (increased WBC count as high as $30,000/mm^3$; usually resolves in 48 hours)

      (b) Leukopenia may occur as a side effect of a topical treatment with silver sulfadiazine or because of SIRS

      (c) Local heat may lead to RBC destruction; however, usually increased hematocrit due to hemoconcentration and "third spacing" occurs

      (d) Thrombocytopenia may occur during the first 72 hours as a result of dilution and some microvascular thromboses

   iv. Nutritional parameters

      (a) Serum glucose levels: elevated from stress response

      (b) Total protein and albumin: decreased because of protein loss from increased vascular permeability

   v. Electrolytes

      (a) Hyperkalemia due to tissue destruction, RBC hemolysis, and increased intracellular sodium concentration from osmotic changes

      (b) Sodium imbalance

        (1) Hypernatremia resulting from intravascular fluid loss and hemoconcentration

        (2) Hyponatremia resulting from sodium loss and hemodilution

   vi. Coagulation studies: elevations in prothrombin and partial thromboplastin time during the first 3 days after burn injury because of leakage of clotting factors from the intravascular space

   vii. Blood alcohol level and drug toxic screen to identify:

      (a) The circumstances of a burn injury

(b) The risk of withdrawal

(c) The complications of substance use

viii. BUN often is elevated because of increased tissue and RBC destruction and dehydration; creatinine level is normal unless acute renal failure is occurring

4. Nursing diagnoses

a. Ineffective airway clearance related to secretions and obstruction from airway edema (see Chapter 1)

   i. Additional nursing interventions

     (a) Monitor for carbonaceous sputum, hoarseness, and stridor

     (b) Maintain the airway with oral or nasal airway or jaw lift and chin thrust. *Note:* keep the patient's head in neutral position until the cervical spine has been determined to be without injury, or maintain intubation as needed

b. Ineffective breathing pattern related to an inflammatory process, decreased lung expansion, and tracheobronchial obstruction (see Chapter 1)

   i. Additional nursing interventions

     (a) Institute pain control measures rapidly

     (b) Avoid overly aggressive fluid resuscitation, which can lead to increasing pulmonary and peripheral edema

     (c) Monitor for inelastic eschar formation of the upper chest and neck, which impedes adequate respiratory excursion

c. Impaired gas exchange related to alveolar-capillary membrane changes (see Chapter 1 and additional nursing interventions in Table 8–5)

d. Fluid volume deficit related to active loss and maldistribution (see Chapter 2)

   i. Additional nursing interventions (Table 8–7)

     (a) Control any bleeding with pressure

     (b) Use large-bore peripheral catheters or central trauma catheters to initiate rapid fluid resuscitation

     (c) Use an accepted formula and solution to calculate fluid replacement needs

       (1) Do not overresuscitate with fluids

       (2) Use hourly urinary outputs to guide fluid replacement, with a goal of more than 1 ml/kg/hour

e. Risk for infection related to inadequate primary defenses (broken skin, traumatized tissues), inadequate secondary defenses (immunosuppression), and invasive procedures (see Chapter 6)

   i. Additional nursing interventions

     (a) Administer tetanus toxoid as prescribed

     (b) Initial debridement: wash the surface of the wound with a mild soap or antiseptic solution

     (c) Debride the devitalized tissue

     (d) Cover the wound with antibacterial agents and occlusive gauze

     (e) Maintain hand-washing and isolation techniques as appropriate

f. Hypothermia related to exposure (see Hypothermia)

   i. Additional nursing interventions

     (a) Do not cover large burns with saline-soaked dressings, which lower core temperature

TABLE 8–7. Phases of Burn Care Management

Phase	Goals	Management Considerations

Emergent
 	
Resuscitative phase: lasts 48 to 72 hours after injury or until diuresis takes place
	Maintain airway, breathing, and circulation
	Maintain excretory function
	Preserve joint function and mobility
	Prevent complications
	Preserve self-concept
		1. Endotracheal intubation and mechanical ventilation if needed
		2. Fluid resuscitation (formulas vary)
		  a. Typical formula is usually a balanced salt solution, such as lactated Ringer's solution or normal saline: (4 ml) $\times$ (% burn) $\times$ (weight in kg) + 1500 $\times$ m^2 equals volume per 24 hours; 50% is given in first 8 hours, 25% is given in second 8 hours, and 25% is given in third 8 hours
		  b. Other fluids, such as dextrose 5% in water, may be given to replace insensible loss or hypertonic saline to lessen burn edema
		  c. Electrolyte replacement based on laboratory results
		3. Pain and anxiety management
		4. Wound care and ongoing debridement
		  a. Wash burn surface with mild soap; apply silver sulfadiazine or collagenase; cover wounds with sterile dry sheets
		  b. Immerse minor burns in normal saline solution 55°C
		5. Nutritional support (often enteral by nasogastric route)

Acute/Wound Coverage *Middle phase:* characterized by eschar separation; lasts until spontaneous healing of burn wound occurs or until grafts are in place (variable time period lasting weeks to months)	Remove burn eschar Promote wound coverage Prevent complications (sepsis, cardiovascular collapse)	1. Maintenance of hydration and electrolyte balance (monitor for decreased potassium and sodium) 2. Hydrotherapy with wound cleansing 3. Ongoing debridement followed by topical antimicrobial agents (silver sulfadiazine, mafenide acetate, silver nitrate) or debridement with collagenase ointment accompanied by application of polymyxin B sulfate/bacitracin powder 4. Skin grafting 5. Ongoing pain management, emotional support, nutritional support, occupational and physical therapy
Convalescent/ Rehabilitative Time period for inpatient rehabilitation	Promote return (functionally and cosmetically) to usual roles and responsibilities Support patient to adapt emotionally to burn injury Encourage maximum function of body parts	Ongoing pain management, emotional support, nutritional support, occupational and physical therapy, speech therapy if needed

        (b) If the patient is hypothermic, maintain a warm ambient temperature; keep the patient covered

        (c) Limit traffic into the patient's room, to prevent drafts

  g. Altered nutrition, less than body requirements, related to increased metabolic rate and decreased intake of nutrients (see Septic Shock and Gastrointestinal System)

  h. Risk for alterations in tissue perfusion (peripheral) related to fluid shifts (see Chapter 2)

     i. Additional nursing interventions

        (a) Remove constricting jewelry to limit tissue hypoperfusion

        (b) Monitor for the need of escharotomy (incision is made through an encircling eschar to release constricted tissue) or fasciotomy

          (1) Check peripheral pulses hourly and as needed, with a Doppler examination if necessary

          (2) Notify the physician for capillary refill longer than 3 seconds, numbness and tingling of the extremities, or dusky extremities

  i. Risk for self-concept, a disturbance in body image related to powerlessness, and changes in body appearance during a critical illness (see Chapter 9)

  j. Risk for altered family process related to a situational crisis of critical illness (see Chapter 9)

Hypothermia

1. Pathophysiology

  a. Temperature regulation

     i. Core temperature, the temperature of deep tissues of the body, ranges between 36° and 37.5°C (97° to 99.5°F)

     ii. Normal core temperature remains relatively constant, with a range of +/− 1°F (0.6°C) during periods of health

     iii. Body temperature is regulated by neural feedback mechanisms operating through temperature-regulating centers in the hypothalamus

        (a) Anterior hypothalamic-preoptic area of the brain has large numbers of heat-sensitive neurons along with one third as many cold-sensitive neurons

        (b) Heat-sensitive neurons increase the rate of firing as the temperature rises, whereas cold-sensitive neurons increase firing as the temperature drops

        (c) Temperature receptors exist in skin and deep tissues (spinal cord, abdominal viscera, great veins) to detect cold and are thought to protect the body from low temperatures

        (d) Peripheral receptors and temperature sensory signals from the anterior hypothalamic-preoptic areas stimulate the posterior hypothalamus to control heat-producing and heat-conserving reactions

        (e) When the body is too cold, the posterior hypothalamus control system institutes physiologic reactions

(1) Skin vasoconstriction caused by stimulation of posterior hypothalamus SNS centers

(2) Piloerection ("goose flesh"; hairs standing on end); SNS stimulation causes arrector pili muscles attached to hair follicles to contract

(3) Increased heat production by metabolic systems

    a) Shivering

        i) The primary motor center for shivering is located in the dorsomedial portion of the posterior hypothalamus; this center is excited by cold signals from the skin and spinal cord when the body temperature falls below a critical value

        ii) Signals increase the tone of skeletal muscles; when the tone reaches a critical level, shivering begins, which increases body heat production four times the normal

    b) SNS stimulation: chemical *thermogenesis* (production of heat) occurs with an increased release of norepinephrine and epinephrine, which increases the rate of cellular metabolism and heat production by 10% to 15%

    c) Thyroxine secretion

        i) Hypothermia causes the release of thyrotropin-releasing hormone from the hypothalamus

        ii) Further stimulation of thyroid-stimulating hormone (TSH) and subsequent thyroxine production occur

        iii) Thyroxine causes chemical thermogenesis, but changes require several weeks because of the need for the thyroid gland to hypertrophy

iv. Temperature set-point in the hypothalamus

  (a) Core temperature of 37.1°C (98.8°F) is considered the set-point, meaning that all temperature control mechanims continually attempt to bring the body temperature back to this level

  (b) At temperatures above this level, the rate of heat loss is greater than heat production

  (c) At temperatures below this level, the rate of heat production is greater than heat loss

v. Thermoneutral zone

  (a) The ambient temperature at which the basal rate of thermogenesis is sufficient to offset continuing heat loss, that is, 28°C (82.4°F)

  (b) When the ambient temperature is below this point, the body increases heat production by combustion

b. Physiology of hypothermia

  i. Definition: core temperature below 35°C (95°F) (Table 8–8)

  ii. Once the body temperature falls below 34°C (93.2°F), the hypothalamus has an impaired ability to regulate temperature. At temperatures of 29.4°C (85°F) and below, the hypothalamus can no longer regulate temperature at all

    (a) Failure is partly due to a loss of the ability to generate chemical heat production

TABLE 8–8. Classification of Hypothermia*,†

Classification	Range	Accompanying Physiologic Changes
Mild	<35°–32°C <95°–89.6°F	Relatively safe zone with depression of cerebral metabolism, confusion, faulty judgment, and amnesia; tachycardia, increased blood pressure, and increased cardiac output leading to progressive bradycardia and vasoconstriction; tachypnea progressing to decreased minute volume and bronchospasm; diuresis; increased preshivering muscle tone followed by shivering; paralytic ileus
Moderate	<32°–28.0°C <89.6°–82.4°F	Decreased level of consciousness, pupil dilation, hallucinations; decrease in pulse and cardiac output, prolonged systole, increased atrial and ventricular dysrhythmias, conduction disturbances, Osborne wave (hypothermic hump: secondary deflection in QRS in medial and lateral precordial leads and inferior leads; related to delayed ventricular depolarization and early ventricular repolarization, acidosis, and myocardial anoxia) appear on electrocardiogram; coagulopathies; hypoventilation, decreased carbon dioxide production, decreased oxygen consumption, absence of protective airway reflexes; decreased renal blood flow; hyporeflexia, diminished shivering, rigidity
Severe	<28°–20°C <82.4–68°F	Decreased cerebral blood flow, coma; decreased cardiac output, hypotension, bradycardia, ventricular fibrillation; pulmonary edema, apnea; oliguria; 80% decrease in basal metabolism; decreased nerve conduction velocity, peripheral areflexia, hyperkalemia
Profound	<20°–14°C <68°–57.2°F	Asystole, isoelectric electroencephalogram, cell death
Deep	<14°C <57.2°F	Incompatible with life unless therapeutically induced

Data from Collins, J.: Hypothermia. Practitioner 239:22–26, 1995; Cummins, R. O.: Textbook of Advanced Cardiac Life Support. Greenville, Texas, American Heart Association, 1994; Danzl, D. F., and Pozos, R. S.: Accidental hypothermia. N. Engl. J. Med. 331:1756–1760, 1994; Fritsch, D. E.: Hypothermia in the trauma patient. AACN Clin. Issues Adv. Pract. Acute Crit. Care 6:196–211, 1995; Gentilello, L. M.: Advances in the management of hypothermia. Surg. Clin. North Am. 75:243–256, 1995; and Humbli, E. H., and Demling, R. H.: Hypothermia and cold-related injuries. *In* Ayers, S. M. (ed.): Textbook of Critical Care, 3rd ed. Philadelphia, W. B. Saunders, 1995.

*Multiple trauma is complicated by hypothermia. Some sources consider mild hypothermia for trauma patients to be classified as a temperature below 36°C to 34°C, moderate hypothermia as a temperature below 34°C to 32°C, and severe hypothermia as a temperature below 32°C.

†Advanced Cardiac Life Support guidelines classify mild hypothermia as 34°C to 36°C, moderate hypothermia as 30°C to 34°C, and severe hypothermia as below 30°C.

    (b) Failure also is due to sleepiness progressing to coma, which depresses heat control mechanisms and shivering mechanisms

  iii. Once the body temperature falls below 25.0°C (77°F), ventricular fibrillation, asystole, and death occur

  iv. Mechanisms of heat loss

    (a) Radiation: heat passes from warmer to cooler areas through air without direct contact

      (1) The normal response in humans makes up as much as 55% to 65% of the total heat loss

      (2) Depends on the amount of skin exposed to the environment and the degree of vasodilation or vasoconstriction

            (3) Heat loss by conduction is limited by clothing and by warming the environment

      (b) Conduction: transfer of heat through direct contact with cool objects; makes up approximately 15% of the body heat loss

            (1) Heat loss is increased when the body is in contact with water, the ground, or metal

            (2) Heat loss by conduction is limited by placing the body in contact with a poor heat conductor, such as wool

      (c) Convection: heat loss caused by movement of gases or liquids over skin (wing, fans, drafts). Liquids decrease the temperature internally or externally when the body is in contact with wet linens of during baths, irrigations, and blood transfusions

      (d) Evaporation: transfer of heat from moist skin or mucous membranes into the atmosphere; accounts for approximately 30% of the heat loss

            (1) Heat loss by evaporation is decreased if the skin is covered, but it increases with open wounds, wet skin, and increased respirations

            (2) Evaporation increases in conditions of low humidity, high environmental temperature, and increased air flow

2. Etiologic or precipitating factors

  a. Predisposing factors

    i. Environmental: skin exposure, wet clothing, low outside temperature, and air movement (wind, drafts)

    ii. Extremes of age: infancy, old age

    iii. Disease states that decrease metabolism: hypothyroidism, hypoadrenalism, malnutrition, hypoglycemia, circulatory shock

    iv. Cutaneous disruptions: wounds, burns

    v. Iatrogenic: exposure during an examination, fluid resuscitation, blood transfusions, immobilization, or surgery

    vi. Medications and substances: alcohol, phenothiazines, hypnotics, anxiolytics, antidepressants, narcotics, neuromuscular blocking agents, anesthesia

  b. Types of hypothermia

    i. Accidental: when an otherwise healthy person experiences overwhelming environmental cold. Examples: outdoor accidents (associated with hiking, mountaineering, or skiing), cold water immersion, sleeping outdoors in winter (particularly by the homeless), multiple trauma leading to exposure to cold environmental conditions, falls, and immobilization indoors (particularly in older people)

    ii. Primary: associated with an inherent defect of CNS control of thermoregulation. Examples: diencephalic epilepsy, cerebrovascular accidents, head injuries, neoplasms, and degenerative diseases

    iii. Secondary: associated with an underlying disease process, multiple trauma, mental illness, a severe infection, and medication or substance use and abuse; can also be a type of accidental hypothemia

      (a) Diseases: hypothyroidism, hypopituitarism, malnutrition, myocardial infarction, vascular insufficiency, pancreatitis, uremia, and carcinoma

(b) Multiple trauma: hypovolemic shock, burns, and near drowning

(c) Mental illness: dementia, self-neglect

(d) Infection: bacterial, viral, parasitic

(e) Medications and substance use as mentioned previously

iv. Therapeutic hypothermia: used during operative procedures to reduce tissue oxygen and nutrient demands

3. **Nursing assessment data base**

a. Nursing history

i. Patient health history

(a) Current history of exposure or trauma, including length of time of exposure and ambient or outdoor temperature

(b) Significant past medical and surgical history, with review of all major systems and of past traumatic injuries

(c) Medication history: prescribed and over-the-counter medications, particularly phenothiazines, hypnotics, anxiolytics, and antidepressants

(d) Relevant family history

(e) Social history

(1) Living situation: older people who live alone on limited incomes are at high risk for hypothermia during winter or after falling

(2) Alcohol use: daily and weekly patterns

(3) Outdoor activities, hobbies, and occupations

(4) Relationships with significant others

(5) Nutrition, daily patterns of eating, and ability to afford adequate nutrition

b. Nursing examination of patient (see Multisystem Trauma for guidelines on Primary and Secondary Surveys)

i. Vital signs: core temperature determines extent of hypothermia. *Note:* Use core temperature measurement with a PA thermistor if available; if no PA catheter is in place, use a rectal, urinary bladder, esophageal, or tympanic route. A diffference of 1° to 2°C may be present between the esophageal, PA, rectal, and bladder temperatures. Whichever method is chosen should be used consistently to enhance precision

(a) Mild hypothermia is usually accompanied by:

(1) Tachycardia

(2) Increased blood pressure and cardiac output

(3) Increased respirations

(b) Moderate hypothermia is associated with:

(1) Bradycardia

(2) Hypotension

(3) Decreased cardiac output

(c) Severe and profound hypothermia is associated with:

(1) Ventricular dysrhythmias

(2) Asystole

(3) Apnea

ii. Inspection

(a) Respiratory: assesses the adequacy of the airway and breathing. Expect tachypnea progressing to bradypnea, hypoventilation, and apnea; the more severe the hypothermia, the more depressed

the respiratory drive and the higher the risk for inadequate
maintenance of the airway and breathing

(b) Circulatory: pallor and increased bleeding tendencies

(c) Neurologic: confusion, anxiety, and apathy progressing to a
decreased level of consciousness, pupil dilation, and coma

(d) Musculoskeletal: increased preshivering muscle tone progressing
to shivering and then rigidity

(e) Renal: cold-induced diuresis progressing to oliguria

(f) Skin: piloerection

(g) Terminal burrowing behavior: a paradoxical reaction of severely
hypothermic patients who undress and find a position of
protection because of vasodilation and feelings of warmth

(1) Final mechanism of protection, with slowly developing lethal
hypothermia

(2) Autonomous process of the brain stem; triggered in final,
lethal hypothermia

iii. Palpation

(a) Circulation: weak, rapid pulses progressing to a slow or absent
pulse, diminished capillary blanching, and cold skin

(b) Gastrointestinal: distention from paralytic ileus

(c) Musculoskeletal: as shivering diminishes at lower temperatures,
hyporeflexia occurs, followed by rigidity and finally peripheral
areflexia

iv. Percussion

(a) Gastrointestinal: increased tympany accompanied by upper
abdominal distention indicates paralytic ileus

(b) Respiratory: with severe hypothermia, dullness may indicate lung
congestion and pulmonary edema

v. Auscultation

(a) Circulatory: rapid heart rate progressing to slow and then absent
heart sounds; hypertension progressing to hypotension and an
absence of blood pressure

(b) Respiratory: decreased air flow, diminished or absent breath
sounds, and crackles and gurgles from pulmonary congestion
and pulmonary edema

(c) Gastrointestinal: diminished bowel sounds progressing to absent
bowel sounds

c. Diagnostic study findings

i. Electrocardiogram (ECG): tachycardia progressing to bradycardia,
atrial and ventricular dysrhythmias, and asystole; conduction
disturbances with prolongation of PR, QRS, and QT intervals, At
temperatures above 29°C, an Osborn or J wave (hypothermic hump)
develops; secondary deflection in the QRS is best seen in medial and
lateral precordial leads and inferior leads

ii. Laboratory findings

(a) ABGs and derived hemodynamic parameters: hypoxemia,
hypocapnia progressing to hypercapnia, metabolic acidosis, and
decreased oxygen delivery and consumption

(b) Hematocrit: increases approximately 2% for every 1°C decrease
in body temperature

(c) Coagulation profile: prothrombin time and partial

thromboplastin time may appear to be normal in spite of coagulopathies because tests are performed at 37°C in the laboratory. At lower temperatures, decreased fibrinogen levels and thrombocytopenia may occur

(d) Serum electrolytes: hypothermia masks ECG changes associated with hyperkalemia. Hyperkalemia and hyponatremia may occur with damage to the sodium-potassium-adenosine triphosphatase (ATPase) pump

(e) Blood ethanol level: blood or urine toxic screen to detect the presence of alcohol or other drugs of abuse

(f) BUN and creatinine: elevated as renal function deteriorates

(g) Urine myoglobin: caused by muscle damage from excessive shivering (rhabdomyolysis)

4. **Nursing diagnoses**
   a. Hypothermia related to exposure to cold, inadequate clothing, evaporation from skin, or inactivity
      i. Assessment for defining characteristics: core temperature below 35°C, shivering, cold skin, pallor, delayed capillary refill, tachycardia progressing to bradycardia, hypertension progressing to hypotension, and piloerection
      ii. Expected outcomes: temperature 37°C within 24 hours
      iii. Nursing interventions
         (a) Institute passive rewarming (relies on endogenous heat generation and ambient temperature to increase the core body temperature slowly at a rate of 0.5° to 2°C/hour) until normothermia is restored
            (1) Remove the patient from a cold environment
            (2) Remove wet clothing
            (3) Increase the ambient room temperature
            (4) Decrease the air flow in rooms
            (5) Cover the patient with blankets; cover the patient's head
            (6) Passive rewarming is reserved for relatively healthy, mildly hypothermic (temperature > 32°C), and hemodynamically stable patients
         (b) Institute active rewarming with both external and internal methods (Table 8–9)
            (1) Active external rewarming (use of a heat source outside the patient's body to raise the core body temperature). Used in patients with temperatures between 32° and 34°C as well as an adjunct to active internal rewarming with temperatures below 32°C
            (2) Active internal rewarming (use of a heat source inside the patient's body to raise the core body temperature). Used in the hospital for core temperatures below 32°C
         (c) Monitor for afterdrop (decrease in the core temperature of up to 2°C) after internal active rewarming is discontinued. Occurs when blood circulates to peripheral tissues, recools, and returns to body's core
         (d) Monitor for rewarming shock (vascular collapse due to decreased cardiac output, hypotension, cardiac dysrhythmias); consequence of warming the periphery before the core

TABLE 8–9. Interventions for Active Rewarming

Type of Rewarming	Intervention	Rationale and Discussion
Active External	Fluid-circulating heating blanket	Heating blankets below patient are in contact with the occiput, shoulder, presacral region, and heels, only 20% to 30% of the body surface when placed beneath patient; place blanket on top of patient because patient loses most heat through radiation/convection to overlying air Warms by decreasing heat loss from radiation/convection Disadvantage: burns at areas of pressure points
	Convective air blanket	Creates an environment of 43°C to prevent further heat loss into environment through convection Blanket must cover substantial portion of patient's body (neck to toes) and have borders fastened tightly
	Aluminum space blanket	Is a radiant blanket that increases insulating capacity of standard blanket coverage Blanket must be wrapped closely around the patient with additional standard blanket on top to minimize convective and conductive heat loss Patient's head must be covered with reflective material to decrease radiant heat loss
	Radiant warmer	Produces intense local heat close to skin Disadvantage: may cause burns if not enough local circulation to carry heat away from skin
Active Internal	Airway rewarming	Humidified, warmed gases (42°–46°C) are often provided through endotracheal tube via mechanical ventilation or through warmed gas via a mask With airway rewarming, only a modest core temperature rise and an afterdrop occur until body temperature begins to equilibrate with surroundings

	Body cavity lavage	Irrigation of body cavities (peritoneal, pleural, mediastinal) with warmed solution raises body temperature on average of 2°C/hour
		Gastric or colonic irrigations may also be used
		Potassium-free solution is used to prevent hyperkalemia
		Disadvantages:
		  Peritoneal lavage may not be an option for patients with abdominal trauma
		  Mediastinal lavage is associated with high morbidity because of a need for median sternotomy
		  Infection is a risk

Table continued on following page

TABLE 8–9. Interventions for Active Rewarming *Continued*

Type of Rewarming	Intervention	Rationale and Discussion

	Warm intravenous infusions	Prewarmed (43°C) fluids and blood products (37°C) prevent further heat loss and help correct hypothermia
		Methods to warm fluid include warm water baths, microwaving (treatment is controversial; do not use for blood products or dextrose-containing solutions), fluid warmers (may provide a flow too slow to correct fluid deficit), and rapid volume infusers
		Disadvantages:
		  Must be used rapidly, or fluids will lose heat to environment
		  If blood is warmed to a temperature above 40°C, cells will hemolyze
		  If flow is too slow, patients will be underresuscitated for hypovolemia
		  Considerable expertise needed to manage techniques

	Extracorporeal circulatory rewarming	Continuous arteriovenous rewarming uses arterial (femoral) and venous (femoral or subclavian) pressure difference to create circulation through a heparin-bonded tubing circuit to a countercurrent fluid warmer
		Increases core temperature approximately 4°C/hour
		Other techniques include extracorporeal venovenous rewarming and cardiopulmonary bypass
		Disadvantages:
		  Bleeding tendencies from heparin
		  High cost
		  Need for expertise for high-technology equipment

        (1) When the periphery is warmed before the core, cold, hyperkalemic, lactate-rich blood is shunted to the core of the body, leading to shock

        (2) Limit rewarming to 2°C/hour to decrease the risk of rewarming shock

     (e) Teach preventive strategies to at-risk patients and to staff caring for them:

        (1) Limit exposure to cold temperatures

        (2) Maximize body coverage

        (3) Monitor the intake of cold or room-temperature fluids

   iv. Evaluation of nursing care

     (a) Core temperature is 37°C

     (b) Patient has no complications of rewarming (afterdrop, bleeding tendencies, or burns)

  b. Hypothermia related to consumption of alcohol

i. Assessment for defining characteristics: core temperature below 35°C, with evidence of alcohol or drug intoxication (assessment findings depend on the toxic substance; Table 8–10, Toxic Ingestion) and hypotension

ii. Expected outcomes

    (a) Temperature returns to 37°C within 24 hours

    (b) Patient experiences no symptoms of alcohol or substance abuse withdrawal

iii. Nursing interventions

    (a) Institute rewarming techniques described previously

    (b) Monitor blood alcohol concentration (BAC) to determine the degree of alcohol intoxication. A BAC of 100 mg/dl or greater indicates legal intoxication in most states

        (1) Alcohol impairs thermoregulation by diminished shivering, decreased cold perception, and suppression of the hypothalamus

        (2) Monitor for hypotension related to depression of vasomotor center and vasodilation

    (c) Malnourished or alcoholic patients should receive thiamine intravenously during rewarming to limit the risk of neurologic impairment from thiamine deficiency

    (d) Institute alcohol and substance abuse assessment and appropriate therapeutic strategies to limit substance use and abuse in the future

iv. Evaluation of nursing care

    (a) Core temperature is 37°C

    (b) Patient has no complications of alcohol or substance abuse withdrawal

c. Ineffective airway clearance related to tracheobronchial obstruction or cognitive impairment from hypothermia (see Chapter 1)

i. Additional nursing interventions

    (a) Decreased mental status that accompanies hypothermia may result in airway obstruction from the patient's tongue

    (b) Endotracheal intubation can be managed safely in most hypothermic patients without inducing cardiac dysrhythmias

    (c) Use care in airway management to immobilize the cervical spine until cervical spine injury, which may accompany hypothermia, is ruled out

d. Ineffective breathing pattern related to neuromuscular impairment (see Chapter 1)

i. Additional nursing interventions

    (a) Monitor respirations; a respiratory rate of four or more breaths/minute may be sufficient for a hypothermic patient with adequate airway protection

    (b) Increase the usual time to determine breathlessness to up to 45 seconds prior to initiating cardiopulmonary resuscitation (CPR) because the presence of breathing may be difficult to detect in hypothermic patients

    (c) Administer warm (42° to 46°C), humidified oxygen

e. Decreased cardiac output related to decreased inotropic changes or alteration in electrical rate, rhythm, or conduction (see Chapter 2)

Text continued on page 779

TABLE 8–10. Symptoms and Toxicology Ranges for Commonly Ingested Toxic Substances

Substance	Therapeutic Level	Toxic Level	Vital Signs	Symptoms	Diagnostic Findings
Acetaminophen	10–20 µg/ml	>150 µg/ml at 4 hours; fatal hepatic necrosis can occur with 30 to 60 regular-strength tablets (10–20 g)	Normal (early) hypotension may be present	Anorexia, nausea, vomiting, diaphoresis, and malaise, followed by right upper quadrant abdominal pain and tenderness; bleeding	Abnormal liver function tests: AST, ALT, PT, bilirubin
Amphetamines	None	Varies by compound	Hypertension, tachycardia, hyperthermia, tachypnea	Hyperactivity, agitation, psychoses, paranoia, headache, hyperreactive reflexes, tremor, seizures, diaphoresis, hyperactive bowel sounds, flushing, and mydriasis	Increased CK; rhabdomyolysis (from hyperthermia or agitation); ECG: dysrhythmias; acidosis
Anticholinergics	Varies by compound	Varies by compound	Hyperthermia, labile blood pressure, circulatory collapse, tachycardia	Variable ranging from anxiety, agitation, mydriasis, confusion, hyperactivity, seizures, and delirium to lethargy, decreased mental status, and coma; urinary retention; dry skin and mouth; vasodilation	ECG: tachycardia, heart block
Arsenic	<100 µg/day	>100 µg/day	Hypotension and tachycardia	Nausea, vomiting, abdominal pain, difficulty swallowing, diarrhea, dehydration	Elevated BUN and creatinine; ECG: tachycardia and other dysrhythmias
Barbiturates (phenobarbital)	10–25 µg/ml	>30 µg/ml	Hypothermia, hypotension, and bradypnea progressing to apnea; bradycardia	Decreased level of awareness, lethargy, slurred speech, sleepiness progressing to confusion, ataxia, decreased reflexes, coma, blisters (bullae)	Hypercapnea; ECG: tachycardia, hypoglycemia
Benzodiazepines (diazepam)	300–400 ng/ml	Unknown	With parenteral but not oral doses: hypotension and bradypnea progressing to apnea	Lethargy, slurred speech, weakness, headache, and vertigo progressing to coma; diminished or absent bowel sounds, nausea, diarrhea, decreased reflexes	Hypercapnia (mild with oral doses)

774

Carbamazepine (Tegretol)	4–12 µg/ml	>12 µg/ml	CNS stimulation, hallucinations, seizures, mydriasis, nystagmus	Hypotension, hypothermia, bradypnea, tachycardia	ECG: tachycardia; leukopenia
Cocaine	None	Variable	Hyperactivity, restlessness, anxiety, agitation, delirium, mydriasis, headache, diaphoresis, nausea, vomiting, chest pain seizures, coma	Hypertension, tachycardia hyperthermia, tachypnea to apnea	Increased CK; ECG: tachycardia, ventricular fibrillation, ventricular tachycardia; acidosis
Cyclic antidepressants	Varies by compound	Varies by compound	Lethargy, confusion, dizziness, somnolence, coma	Hypotension, tachycardia, bradypnea	ECG: prolonged QRS, dysrhythmias such as bundle branch blocks, torsade de pointes
Cyanide	<1 µg/ml	Oral: 200 mg potassium cyanide: immediately fatal > 270 ppm and life-threatening 30 minutes at 110 ppm	Smell of bitter almonds, anxiety, agitation, lethargy, headache, seizures, abdominal pain, vomiting, cherry-red color or cyanosis	Variable but may follow pattern: first, hypertension and bradycardia; second, hypotension and tachycardia; third, hypotension and bradycardia; bradypnea and apnea	ECG: variable; acidosis with elevated lactate levels
Digoxin	0.8–2 ng/ml	>2 ng/ml	Patient may be asymptomatic; nausea, vomiting, anorexia, visual changes (colored lights, blurred vision)	Hypotension, bradycardia, or tachycardia	Hyperkalemia; ECG: heart block, tachydysrhythmias; bradydysrhythmias
Ethanol	None	50–100 mg/dl	Agitation, released inhibitions progressing to depressed mental status, nausea, vomiting, ataxia, poor motor coordination, poor decision-making ability, slurred speech, stupor, coma	Bradycardia or tachycardia; hypertension or hypotension; hypothermia; tachypnea leading to apnea	Respiratory alkalosis progressing to respiratory acidosis; hyperosmolarity of blood
Ethylene glucol (antifreeze)	None	50–100 mg/dl	Decreased mental status, lethargy, seizures, slurred speech, coma, abdominal pain, nausea, vomiting	Tachypnea	Hypoglycemia, metabolic acidosis, hypocalcemia, calcium oxalate crystals in urine

Table continued on following page

TABLE 8–10. Symptoms and Toxicology Ranges for Commonly Ingested Toxic Substances *Continued*

Substance	Therapeutic Level	Toxic Level	Vital Signs	Symptoms	Diagnostic Findings
Iron	<100 µg/dl	350 µg/dl	Hypotension, tachycardia	Nausea, vomiting (hematemesis), diarrhea, abdominal pain and tenderness; late: lethargy	Hyperglycemia, leukocytosis, metabolic acidosis, and blood in stool and vomitus
Isoniazid	3–5 µg/ml 1 to 2 hours after dose	Variable	Tachycardia, hypotension, and hyperthermia	*Note:* One of the most common causes of drug-induced seizures in the United States; nausea, vomiting, dizziness, ataxia, hyperreflexia, slurred speech; hallucinations, seizures, coma, oliguria	Metabolic acidosis, hyperglycemia, leukocytosis, and eosinophilia
Isopropyl alcohol (rubbing alcohol)	None	Variable	Hypotension, bradypnea, and hypothermia	Ataxia, areflexia, dizziness, headache, muscle weakness, abdominal pain and cramping, gastritis, hematemesis, poor peripheral tissue perfusion	Ketones (blood and urine) without acid base disorder; hyperosmolarity of blood
Lead	<10 µg/dl	>10 µg/dl	Hypertension and tachycardia	Anorexia, constipation, abdominal pain, vomiting, lethargy, fatigue, hyperactivity, ataxia, seizures, coma, numbness and tingling of extremities	Anemia, abdominal x-ray changes, increased urinary coproporphyrins, hemolysis, and proteinuria
Lithium	0.5–1.5 mEq/L	>2 mEq/L	Hypotension (late)	Weakness, fatigue, tremor, muscle twitching, ataxia, slurred speech, confusion, restlessness, hyperreflexia, stupor, coma, diuresis, dehydration, diarrhea	ECG: prolonged QT interval, ST segment, and T wave abnormalities; if diabetes insipidus occurs: increased serum osmolarity and decreased urine osmolarity

Mercury	<10 µg/L	>35 µg/L	Hypotension (late), tachypnea (inhaled mercury)	Tremor ataxia, paresthesias, tunnel vision, dyspnea, increased salivation, diarrhea, abdominal pain	Proteinuria, increased BUN and creatinine
Methanol (antifreeze)	None	Variable	Hypotension, tachypnea, temperature variations	Visual disturbances, blindness, blurred vision, dimmed vision (snow storm), inebriation, headache, dizziness, seizures, coma, nausea, vomiting, and abdominal pain	Metabolic acidosis, hyperosmolarity, hypophosphatemia, elevated CK and amylase
Opioids	None	Variable	Hypotension, bradypnea, hypothermia, bradycardia	Respiratory depression, drowsiness, and mood changes progressing to unresponsiveness, seizures, ataxia, nausea, vomiting, hyporeflexia, miosis, and absent bowel sounds	Hypercapnia
Phencyclidine (PCP)	None		Tachycardia, hypertension, tachypnea, hyperthermia	Range of neurologic behaviors: calm and unresponsive to excited, paranoid behavior, tremor, hyperactivity, myoclonic or dystonic movements; blank stare, dysconjugate gaze, nystagmus, blurred vision, miosis	Leukocytosis, hyperkalemia, metabolic acidosis; elevated CK, LDH, and AST; ketonuria, myoglobinuria, EEG changes
Phenothiazines	Variable		Hypotension, tachycardia, temperature variations	Memory deficits, confusion, dizziness, lethargy progressing to coma, decreased bowel sounds, and miosis or mydriasis	ECG: heart block, supraventricular and ventricular tachycardias

Table continued on following page

TABLE 8–10. Symptoms and Toxicology Ranges for Commonly Ingested Toxic Substances *Continued*

Substance	Therapeutic Level	Toxic Level	Vital Signs	Symptoms	Diagnostic Findings
Salicylates	15–30 mg/dl	>30 mg/dl	Hyperthermia, tachypnea, tachycardia	Tinnitus, diminished hearing, vertigo, agitation, hyperactivity, stupor, coma, increased bleeding tendencies, diaphoresis, nausea, vomiting	Increased anion gap, mixed acid-base disturbances with metabolic acidosis, prolonged PT, hypoglycemia or hyperglycemia
Sedatives	Variable	Variable	Hypotension, hypothermia, bradypnea progressing to apnea, bradycardia	Slurred speech, ataxia, incoordination, paradoxical excitement, skin bullae	Hypercapnia
Theophylline	10–20 μg/ml	>20 μg/ml	Hypotension, tachycardia, tachypnea	Hyperactivity, confusion, restlessness, agitation, seizures, nausea, vomiting, diaphoresis	Hypokalemia, ECG: tachycardias, metabolic acidosis, respiratory alkalosis, leukocytosis, hyperglycemia

ALT = alanine aminotransferase; AST = aspartate aminotransferase; BUN = blood urea nitrogen; CK = creatinine phosphokinase; CNS = central nervous system; ECG = electrocardiogram; GI = gastrointestinal; LDH = lactic dehydrogenase; ppm = parts per million; PT = prothrombin time.

    i. Additional nursing interventions

      (a) Handle hypothermic patients gently to prevent stimulation to an irritable myocardium that may lead to lethal ventricular dysrhythmias

        (1) Physical manipulation during endotracheal or nasotracheal intubation may precipitate ventricular fibrillation; intubation should occur only when essential to maintain the airway

        (2) Temporary transvenous pacemaker and PA catheter insertion may precipitate ventricular fibrillation and should be avoided unless essential

      (b) Move and maintain patients in a horizontal position to avoid aggravating hypotension and to prevent orthostasis

      (c) Increase the usual time to determine pulselessness to up to 45 seconds prior to initiating CPR because the presence of a pulse may be difficult to detect in hypothermic patients

      (d) Consider using IV fluids other than lactated Ringer's solution to support circulation because the hypothermic liver may have trouble metabolizing lactate in the solution

      (e) Consider withholding potassium-containing solutions to prevent hyperkalemia

      (f) Use defibrillation at 200, 300, and 360 joules (up to a total of only three shocks) until the patient's temperature exceeds 30°C; then attempt defibrillation again

      (g) Use IV vasoactive medications cautiously because toxicities may occur during rewarming. Increase the interval (longer than standard intervals as recommended by Advanced Cardiac Life Support) between medications. Note that:

        (1) Bradydysrhythmias may be atropine-resistant; slow heart rates are usually not corrected with medications or pacemakers unless the rhythm persists after rewarming

        (2) As long as the temperature is below 30°C, following three defibrillations, medications are withheld until the patient's temperature exceeds 30°C

        (3) Lidocaine and procainamide are often ineffective in hypothermia complicated by ventricular fibrillation, but bretylium may be more useful

        (4) If inotropic support is needed, dopamine or dobutamine is less likely than epinephrine or levarterenol to cause ventricular dysrhythmias

Toxic Ingestion

1. **Pathophysiology**

    a. Definitions

      i. Toxicology: the study of adverse effects of chemicals on living organisms

      ii. Toxicant: any poison

      iii. Absorption: extent and rate of substance movement from outside the body to an intravascular compartment (blood). Factors affecting absorption:

        (a) Route: subcutaneous, oral, intravenous, cutaneous, inhaled, intranasal, intramuscular, rectal

        (b) Bioavailability: solubility, molecular weight, dissolution rate, presence of adsorbent substances, gastric emptying time, intestinal motility, spontaneous vomiting, tissue perfusion, metabolism

   iv. Distribution: way in which a substance disseminates throughout the body. Factors affecting distribution:

        (a) Tissue perfusion

        (b) pH

        (c) Protein and tissue binding

        (d) Lipid solubility

   v. Clearance: measurement of the body's ability to eliminate a substance from blood or plasma over time

        (a) Expressed as the volume of blood or plasma completely cleared of a drug per unit of time

        (b) Elimination results from several processes

            (1) Metabolic processes, renal excretion, respiratory excretion, and excretion in sweat

            (2) Chelation: combining of metallic ions with molecular ring structures so that the ion is held by chemical bonds from each of the participating rings

            (3) Binding to activated charcoal

            (4) Extracorporeal drug removal through processes such as hemodialysis and hemoperfusion

   vi. Median lethal dose (LD_{50}) concentration of a drug that is lethal in 50% of the population

  b. Epidemiology

   i. Between 1.5 and 2 million exposures to potential poisons are reported to poison control centers each year

   ii. Approximately 0.5% of poisoned individuals suffer life-threatening effects, major disabilities, or death

   iii. Approximately 700 people die each year of poisoning reported to poison control centers

   iv. Approximately 5000 people die each year of suicide poisoning from solids, liquids, gas, and vapors

        (a) Another 1500 people die of poisonings of undetermined causes

        (b) It is unknown whether some of these deaths are intentional or unintentional

  c. Physiologic response to toxins: if the concentration of a chemical in tissues does not exceed a critical level, the effects of toxic ingestion are usually reversible

   i. Local toxicity: effects that occur at the site of first contact between a biologic system and a toxicant

   ii. Systemic toxicity: effects that occur after the absorption and distribution of a toxicant.

        (a) Most toxins affect one or two organs predominantly, but a target organ for toxicity is not always where a substance accumulates

        (b) The CNS is involved most frequently, followed by the cardiovascular system, blood and hematopoietic organs, visceral organs (liver, kidney, lung), and skin

TABLE 8–11. Ten Most Common Substances in Human Poison Exposure

Rank	Substance	% of Total
1	Cleaning substances	10.6
2	Analgesics	9.4
3	Cosmetics	8.5
4	Plants	5.4
5	Cough and cold drugs	5.2
6	Animal bites	4.3
7	Pesticides	3.7
8	Topical preparations	3.7
9	Foreign bodies	3.7
10	Food poisoning	3.5

Data from Litovitz, T. L., Felberg, L., Soloway, R. A., et al.: 1994 annual report of the American Association of Poison Control Centers Toxic Exposure Surveillance System. Am. J. Emerg. Med. 13:551–597, 1995.

(c) Muscle and bone are least often affected
   iii. Physiologic effect of a toxicant depends on the particular nature of a poison (Table 8–10)

2. Etiologic or precipitating factors
  a. Common substances
    i. Cleaning substances are the most frequently involved substances in accidental human poison exposure reported to poison control centers (Table 8–11)
    ii. Analgesics are a category of substances with the largest number of deaths from poisoning reported to poison control centers (Table 8–12)
    iii. Local community trends dictate the epidemiology of toxic ingestion by substance abusers for recreational use. Common drugs of abuse:
      (a) Cocaine
      (b) Heroin
      (c) Methamphetamine
      (d) Inhalants
  b. Designer drugs (Table 8–13)

TABLE 8–12. Ten Most Common Causes of Lethal Poison Ingestion

Rank for All People	Rank for Older Adults (>60 Years)	Substance
1	1	Analgesics
2	4	Antidepressants
3	5	Sedatives/hypnotics/psychotics
4		Stimulants and street drugs
5	2	Cardiovascular drugs
6		Alcohols
7		Gases and fumes
8	3	Asthma therapies
9		Automotive products
10		Chemicals

Data from Haselberger, M. B., and Kroner, B. A.: Drug poisoning in older patients. Drugs Aging 7:292–297, 1995; and Litovitz, T. L., Felberg, L., Soloway, R. A., et al.: 1994 annual report of the American Association of Poison Control Centers Toxic Exposure Surveillance System. Am. J. Emerg. Med. 13:551–597, 1995.

TABLE 8–13. Designer Drugs

Street Name	Chemical Name	Characteristics
Amphetamines		
Serenity, tranquility, peace	4-Methyl-2,5-dimethoxyamphetamine	2–3 mg causes euphoria 5 mg causes sympathetic nervous system stimulation and hallucinations
Ecstacy, "E," Adam XTC	3,4-Methylenedioxymethamphetamine	Euphoria, empathy Nausea, anorexia, anxiety Insomnia, sympathetic nervous system stimulation Enhanced pleasure, heightened sexuality, expanded consciousness
Love drug	3,4-Methylenedioxyamphetamine	Relaxation, sensory distortion Agitation, hallucinations
Fentanyl		
China white	α-Methyl fentanyl	Signs of opioid toxicity Lethargy to coma
Meperidine		
New heroin, synthetic heroin	1-Methyl-4 phenyl-4 propionoxy-piperidine and N-methyl-4-phenyl-2,3,5,6-tetrahydropyridine	Euphoria similar to that produced by heroin Parkinson-like syndromes

    i. Active compounds synthesized for legitimate and illicit use
    ii. Most are analogs of phenylethylamine, fentanyl, meperidine, and phencyclidine
  c. Factors associated with poisoning
    i. Physical factors
      (a) Life span considerations
        (1) Children younger than 6 years of age account for 54% of poisoning incidents but only 3% of deaths reported to poison control centers
        (2) Children between ages of 1 and 2 years have the highest incidence of accidental poisonings reported to poison control centers
        (3) People between 20 and 49 years of age account for 59% of poison fatalities
        (4) Most common substances taken as fatal poisons in older adults are analgesics and cardiovascular drugs
        (5) People older than 60 years of age are more likely to require hospitalization and to die of poisonings than younger people
      (b) Gender
        (1) Boys younger than 13 years of age are more likely to be affected than girls
        (2) Teenagers and adults with toxic ingestion are more likely to be female than male
        (3) Females account for 60% of intentional toxic ingestions
      (c) Mode of ingestion

(1) Inhaled and IV routes are usually more rapidly acting than oral routes

(2) "Body packing": the act of swallowing containers, condoms, balloons, or plastic bags filled with illegal drugs for the purpose of smuggling; dugs are carefully packaged to prevent absorption

   a) An individual transporting a substance is known as a "mule"

   b) This practice is more dangerous when a person ingests drugs in an unplanned and hurried manner to conceal evidence ("body stuffing"). Deaths have occurred in cocaine body stuffers when a package reaches the alkaline milieu of the small intestine and the contents burst, causing cardiopulmonary arrest

  ii. Environmental factors

   (a) About 90% of poison exposures are in the home

   (b) About 3% of poison exposures are in the workplace

d. Reason and incidence of exposure (Litovitz et al., 1995): almost 70% of poison exposures are classified as *general* (undefined in contrast to the following list). Other types of exposure:

  i. Environmental (2.5% of total): any passive, nonoccupational exposure resulting from the contamination of air, water, or soil

  ii Occupational (2.2% of total): exposure that occurs as a direct result of being in the workplace or on the job

  iii. Therapeutic error (4.6% of total): unintentional deviation from a proper therapeutic regimen that results in the wrong dose, incorrect route, or wrong substance

  iv. Unintentional misuse (3.6% of total): improper or incorrect use of nonpharmaceutical substances

  v. Bite or sting (3.6% of total): animal bites and stings

  vi. Food poisoning (2.2%): suspected or confirmed ingestion of contaminated food

  vii. Suspected suicide (7.7% of total): exposure resulting from inappropriate use of substances for reasons that are suspected to be self-destructive

  viii. Intentional misuse (1.4% of total): improper use of a substance for reasons other than pursuit of a psychotropic effect

3. Nursing assessment data base

a. Nursing history

  i. Source: patient, family, partner, significant other, prehospital personnel, or bystander

  ii. Description of the event

   (a) Location and time

   (b) Substances involved

    (1) Where a substance is routinely kept

    (2) Type of container: ask for a pill container if available, but many people carry multiple medications in one container. The container label may lead to inaccurate conclusions about a substance ingested

    (3) Volume or number of substances in a container

    (4) Amount ingested

        (5) Patient's symptoms after ingestion

        (6) Home first aid or prehospital treatment

    (c) Body packing or body stuffing: if the patient was confronted by police for illegal substance use or transport, suspect hurried substance ingestion

  iii. Regular pattern of alcohol and substance use

    (a) Suspect polydrug use in substance users and abusers, which is far more common than single drug or alcohol use

    (b) Attempt to obtain collateral reports of substance use patterns from significant others

  iv. Past health history: AMPLE

    (a) *A*: allergies

    (b) *M*: medications

        (1) Prescription and over-the-counter drugs

        (2) Tetanus immunization

    (c) *P*: past illnesses (medical and surgical)

    (d) *L*: last meal (time, quantity, type)

    (e) *E*: events preceding ingestion

  v. Social

    (a) Partner, spouse, housemates, roommates, significant others, or contact person

    (b) Occupation and education

    (c) Dependents, children

    (d) Religion

    (e) Financial considerations: ability to maintain income and insurance coverage

  vi. Other

    (a) Height, weight

    (b) Last menstrual period and potential for pregnancy

b. Nursing examination of patient

  i. Primary survey: rapid assessment (30 seconds to 2 minutes) that simultaneously identifies and manages life-threatening injuries: ABCDE

    (a) *A*: airway; maintain a patent airway. *Note*: stabilizing the cervical spine (cervical collar, foam blocks, rolled sheets, manual stabilization, taping) is mandatory during airway assessment and interventions if injury accompanies toxic ingestion

    (b) *B*: breathing; maintain adequate breathing

    (c) *C*: circulation; maintain adequate circulation

    (d) *D*: disability; monitor the level of consciousness

    (e) *E*: exposure; completely undress the patient to perform a thorough visual examination

    (f) Early consultation with a poison control center is essential when ABCDE is established

  ii. Secondary survey: complete physical examination is begun as soon as a primary survey and emergency, life-saving interventions are completed

    (a) If the patient is suspected of body stuffing or body packing, monitor for cardiovascular compromise in intensive care

    (b) Use a nonjudgmental and honest approach to evaluate

symptoms, and obtain a precise count of the number of bags ingested
   iii. Vital signs are widely variable, depending on the compound (see Table 8–10)
   iv. Inspection
      (a) Inspect all areas of the skin and mucous membranes for needle marks or abscesses
      (b) Know the practices of the substance-abusing population to identify symptoms of unusual routes of administration
   v. Palpation, percussion, and auscultation techniques depend on substances involved
      (a) Assess for multiple trauma
      (b) Assess for hypothermia
  c. Diagnostic study findings: *do not delay treatment while awaiting results*
   i. Urine, blood (rarely gastric contents for toxic screen); acetaminophen level indicated in all patients with intentional overdose
   ii. CBC
   iii. Serum electrolytes and glucose
   iv. Prothrombin and partial thromboplastin time
   v. Liver function tests
   vi. BUN, creatinine levels
   vii. ABGs
   viii. Chest x-ray, ECG
   ix. Pregnancy test: performed on all girls 12 to 17 years of age and women of childbearing age

4. Nursing diagnoses
  a. Ineffective airway clearance related to tracheobronchial obstruction (see Chapter 1)
  b. Ineffective breathing pattern related to neurologic impairment (see Chapter 1)
   i. Additional nursing interventions
      (a) Determine whether respirations are "adequate"
         (1) Adult: 5 to 10 ml/kg per breath at a rate of 12 to 18 breaths/minute (100 ml/kg/minute)
         (2) Child older than 5 years of age: "adequate" rate increases to 20 breaths/minute
      (b) If respirations are not deemed "adequate," hyperventilate with bag-valve-mask and 100% oxygen followed by intubation
      (c) 100% oxygen may be considered an antidote for carbon monoxide poisoning while COHb results are awaited (*do not* rely on PaO$_2$ or SaO$_2$ determinations for carbon monoxide poisoning)
  c. Risk for injury related to toxic ingestion (Fig. 8–10)
   i. Assessment for defining characteristics
      (a) Self-report or collateral report by significant others of toxic ingestion
      (b) Impaired airway, breathing, and circulation
      (c) Decreased mental status
      (d) Nausea, vomiting, diarrhea
      (e) Hypothermia/hyperthermia

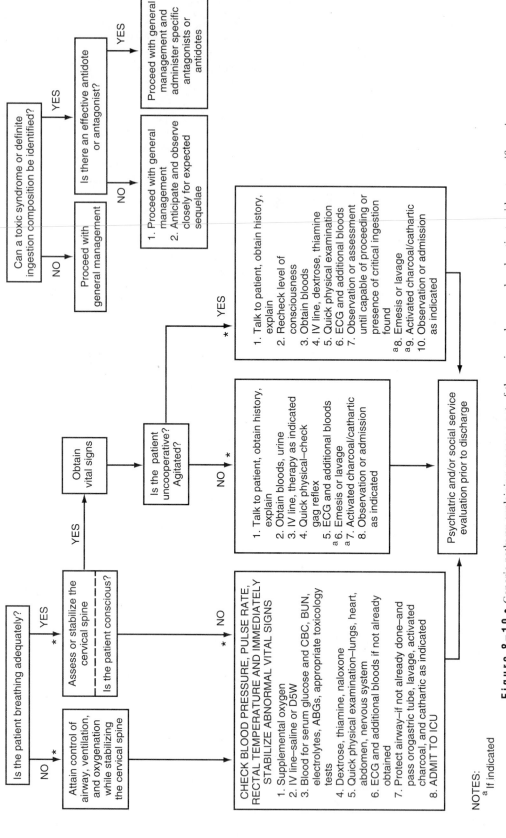

Figure 8–10 • Generic pathway explaining management of the poisoned or overdosed patients without specific toxic symptoms. The asterisks refer to the smaller algorithm, which reminds the clinician to consider antidotal intervention when appropriate throughout to toxicologic care. ABG = arterial blood gas; BUN = blood urea nitrogen; CBC = complete blood count; D5W = 5% dextrose in water; ECG = electrocardiogram; IV = intravenous. (From Goldfrank, L. R., Flomenbaum, N. E., Lewin, N. A., et al.: Toxicologic emergencies, 5th ed. Norwalk, Conn., Appleton & Lange, 1994, pp. 28–29.)

NOTES:
ᵃ If indicated

ii. Expected outcomes
    (a) Airway, breathing, and circulation are adequate
    (b) The toxic substance is removed, reversed, or eliminated
    (c) The preingestion level of consciousness is restored
    (d) Organ function is preserved
    (e) Normothermia is attained
iii. Nursing interventions (see Tables 8–8 and 8–9)
    (a) Monitor core temperature with a rectal or PA catheter thermistor, if available, and manage hypothermia and hyperthermia
    (b) Monitor cardiac rhythm and manage dysrhythmias and hypovolemia with IV crystalloids
    (c) In all comatose adult and adolescent patients, even those without pinpoint pupils, be prepared to give the following drugs if they are prescribed (keeping in mind that routine use of these drugs is *not* recommended):
        (1) Dextrose, 100 ml IV 50% in water (50 g dextrose) to rule out hypoglycemia as a cause for coma (except patients *known* to be hyperglycemic)
            a) Hypoglycemia may result from exposure to insulin, oral hypoglycemic agents, ethanol, and salicylates
            b) If the blood glucose level can be determined rapidly, administer hypertonic dextrose only to patients with a blood glucose level below 60 mg/dl
            c) If the glucose level cannot be determined rapidly, consider hypertonic dextrose for patients with altered consciousness and nonfocal neurologic examinations
        (2) Thiamine, 100 mg IV to prevent precipitation of Wernicke-Korsakoff syndrome
            a) Routine use is warranted
            b) Administer at the same time as hypertonic dextrose
        (3) Naloxone 2 mg IV, intramuscularly, or endotracheally to antagonize narcotics
            a) Use smaller doses (0.1 or 0.2 mg) for opioid-dependent patients who are not apneic to avoid withdrawal
            b) Use routinely for patients with CNS or respiratory depression and who have a low likelihood of opioid addiction and polydrug addiction
            c) Administer routinely to patients with respiratory rates below 12 breaths/minute
            d) Half-life is 30 minutes; symptoms may recur after that time period, indicating a need for continuous infusion
        (4) Do not administer physostigmine (Antilirium), analeptics (amphetamines, caffeine), or flumazenil routinely until the toxicant is identified and these drugs are warranted
    (d) Provide an antidote (Table 8–14)
    (e) If no antidote is available, maintain vital functions, remove the toxic substance, and limit the absorption of any remaining substance
    (f) General management strategies for decontamination
        (1) Orogastric lavage: elimination of unabsorbed toxins; usually

Text continued on page 792

TABLE 8–14. Management Considerations for Ingestion of Toxic Substances

Substance	Antidote	Management
Acetaminophen	NAC (Mucomyst); loading: 140 mg/kg p.o.; maintenance: 70 mg/kg p.o. every 4 hours for 17 doses	Apply gastric emptying if less than 2 hours since ingestion Give activated charcoal if less than 4 hours since ingestion Use NAC if levels are toxic even if ingestion was over 24 hours ago Repeat dose if patient vomits within 1 hour If vomiting persists, use nasogastric decompression and metoclopramide Dilute dose of NAC 1 part to 4 in chilled soft drink or juice
Amphetamines	None	Consider administration of 100 ml 50% glucose if warranted after fingerstick glucose and 100 mg thiamine IV Give activated charcoal for oral ingestion Supportive therapy: benzodiazepines (for agitation or seizures), external cooling (for hyperthermia), phentolamine (for hypertension), IV hydration (replace fluid losses and prevent myoglobin damage in renal tubules) Keep patient in a cool, quiet room Implement hemodialysis for patients with acute renal failure, acidosis, and hyperkalemia, but do not use it to remove drug
Arsenic	None	Give chelating agents, such as British antilewisite (BAL), D-penicillamine, and dimercaptosuccinic acid (DMSA). *Note: these drugs have many side effects* Support circulation with crystalloids and pressor agents as needed Administer blood if GI hemorrhage occurs Treat ventricular dysrhythmia with lidocaine and defibrillation Monitor for seizure activity Determine whether patient needs gastric suction or whole bowel irrigation, depending on exposure
Barbiturates	None	Administer sodium bicarbonate to enhance elimination of phenobarbital only GI evacuation: lavage with large-bore orogastric tube followed by multiple-dose activated charcoal (MDAC) therapy Consider giving adults with altered mental status 100 ml dextrose 50% if warranted after fingerstick glucose, 2 mg naloxone, and 100 mg thiamine Withdrawal symptoms may lead to vomiting and risk for aspiration; maintain patient in left lateral position
Benzodiazepines	Flumazenil; *use caution:* severe withdrawal risk exists	GI evacuation: lavage with large-bore orogastric tube followed by MDAC Consider giving adults with altered mental status 100 ml dextrose 50% if warranted after fingerstick glucose, 2 mg naloxone, and 100 mg thiamine

Carbamazepine (Tegretol)	None	GI evacuation: lavage with large-bore orogastric tube followed by MDAC Implement whole bowel irrigation if medication is enteric coated Give cathartics Monitor for seizures
Cocaine	None	Consider administration of 100 ml 50% glucose if warranted after fingerstick glucose and 100 mg thiamine IV Administer high-flow oxygen immediately For oral ingestion, irrigate through a large-bore orogastric tube, with MDAC and a single dose of cathartic Supportive therapy: benzodiazepines (for sedation); vasodilators (for hypertension); nitrates, phentolamine, and calcium channel blockers (for myocardial ischemia); aspirin, heparin, calcium channel blockers, opioids, and possibly thrombolytic therapy (for myocardial infarction); lidocaine or sodium bicarbonate (for ventricular dysrhythmias) Provide cooling for hyperthermia, a quiet environment, and reassurance Monitor for seizures
Cyclic antidepressants	Sodium bicarbonate	Administer sodium bicarbonate to prevent and treat dysrhythmias GI evacuation: irrigation with large-bore orogastric tube, followed by MDAC Consider giving adults with altered mental status 100 ml dextrose 50% if warranted after fingerstick glucose, 2 mg naloxone, and 100 mg thiamine Withdrawal symptoms may lead to vomiting and risk for aspiration; maintain patient in left lateral position Monitor heart rhythm continuously Administer sodium bicarbonate, and consider hyperventilation to keep pH at 7.50–7.55 Correct hypotension with crystalloids and norepinephrine if needed; avoid dopamine, which may increase dysrhythmias and may not correct hypotension because catecholamine stores have been depleted by overdose
Cyanide	Amyl nitrate: crushed into gauze and inhaled (may place over intake valve of manual resuscitator bag or between oxygen source and endotracheal tube); sodium nitrate 3% IV 10 ml over 4 minutes; sodium thiosulfate IV 25% 50 ml	Administer 100% oxygen Administer crystalloids and vasopressors for hypotension Give sodium bicarbonate to correct acidosis Administer amyl nitrate (patient should inhale while the nurse prepares sodium nitrate), sodium nitrate, and sodium thiosulfate; all drugs are needed in combination for synergistic effects and are prepared as a cyanide kit Suspect cyanide poisoning with any serious smoke inhalation injury

Table continued on following page

TABLE 8–14. Management Considerations for Ingestion of Toxic Substances *Continued*

Substance	Antidote	Management
Ethanol (acute intoxication)	None	Never assume that decreased mental status is a reflection of intoxication alone, since alcohol intoxication is often associated with traumatic injuries; threshold for CT of the head should be low Treat recent (within 1 hour) ingestion with gastric lavage and activated charcoal in severely intoxicated patients Perform fingerstick glucose, and administer 50 ml 50% glucose if indicated Administer 100 mg thiamine IV Consider magnesium and potassium administration to counteract electrolyte depletion, often seen in chronic alcoholics Supportive management: multivitamins with folate (for nutrition), blood products (for coagulopathies), benzodiazepines (for withdrawal)
Ethylene glycol (antifreeze) and methanol	None	Administer ethanol 100–150 mg/dl IV to prevent formation of toxic metabolites by competitive inhibition; maintain blood alcohol level of 100–150 mg/dl Maintain normal pH with sodium bicarbonate administration Maintain hydration Consider hemodialysis as an option Administer thiamine 100 mg IV and pyridoxine 50 mg every 6 hours
Isoniazid (INH)	Pyridoxine	Control seizures with pyridoxine 1 g for every gram of INH ingested (give 1 g over 2–3 minutes) along with diazepam Phenytoin is ineffective and not recommended Implement peritoneal dialysis, hemodialysis, and hemoperfusion
Isopropyl alcohol (rubbing alcohol)	None	Provide supportive treatment, with attention to cardiorespiratory problems Controversial: activated charcoal lavage used early in the overdose; hemodialysis for patients with high levels (400–500 mg/dl)
Lithium	None	GI evacuation: lavage with large-bore orogastric tube, followed by MDAC, cathartic (sorbitol, magnesium citrate) Administer normal saline to enhance elimination Implement hemodialysis Monitor for seizures

Opioids	Naloxone	Naloxone 2 mg (may be repeated, up to a total of 20 mg); if opioid dependence is suspected, give 0.1–0.2 mg naloxone; *duration of action of most opioids exceeds duration of action of naloxone* (repeated doses may be necessary) Monitor for opioid withdrawal in dependent patients: vomiting, abdominal pain, agitation, diaphoresis, piloerection; aspiration of stomach contents is a risk for comatose patients *Note:* higher doses may be needed to reverse propoxyphene, pentazocine, methadone, and fentanyl Position patient to limit risk of aspiration, since vomiting is consequence of withdrawal
Phencyclidine (PCP)	None	GI evacuation for oral ingestion: lavage with large-bore orogastric tube, followed by MDAC, cathartic (sorbitol, magnesium citrate) Supportive care: benzodiazepines (for agitation); IV hydration, diuretics, mannitol (to limit damage from rhabdomyolysis); cooling blanket (for hyperthermia)
Phenothiazines	None	GI evacuation: lavage with large-bore orogastric tube, followed by MDAC, cathartic (sorbitol, magnesium citrate) Implement cardiac monitoring
Salicylates	None	GI evacuation: lavage with large-bore orogastric tube, followed by MDAC, cathartic Cooling: provide hypothermia blanket, ice packs, and a cool environment Provide alkalization of urine with sodium bicarbonate Implement hemodialysis Monitor for and treat hypokalemia
Theophylline	None	Implement charcoal hemoperfusion or hemodialysis GI evacuation: lavage with large-bore orogastric tube, followed by MDAC, cathartics Implement cardiac monitoring

CT = computed tomography; GI = gastrointestinal; IV = intravenous; MDAC = multiple-dose activated charcoal; NAC = *N*-acetylcysteine; p.o. = by mouth.

performed in the emergency department rather than the ICU

a) Indications: generally accepted instead of emesis in comatose patients *except* in cases of caustic ingestion (chemical injury, including acetic acid [permanent wave solution], ammonia [cleaning agents], phosphorus [matches, fireworks], benzalkonium chloride [detergents], oxalic acid [disinfectants, bleach], formaldehyde, iodine [antiseptics], and sulfuric acid [batteries, drain cleaners]). Management of caustics:

    i) Intubation if needed

    ii) Examine for splash injuries to skin and eyes

    iii) If there are no signs of visceral perforation and the patient can swallow, dilute the toxicant with cool milk or tap water

    iv) No emetics or gastric lavage

b) Procedure

    i) Intubate and inflate the cuff to protect the airway if the patient is unable to do so

    ii) Use a 36 to 40 French tube, which is large enough to be able to remove particulate matter

    iii) Pass the tube orally to limit epistaxis and trauma to the nasal mucosa

    iv) If necessary, use the oral airway to prevent the patient from biting the tube

    v) Verify tube placement in the stomach, place the patient in the left lateral decubitus position with the head lower than the feet, attach the lavage funnel to the end of the orogastric tube, and administer 150 to 200 ml (to adults) of tap water or normal saline. In some protocols, a catheter-tipped syringe is used to irrigate and withdraw fluid until it is clear

    vi) Allow the tube to drain by gravity

    vii) Monitor for complications: aspiration, esophageal or gastric perforation, and laryngospasm

c) Other contraindications to lavage: hemorrhagic diathesis, nontoxic ingestion, ingestion of sharp materials, and drug packets

(2) Emetics: ipecac is the emetic of choice for home first aid; very rarely recommended for emergency department use

a) Dose: 15 ml of syrup with 16 to 21 mg of cephaeline and emetine at a ratio of 1:1 to 2.1:1; mix with warm water

b) Causes vomiting by local activation of peripheral sensory receptors in the gastrointestinal tract and central stimulation of the chemoreceptor trigger in the central vomiting center of the brain

c) Vomiting usually begins in 20 minutes, occurs at least three times, and lasts about 30 to 60 minutes

d) Implications:

    i) Do not give with milk, which may slow action

    ii) May be inactivated by activated charcoal

       iii) In the emergency department, gastric decontamination is preferable if gastric emptying is required

       iv) Toxicity: protracted vomiting, diarrhea, seizures, cardiac toxicity, and neuromuscular weakness

(3) Activated charcoal: administer after several liters of gastric lavage produce a clear effluent; administer as a slurry

  a) Dose: 1 g/kg of body weight or 10:1 ratio of activated charcoal to drug (whichever is greater); mix with water or a cathartic via a tube or orally

  b) Often given with a cathartic in an appropriate dose; premixed solutions are available; do not use multiple-dose cathartics

       i) Magnesium citrate, magnesium sulfate, sorbitol

       ii) Contraindications to cathartics: trivial ingestion in children, adynamic ileus, diarrhea, abdominal trauma, intestinal obstruction, renal failure

  c) Composition

       i) Produced from destructive distillation of organic materials such as wood and petroleum; treated at high temperatures to increase its ability to adsorb toxins

       ii) Adsorption relies on external pore size and internal surface area; adsorbs (sticks) by ionic binding and molecular forces

       iii) Adsorption begins 1 minute after administration

  d) Treatment is controversial. For a recent (2–4 hours) acetaminophen overdose because the charcoal does not absorb a clinically significant amount of the antidote (*N*-acetylcysteine); always give for mixed acetaminophen and other drug overdose

  e) May give in multiple doses every 1 to 4 hours, but do not repeat the cathartic; discontinue after the first charcoal stool

  f) Other uses: digitalis, phenobarbital, carbamazepine (Tegretol), phenytoin (Dilantin), theophylline, salicylate, propoxyphene (Darvon), cyclic antidepressants, isoniazid (INH), amphetamines, cocaine, amitryptyline, phenylbutazone

  g) Not useful for alcohol, caustics, iron, or lithium

  h) Hazards: diarrhea, constipation, vomiting, aspiration, intestinal obstruction, reduction of therapeutic levels of prescribed drugs

(4) Whole-bowel irrigation: polyethylene glycol and electrolytes for oral solution

  a) Dose: 2 L/hour orally or by nasogastric tube for 4 to 6 hours until the effluent is clear

  b) Clears the entire gastrointestinal tract without inducing emesis or causing a fluid and electrolyte disturbance

  c) Indications: sustained-release drugs, slowly dissolving

agents (iron tablets, paint chips), ingested "crack" vials, drug (cocaine, heroin) packets for smuggling purposes
  d) Indications: not indicated for quickly absorbing drugs, liquids, parenterally administered drugs, or caustics
  e) Complications: rectal itching, vomiting
  f) Contraindications: Ileus, obstruction, perforation, gastrointestinal bleeding
(5) Hemodialysis, hemoperfusion, and hemofiltration (Table 8–15)
  a) Hemodialysis is usually performed for 4 to 6 hours in poisoned patients
  b) Hemodialysis also corrects for metabolic acid-base disturbances, hyperkalemia, and fluid overload
  c) Hemoperfusion is better than hemodialysis for clearing blood of substances that bind to plasma proteins
  d) Cartridge needs to be changed every 6 hours because its adsorptive capacity decreases
  e) Hemofiltration is mostly experimental; dialysis is usually used
      i) Hemofiltration can remove larger molecules, such as aminoglycoside antibiotics
      ii) Can be used after the other two techniques to prevent a rebound of toxic levels
  f) Hypotension makes all three techniques difficult
(g) Treatment for body stuffing and body packing:
  (1) If the patient becomes symptomatic while in police custody, suspect body stuffing unless proven otherwise
  (2) Treatment is controversial and should be guided by the poison control center; some possibilities include oral activated charcoal, polyethylene glycol and electrolyte solutions, surgical intervention, and laparotomy

TABLE 8–15. Hemodialysis and Hemoperfusion

Technique	Characteristics	Toxic Compounds
Hemodialysis		
Toxic compounds diffuse down the concentration gradient through semipermeable membrane from blood into dialysis solution	Molecular weight < 500 daltons Water-soluble Low volume of distribution Poor protein binding Low body clearance 　(<4 ml/minute/kg)	Bromide Ethylene glycol Lithium Methanol Salicylate Chloral hydrate Ethanol
Hemoperfusion		
Blood pumped through cartridge containing activated charcoal and/or carbon, which absorbs toxin	Absorbed by charcoal or carbon Low volume of distribution Low body clearance 　(<4 ml/minute/kg) Not limited by protein binding (as is hemodialysis)	Carbamazepine Phenobarbital Phenytoin Theophylline Procainamide

iv. Evaluation of nursing care
    (a) A patent airway, regular breathing, and adequate circulation are attained
    (b) The toxic substance is removed or effects are reversed
    (c) The preingestion level of consciousness is restored
    (d) Patient's temperature is 36° to 38°C
d. Self-concept disturbance related to negative self-appraisal (see Chapter 9)
    i. Make appropriate referrals to a social worker or psychiatric clinical nurse specialist
    ii. Monitor the environment for items that could be used for self-inflicted injury
    iii. Implement suicide precautions if appropriate

References

SIRS AND SEPTIC SHOCK

Ackerman, M., Hazinski, M. F., MacIntyre, N., et al.: Sepsis and septic shock across the life span: Epidemiology, clinical recognition and state-of-the-art-management. AACN Pre-NTI Conference Proceedings, 1996.

Beutler, B.: Endotoxin, tumor necrosis factor, and related mediators: New approaches to shock. New Horiz. 1:3–12, 1993.

Bjornson, H. S.: Pathogenesis, prevention, and management of catheter-associated infections. New Horiz. 1:271–278, 1993.

Bone, R. C.: Toward a theory regarding the pathogenesis of the systemic inflammatory response syndrome: What we do and do not know about cytokine regulation. Crit. Care Med. 24:163–172, 1996.

Bone, R. C., Balk, R. A., Cerra, F. B., et al.: Definitions for sepsis and organ failure and guidelines for the use of innovative therapies in sepsis. Chest 101:1644–1655, 1992.

Bower, R. H.: Nutrition during critical illness and sepsis. New Horiz. 1:248–352, 1993.

Braley, S. E., Groner, T. R., Fernandez, M., et al.: Overview of diagnostic imaging in sepsis. New Horiz. 1:214–230, 1993.

Brooks, G. F., Butel, J. S., and Ornston, L. N.: Medical Microbiology. Norwalk, Conn., Appleton & Lange, 1995.

Brun-Buisson, C., Doyon, F., Carlet, J., et al.: Incidence, risk factors, and outcome of severe sepsis and septic shock in adults. J.A.M.A. 274:968–974, 1995.

Cook, D. J., Brun-Buisson, C., Guyatt, G. H., et al.: Evaluation of new diagnostic technologies: Bronchoalveolar lavage and the diagnosis of ventilator-associated pneumonia. Crit. Care Med. 22:1314–1322, 1994.

Cook, J. A., Geisel, J., Halushka, P. V., et al.: Prostaglandins, thromboxanes, leukotrienes, and cytochrome P-450 metabolites of arachidonic acid. New Horiz. 1:60–69, 1993.

Cronin, L., Cook, D. J., Carlet, J., et al.: Corticosteroid treatment for sepsis: A critical appraisal and meta-analysis of the literature. Crit. Care Med. 23:1430–1439, 1995.

Crowley, S. R.: The pathogenesis of septic shock. Heart Lung 25:124–134, 1996.

Fink, M. P.: Failure of the gastrointestinal tract barrier. In Ayers, S. M. (ed.): Textbook of Critical Care, 3rd ed. Philadelphia, W. B. Saunders, 1995.

Ganz, T.: Macrophage function. New Horiz. 1:23–27, 1993.

Goldsberry, D. T., and Hurst, J. M.: Adult respiratory distress syndrome and sepsis. New Horiz. 1:342–346, 1993.

Hazinski, M. F.: Mediator-specific therapies for the systemic inflammatory response syndrome, sepsis, severe sepsis, and septic shock. Crit. Care Nurs. Clin. North Am. 6:309–318, 1994.

Hazinski, M. F., Iberti, T. J., MacIntyre, N. R., et al.: Epidemiology, pathophysiology and clinical presentation of gram-negative sepsis. Am. J. Crit. Care 2:224–237, 1993.

Heumann, D., and Glauser, M. P.: Pathogenesis of sepsis. Sci. Am. 1:28–37, 1994.

Kim, M. J., McFarland, G. K., and McLane, A. M.: Pocket Guide to Nursing Diagnoses, 6th ed. St. Louis, Mosby–Year Book, 1995.

Koltai, M., Hosford, D., and Braquet, P. G.: Platelet-activating factor in septic shock. New Horiz. 1:87–95, 1993.

Lefering, R., and Neugebauer, E. A.: Steroid controversy in sepsis and septic shock: A meta-analysis. Crit. Care Med. 23:1294–1303, 1995.

Lowry, S. F.: Anticytokine therapies in sepsis. New Horiz. 1:120–126, 1993.

Martin, M. A.: Nosocomial infections in intensive care units: An overview of their epidemiology, outcome, and prevention. New Horiz. 1:162–171, 1993.

McCord, J. M.: Oxygen-derived free radicals. New Horiz. 1:70–76, 1993.

Moore, E. E., Moore, F. A., Francoise, R. J., et al.: The postischemic gut serves as a priming bed for circulating neutrophils that provoke multiple organ failure. J. Trauma 37:881–887, 1994.

Palmer, R. M. J., Bridge, L., Foxwell, N. A., et al.: The role of nitric oxide in endothelial cell damage and its inhibition of glucocorticoids. Br. J. Pharmacol. 105:11–12, 1992.

Parker, M. M.: The heart in sepsis. In Ayers, S. M. (ed.): Textbook of Critical Care, 3rd ed. Philadelphia, W. B. Saunders, 1995.

Rangel-Frausto, M. S., Pittet, D., Costigan, M., et al.: The natural history of the systemic inflammatory response syndrome (SIRS). J.A.M.A. 273:117–123, 1995.

Shapiro, L., and Gelfand, J. A.: Cytokines. In Ayers, S. M. (ed.): Textbook of Critical Care, 3rd ed. Philadelphia, W. B. Saunders, 1995.

Shapiro, L., and Gelfand, J. A.: Cytokines and sepsis: Pathophysiology and therapy. New Horiz. 1:13–22, 1993.

Shoemaker, W. C., Appel, P. L., Kram, H. B., et al.: Hemodynamic and oxygen transport monitoring to titrate therapy in septic shock. New Horiz. 1:145–159, 1993.

Steuble, B. T.: Shock: Septic and anaphylactic. *In* Swearingen, P. L., and Keen, J. H. (eds.): Manual of Critical Care Nursing, 3rd ed. St. Louis, Mosby–Year Book, 1995.

Vallance, P., and Moncada, S.: Role of endogenous nitric oxide in septic shock. New Horiz. 1:77–86, 1993.

Wiessner, W. H., Casey, L. C., and Zbilut, J. P.: Treatment of sepsis and septic shock. Heart Lung 24:380–392, 1995.

Zeni, F., Pain, P., Vindimian, M., et al.: Effects of pentoxifylline on circulating cytokine concentrations and hemodynamics in patients with septic shock: Results from a double-blind, randomized, placebo-controlled study. Crit. Care Med. 24:207–214, 1996.

MODS

Aragon, D., and Parson, R.: Multiple organ dysfunction syndrome in trauma patients. Crit. Care Clin. North Am. 6:873–881, 1994.

Bare, P. S., Hydo, L. J., and Fischer, E.: Development of multiple organ dysfunction syndrome in critically ill patients with perforated viscus. Arch. Surg. 131:37–43, 1996.

Beal, A. L., and Cerra, F. B.: Multiple organ failure syndrome in the 1990s. J.A.M.A. 271:226–233, 1994.

Bone, R. C., Balk, R. A., Cerra, F. B., et al.: Definitions for sepsis and organ failure and guidelines for the use of innovative therapies in sepsis. Chest 101:1644–1655, 1992.

Bone, R. C.: Toward a theory regarding the pathogenesis of the systemic inflammatory response syndrome: What we do and do not know about cytokine regulation. Crit. Care Med. 24:163–172, 1996.

Botha, A. J., Moore, F. A., Moore, E. E., et al.: Early neutrophil sequestration after injury: A pathogenic mechanism for multiple organ failure. J. Trauma 39:411–417, 1995.

Brass, N. J.: Predisposition to multiple organ dysfunction. Crit. Care Nurs. Q. 16:1–7, 1994.

Dunham, C. M., Damiano, A. M., Wiles, C. E., et al.: Posttraumatic multiple organ dysfunction syndrome–infection is an uncommon antecedent risk factor. Injury 26:373–378, 1995.

Fink, M. P.: Failure of the gastrointestinal tract barrier. *In* Ayers, S. M. (ed.): Textbook of Critical Care, 3rd ed. Philadelphia, W. B. Saunders, 1995.

Fitzsimmons, L.: Consequences of Trauma: Systemic inflammation and multiple organ dysfunction. Crit. Care Nurs. Q. 17:74–90, 1994.

Fry, D. E.: Multiple system organ failure. In Fry, D. E. (ed.): Multiple system organ failure. St. Louis, 1992, Mosby–Year Book.

Hazinski, M. F., Iberti, T. J., MacIntyre, N. R., et al.: Epidemiology, pathophysiology and clinical presentation of gram-negative sepsis. Am. J. Crit. Care 2:224–237, 1993.

Kim, M. J., McFarland, G. K., and McLane, A. M.: Pocket Guide to Nursing Diagnoses, 6th ed. St. Louis, 1995, Mosby–Year Book.

Livingston, D. H., and Deitch, E. A.: Multiple organ failure: A common problem in surgical intensive care unit patients. Ann. Med. 27:13–20, 1995.

Marshall, J. C., Cook, D. J., Christou, N. V., et al.: Multiple organ dysfunction score: A reliable descriptor of a complex clinical outcome. Crit. Care Med. 23:1638–1657, 1995.

Moore, F. A., and Moore, E. E.: Evolving concepts in the pathogenesis of postinjury multiple organ failure. Surg. Clin. North Am. 75:257–277, 1995.

Moore, F. A., Sauaia, A., Moore, E. E., et al.: Postinjury multiple organ failure: A bimodal phenomenon. J. Trauma 40:501–510, 1996.

Moore, E. E., Moore, F. A., Francoise, R. J., et al.: The postischemic gut serves as a priming bed for circulating neutrophils that provoke multiple organ failure. J. Trauma 37:881–887, 1994.

Parker, M. M.: The heart in sepsis. *In* Ayers, S. M. (ed.): Textbook of Critical Care, 3rd ed. Philadelphia, W. B. Saunders, 1995.

Reilly, E. R., and Yucha, C. B.: Multiple organ failure syndrome. Crit. Care Nurse 14:25–26; 28–31, 1994.

Sauaia, A., Moore, F. A., Moore, E. E., et al.: Early predictors of postinjury multiple organ failure. Arch. Surg. 129:39–45, 1994.

Shapiro, L., and Gelfand, J. A.: Cytokines. *In* Ayers, S. M., (ed.): Textbook of Critical Care, 3rd ed. Philadelphia, W. B. Saunders, 1995.

Shapiro, L., and Gelfand, J. A.: Cytokines and sepsis: Pathophysiology and therapy. New Horiz. 1:13–22, 1993.

Shoemaker, W. C., Appel, P. L., Kram, H. B., et al.: Hemodynamic and oxygen transport monitoring to titrate therapy in septic shock. New Horiz. 1:145–159, 1993.

Smail, N., Messiah, A., Edouard, A., et al.: Role of systemic inflammatory response syndrome and infection in the occurrence of early multiple organ dysfunction syndrome following severe trauma. Intens. Care Med. 21:813–816, 1995.

Steuble, B. T.: Shock: Septic and anaphylactic. *In* Swearingen, P. L., and Keen, J. H. (eds.): Manual of Critical Care Nursing, 3rd ed. St. Louis, Mosby–Year Book, 1995.

Waydhas, C., Nast-Kolb, D., Trupka, A., et al.: Posttraumatic inflammatory response, secondary operations, and late multiple organ failure. J. Trauma 40:624–631, 1996.

MULTISYSTEM TRAUMA

Bayley, E. W., and Turcke, S. A. (eds.): A Comprehensive Curriculum for Trauma Nursing. Boston, Jones and Bartlett, 1992.

Border, J. R.: Death from severe trauma: Open fractures to multiple organ dysfunction syndrome. J. Trauma 39:12–22, 1995.

Cooper, C., and Militello, P.: The multi-injured patient: The Maryland shock trauma protocol approach. Semin. Thorac. Cardiovasc. Surg. 4:163–167, 1992.

Hinkle, J., and Betz, S.: Gunshot injuries. AACN Clin. Issues Adv. Pract. Acute Crit. Care 6:175–186, 1995.

Keen, J.: Major trauma. *In* Swearingen, P. L., and Keen, J. H. (eds.): Manual of Critical Care Nursing, 3rd ed. St. Louis, Mosby–Year Book, 1995.

Kelleher, D. L., and Trask, A. L.: Epidemiology of trauma. *In* Ayers, S. M. (ed.): Textbook of Critical Care, 3rd ed. Philadelphia, W. B. Saunders, 1995.

Kim, M. J., McFarland, G. K., and McLane, A. M.: Pocket Guide to Nursing Diagnoses, 6th ed. St. Louis, Mosby–Year Book, 1995.

McQuillan, K. A.: Initial management of traumatic shock. *In* Cardona, V. D., Hurn, P. D., Mason, P. J., et al. (eds.): Trauma Nursing: From Resuscitation Through

Rehabilitation, 2nd ed. Philadelphia, W. B. Saunders, 1994.

National Safety Council: Accident Facts. Itasca, Ill., National Safety Council, 1995.

Rostenberg, P.: Alcohol and Other Drug Screening of Hospitalized Trauma Patients. Rockville, Md., Department of Health and Human Services (SMA 95–3041), 1995.

Rutherford, E. J., and Nelson, L. D.: Initial assessment of the multiple trauma patient. *In* Ayers, S. M. (ed.): Textbook of Critical Care, 3rd ed. Philadelphia, W. B. Saunders, 1995.

Sauaia, A., Moore, F. A., Moore, E. E., et al.: Epidemiology of trauma deaths: A reassessment. J. Trauma 38:185–193, 1995.

Shabot, M. M., and Johnson, C. L.: Outcome from critical care in the "oldest old" trauma patients. J. Trauma 39:254–260, 1995.

Sluis, C. K., Duis, H. J., and Geertzen, J. H. B.: Multiple injuries: An overview of the outcome. J. Trauma 38:681–686, 1995.

Sluis, C. K., Klasen, H. J., Eisma, W. H., et al.: Major trauma in young and old: What is the difference? J. Trauma 40:78–82, 1996.

Sommers, M. S.: Missed injuries: A case of trauma hide and seek. AACN Clin. Issues Adv. Pract. Acute Crit. Care 6:187–195, 1995.

Vane, D. W., and Shackford, S. R.: Epidemiology of rural traumatic death in children: A population-based study. J. Trauma 38:867–870, 1995.

Wan, G. J., and Neff-Smith, M.: The impact of demographics, injury severity, and trauma type on the likelihood of survival in child and adolescent trauma patients. J. Trauma 40:412–416, 1996.

Waxman, K.: Physiologic response to injury. *In* Ayers, S. M. (ed.): Textbook of Critical Care, 3rd ed. Philadelphia, W. B. Saunders, 1995.

Weigelt, J. A., and Klein, J. D.: Mechanism of injury. *In* Cardona, V. D., Hurn, P. D., Mason, P. J., et al. (eds.): Trauma Nursing: From Resuscitation Through Rehabilitation. Philadelphia, W. B. Saunders, 1994.

BURNS

Advanced Burn Life Support Curriculum. Lincoln, Neb., 1993.

Bayley, E. W., and Turcke, S. A.: A Comprehensive Curriculum for Trauma Nursing. Boston, Jones and Bartlett, 1992.

Caine, R. M.: Patients with burns. *In* Clochesy, J. M., Breu, C., Cardin, S., et al. (eds.): Critical Care Nursing, 2nd ed. Philadelphia, W. B. Saunders, 1996.

Darling, G. E., Keresteci, M. A., Ibanez, D., et al.: Pulmonary complications in inhalation injuries with associated cutaneous burn. J. Trauma 40:83–89, 1996.

Demling, R. H.: Management of the burn patient. *In* Ayers, S. M. (ed.): Textbook of Critical Care, 3rd ed. Philadelphia, W. B. Saunders, 1995.

Gamelli, R. L., George, M., Sharp-Pucci, M., et al.: Burn-induced nitric oxide release in humans. J. Trauma 39:869–878, 1995.

Gore, D. C., Dalton, J. M., and Gehr, T. W. B.: Colloid infusions reduce glomerular filtration in resuscitated burn victims. J. Trauma 40:356–360, 1996.

Hansbrough, J. F., Achauer, B., Dawson, J., et al.: Wound healing in partial-thickness burn wounds treated with collagenase ointment versus silver sulfadiazine cream. J. Burn Care Rehabil. 16:241–247, 1995.

Johnson, J.: Burns. *In* Swearingen, P. L., and Keen, J. H. (eds.): Manual of Critical Care Nursing, 3rd ed. St. Louis, Mosby–Year Book, 1995.

Kerr, M. E., Bender, C. M., and Monti, E. J.: An introduction to oxygen free radicals. Heart Lung 25:200–209, 1996.

Kim, M. J., McFarland, G. K., and McLane, Am. M.: Pocket Guide to Nursing Diagnoses, 6th ed. St. Louis, Mosby–Year Book, 1995.

Marvin, J.: Thermal injuries. *In* Cardona, V. D., Hurn, P. D., Mason, P. J., et al. (eds.): Trauma Nursing: From Resuscitation Through Rehabilitation, 2nd ed. Philadelphia, W. B. Saunders, 1994.

McGill, V., Kowal-Vern, A., Fisher, S. G., et al.: The impact of substance use on mortality and morbidity from thermal injury. J. Trauma 38:931–934, 1995.

Priser, J., Reper, P., Vlasselaer, D., et al.: Nitric oxide production is increased in patients after burn injury. J. Trauma 40:368–371, 1996.

Reagan, B., Staiano-Coico, L., LaBruna, A., et al.: The effects of burn blister fluid on cultured keratinocytes. J. Trauma 40:361–367, 1996.

Sadowski, D.: Burns. *In* Sommers, M. S., and Johnson, S. (eds.): Davis's Manual of Nursing Therapeutics for Disease and Disorders. Philadelphia, F. A. Davis, 1997.

Solotkin, K. C., and Knipe, C. J.: Burn patient. *In* Lewis, S. M., Collier, I. C., and Heitkemper, M. M. (eds.): Medical-Surgical Nursing: Assessment and Management of Clinical Problems. St. Louis, Mosby–Year Book, 1996.

Vindenes, H., Ulvestad, E., and Bjerknes, R.: Increased levels of circulating interleukin-8 in patients with large burns: Relation to burn size and sepsis. J. Trauma 39:635–640, 1995.

HYPOTHERMIA

Barker, S. J.: Anesthesia in the high-risk patient. *In* Ayers, S. M. (ed.): Textbook of Critical Care, 3rd ed. Philadelphia, W. B. Saunders, 1995.

Collins, J.: Hypothermia. Practitioner 239:22–26, 1995.

Cummins, R. O.: Textbook of Advanced Cardiac Life Support. Greenville, Tex., American Heart Association, 1994.

Danzl, D. F., and Pozos, R. S.: Accidental hypothermia. N. Engl. J. Med. 331:1756–1760, 1994.

Dennison, D.: Thermal regulation of patients during the perioperative period. AORN J. 61:827–828, 831–832, 1995.

Fritsch, D. E.: Hypothermia in the trauma patient. AACN Clin. Issues Adv. Pract. Acute Crit. Care 6:196–211, 1995.

Ganong, W. F.: Review of Medical Physiology, 17th ed. Norwalk, Conn., Appleton & Lange, 1995.

Gentilello, L. M.: Advances in the management of hypothermia. Surg. Clin. North Am. 75:243–256, 1995.

Gunning, K. A., Sugreu, M., Sloane, D., et al.: Hypothermia and severe trauma. Aust. N. Z. J. Surg. 65:80–82, 1995.

Guyton, A. C., and Hall, J. E.: Textbook of Medical Physiology, 9th ed. Philadelphia, W. B. Saunders, 1996.

Hislop, L. J., Wyatt, J. P., McNaughton, G. W., et al.: Urban hypothermia in the west of Scotland, BMJ 311:725, 1995.

Humbli, E. H., and Demling, R. H.: Hypothermia and cold-related injuries. *In* Ayers, S. M. (ed.): Textbook of

Critical Care, 3rd ed. Philadelphia, W. B. Saunders, 1995.

Kim, M. J., McFarland, G. K., and McLane, A. M.: Pocket Guide to Nursing Diagnoses, 6th ed. St. Louis, Mosby–Year Book, 1995.

Johnston, T. D., Chen, Y., and Reed, R. L.: Functional equivalence of hypothermia to specific clotting factor deficiencies. J. Trauma 37:413–417, 1994.

Marion, D. W., Leonov, Y., Ginsberg, M., et al.: Resuscitative hypothermia. Crit. Care Med. 24(2 Suppl.):S81–S89, 1996.

Rothschild, M. A., and Schneider, V.: Terminal burrowing behavior: A phenomenon of lethal hypothermia. Int. J. Legal Med. 107:250–256, 1995.

Scalise, P. J., Mann, M. C., Votto, J. J., et al.: Severe hypothermia in the elderly. Conn. Med. 59:515–517, 1995.

Vretenar, D. F., Urschel, J. D., Parrott, J. C. W., et al.: Cardiopulmonary bypass resuscitation for accidental hypothermia. Ann. Thorac. Surg. 58:895–898, 1994.

TOXIC INGESTION

Barton, E. N., Gilbert, D. T., Raju, K., et al.: Arsenic: The forgotten poison? W. I. Med. J. 41:36–38, 1992.

Bernstein, J.: Common plant ingestions. Fla. M. A. 81:745–746, 1994.

Bevans, D.: Chemical and drug overdose. In Clochesy, J. M., Breu, C., Cardin, S., et al. (eds.): Critical Care Nursing, 2nd ed. Philadelphia, W. B. Saunders, 1996.

Clancy, C., and Litovitz, T. L.: Poisoning. In Ayers, S. M. (ed.): Textbook of Critical Care, 3rd ed. Philadelphia, W. B. Saunders, 1995.

Goldfrank, L. R., Flomenbaum, N. E., Lewin, N. A., et al.: Toxicologic Emergencies, 5th ed. Norwalk, Conn., Appleton & Lange, 1994.

Haselberger, M. B., and Kroner, B. A.: Drug poisoning in older patients. Drugs Aging 7:292–297, 1995.

Hoffman, R. S., and Goldfrank, L. R.: The poisoned patient with altered consciousness: Controversies in the use of a "coma cocktail." J.A.M.A. 274:562–569, 1995.

Keen, J.: Major trauma. In Swearingen, P. L., and Keen, J. H. (eds.): Manual of Critical Care Nursing, 3rd ed. St. Louis, Mosby–Year Book, 1995.

Klaassen, C. D.: Principles of toxicology and treatment of poisoning. In Hardman, J. G., and Limbird, L. E. (eds.): Goodman & Gilman's The Pharmacologic Basis of Therapeutics, 9th ed. New York, McGraw-Hill, 1996.

Kim, M. J., McFarland, G. K., and McLane, A. M.: Pocket Guide to Nursing Diagnoses, 6th ed. St. Louis, Mosby–Year Book, 1995.

Liebelt, E. L., Fransic, P. D., and Woolf, A. D.: ECG lead aVr versus QRS interval in predicting seizures and arrhythmias in acute tricyclic antidepressant toxicity. Ann. Emerg. Med. 26:195–210, 1995.

Litovitz, T. L., Felberg, L., Soloway, R. A., et al.: 1994 annual report of the American Association of Poison Control Centers Toxic Exposure Surveillance System. Am. J. Emerg. Med. 13:551–597, 1995.

Olson, K. R., Kearney, T. E., Dyer, J. E., et al.: Seizures associated with poisoning and drug overdose. Am. J. Emerg. Med. 11:565–568, 1993.

National Safety Council: Accident Facts. Itasca, Ill. National Safety Council, 1995.

Weisman, R. S., Smith, L., and Goldfrank, L. R.: Toxicokinetics. In Hoffman, R. S., and Goldfrank, L. R. (eds.): Critical Care Toxicology. New York, Churchill Livingstone, 1991.

Wigder, H. N., Erickson, T., Morse, T., et al.: Emergency department poison advice telephone calls. Ann. Emerg. Med. 25:349–352, 1995.

Wren, K., Rodewald, L., and Dockstader, L.: Potential misuse of ipecac. Ann. Emerg. Med. 22:1408–1412, 1993.

chapter

9

....Psychosocial Aspects of Critical Care

John L. Carty, R.N.C., D.N.Sc., ARNP

GROWTH AND DEVELOPMENT

Definition

Growth and development refers to repeated cumulative behaviors frequently exhibited by persons as they confront and deal with issues that typically arise during the life cycle

Discussion

1. Some types of growth seem to occur automatically, whereas others take place through focused effort
2. Because growth and development processes are constantly operating within a person, they have an influence on behavior
3. In the ongoing process of evaluating oneself, one measure frequently used is one's success in mastering developmental tasks. For example, during adolescence, many persons measure their adequacy in part by evaluating their success in forming relationships with members of the opposite sex
4. If one does not master the developmental tasks of a particular life stage, one will have increased difficulty in mastering the developmental tasks of future stages
5. Erikson's Eight Stages of Life Cycle (Table 9–1)

Example

A 15-year-old Caucasian female, found by a neighbor in the front yard and transported by police to the emergency department, transferred to the critical care unit. Police report that patient seems to have been raped and physically abused: large abrasions on both wrists and ankles are present, as are dark contu-

TABLE 9–1. Erik H. Erikson's Eight Stages of Life Cycle

Stage*	Developmental Tasks	Approach
	Acquisition of Hope	
Trust versus mistrust (0–2 years)	Incorporative stage by oral, tactual, and visual senses Needs are met, sense of trust of self and others develops Mother figure important	Provide oral gratification Provide soft touch, cuddling Use gentle voice Provide safe, warm enviroment Physical and emotional safety: enable mother to stay with patient Supply special toys and blanket Be a consistent care provider
	Acquisition of Will	
Autonomy versus shame (2–3 years)	Muscle system maturation Coordinating holding on and letting go Beginning of autonomous will Self-control without loss of self-esteem Illness may be seen as shameful and/or dirty or bad	Use gentle firmness and reassurance by word and act Talk to patient before performing procedures Ehance self-esteem Foster autonomy and self-reliance Take time to explain in simple terms; use touch and gentle words
	Acquisition of Purpose	
Initiative versus guilt (3–6 years)	Becomes part of family relationships: *I am a person,* but what kind of person? Identifies with parents Social circles widen; makes friends Has enough language skills to understand and *misunderstand* Imagination increases to point of frightening self Child locomotor skills, mental curiosity, social nature are intrusive on how child thinks Curious about sexuality Early sense of responsibility and conscience	Satisfy curiosity with simple and practical information Provide comfort when child has bad dreams (loss of life, limb) Dispel fantasies; encourage questions Answer within child's understanding Make patient a partner in treatment, within child's limits Enable family to visit or stay with patient Be a consistent provider
	Acquisition of Competence	
Industry versus inferiority (6–12 years)	Active period of socialization Period of learning: *I am what I learn* Balance between *what I want to do* and *what I am told to do* If child is too rigid, develops overly strict sense of duty, restricts socilization and creativity Needs to work and learn to feel good about self Wants to be recognized by doing things well Needs time for self and others	Respect child's need for privacy Provide balance of social time and alone time Let patient help with care Teach about what is going on around area Use gentle firmness Engage in conversation about school activities, sports, classes, hobbies Engage in active listening Recognize importance of respect and dignity Recognize importance for friends to communicate and visit

Example   801

TABLE 9–1. Erik H. Erikson's Eight Stages of Life Cycle *Continued*

Stage*	Developmental Tasks	Approach
	Acquisition of Fidelity	
Identity versus role confusion (13–20 years)	Searches for self, *new self emerging*, with physical growth and secondary sex characteristics development Takes very seriously how he or she thinks others see him or her, in comparison with what he or she feels about self Needs to incorporate new changes and old roles and skills into a person that fits with image of today Identity equals how he or she thinks others see him or her Identity diffusion is confusion between what patient thinks others see and what patient believes about self	Use name of patient Recognize that peers are important and have a powerful influence on patient's identity Foster decision making by patient within safety parameters Encourage patient to believe that he or she is part of the treatment process Encourage patient to talk about plans and dreams, what he or she wants to do Recognize importance of personal grooming Focus on strengths Provide information to patient Make patient's input part of treatment process
	Acquisition of Love	
Intimacy versus isolation (21–45 years)	Increased importance of human closeness Work and study for life's role Interpersonal intimacy with another adult Endless talking about what one feels, what others seem to feel, expectations and hopes If intimacy not accomplished, will isolate self and lack spontaneity	Recognize importance of patient's family Allow involvement of significant others Encourage patient to talk about plans of life, what he or she does and hopes to accomplish Make patient's input part of treatment planning Share information, involve family Talk about children, work, hobbies Communicate openly and honestly about patient's condition
	Acquisition of Care	
Generativity versus stagnation (45–65 years)	Individuals combine their personalities and energies in producing fulfilling relationships, possiblly common offspring, creativity, job fulfillment Believes in self; enhanced self-esteem/ concept allows for closeness of relationships When unable to develop relationships, become self-absorbed or withdrawn	Show respect and concern Recognize patient's need to be involved in treatment along with significant others Provide information about patient and family Engage in information sharing Even if patient is unconscious, talk to him or her Explain what is happening
	Acquisition of Wisdom	
Ego integrity versus despair (≥65 years)	Acceptance of one's own life as significant and others' as important Feels responsible for own life, *I accept what I am* (responsible for own life), life has dignity and love Emotional integration provides the strength to deal with life as it is *right now*	Treat with respect and dignity Address as Mr./Mrs./Ms. or title Involve patient in treatment planning Encourage expressions of life experiences Recognize that significant others are very important in the decision-making process Provide control of pain to enhance dignity and *clarity of mind*

*Ages denoted are only approximations and are offered only as a guide.

sions on face and chest, fractures of ribs on the left with puncture of the lung, fracture of the left arm, and possible closed-head injury. Patient's eyes are open and filled with tears; pupils are equal and reactive; patient does not look at staff and cringes when staff members (especially males) approach. Patient responds to painful stimuli by body movement, makes no verbal responses, not even to name (see Table 9–1, identity versus identity diffusion)

Nursing Assessment Data Base

Nursing History

1. Obtain medical diagnosis and prognosis
2. Note history of prior hospitalization and/or emergency department visits, specifically musculoskeletal and/or internal injuries. Also note whether there were questions about cause of those injuries
3. Assess history of prior disturbed growth and development
4. Assess impact of patient's condition on normal growth and development tasks for age
5. Determine whether mother and father are divorced, number of siblings
6. Determine who lives with the patient, who visits, and whether there are school problems

Nursing Examination of Patient

1. Assessment is geared to identifying the biopsychosocial responses to the illness and the intensive care unit (ICU) environment
2. Note whether patient is fighting equipment, such as ventilator, oxygen mask, nasal sponges, or intravenous lines, and whether such fighting is unrelated to physiologic causes
3. Note withdrawal and/or cringing when the staff approaches
4. Note whether patient has tears in eyes, is unresponsive (but conscious), pulls away, looks frightened
5. Note consistent demands for pain medication or attention
6. Note refusal to accept staff's help or medication
7. Meet needs for privacy and maintenance of human dignity
8. Determine whether patient is afraid, blames self, avoids interactions as if ashamed
9. Note whether patient refuses to look at staff or to see family and friends

Commonly Encountered Nursing Diagnosis: Altered Growth and Development

1. **Assessment for defining characteristics**
   a. Altered physical and/or psychologic growth
   b. Difficulty performing age-appropriate skills (motor, social, or expressive)
   c. Difficulty performing self-care and/or self-control activities appropriate for age

    d. Listlessness, decreased responses

    e. Cringes and stares when males approach; tearful, frightened look on face

2. Expected outcomes

    a. Patient initiates age-appropriate expression of feeling or concerns and practices self-care skills

    b. Patient complies with procedures

3. Nursing interventions

    a. The assessment phase itself is the first step in the implementation phase

    b. Give clear, concise information about equipment

    c. Engage in frequent interaction at specific times, such as, "I'll be back in 15 minutes"; then return at said time

    d. Introduce self: "My name is . . . and I'll be caring for you today"

    e. Female staff can use a light touch when speaking softly to patient, especially when you are *not* going to adjust or change dressings or equipment. Male staff should never be alone with patient. Talk in a calm and caring voice (softly) before performing any procedure

    f. Encourage verbalization of fears, concerns, likes and dislikes

    g. Be aware that modesty and privacy are extremely important at this age

    h. Let patient know you can get someone (e.g., a mental health team) to talk with her

    i. Encourage patient to be involved in own care within safe limits

    j. Family member and/or female staff should stay with patient as much as possible to enhance sense of safety

4. Evaluation of nursing care

    a. Patient is increasingly cooperative with procedures, asks for help when needed

    b. Patient has age-appropriate expression of feelings and concerns (i.e., mixture of tearfulness and fear)

    c. Appropriate use of pain medication

    d. Patient has decreased verbalization of fear and anxiety

    e. Patient is able to verbalize concerns about sexually transmitted disease

    f. Patient expresses needs in age-appropriate manner

PERCEPTION

Definition

The experience of sensory input; that is, all stimuli experienced through sight, hearing touch, taste, and smell

Discussion

1. Perceptions are regulated by past experiences, which act as filters that allow some perceptions to make an impression on a person and others to be kept out of the person's awareness

2. The degree of impact that the person experiences depends on

    a. The meaning the stimuli have for the person at a given moment.

b. How the person feels about himself or herself at a given moment (e.g., weak or strong, overwhelmed or in control, peaceful or agitated)
c. The unfulfilled needs operating in a person when stimuli are experienced
3. Perceptions lead to thoughts and often to feelings. A person's thoughts and feelings influence the way in which the next perception is received
4. Therefore, two persons who experience the same event may perceive it very differently and may have different thoughts and feelings about the shared experience. Perceptions are unique to each individual

Example

You are visiting a long-time, close friend and see her 10-year-old son; as he is leaving, the boy says "Hi" and waves. Your friend says, "He never is in one place long," and both of you laugh. About 3 weeks later, when you return to work after a vacation, you notice a small child in a bed with face bandaged and several tubes hooked up. You look at the chart and find out that the child is your close friend's son. From that moment on, what you perceive is colored by your friendship. For example, your friendship (emotional attachments) may interfere with perception of the child's respirations, skin condition, or pupil response

Nursing Assessment Data Base

Nursing History

1. Medical diagnosis and/or type of surgery
2. Whether the medical diagnosis has a social stigma, such as suicide attempt, acquired immunodeficiency syndrome (AIDS), or a disfiguring type of surgery
3. Whether the person has the ability to hear, see, and talk
4. Taking consciousness-altering chemicals either before or after admission (prescribed or nonprescribed)
5. Availability of significant other support

Nursing Examination of Patient

1. Determine whether patient is under the influence of central or peripheral anesthetic agents
2. Assess for the presence of perception- or sense-altering equipment or dressings, such as ventilator, eye patch, or arm or leg restraints
3. Check for abnormal physiologic parameters, such as fluid volume, electrolytes, and air exchange, which may alter perceptions

Commonly Encountered Nursing Diagnosis: Sensory-Perceptual Alterations

1. **Assessment for defining characteristics**
   a. Using a quiet, calm voice, introduce yourself; orient patient to place and time; reassure his or her safety

    b. Allow patient to respond; use gentle touch to reinforce safety

    c. Listen for remarks disclosing self-perception ("Did I do something wrong?" "When can I go home?" "Can I walk?")

    d. Clarify the remarks if you see the need; determine whether patient feels unsure, helpless, afraid, or worried or thinks he going to die (to correct any misperceptions)

    e. Note alterations of emotional responses, such as extreme anger or laughter in inappropriate situations

    f. Note decreased ability to concentrate

    g. Note altered communication patterns

2. Expected outcomes

    a. Patient explores environment: asks situation- and age-appropriate questions

    b. Patient seeks to experience things and events

    c. Patient asks reality-oriented questions about treatment, condition, prognosis

    d. Patient expresses positive feelings about self

    e. Patient expresses situation-appropriate emotions and behavior: when happy, laughs; when afraid, states being afraid and asks appropriate questions about fearful situations

3. Nursing interventions

    a. Building rapport begins during assessment, with the nurse validating and clarifying data. Process itself shows concern and increases closeness

    b. Validate and reinforce accurate perceptions and positive self-worth by providing clear, concise information and an attitude of caring and concern

    c. Focus on strengths rather than limitations

    d. Take time to validate perceptions: when giving information about a treatment or procedure, have patient tell you in his or her own words what you have said

    e. Always forewarn patient before giving treatment or performing a procedure

    f. Help patient take part in treatment process in an age-appropriate manner

    g. Engage in conversation about hobbies, school

4. Evaluation of nursing care

    a. Patient has positive and accurate perceptions of situation and self

    b. Patient asks questions or makes requests in a positive mode; for example, "Can I have some water?" and "I would like to see my Mom."

    c. Patient has a more positive perception of situation and self, as reflected in the patient's assertive rather than aggressive approach to fulfilling needs

    d. Patient's emotional response is appropriate for situation

    e. Patient spontaneously talks about school, hobbies, sports, friends, and future; sees self doing better and can focus on age-appropriate interests

SELF-CONCEPT

Definition

All that a person can identify as being characteristic of oneself. The components of self-concept are the things that one believes about oneself on the basis of past experiences and experiences currently being confronted. Self-concept is reinforced or harmed in different ways throughout the life cycle (see Table 9–1)

Discussion

1. Self-concept is formed over time in the context of other people and in the presence of the beliefs, values, and norms of the culture. It consists of what a person *believes* others think of him or her (not to be confused with what others may *actually* think of the person) in light of his or her own beliefs and value system
2. Self-concept is always seeking consistency: a person is continually attempting to find information to reinforce beliefs about oneself, even if those beliefs are negative or incorrect
3. When self-concept is threatened, a person will fight to hold on to beliefs about himself or herself
4. A person behaves in a manner that is consistent with one's self-concept: in a way that demonstrates one's beliefs about oneself
5. The state of a person's self-concept is one of the most important influences on behavior
6. The more positive one feels about oneself, the more comfortable one will feel and the more open one will be to new perceptions and new information

Example

A 45-year-old man was admitted to the ICU for observation after an accidental overdose of antihypertensive medication. This occurrence took place 2 days after his wife of 20 years had her lawyer send him papers asking for a divorce. Last week the patient was told that he would have to move across the country to continue working for his employer. There is some question of suicidal attempt. The patient is now experiencing cardiac arrhythmias and is unresponsive to questions or requests of staff. He repeats at intervals, "I can't win; nothing good ever happens to me"; "I am a loser; I may lose my job; my wife is leaving me"; "You think I am a loser, too." Despite much encouragement, the patient relates that everyone sees him as a loser. He believes that everything that he has ever hoped for is now gone

Nursing Assessment Data Base

Nursing History

1. Review chart for medical concerns, such as serious health problems that might alter self-concept
2. Talk to significant others, such as family, friends, and/or patient's co-workers
3. Assess whether patient received any conciousness-altering drugs (prescribed or nonprescribed)
4. Determine actual cardiac disability and/or limitations secondary to medication overdose

5. Note any history of depression and suicidal thoughts and/or attempts
6. Assess how significant others respond to this situation: with anger, worry, guilt, or indifference

Nursing Examination of Patient

1. Assess the physiologic parameters (exertion limitations, cardiac changes) that may interfere with ability to work
2. Ask the same type of questions as used when assessing perceptions
3. Determine whether patient passively accepts or resists procedures
4. Note patient's specific remarks and/or attitude toward self
5. Note the mood or affect expressed by patient: depressed, angry, sad, inappropriate (laughing), or flat
6. Determine whether patient is able to verbalize emotions appropriate to the situation

Commonly Encountered Nursing Diagnosis: Self-Concept Disturbance

1. **Assessment for defining characteristics**
   a. Listen for self-disclosing remarks concerning self as an individual, a worker, and an opinion giver and what the patient sees happening to self
   b. Listen for self-devaluating remarks, inability to see self as positive
   c. Determine whether patient believes others see him or her as worthless or bad
   d. Note poor eye contact
   e. Note extremely aggressive behavior, use of a demanding, angry voice
   f. Note overemphasis on powerfulness and achievements
2. **Expected outcomes**
   a. Patient initiates conversations, questions procedures, and listens
   b. Patient responds in a positive manner to suggestions and explanations
   c. Body posture and facial features are relaxed
   d. Patient participates in own treatment
   e. Patient is able to make decisions about timing of care ("I need my pain medication before morning care")
   f. Patient is more assertive rather than aggressive
   g. Patient's emotions and behaviors are appropriate for situation
3. **Nursing interventions**
   a. Note changes in patient's self-concept by comparing your original assessment with the current assessment
   b. Use interpersonal interactions with patient to build rapport and obtain clear, concise information
   c. Reinforce the positives; show interest in subjects initiated by patient, such as work, family, hobbies, and expressed opinions
   d. Explain procedures and treatment. Encourage questions, and give clear, concise responses
   e. Allow and encourage patient to make decisions about own care within safe medical and nursing care (e.g., "I want pain medication before the treatment"; "Wake me when my visitors arrive")

   f. Encourage and listen to both positive and negative opinions and remarks of patient
   g. Use comfort measures (e.g., back rub, arm massage) to increase touch, thus accomplishing physical relaxation and conveying acceptance of patient as important
   h. Demonstrate acceptance of patient as a worthwhile person
   i. Give honest praise; avoid false hope
   j. Initiate personal grooming measures (e.g., washing face, combing hair, and brushing teeth) and encourage patient to undertake these activities within his or her physical limits
   k. Evaluate impact of losses on the patient's perception of self (see Table 9–1, generativity versus self-absorption)
4. **Evaluation of nursing care**
   a. Patient spontaneously initiates conversations, asks questions, and listens positively with responses, such as "Is that going to help me?" rather than "Is that going to hurt? What are you doing to me?"
   b. Patient is future-oriented; initiates and participates in own treatment
   c. Patient exhibits decreased passiveness and/or aggressiveness with concomitant increase in assertiveness
   d. Patient's body posture and facial expression indicate sense of relaxation, such as relaxed muscles (less rigid), maybe a smile, and eyes bright; acknowledges surrounding activity
   e. Initiate contracts in writing (if possible) or verbally not to harm self

SELF-ESTEEM

Definition

Feelings one has about oneself: one's perceived self-worth. As such, it is a part of self-concept. As a part of self-concept, it is developed and influenced in different ways throughout all the stages of the life cycle

Discussion

1. Self-esteem is based on personal goals measured against perceived successes, in interaction with the beliefs and values of the culture or society
2. Self-esteem is derived from a comparison between the strengths and the limitations that a person believes he or she possesses
3. The amount of a person's self-esteem influences how that person behaves. The impact is seen through demonstrations of self-confidence and the level of comfort with oneself
4. When self-concept is improved, self-esteem is enhanced and a greater degree of comfort is experienced
5. How much a particular event or situation influences self-esteen (positively or negatively) depends on a person's stage of life and the meaning of the event in that life stage

Examples

Case 1

A 52-year-old man with a healthy self-concept and a high level of self-esteem is admitted to the ICU for observation after being involved in an automobile accident (his truck was hit by a drunk driver). He has lost his left leg below the knee, and he possibly sustained a closed-head injury. He was wounded in Vietnam and had a prognosis of partial paralysis of the left arm, which he has overcome. He now is part owner and driver of a small trucking company. He is seen reacting with spontaneous signs of grief (nervousness, sadness, anxiousness) but does not report feelings of helplessness or devastation. He appears to be able to maintain belief in himself and to find sufficient strength to cope with the situation, much as he remembers having done with his previous situation. He is overheard remarking to a doctor in the ICU, "I am stubborn as a mule and a survivor. I've gotten through some pretty difficult times in the past, and I guess I've got what it takes to deal with this one too, but I'm worried about how long it will take and how much it will cost."

Case 2

A 13-year-old girl on vacation with her family is hurt in a department store explosion. Her mother and younger brother are seriously hurt in the same explosion. She repeatedly states her beliefs that the "nurses are mean" and "It's not my fault my mom and brother were hurt, but they will blame me anyhow." She refuses to cooperate in having vital signs taken and yells for help rather than using her call light. Spending the night in the unit is obviously difficult for her, and she is unable to sleep. A night nurse spends some time with her and begins to explore her behavior to try to find out what the patient is feeling and to see whether she herself can be of assistance. She finds that the patient feels ashamed because she has "caused trouble" for her family twice during the past year; she views herself as "selfish with no concern for others, like my father said I was." The patient acts the role of a selfish, self-centered kid.

Nursing Assessment Data Base

Nursing History

1. Use the same assessment material as for self-concept. Self-esteem is assessed at the same time as self-concept
2. Determine availability of family or significant others' support
3. Obtain medical diagnosis and prognosis
4. Check for impaired senses: inability to speak or to see; whether touch is impaired by bandages or restraints
5. Note any disfigurement or physical disability that may influence self-esteem or self-concept

Nursing Examination of Patient

1. Assess whether the patient sees self as adequate or inadequate in current situation
2. Note self-devaluation remarks and negative responses, such as, "I'll never get out of here," "No one cares about me," "Nothing will help me"
3. Assess whether the patient is passive or questions what is being done to him or her

Commonly Encountered Nursing Diagnosis: Disturbances in Self-Esteem

1. **Assessment for defining characteristics**
   a. Patient does not accept positive reinforcement, describes self in negative terms
   b. Patient is very passive, will not participate in own care, makes poor eye contact
   c. Patient's responses are limited; says one or two words or turns head and eyes away
   d. Patient does not initiate personal grooming or ask for help with personal hygiene
2. **Expected outcomes**
   a. Patient participates in own care, asks for medication
   b. Patient initiates requests for personal hygiene care
   c. Patient requests explanation of procedures before they are performed
   d. Patient shows increase in positive remarks about self in current situation
   e. Patient initiates age-appropriate conversations with staff and others
3. **Nursing interventions**
   a. Convey acceptance of the patient as worthwhile; emphasize strengths
   b. Build rapport with interventions in age-appropriate terms (see Table 9–1)
   c. Involve patient in decision making about own care
   d. Give positive reinforcement for accomplishments, but do not give false praise
4. **Evaluation of nursing care**
   a. Patient demonstrates positive self-worth by words and/or behavior
   b. Patient perceives self as adequate in current situation
   c. Patient expresses both limitations and strengths about self: "Not knownig scares me. Please tell me what is planned for me today."
   d. Patient participates in own care within physical limitations
   e. Patient's emotions are appropriate for the situation

NEEDS

Definition

A person's perceived physical and psychosocial requirements for developing, maintaining, and enhancing self. As people go through the stages of the life cycle (see Table 9–1), needs change

Discussion

1. Maslow (1968) categorized human needs according to the following levels, with the first level being the most basic:
   a. Physiologic
   b. Safety and security
   c. Love and belonging
   d. Self-esteem
   e. Self-actualization
2. Satisfying of needs progresses from that of basic needs to that of higher level needs: people do not become preoccupied with meeting higher level needs until basic needs are satisfied
3. Unfulfilled needs are constantly operating in humans and influence their behavior. A person consistently strives to fulfill perceived needs in an ongoing dynamic process throughout the life cycle. The influence of needs on behavior is sometimes a conscious process and at other times unconscious; that is, people are sometimes aware of their unfulfilled needs and at other times unaware of them. Even when unfulfilled needs are not recognized consciously, those needs continue to influence one's behavior
4. One of the most important human needs is to perceive the self as an adequate person
5. Major life changes (e.g., illness) may necessitate a refocusing of energies to meet a more basic need
6. The fulfillment of needs at different stages of the life cycle is influenced by how well the more basic needs have been and are being met (e.g., meeting self-esteem needs is influenced by how well the more basic safety and security needs have been met)

Example

A 70-year-old male is admitted to ICU because of respiratory difficulty, possibly resulting from return of cancer and/or medication reaction. According to history, patient has survived cancer for 10 years, wife is deceased, no immediate family is available, three of four children are alive (two sons, aged 50 years and 48 years, and one daughter, aged 45 years). The fourth child, a son, was killed in Vietnam. All living children are married, with eight grandchildren among them. Patient's eyes are bright and alert, and he responds by touching your hand with his hand or by pointing. He is on a respirator and cannot verbalize, but his eyes let you know when he needs something or has a question. There is a sense of calmness and strength in his face and movements

Nursing Assessment Data Base

Nursing History

1. Medical diagnosis and prognosis
2. Availability of significant other

3. Work history
4. Whether illness will influence relationships with family or significant others, ability to work, or ability to take care of self
5. Effect of the patient's physiologic and psychologic condition on sensory ability (sight, taste, hearing, touch)
6. Effect of the patient's physiologic and psychologic condition on self-concept, self-esteem, and communication

Nursing Examination of Patient

1. **Assess physiologic needs,** such as airway, nutrition, general physical condition, mobility, and skin integrity
2. **Assess safety and security needs,** such as equipment safety; whether the person sees the equipment as hazardous to physical safety; need for safety measures (bed rails); whether the patient understands function and sounds of machines, use of catheters, intravenous lines, and so forth.
3. **Assess belonging needs** (love): whether patient feels as though he or she is a number, a diagnosis, or a human being. Listen for questions and requests of patient. Determine whether patient still identifies self as part of family and community
4. **Assess self-esteem needs** under concepts of self-esteem and self-concept
5. **Assess self-actualization:** listen for self-description in relation to having a future, sense of control, and meaning
6. **Assess whether individual is future- or past-oriented**
7. **Assess patient's responses for age appropriateness.** In the earlier example, the 70-year-old patient is coping well with what Maslow called the need for self-actualization, which in Erikson's terms is the "integrity versus despair" stage of the life cycle (see Table 9–1)

Commonly Encountered Nursing Diagnosis: Need Disturbance

1. **Assessment for defining characteristics**
   a. Threat to health status, to self-preservation, to self-esteem or self-concept
   b. Threat to relationships and to normal role function (as student, as worker, as parent, as spouse)
   c. Age appropriateness of responses
2. **Expected outcomes**
   a. Patient is able to meet physiologic needs within limits of condition
   b. Patient accepts environment as necessary for well-being
   c. Patient sees self as part of family and community and as a participant in relationships
   d. Patient views self as a person with worth and dignity (has achieved self-actualization, or has reached the life cycle stage of integrity)
   e. Patient talks about self in future terms: going back home to family, being with friends, and being involved in hobbies
3. **Nursing interventions**
   a. Implementation starts at the first meeting and interaction with the patient
   b. Sharing of clear, concise information with the patient is necessary for meeting physiologic needs. For example, use of endotracheal tube to allow and enhance breathing needs should be explained. The use of intravenous

lines or other modes for nutrients, medication, and fluids is essential for physiologic survival but also must be explained

c. Use of all safety measures, such as bed rails and alarms, needs to be explained. At the same time, the security needs should also be addressed. Reassurance and optimal meeting of needs along with shared information and a sense of caring expressed by words, touch, and concern will help answer security needs

d. Self-esteem needs are best answered by showing concern, etc. (See Discussion sections on self-esteem and self-concept)

4. Evaluation of nursing care

a. Physiologic parameters indicate that physical needs are being met (e.g., respiratory, nutritional, excretory)

b. Psychologic parameters (e.g., positive self-esteem, self-concept) indicate that psychologic needs are being met

c. Necessary physical safety and security measures (e.g., bed rails, alarms, monitors) are in place

d. Love and belonging: patient refers to self as an important person rather than a diagnosis or number. Patient still identifies self as part of a family and community. Family's or friends' visits are positive events

e. Self-esteem: patient sees self as important and as having value. (See section on self-esteem)

f. Self-actualization (future-oriented): patient takes control of some event, such as requesting specific time for medication or bath

STRENGTHS, POTENTIALS, AND LIMITATIONS

Definition

Strengths are perceived as positive attributes believed to be characteristic of oneself or others. *Potentials* are perceived as latent strengths believed to be characteristic of oneself or others. *Limitations* are perceived as inadequacies or shortcomings believed to be characteristic of oneself or others. Where the individual is in the life cycle will to a great extent influence whether an actualized potential is seen as a strength or a limitation. For example, a 16-year-old has the potential to cope with certain stressful situations, whereas a 30-year-old will, through life experiences, have translated that potential into the strength to cope

Discussion

1. In general, persons are more aware of their perceived limitations than of their perceived strengths

2. People often desperately attempt to hide the limitations that they believe they possess, in an effort to protect their self-concept and self-esteem

3. Humans consciously and unconsciously choose the boundaries of their lives

a. The strengths they choose to maintain

b. The potentials they choose to develop or not to develop

c. The limitations they choose to maintain

4. Because all humans struggle to maintain the "self" as adequate, focusing on their strengths and potentials (instead of their shortcomings) enables them to feel more competent and to deal more effectively with perceived or actual limitations. Learning and growth also are greatly facilitated by recognizing strengths in oneself and in others
5. Poor self-concept and poor self-esteem result from focusing only on limitations and ignoring the potential to develop strengths
6. Strengths and limitations need to be assessed in terms of where the individual is in the life cycle. Time and experience are necessary elements for actualization of potential

Example

A 29-year-old mother of two (7-year-old son, 5-year-old daughter) and 8 months pregnant is admitted to the ICU after being involved in an automobile accident. The patient suffered a dislocated left shoulder, fractured right arm, and impact to the chest area. The baby (female) was born with no severe damage. The patient wants to breast-feed the baby, as she did her other two children; The patient has been told that breast-feeding is currently not possible. The patient believes that her relationships with her other children are stronger because of the breast-feeding and wants to know whether there is any way she could at least feed her baby breast milk. By using a breast pump, the patient can hold and feed the baby and to a large extent achieve what she perceives as one of her strengths: breast-feeding to enhance bonding

Nursing Assessment Data Base

Nursing History

1. Identification of strengths, potentials, and limitations can be accomplished by interpersonal interaction and validated observations. Other sources of information are records (e.g., nursing history to include work, social, medical, and family history) and information from family and friends
2. Medical diagnosis and prognosis
3. Limitations secondary to condition and their influence on sensory organs
4. Availability of family or significant others

Nursing Examination of Patient

1. Assess whether patient sees self as important, being of value
2. Obtain history of coping with illness in past, general state of health, work history
3. Verify marital status, availability of friends, and whether patient sees self as important or unimportant to family and friends
4. Note involvement in community, school activities, kinds of hobbies
5. Note presence or absence of positive self-esteem and self-concept

Commonly Encountered Nursing Diagnosis: Disturbance in Perception, Self-Concept, Self-Esteem, or Needs

1. **Assessment for defining characteristics**
   a. Emotional responses are altered (e.g., extremes in emotions, emotions inappropriate for situation)
   b. Condition of patient restricts involvement in relationships, family, community, and work
   c. Degree of independence is limited by condition
   d. Needs are not met; patient is not participating in self-care
2. **Expected outcomes**
   a. Patient is able to identify strengths, potentials, and limitations in a realistic manner
   b. Patient shows increased involvement in own care
   c. Patient shows increased interest and involvement in relationships, family, and community
   d. Patient is future-oriented: talks about returning to school, job, and family
   e. Patient demonstrates return to premorbid health
3. **Nursing interventions**
   a. Begin implementation at the time of assessment, when attributes are identified and should be reinforced
   b. Support identified strengths and enhance potential strengths by verbal and nonverbal encouragement
   c. Note limitations but do not overemphasize them
   d. Encourage patient to use already developed coping mechanisms
   e. Reinforce outside interests, such as family, work, and hobbies
   f. Give honest, timely compliments that will reinforce strengths
   g. Involve patient in own care as much as possible, from as little as nodding of head for "yes" or "no" to actual hands-on self-care. Encourage patient's taking charge of own life within physical and safety limits
4. **Evaluation of nursing care**
   a. Patient identifies strengths, potentials, and limitations realistically
   b. Patient increases interactions with family, job, community, and hobbies
   c. Show increased concern, love, and care toward family and friends
   d. Patient increases involvement in own care within physical and safety limits

STRESS

Definition

The condition that exists in an organism when it encounters stimuli. Selye (1974) identified two types of stress: (1) distress—the condition that exists in an organism when it meets with *noxious* stimuli; that is, when an individual encounters threatening stimuli—and (2) eustress—the condition that exists in an organism when it meets with *nonthreatening* stimuli. Where an individual is in the life cycle in part influences whether stimuli are experienced as eustress or distress

Discussion

1. Persons may experience the same stressors differently. Stressors that may cause distress in one person may evoke eustress in another
2. Persons respond to stressors differently because their perceptions of the stressful event may be different and because they may possess different coping abilities
3. A person experiencing distress feels uncomfortable. The discomfort provides the motivation to find a way to deal effectively with the stressor
4. If people perceive themselves as adequate in the presence of stressors, self-concept is maintained and may even be enhanced; growth is experienced and self-esteem is heightened. People then function out of strength
5. If people perceive themselves as inadequate in the presence of stressors, they may use defensive mechanisms (e.g., denial, projection) to mask the fact that they view their handling of the stressor as inadequate; however, they will feel overwhelmed and helpless. They then function out of a sense of frustration and helplessness
6. If people continue to experience themselves as inadequate in the presence of stressors for a prolonged period, crisis will result

Example

Two women are admitted to the ICU for observation; both are victims of the same robbery. The first victim is 29 years old, is the clerk at the store, and is the mother of two (a 7-year-old son and a 5-year-old daughter); she was also a victim of robbery 2 years ago and was beaten by the robber at that time. The second victim is 32 years old. She is a mother of two (daughters, aged 8 and 9 years) and has never been involved in anything like this before. Both victims were beaten around their heads until unconscious. The first victim is awake and asking questions (about her children and her husband and how badly she is hurt). The second victim is awake but does not answer questions; at each loud noise, her body tenses, her hands shake, and her eyes close

Nursing Assessment Data Base

Nursing History

1. Medical diagnosis and prognosis
2. Availability of significant other
3. When appropriate, social and work history and prior illness
4. Condition's impact on sensory organs and communication ability
5. Previous experience with similar events

Nursing Examination of Patient

1. Base your assessment on observation, daily interaction, and patient's response to environment (e.g., ICU, equipment, staff)

2. Remember that any change in a patient's normal environment will affect the patient and can be considered stressful; therefore, by assessing perceptions, self-esteem, self-concept, strengths, potentials, and limitations along with growth and development, you are actually assessing the degree of stress experienced by a patient

3. Assess the patient's perception of self, of situation, and of status of self in situation

4. Assess how the person sees self and whether he or she feels adequate to cope

5. Determine whether the patient's interactions emphasize limitations rather than strengths

6. Assess what the patient identifies as stressful; remember that stress for one person may not be stress for another, or at least not to the same degree

7. Remember that stress is expressed by both emotional and physical signs: pulse is increased, blood pressure is elevated, respiration is increased, headache and/or stomachache may be present

8. Note whether responses to stressor are age-appropriate (see Table 9–1)

. . . .

Commonly Encountered Nursing Diagnosis: Alteration in Stress Level

1. **Assessment for defining characteristics**
   a. Hypervigilance or hypovigilance
   b. Impaired problem-solving ability, impaired decision making
   c. Feeling inadequate in situation, uncomfortable with self
   d. Increased tension and sense of helplessness or powerlessness

2. **Expected outcomes**
   a. Patient demonstrates increased initiation of requests and involvement in own care
   b. Patient explores environment: asks situation- and age-appropriate questions
   c. Patient's questions are reality-oriented and express positive aspects about self
   d. Patient is future-oriented, talks (in realistic terms) about return to work, family, community
   e. Patient's responses, questions, and problem solving are age-appropriate

3. **Nursing interventions**
   a. Start implementation with assessment by building rapport and conveying concern and caring
   b. Include frequent interactions at an age-appropriate level; clear, concise information; and timely explanations of equipment, sounds, and sights. Use touch to convey caring
   c. Provide for privacy; decrease noise level (e.g., monitor outside sounds and conversations)
   d. Encourage the patient to make age-appropriate decisions about his or her daily care (e.g., medication, personal hygiene care); increase feelings of control

4. **Evaluation of nursing care**
   a. Patient exhibits behavioral signs of decreased stress reaction (e.g., increased initiation of requests, making decisions)
   b. Patient is able to express needs either verbally or nonverbally; able to disagree with staff in positive, constructive manner

c. Patient shows increased ability to express doubts, fears, and concerns to staff
d. Patient shows increased self-esteem and self-concept, along with expression of strengths (e.g., talking about work, hobbies, family)
e. Patient demonstrates increased interaction with family or significant others (e.g., supporting each other)
f. Patient exhibits decrease in physical signs of stress: pulse, blood pressure, and respiration no longer rise drastically when monitor sounds are heard or when procedures are performed

PAIN

Definition

A concept denoting the experience of multiple stimuli, all perceived as unpleasant by the person involved. It is a multidimensional perception that has an influence on all aspects of one's life. Pain is experienced at all ages, but its meaning and expression are influenced by where the individual is in the life cycle

Discussion

1. Pain is an individual and personal experience. Behavioral expressions of pain are socially and culturally determined. Because of the complexity of pain phenomena, no single theory takes into account all the ramifications. Scientists and clinicians view pain from as many perspectives as there are clinical specialties. However, three elements appear to be common to most definitions of pain:
   a. There is a break in the protective barrier of the person
   b. It is perceived as a danger signal
   c. The meaning of pain is influenced by previous pain experiences
2. Painful stimuli and their associated responses are composed of both physiologic and psychosocial elements. Almost all humans are born with the physiologic ability to experience pain
3. Behavioral responses to pain are developed within the psychosocial realm. Humans are both blessed and cursed by the fact that they can experience pain and remember it. The moment an unpleasant (painful) stimulus is experienced, the experience is integrated with memories of previous painful experiences, and a response occurs. People respond not only to the immediate painful stimulus but also to the memories of other experiences. In fact, the ability to think and remember allows people to feel discomfort without currently experiencing a physiologically unpleasant stimulus
4. The meaning that is placed on an unpleasant sensation is determined by a person's beliefs and values within the context of societal beliefs, values, and norms
5. Pain, like beauty, is in the eye of the beholder. It is whatever the person experiencing it says it is, whenever it is being experienced

Example

A 48-year old man has been admitted for the fourth time to the ICU with chest pain and shortness of breath. Four months ago, he experienced a myocardial infarction with residual heart damage. The patient describes events before admission as follows: "I started to breathe more rapidly, felt dizzy, lightheaded, and faint with increasing chest pain. I felt like this while I was driving to a job interview." While the nurse is talking to the patient, he reports that he is becoming more nervous and anxious. His breathing becomes more rapid, and he mentions that his dizziness is more pronounced. The following diagnosis is made: angina (normal for this patient) and hyperventilation secondary to anxiety. The patient's memories of the heart attack and feelings of anxiety about the job interview are expressed behaviorally as hyperventilation and its sequelae. He perceives his symptoms of hyperventilation as chest "pain" and associates it with a heart attack

Nursing Assessment Data Base

Nursing History

1. History of prior painful conditions or situations
2. Medical diagnosis and prognosis
3. Duration of this episode of pain
4. Whether pain interferes with work, family or social interactions
5. History of pain medication and what being taken now
6. Whether family or significant others have had a painful condition in the past
7. A good pain history should include but not be limited to the following: accidents, fractures, surgeries, and how the patient coped with the pain (by laughing, crying, ignoring the pain, overusing medications, screaming, appropriately using medications, or combination of these)
8. Pain history gives information on meaning of pain and patient's coping style

Nursing Examination of Patient

1. Assessment is aimed at identifying what the patient is experiencing and what it means to the patient
2. Determine what these painful situations mean to the patient: "Pain is a normal response"; "I am critically hurt"; "I am dying"
3. Assess the degree of pain felt: use scale of 1 (the least severe) to 10 (the most severe)
4. Determine location and description of pain and whether it is age appropriate
5. Assess whether pain medications have adequately controlled the pain

Commonly Encountered Nursing Diagnosis: Pain

1. **Assessment for defining characteristics**
   a. Communication (verbal or nonverbal) of pain description
   b. Guarding behavior, protective, self-focusing

      c. Narrowed focus (withdrawal from social contact, impaired perception and thought process)

      d. Restlessness, moaning, crying, pacing, grimacing, lackluster eyes

      e. Flaccid to rigid muscle tone

2. Expected outcomes

      a. Patient reports increased periods of uninterrupted sleep at night

      b. Patient demonstrates decreased signs of anxiety with increased self-esteem and self-concept

      c. Patient experiences increased periods of being pain-free

      d. Patient's expression of pain is appropriate for stage in the life cycle. In the stage of trust versus mistrust, the child may cry in pain. In the stage of intimacy versus isolation, the patient has the ability to verbally express pain

3. Nursing interventions

      a. Assessment is starting point of the pain plan: shows concern and caring

      b. When appropriate, use and reinforce familiar modes of coping with pain

      c. Give clear, concise information about pain. For example, postoperative incisional pain does not mean sutures have broken or patient is dying

      d. Reassure patient that when he or she says "I am in pain," you believe it

      e. Use touch whenever possible; perform frequent and consistent checks for pain relief

      f. Whenever possible, administer pain medication routinely rather than on an as-needed (p.r.n.) basis

      g. Interactions with the patient will be guided by where the patient is in the life cycle. The terms used, depth of explanation, description of treatment used, and other explanations need to be presented at a level equal to the patient's level of understanding

4. Evaluation of nursing care

      a. Patient participates in own treatment within physical limitations

      b. Pain concerns and fears are expressed in age-appropriate terms

      c. Signs of anxiety and requests for pain medication are decreased

      d. Interactions with family or with significant others are increased

      e. When pain is under control, patient feels in control and thereby experiences an increase in positive self-esteem and self-concept

INTERPERSONAL COMMUNICATION

. . . .

Definition

A dynamic process involving verbal and nonverbal means of conveying and receiving information. These forms of communication exist at all age levels and need to be understood in terms of where the individual is in the life cycle

. . . .

Discussion

1. One of the most important aspects of interpersonal communication is that a person cannot *not* communicate. Interpersonal interactions means that every word (spoken or written), movement, facial expression and body posture conveys information. This begins the circular process of communication

2. The receiver accepts information conveyed through the words, gestures, facial expressions, and postures of the sender and assigns meaning to that information. The meaning assigned is understood in context of the situation and in light of the beliefs, values, knowledge, and self-concepts of both sender and receiver. The meaning and significance of the information influences how the receiver responds. The response is based on the meaning the receiver has given the information. The sender then receives the response

3. The response may not be what the sender desired to know, and a breakdown in communication could result. This can be forestalled by verification (e.g., verifying the information received and its meaning with the sender). Verification can be accomplished in a variety of ways (e.g., directly questioning, restating, and reflecting the information received). Through verification, both the receiver and sender achieve a clearer understanding of the information conveyed. In order to accomplish effective communication, it is not necessary to agree with what another says—only that both parties understand what is communicated

Example

A 25-year old man is admitted to the ICU after experiencing cardiac complications while undergoing knee surgery. Patient required multiple intravenous (IV) lines, multiple medications, and placement on respirator. Patient is unable to verbally communicate or write. Therefore, communication must be undertaken by the nurse, letting him know where he is, that he is safe, and, by using a gentle touch, signalling the nurse's concern and support. The nurse must attempt to develop a method of communication; for example, one eye blink equals *yes*, two eye blinks equals *no*. Then by observation of the patient's face and body posture, the nurse must identify possible concerns of the patient and validate (e.g., by use of the eye blink method or some other method that the staff develops). The patient stares at the tube coming out of his mouth and then shifts his eyes toward the respirator. The nurse observes the patient's staring, shares with him the meaning that she assigned to his behavior, and attempts to verify by use of the eye blink method

Nursing Assessment Data Base

Nursing History

1. Review chart, talk to family or significant other to gain understanding of how patient normally communicates
2. Determine whether the patient's condition alters ability to communicate
3. Assess whether patient and staff speak same language (e.g., staff speaks English, patient speaks only Polish)
4. Identify any prior condition that affects the patient's ability to communicate (e.g., mentally retarded, stroke, hearing-impaired)

. . . .

Nursing Examination of Patient

1. Assessment of communication begins at the first interaction with the patient
2. Assessing the communication process involves at least two persons (e.g., health care provider and health care receiver)
3. Assess nonverbal and verbal communication by validating the meaning of what you (staff) perceive and what the patient may perceive; that is, assess the meaning of nonverbal and verbal communication
4. By assessing the preceding concepts of perception, self-esteem, self-concept, and others, you begin the assessment of interpersonal communication
5. Evaluate the congruence between nonberbal clues and verbal responses: for example, saying "I am fine" at the same time the face is white and the body rigid. The incongruence between verbal and nonverbal communication gives clues on how the patient really feels (e.g., feels scared, self-esteem/self-concept threatened, feels alone, decreased trust, and feeling of weakness)
6. Identify not only verbalized needs but also nonverbalized needs
7. Identify how you and staff members are being perceived by the patient (validate either verbally or nonverbally)

. . . .

Commonly Encountered Nursing Diagnosis: Impaired Communication

1. **Assessment for defining characteristics**
   a. Unable to speak dominant language
   b. Will not or cannot speak; medical conditions impinge on ability to communicate
   c. Chronic condition (e.g., mental retardation) affects communication
   d. Incongruence between verbal communication and nonverbal communication (e.g., patient smiles with body rigid, no eye contact)
2. **Expected outcomes**
   a. Patient actively listens and responds to relevant stimuli
   b. Patient demonstrates congruent verbal and nonverbal communication
   c. Patient asks for and receives feedback
3. **Nursing interventions**
   a. When the assessment process is initiated in a positive manner, enhancement of interpersonal communication is part of that process
   b. For the health care provider, there must be congruence between the verbal and nonverbal communication before trust can be initiated and enhanced
   c. Give clear information with adequate time allowed for clarification by patient
   d. Visit patient frequently to check status and needs not just to check equipment. Uses touch and facial expressions of warmth and concern along with words
   e. Clarify your own perceptions. Ask questions; do not assume
   f. Use all modes of communication. If patient is unable to use verbal route, use writing, sign language, eye blinks, or any other mode that will foster the link between health care provider and health care receiver. Trust is enhanced; therefore, compliance and communication are increased
   g. Provide privacy, clarify questions and misperceptions, be open and honest

Example   823

4. **Evaluation of nursing care**
   a. Patient responds willingly
   b. Congruence exists between verbal and nonverbal modes of communication
   c. Patient becomes involved in own care within physical limitations
   d. Questions for clarification are stated in positive terms
   e. Patient demonstrates increased trust, increased compliance, increased self-esteem and self-concepts

BODY IMAGE

Definition

The concept of a person's own body. This concept is formed through an accumulation of all perceptions, information, and feelings incorporated about a person's body as different and apart from all others. The body image evolves and changes as the person moves through Erikson's stages of the life cycle.

Discussion

1. People are not born with a body image. The concept of body is built slowly over a period of time as an integral part of growth and development. Body image is an essential component of the self-concept and as such is grounded in interactions occurring between persons and their environment
2. Like self-concept, body image reflects sociocultural beliefs and values. Body image evolves in a dynamic, ever-changing process that incorporates not only the body but also devices attached to it (e.g., clothes, rings, watches, dialysis machine, pacemaker)
3. Body image is social in nature, yet is individually experienced. If a person experiences a positive body image, self-concept and self-esteem are likely to be influenced favorably. Conversely, a negative body image could lead to a less-than-favorable self-concept and self-esteem. Changes in body image influence a person's perception of consequential events

Example

A 13-year-old female is admitted to unit with multiple contusions, broken nose and jaw, fracture of right arm, and possible internal injuries. She appears malnourished with pale, dry skin and poor general hygiene. She is the youngest of three children and lives with her stepfather and biological mother; both have history of drug abuse. She has a history of being seen in the emergency department three times in the past 7 to 8 months with bruises and contusions reported to be the result of falls downstairs and play accidents. Two older siblings also have seen in the emergency department a number of times in the past 2 years with bruises and fractures (reported to be from falls). The patient is not verbalizing; she has a frightened look on her face; her body is stiff; she makes no eye contact and no verbal complaints of pain; she will not let anyone know when she has to move her bowels or urinate (see Table 9–1)

Nursing Assessment Data Base

Nursing History

1. Verbal responses to actual or perceived changes in body structure and function
2. Nonverbal (behavioral) responses to perceived or actual changes in body structure and function
3. Impact of medical condition on body image
4. Influence of medical conditions on patient's ability to learn, socialize, or relate to family, significant others, friends
5. History of school and social involvement; possible emotional, physical, or sexual abuse

Nursing Examination of Patient

1. Body image assessment starts with assessments of self-concept and self-esteem
2. Observe the impact of any invasive procedures, such as intravenous lines, cutdowns, or central lines on body image
3. Listen to how patient describes and perceives the machines (e.g., monitors, ventilators); determine whether these impinge on body image. For example, a cardiac monitor is incorporated into body image, or ventilator becomes extension of lungs, which are necessary for life. Does the patient have names for machines, or does she just call each "that machine"?
4. Assess need for privacy: covering of culturally defined private parts (e.g., breasts, genitals). If they are not covered, body image is impinged on, and self-esteem and self-concept are threatened
5. Identify areas of body most important to patient (e.g., hands of the pianist, legs of the runner, general mobility of the child). Body image is disturbed when these areas are affected. Stress, anxiety, fear, and anger are increased when self-concept and self-esteem are decreased
6. Determine how patient perceives self and body in this situation (e.g., distorted, feeling depersonalized)

Commonly Encountered Nursing Diagnosis: Disturbance in Body Image

1. **Assessment for defining characteristics**
   a. Verbal and nonverbal responses to actual or perceived change in body structure and function
   b. Refraining from looking at or touching actual or perceived body change area
   c. Body boundaries extended to environment (e.g., ventilator, bedside stand)
   d. Feelings of hopelessness, helplessness, and powerlessness

2. Expected outcomes
   a. Patient improves self-care practices; is able to talk about and focus on affected area
   b. Facial expression and body posture reflect sense of relaxation
   c. Patient initiates age-appropriate expression of feelings about perceived or actual change in structure and function
   d. Patient experiences decreased apprehension; asks questions about equipment and procedures

3. Nursing interventions
   a. Encourage patient to participate in own care
   b. Reassure patient of safety; use a calm, gentle voice to overcome bad thoughts and dreams; let patient know what you are doing, when you will be coming back, that someone is always nearby
   c. Help set age-appropriate goals (body image changes as the person goes through the life stages; therefore, body image is influenced by where the person is in the life cycle)
   d. Remember that the object of the treatment plan is to maintain body image in at least a premorbid status with improvement when possible
   e. Provide adequate time (when possible) for quiet talks with patient at the patient's level about what happened, and explain what is happening
   f. Explain in age-appropriate terms clearly and concisely what each machine will do and what the different sounds, lights, and functions of the machines signify

4. Evaluation of nursing care
   a. Patient's perception of self reflects feelings of being in control of body and/or still liking oneself (body image)
   b. Patient demonstrates less resistance to being in the hospital by being more relaxed and having a less frightened facial expression and brighter eyes
   c. Patient experiences decreased apprehension regarding machines (e.g., body is less rigid; patient tells you when he or she needs to move bowels; frequency in use of call button is decreased; anxiety is decreased)
   d. Patient shows increased interest in what is happening

HUMAN SEXUALITY

Definition

A developmental process encompassing a blend of the physiologic and psychosocial aspects of genetic sex; the latter include gender identity, sexual behavior, and sexual attitudes or values. Sexuality is part of self-concept, embodying how people see themselves as sexual beings. The meaning of sexuality has to be defined and understood in terms of where the individual is in the life cycle (see Table 9–1)

Discussion

1. The interaction between the psyche and the soma is nowhere more evident than in the area of sexuality, in which perception, self-concept, self-esteem,

body image, and personal values combine with basic mechanisms of physiologic functioning in a complex system. Although genetic sex is determined by chromosomal factors before birth, the psychosocial impact on gender identity becomes predominant after birth. The concept of sexuality—or, more specifically, the psychosocial aspect of sexuality—involves primarily the quality of a person's interactions with significant others throughout the life cycle. Gender identity, sexual behaviors, and sexual attitudes and values are integrated into self-concept. Sexuality is so closely interwoven with the self-concept that a perceived threat to the self-concept can have an impact on sexuality, which is expressed in both physiologic and psychosocial realms

2. For different reasons, sexuality is as important to a 70-year-old person as it is to a 20-year-old person. Younger persons often are concerned about their sexual attractiveness as well as their ability to reproduce. Older persons usually are concerned with feeling like a sexual being and being perceived by other as such

3. A perceived threat to the self within a critical care environment has an effect on sexuality. The effects can be expressed in a variety of symptomatic behaviors (e.g., depression or anger, a sense of loss, sexual aggressiveness, noncompliance, or demands on others.) Such behavior can result in decreased self-esteem, influencing the person's perception of events occurring in the environment

Example

A 27-year-old woman is admitted with diagnosis of cancer of both breasts and is scheduled for bilateral mastectomy. According to history, her mother, aunt, and grandmother had breast cancer, and the patient had a small lump removed 5 years ago. She had been married 5 years and is a graduate student; her husband is a doctoral candidate, due to receive his Ph.D. degree in 2 months. They had planned to start a family after school. After surgery, the patient appears very apprehensive, restless, and withdrawn, and these symptoms seem to increase after her husband's visits. She discusses her apprehensions with a nurse after her husband's visit: "Things won't be like they have been. I don't know whether he understands what this means to me." She then grimaces and quickly looks away. The nurse says, "Is there something wrong right now?" The patient replies, "I'm just thinking about how he will see me, with the scars where my breasts were. Maybe he won't want me; I won't be attractive anymore; I was going to breast-feed our babies, and now I can't." The bilateral mastectomy is a threat to the patient's self-concept, self-esteem, body image, and sexual identity

Nursing Assessment Data Base

Nursing History

1. Assess medical condition's physiologic impact on the sexuality of the patient; is there a change in the function or structure of the physical sexual characteristics?

2. Assess how patient's medical condition impinges on the gender identity, sexual behavior, and/or sexual attitudes: does the patient perceive the medical condition affecting his or her sexual relationship with significant other?

3. Assess contact between patient and significant other: do they touch softly (hands, arms, shoulders, or cheeks)? Do they talk to each other? Is there eye contact?

. . . .

Nursing Examination of Patient

1. See assessment of self-concept, self-esteem, and body image
2. Assess how this situation will affect sexual identity and/or function
3. Determine whether the patient saw self as attractive or unattractive before the current illness or accident. Identify changes that the patient sees now
4. Note whether the patient feels comfortable with self identity (male or female) and identifies with role
5. Assess how the patient reinforces sexual identity (e.g., use of clothes or perfumes; reproductive ability; anatomic features; strong-muscled or soft or warm)
6. Determine whether the patient's response to sexuality is appropriate for age

. . . .

Commonly Encountered Nursing Diagnosis: Altered Patterns of Human Sexuality

1. **Assessment for defining characteristics**
   a. Actual or perceived limitations imposed by condition and/or therapy
   b. Seeking confirmation of desirability (verbally or nonverbally)
   c. Change of interest in self and others; speaks of self in negative terms
   d. Extreme shyness or exhibitionistic behavior
2. **Expected outcomes**
   a. Patient pays increased attention to personal grooming (e.g., hair combed, make-up on, perfume used; requests use of mirror; shaving; bathing)
   b. Patient demonstrates appropriate use of privacy; performs personal grooming before seeing significant others
   c. Emotional responses to sexual questions and to procedures are age-appropriate
   d. Patients' questions about medical conditions in relation to self-esteem, self-concept, and body image often reflect their questions about their sexuality
3. **Nursing interventions**
   a. Reinforce identified strengths
   b. Address patient as patient desires (e.g., Mr., Mrs., Miss, or Ms.; first name)
   c. Use touch on shoulder or hand when talking to patient or administering treatment
   d. Provide equipment and time for personal hygiene
   e. Provide privacy; cover as patient requires (e.g., culturally defined private parts)
   f. Reinforce sexual identity modes used by the patient and reinforce other modes of being male or female
   g. Clarify with the patient any uncertainties regarding terminology being used: medical terms, slang, or street terms that may have several meanings

    h. Engage patient in conversation about impact of condition on sexual identity and function

4. Evaluation of nursing care

    a. Patient identifies self with words or actions that reinforce sexual identity

    b. Patient requests equipment for enhancing personal appearance (e.g., comb, make-up, perfume, shaving gear)

    c. Patient increases interaction with special friends and/or family

    d. Patient shows increased self-concept and self-esteem with increased emphasis on strengths rather than limitations

    e. Patient talks in positive terms about going home or leaving hospital

ABUSE

Definition

Abuse is causing harm to another person against his or her will, by physical, sexual, and/or psychologic means. This usually happens when one person perceives himself or herself as dominant, by reason of age, size, physical strength, situation, and/or position, and believes he or she can impose his or her will upon another person. The other person involved believes that he or she is dependent and cannot resist, because of age, size, physical strength, situation, and/or position

Discussion

1. There are three common types of abuse that may be inflicted upon persons of all ages, from children to the elderly

    a. *Physical abuse:* when someone against the victim's will causes harm to the victim's physical body by pushing; slapping; biting; kicking; hitting either with hands or with objects; physically restraining with hands or other objects (rope, belts); refusing to help when the victim is sick or injured; withholding food, water, or medicine; abandoning the victim in dangerous places; raping

        i. The usual victims of physical abuse are children, adolescents, women, and the debilitated elderly

        ii. For children and adolescent (male and female) victims, the usual perpetrators are the parental figures and/or other family members or close family friends

        iii. For young adolescent female victims, a common perpetrator is a boyfriend; for older female victims, a common perpetrator is a live-in boyfriend or spouse

        iv. The usual perpetrators of physical abuse on the debilitated elderly are the caretakers (either their adult children or institutional care providers)

    b. *Sexual abuse:* when someone takes sexual advantage of a person against the person's will and wishes. The perpetrator may insist that the victim dress in a more sexual way than the victim wishes; criticize the victim sexually; harass with sexual jokes, touches, or threats; call the victim names such as "whore" or "bitch"; force sex or force the victim to watch others having sex; force unwanted sex acts; force sex with objects; force sadistic sex

    i. The usual victims of sexual abuse are children, adolesent females, and women. Less frequent but of concern is the elderly woman who is sexually assaulted

    ii The usual perpetrators of sexual abuse on children and adolescents are parental figures, other family members, or family friends. The victims are usually female, but males may also be victimized at this age

    iii. Many adolescent females are victims of sexual abuse by date rape

    iv. Older adolescents and adult females are also sexually victimized by live-in boyfriends, spouses, co-workers, work supervisors and other acquaintances

    v. Strangers and care providers are the usual perpetrators of sexual abuse against the elderly

c. *Psychologic* (emotional) *abuse:* someone terrorizes the victim with threats, says slanderous things about the victim, insults the victim, withholds approval or affection as punishment, laughs at the victim, humiliates the victim in public or private, ignores the victim's feelings, controls everything the victim does, does not let the victim have friends, threatens to deny access to the things or persons the victim loves, manipulates the victim with lies and contraditions, and tells the victim how dumb and ugly the victim is

    i. The perpetrators of psychologic (emotional) abuse or neglect for both male and female children and adolescents are usually the parental figures, other care providers, school friends, or acquaintances

    ii. For older adolescents and young adults (both female and male), the perpetrators are family and significant others (boyfriends and girlfriends, spouses, co-workers, work supervisors)

    iii. The perpetrators of psychologic abuse in the elderly and/or debilitated are usually their adult chidren or other care providers

Example

A 72-year-old man from a local nursing home is admitted to the ICU for respiratory difficulty. According to history, the patient is unable to ambulate without assistance, has periods of willfulness and stubbornness, and is very demanding. On admission his voice was very low, almost in a whisper, and he was oriented to person but not to place or time. Patient appears afraid, eyes darting from place to place, body tense and stiff, and he cringes when someone approaches. He has large bruises encircling both upper arms, with a large round bruise on each cheek and long narrow bruises on both legs. The bruise patterns do not appear congruent with a fall or bumping into things

Nursing Assessment Data Base

Nursing History

1. Obtain medical diagnosis and prognosis
2. Note history of prior hospitalization and/or emergency department visits,

specifically for musculoskeletal and/or internal injuries, and whether there were questions about causes of these injuries

3. Determine whether patient is oriented and able to respond to questions
4. Note availability of significant others

Nursing Examination of Patient

1. Patient withdraws or cringes when someone approaches
2. Patient's orientation is faulty (e.g., time, place, person)
3. Patient is able to respond verbally
4. Patient and staff speak the same language
5. Patient's ability to identify what happened to him or her
6. Need for privacy and maintenance of human dignity
7. Need for mental health and/or legal referral

Commonly Encountered Nursing Diagnosis: Post-Trauma Response

1. **Assessment for defining characteristics**
   a. Reexperiencing of traumatic event
      i. Nightmares, repetitive dreams
      ii. Flashbacks, intrusive thoughts
      iii. Excessive or no verbalization about trauma event
   b. Psychic or emotional numbness
      i. Impaired interpretation of reality
      ii. Confusion, dissociation, amnesia
      iii. Constricted affect
   c. Altered life style
      i. Suicide or other acting-out behavior
      ii. Difficulty with interpersonal relationships
      iii. Irritability, explosiveness
2. **Expected outcomes**
   a. Able to talk to staff about what has happened
   b. Expresses feelings in age-appropriate terms
   c. Able to make a realistic, age-appropriate evaluation of situation
   d. Contacts family and/or significant others
   e. Able to talk to family and/or significant others about situation
3. **Nursing Interventions**
   a. The assessment phase is the first step in building the rapport needed for implementation
   b. Engage in frequent interactions at specific times frames (e.g., every-15-minute checks)
   c. Reassure patient of safety by gentle words, soft touch, consistent approach
   d. Always let patient know what you are about to do (e.g., take blood pressure, draw blood)
   e. Address patient with respect and dignity (Mr., Mrs., Miss, or Ms., not by first name unless patient requests)
   f. Encourage verbalization of fears, concerns, likes, dislikes
   g. Encourage patient to take as much control of self as safe care and physical limitations allow

    h. Make available to patient and family or significant others appropriate support personnel (mental health, religious, and legal)

    i. Allow patient to have some of own things near him (e.g., blanket, clock)

4. Evaluation of nursing care

    a. Patient initiates age-appropriate expression of feelings and concerns (anger, tears, fear)

    b. Patient is compliant with procedures

    c. Patient speaks of self in positive terms

    d. Patient participates in own care within physical limitations

    e. Patient talks about how he or she will handle situation

    f. Patient is future oriented in postdischarge plans (place to live)

FAMILY

Definition

A social group with culturally determined characteristics, which include economic cooperation, reproduction, and the rearing and socialization of children. It is an interacting and transacting group in relation to larger society. Each family member's role is, to a large extent, determined by where he or she is in the life cycle

Discussion

1. The family is the conveyor of the beliefs, values, norms, and roles of society. The entire family participates in the socialization process of its members. A child must acquire an immense amount of traditional knowledge and skill and must learn to subject some natural inborn impulses to the discipline prescribed by society before being accepted as an adult member. The family is a primary building block of all societies

2. Within the family, norms are usually modeled after those of the larger society, which prescribes role-appropriate behaviors for family members; each member has a role. The family usually acts to support and protect its members, both collectively and individually. It is the primary support agency for its members

3. Like individuals, families attempt to maintain a steady state. Any perceived threat to the family's function or structure causes members to feel anxious and to close ranks

4. If one family member is in ICU, other members attempt to assume the role behavior of the absent member. If a family feels the threat of losing one of its members, it mobilizes to defend against the loss

5. Each family member experiences the loss of a family member in terms of where they are in the life cycle

6. A patient in an ICU may experience a biologic crisis, and at the same time his family may undergo a psychologic crisis. The provision of effective care for a patient necessarily involves extending care to family members

Example

A 36-year-old married woman with three children: two boys, aged 9 and 10 years, and a 12-year-old girl. She is admitted to the ICU with renal and liver impairment secondary to cancer. During the first week of hospitalization, the husband is present nearly all day every day. He looks tired and behaves as if he is quite anxious. During the second week of hospitalization, the husband visits less frequently and has dark circles under his eyes. His behavior appears increasingly agitated, except when with his wife; when talking to her and holding her hand he seems to relax considerably. While talking to a nurse, husband has tears in eyes and trembles, saying, "We try to carry on, but it's so hard. My daughter tries to be her mother for the other children, and when I am not home, my daughter cooks. But it is so hard"

Nursing Assessment Data Base

Nursing History

1. Observe impact of medical diagnosis and prognosis on family interaction
2. When family visits, assess family interactions
3. Verify that family members are available for support of patient
4. Identify the patient's roles in family (brother, sister, mother, father, husband, wife, financial supporter, homemaker, son, or daughter)
5. Note significant others' descriptions of the patient
6. Assess whether the medical condition is acute or chronic, temporary or permanent
7. Review treatment and medication on normal role function in the family

Nursing Examination of Patient

1. Assess role and status of patient in family
2. Observe the members relating to each other: warmly, with physical sharing of feelings, or reserved, with very little physical demonstration
3. Identify the modes of communication within the family: verbal or nonverbal (e.g., believe what I do, not what I say)
4. Determine who will fill role of hospitalized person within family
5. Identify what expectations the patient has of family members
6. Identify what expectations the family has of the patient
7. Determine the identified strengths within the family (e.g., good communications, strong loving/caring feelings, willingness to give to the other, decision making shared)
8. Identify family resources and needs

Commonly Encountered Nursing Diagnosis: Altered Family Processes

1. Assessment for defining characteristics
   a. Family system unable to meet physical and emotional needs of its members

    b. Rigidity in function and roles

    c. Inability to express or accept feelings of members

    d. Inability of family members to relate to each other

    e. Family unable to cope with traumatic experience constructively

2. Expected outcomes

    a. Patient demonstrates role congruence (acts in age-appropriate manner, cries when hurt, smiles when happy)

    b. Patient demonstrates clear communication and constructive interaction

    c. Patient is future-oriented: talks about returning to previous family role

    d. Patient expresses positive feelings about self, is involved in own care

3. Nursing interventions

    a. Support efforts to clarify the what, who, when, and where among the interactions of family and to identify positive behaviors of family members

    b. Reinforce role and status of patient in family

    c. Support family with encouragement and clear, concise information; mobilize family support resources; maintain frequent contact with family

    d. Maintain and reinforce communication among family, patient, and staff

    e. Clarify for family and patient what they should expect in the hospital

    f. Reinforce identified family and patient strengths

4. Evaluation of nursing care

    a. Patient sees self as a valuable part of the family

    b. Family and patient communicate needs and concerns

    c. Compliance and actual participation of patient in own care increases

    d. Patient and/or family show decrease in projecting blame on staff for family member's problems and patient's lack of improvement

    e. Behavior of family members is age-appropriate

THE CRITICAL CARE ENVIRONMENT

Definition

The sum of interactions among all persons, objects, and circumstances that affect the well-being of patients in an ICU. The ICU environment is strange and unknown to patients and their families; therefore, it is stressful. Expression of stress in the critical care environment will be in terms of the stage of the life cycle

Discussion

1. Stressors within the critical care environment that have an impact on patients include machines, the noise level, spatial structures, person's preconceived ideas, human interactions, thwarted needs and desires, and numerous decisions. Interactions that occur within this environment are significant in that they regulate the amount of distress as well as the amount of control that each person has over the environment

2. In order to deal with the ever-changing demands of the environment, those present use a variety of coping mechanisms to assist them with their struggles to feel adequate. If a patient's coping mechanisms fail to provide sufficient

protection, the environment is usually perceived as overwhelming and dysfunctional behavior can result

3. Dysfunctional behavior is commonly seen in the following ways:
   a. Among patients, by demanding and acutely aggressive behavior, as well as by withdrawn behavior
   b. Among family members, by repetition of questions or statements, putting blame on nurses, making unrealistic demands on staff, and withdrawn behavior
   c. Among staff, by numerous errors; avoiding patients, other staff members, or family members; increased feelings of competitiveness; and emotional lability "for no apparent reason"

Example

A 50-year-old man is admitted directly from operating room, where he experienced cardiac arrest on the table. He was in the operating room for repair of the rotator cuff, left shoulder. According to history, he had been in hospital only once before: 30 years ago for fracture of left arm, for 2 days. The patient has been married 30 years and has five children, aged 22 to 28 years. He was admitted on the respirator. On the second day after admission, the patient appears apprehensive and restless, jumping at all noises and whenever he is touched. He continuously handles his monitor leads and is unable to sleep for more than 2 hours at a time. When an alarm goes off anywhere in the unit, he becomes ashen and pushes the call button every couple of minutes. He repeatedly asks the nurses for reassurance that he is all right; constant reassurance has not helped. The nurses' reactions become characterized by irritation as they grow weary of his demands for their time and attention. As the days wear on, the staff increasingly avoids the patient, who becomes increasingly demanding and symptomatic

Nursing Assessment Data Base

Nursing History

1. Note history of being in critical care environment before
2. If history is positive, note the medical condition and how long patient was in critical care
3. Note whether the patient is married, separated, or single and with whom the patient lives
4. Record patient's occupation and work history
5. Note patient's expected length of stay in critical care unit
6. Document whether medical condition is life-threatening, entails permanent dysfunction, or entails long-term limitations on function
7. Determine whether the patient's medical condition and its treatment influence physiologic parameters and could influence psychosocial function
8. Note where is the individual in the life cycle (see Table 9–1)

Nursing Examination of Patient

1. Assessment is aimed at identifying, clarifying, and making known what the ICU environment is all about

2. Assess the meaning to the patient of the machines, noise, lights, spatial structures, and interactions within this environment
3. Assess the preconceived ideas held by the patient and family members about the ICU
4. Assess impact of ICU on the patient and family. Use previously assessed concepts
5. Assess orientation to person, time, and place, and note age appropriateness of responses
6. Assess patient's perception of self (e.g., speaks of self in negative terms, not future oriented)

Commonly Encountered Nursing Diagnosis: Environmental Interpretation Syndrome

1. **Assessment for defining characteristics**
   a. Increased tension, apprehension, fearfulness, alertness, aggressive behavior, or increased withdrawal
   b. Verbal expressions of having no control over self or influence over situation
   c. Dysfunctional interaction with peers, family, and/or staff
   d. Increased blaming of others for problems
   e. Increased sleep pattern disturbance with jittery movements
   f. Responses not age-appropriate
2. **Expected outcomes**
   a. Patient is less tense, more relaxed in bed
   b. Behavior is more assertive rather than aggressive
   c. Patient verbally expresses feeling in control and being involved in own care
   d. Patient experiences periods of sleep and wakefulness within normal limits; at least 2 hours of uninterrupted sleep
   e. Patient's responses are congruent with stage of life cycle
3. **Nursing interventions**
   a. Clarification of information about ICU is essential, even if the patient is unable to respond. Each procedure should be explained in age-appropriate terms to the patient and, whenever possible, to the family
   b. Clarify functions and purpose of machines and the significance of the noise and lights
   c. Correct and clarify perceptions of ICU as not a place to die, but a special place to enhance life
   d. Support, reinforce, and enhance positive factors identified earlier
   e. Involve family in patient's care
   f. Encourage questions and information sharing
   g. Provide familiar objects (locate nearby): bathrobe, pictures, watch
4. **Evaluation of nursing care**
   a. Patient decreases use of call light; shows less anger and withdrawal
   b. Patient demonstrates decreased anxiety with increased ability to rest and sleep
   c. Patient and family participate more in care
   d. Patient demonstrates increased compliance with treatment
   e. Communication between patient and family is increased

CRISIS

. . . .
Definition

The state of feeling overwhelmed by stressors and struggling unsuccessfully to cope with the situation. It involves an attempt to regain equilibrium. Crisis is not always an illness; it is an opportunity for growth. Different types of crises are experienced, defined, and expressed in relation to where the patient is in the life cycle

. . . .
Discussion

1. Like stress, crisis is a matter of perception: events that trigger crisis in one person may not do so in another
2. Crisis usually lasts from 4 to 6 weeks and is characteristically self-limiting. The reason for this is related to the fact that humans become depleted of energy after enduring significant distress over a prolonged period; they then begin to adapt to the crisis in order to recoup their energies
3. Two identified types of crisis are commonly experienced:
   a. *Situational:* derived from a particular set of circumstances that occasion major changes in a person's life (e.g., role change, illness, divorce, death)
   b. *Maturational:* derived from difficulties in mastering developmental tasks associated with life stages (e.g., going to school, puberty, middle age, involutional changes)
4. Crisis is part of normal growth and development
5. Whether the crisis is experienced by critical care nurses, their patients, or the patients' families, four observable phases can be distinguished. Fink (1967) identified these as follows:
   a. *Shock:* a person perceives a threat to existing familiar structures; views reality as overwhelming; experiences anxiety, helplessness, and thought disorganization
   b. *Defensive retreat:* a person attempts to maintain usual structures; tries to avoid reality by wishful thinking, denial, or repression; and experiences indifference or euphoria, except when challenged. Challenge makes the person angry and resistant to change, because he or she is defensively reorganizing his or her thoughts
   c. *Acknowledgment:* a person gives up the existing, familiar structures; faces reality; and feels depressed. Apathy, agitation, bitterness, mourning, high anxiety, or suicidal thoughts may be experienced if the stressor is too overwhelming. The thought process is disorganized as a result of altered perceptions of reality
   d. *Adaptation and change:* a person establishes a new structure, feels a renewed sense of self-worth, engages in new reality testing, and experiences a gradual increase in satisfaction. The thought process is reorganized in view of current resources and abilities
6. The outcomes of crisis fall into three categories:
   a. Some persons "break down" under the stress and never learn to cope with the traumatic change
   b. Others emerge from the crisis about the same as they were before

    c. Still others learn about themselves and their ability to handle new situations and emerge feeling stronger and with increased self-esteem
7. Persons in crisis are more open than usual to help and growth

Nursing Assessment Data Base

Nursing History

1. Note length of present illness, history of being in critical care
2. Document diagnosis and prognosis of medical condition
3. Study history of previous crisis situation and how patient coped
4. Note supports available: family, co-workers, friends

Nursing Examination of Patient

1. Identify what the patient perceives as stressful
2. Determine whether this crisis is situation, maturational, or a combination of both
3. Assess behavior: responses demonstrating reaction, whether verbal or nonverbal (crying, withdrawal, inappropriate laughter, denial, anger, fear, frequent use of call bell or light, constant need for attention)
4. Determine when crisis situation started, how long the patient has been in crisis, and where the patient is in the crisis (shock, retreat, acknowledgment, or adaptation)
5. Evaluate patient's strengths and whether perceptions are realistic
6. Determine whether crisis response is appropriate for patient's age

Commonly Encountered Nursing Diagnosis: Ineffective Individual Coping

1. **Assessment for defining characteristics**
   a. Inability to cope with stress, increase in tension, apprehension, withdrawal
   b. Inappropriate use of defense mechanisms
   c. Extremes of emotional responses (from euphoria to depths of depression)
   d. Feelings of being overwhelmed, anxious, and helpless as if in a state of shock
   e. Disorganization of thought patterns, impairment of decision-making ability
   f. Focus only on crisis situation: tunnel vision in that only the perceived crisis is of concern
2. **Expected outcomes**
   a. Patient is able to identify the crisis situation in realistic terms
   b. Patient learns about self and develops the ability to handle new situations
   c. Patient is able to mobilize coping resources; self-esteem increases
3. **Nursing interventions**
   a. Using age-appropriate terms, assist patient in sharing ideas and feelings
   b. Discuss your perceptions of crisis with patient
   c. Help patient identify and clarify problem; help correct distortions
   d. Help patient identify coping mechanisms. Give support while patient is trying to use these mechanisms

   e. Mobilize, as necessary, community resources
   f. Involve patient in performing constructive tasks that can be successfully completed. This will enhance self-concept, self-esteem, and sense of control
   g. Assist patient in identifying alternative solutions. It is important to encourage patient to develop or decide which alternative approaches to use
   h. Reinforce strengths identified
4. **Evaluation of nursing care**
   a. Patient exhibits fewer crisis behaviors
   b. Patient uses denial less often, shows decrease in feeling overwhelmed
   c. Patient shows increased ability to make decisions with increase in self-concept and self-esteem
   d. Patient demonstrates increased participation in own care with feelings of being in control
   e. Patient expresses feelings in age-appropriate terms

FEAR AND ANXIETY

Definition

Unpleasant feelings states, precipitated by perceived threats to self and manifested by psychophysiologic symptoms. Fear is the feeling experienced from a known threatening object or situation; anxiety is the fearful anticipation of an unknown but expected harmful object or situation. Where the individual is in the life cycle influences which and how events are experienced as unpleasant and how the fear and/or anxiety is expressed

Discussion

1. The psychophysiologic symptoms of fear are indistinguishable from those of anxiety. Commonly identified symptoms are increased heart rate, increased muscular tension, trembling, increased startle response, perspiration, sinking feeling in stomach, dry mouth and throat, feelings of faintness, nausea, fatigue, restlessness, changes in appetite, insomnia or increased sleep, nightmares, speech pattern changes, and meaningless gestures. Each of these symptoms can be experienced as normal, everyday feelings at a low-intensity level. Some are adaptive in nature, such as
   a. Increased heart rate and respiratory exchange, which result in increased oxygen and blood supply to muscles
   b. Increased oxygen supply, which enhances mental alertness
2. Adaptive functions enable the person to be in peak condition to respond more effectively to stress
3. When the symptoms of fear and anxiety reach a certain level of intensity, they cease being adaptive and become maladaptive. When a person perceives that symptoms are becoming harmful, the person begins to channel energies

toward achievement of a steady state. This process decreases the amount of energy available to cope with incoming stimuli, and increased anxiety and fear may result. The person feels vulnerable and cannot experience himself or herself as safe

4. Critical care nurses often encounter patients who are unable to sleep because of fear related to illness or to the unfamiliarity of their surroundings. The longer patients are unable to sleep, the greater the fear and anxiety become. When fear and anxiety increase, other symptoms are demonstrated (e.g., confusion, restlessness, irritability, and signs of aggression). Patients experience themselves as threatened and may behave in noncompliant ways. They may even hallucinate or speak from a delusional frame of reference

Example

A 22-year-old single woman is admitted to the unit with internal injuries, second to being physically abused by a live-in boyfriend. She has a history of other physical abuse in the past. There is very little verbal response; the patient follows people with eyes; body is rigid; her facial expression is one of fear; she does not sleep, never closes her eyes, refuses medication, and mumbles "No, no." Whenever a visitor comes, she looks fearful and asks who it is; at any loud noise or raised voice, the patient appears apprehensive, nervous, anxious, with hands trembling and her voice shaky and very quiet

Nursing Assessment Data Base

Nursing History

1. Determine whether the diagnosis and prognosis of medical condition cause the patient fear or anxiety
2. Examine medical condition's impact on patient's ability to communicate
3. Document whether the abuse has been reported to authorities and whether there is a history of past abuse
4. Note length of patient's illness and history of being in critical care before
5. Identify available support systems, (friends and family in area)
6. Determine whether patient is able to speak the dominant language

Nursing Examination of Patient

1. When assessing patients who are experiencing high levels of fear and anxiety, the nurse should ascertain:
   a. What the patient is experiencing and what the perceived threat is
   b. What in the environment can be modified to decrease the sense of threat
   c. What support resources (from within patients as well as externally) are available to help decrease their fear and anxiety
   d. What identified needs for help can be met by the nursing staff
   e. The patient's stage of the life cycle, because the nature and etiology of fears and anxieties vary throughout the life cycle

2. Monitor vital signs (manifestations of fear and anxiety include increased heart rate, increased muscular tension, increased startle response, sinking feeling)
3. Assess behavior: look for increased crying, feelings of unrealness, irritability, aggressiveness, an urge to run and hide, a change in sleeping patterns, and nightmares
4. Explore what the patient is experiencing, what the perceived threat is
5. Determine what resources might be mobilized to decrease feelings of fear and anxiety
6. Identify the patient's fears and anxiety

Commonly Encountered Nursing Diagnosis: Fear and Anxiety

1. **Assessment for defining characteristics**
   a. Increase in tension, apprehension, helplessness
   b. Decrease in self-assurance, increase in feelings of inadequacy
   c. Sympathetic stimulation: cardiovascular excitation, superficial vasoconstriction, pupil dilation
   d. Focus on perceived object of fear or unknown source of anxiety
   e. Appropriateness of expressions for patient's age
2. **Expected outcomes**
   a. Patient demonstrates decreased level of anxiety, as evidenced by decreases in tension, apprehension, restlessness
   b. Patient is able to talk about fear and anxiety
   c. Patient demonstrates effective coping skills, as evidenced by increased ability to solve problems, return to normal sleep pattern, and meet self-care needs
   d. Patient verbalizes increased psychologic comfort and coping skills
   e. Patient expresses need for help in age-appropriate terms
3. **Nursing interventions**
   a. Discuss with the patient any distorted perceptions; provide information to reduce distortions
   b. Avoid surprises; tell patient what to expect
   c. Include patient in planning of care
   d. Maintain calm and safe environment; decrease stimuli; reassure patient
   e. Assist patient in identifying coping mechanisms that were successful in decreasing fear and anxiety
   f. Teach relaxation techniques
   g. Involve family or friends in patient's care
   h. Get appropriate staff (legal, social work) involved in protecting the patient
4. **Evaluation of nursing care**
   a. Patient experiences decreased fear- and anxiety-induced behavior
   b. Patient is able to share fears and anxious feelings
   c. Patient experiences increased feelings of being in control of self (from patient's words and actions)
   d. Patient initiates more interaction with family, friends, and staff
   e. Patient expresses need for help with abusive situation

Example   841

LONELINESS

Definition

Uncomfortable feelings of alienation caused by separation from significant relationships, events, and objects: painful aloneness. Loneliness is experienced and expressed in terms of stage of life cycle

Discussion

1. Loneliness often accompanies major life changes in which some familiar structures are lost. Illness and hospitalization are prime precipitators of feelings of loneliness
2. Everyone experiences loneliness at times, but for some it is a characteristic way of life
3. In attempts to assist someone who is lonely, the goal is to facilitate, in an age-appropriate manner, the person's sense of relatedness to
   a. His or her body
   b. His or her psyche
   c. Significant others
   d. Familiar events
   e. The nurse
4. This goal can be accomplished through interventions, such as
   a. Encouraging patients and family members to participate in their care, when appropriate, and to ask question
   b. Initiating and facilitating discussion about patient's pain, surgery, or illness; feelings about self, visitors, environment, or cherished possessions; and other topics of importance to them
   c. Allowing patients to get to know the nurse, insofar as it seems helpful in enabling them to relate to the caregivers on whom they are dependent
   d. Relating on a person-to-person basis that fosters personalized care
5. Promoting relationships, providing familiar activities, and permitting patients to have objects that hold positive meaning for them are the focus of intervention
6. Remember, however, that the nurse can be only a facilitator when working with those who feel lonely. If, during intervention, patients refuse to relate to others or feel too angry or depressed to focus on familiar (usually comforting) activities, they must make their own choice as to what to do to help themselves feel more comfortable
7. Patients base choices on their self-concept, self-esteem, and need levels at the time. It is not helpful for the nurse to attempt to coerce them into feigning interest when they clearly are not interested: coercion makes them feel more alienated and thus more lonely

Example

An 87-year-old woman is admitted for observation for possible closed-head injury, history of hypertension, diabetes, but *no history of dementia.* Se has been in a nursing home for only 2 months and does not want to be there; she has made no friends at nursing home, according to the nursing home staff. She is oriented, uses a walker, and is very strongwilled and demanding. Emergency department personnel think that the patient was attempting to run away from nursing home when she was injured. The patient responds to name but not to time or place, cringes whenever someone approaches her, and yells when someone touches her. Family members have visited; the patient ignored them and will not talk to her daughter or son.

Nursing Assessment Data Base

Nursing History

1. Identify major life events that have happened recently (e.g., new living arrangements, job loss, divorce, illness)
2. Determine impact of patient's medical condition and/or treatment on ability to respond to stimuli
3. Determine whether the patient's medical condition and/or treatment (e.g., pain medication, tranquilizers) influences ability to communicate
4. Assess availability of significant other for support
5. Determine whether medical condition is disfiguring or perceived to be disfiguring
6. Identify influence of medical condition on future social, work, and/or family functions

Nursing Examination of Patient

1. Assess psychosocial impact of recent major life events
2. Note patient's perception of hospitalization
3. Assess patient's resources: strengths, coping mechanisms that helped in the past to deal with loneliness
4. Find out whether patient has own clothing or possessions, to decrease sense of loneliness
5. Assess which family, friend, or community resources are available to meet needs

Commonly Encountered Nursing Diagnosis: Loneliness, Sense of Alienation

1. **Assessment for defining characteristics**
   a. Uncommunicative, withdrawn, sad; has dull affect; makes no eye contact
   b. Seeking to be alone, expressing feelings of aloneness
   c. Absence of supportive significant other: family, friends, co-workers
   d. Observed use of unsuccessful social interaction behaviors
2. **Expected outcomes**
   a. Patient expresses feelings of loneliness, distrust, and sense of self
   b. Patient initiates conversations and focuses on others rather than self
   c. Patient asks questions about treatment; is involved in own care

   d. Patient talks to significant others about self in relation to family, work, and
      other social situations
   e. Patient identifies social supports and expresses feelings of being in control
3. **Nursing interventions**
   a. Encourage patient and family members to participate in care when
      appropriate
   b. Initiate and facilitate discussion about patient's pain, surgery, or illness;
      feelings about self, visitors, environment, and cherished positions; and
      other topics of importance to patient
   c. Relate on a person-to-person basis that fosters personalized care
   d. Facilitate patient's sense of relatedness to his or her body, his or her
      psyche, significant others, familiar events or objects, and staff
   e. Use patient's last name (with Mr., Mrs., and so forth), not just first name,
      to help maintain dignity and respect
4. **Evaluation of nursing care**
   a. Patient communicates feelings, asks questions related to body responses to
      situation
   b. Family and patient are increasing communication and are more supportive
      and involved with treatment
   c. Patient expresses future orientation, whether it is 1 hour or 5 years in the
      future
   d. Patient demonstrates increased sense of belonging with enhanced self-
      esteem
   e. Patient feels in control and important, is involved in deciding on care
      (e.g., when medication is given, when visitors can come in)

POWERLESSNESS

Definition

A perceived lack of control over the outcome of a specific situation. The ability
of an event to engender a sense of powerlessness is influenced by the individual's
self-esteem and self-concept and by where the individual is in the life cycle

Discussion

1. Powerlessness derives from the belief that no matter how one behaves, one is
   unable to influence the outcome of a situation
2. In the process of concluding that they are incapable of effecting a desired
   change, people attempt to solve problems in as many ways as they can.
   However, they consistently run up against obstacles, and all efforts to bring
   about a desired outcome are ineffective
3. As this process is repeated, people begin to feel frustrated, inadequate,
   hopeless, angry, and depressed
4. In the critical care environment, all parties are capable of experiencing
   themselves as powerless: patients, family members, and staff
5. In order to counteract the powerlessness phenomenon, people must believe

that they are able to behave in ways that will make a difference in the resulting outcome

6. In an effort to help patients who feel powerless, a nurse might consider the following interventions:
   a. Assist them in redefining goals that they are unable to accomplish, in the hope that they will consider shorter, more attainable goals
   b. Assist them in identifying ways in which they can be effective in given situations; help them to focus on ways in which they can be powerful, if they choose
   c. Help them by giving information they need in order to be effective in given situations
   d. Support them by attempting to understand their feelings of impotence when they express them
   e. Provide help at age-appropriate level (see Table 9–1)

7. It is helpful to remember that the nurse cannot take away another person's feelings of powerlessness, inasmuch as they grow out of a person's life situation and someone cannot change another person's life. However, patients themselves can work with inner strengths to discover new meaning in life and to solve problems by determining ways in which they can be effective in influencing desired changes

8. A nurse can be helpful by displaying a caring presence, by actively listening, and by using empathy. The nurse can provide feedback in relation to knowledge gaps, strengths, or confusion that is expressed by patients and can let them know that their emotional pain is recognized

9. It does no good to tell patients how to solve their problems; this only reinforces their view of themselves as inadequate and adds to their feelings of powerlessness

Nursing Assessment Data Base

Nursing History

1. Assess medical condition's influence on sense of independence and self-control
2. Assess medical treatment's influence on actual independence and self-control
3. Identify patient's strengths (e.g., whether the patient has a job, goes to school, is married, or is a single parent)
4. Assess patient's ability to speak the dominant language
5. Document history of illness, dependence on medication, medical equipment for control of illness
6. Note availability of significant others for support

Nursing Examination of Patient

1. Assess the patient's perception of self in this situation (e.g., "Everything is so strange here; everyone takes care of me; they tell me what medicines to take and when to take them")
2. Assess perception, self-concept and self-esteem, body image, and loneliness, to provide clues to the patient's feelings of powerlessness

3. Observe nonverbal and verbal behavior for signs of depression, anger, hopelessness, and/or resignation
4. Assess communication ability, language, and influence of equipment, medication, condition on ability to communicate
5. Observe whether patient verbalizes or behaves as if out of control (e.g., never questions treatment)
6. Note whether patient is withdrawn in bed, eyes are closed or darting around, body is rigid
7. Determine whether patient's behavioral responses are age appropriate (see Table 9–1)

Commonly Encountered Nursing Diagnosis: Powerlessness

1. **Assessment for defining characteristics**
   a. Verbal expressions of having no control over self, situation, or outcome
   b. Reluctance to express true feelings, fearing alienation from caregivers
   c. Self-depreciating remarks
   d. Age appropriateness of behavior
2. **Expected outcomes**
   a. Patient verbalizes increased feelings of self-control; is involved in own care
   b. Patient makes appropriate decisions about own care
   c. Patient verbalizes increased self-concept and self-esteem; is future-oriented
3. **Nursing interventions**
   a. Develop a plan to enhance patient's sense of belonging and control, thereby positively influencing outcomes
   b. Assist patient in redefining goals into obtainable ones; stress "realistic goals"
   c. Assist the patient in identifying and using concrete ways to be effective in specific situations; this will enhance sense of being in control
   d. Involve patient in own care within physical limitations
   e. Take time to listen and hear what is said about feelings of powerlessness and being out of control
   f. Identify and reinforce strengths. Encourage sharing of patient's successes
   g. Be empathetic; visualize yourself in the patient's place
   h. Allow the patient to find a solution. Staff can be the guide by exploring alternatives, reinforcing strengths, and encouraging participation
4. **Evaluation of nursing care**
   a. Patient makes decisions affecting self, is able to say no
   b. Patient is more involved in own care within physical limitations
   c. Patient makes requests for information to make decisions (e.g., "I need to know how this procedure will affect my ability to work")
   d. Patient verbalizes positive feelings about self; self-concept and self-esteem are increasing

SENSORY OVERLOAD

Definition

Repeated multisensory experiences that occur with greater intensity than is normally experienced by a person. Often, the excessive stimuli are experienced suddenly. Where the individual is in the life cycle will, to a large extent, influence whether stimuli are experienced as overload or not. Sometimes, the stimuli are not understood by the person but rather are perceived simply as bothersome, meaningless experiences. In general, excessive sensory stimulation is caused by an onslaught of unfamiliar, uncomfortable, unexpected events

. . . .

Discussion

1. Sensory stimuli are stressors. Because ICUs are areas of excessive sensory stimuli for patients, family members, and staff, stress levels are excessively high. Patients may frequently act out in response to high stress levels by creating a noisy environment, which perhaps relieves some of the tension for them but increases stressors for all others in the environment

2. Along with auditory stimuli, the ICU hosts a myriad of visual, tactile, olfactory, and gustatory stimuli 24 hours a day, which are absorbed by those in the environment. Family members and staff are able to change the types and patterns of stimuli to which they are exposed by routinely leaving the critical care area. Patients, of course, are continually subjected to high levels of stimulation for as long as they are housed on the unit. All who encounter this environment are prone to experience sensory overload

3. Some common symptoms of sensory overload include confusion, restlessness, agitation, anger, and sometimes hallucinations

4. In attempting to prevent or minimize sensory overload, the nurse could
   a. Assess the noise level on the unit, particularly at the bedside of patients, inasmuch as it is here that many noise-producing mechanical devices are located (e.g., the bellows of ventilators and the alarm mechanism of cardiac monitors)
   b. Assess the visual intensity generated by the unit lighting
   c. Assess the environment for malodorous stimuli
   d. Assess each patient's level and type of gustatory stimuli
   e. Assess how staff and family members touch individual patients and the amount of pain experienced by each patient
   f. Implement modifications that seem appropriate regarding
      i. Noise levels: attending particularly to the intensity of conversational tones used by staff members; the positioning of noisy machinery in relation to the head of each patient; and loud, banging noises caused by dropped equipment, bedpan hoppers in need of repair, mishandled food trays, and messengers delivering supplies
      ii. Visual intensity: monitoring the light intensity on the unit to ensure that the environment is as safe and comfortable as possible and attemptimg to simulate natural light cycles from morning to night
      iii. Environmental odors: using air deodorizers and disposing of malodorous substances
      iv. Gustatory stimuli: assisting patients with mouth care when needed and offering palatable fluids and foods as appropriate
      v. Tactile communication: each time the nurse makes physical contact with patients, the nurse should be aware of the message that may be conveyed through touching. This can be accomplished by appropriate gentleness as a nurse turns patients, changes dressings, administers injections, gives baths and back rubs, and provides hair care. When a

nurse becomes aware of the amount of invasive tactile stimulation experienced by patients, the method of evaluating their need for pain medication may change. Administering pain medication effectively greatly helps to decrease sensory overload

Nursing Assessment Data Base

Nursing History

1. Medical diagnosis and prognosis have influence on sensory organs: eyes, ears, skin, tongue
2. History of previous critical care hospitalizations
3. Medications' influence on perception of sensory stimuli
4. Availability of significant others: spouse, parents, friends, co-workers

Nursing Examination of Patient

1. Assess indicators of sensory overload such as
    a. Confusion, restlessness, agitation, anger, change in sleep pattern
    b. Hallucinations, delusions, decreased response, or withdrawal
    c. Increased startle response
2. Appraise the noise level of unit, specifically at bedside
3. Assess the environment for malodorous stimuli
4. Evaluate patient's level and type of gustatory stimuli
5. Observe how staff and family touch the patient. Assess what comes in contact with patient (e.g., bed clothes, intravenous and central lines, tubes, leads from monitor)
6. Evaluate pain routinely and frequently
7. Assess sleep pattern, amount of time awake and asleep, and pattern of sleep/awake cycle

Commonly Encountered Nursing Diagnosis: Sensory Overload

1. **Assessment for defining characteristics**
    a. Confusion or disorientation to time, place, and/or person
    b. Restlessness to point of agitation, irritability, anger
    c. Anxiety or fear, mood swings, possible hallucinations
    d. Poor concentration, withdrawal with no response
2. **Expected outcomes**
    a. Patient is oriented to person, time, and place
    b. Patient is more relaxed, decreased anxiety or fear, decreased mood swings or more stable mood
    c. Concentration is increased, and sleep/awake cycle is improved
3. **Nursing interventions**
    a. Assist patient in screening out unrelated stimuli
        i. Dim hall or outside room lights and patient's room lights

        ii. Avoid banging equipment; turn monitor alarms as low as possible at bedside

       iii. Provide soft music, pictures of quiet scenes

       iv. When giving information, do so slowly, quietly, clearly, and unhurriedly

        v. Explain what noises and lights on machines mean

       vi. Get rid of offensive odors

    b. Control pain by positioning, turning, and medication; use gentle touch

4. Evaluation of nursing care

    a. Patient experiences decrease in confusion, restlessness, agitation, and anger

    b. Body is more relaxed

    c. Patient experiences decreased complaints of discomfort or pain

    d. Patient demonstrates increase in appropriate interactions

SENSORY DEPRIVATION

Definition

The opposite of sensory overload; deprivation denotes a lack of sensory input or a lack of variety, intensity, or perceived meaning of sensory stimulation. As in sensory overload, the meaning given stimuli in the ICU is different for a 6-year-old than it is for a 30-year-old. Therefore, the stage of the life cycle influences the interpretation and impact of the lack of stimuli

Discussion

1. Because most critical care patients are immobile, they are generally confined to a limited space in a machine-oriented, totally unfamiliar environment. They often experience consciousness-altering drugs that numb sensory receptors. Sometimes the nature of their illness reduces sensitivity to stimuli. At other times, technical assists are so complex as to require much time and attention from caregivers, perhaps more than are focused on the patient. All of these factors predispose critical care patients to sensory deprivation

2. The goal of nursing interventions is toward preventing or eliminating sensory deprivation, by providing sensory stimuli that patients find meaningful, in order to facilitate their relatedness to themselves and the unfamiliar world of the ICU

3. Communicating through meaningful touch and conversation is one way in which a nurse can assist patients in increasing their ability to relate, thereby decreasing sensory deprivation. Encouraging family members to provide familiar personal items when possible is also helpful, as is the presence of loved ones

4. Usual symptoms of sensory deprivation can mimic symptoms of sensory overload

5. To distinguish between sensory hunger and sensory overload, the nurse must

carefully assess the types and amounts of sensory stimuli experienced by individual patients and make judgments on the basis of the data collected

6. In general, sensory alterations are caused by a variety of factors found within the ICU. Some common factors include:
    a. Abnormal physiologic conditions, prolonged experience of pain
    b. Ingestion of drugs
    c. Lack of familiar persons and objects, fear of the unknown
    d. Lack of understanding about one's condition
    e. Sleep deprivation caused by interruption in sleep time, which denies a person the opportunity to adequately restore depleted energy supplies

7. Effective nursing interventions involving sensory deprivation and overload are crucial for the protection of the patients' compromised health status

Nursing Assessment Data Base

Nursing History

1. Determine whether sensory inputs are influenced by physical condition, medications, treatments, and/or equipment being used
2. Obtain history of past hospitalizations and/or having been in critical care unit before
3. Document patient's cultural influence, marital status, age, education
4. Assess work history, position held, and job security
5. Note availability of significant others and interaction between patient and significant others

Nursing Examination of Patient

1. Assessment can be carried out simultaneously with that for sensory overload assessment
2. In addition, assess whether medications being given can disturb sensory receptors
3. Evaluate physiologic impact of condition on sensory receptors (e.g., tumors that cause blindness, deafness, or paralysis)
4. Monitor laboratory studies (e.g., blood gas analysis) that could affect sensory receptors
5. Assess time with the patient, type of interactions, quality of interactions
6. Observe sleep pattern changes
7. Evaluate possibility of developing a routine (e.g., regular times for treatment and regular times for rest)
8. Determine whether patient's condition necessitates isolation

Commonly Encountered Nursing Diagnosis: Sensory Deprivation

1. **Assessment for defining characteristics**
    a. Disoriented to person, place, and time; behavior pattern change
    b. Noncompliance

c. Lethargy or withdrawal, decreased concentration, daydreaming

d. Difficulty interacting with staff and significant others

2. **Expected outcomes**

a. Patient is more interactive with family and staff; more involved in treatment planning

b. Patient is more assertive; is able to verbalize concerns and questions

c. Patient is able to relax; is less agitated; and sleep/awake pattern is more normal

d. Patient is oriented to reality and to person, time, and place

3. **Nursing interventions**

a. Attempt to prevent or eliminate sensory deprivation: provide sensory stimuli that can be experienced fully by the patient

b. Increase communication; use touch or any other method (writing, sign language, pictures)

c. Encourage relatives to bring special meaning items to patient, such as family pictures and letters

d. Play music or a tape of family members' voices. Have family tape messages or music

e. Encourage frequent verbal interaction by the primary caregiver to enhance rapport building; this helps to give predictability to the environment

4. **Evaluation of nursing care**

a. Patient exhibits decreased agitation and more participation with treatment

b. Patient increases involvement in identifying own needs and treatment

c. Patient increases interactions with staff and/or family

d. Patient demonstrates fewer extremes in emotions such as anger, crying, and sadness

ADDICTION

Definition

Dependence on a chemical substance outside the self that is perceived by the person as being necessary for self-maintenance and for the self to feel complete (e.g., adequate)

Discussion

1. The addiction phenomenon is a maladaptive effort to help the self feel adequate. The process is considered maladaptive because the end result involves the person in spending time and energy numbing the self, so that spontaneous growth-producing doubts, fears, and stressors are not experienced or managed constructively. Growth does not take place, and the person stagnates

2. When a nurse encounters addicts in the ICU, it is important to remember the following:

a. If patients are still under the influence of the addictive substance, their perceptions of reality will be altered

   b. Patients' self-concept and self-esteem are threatened because they do not
      have access to what they believe will make them complete; they probably
      feel incomplete and desperate for the substance
   c. There is usually some concern on the part of addicts regarding how others
      will view them, so again self-concept and self-esteem are threatened
   d. While withdrawing from the substance, patients are acutely reactive to
      physical and emotional stimuli
3. In attempting to deal effectively with addicts, the nurse should remember
   that such patients may feel threatened. Their behavior, therefore, may reflect
   a strong need to defend themselves by keeping other people at a comfortable
   distance
4. Distancing maneuvers include withdrawal behavior as well as actions that tend
   to push others away by evoking feelings of anger, frustration, repulsion, or
   fear
5. The nurse does not want to make addicted patients feel even more
   threatened (which would occasion further acting-out behavior) and so might
   consider the following:
   a. Attempting to understand their suffering and concerns
   b. Communicating in a straightforward manner (e.g., if patient's behavior is
      disruptive to the nurse or to the unit, telling them so and requesting that
      they behave in a specifically different manner)
   c. Assisting patients to feel secure on the unit by providing simple, clear
      explanations regarding what is happening to them
   d. Avoiding power struggles and arguments by approaching conflicts from
      the perspective of understanding patients' feelings about the issues and
      making clear statements about how the nurse views the situation
6. In general, communicating that the nurse cares about addicted patients and
   wants to be of help during this difficult time is an important factor in
   establishing a helping relationship. At times, attempts to help will include
   insisting that patients do things they may not want to do

Nursing Assessment Data Base

Nursing History

1. Identify substances that patient is addicted to and for how long
2. Record time of last dose (hit) of substance taken
3. Document history of being treated for addiction in the past
4. Note patient's normal withdrawal behavior (e.g., agitated, combative,
   withdrawn, physiologic problems)
5. Note availability of significant others

Nursing Examination of Patient

1. Evaluate the effect of the substance on perceptions and how it makes the
   patient feel
2. Evaluate whether behavioral responses are part of withdrawal
3. Observe staff members' and others' reactions to addicted patient

4. Assess what resources are available for short- and long-term help with addiction

. . . .

Commonly Encountered Nursing Diagnosis: Addiction

1. **Assessment for defining characteristics**
   a. Perceptions of reality altered
   b. Self-concept and self-esteem threatened because patient is unable to obtain addictive substances
   c. Physical nervousness, anxiety, shakiness, tremors, sweating, craving for substance
   d. Altered physical and psychologic response to stimuli (e.g., hyperreaction or hyporeaction)
   e. Inability to sleep or to stay awake; restlessness; agitation
2. **Expected outcomes**
   a. Patient is oriented to person, time, and place
   b. Self-concept and self-esteem are less threatened
   c. Reactions are more stable
   d. Patient verbalizes less craving for substance
   e. Patient verbalizes feelings about self and the addiction problem
   f. Patient begins verbalizing need to get help for addiction problem
3. **Nursing interventions**
   a. Do not be judgmental. Addicts are very sensitive to others' acceptance and/or judgment
   b. Decrease physical and emotional stimuli as much as possible during withdrawal (addicts are very sensitive to stimuli during this period)
   c. Communicate in a straightforward manner without communicating staff's own personal views
   d. Avoid power struggles and arguments by approaching conflicts from the perspective of understanding the patient's feelings and making clear staff's own views of situation
   e. Mobilize resources for short-term and long-term help for the addict
   f. Take care of patient's physiologic needs; during withdrawal, keep close watch on vital signs and other parameters
4. **Evaluation of nursing care**
   a. Physical signs of withdrawal decrease (e.g., pupils not dilated or pinpoint, sweating and/or muscle tension decreased)
   b. Patient has less anger and expresses less hostility
   c. Patient has increased self-esteem and self-concept, ability to express needs without self-depreciation
   d. Patient's participation in treatment is increased
   e. Patient seeks help with addiction; community resources are being used

SUICIDAL PHENOMENON

. . . .

Definition

Suicide is an active or passive self-destructive act that results from a perceived, overwhelming threat to oneself. Whether a perceived threat to self is seen as overwhelming is, to a large extent, determined by the individual's stage in the life cycle

Discussion

1. Everyone at one time or another has suicidal thoughts. These can be as casual as a morning wish to cancel the day from lack of interest, which a person generally would not act on because less drastic coping mechanisms can effectively handle the situation
2. Every case of self-destructive behavior involves the pressure of a phenomenologically unbearable threat to oneself. Less drastic and less destructive coping mechanisms are no longer experienced as effective in handling the perceived overwhelming threat. Suicide, therefore, is the ultimate attempt to deal with this threat, is considered, and sometimes is acted on. In a sense, suicidal behavior is seen as an escape from, rather than a movement toward, something
3. A suicidal person experiences many negative emotions (e.g., despair, guilt, shame, dependency, hopelessness, weariness, boredom, depression). There is a point at which despair becomes overwhelming and unbearable. For some people, there is a sense that life is just not worth living anymore: it no longer has meaning. Others feel that someone does not want them around or that their individual problems can never be resolved
4. In providing nursing services to patients who have attempted suicide, nurses should be aware of the following common characteristics of the suicidal phenomenon:
   a. The acute crisis period or high lethality time is of short duration: it can be counted in hours or days
   b. Suicidal patients are usually ambivalent about dying. At the same time that they plan suicide, they have fantasies of rescue
   c. Persons who commit suicide are people who have talked about it as well as those who do not talk about it
   d. Suicidal persons usually give clues about their intentions
   e. Suicidal behavior has no racial, social, religious, cultural, or economic boundaries
   f. Suicide has no characteristic genetic qualities; however, its incidence is higher in families in which there have been previous suicides
   g. Suicidal behavior does not necessarily mean that the person is mentally ill; in some cases, suicide is viewed as a logical last step by someone who is overwhelmed with stress
   h. Most important, directly asking a person about suicidal intent will not cause suicide
5. In addition to knowing about suicide, caregivers must also be aware of their own feelings about it. Dealing with suicidal persons can raise fears and reactions within caregivers (e.g., anger, anxiety about their own suicidal thoughts, dislike of or resentment toward those who have attempted suicide, a wish to avoid the suicidal person in favor of other patients whose conditions do not appear to be self-inflicted, and doubts about their own ability to care for them). It is easier to care for suicidal patients if the nurse is able to understand why they attempted suicide

Nursing Assessment Data Base

Nursing History

1. History of previous suicide attempts and severity
2. Methods used to attempt suicide: gun, drugs, gas fumes, car accident, starving, burning self, jumping from high place
3. History of significant other's successful completion of suicide (brother, sister, mother, father, best friend)
4. Assess presence of other medical conditions, such as AIDS, cancer, disfigurements

Nursing Examination of Patient

1. Assessment is aimed at gathering information that will identify why suicide was attempted, what was used, where attempt was made, and the psychologic condition at present
2. Determine what major life changes have happened recently. (This is what the patient perceives as a major change, such as job loss, loss of status, divorce, or death)
3. Identify strengths, such as good health, hard worker, caring person, good work history, community involvement
4. Assess where suicide attempt was made: in a public place or in privacy. This will give clue to seriousness of the attempt
5. Specify what was used (e.g., 10 aspirin, 40 Valium, knife, gun, rope). This will give clue as to lethality
6. Identify available close friends, family or other resources
7. Evaluate the emotional state at present: tearful, angry, despondent, sad, depressed, euphoric, or withdrawn
8. Note where the individual is in the life cycle
9. Document how suicide is perceived in the individual's culture

Commonly Encountered Nursing Diagnosis: Risk for Self-Mutilation

1. **Assessment for defining characteristics**
   a. Cognitive or emotional difficulties
   b. See common characteristics of suicidal phenomenon
2. **Expected outcomes**
   a. Patient verbalizes need for help
   b. Patient makes no additional attempts of suicide
   c. Patient verbalizes positive feelings about oneself
   d. Patient is able to communicate with significant others
   e. Patient verbalizes desire to recover
   f. Patient is future-oriented
3. **Nursing interventions**
   a. Accept the suicidal behavior as logical from the patient's point of view. Do not pass judgment

b. Reinforce patient's self-esteem by interacting in such a manner as to accord dignity

c. Use all communication modes (verbal and nonverbal) in an attempt to understand how the patient perceives world and self

d. Reinforce positive aspects (strengths) of patient's self-concept

e. Do not place or leave dangerous objects near bedside (e.g., medication, razors)

f. Assist patient in reestablishing supportive relationships with those whom he or she chooses

g. Support significant others so that they can support the patient

h. Avoid power struggles with the person when behavior is noncompliant or belligerent

i. Be aware of and deal with your own fears, feelings, and conflicts related to suicide

j. Contract with person not to harm self

4. **Evaluation of nursing care**

a. Patient communicates with significant others, verbalizes needs and concerns

b. Patient makes no further suicide attempts

c. Patient complies with treatment

d. Patient asks for help from mental health resources or other suicide resources

e. Patient is future-oriented in discussions

f. Patient verbalizations are congruent with nonverbal behavior

THE DYING PROCESS AND DEATH

Definition

Dying is a psychophysiologic process that evokes many stresses and crises and that ultimately terminates in death for the dying and in suffering for significant survivors; death is the antithesis of life. The stage of the life cycle to a great extent determines the meaning of dying and death to the individual

Discussion

1. Death is not amenable to change or intervention. It represents the greatest loss

2. The dying process is part of the life cycle. When a person is conscious of this process, the threat of death unleashes the primordial feelings of hopelessness, helplessness, and abandonment. We identify ourselves in life in terms of what we as human beings think, feel, and experience. But death cannot be understood in the terms we use to identify life. The fear of the unknown of death evokes fears of the annihilation of self, of being, and of identity

3. The dying process imposes a twofold burden

a. Intrapsychic stress: preparing oneself for death

　　b. Interpersonal stress: preparing oneself for death in relation to significant others while simultaneously preparing those others to be survivors

4. This twofold task evokes a pervasive state of grief about the impending death and anger about one's impotence. The anger can be directed toward God, loved ones, or caregivers. In addition, dying persons may experience anxiety related to fear of pain, loss of identity, loneliness and abandonment, powerlessness, fear of the unknown, and fear of annihilation

5. Elizabeth Kübler-Ross (1969) described five psychologic stages of the dying process:
　　a. Denial or isolation: "No, not me"
　　b. Anger, rage, envy, resentment: "Why me?"
　　c. Bargaining: "If you will . . . then I will"
　　d. Depression: "What's the use?"
　　e. Acceptance: the final resting stage before the long journey

6. Some clinicians who are inexperienced in working with the dying may expect patients to follow the exact sequence described. In reality, the dying process may include all the stages (although some patients never get beyond the denial stage), but the stages shift, depending on what the person experiences. A person may fluctuate from depression to anger or may revert to the denial stage

7. Providing care for the dying may evoke strong emotions in caregivers: anger, frustration, or dislike. These reactions may result in a desire to avoid dying patients or their families. Likewise, being with a dying loved one may evoke strong emotions in family members and may cause them to be less and less available as the process continues. The dying process predisposes people to a sense of abandonment

8. Because psychologic states are complicated clusters of intellectual and affective factors that occur in the context of people's perception of their world and of themselves in the world, it is important to remember two important principles when caring for the dying patient: denial and hope
　　a. *Denial can be an important coping mechanism for enabling persons to maintain some control over the most threatening of situations.* Denial can make it possible for them to block out information with which they cannot successfully cope and to begin to deal with reality in smaller, more manageable segments
　　　　i. Because denial operates protectively in persons on the verge of crises, it is important for the nurse to respond to dying patients by:
　　　　　　(a) Listening to find out their perception of their situation
　　　　　　(b) Showing acceptance whenever they are found to be in the dying process
　　　　　　(c) Not encouraging false beliefs
　　　　　　(d) Attempting to understand why they are behaving as they are
　　　　ii. Examples
　　　　　　(a) A man who suffered a life-threatening myocardial infarction 2 days ago says, "I think I'm well enough to go home now." The nurse responds, "I'm trying to appreciate how badly you want to go home, but it would not be beneficial for you now because of your illness"
　　　　　　(b) A 64-year-old, recently retired woman has been told that she has cancer and that she will probably live another 6 months. She tells a nurse that she plans to buy a new Mercedes, "even though it

will probably take me three years to pay for it." The nurse responds, "I can hear how much you want to own that car. I hope you will be able to do it."

b. *Hope is usually present throughout the dying process in some degree.* Hope, a belief in the desirability of survival, is usually found in persons demonstrating a healthy self-concept and self-esteem but can be lost when persons are unable to act in their own behalf and must submit to the influence of others. To a large extent, denial and hope are necessary for a person to experience the dying process with some control. Denial provides a sorely needed locus of control over the primordial feelings unleashed during that process. Hope is the core of strength needed to withstand the pain, suffering, fears, and conflicts encountered throughout the process

9. In order to provide quality care to dying patients, it is helpful for nurses to be aware of the following:

a. Through caring for the dying the nurse is often made aware of the dying process. All the fears, feelings, and conflicts demonstrated in dying patients are also evoked in the nurse, which in turn evokes the nurse's coping mechanisms. It is essential that nurses be aware of and accept their own fears about dying

b. Like all other kinds of nursing assessments, the assessment of dying patients is aimed at achieving an understanding of the needs of the patient and of family members. This can be accomplished by ascertaining

   i. Perception of their situation and the feelings being expressed

   ii. Family perception of situation and the feelings being expressed

   iii. The strengths and supports used by the patient and family to help them cope with the stress

   iv. Needs that the patient wishes to have met and the most appropriate persons to meet those needs

   v. Whether body image and sexual identity are significantly affected; whether intervention can be designed to reaffirm these identities

   vi. Whether loneliness and powerlessness are causing the dying process to be more painful than is necessary; whether these factors can be altered through interventions

10. The goal of intervention is to respond effectively to the patient's identified needs for help. Because dying is an individual experience, the nurse should respond to the needs identified at a given time. The following are suggested interventions for the stages identified by Kübler-Ross:

a. During the denial stage

   i. Attempt to have staff, volunteer, family member, friend stay with dying patient for a time

   ii. Take cues for conversation from the patient

   iii. Listen (the listener need not attempt to provide solutions to the questions raised, unless specifically requested to do so)

   iv. Respond to patients by sharing your reactions when you think it might be helpful to them or to their families

   v. Provide opportunities for continued communication

b. During the anger stage

   i. Allow patients to express their feelings to you and to ask "Why me?"

   ii. Remember, you need not attempt to answer that unanswerable question

iii. The anger that patients are expressing is not directed at you personally but, rather, toward what you represent (continued life) and toward their own painful situation
   c. During the bargaining stage
      i. Find out what kind of help patients need to complete their unfinished business
      ii. Try to make time just to be with dying persons and to listen
   d. During the depression stage, patients mourn all that they are losing. One can help by:
      i. Not interrupting the grieving process
      ii. Supporting patients in their grief
      iii. Sharing your feelings of sadness appropriately, if you feel sad
   e. During the acceptance stage, the issue of letting go of dying persons arises. One can be helpful by:
      i. Not deserting them
      ii. Respecting their acceptance of death
      iii. Assisting the family with their letting go of someone whom they love by listening and by intervening in areas in which family members feel they need help

11. Providing comfort measures for dying patients is reported to be a most important nursing intervention, for the sake of both the patient and the family. Effective verbal and nonverbal communication is essential for evaluating the need for:
   a. Adequate medication for control of pain
   b. Frequent mouth care
   c. Positioning for comfort
   d. Allowing family members to visit more frequently when the patient desires closer contact with loved ones
   e. Supporting the family's involvement in providing comfort measures for the dying person

12. Providing nursing care for dying patients can be one of the most rewarding experiences if critical care nurses are knowledgeable about and prepared to confront the dying process themselves. Knowing that one may experience the ups and downs of the grieving cycle along with the dying patients helps to diminish the fear of getting involved. Recognizing personal strengths and limitations helps prevent burnout. Realizing that one will ultimately learn more about life and about oneself while working with dying patients helps one take advantage of opportunities for growth

Nursing Assessment Data Base

Nursing History

1. Length of time since diagnosis of terminal illness
2. Whether the physician has discussed the diagnosis and prognosis with patient
3. Whether the physician has discussed the diagnosis and prognosis with significant others
4. The medical plan of care: cure-oriented, pain control, returning home to die, entering hospice

5. Supports available to patient and significant others
6. Financial consideration that would require other resources to be brought into situation (social work)

Nursing Examination of Patient

1. Assessment is aimed at achieving and understanding the needs of the individual and of family members so that the dying process can be influenced in a positive manner
2. Using Kübler-Ross' stages, determine where the patient is in the dying process. Remember, these are only guidelines to help understand behavior
3. Assess how the person perceives the situation: what feelings are being expressed
4. Evaluate how the family or significant others perceive the situation: what feelings they are expressing
5. Identify what strengths and supports the patient and family are using to help cope
6. Appraise what needs the patient and family want met and who can meet these needs (e.g., religious worker, mental health worker, financial consultant, lawyer)
7. Determine whether self-esteem, self-concept, body image, and sexuality are significantly affected
8. Evaluate whether loneliness and powerlessness are causing the dying process to be more painful
9. Assess what comfort measures can be used: pain control, positioning, warmth and caring, community resources
10. Assess the caregiver's ability to cope with concerns and fears of own death

Commonly Encountered Nursing Diagnosis: Dysfunctional Grieving

1. **Assessment for defining characteristics**
   a. Medically diagnosed with terminal illness
   b. Verbal expression of distress at loss; labile affect
   c. Denial of loss; anger, sorrow, crying
   d. Alterations in sleep patterns, dreaming patterns, and eating habits
   e. Interference with life functions
2. **Expected outcomes**
   a. The dying process is positively influenced
   b. Pain is controlled
   c. Patient is able to share fears and concerns
   d. Patient is able to communicate with significant others
   e. Patient can bring closure to unfinished business
   f. Needed and available resources are contacted for support of family
   g. Significant others are able to find support with staff, religious worker, or other resources
3. **Nursing interventions**
   a. Goal is to respond effectively to the patient's and family's needs
   b. Follow suggested interventions based on Kübler-Ross' stages
      i. Continue to show respect for and maintain dignity of the patient. Provide good personal hygiene (shaving, hair care, clean clothes)

      ii. Involve all available resources in assisting the patient and family. Encourage communication and allow patient to make decisions

     iii. Maintain good pain control with pain medication administered regularly rather than as needed. Use frequent mouth care and frequent positioning, and encourage more frequent family visits. Support the family so that the family can support their loved one

  c. Nursing staff needs to realize their own abilities to cope with death themselves and that they can experience the ups and downs of the grieving cycle. They should also recognize their strengths and share concerns and feelings with co-workers

  d. Listen intently and respond in age-appropriate terms

4. Evaluation of nursing care

  a. Evaluation is based not on whether the disease or disorder was cured but rather on whether the dying process was positively influenced

  b. Patient's ability to share fears and concerns

  c. Was pain under control? Was the patient comfortable?

  d. Was communication between patient and family accomplished?

  e. Were resources initiated to support the family during the dying process and after?

CAREGIVER ROLE STRAIN

Because nurses who work in critical care environments are exposed to the same environmental stressors as are patients and family members, similar emotional reactions in staff can be expected over a prolonged period. Nurses are subject to additional stresses: responsibility for knowing how to respond appropriately to patients' medical and emotional crises and desiring to be viewed by peers as competent practitioners. The nurse's position in the administrative structure is sometimes a source of further distress. All of this can lead to exhaustion if the nurse is not able to develop effective ways to deal with the distress.

It is helpful for nurses to remember that they are effective in the work setting to the degree that their own needs are met and in accordance with the level of self-esteem experienced at a given moment.

To help promote self-esteem and to provide mechanisms for discharging distress, nurses may find it useful to:

1. Identify your reasons for choosing the critical care setting for practice
2. Identify your strengths, potentials, and limitations as critical care nurses
3. Routinely identify the effect critical care nursing is perceived to have on them individually
4. Develop peer relationships that allow you to feel safe enough to be comfortable in the critical care setting
5. Develop peer relationships that promote open communication (exchanging ideas, complaining, sharing difficult and positive experiences, resolving conflicts)
6. Attend formal and informal multidisciplinary clinical care conferences
7. Participate in staff groups facilitated by a mental health resource leader
8. Devise work plans that allow for sharing responsibilities as needed
9. Use breaks and meal times to replenish energy levels constructively
10. Use moments alone when feeling overwhelmed by excessive stimuli

11. Develop a relationship with supervisors that promotes open communication
12. Use supports available outside the critical care unit (e.g., clinical nurse experts, in-service personnel, staff clergy or other religious personnel)
13. Routinely schedule participation in continuing education events
14. Develop sources of support and areas of enrichment outside their professional lives
15. Recognize that the meaning given to their work is to some degree influenced by where they are in the life cycle

It is suggested that nurses organize the critical care environment in such a way that an area be established for staff use only, out of view of patients and family members

References

GROWTH AND DEVELOPMENT

Erikson, E.: Childhood and Society, 2nd ed. New York, W. W. Norton, 1963.
Erikson, E.: Identity, Youth and Crisis. New York, W. W. Norton, 1968.
Maslow, A. H.: Toward a Psychology of Being. Princeton, Mass., Van Nostrand, 1968.
Stuart, G., and Sundeen, S.: Principles and Practice of Psychiatric Nursing, 4th ed. New York, Harper & Row, 1991, pp. 68–69.

PERCEPTION

Coombs, A., Richards, A. C., and Richards, F.: Perceptual Psychology: A Humanistic Approach to the Study of Persons. New York, Harper & Row, 1976.
Fisher, S., and Cleveland, S.: Personality, body perception, and body image boundary. In Wager, S., and Warner, H. (eds.): The Body Precept. New York, Random House, 1965, pp. 110–115.
Gowan, N. J.: The perceptual world of the intensive care unit: An overview of some environmental considerations in the helping relationship. Heart Lung 8:340–344, 1979.

SELF-CONCEPT AND SELF-ESTEEM

Brissett, D.: Toward a clarification of self-esteem. Psychiatry 35:255–263, 1972.
Coombs, A., Richards, A. C., and Richards, F.: Perceptual Psychology: A Humanistic Approach to the Study of Persons. New York, Harper & Row, 1976.
Coopersmith, S.: The Antecedents of Self-Esteem. San Francisco, W. H. Freeman, 1960.
Satir, V.: Psychology of Self-Esteem. New York, Bantam Books, 1971.

NEEDS

Maslow, A. H.: Toward a Psychology of Being, 2nd ed. Princeton, Mass., Van Nostrand, 1968.
Yura, H., and Walsh, M.B.: Human Needs and the Nursing Process. New York, Appleton-Century-Crofts, 1978.

STRENGTHS, POTENTIALS, AND LIMITATIONS

Murphy, G.: Human Potentialities. New York, Basic Books, 1958.
Otto, H.: The human potentialities of nurses and patients. Nurs. Outlook 13:32–35, 1965.
Otto, H.: New light on human potential. Saturday Review, December 1969, pp. 14–18.

STRESS

Benson, H.: The relaxation response. Psychiatry 37:37–46, 1974.
Carnevale, F. A., Annibale, F., Grenier, A., Guy, E., and Ottoni, L.: Nursing in the ICU: Stress, without distress? Can. Crit. Care Nurs. J. 4(March–April):16–18, 1987.
Crickmore, R.: A review of stress in the intensive care unit. Intens. Care Nurse 3:19–27, 1987.
Kopolow, L. E.: Plain Talk About Handling Stress (DHHS Publication No. [ADM] 91–502). Washington, D.C., U.S. Government Printing Office, 1991.
Selye, H.: Stress Without Distress. Philadelphia, J. B. Lippincott, 1974.
Soupios, M. A., and Kawry, K.: Stress on personnel working in a critical care unit. Psychiatr. Med. 5:187–198, 1987.
Tiernan, P. J.: Independent nursing intervention: Relaxation and guided imagery in critical care. Crit. Care Nurse 10:47–51, 1994.
van der Kolk, B. A.: The body keeps the score: Memory and the evolving psychobiology of posttraumatic stress. Harvard Rev. Psychiatry 3(2):253–265, 1994.

PAIN

Ferrell, B. A.: Pain management in elderly people. J. Am. Geriatr. Soc. 39(1):64–73, 1991.
Guyton-Simmons, J., and Ehrmin, J. T.: Problem solving in pain management by expert intensive care nurses. Crit. Care Nurse 10:37–44, 1994.
Harrison, M., and Cotanch, P. H.: Pain: Advances and issues in critical care. Nurs. Clin. North Am. 9:691–697, 1987.
Jacox, A., Carr, D. B., Payne, R., et al.: Management of Cancer Pain: Adults Quick Reference Guide. No. 9 (AHCPR Publication No. 04–0593). Rockville, Md., Agency for Health Care Policy and Research, 1994.

McCaffery, M.: Pain in the critical care patient. Dimens. Crit. Care Nurs. 4(6):323–325, 1984.

McCaffery, M., and Beebe, A.: Pain: Clinical Manual for Nursing Practice. St. Louis, Mosby–Year Book, 1989.

INTERPERSONAL COMMUNICATION

Allen, A. L., Jackson, D., and Younger, S.: Closing the communication gap between physician and nurses in the intensive care unit setting. Heart Lung 9:836–840, 1980.

Ashworth, P.: Technology and machines—Bad masters but good servants. Intens. Care Nurse 3:19–27, 1987.

Hein, E. C.: Communication in Nursing Practice, 2nd ed. Boston, Little, Brown & Co., 1980.

BODY IMAGE

Billie, D. A.: The role of body image in patient compliance and education. Heart Lung 6:143–146, 1977.

Corbeil, L.: Nursing process for a patient with a body image disturbance. Nurs. Clin. North Am. 6:155–163, 1971.

Costello, A. M.: Supporting the Patient with Problems Related to Body Image (American Cancer Society Professional Education Publication). Washington, D.C., American Cancer Society, 1975.

Shotz, F.: Body image and its disorders. In Lipowski, Z., Lipsitt, D., and Whybrow, P. P. (eds.): Psychosomatic Medicine. Current Trends and Clinical Applications. New York, Oxford University Press, 1977, pp. 122–132.

HUMAN SEXUALITY

Kolodny, R. C., Masters, W. H., Johnson, V. E., et al.: Textbook of Human Sexuality for Nurses. Boston, Little, Brown & Co., 1979, pp. 31–78.

Satterfield, S. B., and Stayton, W. R.: Understanding sexual function and dysfunction. Top. Clin. Nurs. 1:21–32, 1980.

Wernik, U.: The role of the traumatic component in the etiology of sexual dysfunctions and its treatment with eye movement desensitization procedure. J. Sex Educ. Ther. 212–222, July 1993.

Wise, T.: Sexual difficulties with concurrent physical problems. Psychosomatics 18:56–64, 1977.

ABUSE

Davis, L. V.: Violence and families. J. Nat. Assoc. Soc. Workers 36(5):371–373, 1991.

Dietz, C., and Craft, J.: Family dynamics of incest: A new perspective. Soc. Casework J. Contemp. Soc. Work 61:602–609, 1980.

Finkelhor, D.: A Source Book on Child Sexual Abuse. San Francisco, Sage Publications, 1986.

Gilbert, N.: Sexual assault: The phantom epidemic. Public Interest Spring 1991, pp. 54–65.

Gordon, L.: Heroes of Their Own Lives: The Politics and History of Family Violence. New York, Penguin Books, 1988.

Roberts, L.: A Treatment Manual for Therapy Groups with Survivors of Childhood Incest. Madison, Wisc., Rape Crisis Center, 1987.

Russell, D.: The Secret Trauma: Incest in the Lives of Girls and Women. New York, Basic Books, 1986.

Tierney, K. J.: The battered woman movement and the creation of the wife beating problem. Social Problems, 29:207–220, 1982.

Warshaw, R.: I Never Called It Rape: The Ms. Report on Recognizing, Fighting and Surviving Date and Acquaintance Rape. New York, Harper & Row, 1988.

FAMILY

Bozett, F. W., and Gobbons, R.: The nursing management of families in the critical care setting. Crit. Care Update 2:22–27, 1983.

Hardner, D., and Stewart, N.: Staff involvement with families of patients in critical care units. Heart Lung 7:104–110, 1978.

Kerr, M. E., and Bowen, M.: Family Evaluation. New York, W. W. Norton, 1988.

Lammon, C. A.: Reducing family hostility. Dimens. Crit. Care Nurs. 4(1):58–63, 1985.

CRITICAL CARE ENVIRONMENT AND CAREGIVER ROLE STRAIN

Bibbings, J.: The stress of working in intensive care: A look at the research. Nursing 3:367–570, 1987.

Clifford, C.: Patients, relatives and nurses in a technological environment. Intens. Care Nurse 2:67–72, 1986.

Corcoran, L., and Diers, D.: Nursing intensity in cardiac surgical care. Nurs. Manage. 2:801–807, 1989.

Daniels, V.: Stress and the I.C.U.: Is it for you? Imprint September–October: 1987, pp. 32–35.

Fowler, M. D.: Moral distress and the shortage of critical care nurses. Heart Lung 18:314–315, 1989.

Hague, C.: Caring can damage your health. Intens. Care Nurse 3:28–33, 1987.

Huckabay, L. M. D., and Jagla, B.: Nurses' stress factors in intensive care unit. J. Nurs. Admin. 9:21–26, 1979.

Stern, S. B.: Nursing the patient, not the machines. Am. J. Nurs. 10:1310, 1986.

Ulberg, K.: Burned out: Should a battle-weary nurse endure—or find another job? J. Christ. Nurs. 3:20–21, 1986.

West, A. M.: Suggestions for health care providers in critical care units [Letter]. Heart Lung 1:103–104, 1989.

CRISIS

Aquilera, D. C., and Messick, J.: Crisis Intervention: Theory and Methodology. St. Louis, C. V. Mosby, 1980.

Clifford, C.: Patients, relatives and nurses in a technological environment. Intens. Care Nurse 2:67–72, 1986.

Fink, S. L.: Crisis and motivation: A theoretical model. Arch. Phys. Mod. Rehabil. 48:592–597, 1967.

FEAR AND ANXIETY

Felicetta, J. V., and Sowers, J. R.: Endocrine changes with critical illness. Crit. Care Clinician, 10:855–869, 1987.

Johnson, M. N.: Anxiety/stress and the effects on disclosure between nurses and patients. Adv. Nurs. Sci. 1:1–20, 1979.

McCullough, W. B.: The postoperative pain-anxiety circuit: A general surgeon's perspective. Pain Overview, 14–19, June 1980.

LONELINESS AND POWERLESSNESS

Berni, R., and Fordyce, W. E.: Behavior Modification and the Nursing Process. St. Louis, C. V. Mosby, 1973.

Slater, P.: The Pursuit of Loneliness. Boston, Beacon Press, 1970.

West, A. M.: Suggestions for health care providers in critical care units [Letter]. Heart Lung 1:103–104, 1989.

SENSORY OVERLOAD AND SENSORY DEPRIVATION

Barrie-Shevlin, P.: Maintaining sensory balance for the critically ill patient. Nursing 4:596–601, 1987.

Diekstra, R. F., Stubbie, L. T., and Willemsteyn, B.: ICU sensory deprivation. Nurs. Success Today 6:21–25, 1986.

MacKinnon-Kesler, S.: Maximizing your ICU patient's sensory and perceptual environment. Can. Nurse 5:41–45, 1983.

ADDICTION

Baldwin, W. A., Rosenfeld, B. A., Bresslow, M. G., et al.: Substance abuse–related admissions to adult intensive care. Chest 103:21–25, 1993.

Chan, P., Chen, J. H., Lee, M. H., and Deng, J. F.: Fatal and nonfatal methamphetamine intoxication in the intensive care unit. J. Toxicol. Clin. Toxicol. 32:147–155, 1994.

Jones, C., and Owens, D.: The recreational drug user in the intensive care unit: A review. Intens. Care Crit. Nurs. 12:126–130, 1996.

Smith, H. L., Mangelsdorf, K. L., Louderbough, A. W., and Piland, N. F.: Substance abuse among nurses: Types of drugs. Dimens. Crit. Care Nurs. 8:159–168, 1989.

Terry, P. B., and Fessler, H. E.: Should intensive care be limited for patients with self-induced disease? [editorial]. Am. J. Med. Sci. 307:374–377, 1994.

SUICIDAL PHENOMENON

Farberow, N. L., and Shneidman, E. S.: The Cry for Help. New York, McGraw-Hill, 1961.

Hatten, C., Loing, V., McBride, S., et al.: Suicide Assessment and Intervention. New York, Appleton-Century-Crofts, 1977.

Hervie, C., Gaillard, M., Martel, S., and Huguenard, P.: Serious suicides: Short and long-term results. Acta Anaesthesiol. Belg. 35:353–359, 1984.

Shneidman, E. S.: Deaths of Man. Baltimore, Penguin Books, 1973.

Stevens, B. J.: A phenomenological approach to understanding suicidal behavior. J. Psychiatr. Nurs. 9:33–35, 1971.

THE DYING PROCESS AND DEATH

Garfield, C. A.: Psychosocial care of the dying patient. *In* Patterson, M. E. (ed.): The Living-Dying Process. New York, McGraw-Hill, 1978, pp. 54–68.

Herzog, B. B., and Herrin, J. T.: Near-death experience in the very young. Crit. Care Med. 12:1074–1075, 1985.

Kirchling, J. M., and Pierce, P. K.: Nursing and the terminally ill: Beliefs, attitudes and perceptions of practitioners. Issues Ment. Health Nurs. 4:275–286, 1982.

Kübler-Ross, E.: On Death and Dying. New York, Macmillan, 1969.

Oaks, A. R.: Near-death events and critical care nursing. Top. Clin. Nurs. 10:61–78, 1981.

Richmond, T., and Craig, M.: Timeout: Facing death in the ICU. Dimens. Crit. Care Nurs. 5(1):41–45, 1985.

NURSING DIAGNOSIS

Kim, M. J., McFarland, G. K., and McLane, A. M.: Pocket Guide to Nursing Diagnosis, 6th ed. St. Louis, Mosby–Year Book, 1995.

.... Legal and Ethical Aspects of Critical Care Nursing

Ginger Schafer Wlody, R.N., M.S., Ed.D., FCCM

LEGAL ASPECTS

Law

Sum Total of Rules and Regulations

Sources of Law

1. **The Constitution**: provides the framework of U.S. federal and state governments
2. **Common law**: court-made law and interpretation of statutes
3. **Statutory law**: written laws enacted by the state legislatures and Congress. Basic rules for society established by the U.S. Senate and House of Representatives or by the state legislatures
4. **Administrative law**: made by administrative agencies' top officials, who are appointed by the executive branch of the government, by the president, or by governors of the states. Given power by statutory law to propagate rules and regulations

State Nurse Practice Acts

1. **Purpose:** to protect the public
2. **Statutory laws:** written by the individual states

3. **Usual authorization:** board of nursing to oversee nursing (by use of regulations or administrative law)
4. **Scope of practice**: provides guidance for acceptable nursing roles and practices which vary from state to state
   a. Nurses are expected to follow Nurse Practice Act and not deviate from usual nursing activities
   b. Advanced nursing practice: expanded roles for nurses in special positions. The duty of nurses in expanded roles differs from that of nurses working under direct supervision in the clinical setting. Nurses need to be aware of their state Practice Act limitations. Nurses in expanded roles may not be covered by state Practice Acts
      i. Nurse practitioners: may write prescriptions in certain states
      ii. Clinical nurse specialists: may be privileged to order tests, perform certain procedures
      iii. Nurse anesthetists: first specialty group to be involved in advanced and expanded practice
      iv. American Association of Critical-Care Nurses (AACN)/American Nurses Association (ANA) approves scope and standards for Advanced Practitioners in Critical Care/Advanced Clinical Practitioners (AACN, 1993; Mirr, 1993)
         (a) Members have a graduate degree in nursing, advanced clinical specialty education, and experience in nursing
         (b) Members perform the following functions:
            (1) Conduct comprehensive health assessments
            (2) Demonstrate a high level of autonomy and expert skill in the diagnosis and treatment of complex responses of individuals, families, and communities to actual and potential health problems
            (3) Formulate clinical decisions to manage acute and chronic illness and promote wellness
            (4) Integrate education, research, management, leadership, and consultation into clinical role
            (5) Function in collegial relationships with nursing peers, physicians, professionals, and others who influence the health environment
         (c) Outcomes include
            (1) Integration of education, research, management, leadership, and consultation
            (2) Integration of information in the nursing domain when its functions overlap with those of other disciplines
            (3) Contribution to the profession at large
            (4) Display of expert judgment in immediately recognizing, understanding, and responding to phenomena of nursing concern
            (5) Innovation, by seeing new ways of caring for patients; continuous improvement of quality; and prevention of waste of resources
            (6) Development of new clinical knowledge
            (7) Approach to care from a holistic perspective; seeing beyond the individual

. . . .
:
: **Standards of Nursing Care**

Any established measure of extent, quality, quantity, or value; an agreed-upon level of performance or a degree of excellence of care that is established. Standards are established by usual and customary practice, institutional guidelines, association guidelines, and legal precedent. Standards of care, standards of practice, policies, procedures, and performance criteria all establish an agreed-upon level of performance or degree of excellence.

1. **AACN Standards of Care for the Critically Ill** (1989)
2. **ANA Standards**: ANA has generic standards and also specialty standards (e.g., medical-surgical nursing)
3. **Standards of Clinical Practice for Acute Certified Nurse Practitioners** (1995)
4. **National Facility Standards**
    a. **Joint Commission on Accreditation of Healthcare Organizations (JCAHO) Standards**: nationally recognized standards for patient care. Interdisciplinary standards have implications for nursing care
    b. **National Committee on Quality Assurance (NCQA) standards** are quality accreditation standards for ambulatory care
5. **Community and regional standards**: standards prevalent in certain areas of the country or in specific communities
6. **Hospital and medical center standards**: standards developed by institutions for their staff and patients
7. **Unit practice standards, policies, and protocols**: specific standards of care for specific groups or types of patients
8. **Precedent court cases**: standard of "reasonable, prudent nurse" (e.g., what a reasonable, prudent nurse would have done in the same situation)
9. **Specialty organization standards**: standards developed by other nurse specialty organizations (e.g., Association of Operating Room Nurses [AORN] Standards, Neuroscience Nursing Standards, Emergency Nursing Standards of Care)
10. **Certification in a specialty area**
    a. Certification is defined as a means by which a professional organization attests that an individual has attained proficiency in an area of that profession's practice
    b. Guido (1996) defined certification as "the process of granting recognition to individuals who have attained a specific level of knowledge and expertise in a given field of a profession"
    c. A common goal of specialty certification programs is to promote consumer protection
    d. The certified nurse may be held to a higher standard of practice in the specialty than the noncertified nurse
    e. Critical care certification awarded by the AACN Certification Corporation's CCRN Program. The main objectives of the CCRN certification program are
        i. To establish the body of knowledge necessary for CCRN certification
        ii. To test, by examination, the common body of knowledge needed to function effectively within the critical care setting
        iii. To recognize professional competence by granting CCRN status to successful candidates

. . . .

Documentation

1. **Mandated by regulatory agencies**
   a. Federal requirements: related to narcotics, controlled substances, organ transplantation
   b. National voluntary requirements: JCAHO's requirements related to quality improvement activities
   c. State requirements: may exist in specific situations (e.g., in relation to minors)
   d. Community standard: regional or local standards may include enhanced documentation in specific areas of practice (e.g., epidural medication)
   e. Hospital, medical center, or health maintenance organizations' (HMOs') requirements

2. **Purposes of documentation** of nursing care in the patient record
   a. To plan and evaluate care
   b. To show progress of patient care, treatment of and change in condition, and continuity of care and to reflect patient status, appearance, and behavior
   c. To demonstrate use of the nursing process
   d. To reflect nursing observations, interventions, and evaluation
   e. To protect patient; medical record is used in litigation
   f. To protect health care professionals and institutions
   g. To provide clear and concise communication between providers

3. **Documentation requirements**
   a. General requirements
      i. Should contain accurate, factual observations
      ii. Notations and events must be timed
      iii. Reflects patient status and unusual events
      iv. Reflects nursing interventions and evaluation of their effectiveness
      v. Should reflect omissions of care and rationale
      vi. Should reflect that physician was informed of unusual or adverse situations and nature of physician's response
      vii. Should note deviations from standard hospital practice and their rationale
      viii. Should be legible
      ix. Should carefully document method of patient's admission, condition on admission, discharge planning, and condition on discharge
      x. Should reflect documentation of the nursing process on a continuing basis throughout the hospitalization
   b. Specific requirements of JCAHO for patient records
      i. Patient's name, address, and date of birth, and name of any legally authorized representative
      ii. Legal status of patients receiving mental health services
      iii. Emergency care, if any, provided to the patient before arrival
      iv. Record and findings of the patient's assessment
      v. Conclusions or impressions drawn from the medical history and physical examination
      vi. Diagnosis or diagnostic impression
      vii. Reasons for admission or treatment

    viii. Goals of treatment and the treatment plan

    ix. Evidence of known advance directives

    x. Evidence of informed consent, when required by hospital policy

    xi. Diagnostic and therapeutic orders, if any

    xii. Records of all diagnostic and therapeutic procedures and all test results

    xiii. Records of all operative and other invasive procedures performed, with acceptable disease and operative terminology that includes etiology, as appropriate

    xiv. Progress notes made by the medical staff and other authorized persons

    xv. All reassessments and any revisions of the treatment plan

    xvi. Clinical observations

    xvii. Records of patient's response to care

    xviii. Consultation reports

    xix. Records of every medication ordered or prescribed for an inpatient

    xx. Records of every medication dispensed to an ambulatory patient or an inpatient on discharge

    xxi. Records of every dose of medication administered and any adverse drug reaction

    xxii. All relevant diagnoses established during the course of care

    xxiii. Any referrals and communications made to external or internal care providers and to community agencies

    xxiv. Conclusions at termination of hospitalization

    xxv. Discharge instructions to the patient and family

    xxvi. Clinical resumes and discharge summaries, or a final progress note or transfer summary. Discharge summary contains reason for hospitalization, significant findings, procedures performed and treatment rendered, patient's condition at discharge, and instructions to the patient and family, if any

Informed Consent

1. **Definition**: The President's Commission for the Study of Ethical Problems in Medicine and Biomedical and Behavioral Research recommended "that patient and provider collaborate in a continuing process intended to make decisions that will advance the patient's interests both in health (and well-being generally) and in self-determination. Self-determination, sometimes called 'autonomy,' involves a person forming, revising over time and pursuing his or her own particular plan of life."

2. **Doctrine of informed consent**

    a. Based on principle of autonomy of individuals

    b. Includes right of informed refusal

    c. Obligation of health care provider to provide adequate information (what a reasonable, prudent patient would want to know in the same or similar circumstances) to patient regarding

      i. Treatment options

      ii. Risk versus benefit

        iii. Expected or desired outcomes of procedures or therapy

        iv. Complications or undesired side effects

        v. Alternative therapies, including no therapy at all

  d. Four requisites to informed consent:

        i. Patient must have capacity to reason and make judgments (decision-making capacity)

           (a) Competent adults: able to make health care decisions

           (b) Incompetent adults and minors

               (1) Representatives (agents) of incapacitated individuals

                  a) Legal guardian

                  b) Representative or surrogate of incompetent adult

                  c) Emancipated, married minor

                  d) Mature minor (as applicable)

                  e) Parent or legal guardian of a minor

                  f) Minor (for diagnosis and treatment of specific disease states or conditions)

                  g) Court-ordered representative

               (2) Doctrine of substituted judgment: this standard requires that a surrogate attempt to reach the decision that the incapacitated person would make if he or she were able to choose. As a result, the patient's interest in self-determination is preserved to a certain extent. Families or surrogates should follow patient's wishes or what the patient would have wanted

               (3) Best interest test: this standard rests solely on protection of the patient's welfare. Surrogates often lack guidance for making a substituted judgment because they, like many other people, have not given serious thought to how they would want to be treated under particular circumstances or because they have failed to tell others their thoughts. In these cases, the surrogates try to make a choice for the patient that seeks to implement what is that patient's best interest by reference to more objective, societally shared criteria. Conflict and ethical dilemmas may arise when decision making seems not to take account of a child's (or an incapacitated adult's) best interest

               (4) Refer to individual state requirements for various court-appointed guardian or next-of-kin issues

           (c) Competence: the ability to make rational decisions about one's life. Usually determined by courts

           (d) Decision-making capacity: the ability to make decisions about one's health care. Determining whether a patient lacks the capacity to make a decision to forego life-sustaining treatment rests on generally accepted principles for making assessments of decisional capacity in medical care

        ii. The decision must be made voluntarily and without coercion

        iii. The patient must have a clear understanding of risks and benefits of proposed treatment

        iv. Patient must not be sedated at time of consent

  e. Nurses have a special obligation to ensure that the patient receives informed consent. Nurses have the obligation to be knowledgeable about moral and legal rights of all clients and to protect and support those rights

   f. The responsibility for informing the patient is the physician's, although in most hospital settings, the nurse obtains the signature on the consent form. Some attorneys view nurses as merely facilitators of informed consent, whereas nurses see themselves as guardians of informed consent. The trend is to view nurses as sharing some of the physician's responsibility for informed consent if the circumstances warrant. Nurses' advocacy function must be considered. Failure to obtain informed consent may be grounds for malpractice claims and claims of battery

   g. Informed refusal

     i. Right of patient to refuse care and/or treatment

     ii. Duty of practitioner: to ensure that refusal is based on informed choice

   h. Exceptions to informed consent: most hospitals have strict policies that are followed when all of these conditions exist: in a dire emergency, when the patient is unable to give consent, and when no relatives or significant others can be reached

3. Types of consent

   a. Signature consent (written) is equivalent to express consent

   b. Oral consent: consent by word of mouth (express consent). Given freely

   c. Apparent consent: inferred by patient's conduct

   d. Implied consent: normally involved in true emergency situations and when a delay in providing treatment would result in loss of life or permanent injury. Patient is unable to make his or her wishes known and is incapable of refusing the procedure or therapy

Declaring Death

Originally there were no uniform criteria for declaration of death. The Harvard Criteria referred only to a definition of "irreversible coma"

1. Brain death: Uniform Determination of Death Act (UDDA) guidelines developed by the President's Commission for the Study of Ethical Problems in Medicine and Biomedical and Behavioral Research state that "Any individual who has sustained either irreversible cessation of circulatory and respiratory functions, or irreversible cessation of all functions of the entire brain, including the brain stem, is dead"

   a. A determination of death must be made in accordance with accepted medical standards

   b. UDDA guidelines have been adopted in most states

2. Procedural guidelines for the declaration of death

   a. Triggering a neurologic evaluation: as soon as responsible physician has a reasonable suspicion that an irreversible loss of all brain functions has occurred, he or she should perform the appropriate tests and procedures to determine patient's neurologic status

   b. Obligation to declare a patient dead: cardiopulmonary criteria for determining death are recognized in all states; when the physician determines that the patient has experienced an irreversible cessation of cardiopulmonary functions, he or she declares the patient dead

i. Consent of the surrogate, family, or concerned friends is not required

ii. Sensitivity to family or surrogate needs is required, and as always, they have the option to obtain a second opinion about brain death

c. Cessation of treatment after a declaration of death: once the declaration of death has been made, all treatment of the patient ordinarily should cease. Exceptions to this might be efforts to use the body or body parts for purposes stated in Uniform Anatomical Gift Act (education, research, advancement of medical or dental science, therapy, transplantation) or if the patient is pregnant and efforts are being made to save the life of the fetus

d. In cases involving organ donation, health care professionals who make the declaration of death

i. Should not be members of the organ transplantation team

ii. Should not be a member of the patient's family

iii. Should not have malpractice charges pending against them that are related to the case

iv. Should not have any other special interest in declaration of the patient's death (i.e., stand to inherit anything according to patient's will)

3. **Types of Organ Donors**

a. Tissue donor: donor may be alive (e.g., bone marrow) or deceased (e.g., eyes)

b. Heart-beating donor: donor is brain dead, but respiratory function is supported mechanically while cardiac function continues spontaneously

c. Non–heart-beating donor: organs are procured immediately after cessation of cardiorespiratory function

. . . .

Patient Rights

The rationale surrounding the doctrine of informed consent is that competent adult patients have a right of self-determination, which includes the right to refuse care or treatment. These are legal "rights" that have been established by the courts. These are also reflected in the "Patient's Bill of Rights" adopted by the American Hospital Association

1. **"Right to die"**: Term used by lay public. Generally refers to the right to withdraw or refuse treatment. Title is controversial, but right to refuse treatment has emerged through case law in the individual states and is based on the right to self-determination (autonomy)

2. **Right to refuse treatment**: refusal of care by a competent and informed adult should be respected even if that refusal leads to serious harm to that individual

3. **Right to information**: related to rights of informed consent and right to self-determination

4. **Right to privacy**: invasion of the right of privacy traditionally has four separate causes: appropriation of name and likeness; intrusion upon solitude or seclusion; public disclosure of private facts; and false light in the public eye

5. **Right to confidentiality**: many states have statutorily created a physician-patient privilege that protects physicians from being compelled to testify

confidential communications about the patient. Legislation is needed to extend the privilege to nurses, but courts have held that the premise applies by analogy to the nurse-patient relationship

Do Not Resuscitate Orders

1. **A "do not resuscitate"** (DNR) **order** is a signed order directing that no cardiopulmonary resuscitative efforts are to be undertaken in the event of cardiac or respiratory arrest
2. **Cardiopulmonary resuscitation** (CPR) is an array of interventions undertaken at the time of cardiac or respiratory arrest to restore spontaneous pulse and ventilation

Advance Directive

A document in which a person gives advance directions about medical care or designates who should make medical decisions if he or she should lose decision-making capacity. There are two types of advance directives: treatment directives and proxy directives (such as durable power of attorney or living will). Living wills are not recognized by every state

1. **Patient Self-Determination Act** (1991): federal legislation that requires that hospitals and nursing homes
    a. Provide information to patients on admission regarding their rights to make advance directives
    b. Provide written information to patients on admission about institutional policies that may affect their rights (e.g., to refuse treatment)
2. **Treatment directive**: a written statement prepared by a person directing what forms of medical treatment the person wishes to receive or forgo should he or she lack decision-making capacity as a result of medical condition (such as irreversible coma, terminal illness). A "living will" is one type of treatment directive
3. **Durable power of attorney** (DPA): an individual's written designation of another person to act on his or her behalf, when the designation is authorized by the state's durable power of attorney statute. A durable power of attorney does not terminate under state law (as does a regular power of attorney) when a patient loses decision-making capacity. Patients may revoke a DPA at any time while competent. Nurses should be familiar with their specific state laws

Good Samaritan Acts

1. **Various states have enacted Good Samaritan Acts** that provide immunity from civil liability for acts or omissions of a person who provides emergency care in good faith at the scene of an accident
2. **According to traditional common law, there is no duty to render assistance to one who needs medical care**, even in emergency situations, unless there is an

established care relationship or the condition can be attributed to the provider's actions

. . . .
. .
: The Legal Process

1. **Professional liability**
    a. Professional negligence: an unintentional act or omission; the failure to do what the reasonable, prudent nurse would do under similar circumstances, or an act or failure to act that leads to an injury of another. Specific elements are necessary for professional negligence action and must be established by the plaintiff
        i. Duty: to protect the patient from an unreasonable risk of harm
        ii. Breach of duty: failure by a nurse to do what a reasonable, prudent nurse would do under the same or similar circumstances. The breach of duty is a failure to perform within the given standard of care. Standard of care defines the amount of the duty owed
        iii. Proximate cause: proof that the harm caused was foreseeable and that the person injured was a foreseeable victim. Limits the extent of damages for which a provider will be held liable
        iv. Injury: the harm done
        v. Direct cause of injury: it must be proved that the nurse's conduct was the cause of or contributed to the injury to the patient
        vi. Damages: proof of actual loss, damage, pain, or suffering caused by the nurse's conduct
    b. Malpractice: a specific type of negligence that includes the status of the caregiver as well as the standard of care (Guido, 1996). Professional negligence is malpractice. It is differentiated from ordinary negligence (e.g., failure to clean up water from the floor)
        i. Professional misconduct, improper discharge of professional duties, or a failure to meet the standard of care by a professional that results in harm to another person
        ii. Malpractice is the failure of a professional person to act in accordance with prevailing professional standards or a failure to foresee consequences that a professional person who has the necessary skills and education would foresee
        iii. Most common areas of malpractice or negligence in critical care settings include medication errors, failure to prevent patient falls, failure to assess changes in clinical status, and failure to notify primary provider of changes in patient status
    c. Supervision of unlicensed personnel or unlicensed assistive personnel (UAPs)
        i. Definition of unlicensed personnel: caregivers who are not authorized to perform (nursing care) activities in their respective state Nurse Practice Acts (Blouin & Brent, 1995)
        ii. Legal concerns
            (a) Training and orientation of UAPs
            (b) Liability issues if patient is injured as result of negligence by UAP
            (c) Adequate staffing as identified by the hospital's staffing plan

(d) Delegation of patient care: involves licensure ramifications and liability for professional nurse's negligence should an injury occur because of UAP's alleged negligence

(e) Supervision of caregiver by professional nurse

iii. Delegation and supervision of UAPs

(a) California Administrative Code: definition of delegation: a nurse competent in delegating and supervising "delegates tasks to subordinates and on the preparation and capability needed in the tasks to be delegated, and effectively supervises nursing care being given by subordinates" (16 Cal. Code No. 1443.5)

(b) Negligence

(1) Inappropriate work assignment (failure or breach of duty to delegate properly)

(2) Inadequate supervision of person performing the function

iv. Nurse executives must ensure that

(a) Policies and procedures concerning supervision and delegation are in place and consistent with state Nurse Practice Acts

(b) Job descriptions must not include responsibilities that require a license to perform them (whether license is in nursing or another area; e.g., respiratory therapy, physical therapy)

(c) Adequate training and consistent orientation for UAPs

(d) Mechanism for regular evaluation of UAPs

ETHICAL ASPECTS

Ethical Principles

1. **Patient autonomy**: refers to self-determination, freedom of choice for competent patient
2. **Justice**: refers to what a person deserves, what is just, or what is right. A person deserves to be treated fairly and should not be discriminated against on the basis of social contribution or mental capacity
3. **Veracity**: truth telling, honesty, or integrity
4. **Fidelity**: keeping "promises" or professional obligations as professional nurses to care for patients to the best of their ability
5. **Beneficence:** doing good for others, being helpful, being considerate of other's rights. Beneficence involves removing harmful conditions
6. **Non-maleficence**: this is the principle of "do no harm." This principle may conflict with others when treatment decisions are made
7. **Formalism (Emanuel Kant)/deontologic approach**: refers to the "duty" involved; duties are viewed as the basis for morality. Actions are justified, not by the consequences alone, but by the rightness or wrongfulness of the act itself (the ends do not justify the means)
8. **Consequentialism (John Stuart Mill)/teleologic approach**: bases the rightness or wrongfulness of an action on the consequences of that action. It concerns "outcome" or what the result will be (whether the end does justify the means)

9. **Utilitarianism**: approach or theory that states that the morally right thing to do is the act that produces the greatest good (for the most people or for society). Utilitarianism is derived from the teleologic approach
10. **Paternalism**: based on the claim that beneficence should take precedence over autonomy, at least in some cases (e.g., a health care worker makes a decision for a patient according to the rationale "It's in their best interest"; the patient is then denied the right to make his or her decisions)

Moral Concepts and Theories

1. **Respect for persons**: giving due weight to the welfare and wishes of people
   a. People should be treated with caring; the "ethic of care"
   b. People should not be treated as a means to an end
2. **Justice**: justice is a minimal claim on social order: everyone fundamentally deserves equal respect
   a. Distributive justice: allocation of goods and services
   b. Retributive justice: primarily concerned with punishment for wrongdoing
   c. Procedural justice: focuses on how things are done regardless of final outcome
3. **Values**: the foundation of the seriousness and importance of things; what people see as good or bad, right or wrong. Values have different weights or importance, are the basis of ethical decision making, and may reflect an individual's or a society's beliefs
   a. Instrumental values: activity valuable only as a means to an end
   b. Final values: values that have importance in and of themselves
   c. Value conflicts occur when nurses' values are not congruent with patient's, physician's, family's, or institutional values, leading to ethical dilemmas
4. **Rights**
   a. Basic human rights
      i. Protect people from loss of individual freedoms (e.g., the Bill of Rights protects individuals from illegal search and seizure)
      ii. Demand provision of goods and services by the state (e.g., water)
      iii. Are established by systems of law and backed by state
      iv. Involve responsibilities
      v. Moral rights: backed by general opinion of society, culture
   b. Basic human rights include
      i. Legal rights: life, liberty, property, individual freedoms, due process
      ii. Moral rights: decision making about concepts and beliefs
      iii. Entitlements: statutory rights for defined group of recipients (e.g., Medicare, welfare)

American Nurses Association Ethical Code for Nurses

1. **Based on a belief about the nature of individuals, nursing, health, and society**
2. **Provides guidance for conduct and relationships** in carrying out nursing responsibilities that are consistent with ethical obligations of the profession and with high-quality nursing care

3. **Reflects an essential activity of a profession** and provides one means for the exercise of professional self-regulation
4. **Offers general principles to guide and evaluate nursing actions**, informing both the nurse and society of the profession's expectations and requirements in ethical matters
5. Adopted originally in 1950, revised in 1976 adding interpretative statements. Latest revision, 1985
6. **Code statements**
   a. The nurse provides services with respect for human dignity and the uniqueness of the client, unrestricted by considerations of social or economic status, personal attributes, or the nature of health problems
   b. The nurse safeguards the client's right to privacy by judiciously protecting information of a confidential nature
   c. The nurse acts to safeguard the client and the public when health care and safety are affected by incompetent, unethical, or illegal practice by any person
   d. The nurse assumes responsibility and accountability for individual nursing judgments and actions
   e. The nurse maintains competence in nursing
   f. The nurse exercises informed judgment and uses individual competency and qualifications as criteria in seeking consultation, accepting responsibilities, and delegating nursing activities
   g. The nurse participates in activities that contribute to the ongoing development of the profession's body of knowledge
   h. The nurse participates in the profession's efforts to implement and improve standards of nursing
   i. The nurse participates in the profession's efforts to establish and maintain conditions of employment conducive to high-quality nursing care
   j. The nurse participates in the profession's effort to protect the public from misinformation and misrepresentation and to maintain the integrity of nursing
   k. The nurse collaborates with members of the health professions and other citizens in promoting community and national efforts to meet the health needs of the public

. . . .

American Hospital Association: Patient's Bill of Rights

1. **The patient has the right**
   a. To considerate and respectful care
   b. To obtain from the physician information regarding diagnosis, treatment, and prognosis
   c. To give informed consent before the start of any procedure or treatment
   d. To refuse treatment to the extent permitted by law
   e. To privacy concerning own medical care program
   f. To confidential communication and records
   g. To expect that the hospital will make a reasonable response to a patient's request for service
   h. To information regarding the relationship of his or her hospital to other health and educational institutions as far as care is concerned
   i. To refuse to participate in research projects

j. To expect reasonable continuity of care

k. To examine and question the bill

l. To know the hospital rules and regulations that apply to patients' conduct

Role of the Nurse in Addressing Ethical Issues

1. **Nurse as a moral agent**: morality in the broad sense refers to the search for general action-guiding principles

   a. Value clarification for the nurse is an ongoing process of reflection and adoption that is based on beliefs and experiences

      i. Aesthetic considerations

      ii. Demands of etiquette or "proper" behavior

      iii. Selfish wishes

      iv. Sense of morality (basic values)

      v. AACN: An Ethic of Care (1998)*: AACN's mission, vision, and values are framed within an ethic of care and ethical principles. An ethic of care is a moral orientation that acknowledges the interrelatedness and interdependence of individuals, systems, and society and respects individual uniqueness, personal relationships, and the dynamic nature of life. Compassion, collaboration, accountability, and trust are essential to an ethic of care. The following ethical principles provide a basis for deliberation and decision making:

         (a) *Respect for Persons:* a moral obligation to honor the intrinsic worth and uniqueness of each person; to respect self-determination, diversity, and privacy

         (b) *Beneficence:* a moral obligation to promote good and prevent or remove harm; to promote the welfare, health, and safety of society and individuals in accordance with beliefs, values, preferences, and life goals

         (c) *Justice:* a moral obligation to be fair and promote equity, nondiscrimination, and the distribution of benefits and burdens on the basis of needs and resources available; to advocate in another's behalf when necessary

   b. Patient advocacy role: essential component of contemporary nursing practice

      i. Linked with the notion of rights

      ii. Based on the value of human dignity

      iii. Nurses advocate the rights of patients

      iv. Nurses become partisans in conflicts and assume responsibility for presenting rights and interests of clients

      v. Values-based decision model of advocacy: portrays the nurse as helping patients discuss their needs and interests and make choices congruent with their values

      vi. Nurses are expected to prevent others from limiting the freedom of the patient

      vii. The advocacy role may produce conflict for the nurse

      viii. AACN Position Statement: Role of the Critical-Care Nurse as Patient Advocate (1989) states that as a patient advocate, the critical care nurse shall

---

*American Association of Critical-Care Nurses: An Ethic of Care. AACN News 14(10):3, 1997.

(a) Respect and support the right to informed decision making by the patient or designated surrogate
(b) Intervene when the best interest of the patient is in question
(c) Assist the patient in obtaining necessary care
(d) Respect the values, beliefs, and rights of the patient
(e) Assist patients or designated surrogates in the decision-making process through education and support
(f) Represent the patient in accordance with the patient's choices
(g) Support the decisions of the patient or designated surrogate or transfer care to an equally qualified critical care nurse
(h) Intercede for patients who cannot speak for themselves in situations necessitating immediate action
(i) Monitor and safeguard the quality of care that the patient receives
(j) Act as liaison among the patient, family, and health care professionals

c. Nurse creates the ethical environment
   i. Maximizes opportunities for patient advocacy
   ii. Self-educates with regard to ethics
   iii. Acts as moral agent
   iv. Demonstrates sensitivity to patients' values
   v. Understands and identifies own values

d. Role of nurse in research
   i. AACN Position Statement: Ethics in Critical-Care Research (1985)
      (a) Supports conduct of research in manner that assumes that patients give informed consent for study participation
      (b) Supports conduct of research in manner that ensures that patients' rights continue to be safeguarded during conduct of the study
      (c) Recommends that health care institutions establish formal multidisciplinary peer review boards to ensure that ethical principles that underlie conduct of research are followed when research is conducted
      (d) Recommends that at least one professional nurse with equal voting rights be a regular member of all multidisciplinary peer review boards, including Institutional Review Boards (IRBs)
      (e) Recommends that nursing administrators establish procedures that ensure communication between the investigator and nurses involved in conducting the study so that adequate information regarding the research, its risks, and its possible benefits are understood by the critical care nurses, who function as caregivers, assist the researcher, are responsible for unit management, or are asked to answer questions of participating patients regarding study participation
      (f) Recommends that nursing administrators establish mechanisms for addressing nursing concerns about critical care research

e. Role of the nurse participating in futile care
   i. Critical care nurses frequently care for hopelessly ill patients
   ii. Withdrawal of medical therapy does not mean withdrawal of nursing care
   iii. The nurse should participate in team or family decisions to withhold or withdraw care

     iv. When the patient is being treated against his or her will, it is generally the nurse's moral duty to act as patient advocate

     v. It is morally permissible for a nurse to refuse to participate in withdrawing or withholding therapy on grounds of personal beliefs or patient advocacy, as long as a nurse replacement is available and the patient is not abandoned. Supported by Human Resources Management Standards of JCAHO

f. Whistleblowing: role of the nurse in reporting immoral, illegal, or incompetent behavior with a view to stop it

     i. Nurses are required to report incompetence of peers, physicians, and subordinates and to report abuse of patients

     ii. ANA Code of Ethics requires the nurse to safeguard the client and the public when health care and safety are affected by incompetent, unethical, or illegal practice by any person

     iii. State laws may require reporting

g. Individual ethical dilemmas arise from the current health care environment and are related to

     i. Deciding priorities in care in accepting and completing assignments (e.g., aging population, sicker patients)

     ii. Interference of cost consideration in providing patient care and maintaining quality (e.g., reimbursement changes, managed care conflicts, use of technology)

     iii. Being bound by license and conscience to provide safe, appropriate care

     iv. The fact that before rejecting an assignment, the nurse must

        (a) Understand potential consequences

        (b) Document concerns for patient safety

        (c) Document process used to inform management

        (d) Use other strategies such as joint committees to explore issues and increase recruitment and/or retention (at a later time)

h. Addressing ethical issues

     i. Assessment: identify the factors affecting the patient, family, and situation

        (a) Separate assumptions from facts

        (b) Clarify unclear items

        (c) Identify who should be making decision

        (d) Identify own perspective

     ii. Advocacy: identify and use ethical principles, considering dignity and autonomy of the patient

     iii. Action: define problem, determine strategies, identify alternatives, formulate and take action to address ethical dilemma within the multidisciplinary context

i. Resources for addressing ethical issues

     i. ANA Code for Nurses

     ii. ANA Social Policy Statement

     iii. ANA Position Statements

        (a) Foregoing Artificial Nutrition and Hydration

        (b) Promotion of Comfort and Relief of Pain in Dying Patients

     iv. AACN Position Statements

        (a) Clarification of Resuscitation Status in Critical Care Settings requires that there must be written guidelines denoting levels of resuscitation for each patient within the critical care setting. These guidelines must include the following components:

(1) A system and process for classification of patient resuscitation status

(2) A mechanism for documentation and review of resuscitation status and the process used to arrive at this decision

(3) A mechanism for ensuring patient and family rights

(4) Use of clearly defined terms

(5) The critical care nurse will

    a) Ensure quality of patient care regardless of resuscitation status

    b) Review the current resuscitation status daily with the physician

    c) Reflect the resuscitation status in the patient's plan of care

(b) Required Request and Routine Inquiry: Methods to Improve Organ and Tissue Donation Process

(1) AACN strongly supports legislation for required request

(2) AACN strongly recommends that institutions adopt policies that standardize the process of routine inquiry concerning organ and tissue donation

(3) AACN recommends that the critical care nurse, in accordance with personal beliefs and values, participate in the development, implementation, and evaluation of the facility's policy related to required request

(c) Roles and Responsibilities of Critical Care Nurses in Organ and Tissue Transplantation defines the roles and responsibilities related to organ and tissue transplantation and resolves that the critical care nurse shall

(1) Collaborate with health care professionals and patients' families in donor identification and care, the organ and tissue procurement process, and recipient care

(2) Develop knowledge and awareness of personal, professional, cultural, social, religious, and ethical issues related to organ and tissue transplantation

(3) Develop knowledge and awareness of local state and national legislation relevant to organ and tissue transplantation

(4) Provide support needed by families of potential and actual organ and tissue donors

(5) Participate in the implementation of standards for care of potential donors, recipients, and families

(6) Participate in the selection process of potential recipients

(7) Participate in endeavors designed to advance the science and art of transplantation nursing

v. American College of Emergency Physicians Position Statement, Guidelines for DNR Orders in the Prehospital Setting, recommends that a comprehensive DNR policy should be endorsed by the local, regional, or state medical society and that medical treatments limited by a DNR order should be clearly defined, so that these orders can be honored in prehospital care

vi. Institutional Ethics Committees (IECs)

(a) Establishment of IECs

(1) Recommended by President's Commission for the Study of Ethical Problems in Medicine and Biomedical and Behavioral Research

(2) A prognosis committee first recommended by court in Karen Quinlan case (1976)

(3) Current trend is toward establishing IECs in health care facilities

(b) Purposes of IECs

(1) Initiate educational programs related to ethical dilemmas in health care

(2) Formulate institutional policies and guidelines in sensitive areas (e.g., related to DNR, withholding or withdrawing therapy, tissue and organ procurement, advance directives in health care)

(3) Monitor compliance with those policies

(4) Review and revise policies already in effect

(5) Advise and act as consultants on specific case

(6) Act as forum for discussing and resolving issues and disagreements regarding treatment issues

(7) Provide guidance to management and medical staff in relation to organizational ethics

(8) Provide emotional support for staff

(c) Membership of IECs

(1) Multidisciplinary: should have adequate bedside nursing representation

(2) Large enough to represent diverse professional viewpoints

(d) Models or types of committees

(1) Autonomy model: accountable to the competent patient; facilitates decision making by competent patient

(2) Patient benefit model: accountable to incompetent patient; facilitates decision making for incompetent patient

(3) Social justice model: accountable to institutions; considers broad social issues (i.e., hospital policies, health care policy, resource allocation, cost effectiveness)

(e) Confidentiality related to IECs

(1) Of proceedings

(2) Of records

(3) Should be determined by committee at outset

(f) Education and development of IECs

(1) Self-education: communication with others, attendance at workshops

(2) Staff education: forums, ethics rounds, clinical discussions

(3) Consumer and patient education

(g) Policy development (e.g., DNR, case review, nutrition and hydration related to withdrawal of life support)

(1) Develop and disseminate information

(2) Educate staff

(3) Monitor compliance

(h) Review of ongoing cases: procedural guidelines should reflect

(1) Optional versus mandatory consultation

(2) Decision making authority versus options

(3) Source of requests for review

(4) Types of problems for consideration

(5) Members' responsibilities

(6) Mechanisms to assess and evaluate committee role

(i) Advantages and disadvantages of IECs

(1) Advantages

a) Core group of staff knowledgeable about ethical issues

b) Patient is focus of ethical dilemma

c) Forum for multidisciplinary dialogue related to ethical issues of patient care

d) Objective body to consult and provide assistance to staff

(2) Disadvantages

a) May pose threat to traditional decision-making process

b) Committee may not be able to remain nonbiased

c) Committee may become preoccupied with risk management and prevention of litigation

d) Committee involvement raises potential for loss of patient confidentiality

IDENTIFICATION OF ETHICAL AND LEGAL CONFLICTS IN THE CURRENT HEALTH CARE ENVIRONMENT

Allocation of Resources and Scarce Resources

1. **Organ Donation**

   a. Donation versus sale of body parts

   b. Use of anencephalic or fetal tissue

   c. Organ procurement and harvesting

   d. Caring for patients in a "suspended state of being" (potential donor)

   e. Uniform Anatomical Gift Act (1968)

      i. Any individual of sound mind and 18 years of age or older may donate all or any part of his or her body, the gift to take effect upon death

      ii. In the absence of a gift by the deceased, his or her relatives, in a stated order of priority (spouse, adult children, parents, adult siblings) have the power to give away the body or any of its parts

      iii. Recipients are restricted to hospitals, doctors, medical and dental schools, universities, tissue banks, and a specified individual in need of treatment. The purposes are restricted to transplantation, therapy, research, education, and the advancement of medical or dental science

      iv. A gift may be made by will or by a card or other document

      v. A gift may be revoked at any time

      vi. A donee may accept or reject a gift

   f. Donor issues

      i. Presumed consent: routine salvage of donor organs when the deceased has expressed no wish *not* to donate. Thirteen countries have presumed consent (United States does not have presumed consent)

 ii. Sale of organs by unrelated live donors or, after a donor's death, by the next of kin is not dealt with by the Uniform Anatomical Gift Act. The unwritten code of ethics of transplantation surgeons prevents the sale of organs

2. **Transplantation**
 a. Relates to sanctity of life in Western culture
 b. Cost versus benefit
 c. Scarcity of organs versus demand
 d. Number and types of organs and tissues transplanted grow every year
  i. Heart
  ii. Lung
  iii. Heart/lung combination
  iv. Pancreas
  v. Joints
  vi. Kidneys and multiple abdominal organs
  vii. Cornea
  viii. Liver
  ix. Nerves
  x. Bones and skin
  xi. Other tissues and organs
 e. Issues related to nursing staff may cause ethical conflicts
  i. Death of another person makes organ transplantation possible
  ii. Identification of brain death removes hope of survival
  iii. Special meaning of the heart
  iv. Use of non–heart-beating donors

3. **Technologic imperative:** technologic advances force practitioners and health care administrators to opt for technology in spite of cost even when there is little hope for survival of individual patients

4. **Transfer and discharge of patients unable to pay** ("patient dumping"): refers to hospitals not admitting or transferring patients who are unable to pay. Is illegal

5. **DNR orders**
 a. Hopelessly ill patients who assert right to die
 b. Incompetent patients
  i. Who can decide?
  ii. Principle of substituted judgment
 c. No code and slow code issues

6. **Withdrawal of treatment**
 a. Legal responsibilities
 b. Ethical responsibilities

7. **Withholding food and fluids versus forced feeding:** patients in prolonged coma or persistent vegetative state

8. **Advance Directives:** enhance patient autonomy and increase patient involvement in the decision-making process

9. **Euthanasia and assisted suicide**
 a. Legal in Holland
 b. Groups in United States are attempting to modify laws; U.S. circuit court decisions support the right to assisted suicide (1996)

10. Ethical issues in human immunodeficiency virus (HIV) infection
   a. Basic professional ethic: nurses care for patients regardless of their personal attributes or health problems
   b. Acquired immunodeficiency syndrome (AIDS) challenges that basic ethic: being treated differently than patients with other communicable diseases
   c. Conflicts of patient privacy versus nurses' safety
   d. Nurses have moral duty to provide care, but is that obligation absolute? Under all circumstances?
   e. ANA has concluded that a nurse's obligation is limited by degree of personal risk
   f. Nurse has moral obligation to provide care if situation meets criteria (ANA Position Statement)
      i. Patient is at significant risk of harm, loss, or damage if nurse does not assist
      ii. Nurse's intervention is directly related to preventing harm
      iii. The benefit that the patient gains outweighs any harm that the nurse might incur and does not present more than a minimal risk to the nurse

11. Triage decisions
   a. Who gets a bed when the number of potential patients exceeds the number of available beds
   b. Role of the critical care nurse is to provide needed patient care
   c. Role of the unit medical director is to administer unit and facility policies
   d. Policies are developed and include admission and discharge criteria
   e. AACN Guidelines for Admission/Discharge Criteria in Critical Care
      i. Development of admission and discharge criteria is based on
         (a) Standards for critically ill
         (b) Current unit admission and discharge patterns
         (c) Available resources within the critical care unit
         (d) Number and distribution of critical care beds in the institution
         (e) Institutional occupancy trends
         (f) Data provided by existing measurement tools in the institution (e.g., patient classification tools, severity of illness index)
      ii. The admission and discharge criteria contain or address the following:
         (a) Physiologic parameters that define the need for critical care
         (b) Physiologic parameters that define readiness for discharge
         (c) Definition of unit-specific patient population
         (d) Frequency and type of medical evaluation and/or treatment necessitated by patient's condition
         (e) Frequency and type of critical care nursing assessments and interventions needed by patient
         (f) Technologic monitoring and intervention available only in the critical care setting
         (g) Requirements by external regulatory bodies
         (h) Institutional policies that mandate or preclude critical care for specific patient populations

        (i) Designation of the health team member or members accountable for admission and discharge decisions

        (j) A plan for triage when the need exceeds available physical or human resources

        (k) A plan for conflict resolution between health care team members, using the admission and discharge criteria

     iii. The admission and discharge criteria will be approved through appropriate institutional channels and disseminated to all health team members involved in the process

     iv. Compliance with the admission and discharge processes will be regularly monitored and evaluated annually by the multidisciplinary team

Patient Care Dilemmas

1. **Withholding treatment** (e.g., quadriplegic patient with other medical problems such as renal disease necessitating dialysis)
2. **Code versus no-code decision** (e.g., cardiac patient with severe chronic obstructive pulmonary disease who needs ventilator for the rest of life)
3. **Right to die at home** (e.g., cancer patient with morphine drip)
4. **Technology versus cost** (e.g., patient who receives single-chamber [VVI] versus dual-chamber [DDD] pacemaker)
5. **Nutritional dilemmas** (e.g., withdrawal of food and fluids versus tube feeding or total parenteral nutrition)
6. **Resource allocation and triage decisions** (e.g., who gets the last temporary pacemaker when two patients need it)
7. **Technology versus quality of life decisions** (e.g., left ventricular assist device)
8. **Informed consent** (e.g., scheduling for bilateral above-the-knee amputations versus death from infection)
9. **Managed care conflicts** (e.g., patient's refusal to pay for services)

Use of Technology

1. **Increased use of technology escalates ethical conflicts**
2. **High cost of technology**
   a. Personnel
   b. Equipment
   c. Training
3. **Abuse of technology** (inappropriate use)
4. **Types of technology** in health care
   a. Devices
      i. Ventilator
      ii. Left ventricular assist device
      iii. Total artificial heart
      iv. Pacemaker (multiple types)
      v. Artificial feeding devices
      vi. Defibrillators (internal and external)
      vii. Insulin pumps

    b. Procedures
       i. Hemodialysis
       ii. Surrogate motherhood (embryonic transplantation)
       iii. Genetic engineering
       iv. Artificial insemination
       v. Fetal surgery
       vi. Continuous ambulatory peritoneal dialysis
       vii. Amniocentesis and genetic identification
       viii. Hemofiltration
    c. Organ transplantation
       i. Brain-dead donor
       ii. Non–heart-beating donor

Common Ethical Conflicts in Care of the Critically Ill

1. **Autonomy versus paternalism**: conflicts related to rights of the individual
   a. Informed consent
   b. Technology versus quality of life
   c. Code versus no-code decisions
2. **Justice versus utilitarianism**: conflicts related to resource allocation and triage decisions
   a. Nutritional dilemmas
   b. Quality of life decisions
3. **Veracity versus fidelity**: conflicts related to the unique role of the nurse and other health care professionals
   a. Withholding therapy
   b. Right to die at home
   c. Truth telling
4. **Professional integrity** versus one's own ethical and moral beliefs: professional versus personal conflicts
   a. Delivering therapy that contradicts the nurse's own moral and ethical beliefs
   b. Caring for patients whose practices are not accepted by the caregivers

Institutional and Corporate Ethics

1. **Setting**
   a. Hospital as corporate environment
   b. Individual versus corporation, resulting in ethical conflicts
2. **Types of unethical behaviors:** for example, changing documentation, charting inaccurate data or information, providing misinformation or incomplete information to family or patient
3. **Promotion of ethical behavior by the nurse manager**: creating an ethical environment
   a. Recognition of a lack of ethical behavior when it occurs
   b. Standards development: use of current standards, ANA Code of Ethics for Nurses, or development of specific standards by the group
   c. Recognition that responsibility for ethical behavior belongs to all involved in the patient care environment

4. **Managed Care Dilemmas**
   a. Changing health care environment: moving to HMOs
   b. Individual providers versus preferred provider organizations (PPOs)
   c. Ethical conflicts related to limitation of resources and treatments
   d. Denial of access to specialists
   e. Physician gag orders
   f. Financial incentives to physicians to limit or deny care or special treatment

. . . .
References

LEGAL ASPECTS

American Association of Critical-Care Nurses (AACN): Conceptual Model of Critical-Care Nursing. Aliso Viejo, Calif., AACN, 1981.

American Association of Critical-Care Nurses: Clarification of Resuscitation Status in Critical-Care Settings. Aliso Viejo, Calif., AACN, 1985.

American Association of Critical-Care Nurses: Roles and Responsibilities of Critical-Care Nurses in Organ and Tissue Transplantation. Aliso Viejo, Calif., AACN, 1986.

American Association of Critical-Care Nurses: Required Request and Routine Inquiry: Methods to Improve the Organ and Tissue Donation Process. Aliso Viejo, Calif., AACN, 1986.

American Association of Critical-Care Nurses: Guidelines for Admission/Discharge Criteria in Critical Care. Aliso Viejo, Calif., AACN, 1987.

American Association of Critical-Care Nurses: Critical Care: The Nurse of the Future. Aliso Viejo, Calif., AACN, 1990.

American Association of Critical-Care Nurses: The Nurse of the Future. Aliso Viejo, Calif., AACN, 1993.

American Association of Critical-Care Nurses: Unlicensed Assistive Personnel Curriculum. Aliso Viejo, Calif., AACN, 1996.

American Association of Critical-Care Nurses Certification Corporation: CCRN Certification Handbook. Aliso Viejo, Calif., AACN, 1997.

American Nurses Association: Working Definition: Nurses in Advanced Clinical Practice. Washington, D.C.: American Nurses Association, 1992.

Barter, M., & Furmidge, M. L.: Unlicensed assistive personnel: Issues relating to delegation and supervision. J. Nurs. Admin. 24(4):36–40, 1994.

Beffa, M. C.: The legal side: delegation dilemma. Am. J. Nurs. 95(2):70, 1995.

Blouin, A. S., & Brent, N. J.: Unlicensed assistive personnel: Legal considerations. J. Nurs. Admin. 25(11):7–8, 21, 1995.

Fiesta, J.: The Law and Liability: A Guide for Nurses, 2nd ed. New York, John Wiley & Sons, 1994.

Furmidge, M. L., & Barter, M.: Supreme Court decision affects bargaining rights of nurses. J. Nurs. Admin. 24(8):9–11, 1994.

Guido, G. W.: Legal issues in critical care. In Clochesy, J. M., Breu, C., Cardin, S., et al. (eds.): Critical Care Nursing, 2nd ed. Philadelphia, W. B. Saunders, 1996, pp. 25–35.

Joint Commission on Accreditation of Healthcare Organizations (JCAHO): Hospital Accreditation Standards.

The Joint Commission on Accreditation of Healthcare Organizations. Oakbrook Terrace, Ill., JCAHO, 1997.

Mirr, M.: Advanced clinical practice: A reconceptualized role. AACN Clin. Issues 4(4):599–602, 1993.

Northrop, C., & Kelly, M. E.: Legal Issues in Nursing. St. Louis, C. V. Mosby, 1987.

Pohlman, K. J.: Nursing negligence. Focus Crit. Care 16:296–298, 1989.

Tammelleo, A. D.: Nursing notes can be worth their weight in gold. Regan Report Nurs. Law 33(3):1, 1992.

Tammelleo, A. D.: When nurses obtain consent for organ donations. Regan Report Nurs. Law 53(8):1, 1995.

Wlody, G. S.: Informed consent and the law. In Wlody, G. S. (ed.): Managing Clinical Practice in Critical Care Nursing. St. Louis, Mosby-Year Book, 1994, pp. 15–24.

ETHICAL ASPECTS

American Association of Critical-Care Nurses: Ethics in Critical-Care Research. Aliso Viejo, Calif., AACN, 1985.

American Association of Critical-Care Nurses: Role of the Critical-Care Nurse as Patient Advocate. Aliso Viejo, Calif., AACN, 1989.

American Association of Critical-Care Nurses: Withholding and/or Withdrawing Life-Sustaining Treatment. Aliso Viejo, Calif., AACN, 1990.

American Hospital Association: Patient Bill of Rights. Chicago, Ill., American Hospital Association, 1978.

American Nurses Association: Code for Nurses. Kansas City, Mo., American Nurses Association, 1985.

Cobbs vs. Grant: 8 Cal 3d 229, 1972.

Gilfix, M., & Raffin, T. A.: Withholding or withdrawing extraordinary life support: Optimizing rights and limiting liability. West. J. Med. 141:387–394, 1984.

Hastings Center: Guidelines for the Termination of Life Sustaining Treatment and Care of the Dying. Briarcliff Manor, N.Y., Hastings Center, 1987.

Jonsen, A. R., Siegler, M., and Winslade, W: Clinical Ethics, 2nd ed. New York, Macmillan, 1992.

Murphy, P., Gomez, C., & Hill, P.: Healthcare Ethics Forum 1994. Euthanasia and assisted suicide: Critical care perspectives. AACN Clin. Issues Crit. Care 5(3):333–339.

President's Commission for the Study of Ethical Problems in Medicine and Biomedical and Behavioral Research: Defining Death. Washington, D.C., U.S. Government Printing Office, 1981.

President's Commission for the Study of Ethical Problems in Medicine and Biomedical and Behavioral Research: Deciding to Forego Life-Sustaining Treatment: Ethical, Medical and Legal Issues in Treatment Decisions. Washington, D.C., U.S. Government Printing Office, 1983.

Wanzer, S., Adelstein, J., Cranford, R., et al.: The physician's responsibility toward hopelessly ill patients. N. Engl. J. Med. 310:955–959, 1984.

Wlody, G. S.: The critical care nurse as a moral agent. *In* Wlody, G. S. (ed.): Managing Clinical Practice in Critical Care Nursing. St. Louis, Mosby-Year Book, 1994, pp. 25–43.

Wlody, G. S.: Creating the healing environment in critical care. *In* Wlody, G. S. (ed.): Managing Clinical Practice in Critical Care Nursing. St. Louis, Mosby-Year Book, 1994, pp. 2–14.

ETHICAL CONFLICTS

Barber vs. Superior Court: 147 Cal. App 3d 1006, 1986.

Bartling vs. Superior Court: 163 Cal. App 3d 186, 195, 1984.

Hoffman, P., & Banja, J: Exceptions to the right to refuse treatment. AORN J. 54:892–897, 1987.

Johnson, K.: High Court to hear right to die. USA Today, p. 1, October 2, 1996.

Nokes, K. M.: Examining the ethical and legal issues generated by the HIV epidemic. J. Assoc. Nurses AIDS Care 2(1):25–30, 1991.

Rushton, C. H.: Dialogues in ethics and the law. Placebo pain medication: Ethical and legal issues. Pediatr. Nurs. 21(2):166–168, 1995.

Ruark, J., Raffin, T. A., and the Stanford University Medical Center Committee on Ethics: Initiating and withdrawing life support: Principles and practices in adult medicine. N. Engl. J. Med. 318(1):25–28, 1985.

Weiler, K.: Ethical dilemmas that evolve into legal issues. J. Gerontol. Nurs. 21(5):47, 1995.

Index

Note: Page numbers in *italics* refer to illustrations;
page numbers followed by t refer to tables.